THE USE OF ANTIBIOTICS

A Comprehensive Review with Clinical Emphasis

A. KUCERS, MB BS FRACP

and

N. McK. BENNETT, MB BS FRACP

FRCP (Ed.) FACMA

*Physicians Fairfield Hospital, the Queen's Memorial
Infectious Diseases Hospital, Melbourne, Australia,
and the Clinical School for Infectious Diseases in
Melbourne and Monash Universities*

THIRD EDITION

WILLIAM HEINEMANN MEDICAL BOOKS LTD
LONDON

First published 1972
Second edition (reset) 1975
Second edition (reprinted) 1977
Third edition (reset) 1979
Third edition (reprinted) 1982

ISBN 0 433 18877 4

Text set in 11 pt Photon Times Roman, printed and bound
in Great Britain at The Pitman Press, Bath

THE USE OF ANTIBIOTICS
A Comprehensive Review with Clinical Emphasis

Contents

PART I—ANTIBIOTICS

v

PART II—SYNTHETIC ANTIBACTERIAL AND ANTIPARASITIC DRUGS

PART III—DRUGS MAINLY FOR TUBERCULOSIS

PART IV—ANTIFUNGAL DRUGS

PART V—ANTIVIRAL DRUGS

Preface to First Edition

This book aims to provide a concise, systematized description of antibiotics in current use in antibacterial chemotherapy. Commonly used synthetic antibacterial chemotherapeutic agents are included, but compounds used solely for tuberculosis and leprosy have been omitted. Although primarily designed for clinicians, the book may well be useful for bacteriologists, pharmacists, pharmacologists and undergraduates.

The presentation of a personal viewpoint has been consciously avoided, if this is possible, in favour of a balanced account of data and informed opinion from the medical literature. I have accordingly attempted to acknowledge all of my sources of information in the text.

Where conclusions are in doubt or controversial, the known facts and opinions are recorded for the reader to assess and apply in relevant circumstances.

Each chapter is devoted to one or several related drugs and divided into ten standard sections for ease of reference. A brief introductory description is followed by sections relating to the antibacterial spectrum, *in vitro* sensitivities, administration and dosage, serum levels, excretion, body distribution, mode of action, toxicity and clinical application.

Many colleagues, in particular the senior medical staff of Fairfield Hospital, have assisted with the preparation of this book. Dr. John A. Forbes, the Medical Superintendent and Dean of the Hospital Clinical School, encouraged me some six years ago to write, for use in our hospital, systematized notes on antibiotics which form the basis of this book. He has also read all of the manuscript, and has made many valuable suggestions. I would especially like to thank my colleague, Dr. Noel McK. Bennett, Specialist Physician and Deputy Medical Superintendent, who has been of immense assistance to me. He aided in the detailed editing of the text, and has contributed to much of the content of the book. Dr. Joan D. Schiavone, formerly Assistant Pathologist at Fairfield Hospital, now Senior Lecturer in the Department of Microbiology, University of Melbourne, has helped with many bacteriological aspects.

I would also like to thank my secretary, Mrs. Ann Cullen, for typing the manuscript and Miss Jean Foreman, the hospital medical librarian, for collecting much of the medical literature. I am also indebted to my publishers, particularly Mr. Owen R. Evans, Managing Director, for advice on matters pertinent to medical publication, and for undertaking on my behalf the task of obtaining permission from other authors and publishers to reproduce tables and figures in the text.

A. Kucers

Melbourne, Australia
April 1972

Preface to Second Edition

A considerable amount of new information on chemotherapeutic agents has accumulated in the three years since the first edition of this book was published. We have aimed to make this edition an 'up-to-date' reference text, incorporating the significant advances which have occurred. This has entailed a full revision in which many sections and some chapters have been completely re-written. The modest success and generally favourable reviews of the first edition have encouraged us in this task. The responsibility for this publication is now shared by two authors, but this is only an extension of the close working relationship which we enjoyed when the previous edition was written.

The contents of the book have been enlarged by the addition of chapters on drugs used for the treatment of tuberculosis and fungal diseases. There is also a section on those antiviral drugs which on present evidence appear to be of value in human therapeutics. We have tried to retain the 'concise, systematized description' which was the format of the first edition. The main purpose of this book is still to provide clinicians with comprehensive information on the use of individual chemotherapeutic agents. The text does not deal primarily with the treatment of diseases, although this information is available through the Index. Many of the compounds described are synthetic drugs, and not true antibiotics, but nowadays this distinction is of only academic interest to the clinician. Again we have endeavoured to present the comparative value of various drugs in an unbiased fashion according to published experience, though on controversial subjects we have also expressed our opinion.

We are grateful to Dr. Ray S. A. Marshman, The Director of Tuberculosis in Victoria, for his valuable criticism and comments on the chapters concerning drugs used for the treatment of tuberculosis. Our colleagues, the Senior Medical Staff at Fairfield Hospital, have once again been most tolerant and helpful during the period in which this book was written.

We would like to thank our secretaries, Mesdames Ann Cullen, Ann Fumi, Biddy Gibson and Janet Johnson, the medical librarian Miss Jean Foreman and proof reader Mrs. Anda Kucers for their respective contributions to this edition.

Melbourne, Australia   A. Kucers
February 1975   N. McK. Bennett

Preface to Third Edition

Similar to our second edition, this one follows its predecessor within a period of about four years. In this short time there have been considerable changes in the sensitivities of various organisms to chemotherapeutic agents. The appearance of gonococci and pneumococci resistant to penicillin G are two obvious examples. Where possible we have tried to indicate the best possible alternative drug(s) for the treatment of infections due to drug-resistant strains. The spread of multiple-antibiotic resistant strains of Gram-negative organisms, such as Serratia marcescens in hospitals, has also posed therapeutic problems. Treatment of infections due to these bacteria is difficult and often involves the concomitant use of two or more drugs, so that we have frequently included details of synergistic drug combinations which may prove of value.

Further chemical modifications of the penicillin and cephalosporin molecules have led to a bewildering number of new derivatives. In this edition there are descriptions of the newer penicillins and cephalosporins which are already available commercially; included are also some of these drugs which may be marketed in the future. Based on published data we have endeavoured to put these compounds in their proper clinical perspective. The newer aminoglycosidic aminocyclitols such as tobramycin, amikacin, sisomicin and netilmicin have been similarly assessed. New chapters cover the nitroimidazole drugs, in particular metronidazole, which is proving to have an important place for the treatment of bacterial as well as parasitic infections. Other innovations are descriptions of newer macrolides such as josamycin and rosamicin and the antifungal drugs, miconazole and econazole. Nearly every chapter has been extensively revamped so that this edition is virtually a new text-book. For the benefit of clinicians in countries like Australia who now use SI units, biochemical values are expressed additionally in these units. We have collaborated closely on every chapter to ensure accuracy, relevant cross-referencing and to avoid contradictions. This has been a considerable task for two practising clinicians but we feel that our unified approach to each drug would be difficult to retain with further dilution of authorship.

Once again we express our thanks to Dr. Ray S. A. Marshman who until recently was The Director of Tuberculosis in Victoria, for his wise counsel on the use of drugs for the treatment of tuberculosis. We are also extremely grateful to our secretaries, Mesdames Ann Fumi and Kay Munro. They had the mammoth task of typing the manuscript which they accomplished with accuracy and in record time. The hospital's librarian, Miss Jean Foreman, was ever available to obtain the most obscure reference and she with Mrs. Anda Kucers again helped with the tedious task of proof-reading. Our publishers have been most cooperative in expediting the production of this book. Finally we would like to thank the many medical practitioners throughout the world who have expressed their appreciation of our book in various ways. It was solely this response which encouraged us to write this third edition.

Melbourne, Australia
February 1979

Alvis Kucers
Noel Mck. Bennett

Acknowledgements

We are indebted to the owners of the copyright for permission to use illustrations from the following works:

Bailey, R. R.,
Gower, P. E.,
Dash, C. H.
Table 17
Postgraduate Medical Journal Supplement (1970), **46,** 60, 'The Effect of Impairment of Renal Function and Haemodialysis on Serum and Urine Levels of Cephalexin'.

Barber, M.,
Waterworth, P. M.
Table 21
Table 23
British Medical Journal (1966), **1,** 203, 'Activity of Gentamicin Against Pseudomonas and Hospital Staphylococci'.

Benner, E. J.,
Brodie, J. S.,
Kirby, W. M. M.
Fig. 11
Antimicrobial Agents and Chemotherapy (1965), p. 888, 'Laboratory and Clinical Comparison of Cephaloridine and Cephalothin'.

Bond, J. M.,
Lightbown, J. W.,
Barber, M.,
Waterworth, P. M.
Fig. 2
British Medical Journal (1963), **2,** 956, 'A Comparison of Four Phenoxypenicillins'.

Brumfitt, W.,
Faiers, M. C.,
Pursell, R. E.,
Reeves, D. S.,
Turnbull, A. R.
Fig. 33
Fig. 34
Postgraduate Medical Journal Supplement (1969), **45,** 56, 'Bacteriological Pharmacological and Clinical Studies with Trimethoprim-sulphonamide Combinations'.

Brumfitt, W.,
Koshidis, J.,
Hamilton-Miller, J. M. T.,
Gilchrist, J. N. G.
Fig. 15
Fig. 16
Antimicrobial Agents and Chemotherapy (1974), **6,** 290, 'Cefoxitin and Cephalothin: Antimicrobial Activity, Human Pharmacokinetics, and Toxicology'.

Bryan, C. S.,
Stone, W. J.
Table 2
Annals of Internal Medicine (1975), **82,** 189, ' "Comparably Massive" Penicillin G Therapy in Renal Failure'.

Bullowa, J. G. M.,
Ratish, H. D.
Fig. 32
Journal of Clinical Investigation (1944), **23,** 676, 'A Therapeutic and Pharmacological Study of Sulfadiazine, Monomethylsulfadiazine, and Dimethylsulfadiazine in Lobar Pneumonia'.

Burgess, M. A., Bodey, G. P.	Fig. 38	*Antimicrobial Agents and Chemotherapy* (1972), **2**, 423, 'Clotrimazole (Bay b 5097): In Vitro and Clinical Pharmacological Studies'.
Finland, M., Garrod, L. P.	Fig. 31	*British Medical Journal* (1960), **2**, 959, 'Demethylchlortetracycline'.
Gingell, J. C., Waterworth, P. M.	Fig. 21	*British Medical Journal* (1968), **2**, 19, 'Dose of Gentamicin in Patients with Normal Renal Function and Renal Impairment".
Fong, I. W., Ralph, E. D., Engelking, E. R., Kirby, W. M. M.	Fig. 13 Fig. 14	*Antimicrobial Agents and Chemotherapy* (1976), **9**, 65, 'Clinical Pharmacology of Cefamandole as Compared with Cephalothin'.
Foord, R. D.	Fig. 17	*Antimicrobial Agents and Chemotherapy* (1976), **9**, 741, 'Cefuroxime: Human Pharmacokinetics'.
Godtfredsen, W., Roholt, K., Tybring, L.	Fig. 17	*The Lancet* (1962), **1**, 928, 'Fucidin: A New Orally Active Antibiotic'.
Goodwin, C. S., Dash, C. H., Hill, J. P., Goldberg, A. D.	Fig. 18	*The Journal of Antimicrobial Chemotherapy* (1977), **3**, 253, 'Cefuroxime: pharmacokinetics after a short infusion, and *in vitro* activity against hospital pathogens'.
Gower, P. E.	Table 13	*Postgraduate Medical Journal Supplement* (1967), **43**, 92, 'The Effect of Cephaloridine on Renal Function in Patients with Renal Failure'.
Griffith, R. S. Black, H. R.	Fig. 12	*Clinical Medicine* (1968), **75**, 14, 'Cephalexin: A New Antibiotic'.
Griffith, R. S., Black, H. R.	Fig. 26	*Antimicrobial Agents and Chemotherapy* (1962), **12**, 398, 'A Comparison of Blood Levels After Oral Administration of Erythromycin and Erythromycin Estolate'.
Hultberg, E. R., Backelin, B.	Fig. 8	*Scandinavian Journal of Infectious Diseases* (1972), **4**, 149, 'Studies on the absorption of pivampicillin and ampicillin'.
Kabins, S. A., Kelner, B., Walton, E., Goldstein, E.	Table 16	*American Journal of Medical Sciences* (1970), **259**, 133, 'Cephalexin Therapy as Related to Renal Function'.

Kaplan, K., Chew, W. H., Weinstein, L. — Fig. 25 — *American Journal of Medical Sciences* (1965), **250,** 137, 'Microbiological, Pharmacological and Clinical Studies of Linocomycin'.

Khan, G. A., Scott, A. J. — Fig. 28 — *British Journal of Pharmacol. Chemother.* (1967), **31,** 506, 'The Place of Rifamycin-B-diethylamide in the Treatment of Cholangitis Complicating Biliary Obstruction'.

Kirby, W. M. M., Kind, A. C. — Fig. 6 — *Annals of the New York Academy of Sciences* (1967), **145,** 291, 'Clinical Pharmacology of Ampicillin and Hetacillin'.

Knudsen, E. T., Rolinson, G. N. — Fig. 3 — *British Medical Journal* (1960), **2,** 700, 'Absorption and Excretion of a New Antibiotic (BRL 1241)'.

Knudsen, E. T., Rolinson, G. N., Sutherland, R. — Fig. 9 — *British Medical Journal* (1967), **3,** 75, 'Carbenicillin, A New Semisynthetic Penicillin Active Against Pseudomonas pyocyanea'.

Koechlin, B. A., Rubio, F., Palmer, S., Gabriel, T., Duschinsky, R. — Fig. 37 — *Biochemical Pharmacology* (1966), **15,** 435, 'The Metabolism of 5-Fluorocytosine-2^{14}C and of Cytosine-^{14}C in the Rat and the Disposition of 5-Fluorocytosine-2^{14}C in Man'.

McCrumb, F. R., Jr. Snyder, M. J., Hicken, W. J. — Fig. 22 — *Antibiotics Annual* (1957–58), p. 837, "The Use of Chloramphenicol Acid Succinate in the Treatment of Acute Infections'.

McGehee, R. F., Jr. Smith, C. B., Wilcox, C., Finland, M. — Fig. 24 — *American Journal of Medical Sciences* (1968), **256,** 279, 'Comparative Studies of Antibacterial Activity *in Vitro* and Absorption and Excretion of Lincomycin and Clinimycin'.

Ross, S., Puig, J. R., Zaremba, E. A. — Fig. 27 — *Antibiotics Annual* (1959–60), p. 89, 'Colistin: Some Preliminary Laboratory and Clinical Observations in Specific Gastroenteritis in Infants and Children'.

Short, E. I. — Fig. 36 — *Tubercle, London* (1962), **43,** 33, 'Studies on the Inactivation of Isonicotinyl Acid Hydrazide in Normal Subjects and Tuberculous Patients'.

Standiford, H. C., Jordan, M. C., Kirby, W. M. M.	Fig. 10	*Journal of Infectious Diseases* (1970), Vol. 122 (Sept. Supplement), p. 9, 'Clinical Pharmacology of Carbenicillin Compared with Other Penicillins'.
Sutherland, R., Croydon, E. A. P., Rolinson, G. N.	Fig. 4 Fig. 5	*British Medical Journal* (1970), **4,** 455, 'Flucloxacillin, a New Isoxazolyl Penicillin, Compared with Oxacillin Cloxacillin and Dicloxacillin'.
Sutherland, R., Croydon, E. A. P., Rolinson, G. N.	Fig. 7	*British Medical Journal* (1972), **3,** 13, 'Amoxycillin: A new Semi-synthetic Penicillin'.
Verbist, L., Gyselen, A.	Fig. 29	*American Review of Respiratory Diseases* (1968), **98,** 923, 'Antituber- culous Activity of Rifampin *in Vitro* and *in Vivo* and the Concentrations Attained in Human Blood'.
Welch, Henry	Fig. 1 Fig. 19 Fig. 30	*New York Medical Encyclopedia* (1954), pp. 79, 121, 255, 'Principles and Practice of Antibiotic Therapy'.
Welch, Henry, Wright, W. W., Weinstein, H. I., Staffa, A. W.	Fig. 20	*Annals of the New York Academy of Sciences* (1958), **76,** 66, '*In Vitro* and Pharmacological Studies with Kanamycin'.

Part I
Antibiotics

Penicillin G

Description

Penicillin was isolated from Penicillium notatum by Fleming in 1929 and introduced into clinical medicine in 1941 by Florey, Chain and associates (Fleming, 1929; Chain *et al.*, 1940). The history of penicillin, including its early use in treatment of human infections, is recorded in a number of informative monographs such as those by Stewart (1965), Hare (1970) and Bickel (1972).

The pencillin used by early investigators was an amorphous compound containing impurities, which were introduced during the fermentative processes used in its manufacture, and its activity and dosage were expressed in units. The early penicillin was also a mixture of several penicillin compounds, designated as F, G, X and K. Penicillin G (benzylpenicillin) was found to be the most satisfactory, and this is now used in a highly purified and crystalline form for clinical purposes. Penicillin G as such is a rather unstable acid, and currently the following relatively stable salts are used clinically:

1. *Sodium penicillin G or sodium benzylpenicillin.* This is a highly soluble salt, and a dose can be dissolved completely in a few ml of water prior to administration. The dosage of this and other penicillin G preparations is still commonly expressed in units. One unit of activity is equal to $0 \cdot 6 \ \mu$g of pure sodium penicillin G.

2. *Potassium penicillin G* similarly is a very soluble salt. One unit of activity is equal to $0 \cdot 625 \ \mu$g of pure potassium penicillin G.

The term 'crystalline penicillin G' or simply 'crystalline penicillin' is often used as a synonym for either of the above highly soluble benzylpenicillin salts, but all other penicillins in use are also crystalline in form, unlike the early impure amorphous compound.

3. *Procaine penicillin G* (*Procaine benzylpenicillin or procaine penicillin*). This is a much less soluble salt, and it is administered intramuscularly as a suspension of crystal particles. These particles dissolve slowly after administration, so that absorption from the injection site takes place over a prolonged period. One unit of activity is equal to $1 \cdot 0 \ \mu$g of pure procaine penicillin.

4. *Benzathine penicillin G* (*Di-benzyl-ethylene-diamine penicillin or DBED penicillin*). This salt is even less soluble than procaine penicillin, so it is even more slowly absorbed from an intramuscular injection site. One unit of activity is equivalent to $0 \cdot 75 \ \mu$g of the pure substance.

The procaine and benzathine salts of penicillin G are known as the 'long acting', 'depot' or 'repository' forms of penicillin G.

3

Sensitive Organisms

1. *Gram-positive cocci.* Penicillin G is highly active against many of these bacteria. Strep. pyogenes (Group A) has remained very sensitive (Finland *et al.*, 1976a) and routine sensitivity testing is not required. The same was generally true for Strep. pneumoniae, but since about 1970 relatively resistant strains, and more recently also pneumococcal strains with complete penicillin resistance, have been isolated from patients or pneumococcal carriers.

Relatively resistant pneumococcal strains require from five to a hundred times higher penicillin concentrations for inhibition, than sensitive strains (Table 1). These strains were first detected in Papua New Guinea and Australia (Hansman *et al.*, 1971; Hansman, 1972; Hansman *et al.*, 1973; 1974; Hansman, 1974). More recently they have appeared in other countries such as New Mexico (Tempest *et al.*, 1974), North America (Naraqi *et al.*, 1974; Paredes *et al.*, 1976a; Finland *et al.*, 1976b; Cooksey *et al.*, 1978) and Britain (Howes and Mitchell, 1976). Such pneumococcal strains are also relatively resistant to penicillin V (page 55), methicillin (page 64), cloxacillin (page 79) and to cephalothin and cephaloridine (page 199). By contrast they remain either fully ampicillin-sensitive (page 99), or only show a slight decrease in sensitivity (Hansman, 1975). Most human infections caused by these pneumococci probably would respond to penicillin G, provided that sufficiently large doses are used (Hansman, 1976), but this may not be invariable. Already there are several case reports describing serious infections caused by relatively resistant pneumococci, which responded poorly to standard penicillin G regimens. These include meningitis (Naraqi *et al.*, 1974; Paredes *et al.*, 1976a; Howes and Mitchell, 1976; Mace *et al.*, 1977), and severe pneumococcal pneumonia (Devitt *et al.*, 1977) (*see also* pages 32, 33).

More recently pneumococci, completely resistant to penicillin and also to other antibiotics have been detected in South Africa (Appelbaum *et al.*, 1977; Center for Disease Control, 1977c). Type 19a pneumococci, resistant to penicillin G (MIC 4–8 μg per ml), cephalothin (MIC 4–15), chloramphenicol (MIC 9–37) and partially resistant to ampicillin (MIC 1–4) were isolated from five children in a hospital in Durban, South Africa. Three of these patients died from pneumococcal meningitis; the other two who had pneumonia and septicaemia respectively, recovered after prolonged treatment with antibiotics such as ampicillin, erythromycin and rifampicin. Since then carriers of the same resistant pneumococcal strains have been found in several Durban hospitals.

Multiply-resistant pneumococci were also soon found in Johannesburg in South Africa, a city approximately 300 miles inland from Durban. The first patient was a three-year-old boy who developed measles and pneumococcal pneumonia following cardiac surgery. He recovered with cephalothin and ampicillin treatment, although the type 19 pneumococcus isolated from his sputum was relatively resistant to both these drugs. In addition this strain was resistant to penicillin G (MIC 4–8 μg per ml), methicillin, erythromycin, clindamycin, tetracycline, chloramphenicol, co-trimoxazole and the aminoglycosides. This strain was therefore resistant to more antibiotics than the strain detected in Durban; it was fully sensitive only to rifampicin, vancomycin and bacitracin and moderately sensitive to sodium fusidate (MIC 2 μg per ml). Many carriers of this multiply resistant pneumococcus were detected among both patients and staff in the same hospital, and a few serious infections such as septicaemia also occurred, which were difficult to treat. Attempts to eliminate pneumococci from the carriers by using a rifampicin/sodium fusidate combination were complicated by the emergence of rifampicin-resistant pneumococcal strains (page 552). In Johannesburg some patients were also found to harbour penicillin and tetracycline-resistant type 6 pneumococci.

Subsequent surveys in several communities in South Africa showed that antibiotic-resistant pneumococci have at least five resistance patterns: (1) penicillin resistance only; (2) penicillin and tetracycline resistance; (3) penicillin, tetracycline and chloramphenicol resistance; (4) penicillin and chloramphenicol resistance; (5) penicillin, tetracycline, chloramphenicol, erythromycin and clindamycin resistance. Strains from the last group are now referred to as 'multiply-resistant', and some of these have also developed resistance to other antibiotics such as rifampicin (vide supra). The multiply-resistant pneumococci and also those with other resistance patterns were either type 6 or type 19a (Center for Disease Control, 1978a).

A pneumococcus resistant to chloramphenicol and tetracycline and relatively resistant to penicillin G (MIC 0·25 μg per ml, compared with 0·03 μg per ml for sensitive strains) has been isolated in England from a patient who had recently returned from Spain (Meers and Matthews, 1978). A type 14 pneumococcus, resistant to penicillin (MIC 4 μg per ml) has also been isolated from the blood of a five-year-old girl in Minnesota in the United States (Center for Disease Control, 1977d). This patient had pneumonia and because of immunodeficiency she had been frequently treated by penicillin in the past. This pneumococcal strain was sensitive to other antibiotics such as chloramphenicol and erythromycin, so that it differed both in serotype and antibiotic-resistance pattern from the multiply-resistant strains detected in South Africa (vide supra).

The occurrence of penicillin-resistant and multiply-resistant pneumococcal strains, raises fears that they may emerge in other parts of the world. The mechanisms of pneumococcal resistance is unknown, but the isolation in South Africa of serologically identical pneumococci with similar resistance patterns to several unrelated antibiotics, suggests the possibility of transferable drug resistance by R plasmids (page 422). However beta-lactamase production was not demonstrated in any of the resistant pneumococci isolated in Durban (Applebaum et al., 1977).

In view of these reports it is now advisable for all clinical laboratories to routinely test the sensitivities of all pneumococcal isolates (Leading article, 1977d).

Group B beta-haemolytic streptococci, often normally present in the vagina of both pregnant and non-pregnant women (Baker et al., 1977; Baker, 1977), have increasingly been recognized as an important cause of neonatal infections since about 1960 (McCracken, 1973; Berg et al., 1977; Annotation, 1977). More recently they have also been implicated in certain adult infections (Anthony and Concepcion, 1975; Bayer et al., 1976). These streptococci are consistently sensitive to penicillin G, but their degree of sensitivity is about ten-fold less than that of Group A streptococci (Table 1). Most studies show that the penicillin G sensitivity of Group B streptococci has remained unchanged in recent years (Anthony and Concepcion, 1975; Baker et al., 1976). In a survey conducted by Patterson and Hafeez (1976) there was a slight decrease in their susceptibility to penicillin in the period 1973–74, compared to 1962–63. *In vitro* and animal experimental studies indicate that the combination of penicillin G with an aminoglycoside such as gentamicin (page 329), may be synergistic against Group B streptococci (Baker, 1977; Deveikis *et al.*, 1977).

The less common human pathogens, Groups C and G beta-haemolytic streptococci, are consistently sensitive to penicillin G (Finland *et al.*, 1976a). The same is true for most strains of alpha-haemolytic streptococci such as Strep. sanguis, Strep. mitior (mitis), Strep. mutans, Strep. milleri, Strep. salvarius and the remaining unclassified streptococci in this group known as 'Strep. viridans'. Resistant variants of these streptococci may be found in the pharynx and teeth cavities of patients who have been treated by penicillin, or who are taking prophylactic penicillin for prolonged periods (Sprunt *et al.*, 1968; Phillips *et al.*, 1976). Strep. sanguis appears to be a natural 'penicillin-tolerant' bacterial species. Although its cell growth is inhibited by very low penicillin concentrations, the drug is not bactericidal to it. This appears to be because Strep. sanguis is an autolysin-defective organism, and the activity of such bacterial autolysins is essential for the irreversible bactericidal effect of penicillin (Horne and Tomasz, 1977). Strep. sanguis 'tolerance' to penicillin appears similar to that which has been described with some Staph. pyogenes strains (*vide infra*).

Strep. faecalis (Table 1, page 12) and other enterococcal Group D strep-tococci, such as Strep. faecium, are less sensitive to penicillin G than other streptococci. Some enterococcal strains may be highly resistant, and therefore routine sensitivity testing is required; up to 1969 there had been no increase in incidence of these highly resistant strains (Toala *et al.*, 1969). By contrast to Strep. faecalis, nonenterococcal Group D streptococci such as Strep. bovis, which may cause human disease such as endocarditis, appear to be always highly sensitive to penicillin G (Ravreby *et al.*, 1973; Watanakunakorn, 1974; Moellering *et al.*, 1974).

Anaerobic Gram-positive cocci such as the Peptococcus and Peptostrep-tococcus spp. and anaerobic streptococci are nearly always highly susceptible to penicillin G (Sutter and Finegold, 1976; Sutter, 1977).

Many strains of Staph. pyogenes, even outside hospitals, are resistant to penicillin (Bennett and Kucers, 1970; Bengtsson *et al.*, 1977). This resistance is usually due to penicillinase (beta-lactamase) production (*see* page 20), other mechanisms being less common (Chain, 1972). In a second mechanism of resistance termed 'intrinsic', the cell walls of staphylococci appear to be different, rendering them resistant to all penicillins, including the penicillinase-resistant penicillins and cephalosporins ('methicillin-resistant staphylococci', page 64). This is never the sole mechanism for resistance of Staph. pyogenes to penicillin G, because strains with intrinsic resistance invariably also produce penicillinase.

Recently a third mechanism for Staph. pyogenes resistance to the penicillins has been described and called 'tolerance'. These staphylococci have a deficiency of autolytic enzyme activity on their cell surface. This enzyme activity is required to augment the bacterial cell wall damage initiated by penicillin, and their combined action produces a lethal effect on bacteria (Best *et al.*, 1974; Sabath *et al.*, 1977) (*see also* pages 67, 80). As a result, although the penicillins inhibit these organisms in usual concentrations, they are not bactericidal. 'Tolerance' to penicillins appears to be one of degree, some 'tolerant' strains cannot be killed by a penicillin, whereas others can be killed albeit more slowly. A few surveys have indicated that such strains are by no means rare (Mayhall et al., 1976; Leading article, 1977b). They are often probably unrecognized, because milder infections due to these strains are likely to respond to penicillins. However, highly 'tolerant' staphylococci may cause problems with severe staphylococcal infections such as septicaemia or endocarditis. Three patients with staphylococcal septicaemia caused by these organisms, treated by Mayhall et al. (1976), failed to respond to a standard oxacillin (page 80) regimen, but the infection was controlled when gentamicin was used in addition.

Staph. pyogenes strains 'tolerant' to the penicillins usually also show a similar tolerance to cephalosporins (pages 199, 225) and vancomycin (page 646), but the bactericidal effect of gentamicin, cycloserine and rifampicin against them is unaffected (Sabath et al., 1977). 'Tolerant' strains can best be detected in the laboratory if both the minimum inhibitory concentration and minimum bactericidal concentration are estimated (Sabath et al., 1977; Haldane and Affias, 1977). Lacey (1977b) considers that there is still insufficient evidence to conclude that staphylococcal 'tolerance' is a new resistance mechanism, and that other factors may have been responsible for some of the therapeutic failures attributed to it.

Staph. epidermidis may be penicillin G sensitive (Sabath et al., 1976), but resistant strains commonly occur.

2. *Gram-positive bacilli*. C. diphtheriae and B. anthracis are consistently sensitive to penicillin G. Listeria monocytogenes is also usually sensitive, but occasional resistant strains occur (Kalis et al., 1976; Wiggins et al., 1978). Kanamycin (page 308) and gentamicin (page 329) potentiate the action of penicillin G on Listeria monocytogenes (Gordon et al., 1972; Mohan et al., 1977). The Nocardia spp. are penicillin G-resistant.

Anaerobic Gram-positive sporing bacilli such as Clostridium tetani, Cl. perfringens (welchii), Cl. botulinum, Cl. innocum and Cl. ramosum are also nearly always penicillin-sensitive (Sutter and Finegold, 1976; Sutter, 1977; Rood et al., 1978). Resistant strains of Cl. perfringens and other Clostridium spp. have been detected occasionally (Finegold, 1977). Penicillin G is active against nearly all strains of anaerobic Gram-positive asporogenous bacilli such as the Actinomyces, Eubacterium, Arachnia, Propionibacterium, Bifidobacterium and Lactobacillus spp. (Sutter and Finegold, 1976; Sutter, 1977, Holmberg et al., 1977).

3. *Gram-negative cocci*. Neisseria meningitidis is sensitive to penicillin G, and although resistant strains have been reported (Contoyiannis and Adamopoulos, 1974), they still appear to be very rare. L-forms of N. meningitidis insensitive to penicillin G can be produced *in vitro*, but their importance in disease states such as recurrent meningococcal meningitis is still uncertain (Chin and Lawson, 1976).

Neisseria gonorrhoeae was initially always highly sensitive to penicillin G (Table 1, page 12), but now the position has changed considerably. Relatively resistant gonococcal variants appeared about twenty years ago, and not only has their degree of resistance slowly increased, but now they also have become more frequent (Martin *et al.*, 1970; Sparling, 1972; Smithurst, 1974). Their degree of penicillin resistance varies, the majority of strains requiring at least 0·085 μg per ml for inhibition (Smithurst, 1974), whilst the remainder are more resistant and require 0·125–2·0 μg per ml for inhibition (Rodriguez and Saz, 1975). Relatively resistant gonococci have been detected in most countries including North America (Jaffe *et al.*, 1976), Britain (Jackson and Jephcott, 1976) and Australia (Finger and Handke, 1977). They are particularly prevalent in some areas such as South-East Asia (Willcox, 1970; Hart, 1973). These strains are also often relatively resistant to other unrelated antibiotics such as tetracycline, erthromycin, chloramphenicol, streptomycin, rifampicin and spectinomycin. Gonococcal resistance to such chemically and biological diverse drugs, may be caused by the mutation of a single gene (Maness and Sparling, 1973; Maier *et al.*, 1974; Judson *et al.*, 1974; Powell and Bond, 1976) (*see also* tetracyclines, page 596). This type of antibiotic resistance can be transferred in mixed gonococcal cultures, but it does not seem to be mediated by classical R plasmids (page 422). Such *in vitro* transformation may occur via liberated DNA from donor strains into the culture broth. Transfer of genes amongst gonococci may take place in nature by a similar mechanism (Sarubbi and Sparling, 1974). The basic mechanism for decreased susceptibility of relatively resistant strains, is probably a change in the binding capacity of the cell wall, so that they bind 10–15 times less penicillin than susceptible strains (Rodriguez and Saz, 1975). Beta-lactamase activity plays no role in this resistance (Beebe *et al.*, 1976).

These relatively resistant gonococcal strains, although capable of causing uncomplicated gonorrhoea, may have lost their capacity to cause disseminated infection. Indeed gonococcal isolates from patients with septicaemia have been found to be more susceptible to penicillin than isolates from patients with uncomplicated infections (Wiesner *et al.*, 1973; Handsfield *et al.*, 1976; Eisenstein *et al.*, 1977). By contrast, gonococcal strains from women with pelvic inflammatory disease are more resistant to penicillin G than isolates from uncomplicated anogenital infections (Sackel *et al.*, 1977).

More recently beta-lactamase (penicillinase)-producing strains of gonococci, which are completely penicillin-resistant, have emerged (Ashford *et al.*, 1976; Phillips, 1976; Annotation, 1976b; Leading Article, 1976b). These strains are also resistant to ampicillin (page 102), carbenicillin and other penicillins including mecillinam (page 187). Cephaloridine (page 199) is also inactive against these strains, but cephalexin (page 226) and cephradine (page 257) are moderately active, whilst cefamandole (page 269), cefoxitin (page 270) and especially cefuroxime (page 272) are quite active against them (Sparling *et al.*, 1977). Streptomycin is inactive against penicillinase-producing gonococci; but they are usually sensitive to spectinomycin (page 586), cotrimoxazole (page 711) and kanamycin (page 309). They are often moderately resistant to tetracyclines (page 596) and erythromycin (page 498) (Center for Disease Control, 1978b; Siegel *et al.*, 1978).

Beta-lactamase-producing strains of N. gonorrhoeae were first recognized in the Philippines in late 1975. Soon after they were also detected in many other countries, including the United States of America (Ashford *et al.*, 1976), Britain (Phillips, 1976; Wilkinson *et al.*, 1976), Australia (Lindon and Handke, 1976), Holland (Blog *et al.*, 1977) and Africa (Piot, 1977; Hallet *et al.*, 1977).

These reports each described the occurrence of these strains in one or two patients, but two series, with 26 and 45 patients respectively, were reported from Liverpool (Turner *et al.*, 1976; Percival *et al.*, 1976). By May 1977, these resistant gonococci had been identified in sixteen countries, and in the United States alone, 191 cases of infection had been confirmed in military personnel and civilians by the end of June, 1977 (Center for Disease Control, 1977a and b; Siegel, *et al.*, 1978).

It is possible that these resistant strains will become even more widespread, because their beta-lactamase production is R plasmid-mediated (Roberts and Falkow, 1977; Elwell *et al.*, 1977) (*see* page 422). This plasmid is rather similar to the TEM plasmid of ampicillin-resistant H. influenzae (page 102), and it codes for the production of a cell-bound beta-lactamase, which is similar to the TEM-1 enzyme produced by many Gram-negative bacilli (Bergström *et al.*, 1978). This plasmid can be transferred between gonococci and also into Esch. coli (Sparling *et al.*, 1977; Kirven and Thornsberry, 1977). There is now also a possibility that these genes conferring resistance to penicillin, may be transferred to N. meningitidis (page 7), which is a closely related organism (Saunders, 1977). However such plasmid-containing gonococcal strains lose their beta-lactamase plasmids at a rapid rate and revert to penicillin G susceptibility, so that beta-lactamase producing strains may not become the predominant gonococci in the future (Baron *et al.*, 1977).

There appear to be two distinct types of penicillinase-producing N. gonorrhoeae. Most strains isolated in or epidemiologically linked to the Far East are relatively tetracycline-resistant *in vitro* and carry a plasmid with a molecular weight of $5·8 \times 10^6$ daltons. By contrast penicillinase-producing gonococci linked with West Africa and Europe are tetracycline-sensitive and contain a smaller $3·2 \times 10^6$ dalton plasmid, which codes for beta-lactamase production. Approximately 43 per cent of Far Eastern strains, but none of those from West Africa have an additional $24·5 \times 10^6$ dalton conjugative plasmid (*see* page 422), which can transfer R plasmids to other gonococci and to some other Gram-negative bacilli. The presence of this conjugative plasmid therefore probably confers a selective advantage on the Far Eastern gonococcal strain. Penicillinase-producing gonococci from the Far East have spread more readily than those from West Africa (Perine *et al.*, 1977; WHO, 1977). In Liverpool, England in 1976, beta-lactamase-producing strains constituted 9 per cent of gonococcal isolates, but with control efforts their containment was successful by 1977. By contrast in certain areas of the Philippines the reported prevalence of these strains has been 30 to 40 per cent, and this has remained unchanged despite control programmes (Center for Disease Control, 1978b).

The use of penicillin G, even in large doses, is quite ineffective for the treatment of gonorrhoea caused by penicillinase-producing strains (Percival *et al.*, 1976). Because of their penicillinase production an inoculum effect occurs when their sensitivity to penicillin is tested; the minimum inhibitory concentrations may be low if a small inoculum is used, but very high ($>250 \mu g$ per ml) when a large inoculum is used (Percival *et al.*, 1976). Penicillinase-producing gonococci, unlike relatively-resistant strains (*vide supra*) appear to be fully virulent as they have caused salpingitis and disseminated infections in some cases (Wilkinson, 1977; Sparling *et al.*, 1977; Leftik *et al.*, 1978).

A less common human pathogen, Acinetobacter calcoaceticus var. lwoffi

(Mima polymorpha), may be penicillin-sensitive (Goldstein *et al.*, 1965), but it is more commonly resistant (Olafsson *et al.*, 1958). Gram-negative anaerobic cocci such as Veillonella spp. are sensitive to penicillin G (Sutter and Finegold, 1976).

4. *Gram-negative bacilli.* The Enterobacteriaceae, such as Esch. coli and the Salmonella, Shigella, Enterobacter, Klebsiella, Proteus, Serratia, Citrobacter, Providencia, Yersinia, Hafnia, Edwardsiella and Arizona spp. are resistant to penicillin G. The same applies to most other Gram-negative bacilli such as the Brucella spp., Vibrio cholerae, Pseudomonas pseudomallei and Ps. aeruginosa.

Anaerobic Gram-negative bacilli vary in their sensitivity. Those which normally populate the oropharynx such as Bacteroides melaninogenicus and Fusobacterium spp., are usually sensitive to penicillin G. Bacteroides fragilis, habitually present in the gastro-intestinal tract, however is usually penicillin-resistant. Other Bacteroides spp. vary in their sensitivity, but about 50 per cent of strains are inhibited by low penicillin concentrations ($<1\cdot0$ μg per ml) and about 80 per cent of strains by 16–32 μg per ml (Busch *et al.*, 1976; Sutter and Finegold, 1976).

H. influenzae and B. pertussis are usually regarded as penicillin G-resistant, but they are inhibited by relatively low penicillin concentrations (Table 1, page 12). Beta-lactamase producing strains of H. influenzae (page 102) are highly resistant to penicillin G. Haemophilus ducreyi is usually susceptible, but some strains produce beta-lactamase and are penicillin-resistant (Hammond *et al.*, 1978). Pasteurella multocida with an MIC of $0\cdot39$ μg per ml is penicillin G-sensitive (Bell *et al.*, 1969; Johnson and Rumans, 1977). The Legionnaires' disease bacterium appears sensitive to penicillin G *in vitro* (MIC $0\cdot5$–$2\cdot0$ μg per ml), but the drug does not prevent death of guinea pigs inoculated with this agent (Thornsberry *et al.*, 1978; Fraser *et al.*, 1978). Campylobacter fetus is relatively resistant to penicillin G (median MIC 10 μg per ml) (Chow *et al.*, 1978).

The resistance of Gram-negative bacilli to penicillin is one of degree. Weinstein *et al.* (1964) classified them as 'sensitive' if they were susceptible *in vitro* to $2\cdot0$–45 μg per ml, as 'moderately sensitive' if they were inhibited by 90–370 μg per ml, and 'resistant' if they were inhibited by 740 μg per ml or more. On this basis, the salmonellae and shigellae and 83 per cent of Esch. coli strains tested by these authors, were 'sensitive'. All Proteus mirabilis strains were 'sensitive', but Pr. vulgaris was usually 'resistant', and Ps. aeruginosa always 'resistant'. Bacteroides fragilis would fall in the 'sensitive' group, as most strains are inhibited by 32–40 μg per ml (Schoutens and Yourassowsky, 1974; Tally *et al.*, 1975).

There are two main reasons why Gram-negative bacilli are resistant or relatively resistant to penicillin G and certain other beta-lactam antibiotics. Intrinsic resistance is due to the inability of the antibiotic to penetrate the outer membrane of the cell wall (*see* page 19). For instance, Ps. aeruginosa is penicillin G-resistant mainly because of this permeability barrier (Suginaka *et al.*, 1975). The second reason is the presence of cell-bound beta-lactamase enzymes which are found in the periplasmic space of the cell wall (*see* page 20). The characteristics of these beta-lactamases are either chromosomally or R plasmid controlled. All Gram-negative bacteria including the anaerobes such as Bacteroides spp. produce beta-lactamases (Sykes and Matthew, 1976;

Olsson *et al.*, 1976).

5. *Treponema pallidum* and the *Leptospirae* are consistently sensitive to penicillin G. The same is true for Streptobacillus moniliformis and Spirillum minus (the organisms causing rat-bite fever).

6. *Mycobacteria, Mycoplasmas, Rickettsiae, Fungi* and *Protozoa* are all completely penicillin-resistant. The Chlamydia genus is relatively resistant. For instance, penicillin G interferes with the normal growth of Chlamydia trachomatis as evidenced by the production of abnormal non-fluorescent inclusions, but normal growth pattern returns when penicillin is removed (Johnson and Hobson, 1977).

7. *Non-bacterial penicillin inactivating enzymes.* Penicillin G therapy may occasionally fail in certain infections which would normally respond to penicillin. Some recent reports have ascribed some instances of this to a penicillin inactivating substance, apparently derived from the host and not of bacterial origin. This substance has been detected in inflammatory exudates, especially in collections of pus such as pleural empyema (Barnes and Waterworth, 1977; De Louvois and Hurley, 1977). This inactivating agent is probably an enzyme, which may be capable of inactivating most penicillins and some cephalosporins (including penicillinase-resistant drugs). It has no effect on unrelated antibiotics, such as sodium fusidate, clindamycin, chloramphenicol, tetracycline or gentamicin (Barnes and Waterworth, 1977). However, the possible bacterial origin of this enzyme has not yet been definitely excluded (Lacey, 1977a).

In Vitro Sensitivities

The MIC's of penicillin G against some selected bacterial species are shown in Table 1. Penicillin G is still frequently prescribed in units, and MIC's expressed in units per ml are about 1·7 times higher than shown in this table (one unit is equivalent to 0·6 μg per pure sodium penicillin G).

Mode of Administration and Dosage

1. Penicillin G is destroyed by acid in the stomach and therefore absorption after oral administration is irregular and variable. Intramuscular injection is the usual method of administration, but the highly soluble salts of penicillin G can also be given intravenously.

2. *Crystalline penicillin G.* This drug may be administered either intramuscularly or intravenously. The common mode of administration is by the intramuscular route, but there are circumstances in which the intravenous method is preferable. For instance in shocked patients the absorption of penicillin from intramuscular sites may be inadequate. In addition the intravenous route is convenient for patients requiring large doses of parenteral penicillin for prolonged periods, e.g. patients with bacterial endocarditis. The only advantage of intravenous penicillin in this situation is the avoidance of frequent painful intramuscular injections.

Crystalline penicillin G is usually administered every six hours, but intervals of one to two hours between doses may be necessary in severe infections. A common adult dosage is one million units (0·6 g) intramuscularly or in-

12 THE USE OF ANTIBIOTICS

TABLETABLE 1

Compiled from data published by Garrod (1960a and b), Knox (1960), Barber and
Waterworth (1962), Sutherland *et al.* (1970), Watanakunakorn (1974), Rodriguez and
Saz (1975), Tally *et al.* (1975), Baker *et al.* (1976), Percival *et al.* (1976), Sutter and
Finegold (1976), Devitt *et al.* (1977) and Mohan *et al.* (1977)

ORGANISM	MIC (μg per ml)
Gram-positive bacteria	
Staph. pyogenes (non-penicillinase producer)	0·03
Strep. pyogenes (Group A)	0·007
Strep. pneumoniae (Dip. pneumoniae)	0·015
Strep. pneumoniae (relatively resistant)	0·1–2·0
Streptococci, Group B	0·025–0·2
Strep. viridans spp.	0·01
Strep. faecalis (Enterococcus, Group D)	2·0
Strep. bovis (Non-enterococcal, Group D)	0·024
Bacillus anthracis	0·015
Corynebacterium diphtheriae	0·062
Listeria monocytogenes	0·1
Clostridium tetani	0·06
Actinomyces israelii	0·05
Gram-negative bacteria	
Neisseria meningitidis	0·03
Neisseria gonorrhoeae:	
(a) sensitive strains	0·007
(b) relatively resistant strains	0·125–2·0
(c) penicillinase-producing strains	2·0–>250
Haemophilus influenzae	1·0
Bordetella pertussis	0·5
Brucella abortus	6·0
Salmonella typhi	4·0
Shigella spp.	16·0
Escherichia coli	64·0
Proteus mirabilis	32·0
Bacteroides fragilis	32·0
Bacteroides melaninogenicus	0·1–0·5
Other Bacteroides spp.	0·1–32·0

travenously, every six hours. For serious infections much higher doses can be
given, e.g. for bacterial meningitis a common starting dose for adults is three
million units (1·8 g) three-hourly. Doses higher than this are usually unnecessary for infections, however severe, caused by penicillin-sensitive
organisms. 'Massive' penicillin doses of up to 100 million units (60 g) daily, intravenously, have been occasionally used for serious infections due to relatively
resistant organisms, such as those due to Gram-negative bacilli (Weinstein *et
al.*, 1964). Conversely, some authors consider that a dose of one million units
six-hourly, is unnecessarily high for many infections of moderate severity. For
instance Anderson *et al.* (1968) regarded an adult dose of crystalline penicillin
as low as 300 000 units (0·18 g) intramuscularly, twelve-hourly, as satisfactory

for the treatment of pneumococcal pneumonia, a disease in which the blood supply to all diseased areas is very good. These small penicillin doses entail risks and are not now generally advocated. It is interesting that doses now regarded as inadequate (e.g. 15 000 units four-hourly), were lifesaving in very severe infections during the early years of penicillin (Stewart, 1965). More recently Brewin et al. (1974) found that procaine penicillin (vide infra) in a dose of 600 000 units (0·6 g) intramuscularly, twelve-hourly, was as satisfactory as a daily intravenous dose of 20 million units (12 g) crystalline penicillin for the treatment for pneumococcal pneumonia. If the pneumonia is caused by the still uncommon pneumococci, which are relatively resistant to penicillin (page 4), this procaine penicillin regimen may well be inadequate, but crystalline penicillin in a dose of one million units (0·6 g) six-hourly may succeed (Hansman, 1976).

3. *Method of intravenous administration.* Crystalline penicillin G may be administered intravenously by either continuous infusion or by intermittent injections into the intravenous tubing. In emergency treatment of serious infections, an initial direct injection of penicillin G should be given intravenously to achieve a high level of penicillin quickly, and this could then be followed by continuous penicillin infusion. Continuous infusion was once considered preferable because of rapid excretion of the drug and the increased hazard of thrombophlebitis with intermittent administration (Welch, 1954). However, problems arise if penicillin is added to intravenous fluid bottles. It may be incompatible with other additives to intravenous solutions. For instance, penicillin G and semisynthetic penicillins are almost completely inactivated within a few hours in carbohydrate solutions containing sufficient bicarbonate to elevate the pH above 8·0 (Simberkoff et al., 1970). Furthermore, penicilloic acid, which appears to have a role in some of the allergic reactions, is a major product of such inactivation. Most clinicians therefore now prefer intermittent intravenous injections or intermittent rapid infusions of high concentration penicillin solutions via a secondary intravenous bottle or a buretrol (see methicillin, page 68 and ampicillin, page 106).

4. *Procaine penicillin.* During the later stages of treatment of many infections such as scarlet fever and pneumonia, procaine penicillin can be substituted for crystalline penicillin. This penicillin is useful because the absorption of an injected dose continues for up to 24 h, so that injections may be separated by this interval, but lower serum levels are obtained. These injections are also less painful than crystalline penicillin. A common adult dosage for procaine penicillin is one million units (1·0 g) intramuscularly once or twice a day. In milder infections procaine penicillin may be satisfactory for initial treatment. This compound must not be given intravenously (see page 26).

5. *Benzathine penicillin.* This preparation when injected intramuscularly in doses of 600 000 to 1 200 000 units, maintains a low serum concentration of penicillin for a period of one to three weeks. Single injections of benzathine penicillin have been used for treatment of streptococcal pharyngitis (Bass et al., 1976), diphtheria carriers (McCloskey et al., 1974) and syphilis (McCracken, 1974), while monthly injections are sometimes used for rheumatic fever prophylaxis (see page 40).

6. *Children.* The doses of crystalline, procaine or benzathine penicillin should be adjusted to the age and weight of the patient. In general, one quarter

of the adult dose is suitable for children under three years of age and one half the adult dose for older children.

7. *Newborn and premature infants.* The renal clearance of crystalline penicillin G in this age group is reduced. The mean half-life value in infants under six days of age is 3·2 h; in those aged 7–13 days it is 1·7 h and in infants 14 days of age and older, it is 1·4 h (McCracken, 1974). By comparison this half-life in normal adults, is only 30 min (page 16). Therefore small doses of crystalline penicillin given at eight- or twelve-hourly intervals are recommended for infants. A total daily dosage of 50 000 units per kg body weight, given in two or three divided doses, is usually adequate for most infections caused by highly susceptible bacteria (McCracken *et al.*, 1973). However, infants suffering from Group B streptococcal infections (pages 31, 34) should receive 100 000 units per kg per day, divided in two or three doses (McCracken, 1974). For serious infections such as meningitis, infants younger than 7 days may be given 100 000–150 000 units per kg per day, and those aged more than seven days may receive 150 000–250 000 units per kg per day.

Procaine penicillin G in a single daily dose of 50 000 units per kg, appears suitable for the treatment of minor infections. The drug is well tolerated in this age group without evidence of local reactions.

Benzathine penicillin G, if indicated in neonates, is given in a single dose of 50 000 units per kg body weight (McCracken, 1974).

8. *Patients with renal failure.* Penicillin G is often administered in the usual doses to these patients, because with small doses there is no great risk of toxicity. Moderately large intravenous doses may yield toxic levels (page 28) necessitating dosage reduction. If a crystalline penicillin dose of one to two million units six-hourly is normally indicated, then in anuric or severely uraemic patients, the intervals between the doses should be increased to eight or ten hours (Kunin, 1967). If high dose intravenous penicillin therapy is contemplated, equivalent to 24 million units daily for patients with normal renal function, more meticulous dosage adjustment is necessary for those with renal failure. Practical guidelines are shown in Table 2, for the use of large doses and intermittent intravenous penicillin G for such patients. These aim to achieve a mean serum penicillin concentration of approximately 20 μg per ml (Bryan and Stone, 1975).

TABLE 2

Dosage schedule for intermittent intravenous penicillin G therapy for patients with renal failure (After Bryan and Stone, 1975)

Creatinine clearance (ml per min)	Dose (million units)	Interval (h)
125	1·7–2·0	2
	or 2·6–3·0	3
60	1·8–2·0	4
40	1·3–1·5	4
20	0·8–1·0	4
10	0·8–1·0	6
nil	0·5–0·8	6
	or 0·7–1·1	8

These authors suggested that a loading dose of 750 000 to 1·2 million units should be given initially to patients with severe renal failure. If haemodialysis is required, an additional 500 000 units should be given every six hours during this procedure. The penicillin dose should be further reduced to 500 000 units every eight hours if there is also advanced liver disease associated with severe renal failure (see page 70).

9. *Intraperitoneal administration.* Crystalline penicillin G may be added to peritoneal dialysis fluid either to treat or to prevent intraperitoneal infection. Usually a dose of 50 000 units is added to each litre of dialysate resulting in a penicillin concentration of 50 units (31 μg) per ml. If this concentration of penicillin is used continuously, penicillin is absorbed from the peritoneum, and penicillin serum levels of about 25–30 per cent of the concentrations in the dialysate, are attained in patients with renal failure (Bulger *et al.*, 1965).

10. *Oral potassium penicillin G or benzathine penicillin G.* These have been used in children, but the acid stable phenoxypenicillins (page 55) are now preferred for oral therapy. The loose term 'oral penicillin' now usually applies to one of the phenoxypenicillins such as penicillin V or phenethicillin.

Availability

1. *Crystalline penicillin G,* suitable for IM or IV administration, is available as either the sodium or potassium salt of penicillin G. For parenteral therapy the sodium salt is often used, and vials of 0·5, 1·0, 1·5, 2·0, 5·0 and 10·0 mega units (0·3, 0·6, 0·9, 1·2, 3·0 and 6·0 g) are available. Potassium penicillin G is also available for oral administration, e.g. in 250 mg capsules, but this is now rarely used.

2. *Procaine penicillin* for IM use only.
   (a) Aqueous suspension of procaine penicillin is now most commonly marketed in disposable syringes, each containing either 0·6, 1·0 or 1·5 million units or g of procaine penicillin.
   (b) Fortified aqueous suspension, which contains added crystalline penicillin G.
   (c) Oily suspension containing procaine penicillin and aluminium monostearate. The absorption of this product is even more delayed but tissue damage may be a problem. This is now rarely used.

3. *Benzathine penicillin.* Pure benzathine penicillin is available in suspension containing 600 000 units per ml for IM administration. In addition vials of a mixture containing benzathine penicillin 450 mg (600 000 units), procaine penicillin 300 mg (300 000 units) and potassium penicillin 187 mg (300 000 units) ('Bicillin all purpose', Wyeth) are available for IM use. Tablets of benzathine penicillin (e.g. 'Bicillin' Wyeth, 150 mg) are available for oral administration, but like oral potassium penicillin G, these are now rarely used, the phenoxypenicillins (page 55) being preferred for oral penicillin therapy.

Serum Levels in Relation to Dosage

1. *Intravenous crystalline penicillin G.* Immediate high serum levels are attained after rapid intravenous injection of this preparation. If a dose of 1·2 g (2 million units) is administered intermittently, intravenously, every two hours, or 1·8 g (3 million units) every three hours, a mean serum concentration of approximately 20 μg per ml is attained (Bryan and Stone, 1975). This is adequate for the treatment of most severe infections (page 12).

Plaut *et al.* (1969) studied serum levels in ten patients with normal renal function, who received an intravenous injection of 3 g (5 million units) of sodium penicillin G, during a 3 to 5 min period. The resulting mean serum concentration after 5 min was 400 μg per ml and after 10 min, 273 μg per ml.

During the first hour there was a rapid decrease in the serum concentrations (due to both distribution and elimination of the drug), and at the end of the hour the mean serum level was 45 μg per ml. The subsequent fall in serum levels was slower, and presumably this was mainly due to penicillin elimination; at four hours the mean serum level was 3·0 μg per ml. This study also showed that if the same dose of penicillin G was administered by continuous infusion over a six-hour period, two hours were required to achieve a serum level of 12 to 20 μg per ml, which then could only be maintained by the use of a constant infusion pump. If the infusion was given by an ordinary intravenous drip, surprisingly large serum level fluctuations were observed, despite close supervision of the infusions.

2. *Intramuscular crystalline penicillin G.* With this method of administration, a peak serum level is obtained within half an hour. After one million units (0·6 g) this is usually 12 μg per ml (about 20 units per ml); the level thereafter falls rapidly, the usual half-life of the drug being only 30 min, but detectable serum levels remain for 4–6 h. The height of the peak and persistence of serum levels depend on the dose, but the relation is not always linear. There is also an individual variation and even in the same subject the response may vary under different conditions. For instance, the period of sustained therapeutic levels is shorter in healthy ambulatory volunteers than in patients confined to bed (Hussar and Holley, 1954). Diabetic patients may absorb penicillin G relatively poorly from intramuscular sites (Weinstein and Dalton, 1968).

In newborn infants, after an intramuscular dose of 25 000 units per kg body weight of crystalline penicillin, the mean peak serum level one half to one hour later, is approximately 22 μg per ml; this level falls to 1·0–2·0 μg per ml after 12 h. Penicillin does not accumulate if this dose is given every 12 h. Following a dose of 50 000 units per kg, a peak level of approximately 35 μg per ml occurs, but the level at 12 h is similar to that resulting from a dose of 25 000 units per kg. There is also no accumulation of penicillin when a dose of 50 000 units per kg is given every 12 h (McCracken *et al.*, 1973). In general penicillin serum levels are independent of birth weight, except that in infants weighing less than 2000 g at birth, peak serum levels are slightly lower, possibly due to more of the drug being distributed in extracellular fluid (McCracken, 1974). With older infants, mean serum levels become lower, because the penicillin half-life decreases as post-natal age increases (page 14).

3. *Procaine penicillin.* After intramuscular injection of an aqueous suspension of procaine penicillin (Fig. 1), a peak serum level is reached in about two hours and in adults given 600 000 units or more, detectable levels are usually maintained for at least 24 h.

In infants aged less than one week, following intramuscular procaine penicillin in a dose of 50 000 units per kg body weight, the mean serum level 2–12 h later is 7·4–8·8 μg per ml, and the level at 24 h is 1·5 μg per ml. Penicillin does not accumulate in the body if this dose is repeated every 24 h. Lower serum levels (5–6 μg per ml during first four hours, 0·4 μg per ml at 24 h) occur if this dose is given to infants older than one week (McCracken *et al.*, 1973).

4. *Benzathine penicillin.* Therapeutic levels are maintained for more prolonged periods with intramuscular injection of this preparation. In adults, a serum penicillin level of 0·12 μg per ml may be detected at 14 days following a

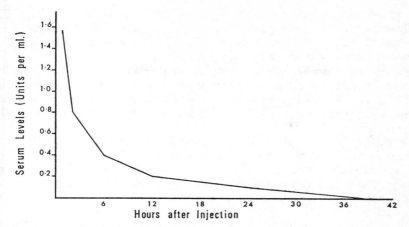

FIG. 1. Serum levels after 300 000 units aqueous suspension of procaine penicillin intramuscularly. (Redrawn from Welch, 1954).

dose of 2·4 million units (Kaplan and McCracken, 1973). In newborn infants, after an intramuscular dose of 50 000 units per kg body weight, a peak level of 1·23 μg per ml is attained 13–24 h after administration, which falls to 0·65–0·92 μg per ml at four days and to 0·07–0·09 μg per ml at 12 days (Klein et al., 1973; Kaplan and McCracken, 1973).

Excretion

URINE: If renal function is normal, over 70 per cent of an injected dose of penicillin G is excreted within six hours, mainly as the active drug, and high urinary concentrations are attained. In healthy adults, only about 10 per cent of an injected dose of penicillin is excreted by glomerular filtration, the remainder predominantly by tubular secretion (McCracken et al., 1973). Animal experiments indicate that this secretion takes place in proximal tubules, and that a small amount (about 10 per cent of the administered dose) then appears to be reabsorbed in the collecting ducts (Bergeron et al., 1975). In newborn infants excretion is predominantly by glomerular filtration, probably because of the immaturity of tubular function at this age (McCracken et al., 1973); this results in a prolonged penicillin serum half-life (page 14).

Renal tubular secretion can be partly blocked by probenecid ('Benemid'), and if it is used with penicillin G, serum concentrations are approximately doubled. It was postulated that probenecid also enhances penicillin serum levels by limiting its distribution to some organs and tissues, causing more penicillin to be confined to the vascular space (Gibaldi and Schwartz, 1968). More recent reports by Nauta et al. (1974), who studied the effect of probenecid on the distribution of cloxacillin (page 85) in anephric patients, and by Barza et al. (1975) who performed animal experiments, indicate that probenecid does not limit the access of penicillin to organs and tissues. Therefore, it appears that probenecid can be used therapeutically to enhance the serum levels of penicillins or cephalosporins and this will not lower the penicillin concentration at the site of infection (Nauta et al., 1974). The recommended adult dose of probenecid for this purpose, is 2·0 g daily. The daily dose for children aged 2–5 years is 0·5–0·75 g, for those aged 5–10 years 0·75–1·25 g, and for those aged 10–14 years it is 1·25–1·5 g. This is administered orally, usually in four divided doses.

Various other drugs, especially organic acids, may compete with penicillin for renal tubular secretion, similar to probenecid. In this way, the penicillin half-life may be prolonged by aspirin, phenylbutazone, sulphonamides, indomethacin, thiazide diuretics, frusemide and ethacrynic acid (Leading article, 1975a).

In patients with impaired renal function, the penicillin serum half-life increases as renal function deterioriates (Plaut et al., 1969), but penicillin still disappears from the blood at a significant, but reduced rate of anuric patients (Kunin, 1967). Elderly subjects also have a diminished renal tubular secretory ability and are liable to penicillin neurotoxicity (page 28), if large doses are given intravenously (Lerner et al., 1967).

BILE: A small amount of the active drug is eliminated by this route. In animals penicillin G is actively secreted into the bile and amounts to about 4·5 per cent of the total dose administered. Probenecid may reduce biliary excretion and possibly also interfere with penicillin inactivation in the liver (vide infra), because probenecid significantly prolongs the cloxacillin half-life in anephric patients (Nauta et al., 1974).

INACTIVATION IN BODY: The remainder of an administered dose of penicillin G which is not excreted in urine or bile (usually less than 30 per cent), is inactivated in the body. This occurs in the liver and penicilloic acid is the major end-product (Cole et al., 1973). Inactivation of penicillin G is more rapid than that of other penicillins such as ampicillin (page 109) and carbenicillin (page 157), so that in anuric patients the serum half-life of penicillin G is only 3 h, but with ampicillin it is 7—8 h and 15 h with carbenicillin. However, serum levels of penicillin G decline very slowly in the absence of both hepatic and renal function (Bryan and Stone, 1975) (see methicillin, page 70).

Distribution of the Drug in Body

Penicillin G diffuses fairly readily into pleural, pericardial, ascitic, and synovial fluids (Hussar and Holley, 1954; Gerding et al., 1977). The drug easily penetrates into inflamed tissues, where it persists longer than in normal tissues (Florey et al., 1946). Its diffusion is poor into avascular areas and abscesses (Fishman and Hewitt, 1970), non-inflamed bone (Smilack et al., 1976) and the cerebrospinal fluid (with uninflamed meninges). Hieber and Nelson (1977) studied serial CSF penicillin concentrations in children with bacterial meningitis, who were treated by intravenous penicillin G in a dose of 250 000 units per kg per day. The mean CSF penicillin concentrations on the first, fifth and tenth days of therapy were 0·8, 0·7 and 0·3 μg per ml, respectively. These decreasing CSF levels correlated with the return of CSF protein concentrations towards normal.

When parenteral penicillin is administered to subjects with normal meninges, CSF penicillin levels are kept low not only by passive CSF flow into the venous system via the arachnoid villi, but also by an active transport system localized in the choroid plexus, which specifically excretes penicillin and other organic acids from the CSF (Hieber and Nelson, 1977). In patients with meningitis there is increased vascular permeability allowing more penicillin to enter the CSF, and also a decreased clearance from the CSF by partial inhibition of the organic acid pump. In animals with normal meninges and in those with experimental bacterial meningitis, CSF penicillin levels increase two to three times, if probenecid is also given. This increase is greater than can be expected from the associated serum level increase (page 17). It appears that probenecid elevates the CSF penicillin concentration by directly inhibiting excretion of organic acids from the cerebrospinal fluid (Dacey and Sande, 1974). This probenecid effect may precipitate encephalopathy (page 28) if penicillin is used in large doses. Probenecid also has the same effect on CSF concentrations of other penicillins and cephalosporins. Occasionally this probenecid action may be useful therapeutically to increase CSF antibiotic levels; in this way it would be possible to increase ticarcillin (page 170) CSF levels to treat Pseudomonas meningitis (Dacey and Sande, 1974).

Penicillin G enters erythrocytes. If it is given by a direct intravenous injection and this is followed by a constant penicillin infusion, the red blood cell penicillin concentration equals or exceeds the serum concentration after two hours. If penicillin administration is then ceased, the erythrocytic penicillin concentration is only halved in 50–60 min, whereas the serum penicillin half-life is 30 min (page 16). This slower rate of efflux of penicillin G from erythrocytes probably helps to maintain high initial drug levels for a longer period (Kornguth and Kunin, 1976). Penicillin G easily crosses the placenta, reaching therapeutic concentrations in both fetus and amniotic fluid, except that levels are low in the amniotic fluid during the first trimester (Wasz-Höckert et al., 1970). Penicillin G is 46–58 per cent protein bound (Kunin, 1967).

Mode of Action

1. *Structure of bacterial cell envelope.* The cell wall is complex and unique to bacteria. Being relatively inelastic, it confers shape on the organism and protects it against lysis due to osmotic pressure differences between the cell cytoplasm and the external environment. Beta-lactam antibiotics (penicillins and cephalosporins) are of comparatively low toxicity to humans because they act by interfering with synthesis of the cell wall, without affecting protein synthesis within the cell.

The cytoplasmic membrane lies immediately beneath the cell wall and is pressed up against it by osmotic forces within the cell. The cell wall and the cytoplasmic membrane together form the cell envelope. These component structures are interdependent and alterations in one may render the other ineffective. The composition of the cell envelope, the complexity of which varies with different bacterial species, has an important role in modifying the action of antibiotics (Costerton and Cheng, 1975). Antibiotics act on protein synthesis within the cell or at a site within the envelope, so that they must pass through part or all of the envelope to reach their target.

In Gram-positive bacteria the major portion of the cell wall consists of a mucopeptide layer (also known as murein or peptidoglycan) which supports the cytoplasmic membrane. This mucopeptide layer consists of a giant molecule, constructed in the form of a net of polysaccharide strands, which are interlinked by short peptide bonds. In the resting cell, this molecule is apparently united in every direction over the cell's surface and there are no free ends available for further growth (Leading article, 1972c). For cell growth to proceed, this mucopeptide lattice must be broken to enable new cell wall material to be inserted. In the dividing cell there is the additional complex process of the formation of a septum or cross-wall (consisting of cytoplasmic membrane and wall), which splits in a special way to produce progeny indentical to the parent cell. Lytic enzymes (autolysins) are involved in both of these processes. Obviously in the normal growing cell, synthesis and lysis must be balanced to allow cell division, without cell destruction. In Gram-positive bacteria the interstices within the mucopeptide net, communicating as they do with the cytoplasmic membrane constitute a periplasmic space. A number of degradative enzymes may occur in this space, which are capable of destroying a variety of antibiotics; these include beta-lactamases (penicillinases and cephalosporinases), which hydrolyse the beta-lactam ring of susceptible penicillins and cephalosporins. The type and amount of the enzymes present in the periplasmic space depend on the bacterial species. In pathogenic Gram-positive bacteria, the bacterial envelope is usually completed by a third component, a protein coat or a carbohydrate capsule, exterior to the mucopeptide layer. Beta-lactam antibiotics bind to proteins on the external surface of the cytoplasmic membrane and these may be their site of action. It follows that with resistant Gram-positive bacteria, beta-lactam antibiotics may at first be subjected to cell-free beta-lactamases and, during penetration of the cell envelope, be confronted by further beta-lactamases before they reach their target on the cytoplasmic membrane.

In Gram-negative bacteria, the envelope is more complex and consists of four layers. A mucopeptide net again is exterior to, and supports the cytoplasmic membrane, but the periplasmic space formed by the niches in the mucopeptide is extended out beyond the mucopeptide layer, by protruding lipoprotein bundles which meet an extra outer membrane. Exterior to this outer membrane there is also usually a protein coat or a carbohydrate capsule. The periplasmic space of Gram-negative bacteria, therefore, consists of an area spreading from the cytoplasmic membrane through the mucopeptide net to the outer membrane. This outer membrane is very important, because it has selective permeability and thereby preserves the micro-environment of the periplasmic space. For instance, it prevents the outward passage of periplasmic enzymes and prevents the inward passage of some antibiotics (*see also* page 10). The penetrability of the outer membrane to various antibiotics is often specific for particular bacterial species, but may be altered by a number of factors, including the acquisition of R plasmids (*see* page 422). Inability to penetrate the various layers of the envelope, is the explanation for the intrinsic resistance of Gram-negative bacteria to antibiotics (*see* page 10). Sometimes antibiotics are used in combination to effect killing of both Gram-negative and Gram-positive bacteria; various beta-lactam antibiotics are used to increase the penetrability of the cell envelope to aminoglycosides, so that these antibiotics can reach their receptor sites within the cell cytoplasm (*see* pages 294, 329). Degradative enzymes in the periplasmic space which are confined within the cell by the outer membrane of Gram-negative bacteria, are also very important in determining antibiotic resistance of Gram-negative bacteria. Of special importance are the beta-lactamases which confer resistance to beta-lactam antibiotics (Sykes and Mathew, 1976). A number of factors influence the efficacy of these beta-lactamases in destroying beta-lactam antibiotics. These include the amount of the beta-lactam antibotic which has penetrated through into the space, the amount of enzyme present, the affinity or specificity of the enzyme for the particular beta-lactam antibiotic involved and its 'efficiency' in hydrolysing the antibiotic. In addition, the amount of beta-lactamase present in the periplasmic space can be altered in many Gram-negative bacteria, by induction, mutation, or by the acquisition of R plasmids.

Therefore, the sensitivity of bacteria to beta-lactam antibiotics varies with the bacterial species involved, which determines the site, type, amount and quality of beta-lactamase produced, and the ability of the antibiotic to penetrate the layers of the bacterial envelope.

2. *Action of beta-lactam antibiotics.* These antibiotics act by selectively inhibiting the synthesis of mucopeptide in the bacterial cell wall of multiplying bacteria. This inhibitory action is incomplete and cell wall construction and cell division continue. Mucopeptide, however, is liable to destruction by the unopposed action of autolytic enzymes so that cells clothed by absent (protoplasts) or defective (spheroplasts) walls are produced. Beta-lactam antibiotics are lethal to susceptible organisms because under most circumstances these progeny, after cell division, are subject to lysis as a result of osmotic forces. Microorganisms such as the Mycoplasmas, which do not possess a mucopeptide cell wall, are not susceptible to beta-lactam antibiotics.

Penicillin inhibits a number of enzymes concerned in the synthesis of cell wall mucopeptide (Blumberg and Strominger, 1974). The exact biochemical mechanisms involved are not yet defined, but it may be a competitive process because there are structural similarities between penicillin and various portions of mucopeptide. Originally, it was believed that the sole action of penicillin was to inhibit the synthesis of cross-linkages (peptide bonds) in mucopeptide, by reacting with an enzyme, transpeptidase (Strominger and Tipper, 1965). Later, Hartmann *et al.* (1972) isolated two cell wall active enzymes from Esch. coli, both of which were inhibited by penicillin. These were autolytic enzymes (mucopeptide hydrolases), which were capable of producing cleavage points in intact mucopeptide walls, thereby providing acceptor sites for incoming new material during cell growth. One of these enzymes, an endopeptidase, has transferase activity and may be identical to the transpeptidase previously thought to be the chief target of penicillin's action. The second enzyme was identified as a glycosidase, which is involved in the synthesis of polysaccharide chains in the cell wall. Hartmann *et al.* (1972) also correlated the action of these two enzymes with morphological changes observed in Esch. coli, exposed to penicillin at different concentrations. At relatively low concentrations of penicillin, endopeptidase activity is inhibited and this affects cross-wall synthesis, concerned with the formation of the septum across the cell. Cell division is therefore inhibited, but the cell continues to elongate resulting in the production of filamentous forms. If Esch. coli are exposed to higher concentrations of penicillin, glycosidase activity is also inhibited, which prevents side-wall synthesis and elongation of the cell. As a result of the combined inhibition of these two enzymes, organisms with defective cell wall (spheroplasts) are produced, the classical penicillin effect. Greenwood and O'Grady (1973a and b) showed that cephalexin (similar to low concentrations of other cephalosporins and penicillins) also produces filamentous changes in Esch. coli, and they suggested that this antibiotic selectively inhibits endopeptidase, which is involved in cross-wall synthesis.

Ampicillin (page 99) also produces filamentous forms of Esch. coli, but by contrast amoxycillin (page 132) produces rapid formation of spheroplasts and lysis of these organisms (Comber et al., 1977). It therefore appears that ampicillin mainly inhibits cross-wall synthesis and amoxycillin predominantly inhibits side-wall synthesis. This may explain why amoxycillin is more rapidly bactericidal than ampicillin in experimental Esch. coli infections in animals (page 133). Peripheral growth and cross-wall formation, also appear to be separable processes in cocci (Lorian and Atkinson, 1976). Cell wall growth only seems to occur at the equatorial plane in Gram-positive cocci and cleavage of cross-walls prior to cell separation is carried out by autolytic enzymes. When Staph. pyogenes is exposed to subinhibitory concentrations of penicillin, the cell divides but the resultant progeny cannot separate normally, because these autolytic enzymes are inhibited by penicillin (Lorian, 1975). Paradoxically, if Staph. pyogenes is exposed to very high concentrations of a beta-lactam antibiotic, its bactericidal action is reduced and this is also apparently due to interference with autolytic enzymes necessary for cell division (Nishino and Nakazawa, 1976). The continuing action of autolysins is therefore important for the lethal action of beta-lactam antibiotics. Descriptions of a newly recognised type of penicillin resistance of Staph. pyogenes (pages 6, 67, 80), supports this view (Sabath et al., 1977). These authors detected strains of Staph. pyogenes which they designated as 'penicillin tolerant'; tests with nafcillin showed that the minimum inhibitory concentrations of these organisms were low (sensitive range) but their minimum bactericidal concentrations were often more than 100 times higher; these strains also showed 'cross-tolerance' to the killing action of cephalosporins and vancomycin, by which they were also only inhibited. The dissociation of these two effects of penicillin disappeared with prolonged incubation of some of these strains, indicating that for some strains penicillin was still lethal but at a slower rate. This 'penicillin tolerance' was associated with a deficiency in these organisms of autolytic enzyme activity which was caused by an inhibitor of autolysin.

The comparatively new class of penicillins, amidino penicillins (see mecillinam, page 187), differ in their mode of action from other penicillins (Greenwood and O'Grady 1973b; Blumberg and Strominger, 1974). Esch. coli exposed to low concentrations of these penicillins, forms large spherical bodies and not the spheroplasts associated with exposure to ampicillin or penicillin G. In addition, the enzymes known to be inhibited by normal penicillins are not inhibited by lethal concentrations of the amidino penicillins. Amidino penicillins bind to a specific penicillin-binding protein which is involved in the shape of bacilli (page 193). They do not affect the proteins which are implicated in cell elongation or septum formation, which are affected by other beta-lactam antibiotics. This differing mechanism has been used to produce synergy by combing an amidino penicillin such as mecillinam (page 189), with other beta-lactam antibiotics, against certain Gram-negative bacteria (Neu, 1976).

That penicillin inhibits cell wall autolytic enzymes with mucopeptide hydrolase activity provides an explanation for bacterial persisters (Greenwood, 1972). Persisters are morphologically normal bacteria which survive lethal concentrations of one of the penicillins, but whose progeny are fully sensitive to these agents. Bacterial persisters may be important clinically in causing recurrence of infection. According to Hartmann *et al.* (1972) penicillin is only lethal to growing cells (the great majority of any cell population), in which the hydrolases have already initiated cell wall growth-points. Greenwood (1972) postulates that the small percentage of bacteria which are not growing at the time, become persisters because they have an intact bacterial cell wall. Penicillin prevents cell wall hydrolases from forming growing-points in these cells and they become 'frozen in suspended animation', as long as they are exposed to the antibiotic. Once the antibiotic is removed persisters revert to normal growth patterns.

In hypertonic media bacterial cells can survive as viable protoplasts, spheroplasts or L-forms, which are stable despite absent or defective cell walls. These forms may occur and persist during penicillin treatment of infections in areas where the surrounding medium is hypertonic, e.g. the renal medulla or even possibly purulent accumulations (Strominger and Tipper, 1965). There is evidence that following cessation of penicillin treatment reversion of L-forms to classical bacteria can cause a recrudescence of infection, but it is uncertain whether L-forms *per se* can cause symptoms of a disease (Feingold, 1969).

Toxicity

1. *Hypersensitivity reactions.* Penicillin is one of the least toxic of all antibiotics, but commonly causes hypersensitivity reactions. Sensitization is usually the result of previous treatment but some subjects have had immediate reactions to penicillin when first treated. In these it is postulated that a 'hidden contact', such as consumption of milk containing penicillin as a result of veterinary treatment, has occurred.

Allergic phenomena were more common with early amorphous penicillin preparations because they contained impurities (page 3), including high molecular weight proteins. The penicillin molecule itself may also evoke allergy by acting as a haptene and combining with body proteins to form an antigenic compound (Idsøe *et al.*, 1972). In addition, various derivatives of the penicillin nucleus, 6-aminopenicillanic acid, often share cross-sensitivity demonstrating that the nucleus itself plays an important role. It was predicted that all penicillins derived from 6-aminopenicillanic acid would cross-react in sensitized individuals (Stewart, 1962). Experience has shown that this is not invariable (*see* methicillin, page 71). The penicillin molecule itself apparently does not combine readily with protein to produce an antigen and the actual haptenes are various penicillin derivatives or breakdown products. The most important of these is the penicilloyl derivative, in which the beta-lactam ring of the penicillin molecule has been opened and a stable attachment can now be formed to protein via an amino group. This penicilloyl derivative can arise directly from penicillin or through an intermediary, penicillenic acid, which is another penicillin degradation product (Parker, 1964). The penicilloyl derivative readily combines with body proteins and this penicilloyl protein conjugate is commonly referred to as the 'major antigenic determinant' (Isbister,

1971; Idsøe *et al.*, 1972). Other penicillin degradation products such as penicilloic acid (pages 13, 18), and penilloic acid, which are also involved in allergy, are grouped together and called 'minor antigenic determinants'. The major antigenic determinant cannot be used for skin-testing procedures because it is itself a potent sensitizing agent. However, when penicilloyl is conjugated with polymerized lysine, penicilloyl-polylysine (PPL) is obtained, which appears to be much safer as a skin-test reagent (page 26).

In the late sixties standard preparations of 6-aminopenicillanic acid and penicillin G were shown still to contain high molecular weight protein impurities (Batchelor *et al.*, 1967; Stewart, 1967). It was thought that if these residual impurities were removed, the prevalence of penicillin allergy would be reduced (Knudsen *et al.*, 1967) and purified penicillin ('Purapen G', Beecham), was produced. Although the purpose of this preparation was to further reduce penicillin sensitization, it was not considered safe for penicillin-allergic patients. Because of this and other limitations, this drug was not widely used, and its manufacture was discontinued.

Another problem with penicillin is that it can become more allergenic after a period in solution. This may occur because it is degraded to more allergenic substances (pages 13, 18), or because of the formation of high molecular weight penicillin polymers (Smith and Marshall, 1971; Dewdney *et al.*, 1971). The factors responsible for polymer formation are unknown, and the clinical implications are still uncertain. It is therefore always wise to use freshly prepared penicillin solutions (Smith *et al.*, 1971).

Penicillin hypersensitivity may take the following forms:
(a) *Anaphylactic reactions.* These occur in previously sensitized patients, are exceedingly rare, but may result in death within a few minutes. The features are nausea, vomiting, abdominal pain, pallor, tachycardia, severe dyspnoea due to bronchospasm, rigors, loss of consciousness and peripheral circulatory failure due to vasodilation and loss of plasma volume. Acute urticaria and angioneurotic oedema which may affect the larynx, can also occur (Austen, 1974). Large scale surveys have shown that these anaphylactic reactions may occur in 0·004 to 0·04 per cent of penicillin treated patients (Idsøe *et al.*, 1968; Rudolph and Price, 1973; Porter and Jick, 1977); the mortality is about 10 per cent (Johnson, 1962). Parenteral penicillin G accounts for nearly all cases of anaphylaxis, but there are occasional reports following the use of oral potassium penicillin G (Spark, 1971). Treatment should include immediate intravenous or intramuscular administration of adrenaline, followed by large doses of corticosteroids given intravenously, If possible a torniquet should be applied proximal to the site of the penicillin injection. Other immediate resuscitative measures such as provision of a clear airway, positive pressure oxygen administration and treatment of cardiac arrhythmias, may be required (Van Arsdel, 1968). Rapid infusion of saline or plasma expanders may be necessary to combat shock (Amer. Acad. Pediatrics, 1973). If hypotension persists intravenous metaraminol (aramine) should be tried. Antihistamines may be administered to relieve urticaria, but this therapy is not life-saving and is only of secondary importance (Greaves and Holti, 1971; Amer. Acad.

Pediatrics, 1973). Penicillinase has little if any place in the emergency treatment of anaphylactic reactions. It rapidly breaks down circulating penicillin G, but probably has no effect on preformed antigen–antibody complexes (Westerman *et al.*, 1966). Furthermore, penicillinase itself may provoke sensitivity reactions (Idsøe *et al.*, 1968).

The anaphylactic reaction in man is largely mediated by IgE (reaginic) antibodies, but certain IgG subclass antibodies may also play a part (Parker, 1975).

(b) *Serum sickness*. This is not uncommon and has occurred in 1–7 per cent of patients treated with penicillin (Levine, 1972; Caldwell and Cluff, 1974). It usually occurs seven to ten days after primary administration of penicillin and is produced by circulating immune complexes. The formation of such antigen–antibody complexes is possible because intravascular antigen is still present at the time when the antibody is first produced (Parker, 1975). Serum sickness is characterized by fever, malaise, urticaria, joint pains, lymphadenopathy, and occasionally angioneurotic oedema. Erythema nodosum is a less common manifestation. Exfoliative dermatitis (which may be serious or even fatal) and Stevens–Johnson syndrome may also rarely occur. 'Accelerated' reactions, occurring within 2 to 48 h, may sometimes happen in previously sensitized patients and take the form of urticaria, but laryngeal oedema may also occur (Idsøe *et al.*, 1972).

Serum sickness and accelerated reactions are not usually serious and subside when penicillin is withdrawn. Antihistamines may be helpful and in severe cases corticosteroids are justified. Penicillinase has also been effective in severe cases, but as this product itself can cause acute sensitivity reactions (*vide supra*), corticosteroids are preferable.

(c) *Contact dermatitis*. This results from local penicillin application or exposure to penicillin aerosol and is an occupational disease of nurses.

(d) *Local reactions*. Swelling and redness at the site of penicillin injections may occur.

A careful clinical history still remains the main indicator of possible reactors to penicillin. Idsøe *et al.* (1968) analysed 151 deaths due to penicillin, reported from 1951 to 1965. Thirty-eight of these had a history of previous reaction and in 74 others the history was not recorded. Some authors consider that patients with a history of asthma, hay fever and other allergies are also more likely to react to penicillin (Hewitt, 1963; Smith, 1974), but others have found no correlation between penicillin reactions and family or personal history of other allergies (Horowitz, 1975). In any case, the increased risk of penicillin reactions in patients with other allergies appears to be small and penicillin may be given to them whenever it is indicated.

Routine testing for sensitive individuals prior to penicillin administration is not yet practicable. Certainly skin tests using penicillin G as the antigen, are inadvisable, because even the small doses used may cause serious reactions or sensitize some patients. In addition, this method of testing is unreliable for detecting the rare patient liable to severe anaphylaxis (NHMRC, 1965).

Other tests have been investigated for both safety and reliability, and they may be warranted in special instances, if facilities are available. The penicilloyl-polylysine skin-test (page 23) appears considerably safer, in spite of occasional reports of anaphylaxis (Parker, 1963; Finke *et al.*, 1965; Smith *et al.*, 1966; Resnik and Shelley, 1966). However, this test also does not detect all potential candidates for anaphylactic reactions (Voss *et al.*, 1966; Levine *et al.*, 1967; Van Arsdel, 1968). The predictive value of skin testing is increased if in addition to the penicilloyl-polylysine test, another test is performed using a 'minor determinant mixture', which contains various penicillin metabolites (page 24) and some crystalline penicillin G (Levine *et al.*, 1967; Levine and Zolov, 1969; Levine and Redmond, 1969). It appears that the combined use of these two skin tests (sometimes preceded by scratch tests as an additional precaution) are safe and helpful, because if both are negative in a patient with a history of possible penicillin allergy, the risk of an immediate reaction to penicillin is very low (Levine and Zolov, 1969; Adkinson *et al.*, 1971). Also in such patients the frequency of late reactions to penicillin are not much greater than that in patients with no history of previous penicillin hypersensitivity (Levine, 1972).

In the United States of America, penicilloyl-polylysine (PPL) is now available commercially under the trade name of 'Pre-Pen'. Parker (1975) considers that this preparation may be used to screen patients with no history of penicillin allergy, and that this will markedly reduce the incidence of penicillin reactions. Unfortunately, the testing of patients with a history of penicillin allergy is still unsatisfactory, as the more important antigen, the 'minor determinant mixture', which identifies those liable to anaphylaxis, is still not available commercially (Shapiro *et al.*, 1977).

A number of *in vitro* tests have been used to investigate penicillin hypersensitivity. Serological tests have been developed but these usually only estimate IgM and IgG antibodies, and not reaginic (IgE) antibodies, which mediate the anaphylactic reaction (Schwartz and Vaughan, 1963). Other *in vitro* tests include indirect basophil degranulation (Shelley, 1963; Katz *et al.*, 1964), lymphocyte transformation (Halpern *et al.*, 1967) and the use of bacteriophages (Chain, 1970). Radioimmunoassay can also be used to demonstrate the presence of circulating IgG and IgE antibodies, specific for a penicillin antigen (Parker, 1975). However, none of these tests has so far proved to be suitable for routine clinical use.

Desensitization of penicillin-allergic patients has not proved to be practicable and effective alternative antibiotics can be usually selected. In serious infections such as pneumococcal meningitis, penicillin G, the drug of first choice, can often be used in penicillin-allergic patients if it is administered in conjunction with corticosteroids. A novel approach, still in the experimental stage, is the induction of specific immunological tolerance to the penicilloyl haptene (page 23). Animals rendered specifically tolerant to this antigenic determinant, do not produce anti-penicilloyl haptene antibodies of either IgE or IgG class. It is possible that this work may be extended so that immunological tolerance can be similarly induced in penicillin-allergic humans (Annotation, 1976a).

2. *Reactions peculiar to procaine penicillin.* Occasionally very severe reactions and even death, occurring during or shortly after an 'intramuscular' injection of procaine penicillin, may result from accidental intravenous injection. These reactions are partly caused by micro-embolization of procaine penicillin particles to the lungs and brain, which produces hyperventilation, dilation of

pupils, convulsions and coma (Galpin *et al.*, 1974). However, direct procaine toxicity is also contributory. Early manifestations of this toxicity include marked anxiety, fever, hypertension, tachycardia, vomiting and audio-visual hallucinations. In severe cases, there may be convulsions, abrupt hypotension and cardio-respiratory arrest (Lewis, 1957; Galpin *et al.*, 1974). These severe acute reactions may simulate anaphylaxis. Galpin *et al.* (1974) described three patients to whom aqueous procaine penicillin G was administered inadvertently by intravenous infusion. Within 15 min one patient developed a generalized seizure and cardio-respiratory arrest with slow idioventricular rhythm, but recovered with resuscitation. In the other two patients, sudden acute anxiety, tachypnoea, dizziness and tinnitus were the main symptoms.

Procaine penicillin may also cause less severe side-effects. The occasional patient may experience extreme anxiety and a sensation of impending death after an intramuscular injection of aqueous procaine penicillin, but show no major abnormal physical signs, such as shock or bronchospasm. In addition, some develop hallucinations, disorientation, acute depersonalization or frank pyschotic behaviour. Minor physical abnormalities such as tachycardia, hypertension or twitching of extremities are sometimes observed. These attacks are self-limiting, subsiding after 15–30 min, but some patients may exhibit some mental lability for several months after the reaction. Furthermore, according to some authors this complication may occur more commonly in patients with a past history of mental instability (Menke and Pepplinkhuizen, 1974). These minor reactions to procaine penicillin occur in about 0·1–0·3 per cent of treated patients. They are probably caused by direct procaine toxicity. *In vivo*, procaine is quickly liberated from procaine penicillin, because free procaine can be detected in the serum immediately after an intramuscular injection, and measurable levels persist for about 30 min (Green *et al.*, 1974). Accidental intravenous injection of part of the dose may also sometimes be a factor (Downham and Ramos, 1973). Patients exhibiting this side-effect may be regarded as hysterical by doctors or nurses who are unaware of this clinical entity.

3. *Jarisch–Herxheimer reaction.* This may be evoked when patients with syphilis are treated with penicillin G (page 38) and it appears to be due to the release of endotoxins (lipopolysaccharides) from large numbers of killed treponemes (Gelfand *et al.*, 1976). The reaction usually occurs 6–8 h after commencement of penicillin and subsides within 12–24 h. Features include malaise, chills, fever, sore throat, myalgia, headache and tachycardia; there may also be an exacerbation of existing syphilitic lesions e.g. flaring of the rash of secondary syphilis (Bryceson, 1976; Gelfand *et al.*, 1976). Such reactions in early syphilis, are unpleasant but not serious. In late cardiovascular or neurosyphilis, serious reactions, although rare, are possible due to aggravation of local lesions. For instance, patients with late cardiovascular syphilis may die during a reaction (Leading article, 1977a) and those with cerebral syphilis may develop increased mental disturbance (Bryceson, 1976).

The Jarisch–Herxheimer reaction is quite common during penicillin treatment of syphilis. It may occur in about 50 per cent of patients treated for primary syphilis, 75 per cent of those with secondary syphilis and 30 per cent of those with neurosyphilis (Gelfand *et al.*, 1976). Corticosteroids may modify this reaction, but even large doses do not abolish most of the clinical and pathological changes, so their role in treatment is controversial and probably minimal (Leading article, 1977a). It is now generally accepted that all patients with early syphilis and most with late cardiovascular and neurosyphilis, can be treated from the outset with therapeutic doses of penicillin G. Initial treatment with small doses or the concomitant use of corticosteroids is indicated only in patients in whom there is a serious risk of increased local damage, e.g. syphilitic optic atrophy (Idsøe et al., 1968).

Jarisch–Herxheimer reactions may also occur when certain other infections are treated by penicillin G. They are frequent in leptospirosis (page 39) following initiation of penicillin therapy, and are characterized by fever, hypotension and precipitation or aggravation of signs and symptoms of the disease (Center for Disease Control, 1975a). Similarly this reaction may follow the use of penicillin G for the treatment of yaws (page 39), rat-bite fever (page 40) and anthrax (page 36). Furthermore a Jarisch–Herxheimer reaction may occur when antibiotics other than penicillin are used to treat certain infections. A most severe form of this reaction may be provoked by the use of tetracyclines in louse-borne relapsing fever (pages 614, 625), and this may be fatal (Bryceson, 1976). The reaction also occasionally follows tetracycline treatment of brucellosis and tularaemia (page 614) and chloramphenicol treatment of typhoid fever (page 440).

4. *Direct penicillin toxicity.* Penicillin is of very low toxicity to humans, but when 'massive doses' of 100 million units (60 g) daily or more, are given intravenously, central nervous system irritation with convulsions and coma may result (Weinstein et al., 1964; Lerner et al., 1967; Conway et al., 1968). These very high doses of penicillin G are rarely indicated nowadays. Such toxicity is more likely to occur in patients with impaired renal function and in elderly patients. In one patient who developed convulsions, the serum penicillin concentration was 737 units (433 μg) per ml, two hours after intravenous administration of 10 million units (6 g) (Weinstein et al., 1964). The CSF penicillin level appears to be more important than serum levels, and apparently there is little danger of convulsions unless CSF penicillin levels exceed 8 units (5 μg) per ml; higher CSF levels are achieved by a continuous infusion than by intermittent rapid intravenous injections of the same daily penicillin dose (Lerner et al., 1967). The latter method is therefore preferable when administering large doses.

Since the permeability of the 'blood-brain barrier' to penicillin increases in meningitis (Conway et al., 1968), smaller doses may precipitate encephalopathy in patients with this disease (*see also* page 19). Cardiopulmonary bypass may also in some manner predispose patients to penicillin neurotoxicity. Convulsions, apparently due to intravenous penicillin, have been observed in patients undergoing open heart surgery (Seamans et al., 1968; Leading article, 1968b). If massive doses of penicillin are administered, probenecid should not be given (Lerner et al., 1967). Apart from its action of blocking renal tubular secretion (page 17), probenecid also inhibits efflux of the drug from the cerebrospinal fluid causing an accumulation of penicillin in the CSF (Dacey and Sande, 1974; Leading article, 1976c) (*see also* page 19). In animals, penicillin encephalopathy can be reversed by systemically administered penicillinase (Raichle et al., 1971). The administration of much smaller doses of penicillin intrathecally can cause encephalopathy, but such treatment for meningitis is unnecessary (Forbes, 1962). If penicillin G is given intrathecally, the adult dose must not exceed 10 000 to 20 000 units daily. In infants a daily intraventricular dose of 5000 units penicillin G has been used with no side-effects (Lee *et al.*, 1977).

5. *Nephropathy*. Interstitial nephritis can occur in association with the administration of large doses of penicillin G (20–60 million units daily) intravenously (Schrier *et al.*, 1966; Baldwin *et al.*, 1968). This complication usually occurs after about eight days treatment, and is manifested by fever, eosinophilia, occasional rashes, albuminuria and a rise in blood urea. Renal biopsy shows interstititial nephritis without glomerular abnormalities or arteritis. The majority of patients recover when penicillin is stopped. Associated clinical features of an allergic reaction, and the results of immunological studies performed by Baldwin *et al.* (1968), strongly suggest a hypersensitivity mechanism for this nephropathy (*see also* methicillin, page 72).

A milder form of penicillin-hypersensitivity nephritis may occur in which the presenting symptoms of dysuria, pyuria, proteinuria and eosinophilia suggest a urinary tract infection, and there is usually no azotaemia. Symptoms soon cease when penicillin is withdrawn, but they promptly recur on readministration of the drug (Orchard and Rooker, 1974).

Rare cases of renal disease characterized by glomerulonephritis or periarteritis occurring soon after the administration of relatively low doses of penicillin have been reported. The causal role of penicillin in these cases is doubtful (Baldwin *et al.*, 1968).

6. *Penicillin-induced haemolytic anaemia*. This uncommon complication may occur in patients who are treated with intravenous penicillin G, in a dose usually greater than 10 million units per day, and who have previously received large doses of the drug (White *et al.*, 1968; Leading article, 1968a). A falling haemoglobin level and rising reticulocyte count are characteristic. A strongly positive direct antiglobulin reaction (Coombs test) is the main diagnostic feature, which is due to induced IgG antibody reacting with penicillin coated red cells (Garratty and Petz, 1975). The IgG Coombs test is therefore positive but the C3 Coombs test is usually negative, and the pathogenic mechanism of this penicillin-induced haemolytic anaemia is of the haptene type (Abramson and Lee, 1974). Erythrocytes not coated with penicillin may also be destroyed because such cells may bind activated complement components, rendering them susceptible to premature destruction by the reticuloendothelial system (Kerr *et al.*, 1972).

Penicillin-induced haemolytic anaemia should be suspected in patients who develop anaemia while receiving high doses of penicillin G. Patients with severe infections such as bacterial endocarditis, often develop anaemia due to infection and the haemolytic component may be overlooked. On withdrawing penicillin, the haemoglobin value usually rises quickly, and the direct antiglobulin test becomes negative in one to three months. White *et al.* (1968) showed that IgG antibody to penicillin G cross-reacts with red cells sensitized with the semisynthetic penicillins and cephalosporins, so that these drugs are not safe alternatives.

More rarely, penicillin administered in ordinary therapeutic doses may cause a haemolytic anaemia. In these cases IgG antibody cannot be detected but an

IgM antibody is present (Dove *et al.*, 1975). Penicillin has also been suggested as a possible cause of microangiopathic haemolytic syndrome (thrombotic thrombocytopenic purpura) in one patient (Parker and Barrett, 1971). Penicillin-induced haemolytic anaemia has also been described in another patient who presented with post-partum disseminated intravascular coagulation and microangiopathy. She had only been given 5 million units of penicillin daily, and haemolysis occurred at a time when she had received nine days treatment with heparin and the coagulation disorder had been controlled (McPherson *et al.*, 1976).

7. *Other haematological side-effects.* Penicillin in large doses has been reported to cause pancytopenia due to an apparent blockade of the release of mature cells from the bone marrow (Joorabchi and Kohout, 1973). If administered in doses of 10 million units daily to uraemic patients or in a dose of 40 million units daily to those with normal renal function, penicillin G can induce a coagulation disorder. This may appear soon after penicillin administration is commenced and persist for four days after it is stopped. The coagulation abnormality is due to platelet dysfunction (*see also* carbenicillin, page 159), disturbed conversion of fibrinogen to fibrin and increased antithrombin-III activity (Andrassy *et al.*, 1976). A coagulation disorder has also been described due to production of Factor VIII inhibitors, which are apparently initiated as a result of the altered immunologic state induced by an allergic reaction to penicillin (Green, 1968).

8. *Cation intoxication.* One million units (0·625 g) of the potassium salt of crystalline penicillin G contains 1·5 milliequivalents of potassium ion (or 0·066 g potassium). If 'massive doses' of this preparation are given intravenously, potassium intoxication may occur. The sodium salt, which contains 1·7 mEq or 0·039 g of sodium in one million units (0·6 g) is unlikely to cause complications, unless 'massive doses' are used in patients with renal or cardiac failure. Brunner and Frick (1968) described hypokalaemia, metabolic alkalosis and hypernatraemia in a few patients treated with 100 million units of sodium penicillin G daily. In these patients hypernatraemia was probably aggravated by insufficient fluid administration. Despite this, their daily urine output exceeded one litre, due to the osmotic diuretic action of 100 million units of penicillin, which is equivalent to about 600 ml of 10 per cent mannitol. Penicillin probably induces an excessive renal potassium loss by direct action on distal renal tubules, thereby producing hypokalaemia and metabolic alkalosis. There is also some evidence that antibiotics may cause a redistribution of potassium within the body rather than a potassium loss (Tattersall *et al.*, 1972).

9. *Other rare side-effects.* Penicillin has occasionally been reported as the cause of pericarditis, myocarditis, intestinal haemorrhage, liver necrosis and gangrene (Idsøe *et al.*, 1968). Its use has been associated with drug-induced lupus syndromes (Alarcón-Segovia, 1969), but no definite causal relationship has been established. Intravenous penicillin injections may rarely cause attacks of colicky abdominal pain (Davies *et al.*, 1974). Schmitt and Krivit (1969) reported a case of a nine-year-old girl in whom benign intracranial hypertension, presumably due to vasculitis, appeared to be a manifestation of penicillin sensitivity. Another patient, who experienced a severe serum sickness following penicillin, later developed increased intracranial pressure due to a marked

pachymeningitis of the dura mater, and this also was thought to be the result of an allergic reaction to penicillin. This meningitis responded to corticosteroid therapy (Farmer *et al.*, 1960).

10. *Nerve and muscle injury.* The danger of sciatic nerve injury from intramuscular penicillin injections in the buttock is well known and in most hospitals the drug is given in the lateral aspect of the thigh. Muscle necrosis and abscess formation can also occur after intramuscular injection, and rarely muscle contractures may be a sequel to repeated intramuscular injections in the thigh.

11. *Intra-arterial injection of penicillin.* This is less recognized and a more serious complication of intramuscular injections of viscid procaine penicillin. Atkinson (1969) described a seven-month-old girl in whom procaine-benzathine penicillin was injected into the gluteal artery, causing transverse myelopathy with apparently permanent paraplegia. This was presumably due to occlusive vascular disease caused by the intra-arterial penicillin. These injections are given under pressure, and it is likely that retrograde distribution to vessels supplying the spinal cord occurred. In the case reported the injection was given in the upper and outer quadrant. More recently Sengupta (1976) described a one-year-old child, who developed irreversible ischaemic gangrene of the upper limb after an unintentional intra-arterial injection of procaine penicillin.

Clinical Uses of the Drug

Penicillin G is still one of the most effective antibiotics, and it remains the drug of first choice for most infections due to bacteria sensitive to penicillin in low concentrations.

1. *Strep. pyogenes infections.* Penicillin is very effective for infections due to Group A beta-haemolytic streptococci, such as pharyngitis, scarlet fever, cellulitis, septic arthritis, puerperal infections (page 35) and septicaemia. For severe infections intramuscular or intravenous crystalline penicillin G (one to two million units for adults) every 3–6 h is required. Streptococcal pharyngitis should be treated for at least ten days to ensure eradication of the organisms from the pharynx. This is important for the prevention of subsequent rheumatic fever (Peter and Smith, 1977). Mild to moderate streptococcal pharyngitis in children can be treated satisfactorily by a single intramuscular injection containing 900 000 units of benzathine and 300 000 units of procaine penicillin (Bass *et al.*, 1976).

2. *Group B streptococcal infections.* Since about 1960, these organisms have been recognized as an increasingly important cause of neonatal infections (Patterson and Hafeez, 1976; Berg *et al.*, 1977; Annotation, 1977). In recent years they have also become a prevalent cause of adult infections (Anthony and Concepcion, 1975; Bayer *et al.*, 1976; Patterson and Hafeez, 1976). In infants, Group B streptococci may cause an acute early-onset type of disease presenting with sepsis, acute respiratory distress, apnoea, shock, meningitis and septicaemia, usually within 24 h of delivery or within the first five days after birth. The mortality of this disease may be 60–75 per cent. Other infants may develop a disease of later onset and present with meningitis with or without septicaemia, usually after the age of 10 days. The mortality in this

group is only 14–18 per cent. In adults, Group B streptococci have been implicated most commonly in post-partum infections (page 35), urinary tract infections, pneumonia and septicaemia, but meningitis, endocarditis, osteomyelitis and peritonitis have also occured.

Penicillin G is the drug of choice for the treatment of all of these infections, and most cases require parenteral therapy with crystalline penicillin. In neonates, a dose double that recommended for other infections (page 14) is advocated. In addition, therapy by penicillin G plus an aminoglycoside such as gentamicin may be more effective (page 329), so that initial treatment by both drugs should be considered for severe infections (Baker, 1977).

Although penicillin G is very effective for the treatment of Group B streptococcal infections, its role in chemoprophylaxis of neonatal infections is not well defined. In the United States approximately 25–35 per cent of pregnant women at term have Group B streptococci in their vaginal flora. It appears that the Group B streptococcus responsible for neonatal sepsis is acquired from the female genital tract (Baker, 1977; Young et al., 1977). Nevertheless, prophylactic chemotherapy for eradication of genital Group B streptococcal colonization state during pregnancy is not practicable. Penicillin G treatment of all asymptomatically colonized infants is also not recommended. Although effective for the treatment of Group B streptococcal disease, penicillin G often fails to eradicate the carrier state of these organisms in infants from sites such as the throat, umbilicus and rectum (Paredes et al., 1976b). Penicillin G prophylaxis has been advocated for neonates with evidence of Group B streptococcal colonization when there are also special risk factors, such as prematurity, prolonged rupture of membranes and maternal fever (Young et al., 1977). In addition, it has been suggested that a single intramuscular injection of 50 000 units of crystalline penicillin given at birth in the delivery room to all live-born babies, may avoid early-onset invasive Group B streptococcal disease (Steigman et al., 1978). However, the efficacy of any form of chemoprophylaxis has not been determined by prospective controlled studies (Baker, 1977).

3. *Respiratory tract infections in adults*. For pneumococcal lobar pneumonia, penicillin is the best treatment, and at least one million units crystalline penicillin every six hours should be used initially, though severely ill patients may respond to as little as 1 200 000 units procaine penicillin, daily (Brewin et al., 1974). If relatively penicillin-resistant pneumococcal strains (page 4) are involved, a crystalline penicillin dose of one million units six-hourly or more is likely to be required for successful treatment (Hansman, 1976). Pneumococcal empyema may not respond to penicillin because it either needs surgical drainage, or because there are penicillin inactivating enzymes in the empyema fluid (page 11). It is not advisable to use penicillin G alone in cases of life-threatening pneumonia, where the correct bacterial aetiology cannot be immediately determined. The combination of penicillin G and chloramphenicol may be very satisfactory in this situation, provided that the infection is not hospital acquired (page 444). Nowadays the possibility of Legionnaires' disease may also need to be considered, and appropriate antibiotics (pages 509, 575) instituted.

In acute bronchitis and bronchopneumonia the pneumococcus may be the major pathogen, necessitating the use of penicillin. In chronic bronchitis, H. influenzae may also be an important pathogen, and treatment by penicillin G alone may not be satisfactory. In this disease, another drug such as ampicillin (page 115), amoxycillin (page 142), chloramphenicol (page 442), a tetracycline (page 621) or co-trimoxazole (page 709) may be needed. Penicillin G is the antibiotic of choice for pulmonary infections involving anaerobic bacteria, such as lung abscess and aspiration pneumonia. In severe life-threatening cases gentamicin and/or chloramphenicol should also be added, as penicillin-resistant organisms such as Bacteroides fragilis or Klebsiella spp. may occasionally be involved in a mixed infection with penicillin-sensitive anaerobes (page 443).

4. *Childhood respiratory infections.* In syndromes which are primarily viral in origin, such as croup and bronchiolitis, pneumococci are the commonest secondary invaders, so that penicillin G may be sometimes of value. H. influenzae and Staph. pyogenes may also be secondary invaders, so that other drugs may be necessary in some cases. Most childhood pneumonias are pneumococcal and respond well to penicillin G, but H. influenzae type b (pages 117, 442) and Mycoplasma pneumoniae infections (pages 508, 623) and less frequently staphylococcal pneumonia (pages 74, 88, 96) are important entities in this age group, so other drugs are necessary when these are suspected or confirmed bacteriologically.

5. *Otitis media.* Since either Strep. pneumoniae or Strep. pyogenes are frequently responsible for this disease, penicillin G alone will be effective for the majority. However, in children H. influenzae is also a common pathogen (Feingold *et al.*, 1966) and other drugs such as ampicillin (page 116), amoxycillin (page 142) or erythromycin (page 507) may be necessary (McCracken and Eichenwald, 1974).

6. *Bacterial meningitis.* With the exception of neonatal meningitis, a combination of penicillin G and chloramphenicol has been used at Fairfield Hospital for the initial treatment (before the organism is identified) of acute bacterial meningitis, since 1955. This therapy covers nearly all causal organisms and has proved very satisfactory (*see also* page 441). The crude mortalities at Fairfield Hospital from the institution of this treatment to 1976, for pneumococcal, meningococcal and H. influenzae meningitis are 11·2 (22/195), 0·9 (2/219) and 2·7 (9/337) per cent, respectively. Once the organism is identified, penicillin G alone is still the drug of choice for meningococcal and pneumococcal meningitis (Forbes, 1962). The antibiotic may also be satisfactory for the treatment of Listeria monocytogenes meningitis, but occasional strains are penicillin G-resistant (page 7), and ampicillin (page 118) seems to be preferable (Kalis *et al.*, 1976). For bacterial meningitis, we usually advocate parenteral penicillin for a minimum of two weeks, although for milder cases of meningococcal meningitis shorter courses may suffice. The initial adult dose used is 16–24 million units (10–15 g) daily, given intravenously or intramuscularly in six or eight divided doses. Cases of pneumococcal meningitis in which the disease is caused by relatively penicillin-resistant organisms (page 4), may fail to respond satisfactorily even to these high penicillin doses (Naraqi *et al.*, 1974; Paredes *et al.*, 1976a; Howes and Mitchell, 1976; Mace *et al.*, 1977). A response may be obtained if the penicillin dose is further increased, or if treatment is changed to either chloramphenicol (page 441) or ampicillin (page 117). We do not use intrathecal penicillin (page 29) under any circumstances, and it seems that most clinicians are now in agreement with this.

For neonatal meningitis the preferred initial chemotherapy is ampicillin combined with gentamicin (McCracken and Eichenwald, 1974; Lewis and Gupta, 1977), but penicillin G is the drug of choice for continuation therapy if the organism is a Group B streptococcus (page 31).

Penicillin G is also an important antibiotic for the treatment of cerebral abscess. Abscesses in the frontal lobe which arise from the sinuses may respond to penicillin G alone, as these are usually caused by various types of penicillin G-sensitive streptococci. Abscesses of otitic origin, which occur in the temporal lobe, usually yield a mixed flora, often including anaerobic bacteria, and for these infections penicillin G should be combined with other drugs such as chloramphenicol (page 442), clindamycin (page 484) or metronidazole (page 773) (De Louvois et al., 1977a and b). However, because of the seriousness of the disease it is advisable to use combination chemotherapy for most cerebral abscesses initially (De Louvois, 1978) (see also page 442).

7. *Bacterial endocarditis*. Penicillin G is the most satisfactory treatment for endocarditis caused by alpha-haemolytic streptococci of the 'viridans' group (page 6). For endocarditis due to Group D enterococci, such as Strep. faecalis, penicillin G is used in combination with an aminoglycoside such as streptomycin (page 302), kanamycin (page 318), gentamicin (page 344), or tobramycin (page 361). By contrast endocarditis, cause by nonenterococcal group D streptococci such as Strep. bovis, can be treated by penicillin G alone (Moellering et al., 1974), because these organisms are as sensitive to penicillin G as the 'viridans' group (page 6). A six weeks course of penicillin G in a dose ranging from 8 to 24 million units (5–15 g) daily, is usually advocated for patients with endocarditis. Patients with Strep. faecalis endocarditis in general need the higher doses (Bryan and Stone, 1975), and some authors consider that most patients with endocarditis require at least 20 million units of penicillin G daily (Baron and Hickie, 1977).

A penicillin G/streptomycin combination is also sometimes advocated for the treatment of endocarditis caused by highly sensitive 'viridans' streptococci. The results of such treatment are no better than those with penicillin G alone, but the duration of therapy is reduced. In this way, Wolfe and Johnson (1974) obtained good results by using a penicillin G/streptomycin combination for two weeks, followed by penicillin G alone for another two weeks. Others have used only a two weeks' course of penicillin plus streptomycin for 'viridans' endocarditis (see page 302).

Penicillin G is effective in Staph. pyogenes endocarditis if the organism does not produce penicillinase. With penicillinase-producing staphylococci, penicillin therapy alone is quite unreliable even if massive doses are used. Penicillin G is probably also of no value in such infections, if used in combination with other drugs such as sodium fusidate (page 467).

8. *Endocarditis chemoprophylaxis*. Penicillin G is recommended before dental procedures and surgery involving the upper respiratory tract in those patients who are at risk of developing bacterial endocarditis. This treatment should be started only just prior to the dental procedure. Sometimes a single injection of crystalline penicillin is given, but prophylaxis is likely to be more effective if a therapeutic penicillin level is maintained for two days. This can be achieved by following the initial injection with oral penicillin V (page 55) for two days, or by giving a single intramuscular injection of a mixture of crystalline and benzathine penicillin (page 13). Currently it is recommended

that an intramuscular injection of a mixture of procaine and crystalline penicillin should be given 30–60 min before the procedure (Garrod, 1975; Leading article, 1975b; Kaplan et al., 1977). For adults crystalline penicillin G 1 000 000 units mixed with procaine penicillin 600 000 units is suitable for this purpose. This should then be followed by oral penicillin V in a dose of 500 mg six-hourly for two days.

Endocarditis apparently developing despite two days of penicillin chemoprophylaxis in adequate doses has been reported in one patient (Durack and Littler, 1974). However, in this case the disease was probably present before the dental procedure, because features of endocarditis followed within three days.

If streptomycin in an adult dose of 1·0 g intramuscularly is added to the above penicillin G/penicillin V regimen and administered at the same time as intramuscular penicillin G, this combined regimen has greater bactericidal activity and is more effective than penicillin alone in experimental animals (Leading article, 1976a). Similarly vancomycin is more bactericidal, and if this is used for chemoprophylaxis in penicillin-allergic patients, it should be followed by erythromycin for two days (see pages 506, 650).

These two more bactericidal regimens have disadvantages and it is unlikely that they will be used frequently for humans. However, they are recommended for patients considered to belong to a 'high risk' group such as those with prosthetic heart valves (Kaplan et al., 1977; Shanson, 1978). For most others the penicillin G/penicillin V regimen seems adequate and for most penicillin-allergic patients prophylaxis with erythromycin alone (page 506) is sufficient.

Because penicillin-resistant Strep. viridans strains are often present in patients receiving long-term rheumatic fever prophylaxis with one of the penicillins, penicillin G is usually not suitable prophylaxis against endocarditis under these circumstances (page 60).

For patients at risk of developing bacterial endocarditis, who are undergoing gastro-intestinal or genito-urinary tract surgery or instrumentation, it is recommended that chemoprophylaxis should consist of crystalline penicillin G 2 000 000 units given intramuscularly or intravenously (or ampicillin 1·0 g IM or IV) plus gentamicin 1·5 mg per kg body weight intramuscularly or intravenously. The initial dose should be given 30 to 60 min prior to procedure, and then the same dose of both drugs is repeated every eight hours for two additional doses. For penicillin-allergic patients vancomycin 1 g intravenously and streptomycin 1 g intramuscularly may be given before the procedure and both doses repeated once in 12 h (Kaplan et al., 1977).

9. *Puerperal infections.* These infections are often caused by Strep. pyogenes, Group B streptococci or anaerobic streptococci, for which penicillin G is optimal treatment. If Gram-negative bacilli or staphylococci are involved, other antibiotics are indicated. Seriously ill patients in whom bacteriological diagnosis has not been established should receive large doses of intravenous penicillin combined with an aminoglycoside such as kanamycin (page 308) or gentamicin (page 325). In many cases the addition of chloramphenicol (page 443), clindamycin (page 485) or metronidazole (page 773) may be advisable to provide a cover for anaerobic Gram-negative bacilli such as Bacteroides species (Wilkowske and Hermans, 1974).

10. *Clostridium perfringens (welchii) infections.* For treatment of gas

gangrene and post-abortal Cl. perfringens septicaemia, penicillin G is the best antibiotic. Large doses are recommended such as two to three million units intravenously every hour, with appropriate dosage reduction in children, elderly patients and those with impaired renal function (Deveridge and Unsworth, 1973). The use of polyvalent gas gangrene antitoxin as an adjunct to penicillin G has been controversial, but most authorities advise against its use (Leading article, 1972d; Roding et al., 1972). Gas gangrene may occur in patients with occlusive arterial disease undergoing lower limb amputation and prophylactic penicillin G should be used for five days, starting immediately before the operation (Leading article, 1970; Brumfitt and Hamilton-Miller, 1975). For penicillin-allergic patients, erythromycin (page 508) is probably the best alternative.

11. *Tetanus*. Penicillin G is used in conjunction with antitoxin in the treatment of tetanus. Although Cl. tetani is sensitive to penicillin, the nature of the infected wound is often such that the organism is inaccessible to antibiotics. The main principles in the treatment of a tetanus wound are surgical débridement and prevention or treatment of associated infection. The latter may lead to activation of spores and create an anaerobic environment (particularly if an undetected foreign body is present) for the proliferation of Cl. tetani. Penicillin G is not necessarily the most suitable antibiotic for this purpose. Similar to diphtheria, the early establishment of adequate circulating levels of antitoxin is the essential measure in preventing tetanus. It was suggested that penicillin may replace antitoxin in tetanus prophylaxis, but the efficacy of such antibiotic prophylaxis has not been demonstrated (Rubbo, 1966).

12. *Anthrax*. Penicillin G is the mainstay of treatment for this disease. Antianthrax serum is used as an adjunct to penicillin in the treatment of severe, very toxic patients, but its efficacy is controversial (Christie, 1974).

13. *Diphtheria*. Penicillin is used to eradicate the organisms in this disease, but the timely administration of diphtheria antitoxin remains the essential measure. Penicillin G can also be used to eradicate the diphtheria carrier state. McCloskey et al. (1974) found that a single injection of benzathine penicillin was effective in 84 per cent of carriers, but oral erythromycin (page 508) or clindamycin (page 485) was superior.

14. *Gonorrhoea*. Ever since the discovery of penicillin it has been the preferred drug for the treatment of this disease. Even in recent years, despite the emergence of N. gonorrhoeae strains relatively resistant to penicillin (page 7), penicillin has remained the most useful antibiotic (Litt et al., 1974; Center for Disease Control, 1974; 1975b). However, penicillin is ineffective for infections caused by penicillinase-producing gonococci (page 8). At present penicillin is still retained for the treatment of gonorrhoea in countries such as the United States of America and Great Britain, because there these strains are not yet widely prevalent. If penicillinase-producing gonococci become more widespread, then other drugs such as spectinomycin (page 589), cotrimoxazole (page 710) or cefuroxime (page 286) will need to be used more extensively for gonorrhoea (Leading article, 1977c; McCormack, 1977; Willcox, 1977).

(a) *Uncomplicated genital gonorrhoea*. For this the so-called 'single-dose' treatment with penicillin, has been extensively used. This may have contributed to the emergence of relatively resistant strains, and the single dose recommended has risen steadily over the years. Not so very long ago, commonly advocated 'single-dose' treatments for men and women with uncomplicated gonorrhoea, were 2·4 and 4·8 million units of procaine penicillin, respectively. Such regimens were used extensively in Britain and North America (Caldwell et al., 1971; Leading article, 1973b), but treatment failures still occurred. Results were improved when the penicillin injection was preceded by an oral dose of 1–2 g of probenecid (page 17), to delay penicillin excretion (Leading article, 1972a; Homes et al., 1973). Subsequently a dose of 4·8 million units of procaine penicillin plus 1 g probenecid, was recommended for the treatment of both men and women with gonorrhoea, in North America (Sparling et al., 1973; Judson et al., 1974; Center for Disease Control, 1974; 1975b). Although this penicillin G regimen has been regarded as the one of choice, other recommended 'single-dose' regimens such as ampicillin-probenecid (page 119), or spectinomycin (page 588) produce similar 'cure rates' in uncomplicated gonorrhoea (Kaufman et al., 1976). Several other drugs are also effective, including tetracyclines (page 625), co-trimoxazole (page 710) and cephaloridine (page 215), but these cannot be used as 'single-dose' therapy. There is a correlation between the increasing frequency of treatment failures with penicillin G and the development of greater in vitro resistance of gonococci to the drug (Jaffe et al., 1976). In some Asian areas, where strains highly resistant to penicillin have been common (page 8), the recommended dose for 'single-session' treatment has reached as high as 6·4 million units of procaine penicillin (Leading article, 1972a). 'Single-session' treatment is convenient for the treatment of a large number of patients, and it also copes with those who are likely to default from further treatment. In ideal circumstances an adequate course of chemotherapy, related to the duration and severity of the infection, should be used. A course of procaine penicillin for one to two weeks, in a daily dose of one million units, would be satisfactory for most patients. In areas where gonococcal strains relatively resistant to penicillin are common, other drugs may be preferable. If penicillinase-producing strains which are completely penicillin-resistant are involved, other drugs are essential (see pages 286, 319, 589, 710).

(b) *Other forms of gonorrhoea.* The usually recommended 'single session' treatment regimens for uncomplicated genital gonorrhoea, also appear effective for anorectal gonorrhoea in females. The response of anorectal disease in males is not as satisfactory and daily procaine penicillin G for five to seven days may be needed (Klein et al., 1977). Gonococcal pharyngeal infection is also difficult to eradicate, and a course of penicillin G for five to seven days or a course of tetracycline is recommended (Center for Disease Control, 1975b).

A satisfactory treatment for gonococcal salpingitis is a 10–14 day course of crystalline penicillin G, in a dose of 10–20 million units daily (Litt et al., 1974; Center for Disease Control, 1975b). In patients who respond well, oral ampicillin may be substituted for penicillin after three to five days of treatment and be used to complete a total of 10–14 days chemotherapy. Disseminated gonococcal infection, which most commonly is manifested by arthritis, tenosynovitis and dermatitis, has been cured with only three days of parenteral penicillin G in high dosage (Blankenship *et al.*, 1974). However, most authorities recommend a 10–14 days course, similar to that used for salpingitis (Litt *et al.*, 1974; Center for Disease Control, 1975b; Handsfield *et al.*, 1976). For the less common gonococcal endocarditis or meningitis, prolonged treatment for three to six weeks with intravenous penicillin G (10–20 million units daily) is necessary (Handsfield *et al.*, 1976).

Gonococcal ophthalmia neonatorum should be treated by parenteral penicillin G in combination with topical therapy with other antibiotic eye drops (Center for Disease Control, 1975b). One per cent silver nitrate is useful for the prevention of this disease, but it may cause allergic conjunctivitis. It is important to establish the correct bacteriological diagnosis in neonatal eye infections, as chlamydial ophthalmia (page 626) may present with similar clinical features (Armstrong *et al.*, 1976).

15. *Syphilis.* Penicillin G is an excellent drug for the treatment of this disease and there has been no apparent change in the sensitivity of T. pallidum over the years (Schroeter, 1972; Idsøe *et al.*, 1972). It is commonly stated that the aim of treatment is to maintain sustained comparatively low penicillin serum and tissue levels of at least 0·02 μg per ml, for 7–10 days. The reasons given are that Treponema pallidum is sensitive to such penicillin levels, and that it multiplies slowly by dividing once every 30 h, and only actively dividing organisms are susceptible to penicillin (Leading article, 1973a). However, to attain such levels in the tissues, doses of penicillin are necessary which produce much higher serum levels. As with gonorrhoea, 'single-session' treatment has been extensively used, and primary and secondary syphilis have been treated with single injections of 2·4 million units of long-acting benzathine penicillin G, with reasonably good results (Center for Disease Control, 1976). Similar to gonorrhoea (*vide supra*), such single dose methods cannot be regarded as ideal treatment, and a 10–14 days course of procaine penicillin in daily doses of one million units, is preferable (Smithurst, 1971). Many patients with secondary syphilis, especially those with early central nervous system involvement in the form of meningitis, are best treated by intravenous crystalline penicillin in a dose of 5–20 million units daily for two to four weeks.

For tertiary syphilis more prolonged courses of penicillin are also desirable. Injectable penicillin G for two to four weeks is usually required, and additional courses of treatment may be necessary in individual patients. It may be satisfactory to treat many of these patients by daily injections of one million units of procaine penicillin, but crystalline penicillin in a dose of 5–20 million units daily is more reliable. Patients with neurosyphilis should certainly be given such doses of crystalline penicillin, usually intravenously, for three to four weeks. These penicillin doses are considerably higher than those commonly recommended (Center for Disease Control, 1976; Newnham, 1978), because there is evidence that lower doses may be inadequate in all but primary syphilis (Levit, 1976). Mohr *et al.* (1976) studied CSF penicillin levels in 15 patients with neurosyphilis. Two received crystalline penicillin G intravenously (5 and 10 million units daily, respectively) and their CSF penicillin levels were 0·3 and 2·4 μg per ml, respectively. The other received benzathine penicillin G in a dose of 3·6 million units per week, intramuscularly for four weeks. One of these patients had a level of 0·1 μg per ml, but all of the others had no detectable penicillin in the cerebrospinal fluid. Furthermore, Tramont (1976) reported the isolation of Treponema pallidum from the CSF of two patients, both of whom had recently received 'standard' penicillin courses. One had received benzathine penicillin 1·2 million units intramuscularly, three times weekly for three weeks (recommended for neurosyphilis) and the other a single injection of 4·8 million units of benzathine penicillin (recommended for secondary syphilis). After these patients were re-treated by large doses of intravenous crystalline penicillin G, Treponema pallidum could no longer be detected in their CSF.

Some patients with tertiary syphilis have remained seropositive after 'standard courses' of treatment. Whilst this may be due to persistence of treponemes, probably inactive, in the body, more prolonged penicillin treatment may be advisable (Hatos, 1972). So far there is no evidence to suggest that the prognosis of these patients is improved by such treatment (Annotation, 1973).

The treatment of syphilis during pregnancy is identical to that in nonpregnant patients (Holder and Knox, 1972).

Congenital neurosyphilis should be treated by intramuscular or intravenous crystalline penicillin G for a minimum of two weeks. In newborn infants adequate levels of penicillin cannot be achieved in the CSF after benzathine penicillin G administration (Speer et al., 1977). Although benzathine penicillin G in a single dose has been advocated for congenital syphilis without central nervous system involvement (McCracken, 1974), a two weeks course of crystalline penicillin is definitely preferable (Kaplan and McCracken, 1973).

If a patient suffering from gonorrhoea is also incubating syphilis, it appears that a single dose of 2·4 or 4·8 million units of procaine penicillin (a dose commonly used in gonorrhoea) is also effective therapy for incubating syphilis (Schroeter et al., 1971).

For the treatment of syphilis in penicillin-allergic patients, tetracyclines (page 627) are recommended currently in the United States, except for pregnant patients who should receive erythromycin (page 509).

16. *Yaws.* Similar to syphilis, penicillin G is the treatment of choice for this disease.

17. *Leptospirosis.* This is an acute disease which is often mild and self-limited, so that the efficacy of antibiotic treatment is difficult to assess. Although leptospirae are sensitive to penicillin *in vitro*, some consider that penicillin G (or any other antibiotic) is of little value for treatment of human infections. In one controlled trial in leptospirosis, no benefit was obtained from the administration of penicillin G or chloramphenicol (Fairburn and Semple, 1956). However, Kocen (1962) found that penicillin G reduced the duration of pyrexia in patients treated within four days of the onset of their illness, and also in those treated later. Penicillin treatment also reduced the frequency of jaundice and renal involvement. Doherty (1955; 1960) also claims that the early administration of high doses of penicillin G is beneficial. It seems that most authors advocate the use of penicillin G in severe leptospiral infections such as those due to L. icterohaemorrhagiae (Turner, 1969; Clein, 1973; Lawson, 1973).

18. *Actinomycosis.* Penicillin G is the drug of choice but, owing to the

fibrotic nature of the lesions, large doses for several months are necessary.

19. *Rat-bite fever*. Penicillin G is effective for both Streptobacillus moniliformis (Actinobacillus muris) and Spirillum minus infections (Gilbert *et al*., 1971). If endocarditis is present, at least six weeks chemotherapy is advisable.

20. *Pasteurella multocida infections*. This organism may cause wound infections following animal bites. Less commonly it can cause septic arthritis, osteomyelitis, septicaemia, meningitis, endocarditis, puerperal sepsis, renal infection, acute epiglottitis or pleuro-pulmonary infections (Bell *et al*., 1969; Johnson and Rumans, 1977; Lehmann *et al*., 1977).Penicillin G is the best drug for all of these infections, as this Gram-negative bacillus, unlike others, is highly sensitive to penicillin G (page 10).

21. *Infections due to other Gram-negative bacilli*. Serious infections such as Esch. coli septicaemia, have been successfully treated with 'massive' doses of penicillin G (up to 60 million units per day) intravenously (Weinstein *et al*., 1964). There are certain dangers with such high doses (*see* page 28), and other drugs are usually preferred for such infections.

Inconclusive results were obtained when a large dose of intravenous penicillin (10 million units) was given immediately before large bowel surgery in an attempt to reduce the frequency of wound infections (Batchelder *et al*., 1970; Hughes *et al*., 1970).

Penicillin G in commonly prescribed doses can often be used successfully for the treatment of urinary tract infections, because it is excreted in high concentrations in the urine. In one trial even potassium penicillin G, given in an oral dose of 500 mg six-hourly, was as satisfactory as other established regimens for the treatment of these infections (Hulbert, 1972).

22. *Chemoprophylaxis of rheumatic fever*. In some patients who cannot or will not take tablets, benzathine penicillin G in a dosage of 600 000 to 1 200 000 units intramuscularly, once a month, may be used successfully. Otherwise penicillin G is not used for this purpose and one of the oral acid-stable phenoxypenicillins (e.g. penicillin V), is usually selected (page 60).

23. *Whipple's disease*. Bacterial infection with atypical beta-haemolytic enterococci may be involved in the aetiology of this disease. For this reason, penicillin has been advocated for treatment and a two weeks course of crystalline penicillin followed by oral phenoxymethylpenicillin (page 55) for three months has been recommended (Comments, 1974). Other evidence has implicated cell wall deficient forms of alpha-haemolytic streptococci in this disease, in which case tetracyclines may be preferable (page 630).

24. *Botulism*. Penicillin G therapy has been suggested as an adjunct to other treatment in this disease to prevent Clostridium spore germination and release of more toxin in the bowel (Eisenberg and Bender, 1976).

REFERENCES

Abramson, N. and Lee, D. P. (April, 1974), 'Immune hemolytic anemias', *Disease-a-Month*. Year Book Medical Publishers inc. Chicago.

Adkinson, N. F. Jr., Thompson, W. L., Maddrey, W. C. and Lichtenstein, L. M. (1971). 'Routine use of penicillin skin testing on an inpatient service', *New Engl. J. Med*., **285**: 22.

Alarcon-Segovia, D. (1969), 'Drug-induced lupus syndromes', *Mayo Clin. Proc.*, **44**, 664.

American Academy of Pediatrics Committee on Drugs (1973), 'Anaphylaxis', *Pediatrics*, **51**, 136.

Anderson, R., Bauman, M. and Austrian, R. (1968), 'Lincomycin and penicillin G in the treatment of mild and moderately severe pneumococcal pneumonia', *Amer. Rev. Resp. Dis.*, **97**, 914.

Andrassy, K., Scherz, M., Ritz, E., Walter, E., Hasper, B., Storch, H. and Wömel, W. (1976), 'Penicillin-induced coagulation disorder', *Lancet*, **2**, 1039.

Annotation (1973), 'Penicillin and syphilis', *Lancet*, **1**, 649.

Annotation (1976a), 'Immunological tolerance to treat penicillin allergy?', *Lancet*, **2**, 943.

Annotation (1976b), 'Penicillinase-producing Gonococci', *Lancet*, **2**, 725.

Annotation (1977), 'Group-B streptococci in the newborn', *Lancet*, **1**, 520.

Anthony, B. F. and Concepcion, N. F. (1975), 'Group B streptococcus in a general hospital, *J. Infect. Dis.*, **132**, 561.

Appelbaum, P. C., Scragg, J. N., Bowen, A. J., Bhamjee, A., Hallet, A. F. and Cooper, R. C. (1977), 'Streptococcus pneumoniae resistant to penicillin and chloramphenicol', *Lancet*, **2**, 995.

Ashford, W. A., Golash, R. G. and Hemming, V. G. (1976), 'Penicillinase-producing Neisseria gonorrhoeae', *Lancet*, **2**, 657.

Armstrong, J. H., Zacarias, F. and Rein, M. F. (1976). 'Opthalmia neonatorum: a chart review', *Pediatrics*, **57**, 884.

Atkinson, J. P. (1969), 'Transverse myelopathy secondary to injection of penicillin', *J. Pediatrics*, **75**, 867.

Austen, K. F. (1974), 'Current concepts. Systemic anaphylaxis in the human being', *New Engl. J. Med.*, **291**, 661.

Baker, C. J., Webb, B. J. and Barrett, F. F. (1976), 'Antimicrobial susceptibility of Group B streptococci isolated from a variety of clinical sources, *Antimicrob. Ag. Chemother.*, **10**, 128.

Baker, C. J., Goroff, D. K., Alpert, S., Crockett, V. A., Zinner, S. H., Evrard, J. R., Rosner, B. and McCormack, W. M. (1977), 'Vaginal colonization with Group B streptococcus: a study in college women', *J. Infect. Dis.*, **135**, 392.

Baker, C. J. (1977), Summary of the workshop on perinatal infections due to Group B streptococcus', *J. Infect. Dis.*, **136**, 137.

Baldwin, D. S., Levine, B. B., McClusky, R. T. and Gallo, G. R. (1968), 'Renal failure and interstitial nephritis due to penicillin and methicillin', *New Engl. J. Med.*, **279**, 1245.

Barber, M. and Waterworth, P. M. (1962), 'Antibacterial activity of the penicillins', *Brit. med. J.*, **1**, 1159.

Barnes, P. and Waterworth, P. M. (1977), 'New cause of penicillin treatment failure', *Brit. med. J.*, **1**, 991.

Baron, D. W. and Hickie, J. B. (1977), 'Changing concepts in management of infective endocarditis', *Med. J. Aust.*, **1**, 767.

Baron, E. S., Saz, A. K., Kopecko, D. J. and Wohlhieter, J. A. (1977), 'Transfer of plasmid-borne beta-lactamase in Neisseria gonorrhoeae', *Antimicrob. Ag. Chemother.*, **12**, 270.

Barza, M., Brusch, J., Bergeron, M. G., Kemmotsu, O. and Weinstein, L. (1975), 'Extraction of antibiotics from the circulation by liver and kidney: effect of probenecid', *J. Infect. Dis.* (Suppl.), **131**, 86.

Bass, J. W., Crast, F. W., Knowles, C. R. and Onufer, C. N. (1976), 'Streptococcal pharyngitis in children. A comparison of four treatment schedules with intramuscular penicillin G benzathine', *JAMA*, **235**, 1112.

Batchelder, E. J., Rubbo, S. D., Hardy, K. J. and Hughes, E. S. R. (1970),

'Chemoprophylaxis in large bowel surgery: 2. Effect of penicillin on penicillin-resistant organisms', *Med. J. Aust.,* **1,** 367.

Batchelor, F. R., Dewdney, J., Feinberg, J. G. and Weston, R. D. (1967), 'A penicilloylated protein impurity as a source of allergy to benzylpenicillin and 6-aminopenicillanic acid', *Lancet,* **1,** 1175.

Bayer, A. S., Chow, A. W., Anthony, B. F. and Guze, L. B. (1976), 'Serious infections in adults due to Group B streptococci. Clinical and serotypic characterization', *Amer. J. Med.,* **61,** 498.

Beebe, J. L., Ligeti, P. and Wlodkowski, T. J. (1976), 'Abesence of penicillin-degrading enzymes in penicillin-resistant strains of Neisseria gonorrhoeae, *Antimicrob. Ag. Chemother.,* **10,** 179.

Bell, D. B., Marks, M. I. and Eickhoff, T. C. (1969), 'Pasteurella multocida arthritis and osteomyelitis', *JAMA,* **210,** 343.

Bengtsson, S., Forsgren, A. and Mellbin, T. (1977), 'Penicillinase production in community strains of Staphylococcus aureus', *Scand, J. Infect. Dis.,* **9,** 23.

Bennett, N. McK. and Kucers, A. (1970), 'Staphylococcal and Gram-negative septicaemia', *Aspects of Infection, Proc. Symp. Auckland, Sydney and Melbourne,* p. 123.

Berg, T., Hallander, H. O., Nathorst-Windahl, G. and Nordlander, I.-M. (1977), 'Group B beta-hemolytic streptococci as an important cause of perinatal mortality', *Scand. J. Infect. Dis.,* **9,** 19.

Bergeron, M. G., Gennari, F. J., Barza, M., Weinstein, L. and Cortell, S. (1975), 'Renal tubular transport of penicillin G and carbenicillin in the rat', *J. Infect. Dis.,* **132,** 374.

Bergström, S., Norlander, L., Norqvist, A. and Normark, S. (1978), 'Contribution of a TEM-1-like beta-lactamase to penicillin resistance in Neisseria gonorrhoeae', *Antimicrob. Ag. Chemother.,* **13,** 618.

Best, G. K., Best, N. H. and Koval, A. V. (1974), 'Evidence for participation of autolysins in bactericidal action of oxacillin on Staphylococcus aureus', *Antimicrob. Ag. Chemother.,* **6,** 825.

Bickel, L. (1972), *Rise up to life. A biography of Howard Walter Florey who gave penicillin to the world,* Angus and Robertson (UK) Ltd.

Blankenship, R. M., Holmes, R. K. and Sanford, J. P. (1974), 'Treatment of disseminated Gonococcal infection', *New Engl. J. Med.,* **290,** 267.

Blog, F. B., Chang, A., DeKoning, G. A. J., Oranje, A. P., Stolz, E., Bosscher-Koetsier, G., De-Jonge-Suy, M. P. E., Michel, M. F., O'Neil, E., De Weerdt-Van Ameyden, S. and Gaastra, L. (1977). Penicillinase-producing strains of Neisseria gonorrhoeae isolated in Rotterdam', *Brit. J. vener, Dis.,* **53,** 98.

Blumberg, P. M. and Strominger, J. L. (1974), 'Interaction of penicillin with the bacterial cell: penicillin-binding proteins and penicillin-sensitive enzymes', *Bacteriol. Rev.,* **38,** 291.

Brewin, A., Arango, L., Hadley, W. K. and Murray, J. F. (1974), 'High-dose penicillin therapy and pneumococcal pneumonia', *JAMA,* **230,** 409.

Brumfitt, W. and Hamilton-Miller, J. M. T. (1975), 'The place of antibiotic prophylaxis in medicine', *J. Antimicrob. Chemother.,* **1,** 163.

Brunner, F. P. and Frick, P. G. (1968), 'Hypokalaemia, metabolic alkalosis, and hypernatraemia due to 'massive' sodium penicillin therapy', *Brit. med. J.,* **4,** 550.

Bryan, C. S. and Stone, W. J. (1975), 'Comparably massive penicillin G therapy in renal failure', *Ann. Intern. Med.,* **82,** 189.

Bryceson, A. D. M. (1976), 'Clinical pathology of the Jarisch-Herxheimer reaction', *J. Infect. Dis.,* **133,** 696.

Bulger, R. J., Bennett, J. V. and Boen, S. T. (1965), 'Intraperitoneal administration of broad-spectrum antibiotics in patients with renal failure', *JAMA,* **194,** 1198.

Busch, D. F., Kureshi, L. A., Sutter, V. L. and Finegold, S. M. (1976), 'Susceptibility of respiratory tract anaerobes to orally administered penicillins and cephalosporins',

Antimicrob. Ag. Chemother., **10**, 713.

Caldwell, J. G., Wessler, S. and Avioli, L. V. (1971), 'Current therapy of gonorrhea', *JAMA*, **218**, 714.

Caldwell, J. R. and Cluff, L. E. (1974), 'Adverse reactions to antimicrobial agents', *JAMA*, **230**, 77.

Center for Disease Control (1974), 'Gonorrhea-CDC recommended treatment schedules, 1974', *Morbidity and Mortality Weekly Report*, **23**, 341.

Center for Disease Control (1975a), 'Leptospirosis surveillance', *Annual Summary, 1974*.

Center for Disease Control (1975b), 'Gonorrhoea: recommended treatment schedules., *Ann. Intern. Med.*, **82**, 230.

Center for Disease Control (1976), 'Syphilis—CDC recommended treatment schedules, 1976', *J. Infect. Dis.*, **134**, 97.

Center for Disease Control (1977a) 'Follow-up on antibiotic resistant Neisseria gonorrhoeae', *Morbidity and Mortality Weekly Report*, **26**, 29.

Center for Disease Control (1977b) 'Follow-up on penicillinase-producing Neisseria gonorrhoeae-worldwide', *Morbidity and Mortality Weekly Report*, **26**, 153.

Center for Disease Control (1977c), 'Multiple-antibiotic resistance of pneumacocci—South Africa', *Morbidity and Mortality Weekly Report*, **26**, 285.

Center for Disease Control (1977d), 'Penicillin-resistant Streptococcus pneumoniae-Minnesota', *Morbidity and Mortality Weekly Report*, **26**, 345.

Center for Disease Control (1978a), 'Follow-up on multiple-antibiotic-resistant pneumococci—South Africa', *Morbidity annd Mortality Weekly Report*, **27**, 1.

Center for Disease Control (1978b), 'Penicillinase-(beta-lactamase-)producing Neisseria gonorrhoeae-worldwide', *Morbidity and Mortality Weekly Report*, **27**, 10.

Chain, E., Florey, H. W., Gardner, A. D., Heatley, N. G., Jennings, M. A., Orr-Ewing, J. and Sanders, A. G. (1940), 'Penicillin as a chemotherapeutic agent', *Lancet*, **2**, 226.

Chain, E. B. (1970), 'Advances in the understanding of the mechanism of penicillin allergy', *Aspects of Infection, Proc. Symp. Auckland, Sydney and Melbourne*, p. 89.

Chain, E. (1972), 'Thirty years of penicillin therapy', *J. Roy. Coll. Phycns. Lond.*, **6**, 103.

Chin, W. L. and Lawson, J. W. (1976), 'Effect of antibiotics on L-form induction of Neisseria meningitidis', *Antimicrob. Ag. Chemother.*, **9**, 1056.

Chow, A. W., Patten, V. and Bednorz, D. (1978), 'Susceptibility of Campylobacter fetus to twenty-two antimicrobial agents', *Antimicrob. Ag. Chemother.*, **13**, 416.

Christie, A. B. (1974), *Infectious diseases: epidemiology and clinical practice*, 2nd Edn., Churchill Livingstone, Edinburgh, London and New York, p. 808.

Clein, L. (1973), 'Penicillin in leptospirosis', *Brit. med. J.*, **3**, 354.

Cole, M., Kenig, M. D. and Hewitt, V. A. (1973), 'Metabolism of penicillins to penicilloic acids and 6-aminopenicillanic acid in man and its significance in assessing penicillin absorption', *Antimicrob. Ag. Chemother.*, **3**, 463.

Comber, K. R., Boon, R. J. and Sutherland, R. (1977), 'Comparative effects of amoxycillin and ampicillin on the morphology of Escherichia coli *in vivo* and correlation with activity', *Antimicrob. Ag. Chemother.*, **12**, 736.

Comments (1974), 'Whipple's disease', *Med. J. Aust.*, **1**, 646.

Contoyiannis, P. and Adamopoulos, D. A. (1974), 'Penicillin-resistant Neisseria meningitidis', *Lancet*, **1**, 462.

Conway, N., Beck, E. and Sommerville, J. (1968), 'Penicillin encephalopathy', *Postgrad. Med. J.*, **44**, 891.

Cooksey, R. C., Facklam, R. R. and Thornsberry, C. (1978), 'Antimicrobial susceptibility patterns of Streptococcus pneumoniae', *Antimicrob. Ag. Chemother.*, **13**, 645.

Costerton, J. W. and Cheng, K.-J. (1975), 'The role of the bacterial cell envelope in antibiotic resistance', *J. Antimicrob. Chemother.*, **1**, 363.

Dacey, R. G. and Sande, M. A. (1974), 'Effect of probenecid on cerebrospinal fluid concentrations of penicillin and cephalosporin derivatives', *Antimicrob. Ag. Chemother.*, **6**, 437.

Davies, G. K., Turner, P. and Spencer, B. T. (1974), 'Abdominal pain after intravenous benzylpenicillin', *Lancet*, **2**, 167.

De Louvois, J., Gortvai, P. and Hurley, R. (1977a), 'Bacteriology of abscesses of central nervous system: a multicentre prospective study', *Brit. med. J.*, **2**, 981.

De Louvois, J., Gortvai, P. and Hurley, R. (1977b), 'Antibiotic treatment of abscesses of the central nervous system', *Brit. med. J.*, **2**, 985.

De Louvois, J. and Hurley, R. (1977), 'Inactivation of penicillin by purulent exudates', *Brit. med. J.*, **1**, 998.

De Louvois, J. (1978), 'The role of Bacteroides fragilis in abscesses of the central nervous system: implications for therapy', *J. Antimicrob. Chemother.*, **4**, 97.

Deveikis, A., Schauf, V., Mizen, M. and Riff, L. (1977), 'Antimicrobial therapy of experimental Group B streptococcal infection in mice', *Antimicrob. Ag. Chemother.*, **11**, 817.

Deveridge, R. J. and Unsworth, I. P. (1973), 'Gas gangrene', *Med. J. Aust.*, **1**, 1106.

Devitt, L., Riley, I. and Hansman, D. (1977), 'Human infection caused by penicillin-insensitive pneumococci', *Med. J. Aust.*, **1**, 586.

Dewdney, J. M., Smith, H. and Wheeler, A. W. (1971), 'The formation of antigenic polymers in aqueous solutions of β-lactam antibiotics', *Immunology*, **21**, 517.

Doherty, R. L. (1955), 'A clinical study of leptospirosis in North Queensland', *Aust. Ann. Med.*, **4**, 53.

Doherty, R. L. (1960), 'Penicillin in leptospirosis', *Lancet*, **1**, 58.

Dove, A. F., Thomas, D. J. B., Aronstam, A. and Chant, R. D. (1975), 'Haemolytic anaemia due to penicillin', *Brit. med. J.*, **3**, 684.

Downham, T. F. II and Ramos, D. P. (1973), 'Non-allergic adverse reactions to aqueous procaine penicillin G', *Michigan Medicine*, **72**, 223.

Durack, D. T. and Littler, W. A. (1974), 'Failure of "adequate" penicillin therapy to prevent bacterial endocarditis after tooth extraction', *Lancet*, **2**, 846.

Eisenstein, B. I., Lee, T. J. and Sparling, P. F. (1977), 'Penicillin sensitivity and serum resistance are independent attributes of strains of Neisseria gonorrhoeae causing disseminated gonococcal infection', *Infect. Immunity*, **15**, 834.

Eisenberg, M. S. and Bender, T. R. (1976), 'Botulism in Alaska, 1947 through 1974', *JAMA*, **235**, 35.

Elwell, L. P., Roberts, M., Mayer, L. W. and Falkow, S. (1977), 'Plasmid-mediated beta-lactamase production in neisseria gonorrhoeae', *Antimicrob. Ag. Chemother.*, **11**, 528.

Fairburn, A. C. and Semple, S. J. G. (1956), 'Chloramphenicol and penicillin in the treatment of leptospirosis among British troops in Malaya', *Lancet*, **1**, 13.

Farmer, L., Echlin, F. A., Loughlin, W. C., Breakey, A. S. and Duvoisin, R. (1960), 'Pachymeningitis apparently due to penicillin hypersensitivity', *Ann. Intern. Med.*, **52**, 910.

Feingold, D. S. (1969), 'Biology and pathogenicity of microbial spheroplasts and L-forms', *New Engl. J. Med.*, **281**, 1159.

Feingold, M., Klein, J. O., Haslam, G. E., Jr., Tilles, J. G., Finland, M. and Gellis, S. S. (1966), 'Acute otitis media in children', *Amer. J. Dis. Child.*, **111**, 361.

Finegold, S. M. (1977), 'Therapy for infections due to anaerobic bacteria: an overview', *J. Infect. Dis.* (Suppl.), **135**, 25.

Finger, A. and Handke, G. (1977), 'Antibiotic sensitivity of gonococci in South Australia, 1974 to 1975', *Med. J. Aust.*, **1**, 133.

Finke, S. R., Grieco, M. H., Connell, J. T., Smith, E. C. and Sherman, W. B. (1965), 'Results of comparative skin tests with penicilloyl-polylysine and penicillin in patients with penicillin allergy', *Amer. J. Med.*, **38**, 71.

Finland, M., Garner, C., Wilcox, C. and Sabath, L. D. (1976a), 'Susceptibility of beta-hemolytic streptococci to 65 antibacterial agents', *Antimicrob. Ag. Chemother.*, **9**, 11.

Finland, M., Garner, C., Wilcox, C. and Sabath, L. D. (1976b), 'Susceptibility of pneumococci and Haemophilus influenzae to antibacterial agents', *Antimicrob. Ag. Chemother.*, **9**, 274.

Fleming, A. (1929), 'On the antibacterial action of cultures of a penicillium with special reference to their use in the isolation of B. influenzae', *Brit. J. Exper. Path.*, **10**, 226; quoted by Welch (1954).

Florey, M. E., Turton, E. C. and Duthrie, E. S. (1946), 'Penicillin in wound exudates', *Lancet*, **2**, 405; quoted by Hussar and Holley (1954).

Forbes, J. A. (1962), 'Purulent meningitis; Principles and results of revised standardized treatment in 281 cases', *Aust. Ann. Med.*, **11**, 92.

Fraser, D. W., Wachsmuth, I. K., Bopp, C., Feeley, J. C. and Tsai, T. F. (1978), 'Antibiotic treatment of guinea-pigs infected with agent of legionnaires' disease', *Lancet*, **1**, 175.

Gale, E. F. (1973), 'Perspectives in chemotherapy', *Brit. med. J.*, **4**, 33.

Galpin, J. E., Chow, A. W., Yoshikawa, T. T. and Guze, L. B. (1974), 'Pseudoanaphylactic reactions from inadvertent infusion of procaine penicillin G', *Ann. Intern. Med.*, **81**, 358.

Garratty, G. and Petz, L. D. (1975), 'Drug-induced immune hemolytic anemia', *Amer. J. Med.*, **58**, 398.

Garrod, L. P. (1960a), 'Relative antibacterial activity of three penicillins', *Brit. Med. J.*, **1**, 527.

Garrod, L. P. (1960b), 'The relative antibacterial activity of four penicillins', *Brit. med. J.*, **2**, 1695.

Garrod, L. P. (1975), 'Chemoprophylaxis', *Brit. med. J.*, **4**, 561.

Gelfand, J. A., Elin, R. J., Berry, F. W., Jr. and Frank, M. M. (1976), 'Endotoxemia associated with the Jarisch-Herxheimer reaction', *New Engl. J. Med.*, **295**, 211.

Gerding, D. N., Hall, W. H. and Schierl, E. A. (1977), 'Antibiotic concentrations in ascitic fluid of patients with ascites and bacterial peritonitis', *Ann. Intern. Med.*, **86**, 708.

Gibaldi, M. and Schwartz, M. A. (1968), 'Apparent effect of probenecid on the distribution of penicillins in man', *Clin. Pharmacol. Ther.*, **9**, 345.

Gilbert, G. L., Cassidy, J. F. and Bennett, N. McK. (1971), 'Rat-bite fever', *Med. J. Aust.*, **2**, 1131.

Goldstein, G., Cowling, D. C. and Wall, A. J. (1965), 'Infection with Mima polymorpha: Fatal meningitis and septicaemia', *Aust. Ann. Med.*, **14**, 167.

Gordon, R. C., Barrett, F. F. and Clark, D. J. (1972), 'Influence of several antibiotics, singly and in combination on the growth of Listeria monocytogenes', *J. Pediatrics*, **80**, 667.

Greaves, M. W. and Holti, G. (1971), 'Treatment of anaphylactic shock', *Brit. med. J.*, **2**, 398.

Green, D. (1968), 'Spontaneous inhibitors of factor VIII', *Brit. J. Haemat.*, **15**, 57.

Green, R. L., Lewis, J. E., Kraus, S. J. and Frederickson, E. L. (1974), 'Elevated plasma procaine concentrations after administration of procaine penicillin G', *New Engl. J. Med.*, **291**, 223.

Greenwood, D. (1972), 'Mucopeptide hydrolases and bacterial "persisters"', *Lancet*, **2**, 465.

Greenwood, D. and O'Grady, F. (1973a), 'Comparison of the responses of Escherichia coli and Proteus mirabilis to seven beta-lactam antibiotics', *J. Infect. Dis.*, **128**, 211.

Greenwood, D. and O'Grady, F. (1973b), 'The two sites of penicillin action in Escherichia coli', *J. Infect. Dis.*, **128**, 791.

Haldane, E. V. and Affias, S. (1977), 'Penicillin-tolerant staphylococcus aureus',

Lancet, **2,** 39.

Hallett, A. F., Appelbaum, P. C., Cooper, R., Mokgokong, S. and Monale, D. (1977), 'Penicillinase-producing Neisseria gonorrhoeae from South Africa', *Lancet,* **1,** 1205.

Halpern, B., Ky, N. T. and Amache, N. (1967), 'Diagnosis of drug allergy in vitro with the lymphocyte transformation test', *J. Allergy,* **40,** 168.

Hammond, G. W., Lian, C. J., Wilt, J. C. and Ronald, A. R. (1978), 'Antimicrobial susceptibility of Haemophilus ducreyi', *Antimicrob. Ag. Chemother.,* **13,** 608.

Handsfield, H. H., Wiesner, P. J. and Holmes, K. K. (1976), 'Treatment of the gonococcal arthritis-dermatitis syndrome', *Ann. Intern. Med.,* **84,** 661.

Hansman, D., Glasgow, H., Sturt, J., Devitt, L. and Douglas, R. (1971), 'Increased resistance to penicillin of pneumococci isolated from man', *New Engl. J. Med.,* **284,** 175.

Hansman, D. (1972), 'Type distribution and antibiotic sensitivity of pneumococci from carriers in Kiriwina, Trobriand Islands (New Guinea)', *Med. J. Aust.,* **2,** 771.

Hansman, D. Devitt, L. and Riley, I. (1973), 'Pneumococci with increased resistance to penicillin', *Brit. med. J.,* **3,** 405.

Hansman, D., Devitt, L., Miles, H. and Riley, I. (1974), 'Pneumococci relatively insensitive to penicillin in Australia and New Guinea', *Med. J. Aust.,* **2,** 353.

Hansman, D. (1974), 'Type distribution and antibiotic sensitivity of Diplococcus pneumoniae: a five-year study in Sydney', *Med. J. Aust.,* **2,** 436.

Hansman, D. (1975), 'Antibiotic sensitivity pattern of pneumococci relatively insensitive to penicillin and cephalosporin antibiotics', *Med. J. Aust.,* **2,** 740.

Hansman, D. (1976), 'Penicillin-insensitive pneumococci and pneumococcal infections', *Med. J. Aust.,* **1,** 132.

Hare, R. (1970), *The Birth of Penicillin and the Disarming of Microbes,* George Allen and Unwin, Ltd.

Hart, G. (1973), 'Penicillin resistance of Gonococci in South Vietnam', *Med. J. Aust.,* **2,** 638.

Hartmann, R., Höltje, J. and Schwarz, U. (1972), 'Targets of penicillin action in Escherichia coli', *Nature,* **235,** 426.

Hatos, G. (1972), 'Evaluation of 460 cases of treated syphilis', *Med. J. Aust.,* **2,** 415.

Hewitt, W. L. (1963), 'The penicillins', *JAMA,* **185,** 264.

Hieber, J. P. and Nelson, J. D. (1977), 'A pharmacologic evaluation of penicillin in children with purulent meningitis', *New Engl. J. Med.,* **297,** 410.

Holder, W. R. and Knox, J. M. (1972), 'Syphilis in pregnancy', *Med. Clin. North Amer.,* **56,** 1151.

Holmberg, K., Nord, C.-E. and Dornbusch, K. (1977), 'Antimicrobial *in vitro* susceptibility of Actinomyces israelii and Archnia propionica', *Scand. J. Infect. Dis.,* **9,** 40.

Holmes, K. K., Karney, W. W., Harnisch, J. P., Wiesner, P. J., Turck, M. and Pedersen, A. H. B. (1973), 'Single-dose aqueous procaine penicillin G therapy for gonorrhea: Use of probenecid and cause of treatment failure', *J. Infect. Dis.,* **127,** 455.

Horne, D. and Tomasz, A. (1977), 'Tolerant response of Streptococcus sanguis to beta-lactams and other cell wall inhibitors', *Antimicrob. Ag. Chemother.,* **11,** 888.

Horowitz, L. (1975), 'Atopy as factor in penicillin reactions', *New Engl. J. Med.,* **292,** 1243.

Howes, V. J. and Mitchell, R. G. (1976), 'Meningitis due to relatively penicillin-resistant pneumococcus, *Brit. med. J.,* **1,** 996.

Hughes, E. S. R., Hardy, K. J., Cutherbertson, A. M. and Rubbo, S. D. (1970), 'Chemoprophylaxis in large bowel surgery: 1. Effect on incidence of postoperative infection', *Med. J. Aust.,* **1,** 305.

Hulbert, J. (1972), 'Gram-negative urinary infection treated with oral penicillin G', *Lancet,* **2,** 1216.

Hussar, A. E. and Holley, H. L. (1954), *Antibiotics and Antibiotic Therapy,* The Macmillan Company, New York, pp. 61 and 73.

Idsøe, O., Guthe, T., Willcox, R. R. and de Weck, A. L. (1968), 'Nature and extent of penicillin side-reactions, with particular reference to fatalities from anaphylactic shock', *Bull. Wld. Hlth. Org., 38*, 159.

Idsøe, O., Guthe, T. and Willcox, R. R. (1972), 'Penicillin in the treatment of syphilis. The experience of three decades', *Bull. Wld. Hlth. Org., Suppl.* Vol. 47, pp. 1–68.

Isbister, J. P. (1971), 'Penicillin allergy: A review of the immunological and clinical aspects', *Med. J. Aust., 1*, 1067.

Jackson, D. H. and Jephcott, A. E. (1976), 'Penicillin sensitivity of gonococci. An evaluation of monitoring as an index of epidemiological control', *Brit. J. vener, Dis., 52*, 253.

Jaffe, H. W., Biddle, J. W., Thornsberry, C., Johnson, R. E., Kaufman, R. E., Reynolds, G. H., Wiesner, P. J. and The Cooperative Study Group (1976), 'National gonorrhea therapy monitoring study. *In vitro* antibiotic susceptibility and its correlation with treatment results', *New. Engl. J. Med., 294*, 5.

Johnson, A. (1962), 'Hypersensitivity to penicillin: A short review', *Med. J. Aust., 2*, 432.

Johnson, F. W. A. and Hobson, D. (1977), 'The effect of penicillin on genital strains of Chlamydia trachomatis in tissue culture', *J. Antimicrob. Chemother., 3*, 49.

Johnson, R. H. and Rumans, L. W. (1977), 'Unusual infections caused by Pasteurella multocida', *JAMA, 237*, 146.

Joorabchi, B. and Kohout, E. (1973), 'Apparent penicillin-induced arrest of mature bone marrow elements', *Brit. Med. J., 2*, 26.

Judson, F. N., Allaman, J. and Dans, P. E. (1974), 'Treatment of gonorrhea. Comparison of penicillin G procaine, doxycyline, spectinomycin, and ampicillin', *JAMA, 230*, 705.

Kalis, P., Le Frock, J. L., Smith, W. and Keefe, M. (1976), 'Listeriosis', *Amer. J. Med. Sci., 271*, 159.

Kaplan, J. M. and McCracken, G. H. Jr. (1973), 'Clinical pharmacology of benzathine penicillin G in neonates with regard to its recommended use in congenital syphilis', *J. Pediatrics, 82*, 1069.

Kaplan, E. L., Anthony, B. F., Bisno, A., Durack, D., Houser, H., Millard, H. D., Sanford, J., Shulman, S. T., Stillerman, M., Taranta, A. and Wenger, N. (1977), 'Prevention of bacterial endocarditis', *Circulation, 56*, 139A.

Katz, H. I., Gill, K. A., Baxter, D. L. and Moschella, S. L. (1964), 'Indirect basophil degranulation test in penicillin allergy', *JAMA, 188*, 351.

Kaufman, R. E., Johnson, R. E., Jaffe, H. W., Thornsberry, C., Reynolds, G. H., Wiesner, P. J. and The Cooperative Study Group (1976), 'National gonorrhea therapy monitoring study. Treatment results', *New Engl. J. Med., 294*, 1.

Kerr, R. O., Cardamone, J., Dalmasso, A. P. and Kaplan, M. E. (1972), 'Two mechanisms of erythrocyte destruction in penicillin-induced hemolytic anemia', *New Engl. J. Med., 287*, 1322.

Kirven, L. A. and Thornsberry, C. (1977), 'Transfer of beta-lactamase genes of Neisseria gonorrhoeae by conjugation', *Antimicrob. Ag. Chemother., 11*, 1004.

Klein, J. O., Schaberg, M. J., Buntin, M. and Gezon, H. M. (1973), 'Levels of penicillin in serum of newborn infants after single intramuscular doses of benzathine penicillin G', *J. Pediatrics, 82*, 1065.

Klein, E. J., Fisher, L. S., Chow, A. W. and Guze, L. B. (1977), Anorectal gonococcal infection', *Ann. Intern. Med., 86*, 340.

Knox, R. (1960), 'A new penicillin (BRL 1241) active against penicillin-resistant staphylococci', *Brit. med. J., 2*, 690.

Knudsen. E. T., Robinson. O. P. W., Croydon, E. A. P. and Tees, E. C. (1967), 'Cutaneous sensitivity to purified benzylpenicillin', *Lancet, 1*, 1184.

Kocen, R. S. (1962), 'Leptospirosis', *Brit. med. J., 1*, 1181.

Kornguth, M. L. and Kunin, C. M. (1976), 'Uptake of antibiotics by human erythrocytes', *J. Infect. Dis.*, **133**, 175.

Kunin, C. M. (1967), 'A guide to use of antibiotics in patients with renal disease', *Ann. Intern. Med.*, **67**, 151.

Lacey, R. W. (1977a), 'Inactivation of penicillins and cephalosporins by enzymes', *Brit. med. J.*, **1**, 1285.

Lacey, R. (1977b), 'A new type of penicillin resistance of Staphylococcus aureus?', *J. Antimicrob. Chemother.*, **3**, 380.

Lawson, J. H. (1973), 'Penicillin in leptospirosis', *Brit. med. J.*, **4**, 109.

Leading Article (1968a), 'Penicillin-induced haemolytic anaemia', *Brit. med. J.*, **3**, 4.

Leading Article (1968b), 'Encephalopathy from penicillin', *Brit. med. J.*, **3**, 198.

Leading Article (1970), 'Prophylactic antibiotics', *Lancet*, **2**, 1231.

Leading Article (1972a), 'Single-dose treatment of gonorrhoea', *Lancet*, **1**, 885.

Leading Article (1972b), 'Treatment of gonorrhoea', *Brit. med. J.*, **2**, 421.

Leading Article (1972c), 'How bacteria knit their overcoats and penicillins make them drop stitches', *Lancet*, **2**, 468.

Leading Article (1972d), 'Gas gangrene and hyperbaric oxygen', *Brit. med. J.*, **3**, 715.

Leading Article (1973a), 'Penicillin in the treatment of syphilis', *Brit. med. J.*, **2**, 259.

Leading Article (1973b), 'Single-dose treatment of gonorrhoea', *Brit. med. J.*, **4**, 65.

Leading Article (1975a), 'Drug interactions', *Lancet*, **1**, 904.

Leading Article (1975b), 'Antibiotic cover for dental extraction', *Brit. med. J.*, **3**, 191.

Leading Article (1976a), 'Prophylaxis of bacterial endocarditis. Faith, hope and charitable interpretations', *Lancet*, **1**, 519.

Leading Article (1976b), 'Penicillinase-producing gonococci', *Brit. med. J.*, **2**, 963.

Leading Article (1976c), 'Clinical aspects of the blood-brain barrier', *Brit. med. J.*, **2**, 133.

Leading Article (1977a), 'The Jarisch-Herxheimer reaction', *Lancet*, **1**, 340.

Leading Article (1977b), 'New light on penicillin', *Brit. med. J.*, **1**, 986.

Leading Article (1977c), 'Control of penicillinase-producing gonococci, *Brit. med. J.*, **1**, 1618.

Leading Article (1977d), 'Resistant pneumococci', *Lancet*, **2**, 803.

Lee, E. L., Robinson, M. J., Thong, M. L., Puthucheary, S. D., Ong, T. H. and Ng, K. K. (1977), 'Intraventricular chemotherapy in neonatal meningitis', *J. Pediatrics*, **91**, 991.

Leftik, M. I., Miller, J. W. and Brown, J. D. (1978), 'Penicillin-resistant gonococcal polyarthritis', *JAMA*, **239**, 134.

Lehmann, V., Knutsen, S. B., Ragnhildstveit, E., Skagseth, E. and Solberg, C. O. (1977), 'Endocarditis caused by Pasteurella multocida', *Scand. J. Infect. Dis.*, **9**, 247.

Lerner, P. I., Smith, H. and Weinstein, L. (1967), 'Penicillin neurotoxicity', *Ann. N.Y. Acad. Sci.*, **145**, 310.

Levine, B. B., Redmond, A. P., Voss, H. E. and Zolov, D. M. (1967), 'Prediction of penicillin allergy by immunological tests', *Ann. N.Y. Acad. Sci.*, **145**, 298.

Levine, B. B. and Redmond, A. P. (1969), 'Minor haptemic determinant specific reagin of penicillin hypersensitivity in man', *Inter. Arch. Allerg.*, **35**, 445; quoted by Fishman and Hewitt (1970).

Levine, B. B. and Zolov, D. M. (1969), 'Prediction of penicillin allergy by immunological tests', *J. Allergy*, **43**, 231.

Levine, B. B. (1972), 'Editorial. Skin rashes with penicillin therapy: Current management', *New Engl. J. Med.*, **286**, 42.

Levit, F. (1976), 'Syphilis therapy still imperfect', *JAMA*, **236**, 2213.

Lewis, G. W. (1957), 'Acute immediate reactions to penicillin', *Brit. med. J.*, **1**, 1153.

Lewis, B. R. and Gupta, J. M. (1977), 'Present prognosis in neonatal meningitis', *Med. J. Aust.*, **1**, 695.

Lindon, M. and Handke, G. (1976), 'Penicillinase-producing Neisseria gonorrhoeae in Adelaide', *Med. J. Aust.*, **2**, 660.

Litt, I. F., Edberg, S. C. and Finberg, L. (1974), 'Gonorrhea in children and adolescents: a current review', *J. Pediatrics*, **85**, 595.

Lorian, V. (1975), 'Some effects of subinhibitory concentrations of penicillin on the structure and division of staphylococci', *Antimicrob. Ag. Chemother.*, **7**, 864.

Lorian, V. and Atkinson, B. (1976), 'Effects of subinhibitory concentrations of antibiotics on cross walls of cocci', *Antimicrob. Ag. Chemother.*, **9**, 1043.

Mace, J. W., Janik, D. S., Sauer, R. L. and Quilligan, J. J. Jr. (1977), 'Penicillin-resistant pneumococcal meningitis in an immunocompromised infant', *J. Pediatrics*, **91**, 506.

Maness, M. J. and Sparling, P. F. (1973), 'Multiple antibiotic resistance due to a single mutation in Neisseria gonorrhoeae', *J. Infect. Dis.*, **128**, 321.

Martin, J. E., Jr., Lester, A., Price, E. V. and Schmale, J. D. (1970), 'Comparative study of gonococcal susceptibility to penicillin in the United States, 1955–1969', *J. Infect. Dis.*, **122**, 459.

McCloskey, R. V., Green, M. J., Eller, J. and Smilack, J. (1974), 'Treatment of diphtheria carriers: benzathine penicillin, erythromycin, and clindamycin', *Ann. Intern. Med.*, **81**, 788.

McCormack, W. M. (1977), 'Treatment of gonorrhoea—is penicillin passé?', *New Engl. J. Med.*, **296**, 934.

McCracken, G. H. Jr., Ginsberg, C., Chrane, D. F., Thomas, M. L. and Horton, L. J. (1973), 'Clinical pharmacology of penicillin in newborn infants', *J. Pediatrics*, **82**, 692.

McCracken, G. H. Jr. (1973), 'Group B Streptococci: The new challenge in neonatal infections', *J. Pediatrics*, **82**, 703.

McCracken, G. H., Jr. (1974), 'Pharmacological basis for antimicrobial therapy in new-born infants', *Am. J. Dis. Child.*, **128**, 407.

McCracken, G. H., Jr. and Eichenwald, H. F. (1974), 'Antimicrobial therapy; therapeutic recommendations and a review of newer drugs. Part 1. Therapy of infectious conditions', *J. Pediatrics*, **85**, 297.

McPherson, A. J., Parkin, J. D. and Hope, R. (1976), 'Penicillin-induced haemolytic anaemia associated with microangiopathy', *Aust. N.Z. J. Med.*, **6**, 152.

Maier, T. W., Beilstein, H. R. and Zubrzycki, L. (1974), 'Multiple antibiotic resistance in Neisseria gonorrhoeae', *Antimicrob. Ag. Chemother.*, **6**, 22.

Mayhall, C. G., Medoff, G. and Marr, J. J. (1976), 'Variation in the susceptibility of strains of Staphylococcus aureus to oxacillin, cephalothin, and gentamicin', *Antimicrob. Ag. Chemother.*, **10**, 707.

Meers, P. D. and Matthews, R. B. (1978), 'Multiply resistant pneumococcus', *Lancet*, **2**, 219.

Menke, H. E. and Pepplinkhuizen, L. (1974), 'Acute non-allergic reaction to aqueous procaine penicillin', *Lancet*, **2**, 723.

Moellering, R. C., Jr., Watson, B. K. and Kunz, L. J. (1974), 'Endocarditis due to group D streptococci. Comparison of disease caused by Streptococcus bovis with that produced by the enterococci', *Amer. J. Med.*, **57**, 239.

Mohan, K., Gordon, R. C., Beaman, T. C., Belding, R. C., Luecke, D., Edmiston, C. and Gerhardt, P. (1977), 'Synergism of penicillin and gentamicin against Listeria monocytogenes in *ex vivo* hemodialysis culture', *J. Infect. Dis.*, **135**, 51.

Mohr, J. A., Griffiths, W., Jackson, R., Saadah, H., Bird, P. and Riddle, J. (1976), 'Neurosyphilis and penicillin levels in cerebrospinal fluid', *JAMA*, **236**, 2208.

Nauta, E. H., Mattie, H. and Goslings, W. R. O. (1974), 'Effect of probenecid on the apparent volume of distribution and elimination of cloxacillin', *Antimicrob. Ag. Chemother.*, **6**, 300.

Naraqi, S., Kirpatrick, G. P. and Kabins, S. (1974), 'Relapsing pneumococcal meningitis: isolation of an organism with decreased susceptibility to penicillin G', *J. Pediatrics*, **85,** 671.

Neu, H. C. (1976), 'Synergy of mecillinam, a beta-amidinopenicillanic acid derivative, combined with beta-lactam antibiotics', *Antimicrob. Ag. Chemother.*, **10,** 535.

N.H.M.R.C. Report (1965), 'Penicillin anaphylaxis and skin tests', *Med. J. Aust.*, **2,** 42.

Nishino, T. and Nakazawa, S. (1976), 'Bacteriological study on effects of beta-lactam group antibiotics in high concentrations', *Antimicrob. Ag. Chemother.*, **9,** 1033.

Newnham, W. A. (1978), 'Editorial. The penicillin treatment of syphilis', *Med. J. Aust.*, **1,** 369.

Olafsson, M., Lee, Y. C. and Abernethy, T. J. (1958), 'Mima polymorpha meningitis: Report of a case and review of the literature', *New Engl. J. Med.*, **258,** 465.

Olsson, B., Nord, C.-E. and Wadström, T. (1976), 'Formation of beta-lactamase in Bacteroides fragilis: cell-bound and extracellular activity', *Antimicrob. Ag. Chemother.*, **9,** 727.

Orchard, R. T. and Rooker, G. (1974), 'Penicillin-hypersensitivity nephritis', *Lancet,* **1,** 689.

Paredes, A., Taber, L. H., Yow, M. D., Clark, D. and Nathan, W. (1976a), 'Prolonged pneumococcal meningitis due to an organism with increased resistance to penicillin', *Pediatrics,* **58,** 378.

Paredes, A., Wong, P. and Yow, M. D. (1976b), 'Failure of penicillin to eradicate the carrier state of group B streptococcus in infants', *J. Pediatrics,* **89,** 191.

Parker, C. W. (1963), 'Editorial. Penicillin allergy', *Amer. J. Med.*, **34,** 747.

Parker, C. W. (1964), 'The immunochemical basis for penicillin allergy', *Postgrad. Med. J.* (Suppl.), **40,** 141.

Parker, J. C. and Barrett, D. A. II (1971), 'Microangiopathic hemolysis and thrombocytopenia related to penicillin drugs', *Arch. Intern. Med.*, **127,** 474.

Parker, C. W. (1975), 'Drug allergy', *New Engl. J. Med.*, **292,** 511, 732 and 957.

Patterson, M. J. and Hafeez, A. E. B. (1976), 'Group B streptococci in human disease', *Bacteriol. Rev.*, **40,** 774.

Percival, A., Rowlands, J., Corkill, J. E., Alergant, C. D., Arya, O. P., Rees, E. and Annels, E. H. (1976), 'Penicillinase-producing gonocci in Liverpool.', *Lancet,* **2,** 1379.

Perine, P. L., Schalla, W., Siegel, M. S., Thornsberry, C., Biddle, J., Wong, K. and Thompson, S. E. (1977), 'Evidence for two distinct types of penicillinase-producing Neisseria gonorrhoeae', *Lancet,* **2,** 993.

Peter, G. and Smith, A. L. (1977), 'Group A streptococcal infections of the skin and pharynx. (Second of two parts)', *New Engl. J. Med.*, **297,** 365.

Phillips, I. (1976), 'Beta-lactamase-producing, penicillin-resistant gonococcus', *Lancet,* **2,** 656.

Phillips, I., Warren, C., Harrison, J. M., Sharples, P., Ball, L. C. and Parker, M. T. (1976), 'Antibiotic susceptibilities of streptococci from the mouth and blood of patients treated with penicillin or lincomycin and clindamycin', *J. Med. Microbiol.*, **9,** 393.

Piot, P. (1977), 'Resistant gonococcus from the Ivory Coast', *Lancet,* **1,** 857.

Plaut, M. E., O'Connell, C. J., Pabico, R. C. and Davidson, D. (1969), 'Penicillin handling in normal and azotemic patients', *J. Lab. Clin. Med.*, **74,** 12.

Porter, J. and Jick, H. (1977), 'Drug-induced anaphylaxis, convulsions, deafness, and extrapyramidal symptoms', *Lancet,* **1,** 587.

Powell, J. T. and Bond, J. H. (1976), 'Multiple antibiotic resistance in clinical strains of Neisseria gonorrhoeae isolated in South Carolina', *Antimicrob. Ag. Chemother.*, **10,** 639.

Raichle, M. E., Kutt, H., Louis, S. and McDowell, F. (1971), 'Neurotoxicity of intravenously administered penicillin G', *Arch. Neurol.*, **25,** 232.

Ravreby, W. D., Bottone, E. J. and Keusch, G. T. (1973), 'Group D streptococcal bacteremia, with emphasis on the incidence and presentation of infections due to Streptococcus bovis', *New Engl. J. Med.*, **289**, 1400.

Resnik, S. S. and Shelley, W. B. (1966), 'Penicilloyl-polylysine skin test: Anaphylaxis in absence of penicillin sensitivity', *JAMA*, **196**, 740.

Roberts, M. and Falkow, S. (1977), 'Conjugal transfer of R plasmids in Neisseria gonorrhoeae', *Nature*, **266**, 630.

Roding, B., Groenveld, P. H. and Boerema, I. (1972), 'Ten years' experience in the treatment of gas gangrene in hyperbaric oxygen', *Surg. Gynec. Obstet.*, **134**, 579; quoted by Deveridge and Unsworth (1973).

Rodriguez, W. and Saz, A. K. (1975), 'Possible mechanism of decreased susceptibility of Neisseria gonorrhoeae to penicillin', *Antimicrob. Ag. Chemother.*, **7**, 788.

Rood, J. I., Maher, E. A., Somers, E. B., Compos, E. and Duncan, C. L. (1978), 'Isolation and characterization of multiply antibiotic-resistant Clostridium perfringens strains from porcine feces', *Antimicrob. Ag. Chemother.*, **13**, 871.

Rubbo, S. D. (1966), 'New approaches to tetanus prophylaxis', *Lancet*, **2**, 449.

Rudolph, A. H. and Price, E. V. (1973), 'Penicillin reactions among patients in venereal disease clinics', *JAMA*, **223**, 499.

Sabath, L. D., Garner, C., Wilcox, C. and Finland, M. (1976), 'Susceptibility of Staphylococcus aureus and Staphylococcus epidermidis to 65 antibiotics', *Antimicrob. Ag. Chemother.*, **9**, 962.

Sabath, L. D., Wheeler, N., Laverdiere, M., Blazevic, D. and Wilkinson, B. J. (1977), 'A new type of penicillin resistance of Staphylococcus aureus', *Lancet*, **1**, 443.

Sackel, S. G., Alpert, S., Rosner, B., McCormack, W. M. and Finland, M. (1977), '*In vitro* activity of *p*-hydroxybenzyl penicillin (penicillin X) and five other penicillins against Neisseria gonorrhoeae: comparisons of strains from patients with uncomplicated infections and from women with pelvic inflammatory disease', *Antimicrob. Ag. Chemother.*, **12**, 31.

Sarubbi, F. A., Jr. and Sparling, P. F. (1974), 'Transfer of antibiotic resistance in mixed cultures of Neisseria gonorrhoeae', *J. Infect. Dis.*, **130**, 660.

Saunders, J. R. (1977), 'Transferable drug resistance in the gonococcus', *Nature*, **266**, 586.

Schmitt, B. D. and Krivit, W. (1969), 'Benign intracranial hypertension associated with a delayed penicillin reaction', *Pediatrics*, **43**, 50.

Schoutens, E. and Yourassowsky, E. (1974), 'Speed of bactericidal action of penicillin G, ampicillin and carbenicillin on Bacteroides fragilis', *Antimicrob. Ag. Chemother.*, **6**, 227.

Schrier, R. W., Bulger, R. J. and van Arsdel, P. P. Jr. (1966), 'Nephropathy associated with penicillin and homologues', *Ann. Intern. Med.*, **64**, 116.

Schroeter, A. L., Turner, R. H., Lucas, J. B. and Brown, W. J. (1971), 'Therapy for incubating syphilis. Effectiveness of gonorrhea treatment', *JAMA*, **218**, 711.

Schroeter, A. L., Lucas, J. B., Price, E. V. and Falcone, V. H. (1972), 'Treatment for early syphilis and reactivity of serologic tests', *JAMA*, **221**, 471.

Schwartz, R. H. and Vaughan, J. H. (1963), 'Immunologic responsiveness of man to penicillin', *JAMA*, **186**, 1151.

Schwartzman, J. D., Reller, L. B. and Wang, W. L. (1977), 'Susceptibility of Clostridium perfringens isolated from human infections to twenty antibiotics', *Antimicrob. Ag. Chemother.*, **11**, 695.

Seamans, K. B., Gloor, P., Dobell, A. R. C. and Wyant, J. D. (1968), 'Penicillin-induced seizures during cardio-pulmonary bypass', *New Engl. J. Med.*, **278**, 861.

Sengupta, S. (1976), 'Gangrene following intra-arterial injection of procaine penicillin', *Aust. N.Z. J. Med.*, **6**, 71.

Shanson, D. C. (1978), 'The prophylaxis of infective endocarditis', *J. Antimicrob. Chemother.*, **4**, 2.

Shapiro, G. G., Bierman, C. W., Furukawa, C. T. and Pierson, W. E. (1977), 'Allergy skin testing: science or quackery?', *Pediatrics*, **59**, 495.

Shelley, W. B. (1963), 'Indirect basophil degranulation test for allergy to penicillin and other drugs', *JAMA*, **184**, 171.

Siegel, M. S., Thornsberry, C., Biddle, J. W., O'Mara, P. R., Perine, P. L. and Wiesner, P. J. (1978), 'Penicillinase-producing Neisseria gonorrhoeae: results of surveillance in the United States', *J. Infect. Dis.*, **137**, 170.

Simberkoff, M. S., Thomas, L., McGregor, D., Shenkein, I. and Levine, B. B. (1970), 'Inactivation of penicillins by carbohydrate solutions at alkaline pH', *New Engl. J. Med.*, **283**, 116.

Smilack, J. D., Flittie, W. H. and Williams, T. W. Jr. (1976), 'Bone concentrations of antimicrobial agents after parenteral administration', *Antimicrob. Ag. Chemother.*, **9**, 169.

Smith, J. W., Johnson, J. E. and Cluff, L. E. (1966), 'Studies on the epidemiology of adverse drug reactions. II. An evaluation of penicillin allergy', *New Engl. J. Med.*, **274**, 998.

Smith, H., Dewdney, J. M. and Wheeler, A. W. (1971), 'A comparison of the amounts and the antigenicity of polymeric materials formed in aqueous solution by some β-lactam antibiotics', *Immunology*, **21**, 527.

Smith, H. and Marshall, A. C. (1971), 'Polymers formed by some β-lactam antibiotics', *Nature*, **232**, 45.

Smith, J. M. (1974), 'Incidence of atopic disease', *Med. Clin. North Amer.*, **58**, 3.

Smithurst, B. A. (1971), 'Penicillin therapy in primary and secondary syphilis', *Med. J. Aust.*, **2**, 248.

Smithurst, B. A. (1974), 'Resistance of Neisseria gonorrhoeae to penicillin in 199 gonococcal infections in women and the response of those infections to penicillin treatment', *Med. J. Aust.*, **1**, 585.

Spark, R. P. (1971), 'Fatal anaphylaxis due to oral penicillin', *Amer. J. clin. Path.*, **56**, 407.

Sparling, P. F. (1972), 'Antibiotic resistance in Neisseria gonorrhoeae', *Med. Clin. North Amer.*, **56**, 1133.

Sparling, P. F., Wiesner, P. J., Holmes, K. K. and Kass, E. H. (1973), 'Editorial. Treatment of gonorrhea', *J. Infect. Dis.*, **127**, 578.

Sparling, P. F., Holmes, K. K., Wiesner, P. J. and Puziss, M. (1977), 'Summary of the conference on the problem of penicillin-resistant gonococci', *J. Infect. Dis.*, **135**, 865.

Speer, M. E., Taber, L. H., Clark, D. B. and Rudolph, A. J. (1977), 'Cerebrospinal fluid levels of benzathine penicillin G in the neonate', *J. Pediatrics*, **91**, 996.

Sprunt, K., Redman, W. and Leidy, G. (1968), 'Penicillin-resistant alpha streptococci in pharynx of patients given oral penicillin', *Pediatrics*, **42**, 957.

Steigman, A. J., Bottone, E. J. and Hanna, B. A. (1978), 'Control of perinatal group B streptococcal sepsis: efficacy of single injection of aqueous penicillin at birth', *in press*.

Stewart, G. T. (1962), 'Cross-allergenicity of penicillin G and related substances', *Lancet*, **1**, 509.

Stewart, G. T. (1965), *The Penicillin Group of Drugs*, Elsevier Publishing Company.

Stewart, G. T. (1967), 'Allergenic residues in penicillins', *Lancet*, **1**, 1177.

Strominger, J. L. and Tipper, D. J. (1965), 'Bacterial cell wall synthesis and structure in relation to the mechanism of action of penicillins and other antibacterial agents', *Amer. J. Med.*, **39**, 708.

Suginaka, H., Ichikawa, A. and Kotani, S. (1975), 'Penicillin-resistant mechanisms in Pseudomonas acruginosa: binding of penicillin to Pseudomonas aeruginosa KM 338', *Antimicrob. Ag. Chemother.*, **7**, 629.

Sutherland, R., Croydon, E. A. P. and Rolinson, G. N. (1970), 'Flucloxacillin, a new isoxazolyl penicillin, compared with oxacillin, cloxacillin and dicloxacillin', *Brit.*

med. J., **4,** 455.

Sutter, V. L. and Finegold, S. M. (1976), 'Susceptibility of anaerobic bacteria to 23 antimicrobial agents', *Antimicrob. Ag. Chemother.,* **10,** 736.

Sutter, V. L. (1977), '*In vitro* susceptibility of anaerobes: comparison of clindamycin and other antimicrobial agents', *J. Infect. Dis.* (Suppl.), **135,** 7.

Sykes, R. B. and Matthew, M. (1976), 'The beta-lactamases of Gram-negative bacteria and their role in resistance to beta-lactam antibiotics', *J. Antimicrob. Chemother.,* **2,** 115.

Tally, F. P., Jacobus, N. V., Bartlett, J. G. and Gorbach, S. L. (1975), '*In vitro* activity of penicillins against anaerobes', *Antimicrob. Ag. Chemother.,* **7,** 413.

Tattersall, M. H. N., Battersby, G. and Spiers, A. S. D. (1972), 'Antibiotics and hypokalaemia', *Lancet,* **1,** 630.

Tempest, B., Carney, J. P. and Eberle, B. (1974), 'Distribution of the sensitivities to penicillin of types of Diplococcus pneumoniae in an American Indian population', *J. Infect. Dis.,* **130,** 67.

Thornsberry, C., Baker, C. N. and Kirven, L. A. (1978), '*In vitro* activity of antimicrobial agents on Legionnaires' Disease bacterium', *Antimicrob. Ag. Chemother.,* **13,** 78.

Toala, P., McDonald, A., Wilcox, C. and Finland, M. (1969), 'Susceptibility of Group D streptococcus (Enterococcus) to 21 antibiotics *in vitro,* with special reference to species differences', *Amer. J. Med. Sci.,* **258,** 416.

Tramont, E. C. (1976), 'Persistence of Treponema pallidum following penicillin G therapy. Report of two cases', *JAMA,* **236,** 2206.

Turner, L. H. (1969), 'Leptospirosis', *Brit. med. J.,* **1,** 231.

Turner, G. C., Ratcliffe, J. G. and Anderson, D. (1976), 'Penicillinase-producing Neisseria gonorrhoeae', *Lancet,* **2,** 793.

van Arsdel, P. P. Jr. (1968), 'Editorial. The risk of penicillin reactions', *Ann. Intern. Med.,* **69,** 1071.

Voss, H. E., Redmond, A. P. and Levine, B. B. (1966), 'Clinical detection of the potential allergic reactor to penicillin by immunologic tests', *JAMA,* **196,** 679.

Wasz-Höckert, O., Nummi, S., Vuopala, S. and Järvinen, P. A. (1970), 'Transplacental passage of azidocillin, ampicillin and penicillin G during early and late pregnancy', *Scand. J. Infect. Dis.,* **2,** 125.

Watanakunakorn, C. (1974), 'Streptococcus bovis endocarditis', *Amer. J. Med.,* **56,** 256.

Weinstein, L. and Dalton, A. C. (1968), 'Host determinants of response to antimicrobial agents', *New Engl. J. Med.,* **279,** 524.

Weinstein, L., Lerner, P. I. and Chew, W. H. (1964), 'Clinical and bacteriologic studies of the effect of "massive" doses of penicillin G on infections caused by Gram-negative bacilli', *New Engl. J. Med.,* **271,** 525.

Welch, H. (1954), *Principles and Practice of Antibiotic Therapy,* Med. Encyc. Inc., New York, pp. 46, 66 and 74.

Westerman, G., Gorman, A., Stelos, P. and Nodine, J. H. (1966), 'Adverse reactions to penicillin. A review of treatment', *JAMA,* **198,** 173.

White, J. M., Brown, D. L., Hepner, G. W. and Worlledge, S. M. (1968), 'Penicillin induced haemolytic anaemia', *Brit. Med. J.,* **3,** 26.

WHO (1977), 'Neisseria gonorrhoeae producing beta-lactamase (penicillinase)' *Wkly Epidem. Rec.,* **52,** 357.

Wiesner, P. J., Handsfield, H. H. and Holmes, K. K. (1973), 'Low antibiotic resistance of gonococci causing disseminated infection', *New Engl. J. Med.,* **288,** 1221.

Wiggins, G. L., Albritton, W. L. and Feeley, J. C. (1978), 'Antibiotic susceptibility of clinical isolates of Listeria monocytogenes', *Antimicrob. Ag. Chemother.,* **13,** 854.

Wilkinson, A. E., Seth, A. D. and Rodin, P. (1976), 'Infection with penicillinase-producing gonococcus', *Brit. med. J.,* **2,** 1233.

Wilkinson, A. E. (1977), 'The sensitivity of gonococci to penicillin', *J. Antimicrob. Chemother.*, **3,** 197.

Wilkowske, C. J. and Hermans, P. E. (1974), 'Antimicrobial agents in the treatment of obstetric and gynecologic infections', *Med. Clin. North Amer.*, **58,** 711.

Willcox, R. R. (1970), 'A survey of problems in the antibiotic treatment of gonorrhoea with special reference to South-East Asia', *Brit. J. Vener. Dis.*, **46,** 217.

Willcox, R. R. (1977), 'How suitable are available pharmaceuticals for the treatment of sexually transmitted diseases? 1: Conditions presenting as genital discharges', *Brit. J. Vener. Dis.*, **53,** 314.

Wolfe, J. C. and Johnson, W. D. Jr. (1974), 'Penicillin-sensitive streptococcal endocarditis. *In-vitro* and clinical observations on penicillin-streptomycin therapy', *Ann. Intern. Med.*, **81,** 178.

Young, P. S., Smith, D. D. and Walsingham, B. (1977), 'Group B streptococcal infection in neonates', *Med. J. Aust.*, **2,** 497.

Phenoxypenicillins

Description

Four different acid-stable phenoxypenicillins have been developed, which are all suitable for oral administration.

Phenoxymethylpenicillin (*Penicillin V*) was introduced in 1953 (Spitzy, 1953), and since then has been widely used as an 'oral penicillin'. Penicillin V, like G, is a natural penicillin produced biosynthetically, and it is obtained if the precursor, phenoxyacetic acid, is added to the fermentation medium, while addition of phenylacetic acid results in production of pencillin G. Pencillin V, unlike G, is acid-stable and it is therefore more suitable for oral administration.

With the discovery of the penicillin nucleus (6-aminopenicillanic acid) (Batchelor *et al.*, 1959) it became possible to synthetize new penicillins by the introduction of side chains. Since then a number of semisynthetic pencillins analogous to phenoxymethylpenicillin have been produced:

1. *Phenoxyethylpenicillin* (*Phenethicillin*) was introduced by Beecham Research Laboratories in 1959.

2. *Phenoxypropylpenicillin* (*Propicillin*) was introduced in 1961 (Williamson *et al.*, 1961; Nagley, 1961).

3. *Phenoxybenzylpenicillin* (*Phenbenicillin*) became available in 1962 (Rollo *et al.*, 1962; Carter and Brumfitt, 1962).

These four compounds are similar, but they differ somewhat in antibacterial activity, stability in the presence of staphylococcal penicillinase, absorption from the gastro-intestinal tract and serum protein binding. They are all usually marketed as potassium salts, but a benzathine (DBED) salt of phenoxymethylpenicillin (benzathine penicillin V, 'Bicillin-V') is also available. This preparation is not as well absorbed from the gastro-intestinal tract as potassium phenoxymethylpenicillin (Palatsi and Kaipainen, 1971), and as it has no special advantages, it is not widely used.

Sensitive Organisms

The range of antimicrobial activity of the phenoxypenicillins is generally similar to that of penicillin G (page 4).

These compounds are active against Gram-positive cocci, such as Strep. pyogenes, Strep. pneumoniae, non-penicillinase producing Staph. pyogenes, alpha-haemolytic streptococci such as the 'viridans' group and anaerobic streptococci.

Gram-positive bacilli, such as Cl. tetani, Cl. perfringens, C. diphtheriae and B. anthracis, are also sensitive to the phenoxypenicillins.

Among Gram-negative bacteria, both N. meningitidis and N. gonorrhoeae are sensitive to a degree, H. influenzae is moderately resistant, and all other aerobic Gram-negative bacilli are highly resistant. The anaerobic Gram-negative bacilli which reside in the upper respiratory tract, may be sensitive to these penicillins, but Bacteroides fragilis is resistant (Busch *et al.*, 1976).

There are some important differences between the antibacterial activity of penicillin G and these compounds, and also between individual phenoxypenicillins.

Against streptococci, pneumococci and non-penicillinase producing staphylococci penicillin G is the most active, and the activity of the phenoxypenicillins against these organisms declines in the order, penicillin V, phenethicillin, propicillin and phenbenicillin. However, because phenethicillin, propicillin and phenbenicillin are slightly less susceptible to penicillinase, they are more active than penicillin G and V against penicillinase-producing staphylococci *in vitro* (Jackson and Rao, 1961). Nevertheless these drugs are not useful for treatment of resistant staphylococcal infections, unlike the fully penicillinase-resistant penicillins such as methicillin (page 64), the isoxazoly penicillins (page 79) and nafcillin (page 93).

Penicillin G is about four times more active than penicillin V against meningococci and gonococci, and the newer phenoxypenicillins are even less active than penicillin V (Garrod, 1960b). The activity of penicillin G against H. influenzae is four to eight times greater than that of penicillin V or phenethicillin (Garrod, 1973).

In Vitro Sensitivities

Table 3 shows the MIC's of penicillin G and the four phenoxypenicillins against some selected bacteria. As each subsequent compound has become available, it has usually had a diminished order of activity to the preceding one. Bond *et al.* (1963) have shown that the MIC's of all these drugs are higher, if the test is done in serum rather than in broth because of serum binding of these antibiotics (page 59). These authors estimated the MIC's of each of these penicillins against Strep. pyogenes in both broth and serum. The MIC's in serum compared to broth were increased four-fold with penicillin G and V, eight-fold with phenethicillin and propicillin and thirty-two fold in the case of phenbenicillin.

Mode of Administration and Dosage

These drugs are administered by the oral route. The dosage for children under five years is 125 mg (200 000 units), and for children over five years and adults 250 mg or 500 mg administered six-hourly. These drugs should be given when fasting, preferably about one hour before meals (Bell, 1970).

Higher doses can be used for the treatment of more serious infections. Gray *et al.* (1964) used propicillin 500–1000 mg four-hourly for treatment of bacterial endocarditis.

TABLE 3

Compiled from data published by Garrod (1960a and b) and Barber and Waterworth (1962)

ORGANISM	MIC (μg per ml)				
	Peni-cillin G	Peni-cin V	Phene-thicillin	Propi-cillin	Phenbeni-cillin
Gram-positive bacteria					
Staph. pyogenes (non-penicillinase producer)	0·03	0·03	0·03	0·06	0·12
Strep. pyogenes	0·007	0·015	0·03	0·03	0·03
Strep. pneumoniae (Dip. pneumoniae)	0·015	0·03	0·06	0·06	0·015
Strep. faecalis (Enterococcus, Group D)	2·0	4·0	4·0	—	4·0
Bacillus anthracis	0·015	0·015	0·06	—	0·06
Corynebacterium diphtheriae	0·06	0·03	0·12	—	—
Gram-negative bacteria					
Escherichia coli	64·0	128·0	512·0	—	64·0
Salmonella typhi	4·0	64·0	256·0	—	64·0
Neisseria gonorrhoeae	0·007	0·03	0·12	—	0·12
Neisseria meningitidis	0·03	0·25	1·0	0·50	0·12
Haemophilus influenzae	1·0	4·0	4·0	—	4·0

Availability

Penicillin V and phenethicillin are available as:

(a) capsules or tablets: 125 mg, 250 mg and 500 mg.
(b) paediatric syrup: 125 mg or 250 mg in 5 ml.

Serum Levels in Relation to Dosage

After oral administration of these compounds (Fig. 2), peak serum levels are obtained within half to one hour. The newer drugs give higher and more prolonged levels than penicillin V. Doubling the usual doses of these four penicillins, approximately doubles the serum concentrations obtained. The absorption of phenethicillin, when taken in the form of the recently introduced aqueous paediatric syrup, is superior to that obtained when the older oily paediatric suspension is used (Marty and Hersey, 1975).

There is considerable variation in the absorption of oral penicillins, and some patients for reasons unexplained, absorb them poorly. Diarrhoea of short duration does not influence the absorption of oral penicillins, but if diarrhoea persists for a week, absorption is usually reduced (Bolme and Eriksson, 1975). Similarly, oral penicillin absorption is reduced in patients with malabsorption (Prescott, 1974). Peak serum levels are lower, but more sustained when these drugs are taken with meals than when fasting (McCarthy and Finland, 1960), but it was generally considered that the same total amount is eventually absorbed (Stewart, 1965). However, peak serum levels can be as much as three times higher if the dose is taken one hour before meals, suggesting that oral penicillins as well as some other antibiotics should be prescribed accordingly (Bell, 1970). If this timing of antibiotic administration is strictly supervised, the results of treatment of patients with chronic osteomyelitis are improved (Bell, 1968; 1976).

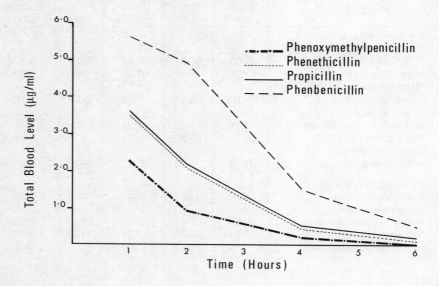

FIG. 2. Mean blood levels of total antibiotic after a single oral dose of 250 mg in 19 subjects. (After Bond *et al.*, 1963.)

Excretion

URINE: Oral penicillins are excreted in urine. Depending on the penicillin used, about 20 to 40 per cent of a given dose can be recovered from urine during the first six hours. That urinary excretion is lowest in the case of phenbenicillin appears paradoxical in view of the high blood levels achieved with this drug. Chromatographic analysis has shown that each of these four penicillins is excreted in urine partly unchanged and also as biologically active metabolites (Bond *et al.*, 1963). Phenbenicillin for instance is excreted mainly in its original form, but two other associated unidentified compounds account for 20 per cent of its urinary activity (Rollo *et al.*, 1962). Some 25–30 per cent of a dose of propicillin is excreted in the urine as an active metabolite, but with penicillin V and phenethicillin, the proportion of active breakdown products in urine is small. The fact that phenoxypenicillins are found in altered but biologically active forms in the urine, raises the possibility that these forms may exist also in blood (Bond *et al.*, 1963). Renal tubular secretion of the phenoxypenicillins can be partially blocked by probenecid ('Benemid').

BILE: Only small amounts of these drugs are excreted in the bile, mainly in the unchanged form.

Distribution of the Drugs in Body

Phenoxypenicillins, like penicillin G, diffuse readily into pleural, pericardial, ascitic and synovial fluids and pass into the fetal circulation. However, penicillin V penetrates poorly into maxillary sinus secretions (Lundberg and Malmborg, 1973). There is a very little penetration of any of the phenoxypenicillins into the CSF if the meninges are uninflamed.

All phenoxypenicillins are bound to serum proteins to some extent, and their protein binding percentages are penicillin V 80, phenethicillin 75, propicillin 89 and phenbenicillin 97 (Bond et al., 1963). These values are higher than other reported figures, but in this study human sera with low penicillin concentrations, similar to those which would be found in vivo, were used. If serum protein binding is estimated at a very high penicillin concentration, lower percentages of serum binding would be obtained. The clinical significance of the protein binding of these and other penicillins is discussed on page 85.

Mode of Action

The mode of action of the phenoxypenicillins is similar to penicillin G (see page 19).

Toxicity

1. *Gastro-intestinal side-effects*. Transient disturbances such as nausea and diarrhoea can follow the oral administration of these drugs. Moniliasis may also occur. Pseudomembranous colitis (page 481) developed in one 12-year-old girl following a four days course of oral phenoxymethylpenicillin (Larson et al., 1977).

2. *Hypersensitivity reactions*. These may occur in penicillin-sensitive patients. Phenoxypenicillins may be cross-allergenic with penicillin G and also with all other penicillins.
   (a) *Anaphylaxis*. This is much less common with the oral phenoxypenicillins than with parenteral penicillin G (page 24). In one patient, symptoms started 30 min after ingestion of 500 mg of penicillin V (Coates, 1963).
   (b) *Serum sickness*. This is quite common, and the reactions are similar to those which occur after penicillin G (page 25).

3. *Direct toxicity*. The oral penicillins are of low toxicity, but massive doses, like those used with penicillin G (page 28), have not been administered to humans. Penicillin V and phenethicillin are well tolerated orally in doses of 6 g per day.

4. *Haemolytic anaemia*. One case has been reported in a three-year-old boy who was treated by penicillin V in a dose of 125 mg six-hourly (Bird et al., 1975). This was an immune haemolytic anaemia due to a penicillin antibody of the IgM class. Antibodies of the IgM class may also be implicated in haemolytic anaemias following penicillin G administration in ordinary doses, but more commonly haemolytic anaemia induced by penicillin G is a sequel to large doses and antibody of the IgG class is involved (page 29).

5. *Jaundice*. Beeley et al. (1976) reported one adult patient, who developed liver damage as part of a severe hypersensitivity reaction to penicillin V.

6. *Cation toxicity.* All the phenoxypenicillins are usually marketed as potassium salts. The doses so far employed (up to 8 g per day) would not cause potassium intoxication, unless there is a serious renal insufficiency, or if a tubular blocking agent is given (*see also* penicillin G, page 30).

Clinical Uses of the Drugs

1. *Respiratory infections.* Phenoxypenicillins are suitable for the oral treatment of mild or convalescent infections due to Strep. pyogenes such as pharyngitis, scarlet fever and cellulitis, and those due to pneumococci such as bronchitis, pneumonia, sinusitis and otitis media. Mild or moderate acute streptococcal pharyngitis in children can usually be successfully treated by one of these drugs, provided that parents are instructed on the importance of regular medication (Colcher and Bass, 1972). In young children, bronchitis and especially otitis media is frequently caused by H. influenzae, and in these cases results of treatment with oral phenoxypenicillins are poor (Kamme and Lundgren, 1971). Serum levels attained following usual doses of these penicillins are rarely high enough to inhibit this pathogen (Oakes *et al.*, 1973). Parenteral penicillin G is a more reliable drug for the treatment of severe streptococcal and pneumococcal infections, as absorption of oral phenoxypenicillins is variable (page 57). Oral therapy with penicillin V or one of its analogues is therefore only recommended for relatively mild infections, or for late treatment of more severe infections, after a favourable clinical response has been obtained with intramuscular penicillin G. Long-term oral penicillin prophylaxis may be useful in some patients who are prone to recurrent streptococcal cellulitis, such as those with lymphoedema of the arms or legs.

2. *Bacterial meningitis.* Oral phenoxypenicillins are not recommended for treatment of any stage of this disease, but it appears that recurrence of pneumococcal meningitis related to a previous head injury, can be prevented sometimes by long-term oral penicillin prophylaxis (Forbes, 1962; Levin *et al.*, 1972). Data from controlled studies on the efficacy of such chemoprophylaxis, however, are not available.

3. *Strep. 'viridans' endocarditis.* This disease has been treated successfully by large doses of an oral phenoxypenicillin e.g. 500 to 1000 mg every four hours with or without probenecid (Gray *et al.*, 1964). A combination of oral penicillin V and intramuscular streptomycin has also been used with success (Hamburger *et al.*, 1961; Tan *et al.*, 1971). Nevertheless, most clinicians prefer to use intramuscular or intravenous penicillin G for the treatment of this serious infection.

4. *Rheumatic fever chemoprophylaxis.* Long-term administration of one of the penicillins is recommended for patients who have had prior rheumatic fever to prevent recurrence of the disease. Monthly injections of 1·2 million units of benzathine penicillin G or 'Bicillin' (pages 13, 40) can be used for this purpose (Krause, 1975), but oral chemotherapy is often preferred, in which case penicillin V or one of its analogues is recommended (Garrod, 1975). The usual dose of these is 500 mg daily given in two divided doses.

Patients with rheumatic heart disease receiving such long-term prophylaxis require additional chemotherapy for short-term protection against bacterial endocarditis during dental procedures. In these patients their oral Strep. 'viridans' strains may become relatively penicillin-resistant (Garrod and Waterworth, 1962; Sprunt *et al.*, 1968). The dose of penicillin may be increased to overcome the resistant strains; intramuscular crystalline penicillin G in a dose of 1–2 million units may be given just before the dental procedure and the same dose repeated six-hourly for the following 12–24 h. The findings by Garrod and Waterworth (1962) indicate that in some patients even these large doses of penicillin G may be inadequate, and another antibiotic such as erythromycin or cephaloridine in full dosage is preferable on a short-term basis (Tozer *et al.*, 1966).

5. *Urinary tract infections.* Acute uncomplicated urinary tract infections caused by Gram-negative bacilli such as Esch. coli, may respond well to penicillin V given to adults in an oral dosage of 500 mg four times daily (Gower *et al.*, 1975). This is because high urine levels of penicillin V are attained. However, other drugs are usually selected for these infections. Penicillin V is not suitable for the treatment of any systemic infections caused by Gram-negative bacilli.

6. *Gonorrhoea.* Oral penicillin V is relatively ineffective in this disease and its use is not recommended (Leading article, 1971). This drug has a lesser intrinsic activity against the gonococcus compared to penicillin G (page 56).

7. *Syphilis and leptospirosis.* The treatment of these diseases with oral penicillins is not recommended.

8. *Comparative efficacy of phenoxypenicillins.* This has not been determined by clinical trials, and soon after the introduction of the three semisynthetic drugs there was uncertainty about the oral penicillin of choice (Leading article, 1962). The semisynthetic drugs are better absorbed than penicillin V, but they have a lower intrinsic antibacterial activity. Propicillin and phenbenicillin are also more highly bound to serum proteins. A critical *in vitro* comparison of these four compounds was made by Bond *et al.* (1963). It appeared that penicillin V and phenethicillin would be about equally effective against streptococcal and staphylococcal infections, and that both would be superior to either propicillin or phenbenicillin. Thus the last two drugs are not widely used. In clinical practice there is probably little difference between penicillin V and phenethicillin.

REFERENCES

Barber, M. and Waterworth, P. M. (1962), 'Antibacterial activity of the penicillins', *Brit. med. J.*, **1**, 1159.

Batchelor, F. R., Doyle, F. P., Nayler, J. H. C. and Rolinson, G. N. (1959), 'Synthesis of penicillin: 6-aminopenicillanic acid in penicillin fermentation', *Nature (Lond.)*, **183**, 257.

Beeley, L., Gourevitch, A. and Kendall, M. J. (1976), 'Jaundice after oral penicillin', *Lancet*, **2**, 1297.

Bell, S. M. (1968), 'Oral penicillins in the treatment of chronic staphylococcal osteomyelitis', *Lancet*, **2**, 295.

Bell, S. M. (1970), 'Supervision of antibiotic treatment—an important medical responsibility', *Aspects of Infection. Proc. Symp. Auckland, Sydney and Melbourne*, p. 107.

Bell, S. M. (1976), 'Further observations on the value of oral penicillins in chronic staphylococcal osteomyelitis', *Med. J. Aust.*, **2**, 591.

Bird, G. W. G., McEvoy, M. W. and Wingham, J. (1975), 'Acute haemolytic anaemia due to IgM penicillin antibody in a 3-year-old child: a sequel to oral penicillin', *J. clin. Path.*, **28**, 321.

Bolme, P. and Eriksson, M. (1975), 'Influence of diarrhoea on the oral absorption of penicillin V and ampicillin in children', *Scand. J. Infect. Dis.*, **7**, 141.

Bond, J. M., Lightbown, J. W., Barber, M. and Waterworth, P. M. (1963), 'A comparison of four phenoxypenicillins', *Brit. med. J.*, **2**, 956.

Busch, D. F., Kureschi, L. A., Sutter, V. L. and Finegold, S. M. (1976), 'Susceptibility of respiratory tract anaerobes to orally administered penicillins and cephalosporins', *Antimicrob. Ag. Chemother.*, **10**, 713.

Carter, M. J. and Brumfitt, W. (1962), "Bacteriological and clinical studies with phenoxybenzylpenicillin', *Brit. med. J.*, **1**, 80.

Coates, W. H. (1963), "Anaphylactic shock following the administration of oral penicillin", *Med. J. Aust.*, **1**, 967.

Colcher, I. S. and Bass, J. W. (1972), "Penicillin treatment of streptococcal pharyngitis', *JAMA*, **222**, 657.

Forbes, J. A. (1962), 'Purulent meningitis: Principles and results of revised standardized treatment in 281 cases', *Aust. Ann. Med.*, **11**, 92.

Garrod, L. P. (1960a), 'Relative antibacterial activity of three penicillins', *Brit. med. J.*, **1**, 527.

Garrod, L. P. (1960b), 'The relative antibacterial activity of four penicillins', *Brit. med. J.*, **2**, 1695.

Garrod, L. P. and Waterworth, P. M. (1962), 'The risks of dental extraction during penicillin treatment', *Brit. Heart J.*, **24**, 39.

Garrod, L. P. (1973), 'Penicillins for haemophilus infections', *Brit. med. J.*, **3**, 290.

Garrod, L. P. (1975), 'Chemoprophylaxis', *Brit. med. J.*, **4**, 561.

Gower, P. E., Marshall, M. J. and Dash, C. H. (1975), 'Clinical, pharmacokinetic and laboratory study of penicillin V in the treatment of acute urinary infection', *J. Antimicrob. Chemother.*, **1**, 187.

Gray, I. R., Tai, A. R., Wallace, J. G. and Calder, J. H. (1964), 'Oral treatment of bacterial endocarditis with penicillins', *Lancet*, **2**, 110.

Hamburger, M., Kaplan, S. and Walker, W. F. (1961), 'Subacute bacterial endocarditis caused by penicillin-sensitive streptococci', *JAMA*, **175**, 554.

Jackson, F. L. and Rao, K. K. (1961), 'Comparative *in-vitro* activities of five penicillins against penicillinase-producing staphylococci', *Lancet*, **1**, 850.

Kamme, C. and Lundgren, K. (1971), 'Frequency of typable and non-typable Haemophilus influenzae strains in children with acute otitis media and results of penicillin V treatment', *Scand. J. Infect. Dis.*, **3**, 225.

Krause, R. M. (1975), 'Prevention of streptococcal sequelae by penicillin prophylaxis: a reassessment', *J. Infect. Dis.*, **131**, 592.

Larson, H. E., Parry, J. V., Price, A. B., Davies, D. R., Dolby, J. and Tyrrell, D. A. J. (1977), 'Undescribed toxin in pseudomembranous colitis', *Brit. med. J.*, **1**, 1246.

Leading article (1962), 'Some new penicillins', *Brit. Med. J.*, **1**, 99.

Leading Article (1971), 'Choice of penicillins for gonorrhoea', *Brit. med. J.*, **2**, 485.

Levin, S., Nelson, K. E., Spies, H. W. and Lepper, M. H. (1962), 'Pneumococcal meningitis: The problem of the unseen cerebrospinal fluid leak', *Amer. J. Med. Sci.*, **264**, 319.

Lundberg, C. and Malmborg, A. S. (1973), 'Concentration of penicillin V and tetracycline in maxillary sinus secretion after repeated doses', *Scand. J. Infect. Dis.*, **5**, 123.

McCarthy, C. G. and Finland, M. (1960), 'Absorption and excretion of four penicillins: penicillin G., penicillin V., phenethicillin and phenylmercaptomethyl penicillin', *New Engl. J. Med.*, **263**, 315.

Marty, J. J. and Hersey, J. A. (1975), 'Absorption of phenethicillin from oral paediatric formulations', *Med J. Aust.,* **1,** 382.

Nagley, M. (1961), 'Clinical use of a new synthetic penicillin: PA-248', *Lancet,* **1,** 851.

Oakes, M., Human, R. P. and Meers, P. D. (1963), 'Serum-lvels of four antibiotics administered orally to patients in general practice', *Lancet,* **1,** 222.

Palatsi, I. and Kaipainen, W. (1971), 'A comparative study of blood concentrations after peroral benzathine (DBED) penicillin V and potassium penicillin V', *Scand. J. Infect. Dis.,* **3,** 71.

Prescott, L. F. (1974), 'Gastrointestinal absorption of drugs', *Med. Clin. North Amer.,* **58,** 907.

Rollo, I. M., Somers, G. F. and Bruley, D. M. (1962), 'Bacteriological and pharmacological properties of phenoxybenzylpenicillin', *Brit. med. J.,* **1,** 76.

Spitzy, K. H. (1953), *Wein Klin. Wschr.,* **65,** 583; quoted by Bond *et al.* (1963).

Sprunt, K., Redman, W. and Leidy, G. (1968), 'Penicillin-resistant alpha streptococci in pharynx of patients given oral penicillin', *Pediatrics,* **42,** 957.

Stewart, G. T. (1965), *The Penicillin Group of Drugs,* Elsevier Publishing Company.

Tan, J. S., Terhune, C. A. Jr., Kaplan, S. and Hamburger, M. (1971), 'Successful two-week treatment schedule for penicillin-susceptible Streptococcus viridans endocarditis', *Lancet,* **2,** 1340.

Tozer, R. A., Boutflower, S. and Gillespie, W. A. (1966), 'Antibiotics for prevention of bacterial endocarditis during dental treatment', *Lancet,* **1,** 686.

Williamson, G. M., Morrison, J. K. and Stevens, K. J. (1961), 'A new synthetic penicillin PA-248', *Lancet,* **1,** 847.

Methicillin

Description

Methicillin is a penicillinase-resistant semisynthetic penicillin derived from the penicillin nucleus, 6-aminopenicillanic acid (Knudsen and Rolinson, 1960). The drug was discovered at Beecham Research Laboratories, and marketed as 'Celbenin'. Other trade names are 'Staphcillin' (America) and 'Metin' CSL, (Australia).

Sensitive Organisms

1. *Antibacterial spectrum.* This is similar to that of penicillin G. Methicillin is active against the Gram-positive bacteria, and also against the Gram-negative cocci such as meningococci and gonococci. Being both stable and active in the presence of staphylococcal penicillinase (Rolinson *et al.*, 1960), methicillin is active against penicillin G—resistant staphylococci. Stability of the penicillinase-resistant penicillins in the presence of this enzyme is one of degree. Methicillin and nafcillin (page 93) are the most stable and are followed closely by oxacillin, cloxacillin and dicloxacillin (page 80), whereas flucloxacillin (page 80) is inactivated by penicillinase somewhat more readily (Sabath *et al.*, 1975; Lacey and Stokes, 1977). Although methicillin is not hydrolysed by penicillinase it has a high affinity for this enzyme, and in sub-inhibitory concentrations it actually acts as a penicillinase inducer (Stewart, 1965). This observation is of doubtful clinical significance.

2. *Methicillin-resistant staphylococci.* Staphylococcal resistance to methicillin is not due to the destruction of the antibiotic by a bacterial enzyme (Leading article, 1968). The resistance is of the intrinsic type (page 6) and cell walls of resistant strains appear to differ from those of susceptible strains (Sabath *et al.*, 1970a and b). The first methicillin-resistant staphylococcal isolates seemed to consist of mixed populations, in which only a very small proportion of cells were resistant (Rolinson, 1961), and it was considered that these would not be clinically important. Later reports showed that significant infections due to methicillin-resistant staphylococci can occur (Barrett *et al.*, 1968; Benner and Kayser, 1968). Some evidence suggested that these staphylococci may be less pathogenic. They were often isolated only from the flora of hospitalized patients or from surgical wounds, and serious conditions such as septicaemia appeared to be less common, except in debilitated patients (Rountree and Beard, 1968; Blackwell and Feingold, 1975). There have been other reports of methicillin-resistant staphylococci producing serious diseases such as pneumonia, empyema, osteomyelitis, enterocolitis and septicaemia

(Rountree and Vickery, 1973; Klimek *et al.,* 1976). Methicillin resistance has so far been found mainly in hospital acquired infections (Kayser and Mak, 1972; Kayser, 1975). These staphylococci are also penicillinase producers and are therefore resistant to penicillin G (page 6). It is probable that only penicillinase-producing staphylococcal strains could survive in the hospital environment for a prolonged period (Kayser, 1975).

When methicillin was first introduced, staphylococcal strains resistant to it appeared to be rare; about 5000 strains were examined in Britain before a naturally occurring resistant strain was found (Jevons, 1961). In subsequent surveys in London, the percentage of resistant strains rose from 0·06 in 1960 to 0·97 in 1964 (Dyke *et al.*, 1966). Since then the incidence of methicillin-resistant staphylococci has varied in different parts of the world. They have been common in some hospitals in Britain and in certain other European countries (Parker and Hewitt, 1970; Kayser and Mak, 1972). In the United States methicillin-resistant staphylococci have been uncommon and only isolated instances were reported (Bran *et al.*, 1972; Finland, 1972; Wise, 1973). More recently these staphylococci appear to be more prevalent in America; Blackwell and Feingold (1975) reported the isolation of 13 methicillin-resistant strains, Klimek *et al.* (1976) reported 61 strains and Richmond *et al.* (1977) reported another six strains. All isolates were made from hospitalized patients, and in several instances they caused severe infections.

The spread of methicillin-resistant strains appears to be related to the use of all penicillins and perhaps other antibiotics, and not specifically to the use penicillinase-resistant penicillins, such as methicillin. These staphylococci have been detected in areas where methicillin and other penicillinase-resistant penicillins have been used very little, if at all (Parker and Hewitt, 1970; Klimek *et al.,* 1976). In this context, observations on the incidence of methicillin resistance in hospitals in the Zurich area are of interest. By the year 1971, about 20 per cent of all staphylococcal infections were caused by methicillin-resistant strains, but after 1972 they gradually decreased so that by 1975 only 3 per cent were caused by these strains. The reasons for this decrease were not apparent, as the use of penicillinase-resistant penicillins and cephalosporins had remained unrestricted in the hospitals concerned (Kayser, 1975). Methicillin-resistant Staph. pyogenes strains may revert to sensitive ones during *in vitro* culture. There is a report suggesting that this may also occur *in vivo*; a patient with chronic empyema initially yielded a methicillin-resistant staphylococcus but a sensitive organism was obtained from the same empyema seven years later (Annear and Baron-Hay, 1976).

Resistant strains grow much better in the presence of methicillin at 30°C, than at the usual 37°C (Annear, 1968). Methicillin resistance therefore can be overlooked by routine laboratory sensitivity tests, such as disc diffusion tests performed at 37°C. At this temperature growth is heterogeneous yielding many sensitive and very few resistant bacterial cells, so that methicillin causes lysis and death of a large proportion of bacterial cells, whereas such lysis does not occur at 30°C (Hewitt and Sanderson, 1974). In addition, the temperature at which the culture is subjected to methicillin is more important than the temperature used to grow the culture (Vernon and Russell, 1976). Annear (1968) recommends that methicillin resistance is best detected by incubating cultures for 18 h at 30°C or perhaps for 48 h at 37°C, but the former appears preferable because it detects all staphylococci with temperature-dependent heterogeneous resistance (Hallender *et al.*, 1969; Hewitt and Sanderson, 1974). The pH of the medium also seems critical for the test, because acidity (pH 5·2) seems to abolish methicillin resistance. This probably has no clinical significance, but it raises the interesting possibility that the expression of methicillin resistance by these staphylococci may be inhibited by both heat and acid (Sabath *et al.*, 1972). By contrast, this resistance is enhanced and more easily detected if 5 per cent sodium chloride is added to the testing medium (Sabath and Wallace, 1971).

The ability of methicillin-resistant staphylococci to grow more readily at 30°C may enable them to survive at common carrier sites in the body, such as the nose. Conversely, it is also possible that methicillin has some inhibiting action against such staphylococci in the blood of patients with a temperature of 37°C or higher, because a high proportion of bacteria which grow at this temperature are sensitive (Parker and Hewitt, 1970). It has, therefore, been suggested that methicillin-resistant staphylococci may not be truly resistant *in vivo*, and that clinical trials are justified to evaluate the efficacy of methicillin and other penicillinase-resistant penicillins for the treatment of diseases due to these strains (Lacey, 1974). Recently Lowbury *et al.* (1977) used flucloxacillin to treat 'methicillin-resistant' staphylococcal burn infections in 17 patients. From nine of these the organisms were eliminated, whereas infection persisted in all of 17 control patients. All staphylococci isolated from these patients were 'methicillin-resistant' when tested at 30°C, but showed a heterogeneous growth of 37°C with many sensitive and very few resistant cells. Furthermore, when these tests were done using cloxacillin or flucloxacillin (page 79) rather than methicillin, the staphylococci appeared even more sensitive at 37°C, as only very few resistant cells were found in a predominantly sensitive culture. Therefore, these authors considered that it may be anomalous to use methicillin as the usual test antibiotic for the penicillinase-resistant penicillins, especially as cloxacillin (page 79) or flucloxacillin (page 79) are now more commonly used clinically. Lacey (1977) considers that the somewhat misleading term of 'methicillin-resistant' staphylococci should be discontinued. An 18 h disc diffusion test with cloxacillin or flucloxacillin performed at 37°C may more accurately indicate the possible clinical value of these drugs for the treatment of moderate staphylococcal infections, than a similar test performed at 30°C (Lowbury *et al.*, 1977). Nevertheless, at present none of the penicillinase-resistant penicillins or cephalosporins can be recommended to be used singly for the treatment of severe staphylococcal infections such as septicaemia, if 'methicillin-resistant' strains as detected by the 18 h test at 30°C are involved. The same applies even if such a strain is found to be 'moderately sensitive' to flucloxacillin by the 18 h disc test at 37°C.

'Methicillin-resistant' staphylococci are always resistant to penicillin G, the cephalosporins and other penicillinase-resistant penicillins such as oxacillin, cloxacillin, flucloxacillin and nafcillin, although there are variations in their degree of resistance to these various drugs (*vide supra*). They are also frequently resistant to streptomycin, tetracycline, chloramphenicol and erythromycin. Some strains are in addition resistant to lincomycin, clindamycin and kanamycin (Rountree and Vickery, 1973; Jordan and Hoeprich, 1977). Thus the treatment of a hospital acquired 'methicillin-resistant' staphylococcal infection may be difficult, especially if the infection is severe. Bulger (1967) reported that combinations of methicillin and kanamycin or cephalothin and kanamycin are synergistic against some of these strains *in vitro* and suggested that these combinations may be valuable *in vivo*. Lincomycin (Rountree and Beard, 1968), a combination of rifampicin and novobiocin (Jensen, 1968), sodium fusidate (Garrod, 1968), and, if necessary, even more toxic but effective antibiotics such as gentamicin (Rountree and Vickery, 1973), and vancomycin (Benner and Morthland, 1967; Bulger *et al.*, 1972) have also been suggested for the treatment of these resistant infections. 'Methicillin-resistant' staphylococci are usually sensitive to gentamicin and to newer aminoglycosides such as tobramycin (page 361) and sisomicin (page 395), but some strains are resistant to amikacin (page 379) (Jordan and Hoeprich, 1977). One hospital outbreak of infection with a staphylococcal strain, resistant to both methicillin and gentamicin, has been described (Shanson *et al.*, 1976). A combination of two effective antibiotics has been advocated for the treatment of 'methicillin-resistant' staphylococcal infections to prevent the emergence of resistance to other drugs (Jensen, 1968).

3. *Methicillin-resistant Staph. epidermidis*. An incidence of methicillin resistance among Staph. epidermidis as high as 10 per cent, was noted in the years 1962–1963 (Kjellander *et al.*, 1963). By contrast with 'methicillin-resistant' Staph. pyogenes strains, the incidence of methicillin-resistant Staph. epidermidis has not altered significantly over the years (Sabath *et al.*, 1969), and they usually remain sensitive to the cephalosporins (Speller and Mitchell, 1973).

4. *Penicillin-tolerant staphylococci*. These Staph. pyogenes strains have a deficiency in an autolytic enzyme activity in the cell wall. The action of this enzyme appears to be necessary before any of the penicillins, including penicillinase-resistant penicillins such as methicillin, can exert a bactericidal effect (*see also* pages 6, 80). The minimum inhibitory concentrations of methicillin against these strains are in the usual low (sensitive) range, but minimum bactericidal concentrations are high. Severe infections such as septicaemia caused by these staphylococci may not respond to an otherwise satisfactory methicillin regimen (Best *et al.*, 1974; Mayhall *et al.*, 1976; Sabath *et al.*, 1977).

5. *Penicillin inactivating enzymes of host origin*. These enzymes which have been found in purulent accumulations such as empyema and which are presumed to be of host and not bacterial origin, can inactivate methicillin similar to penicillin G (*see* page 11).

In Vitro Sensitivities

The MIC's of methicillin and penicillin G against various bacteria are listed in Table 4. Methicillin inhibits the growth of both penicillin-sensitive and penicillinase-producing staphylococci. The activity of penicillin G is approximately fifty times greater than methicillin against penicillin-sensitive staphylococci and streptococci. It can be calculated that a dose of 1 g of methicillin has an effect comparable to about 30 000 units of penicillin G against a streptococcus or non-penicillinase producing staphylococcus (0·6 g of methicillin is equivalent to 1 000 000 units of penicillin G by weight).

TABLE 4

Modified from Knox (1960)

ORGANISM	MIC(μg per ml)	
	Penicillin G	Methicillin
Gram-positive bacteria		
Staph. pyogenes (non-penicillinase-producer)	0·02	1·0
Staph. pyogenes (penicillinase-producer)	125·0	2·0
Strep. pyogenes (Group A)	0·005	0·2
Strep. viridans spp.	0·01	0·1
Gram-negative bacteria		
Escherichia coli	15·0	>250
Salmonella typhi	7·5	>250
Proteus vulgaris	15·0	>250
Neisseria meningitidis	0·2	6·0

Mode of Administration and Dosage

1. Methicillin is not stable in acid medium, so it is ineffective if given orally. Although routinely administered by the intramuscular route, the drug can also be given intravenously, to avoid frequent painful intramuscular injections when large doses are required.

2. *The dosage of methicillin* can be varied widely according to the site and severity of the infection. For infections of moderate severity, a commonly used adult dosage is 1 g four-hourly. The corresponding dosage for children is 100 mg per kilogram body weight per day, given in four or six divided doses.

3. *Serious infections.* For these the dose can be doubled or increased even further. Daily doses of up to 25 g have been given intravenously for several weeks without toxic effect (Stewart, 1965). It has been recommended that adults with staphylococcal endocarditis, should be given methicillin intravenously, in a dosage of 2 g every two to three hours (16–24 g per day), until the infection is controlled (Geraci and Frye, 1966). Probenecid (page 17), which partially blocks its renal tubular secretion may be used in addition, to obtain higher and more sustained serum levels.

4. *Intravenous administration.* Intermittent injection or rapid infusion of a concentrated methicillin solution, rather than continuous intravenous infusion, is now advocated (Knudsen, 1970). Each dose of the drug can be dissolved in 10–20 ml of sterile water in a syringe, and this is then injected directly into the intravenous tubing over a period of five minutes. It now seems preferable to give the drug via a paediatric buretrol which is incorporated into the intravenous set. When a dose of the drug is due, 20–30 ml of intravenous fluid is delivered into the buretrol to which a dissolved methicillin dose is added; this concentrated drug solution is then infused over a period 5–10 min. With this method the antibiotic passes through the buretrol filter before reaching the patient. As a result, a proportion of particulate matter, which is commonly present in the syringe when antibiotics are withdrawn from ampoules or vials, is filtered out. This particulate matter may include minute particles of rubber, glass and undissolved antibiotic.

Intermittent intravenous administration of methicillin or any other antibiotic has no proven therapeutic advantage, but it obviates drug inactivation in intravenous solution bottles (*see* penicillin G, page 13). Intravenous glucose-saline solutions frequently have a pH value of 4–5 and in this acid medium methicillin is slowly inactivated; according to some authors significant inactivation may occur in three to four hours (Kirby and Bulger, 1964). The stability of methicillin in a concentration of 1 mg per ml has been tested in seven different intravenous glucose-saline solutions (Wyatt *et al.*, 1972). The most acid solution tested was 10 per cent dextrose in water (pH 4·4) and after sodium methicillin which is alkaline was added, this pH rose to 6·36. This study indicated that methicillin was stable at 4°C, 25°C and 37°C for at least 24 h in the seven intravenous solutions tested. In alkaline intravenous fluids which result from the addition of sodium bicarbonate, inactivation of the penicillins also occurs (Simberkoff *et al.*, 1970). This process seems to be slower with methicillin than with other penicillins (Lynn, 1971). Methicillin is not stable at room temperature in amino acid mixtures used for hyperalimentation (Feigin *et al.*, 1973). As with other drugs, certain intravenous additives may be incompatible with methicillin. Sometimes a continuous infusion of methicillin has been used at Fairfield Hospital as this may minimize thrombophlebitis. To avoid some of the above pitfalls, this drug alone is added to a small volume of fluid (usually 100 ml) in a paediatric buretrol, and not to a 500 ml intravenous solution flask. This allows the methicillin solution to be infused satisfactorily within one or two hours.

5. *Patients with renal failure*. Methicillin, being relatively non-toxic, is often administered in the normal dosage to patients with mild to moderate renal failure. Because its serum half-life is prolonged by profound renal failure, the dosage should be reduced and an adult dose of 1–2 g administered every eight to twelve hours has been recommended (Bulger *et al.*, 1964; Gilbert and Sanford, 1970). If a patient with renal failure requires intravenous methicillin in large doses (equivalent to 16 g daily for an adult with normal renal function), this dosage can be adjusted in a similar manner to that of penicillin G. This can be estimated by using Table 2 (page 14), and substituting 0·6 g of methicillin for one million units of penicillin G.

6. *Newborn and premature infants*. Renal excretion of methicillin in these patients is slower (Axline *et al.*, 1967), and a dosage as low as 25–50 mg per kilogram body weight, per day, given in two divided doses, may be sufficient (McCracken, 1974). Methicillin excretion increases four to five days after birth, and by the age of one month it should be administered in the dose recommended for older children (Boe *et al.*, 1967).

Availability

The drug, available in vials containing 1 g methicillin as the sodium salt, should be dissolved in 1·5 ml of sterile water for injection. Solutions for injection should be freshly prepared, since about 50 per cent of the activity is lost in five days at room temperature. Being much more unstable in acid solutions, 50 per cent of activity is lost in 20 min at pH 2·0 at 25°C.

Serum Levels in Relation to Dosage

1. *Intramuscular administration*. After a 1 g dose a mean peak serum level

of 18 μg per ml is reached after half an hour (Fig. 3), and this level falls to 3–4 μg per ml after three hours (Knudsen and Rolinson, 1960; Sabath et al., 1962).

Probenecid (page 17) by slowing the rate of renal tubular secretion of methicillin, can greatly enhance the peak serum level and prolong the serum half-life. Using probenecid, a peak serum level of 32–64 μg per ml can be obtained after 1 g intramuscular methicillin, and levels of 4–16 μg per ml may still be detectable after eight hours (Stevenson and Harrison, 1960).

2. *After intravenous injection* of 1 g methicillin over a five-minute period, a peak serum level of about 60 μg per ml is reached. This peak level is doubled by doubling the dose. Subsequently, there is a rapid fall in the serum level to about 7 μg per ml after one hour, and in two to three hours the level is usually less than 1 μg per ml, a therapeutically ineffective concentration. Usually methicillin cannot be detected in the serum after four hours despite the use of probenecid (Kirby and Bulger, 1964).

3. *In newborn infants,* after a single intramuscular methicillin dose of 25 mg per kilogram, the peak serum level is 47 μg per ml in those aged four to five days, 41 μg per ml at eight to nine days, 35 μg per ml at 13–15 days and 25 μg per ml in those aged 25–30 days (McCracken, 1974).

4. *Patients with cystic fibrosis* eliminate methicillin (similar to dicloxacillin, page 85) much faster than normal subjects due to an increase in their tubular secretory capacity. Thus the serum levels attained are lower, and these patients may need larger methicillin doses, especially when serious infections are treated (Yaffe et al., 1977).

Excretion

URINE: The drug is excreted in urine in an unchanged active form (Stewart et al., 1960). Very high urine concentrations of methicillin are attained, provided renal function is normal. It is excreted by both glomerular filtration and tubular secretion, and up to 80 per cent of an injected dose can be recovered from urine (Stewart, 1965). Probenecid delays renal tubular secretion of the drug (*see* penicillin G, page 17).

BILE: Some 2–3 per cent of an injected dose is excreted in bile. The biliary concentration of the drug is somewhat higher than in serum specimens collected simultaneously. The drug which is excreted in the bile is not reabsorbed, but is subsequently destroyed in the gut (Stewart, 1965).

INACTIVATION IN THE BODY: The fraction of methicillin which is not excreted, is inactivated in the body. Although like penicillin G, it is excreted largely through the kidney, it still disappears from the blood at a significant, but reduced, rate in anuric patients. Methicillin is only slowly removed by haemodialysis, so that in anuric patients its disappearance from serum is not appreciably influenced by this procedure (Bulger et al., 1964). Extrarenal mechanisms for the removal of methicillin (Biliary excretion and inactivation) appear to be more effective than haemodialysis. Apart from biliary excretion, the liver is an important extrarenal site for inactivation of the penicillins (*see* penicillin G, page 18). In patients with both severe renal and liver disease, the clearance rate of penicillin G from blood is much slower than in patients with renal failure alone (Kunin and Finland, 1959).

Distribution of the Drug in Body

Methicillin is widely distributed in various body fluids. Antibacterial levels which equate with those in serum have been demonstrated in pleural, pericardial and ascitic fluids (White and Warga, 1961), and in septic joint effusions (Nelson, 1971). The drug also reaches high concentrations in the pus and bone of patients with acute osteomyelitis (Tetzlaff *et al.*, 1978). Compared to penicillin G (page 18), methicillin penetrates much better into normal human bone tissue, where therapeutic levels may be reached when the drug is given intravenously in a dose of 2 g every four hours (Smilack *et al.*, 1976). As with other penicillins, significant concentrations are not attained in normal CSF but these may be moderately high in patients with meningitis.

Methicillin seems to be one of the penicillins least bound to serum proteins. Values for serum protein binding ranging from 17 to 43 per cent have been found by different investigators (46–58 per cent for penicillin G). The clinical significance of antibiotic protein binding is discussed on page 85).

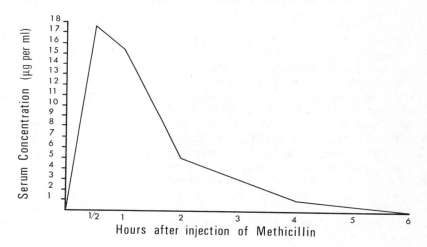

FIG. 3. Mean serum concentration in twelve subjects after intramuscular injection of 1 g methicillin. (Redrawn from Knudsen and Rolinson, 1960.)

Mode of Action

Methicillin acts on bacteria in a similar manner to penicillin G (*see* page 19).

Toxicity

1. *Hypersensitivity reactions.* These should be anticipated in patients known to be sensitive to the penicillins (Stewart *et al.*, 1960). However, not all patients allergic to penicillin G react to methicillin. In a study of eight consecutive patients with histories of penicillin G anaphylaxis, Luton (1964) showed that all tolerated usual intramuscular doses of methicillin without reaction. Prior to methicillin administration, skin testing with penicillin G in these patients gave

positive reactions, while similar tests with methicillin were negative. It appears that severe allergic reactions to methicillin and to other semisynthetic penicillins may be less common than to penicillin G. Nevertheless, in general it should be assumed that patients allergic to other penicillins will be sensitized to methicillin, and it should be avoided in such subjects. All of the hypersensitivity reactions which occur with penicillin G, can be provoked by methicillin (*see* page 24). In a study of 124 children who received methicillin for ten days or longer, the frequency of skin rashes, either maculopapular or urticarial, was 6 per cent (Yow *et al.*, 1976).

2. *Drug fever*. This can occur with methicillin; it is abrupt in onset and the patient usually appears otherwise relatively well despite the fever. This fever rapidly resolves when the drug is stopped, and may recur later if another penicillin analogue is administered (Yow *et al.*, 1976).

3. *Haematological side-effects*. Leucopenia is fairly common during methicillin therapy. Yow *et al.* (1976) observed leucopenia in 16 of 124 children who received methicillin for ten days or longer, and it usually occurred 10–20 days after starting treatment. Some patients developed a decrease in both neutrophils and lymphocytes, others an absolute neutropenia (less than 500 per cmm). The white cell count usually reverted to normal in a few days after cessation of methicillin. The leucopenia may worsen if another penicillin such as oxacillin, is substituted for methicillin. No serious problems resulting from leucopenia have been encountered.

Thrombocytopenia caused by methicillin appears to be rare. Schiffer *et al.* (1976) described a patient with leukaemia who developed a thrombocytopenia during methicillin treatment and again later when the drug was readministered. Methicillin-dependent anti-platelet antibodies were demonstrated in this patient.

Bone marrow depression has been observed occasionally and in each case there was improvement after cessation of methicillin (Simon, 1965). In one patient reported by McElfresh and Huang (1962), a high serum iron level was noted, which fell to normal twelve days after methicillin was stopped, a finding similar to that observed in the early reversible form of bone marrow depression caused by chloramphenicol (*see* page 437). No cases of irreversible aplastic anaemia have been reported.

4. *Nephropathy*. An interstitial nephritis can be caused by large intravenous doses of methicillin (Schrier *et al.*, 1966; Baldwin *et al.*, 1968; Woodroffe *et al.*, 1974). This is characterized by fever, rash, eosinophilia, haematuria, proteinuria and renal insufficiency. Microscopic changes in the kidneys consist of interstitial nephritis without glomerular abnormalities. Cogan and Arieff (1978) reported a patient in whom methicillin-induced interstitial nephritis also resulted in functional impairment specific for the distal tubule. The patient developed dehydration due to a sodium-losing nephropathy, a renal tubular acidosis and hyperkalaemia due to impaired ability to excrete potassium. Sometimes haematuria may be the sole manifestation of nephropathy, and in such cases it may be difficult to distinguish whether this is due to the drug or to the patient's disease such as staphylococcal septicaemia (Gallagher and Wayne, 1971). Haematuria and dysuria may also result in some methicillin treated patients, because the drug occasionally appears to cause a haemorrhagic cystitis, possibly by direct chemical irritation (Yow *et al.*, 1976; Bracis *et al.*, 1977). This complication appears distinct from methicillin-

induced interstitial nephritis, and its presence can be confirmed by cystoscopy. In this condition haematuria may disappear when a few doses of methicillin are omitted, and therapy is resumed with a lower daily dose of the drug in association with an increase in the patient's fluid intake. However, as in the case of methicillin-induced interstitial nephritis, it seems preferable to discontinue methicillin in these patients.

Most patients appear to recover slowly and completely from methicillin interstitial nephritis after cessation of the drug. Jensen *et al.* (1971) reported one patient with this complication, who still had evidence of impaired renal function two years later. The substitution of another penicillin such as oxacillin in these patients is likely to aggravate the nephritis (Yow *et al.*, 1976). A cephalosporin may also not always be a safe substitute antibiotic. Sanjad *et al.* (1974) described thirteen children with methicillin nephritis whose renal abnormalities disappeared when the drug was ceased. Later two of these were treated by cephalothin and in both an identical renal disease recurred.

The clinical picture suggests that a hypersensitivity mechanism may be involved in methicillin nephritis. Immunofluorescent studies in one patient showed that dimethoxyphenyl-penicilloyl, the haptenic group (page 23) of methicillin, was firmly bound to kidney tissue together with immunoglobulin (Baldwin *et al.*, 1968). In another patient a methicillin antigen, assumed to be dimethoxyphenyl-penicilloyl, was fixed in a linear pattern along the renal tubular basement membrane together with IgG and C_3 (a complement constituent). This patient also had an autoantibody in the serum reactive with the tubular basement membranes of normal human and monkey kidneys (Border *et al.*, 1974). Thus methicillin nephritis may be an example of drug-induced autoimmunity; methicillin acts as a haptene and alters the antigenicity of the tubular basement membrane in such a way that the resultant autoantibodies react not only against the drug but also against the tissue antigen (Flax, 1974).

Methicillin nephritis may not be infrequent when large doses of the drug are given (Sanjad *et al.*, 1974). According to Graber and Gluckin (1977), over one hundred cases of methicillin-associated interstitial nephritis have been reported in the medical literature, and this side-effect certainly seems more common with methicillin than with other penicillins (*see* pages 29, 96).

5. *Serum aspartate aminotransferase (SGOT) elevations.* As with the isoxazolyl penicillins (page 87), elevation of this enzyme has been occasionally observed during methicillin therapy (Berger and Potter, 1977).

6. *Encephalopathy*, similar to that seen after 'massive' doses of penicillin G (page 28) would be expected if very large doses (e.g. 50–100 g daily) were given intravenously. This complication could be anticipated with smaller doses in patients with renal failure. Much smaller doses of intrathecally administered methicillin are likely to produce the same effect. Though not advocated, the adult daily intrathecal methicillin dose should not exceed 40 mg.

7. *Coombs positive haemolytic anaemia,* similar to that described with penicillin G (page 29) can apparently also be caused by methicillin (Gilbert and Sanford, 1970).

8. *Intramuscular injections of methicillin are quite painful*, but if given deeply and slowly into the muscle, the pain is no worse than that due to crystalline penicillin G.

9. *Thrombophlebitis due to intravenous methicillin* in our experience is

usually not a major problem. A good way to administer the drug intravenously is to use small needles in peripheral veins with frequent changes of the intravenous site.

Clinical Uses of the Drug

Methicillin is indicated only for the treatment of staphylococcal infections (proven or suspected), due to penicillinase-producing staphylococci which are resistant to penicillin G. Originally this antibiotic was regarded by many as the drug of first choice for severe staphylococcal infections such as septicaemia, endocarditis, pneumonia, meningitis, osteomyelitis and septic arthritis.

In early studies it was effective in the treatment of penicillin-resistant staphylococcal infections (Douthwaite and Trafford, 1960; Douthwaite et al., 1961; White et al., 1961; Sabath et al., 1962), including staphylococcal septicaemia and endocarditis (Allen et al., 1962; Geraci and Frye, 1966). Methicillin, the first penicillinase-resistant penicillin to be discovered, has consequently been used more extensively than other penicillins of this group. Present evidence indicates that, if adequate doses are used, all other parenteral penicillinase-resistant penicillins, such as oxacillin (page 79), cloxacillin (page 79), flucloxacillin (page 79) and nafcillin (page 93), have the same therapeutic efficacy as methicillin (Gilbert and Sanford, 1970; Wise, 1973). The clinician therefore often selects the drug with which he is most familiar.

In recent years many clinicians, including ourselves, prefer one of the isoxazolyl penicillins such as cloxacillin to methicillin. Methicillin seems to cause nephritis (page 72) more commonly than the other penicillins and it can only be administered parenterally, whereas cloxacillin is also suitable for oral administration. For these reasons methicillin will probably be used much less frequently in the future.

Methicillin should not be used for infections caused by organisms susceptible to penicillin G (e.g. Strep. pyogenes and non-penicillinase producing staphylococci), because penicillin G is more effective.

REFERENCES

Allen, J. D., Roberts, C. E. and Kirby, W. M. M. (1962), 'Staphylococcal septicaemia treated with methicillin: report of twenty-two cases', New Engl. J. Med., 266, 111.

Annear, D. I. (1968), 'The effect of temperature on resistance of Staphylococcus aureus to methicillin and some other antibiotics', Med. J. Aust., 1, 444.

Annear, D. I. and Baron-Hay, G. S. (1976), 'Loss of resistance to methicillin and other antibiotics in Staphylococcus aureus associated with a chronic empyema', Med. J. Aust., 1, 399.

Axline, S. G., Yaffe, S. J. and Simon, H. J. (1967), 'Clinical pharmacology of antimicrobials in premature infants: II. Ampicillin, methicillin, oxacillin, neomycin and colistin'', Pediatrics, 39, 97.

Baldwin, D. S., Levine, B. B., McCluskey, R. T. and Gallo, G. R. (1968), 'Renal failure and interstitial nephritis due to penicillin and methicillin', New Engl. J. Med., 279, 1245.

Barrett, F. F., McGehee, R. F. and Finland, M. (1968), 'Methicillin-resistant staphylococcus at Boston City Hospital', New Engl. J. Med., 279, 441.

Benner, E. J. and Morthland, V. (1967), "Methicillin-resistant Staphylococcus aureus', New Engl. J. Med., 277, 678.

Benner, E. J. and Kayser, F. H. (1968), 'Growing clinical significance of methicillin-resistant Staphylococcus aureus', *Lancet*, **2**, 741.

Berger, M. and Potter, D. E. (1977), 'Pitfall in diagnosis of viral hepatitis on haemodialysis unit', *Lancet*, **2**, 95.

Best, G. K., Best, N. H. and Koval, A. V. (1974), 'Evidence for participation of autolysins in bactericidal action of oxacillin on Staphylococcus aureus', *Antimicrob. Ag. Chemother.*, **6**, 825.

Blackwell, C. C. and Feingold, D. S. (1975), 'Frequency and some properties of clinical isolates of methicillin-resistant Staphylococcus aureus', *Amer. J. Clin. Path.*, **64**, 372.

Boe, R. W., Williams, C. P. S., Bennet, J. V. and Oliver, T. K. (1967), 'Serum levels of methicillin and ampicillin in newborn and premature infants in relation to postnatal age', *Pediatrics*, **39**, 194.

Border, W. A., Lehman, D. H., Egan, J. D., Sass, H. J., Glode, J. E. and Wilson, C. B. (1974), 'Antitubular basement-membrane antibodies in methicillin-associated interstitial nephritis', *New Engl. J. Med.*, **291**, 381.

Bracis, R., Sanders, C. V. and Gilbert, D. N. (1977), 'Methicillin hemorrhagic cystitis', *Antimicrob. Ag. Chemother.*, **12**, 438.

Bran, J. L., Levison, M. E. and Kaye, D. (1972) 'Survey for methicillin-resistant staphylococci', *Antimicrob. Ag. Chemother.*, **1**, 235.

Brown, D. M. and Acred, P. (1960), 'Chemotherapeutic studies on a new antibiotic—BRL. 1241', *Lancet*, **2**, 568.

Bulger, R. J., Lindholm, D. D., Murray, J. S. and Kirby, W. M. M. (1964), 'Effect of uremia on methicillin and oxacillin blood levels', *JAMA*, **187**, 319.

Bulger, R. J. (1967), '*In-vitro* activity of cephalothin/kanamycin and methicillin/kanamycin combinations against methicillin-resistant Staphylococcus aureus', *Lancet*, **1**, 17.

Bulger, R. J. (1967), 'A methicillin-resistant strain of Staphylococcus aureus', *Ann. Intern. Med.*, **67**, 81.

Bulger, R. J., Feigl, P. and Nielson, K. (1972), 'Comparison of treatments with several antibiotics in experimental infections due to methicillin-resistant Staphylococcus aureus', *J. Infect. Dis.*, **126**, 674.

Cogan, M. C. and Arieff, A. I. (1978), 'Sodium wasting, acidosis and hyperkalemia induced by methicillin interstitial nephritis. Evidence for selective distal tubular dysfunction', *Amer. J. Med.*, **64**, 500.

Douthwaite, A. H. and Trafford, J. A. P. (1960), 'A new-synthetic penicillin', *Brit. med. J.*, **2**, 687.

Douthwaite, A. H., Trafford, J. A. P., McGill, D. A. F. and Evans, I. E. (1961), 'Methicillin', *Brit. med. J.*, **2**, 6.

Dyke, K. G. H., Jevons, P. and Parker, M. T. (1966), 'Penicillinase production and intrinsic resistance to penicillins in Staphylococcus aureus', *Lancet*, **1**, 835.

Feigin, R. D., Moss, K. S. and Shackelford, P. G. (1973), 'Antibiotic stability in solutions used for intravenous nutrition and fluid therapy', *Pediatrics*, **51**, 1016.

Finland, M. (1972), 'Hospital-acquired infections: The problems of methicillin-resistant Staphylococcus aureus and infections with Klebsiella pneumoniae', *Amer. J. Med. Sci.*, **264**, 207.

Flax, M. H. (1974), 'Editorial. Drug-induced autoimmunity', *New Engl. J. Med.*, **291**, 414.

Gallagher, P. J. and Wayne, D. J. (1971), 'Haematuria during methicillin therapy', *Postgrad. Med. J.*, **47**, 511.

Garrod, L. P. (1968), 'Methicillin-resistant staphylococci', *Lancet*, **2**, 871.

Geraci, J. E. and Frye, R. L. (1966), 'Methicillin and other semi-synthetic penicillins in the therapy of staphylococcal endocarditis', *Antimicrob. Agents Chemother.*—1965, p. 627.

Gilbert, D. N. and Sanford, J. P. (1970), 'Methicillin: Critical appraisal after a decade of experience', *Med. Clin. North America, 54*, 1113.

Graber, M. L. and Gluckin, D. S. (1977), 'Antimicrobials and the kidney', *New Engl. J. Med., 297*, 224.

Hallander, H. O., Laurell, G. and Dornbusch, K. (1969), 'Determination of methicillin resistance of Staphylococcus aureus', *Scand. J. Infect. Dis., 1*, 169.

Hewitt, J. H. and Sanderson, P. J. (1974), 'The effect of methicillin on skin lesions in guinea-pigs caused by "methicillin-sensitive" and "methicillin-resistant" Staphylococcus aureus', *J. Med. Microbiol., 7*, 223.

Jensen, H. A., Halveg, A. B. and Saunamki, K. I. (1971), 'Permanent impairment of renal function after methicillin nephropathy', *Brit. med. J., 4*, 406.

Jensen, K. (1968), 'Methicillin-resistant staphylococci', *Lancet, 2*, 1078.

Jevons, M. P. (1961), ' "Celbenin"-resistant staphylococci', *Brit. med. J., 1*, 124.

Jordan, G. W. and Hoeprich, P. D. (1977), 'Susceptibility of three groups of Staphylococcus aureus to newer antimicrobial agents', *Antimicrob. Ag. Chemother., 11*, 7.

Kayser, F. H. and Mak, T. M. (1972), 'Methicillin-resistant staphylococci', *Amer. J. Med. Sci., 264*, 197.

Kayser, F. H. (1975), 'Methicillin-resistant staphylococci 1965–75', *Lancet, 2*, 650.

Kirby, W. M. M. and Bulger, R. J. (1964), 'The new penicillins and cephalosporins', *Ann. Rev. Med., 15*, 393.

Kjellander, J. O., Klein, J. O., and Finland, M. (1963) '*In vitro* activity of penicillins against Staphylococcus albus', *Proc. Soc. Exptl. Biol. Med., 113*, 1023; quoted by Sabath *et al.* (1969).

Klimek, J. J., Marsik, F. J., Bartlett, R. C., Weir, B., Shea, P. and Quintiliani, R. (1976), 'Clinical, epidemiologic and bacteriologic observations of an outbreak of methicillin-resistant Staphylococcus aureus at a large community hospital', *Amer. J. Med., 61*, 340.

Knox, R. (1960), 'A new penicillin (BRL. 1241) active against penicillin-resistant staphylococci', *Brit. med. J., 2*, 690.

Knudsen, E. T. and Rolinson, G. N. (1960), 'Absorption and excretion of a new antibiotic (BRL. 1241)', *Brit. med. J., 2*, 700.

Knudsen, E. T. (1970), 'Factors influencing penicillin therapy', *Aspects of Infection, Proc. Symp. Auckland, Sydney and Melbourne*, p. 115.

Kunin, C. M. and Finland, M. (1959), 'Persistence of antibiotics in blood of patients with acute renal failure: III Penicillin, streptomycin, erythromycin and kanamycin', *J. Clin. Invest., 38*, 1509; quoted by Bulger *et al.* (1964).

Lacey, R. W. (1974), 'Can methicillin-resistant strains of Staphylococcus aureus be treated with methicillin?', *1*, 88.

Lacey, R. W. (1977), 'Inactivation of penicillins and cephalosporins by enzymes', *Brit. med. J., 1*, 1285.

Lacey, R. W. and Stokes, A. (1977), 'Susceptibility of the "penicillinase-resistant" penicillins and cephalosporins to penicillinase of Staphylococcus aureus', *J. clin. Path., 30*, 35.

Leading Article (1968), 'The staphylococcus and methicillin resistance', *Med. J. Aust., 2*, 1189.

Lowbury, E. J. L., Lilly, H. A. and Kidson, A. (1977), ' "Methicillin-resistant", Staphylococcus aureus: reassessment by controlled trial in burns unit', *Brit. med. J., 1*, 1054.

Luton, E. F. (1964), 'Methicillin tolerance after penicillin G anaphylaxis', *JAMA, 190*, 39.

Lynn, B. (1971), 'Inactivation of methicillin in dextrose solutions at alkaline pH', *New Engl. J. Med., 285*, 690.

McElfresh, A. E. and Huang, N. N. (1962), 'Bone-marrow depression resulting from the administration of methicillin', *New Engl. J. Med.,* **266,** 246.

Mayhall, C. G., Medoff, G. and Marr, J. J. (1976), (Variation in the susceptibility of strains of Staphylococcus aureus to oxacillin, cephalothin and gentamicin', *Antimicrob. Ag. Chemother.,* **10,** 707.

McCracken, G. H., Jr. (1974), 'Pharmacological basis for antimicrobial therapy in newborn infants', *Am. J. Dis. Child.,* **128,** 407.

Nelson, J. D. (1971), 'Antibiotic concentrations in septic joint effusions', *New Engl. J. Med.,* **284,** 349.

Parker, M. T. and Hewitt, J. H. (1970), 'Methicillin resistance in Staphylococcus aureus', *Lancet,* **1,** 800.

Richmond, A. S., Simberkoff, M. S., Schaefler, S. and Rahal, J. J., Jr. (1977), 'Resistance of Staphylococcus aureus to semisynthetic penicillins and cephalothin', *J. Infect. Dis.,* **135,** 108.

Rolinson, G. N., Stevens, S., Batchelor, F. R., Wood, J. C. and Chain, E. B. (1960), 'Bacteriological studies on a new penicillin—BRL. 1241', *Lancet,* **2,** 564.

Rolinson, G. N. (1961), 'Celbenin-resistant staphylococci', *Brit. med. J.,* **1,** 125.

Rountree, P. M. and Beard, M. A. (1968), 'Hospital strains of Staphylococcus aureus, with particular reference to methicillin-resistant strains', *Med. J. Aust.,* **2,** 1163.

Rountree, P. M. and Vickery, A. M. (1973), 'Further observations on methicillin-resistant staphylococci', *Med. J. Aust.,* **1,** 1030.

Sabath, L. D., Barrett, F. F., Wilcox, C., Gerstein, D. A. and Finland, M. (1969), 'Methicillin resistance of Staphylococcus aureus and Staphylococcus epidermidis', *Antimicrob. Agents Chemother.*—1968, p. 302.

Sabath, L. D., Leaf, C. D., Gerstein, D. A. and Finland, M. (1970a), 'Cell walls of methicillin-resistant Staphylococcus aureus', *Antimicrob. Agents Chemother.*—1969, p. 73.

Sabath, L. D., Leaf, C. D., Gerstein, D. A. and Finland, M. (1970b), 'Altered cell walls of Staphylococcus aureus resistant to methicillin', *Nature,* **225,** 1074.

Sabath, L. D., Postic, B. and Finland, M. (1962), 'Laboratory studies on methicillin', *Amer. J. Med. Sci.,* **244,** 484.

Sabath, L. D. and Wallace, S. J. (1971), 'Factors influencing methicillin resistance in staphylococci', *Ann. N.Y. Acad. Sci.,* **182,** 258.

Sabath, L. D., Wallace, S. J. and Gerstein, D. A. (1972), 'Suppression of intrinsic resistance to methicillin and other penicillins in Staphylococcus aureus', *Antimicrob. Ag. Chemother.,* **2,** 350.

Sabath, L. D., Garner, C., Wilcox, C. and Finland, M. (1975), 'Effect of inoculum and of beta-lactamase on the anti-staphylococcal activity of thirteen penicillins and cephalosporins' *Antimicrob. Ag. Chemother.,* **8,** 344.

Sabath, L. D., Wheeler, N., Laverdiere, M., Blazevic, D. and Wilkinson, B. J. (1977), 'A new type of penicillin resistance of Staphylococcus aureus', *Lancet,* **1,** 443.

Sanjad, S., Haddad, G. G. and Nassar, V. H. (1974), 'Nephropathy, an underestimated complication of methicillin therapy', *J. Pediatrics,* **84,** 873.

Schiffer, C. A., Weinstein, H. J., Wiernik, P. H. (1976), 'Methicillin-associated thrombocytopenia', *Ann. Intern. Med.,* **85,** 338.

Schrier, R. W., Bulger, R. J. and van Arsdel, P. P. (1966), 'Nephropathy associated with penicillin and homologues', *Ann. Intern. Med.,* **64,** 116.

Shanson, D. C., Kensit, J. G. and Duke, R. (1976), 'Outbreak of hospital infection with a strain of Staphylococcus aureus resistant to gentamicin and methicillin', *Lancet,* **2,** 1347.

Simberkoff, M. S., Thomas, L. McGregor, D., Shenkein, I. and Levine, B. B. (1970), 'Inactivation of penicillins by carbohydrate solutions at alkaline pH', *New Engl. J. Med.,* **283,** 116.

Simon, H. J. (1965), 'Current status of methicillin, oxacillin and cloxacillin', *Antimicrob. Agents Chemother.*—1964, p. 280.

Smilack, J. D., Flittie, W. H. and Williams, T. W., Jr. (1976), 'Bone concentrations of antimicrobial agents after parenteral administration', *Antimicrob. Ag. Chemother.*, **9,** 169.

Speller, D. C. E. and Mitchell, R. G. (1973), 'Coagulase-negative staphylococci causing endocarditis after cardiac surgery', *J. clin. Path.*, **26,** 517.

Stevenson, F. H. and Harrison, K. J. (1960), 'Celbenin and probenecid', *Brit. med. J.*, **2,** 1596.

Stewart, G. T., Harrison, P. M. and Holt, R. J. (1960) 'Microbiological studies on sodium 6-(2,6-dimethoxybenzamido) penicillanate monohydrate (BRL. 1241) *in vitro* and in patients', *Brit. med. J.*, **2,** 694.

Stewart, G. T. (1965), *The Penicillin Group of Drugs*. Elsevier Publishing Company, p. 70.

Tetzlaff, T. R., Howard, J. B., McCracken, G. H., Jr., Calderon, E. and Lorrondo, J. (1978), 'Antibiotic concentrations in pus and bone of children with osteomyelitis', *J. Pediatrics*, **92,** 135.

Vernon, G. N. and Russell, A. D. (1976), 'Effects of methicillin, cephaloridine and cephalothin on the growth, lysis and viability of some methicillin-resistant strains of Staphylococcus aureus at different temperatures', *J. Antimicrob. Chemother.*, **2,** 41.

White, A. and Varga, D. T. (1961), 'Antistaphylococcal activity of sodium methicillin', *Arch. Intern. Med.*, **108,** 671.

Wise, R. I. (1973), 'Modern management of severe staphylococcal disease', *Medicine*, **52,** 295.

Woodroffe, A. J., Thomson, N. M., Meadows, R. and Lawrence, J. R. (1974), 'Nephropathy associated with methicillin administration', *Aust. N.Z. J. Med.*, **4,** 256.

Wyatt, R. G., Okamoto, G. A. and Feigin, R. D. (1972), 'Stability of antibiotics in parenteral solutions', *Pediatrics*, **49,** 22.

Yaffe, S. J., Gerbracht, L. M., Mosovich, L. L., Mattar, M. E., Danish, M. and Jusko, W. J. (1977), 'Pharmacokinetics of methicillin in patients with cystic fibrosis', *J. Infect. Dis.*, **135,** 828.

Yow, M. D., Taber, L. H., Barrett, F. F., Mintz, A. A., Blankinship, G. R., Clark, G. E. and Clark, D. J. (1976), 'A ten-year assessment of methicillin-associated side-effects, *Pediatrics*, **58,** 329.

Isoxazolyl Penicillins: Oxacillin, Cloxacillin, Dicloxacillin and Flucloxacillin

Description

These semisynthetic compounds, derived from the penicillin nucleus (6-aminopenicillanic acid), are all chemically 3:5 disubstituted 4-isoxazolyl penicillins. They combine the property of resistance to penicillinase with resistance to gastric acidity. Similar to methicillin (page 64), these drugs are effective antistaphylococcal agents, but they may be administered orally. Four such penicillins are available:

1. *Oxacillin,* 'BRL 1400', 'Prostaphlin' or 'Bactocill' (3-methyl-5-phenyl-4-isoxazolyl penicillin). This drug was synthetized in 1961 and has been extensively used in North America.

2. *Cloxacillin,* 3-0-chlorophenyl-5-methyl-4-isoxazolyl penicillin (Knudsen *et al.,* 1962) only differs from oxacillin by having an additional chlorine atom. This drug, rather than oxacillin, has been used in England and Australia. Trade names include 'Orbenin' (Beecham), 'Tegopen' (Bristol, USA) and 'Austrastaph' (CSL, Australia).

3. *Dicloxacillin* or 'BRL 1702' is chemically 3(2,6-dichlorophenyl)-5-methyl-4-isoxazolyl penicillin. It differs from cloxacillin by having two chloride ions attached to the phenyl group. Trade names in the United States include 'Dynapen', 'Pathocil' and 'Veracillin'.

4. *Flucloxacillin* ('Floxapen'), which is chemically 3(2-chloro-6-fluorophenyl)-5-methyl-4-isoxazolyl penicillin, is similar to dicloxacillin but one of the chlorine atoms has been replaced by fluorine (Sutherland *et al.,* 1970).

Sensitive Organisms

1. *Antibacterial spectrum.* This is similar to that of methicillin; isoxazolyl penicillins are active against Gram-positive cocci, such as Staph. pyogenes, Staph. epidermidis, Strep. pyogenes, Strep. pneumoniae, Strep. viridans spp. and the Gram-positive bacilli, but Strep. faecalis is relatively resistant. Marier *et al.* (1975) found that oxacillin and gentamicin often acted synergistically against Strep. faecalis, and at clinically attainable serum levels this combination was synergistically bactericidal against 27 of 34 strains tested. Watanakunakorn and Glotzbecker (1977) studying nafcillin (page 94), oxacillin and methicillin (page 64) each combined with either gentamicin or tobramycin, found that none of these antibiotic combinations demonstrated enhanced killing of all enterococcal strains. Nafcillin/gentamicin (page 94) was superior to oxacillin/gentamicin, and methicillin/gentamicin was the least effective combination. Results with tobramycin were not as good as with gentamicin in all

79

these combinations. Similar conclusions were reached by Glew *et al.* (1975) who found that the combination of oxacillin plus gentamicin was synergistic against only 3 of 14 enterococcal strains tested. A combination of gentamicin with either oxacillin, methicillin or nafcillin is relatively ineffective for the treatment of experimental enterococcal sepsis in animals (Lincoln *et al.*, 1977). It therefore appears that combinations of a penicillinase-resistant penicillin with an aminoglycoside are not reliable for the treatment of severe Strep. faecalis infections.

The Neisseria spp. are the only Gram-negative bacteria sensitive to these drugs. Cloxacillin in a concentration of 10 μg per ml, was shown to be bactericidal to some strains of Mycobacterium tuberculosis (Lorian and Sabath, 1972). This appears of no clinical significance.

2. *Activity against Staph. pyogenes*. The isoxazolyl penicillins are primarily of interest because, being penicillinase-resistant (Knox and Smith, 1963), they are active against staphylococci resistant to penicillin G. Resistance to penicillinase is one of degree. Oxacillin, cloxacillin and dicloxacillin are relatively resistant to this enzyme and their resistance is only slightly exceeded by methicillin (page 64) and nafcillin (page 93). Flucloxacillin, however, compared to all other penicillinase-resistant penicillins, is inactivated by penicillinase to a somewhat greater extent (Sabath *et al.*, 1975; Lacey and Stokes, 1977).

There is cross-resistance between methicillin and all other penicillinase-resistant penicillins, so that methicillin-resistant staphylococci (page 64) are also resistant to isoxazolyl penicillins (Barber and Waterworth, 1964; Turner and Cox, 1967; Sutherland *et al.*, 1970; Richmond *et al.*, 1977). This resistance is also one of degree. Lowbury *et al.* (1977) demonstrated that some strains normally classified as 'methicillin-resistant' may be 'relatively sensitive' to cloxacillin and flucloxacillin (*see also* page 66).

3. *Penicillin-tolerant Staph. pyogenes*. These strains have a deficiency in an autolytic enzyme activity on the cell surface. This enzyme appears to be necessary before any of the penicillins, including penicillinase-resistant penicillins, can exert a bactericidal effect (*see* pages 6, 67). The minimum inhibitory concentrations of oxacillin (and other isoxazolyl penicillins) against these strains are in the usual low range, but minimum bactericidal concentrations are high (Best *et al.*, 1974; Sabath *et al.*, 1977). Three patients with staphylococcal septicaemia caused by these tolerant strains were treated by Mayhall *et al.* (1976). Adequate oxacillin doses failed to control the infection in each case, but treatment with an oxacillin/gentamicin combination was successful.

4. *Penicillin inactivating enzymes of host origin*. Such enzymes have been found in purulent accumulations such as empyema and are presumed to be of host and not bacterial origin. They inactivate cloxacillin and presumably also the other drugs of this group, but varying rates of inactivation of different penicillins has been demonstrated (*see* pages 11, 67, 201).

5. *Comparative antibacterial activity of isoxazolyl penicillins*. Cloxacillin is considerably less active than penicillin G against bacteria which are sensitive to penicillin G. However, it is four to eight times more active than methicillin against Staph. pyogenes. Oxacillin has about the same activity as cloxacillin against these organisms but dicloxacillin is slightly more active. In addition, dicloxacillin is more active than cloxacillin against streptococci and

pneumococci (Gravenkemper *et al.*, 1965). The activity of flucloxacillin against all these organisms is similar to oxacillin and cloxacillin (Sutherland *et al.*, 1970; Bergeron *et al.*, 1976).

In Vitro Sensitivities

Table 5 shows the minimum inhibitory concentrations of the four isoxazolyl penicillins against some selected bacteria, compared to those of penicillin G. The MIC's of cloxacillin, oxacillin and flucloxacillin against staphylococci are increased tenfold if the test is performed in 95 per cent human serum instead of nutrient broth (Barber and Waterworth, 1964; Sutherland *et al.*, 1970). Dicloxacillin is more protein bound than cloxacillin, and its MIC increases 20–25 fold in 95 per cent serum (Hammerstrom *et al.*, 1967).

TABLE 5

Compiled from data published by Hammerstrom *et al.*, (1967) and Sutherland *et al.*, (1970)

ORGANISM	MIC (μg per ml)				
	Peni-cillin G	Oxa-cillin	Cloxa-cillin	Dicloxa-cillin	Flucloxa-cillin
Staph. pyogenes (non-penicillinase producer)	0·02	0·35	0·1–0·25	0·06	0·1–0·25
Staph. pyogenes (penicillinase producer)	50·0	0·40	0·25–0·5	0·12	0·25–0·5
Strep. pyogenes (Group A)	0·01	0·05–0·1	0·05–0·1	0·05	0·05–0·1
Strep. pneumoniae (Dip. pneumoniae)	0·01	0·5	0·25–0·5	0·15	0·25
Strep. faecalis (Enterococcus, Group D)	5·0	>12·5	25·0	>12·5	25·0

Mode of Administration and Dosage

1. *Oral administration.* Isoxazolyl penicillins are acid stable and can be administered orally. The usual oral adult dose of these drugs is 500 mg six-hourly and for children 50 mg per kg per day, given in four divided doses. These drugs should be administered about one hour before meals to ensure better absorption (Bell, 1970; Sutherland *et al.*, 1970) (page 83). In severe infections the dose can be doubled or even further increased. Bell (1968; 1976) obtained good results in chronic osteomyelitis by using oral cloxacillin in a dosage of 1 g four-hourly for prolonged periods. Oral probenecid in a dose of 2 g daily was also used to produce higher serum levels.

2. *Parenteral administration.* Oxacillin, cloxacillin and flucloxacillin can also be administered both intramuscularly or intravenously. In the United States dicloxacillin is also available for intramuscular administration. A dose as small as 250 mg six-hourly may suffice for mild infections, but for infections of moderate severity the usual parenteral dose of these drugs is 1 g every four hours. This dose may be doubled or even further increased for severe infec-

tions. Oxacillin in a dose of 18 g daily intravenously has been used to treat seriously ill patients (Klein *et al.*, 1963). Comparable intravenous doses for children would be 100–300 mg per kg body weight per day.

3. *Method of intravenous administration.* The decision to administer either oxacillin, cloxacillin or flucloxacillin by intermittent injection or continuous intravenous infusion, is governed by principles similar to those which apply to penicillin G (page 13) and methicillin (68). However compared to methicillin, the more acid-stable isoxazolyl penicillins are stable in commonly used acid intravenous solutions for up to six hours, provided other incompatible additives are not present. For intermittent intravenous injection, each dose should be dissolved in 10–20 ml of sterile water and then injected directly into the intravenous tubing over a period of two to three minutes. Alternatively the intermittent rapid infusion method via a paediatric buretrol or a secondary intravenous bottle may be used (*see* methicillin, page 68).

4. *Patients with renal failure.* In the presence of severe renal impairment the dose of cloxacillin, dicloxacillin or flucloxacillin should be reduced as for methicillin (page 69), especially if high parenteral doses are used. Compared to methicillin, the serum half-life of oxacillin in such patients is much shorter, so that a high parenteral dosage of oxacillin (1 g every four to six hours) has been recommended for the treatment of severe infections in anuric patients (Bulger *et al.*, 1964).

5. *Newborn and premature infants.* The renal excretion of oxacillin in these patients is slower (Axline *et al.*, 1967), and this probably applies to all the isoxazolyl penicillins. During the first 14 days of life an oxacillin dose of 25 mg per kg, administered every 12 h, is recommended for infants weighing less than 2000 g; to those weighing more than 2000 g this dose may be given eight-hourly. Infants aged 15–30 days should receive 25 mg per kg eight-hourly if weighing less than 2000 g and the same dose six-hourly if weighing over 2000 g (McCracken and Nelson, 1977).

Availability

1. *Cloxacillin*
   (a) *Capsules:* 250 and 500 mg.
   (b) *Syrup:* 125 mg in 5 ml.
   (c) *Vials:* 250 mg, 500 mg and 1·0 g, suitable for intramuscular and intravenous administration.
   (d) *'Ampiclox'.* This is a 2:1 mixture of ampicillin and cloxacillin, which is advertised for treatment of neonatal infections. Both oral and parenteral preparations are available, and these are described in more detail on page 107.
2. *Oxacillin*
   (a) *Capsules:* 250 and 500 mg.
   (b) *Syrup:* 250 mg in 5 ml.
   (c) *Vials:* 250 and 500 mg and 1·0, 2·0 and 4·0 g, suitable for intramuscular and intravenous administration.
3. *Dicloxacillin*
   (a) *Capsules:* 125, 250 and 500 mg.
   (b) *Syrup:* 62·5 mg in 5 ml.
   (c) *Vials:* 250 mg for intramuscular administration.
4. *Flucloxacillin*
   (a) *Capsules:* 250 mg.
   (b) *Vials:* 250 mg.

Serum Levels in Relation to Dosage

1. *Oral administration.* When a 500 mg oral dose of oxacillin is given, a peak serum level of about 4 μg per ml is reached in 30–60 min (Hammerstrom *et al.*, 1967). Thereafter the serum concentration falls, but significant levels are maintained for 4–6 h.

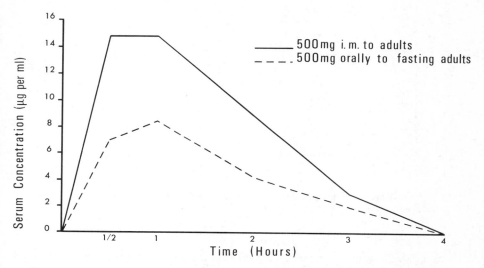

FIG. 4. Serum levels after oral and intramuscular cloxacillin. (Redrawn from Sutherland *et al.*, 1970.)

Most investigators have found that serum levels after oral administration of cloxacillin are about twice as high as those obtained with oxacillin (Fig. 4) (Knox *et al.*, 1962; Turck *et al.*, 1965; Sutherland *et al.*, 1970). Others have found somewhat lower levels after oral cloxacillin administration (Kislak *et al.*, 1965). Oral dicloxacillin produces serum levels approximately twice as high as cloxacillin (Gravenkemper *et al.*, 1965; Marcy and Klein, 1970). Serum levels after oral flucloxacillin are about the same as those obtained with dicloxacillin (Fig. 5).

The differing serum levels obtained with oral administration of these antibiotics are not solely due to differences in their absorption. If they are administered by continuous intravenous infusion, their rates of clearance from the body by both renal and non-renal mechanisms also differ. The clearance of dicloxacillin from the body is slower than that of cloxacillin, which in turn is slower than that of oxacillin (Rosenblatt *et al.*, 1968).

Doubling the dose of all of these penicillins doubles serum concentrations. The presence of food in the stomach interferes with their absorption. The peak serum level of cloxacillin can be fourfold higher if the drug is given whilst fasting (Bell, 1970). Flucloxacillin serum levels also are higher if it is given in the fasting state (Kamme and Ursing, 1974).

2. *Parenteral administration.* Oxacillin and cloxacillin produce satisfactory

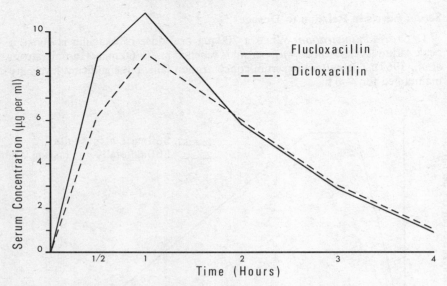

FIG. 5. Serum concentrations of flucloxacillin and dicloxacillin after a single 250 mg oral dose to fasting subjects. (Redrawn from Sutherland *et al.*, 1970.)

serum levels after parenteral administration. The serum level after intramuscular oxacillin is approximately twice that obtained when the same dose is given orally to a fasting subject (Marcy and Klein, 1970). Similarly, intramuscular cloxacillin produces higher serum concentrations than the orally administered drug (Fig. 4). Peak serum levels of oxacillin, cloxacillin, dicloxacillin and flucloxacillin after a single intramuscular injection of 500 mg are similar (14–16 μg per ml). Flucloxacillin levels are considerably more prolonged than those of oxacillin and slightly more prolonged than those of cloxacillin (Sutherland *et al.*, 1970). It appears therefore that flucloxacillin, like dicloxacillin (*vide supra*), is cleared more slowly from the body than cloxacillin.

As with other penicillins, concurrent administration of probenecid (page 17) enhances serum concentrations.

3. *Newborn and premature infants.* After a single intramuscular injection of oxacillin in a dose of 20 mg per kg to newborn infants (aged 8–15 days), the mean peak serum concentration is 51·5 μg per ml and the mean serum half-life is 1·6 h. In infants aged 20–21 days, the peak level is 47·0 μg per ml and the mean serum half-life is 1·2 h (Axline *et al.*, 1967).

Schwartz *et al.* (1976) studied a neonate who failed to achieve therapeutic levels after oral administration of dicloxacillin, even when the dosage was as high as 175 mg per kg per day. Intestinal absorption appeared normal, but there was an abnormally high urinary excretion rate. It was postulated that the renal tubular secretion of the drug was stimulated either by the penicillin derivative itself, or by phenobarbital which the neonate was receiving concurrently. From this experience the authors stressed the importance of antibiotic serum level monitoring in the neonatal period.

4. *Patients with cystic fibrosis.* These patients eliminate dicloxacillin three times faster than normal subjects due to an increase in their tubular secretory capacity. Thus when usual doses of the drug are given, relatively low and unpredictable serum levels result, despite normal absorption of the drug (Jusko *et al.*, 1975). Other isoxazolyl penicillins may be handled in a similar manner. Therefore when patients with cystic fibrosis are treated with these drugs, larger doses and serum level monitoring is necessary (*see also* methicillin, page 70).

Excretion

URINE: Isoxazolyl penicillins are mainly excreted in the urine. After oral administration of cloxacillin about 30 per cent of the dose is excreted in this way (Stewart, 1965); a higher percentage of the dose is recoverable when it is administered intramuscularly. Compared to cloxacillin, oxacillin is excreted to a lesser extent via the kidney, partly because of its poorer absorption, and partly because more oxacillin is cleared by other mechanisms (*vide infra*). Larger amounts of dicloxacillin and flucloxacillin are excreted in urine after oral administration, because the absorption of these drugs is better than cloxacillin (Sutherland *et al.*, 1970).

Antibacterially active metabolites of the isoxazolyl penicillins exist in serum and are excreted in urine (Thijssen and Mattie, 1976). Under normal conditions serum levels of these metabolites are low, representing only 9 per cent of the total antibiotic serum concentration. However in patients with markedly impaired renal function, metabolites may represent up to 50 per cent of the total penicillin serum level. In healthy subjects, 10–23 per cent of the penicillin excreted in urine is in the form of metabolites; the higher percentages occur with oxacillin and the lowest with flucloxacillin. Because only small amounts of active metabolites are formed from the isoxazolyl penicillins and these have similar activity to the parent drug, they have no real clinical significance.

The excretion of isoxazolyl penicillins is by glomerular filtration and tubular secretion. Probenecid can delay their excretion by partly blocking renal tubular secretion (*see* penicillin G, page 17). Nauta *et al.* (1974) studied the effect of probenecid on the volume of distribution of cloxacillin in anephric patients, and showed that it was not significantly changed. This indicates that probenecid does not limit the access of penicillins to tissues. However, these anephric patients did show a significant reduction of drug elimination when probenecid was used. This suggests that probenecid also diminishes the extrarenal elimination of the penicillin via the liver (*vide infra*).

BILE: These penicillins are eliminated by the biliary tract to some extent. This method of excretion is more marked with oxacillin than cloxacillin.

INACTIVATION IN BODY: This occurs with all the isoxazolyl penicillins, and probably takes place in the liver. Oxacillin is more rapidly destroyed in the body than the others, and therefore has little tendency to accumulate in patients with renal failure (Bulger *et al.*, 1964).

Distribution of the Drugs in Body

Cloxacillin and dicloxacillin, which are highly serum protein bound (*vide infra*), penetrate as well as drugs with a low degree of protein binding such as methicillin (page 71) and ampicillin (page 110) into the pus and bone of patients with acute pyogenic osteomyelitis and also into septic joint effusions (Tetzlaff *et al.*, 1978; Nelson *et al.*, 1978). Significant concentrations of cloxacillin have been also detected in pleural fluid (Stewart, 1962), and this drug crosses the placenta (Marcy and Klein, 1970). However these penicillins do not pass into normal cerebrospinal fluid.

In vitro, all of these penicillins are extensively bound to serum proteins. Oxacillin is about 93 per cent serum protein bound, cloxacillin and flucloxacillin 94 per cent and dicloxacillin at 97 per cent is the most highly bound of all the penicillins (Rolinson and Sutherland, 1965; Sutherland *et al.,* 1970; Bergeron *et al.*, 1976). Slightly differing figures have been reported, and results vary according to the laboratory method used (Marcy and Klein, 1970).

The percentage of any drug bound to serum proteins is less when high serum levels are attained, because the binding capacity of serum proteins is exceeded. However, *in vitro* studies with penicillin G and cloxacillin show that the percentage of the unbound drug is only significantly increased when a total serum concentration of 200 μg per ml or higher, is attained (Rolinson and Sutherland, 1965). It has been suggested that the protein bound part of an antibiotic has little or no antibacterial activity (Rolinson, 1964; Rolinson and Sutherland, 1965; Kunin, 1967). The greater intrinsic activity of cloxacillin compared to methicillin would thereby be compromised *in vivo* by its protein binding. This can be demonstrated *in vitro* because the activity of these two drugs is similar when tested in the presence of serum (page 81). On this basis it would seem that for serious staphylococcal infections the minimum dose of cloxacillin should be at least 1 g four-hourly by injection, as in the case of methicillin (page 68).

It is still not absolutely clear to what extent serum binding affects the therapeutic activity of the penicillins, because this binding may be loose and rapidly reversible *in vivo* (Kislak *et al.*, 1964; Barza *et al.*, 1972; Mattie *et al.*, 1973). The protein bound drug may serve as a circulating drug reservoir, which releases more drug as the free drug is excreted or metabolized (Koch-Weser and Sellers, 1976). Thus protein binding may increase the duration of action of many drugs. Antibiotics such as oxacillin and flucloxacillin which are highly bound to serum proteins, certainly diffuse poorly into human interstitial fluid (Tan *et al.*, 1972) and into fibrin clots in experimental animals (Barza *et al.*, 1974). In the latter their penetration is enhanced by probenecid (Lee *et al.*, 1975). The relevance of these experimental findings to human disease with tissue inflammation is not yet known. Isoxazolyl penicillins despite their high degree of serum binding are effective in clinical practice. Furthermore, two other antibiotics which are even more protein bound, sodium fusidate (97·3 per cent) and novobiocin (99·2 per cent) are also effective therapeutically (Leading article, 1966). However Rolinson (1967) has shown that even with some of the highly protein bound antibiotics, the peak serum level of 'free antibiotic', after usual therapeutic doses, still exceeds the concentration necessary to inhibit highly sensitive bacteria.

Mode of Action

These drugs have a mode of action similar to penicillin G (page 19).

Toxicity

1. *Allergic reactions.* These drugs are contraindicated in penicillin allergic patients, because they may evoke all the hypersensitivity reactions caused by penicillin G (page 24).

2. *Gastro-intestinal side-effects.* Oral administration of the isoxazolyl penicillins may cause nausea and diarrhoea, which only occasionally necessitate cessation of treatment.

3. *Hepatotoxicity.* Oxacillin occasionally causes fever, nausea and vomiting associated with abnormal liver function tests, mainly elevated serum aspartate aminotransferase (SGOT) levels (Dismukes, 1973). Liver biopsy in these patients may show the changes of a non-specific hepatitis (Bruckstein and Attia, 1978). Some patients remain asymptomatic and anicteric, the only abnormalities being elevated serum enzymes and sometimes eosinophilia (Olans and Weiner, 1976). Reversible cholestatic hepatitis has been noted in one patient (Ten Pas and Quinn, 1965). Liver function test abnormalities rapidly disappear when oxacillin is ceased. Olans and Weiner (1976) who studied eight children with this complication found that it was safe to substitute another penicillin such as penicillin G or nafcillin, for oxacillin, because liver dysfunction rapidly resolved despite their use. Hepatotoxicity may be more common with oxacillin, because compared to other isoxazolyl penicillins, it is cleared to a greater extent through the liver and biliary tract (Simon, 1965). Elevation of SGOT levels has also been rarely noted with cloxacillin and dicloxacillin (Yow, 1964; Berger and Potter, 1977).

4. *Neurotoxicity.* This may occur if very large doses are given intravenously, especially in patients with renal failure. Conway and Beck (1968) reported a patient who convulsed whilst receiving 18 g of intravenous cloxacillin per day, but who also had renal functional impairment and was concurrently receiving cephaloridine in a dose of 2 g daily. Malone *et al.* (1977) described a patient with acute bacterial endocarditis and impaired renal function, who convulsed while receiving 16 g oxacillin intravenously per day. This patient's pre-dose oxacillin serum level was 270 μg per ml; one hour after a dose it was 340 μg per ml, and the CSF level was 70 μg per ml (*see also* page 28).

5. *Neutropenia.* This has been noted with oxacillin, but it can occur with the other isoxazolyl penicillins. Leventhal and Silken (1976) described four children who developed marked neutropenia while being treated with intravenous oxacillin in a dose of 200 mg or more, per kg per day. Neutropenia appeared after the third week of therapy, and in all cases the white cell count returned to normal when the drug was stopped (*see also* methicillin, page 72). Oxacillin probably exerts a toxic effect on the maturation of neutrophils (Chu *et al.*, 1977). An acute agranulocytosis has been reported in a 79-year-old woman following a 53 day course of oxacillin. This drug was considered as the most likely cause although she was also taking tolbutamide and chlorpromazine (Scalley and Roark, 1977). Agranulocytosis has also been described in one adult patient with cloxacillin therapy. After receiving this drug for 35 days he developed fever, pharyngitis and profound leucopenia, which subsequently resolved upon withdrawal of the drug (Westerman *et al.*, 1978).

6. *Kernicterus.* Animal studies suggest that flucloxacillin, similar to sulphonamides (page 670), may displace bilirubin from its binding sites on albumin.

Thus it is possible that this drug, if used in the jaundiced neonate, may cause kernicterus (Hanefeld and Ballowitz, 1976).

7. *Corneal opacities*. Direct application of cloxacillin to the eye should be avoided, because such opacities have been produced in rabbits when this drug was injected subconjunctivally (Knudsen *et al.*, 1962).

Clinical Uses of the Drugs

1. All these penicillins, like methicillin (page 64) are primarily used for treatment of penicillin-resistant staphylococcal infections. Results comparable to those obtained with methicillin (page 74) or nafcillin (page 96), have been obtained with oxacillin administered in large doses parenterally (6–18 g daily for adults), for the treatment of severe staphylococcal infections (Kirby *et al.*, 1962; Klein *et al.*, 1963; Walker and Standiford, 1967). Parenteral cloxacillin and flucloxacillin are also satisfactory. It now appears that all the penicillinase-resistant penicillins which can be administered parenterally are about equally effective for the treatment of severe staphylococcal disease (Wise, 1973), but the other drugs now seem preferable to methicillin (page 74). Of the isoxazolyl penicillins, cloxacillin appears to be at this time the best drug to be used parenterally because it has pharmacological advantages over oxacillin (page 84). Parenteral flucloxacillin has a slight pharmacological advantage over cloxacillin, but it has not as yet been extensively used for severe infections. Cloxacillin may also be preferable to flucloxacillin because it is somewhat more resistant to staphylococcal beta-lactamase (Selwyn, 1976) (*see also* page 80).

For oral administration, cloxacillin is superior to oxacillin because of its better gastro-intestinal absorption. Early reports indicated that oral cloxacillin was effective for the treatment of staphylococcal infections of moderate severity (Stewart, 1962; Lowbury and Miller, 1962; Turck *et al.*, 1965), but inconsistent results were obtained when it was used for the treatment of severe infections (May *et al.*, 1964). Oral cloxacillin is suitable for the treatment of minor staphylococcal infections, and also for prolonged out-patient treatment of chronic infections such as osteomyelitis (Bell, 1968; 1976).

Dicloxacillin being well absorbed, also gives satisfactory results in staphylococcal infections such as osteomyelitis, when administered by the oral route (Hammerstrom *et al.*, 1967; Hedström, 1975). Flucloxacillin may supersede both cloxacillin and dicloxacillin for oral therapy, because like dicloxacillin its absorption is superior to cloxacillin, but it is less protein bound than dicloxacillin (Leading article, 1970; Bergeron *et al.*, 1976). It is yet to be determined whether flucloxacillin's lesser stability to staphylococcal beta-lactamase (page 80) will be a disadvantage. Oral flucloxacillin has been used with success for the treatment of staphylococcal skin and soft tissue infections as well as for deeper infections such as osteomyelitis, empyema and post-operative abscesses (Kamme and Ursing, 1974; Price and Harding, 1975).

2. Isoxazolyl penicillins such as cloxacillin or dicloxacillin were occasionally used in combination with either ampicillin (Acred and Sutherland, 1967; Sabath *et al.*, 1967a and b), hetacillin (Riff *et al.*, 1970) or one of the cephalosporins (Muggleton and O'Callaghan, 1967) for the treatment of urinary tract infections caused by Gram-negative bacilli. Isoxazolyl penicillins have no activity against these bacteria, but it was hoped that they would

protect the action of ampicillin or a cephalosporin by binding bacterial beta-lactamases which destroy these drugs. Such penicillin combinations have met with very little clinical success (*see* page 103).

REFERENCES

Acred, P. and Sutherland, R. (1967), 'Antibacterial activities of combinations of ampicillin and cloxacillin', *Antimicrob. Agents Chemother.*—1966, p. 53.

Axline, S. G., Yaffe, S. J. and Simon, H. J. (1967), 'Clinical pharmacology of antimicrobials in premature infants. II. Ampicillin, methicillin, oxacillin, neomycin and colistin', *Pediatrics,* **39,** 97.

Barber, M. and Waterworth, P. M. (1964), 'Penicillinase-resistant penicillins and cephalosporins', *Brit. med. J.,* **2,** 344.

Barza, M., Vine, H. and Weinstein, L. (1972), 'Reversibility of protein binding of penicillins: an *in vitro study* employing a rapid diafiltration process', *Antimicrob. Ag. Chemother.,* **1,** 427.

Barza, M., Samuelson, T. and Weinstein, L. (1974), 'Penetration of antibiotics into fibrin loci *in vivo.* II. Comparison of nine antibiotics; effect of dose and degree of protein binding', *J. Infect. Dis.,* **129,** 66.

Bell, S. M. (1968), 'Oral penicillins in the treatment of chronic staphylococcal osteomyelitis', *Lancet,* **2,** 295.

Bell, S. M. (1970), 'Supervision of antibiotic treatment—an important medical responsibility', *Aspects of Infection. Proc. Symp. Auckland, Sydney and Melbourne,* p. 107.

Bell, S. M. (1976), 'Further observations on the value of oral penicillins in chronic staphylococcal osteomyelitis', *Med. J. Aust.,* **2,** 591.

Berger, M. and Potter, D. E. (1977), 'Pitfall in diagnosis of viral hepatitis on haemodialysis unit', *Lancet,* **2,** 95.

Bergeron, M. G., Brusch, J. L., Barza, M. and Weinstein, L. (1976), 'Bactericidal activity and pharmacology of flucloxacillin', *Amer. J. Med., Sci.,* **271,** 13.

Best, G. K., Best, N. H. and Koval, A. V. (1974), 'Evidence for participation of autolysins in bactericidal action of oxacillin on Staphylococcus aureus', *Antimicrob. Ag. Chemother.,* **6,** 825.

Bruckstein, A. H. and Attia, A. A. (1978), 'Oxacillin hepatitis. Two patients with liver biopsy, and review of the literature', *Amer. J. Med.,* **64,** 519.

Bulger, R. J., Lindholm, D. D., Murray, J. S. and Kirby, W. M. M. (1964), 'Effect of uremia on methicillin and oxacillin blood levels', *JAMA,* **187,** 139.

Chu, J.-Y., O'Connor, D. M. and Schmidt, R. R. (1977), 'The mechanism of oxacillin-induced neutropenia', *J. Pediatrics,* **90,** 668.

Conway, N., Beck, E. and Somerville, J. (1968), 'Penicillin encephalopathy', *Postgrad. Med. J.,* **44,** 891.

Dismukes, W. E. (1973), 'Oxacillin-induced hepatic dysfunction', *JAMA,* **226,** 861.

Glew, R. H., Moellering, R. C., Jr. and Wennersten, C. (1975), 'Comparative synergistic activity of nafcillin, oxacillin and methicillin in combination with gentamicin against enterococci', *Antimicrob. Ag. Chemother.,* **7,** 828.

Gravenkemper, C. F., Bennett, J. V., Brodie, J. L. and Kirby, W. M. M. (1965), 'Dicloxacillin. *In vitro* and pharmacologic comparisons with oxacillin and cloxacillin', *Arch. Intern. Med.,* **116,** 340.

Hammerstrom, C. F., Cox, F., McHenry, M. C. and Quinn, E. L. (1967), 'Clinical, laboratory, and pharmacological studies of dicloxacillin', *Antimicrob. Agents Chemother.*—1966, p. 69.

Hanefeld, F. and Ballowitz, L. (1976), 'Flucloxacillin and bilirubin binding', *Lancet*, **1**, 433.

Hedström, S. A. (1975), 'Treatment of chronic staphylococcal osteomyelitis with cloxacillin and dicloxacillin—a comparative study in 12 patients', *Scand. J. Infect. Dis.*, **7**, 55.

Jusko, W. J., Mosovich, L. L., Gerbracht, L. M., Mattar, M. E. and Yaffe, S. J. (1975), 'Enhanced renal excretion of dicloxacillin in patients with cystic fibrosis', *Pediatrics*, **56**, 1038.

Kamme, C. and Ursing, B. (1974), 'Serum levels and clinical effect of flucloxacillin in patients with staphylococcal infections', *Scand. J. Infect. Dis.*, **6**, 273.

Kirby, W. M. M., Rosenfeld, L. S. and Brodie, J. (1962), 'Oxacillin. Laboratory and clinical evaluation', *JAMA*, **181**, 739.

Kislak, J. W., Eickhoff, T. C. and Finland, M. (1965), 'Cloxacillin: Activity *in vitro*, and absorption and urinary excretion in normal young men', *Amer. J. Med. Sci.*, **249**, 636.

Klein, J. O., Sabath, L. D., Steinhauer, B. W. and Finland, M. (1963), 'Oxacillin treatment of severe staphylococcal infections', *New Engl. J. Med.*, **269**, 1215.

Knox, R., Maclaren, D. M., Smith, J. T., Trafford, J. A. P. and Barnes, R. D. S. (1962), 'BRL. 1621: A comparison with other isoxazolyl penicillins', *Brit. med. J.*, **2**, 831.

Knox, R. and Smith, J. T. (1963), 'Stability of methicillin and cloxacillin to staphylococcal penicillinase', *Brit. med. J.*, **2**, 205.

Knudsen, E. T., Brown, D. M. and Rolinson, G. N. (1962), 'A new orally effective penicillinase-stable penicillin—BRL. 1621', *Lancet*, **2**, 632.

Koch-Weser, J. and Sellers, E. M. (1976), 'Binding of drugs to serum albumin (first of two parts)', *New Engl. J. Med.*, **294**, 311.

Kunin, C. M. (1967), 'Clinical significance of protein binding of the penicillins, *Ann. N.Y. Acad. Sci.*, **145**, 282.

Lacey, R. W. and Stokes, A. (1977), 'Susceptibility of the "penicillinase-resistant" penicillins and cephalosporins to penicillinase of Staphylococcus aureus', *J. clin. Path.*, **30**, 35.

Leading Article, (1966), 'Serum binding of antibiotics', *Brit. med. J.*, **1**, 1059.

Leading Article (1970), 'Yet another penicillin', *Brit. med. J.*, **4**, 446.

Lee, R. D., Brusch, J. L., Barza, M. J. and Weinstein, L. (1975), 'Effect of probenecid on penetration of oxacillin into fibrin clots *in vitro*', *Antimicrob. Ag. Chemother.*, **8**, 105.

Leventhal, J. M. and Silken, A. B. (1976), 'Oxacillin-induced neutropenia in children', *J. Pediatrics*, **89**, 769.

Lincoln, L. J., Weinstein, A. J., Gallagher, M. and Abrutyn, E. (1977), 'Penicillinase-resistant penicillins plus gentamicin in experimental enterococcal endocarditis', *Antimicrob. Ag. Chemother.*, **12**, 484.

Lorian, V. and Sabath, L. D. (1972), 'The effect of some penicillins on Mycobacterium tuberculosis', *Amer. Rev. Resp. Dis.*, **105**, 632.

Lowbury, E. J. L. and Miller, R. W. S. (1962), 'Treatment of infected burns with BRL. 1621', *Lancet*, **2**, 640.

Lowbury, E. J. L., Lilly, H. A. and Kidson, A. (1977), ' "Methicillin-resistant" Staphylococcus aureus: reassessment by controlled trial in burns unit', *Brit. med. J.*, **1**, 1054.

Malone, A. J., Jr., Field, S., Rosman, J. and Shemerdiak, W. P. (1977), 'Neurotoxic reaction to oxacillin', *New Engl. J. Med.*, **296**, 453.

McCracken, G. H., Jr. and Nelson, J. D. (1977), *Antimicrobial Therapy for Newborns: Practical Application of Pharmacology to Clinical Usage*, Grune & Stratton, Inc., New York, San Francisco, London, p. 25.

Marcy, S. M. and Klein, J. O. (1970), 'The isoxazolyl penicillins: Oxacillin, cloxacillin and dicloxacillin', *Med. Clin. North America*, **54**, 1127.

Marier, R. L., Joyce, N. and Andriole, V. T. (1975), 'Synergism of oxacillin and gentamicin against enterococci', *Antimicrob. Ag. Chemother.*, **8**, 571.

Mattie, H., Goslings, W. R. O. and Noach, E. L. (1973), 'Cloxacillin and nafcillin: serum binding and its relationship to antibacterial effect in mice', *J. Infect. Dis.*, **128**, 170.

May, J., Rountree, P. M., Beard, M. A. and Loewenthal, J. (1964), 'Cloxacillin in the therapy of staphylococcal infection', *Med. J. Aust.*, **2**, 496.

Mayhall, C. G., Medoff, G. and Marr, J. J. (1976), 'Variation in the susceptibility of strains of Staphylococcus aureus to oxacillin, cephalothin, and gentamicin', *Antimicrob. Ag. Chemother.*, **10**, 707.

Muggleton, P. W. and O'Callaghan, C. H. (1967), 'The antibacterial activities of cephaloridine: laboratory investigation', *Postgrad. Med. J.* (Suppl.), **43**, 17.

Nauta, E. H., Mattie, H. and Goslings, W. R. O. (1974), 'Effect of probenecid on the apparent volume of distribution and elimination of cloxacillin', *Antimicrob. Ag. Chemother.*, **6**, 300.

Nelson, J. D., Howard, J. B. and Shelton, S. (1978), 'Oral antibiotic therapy for skeletal infections of children. 1. Antibiotic concentrations in suppurative synovial fluid', *J. Pediatrics*, **92**, 131.

Olans, R. N. and Weiner, L. B. (1976), 'Reversible oxacillin hepatotoxicity', *J. Pediatrics*, **89**, 835.

Price, J. D. and Harding, J. W. (1975), 'Flucloxacillin in the treatment of infectious conditions in children', *Curr. Med. Res. Opin.*, **3**, 77.

Richmond, A. S., Simberkoff, M. S., Scaefler, S. and Rahal, J. J., Jr. (1977), 'Resistance of Staphylococcus aureus to semisynthetic penicillins and cephalothin', *J. Infect. Dis.*, **135**, 108.

Riff, L., Olexy, V. M. and Jackson, G. G. (1970), 'Therapy with combinations of penicillin analogues in urinary-tract infections', *Antimicrob. Agents Chemother.* —1969, p. 405.

Rolinson, G. N. (1964), 'The significance of protein binding of penicillins', *Postgrad. Med. J.*, (Suppl.), **40**, 20.

Rolinson, G. N. and Sutherland, R. (1965), 'The binding of antibiotics to serum proteins', *Brit. J. Pharmacol.*, **25**, 638.

Rolinson, G. N. (1967), 'The significance of protein binding of antibiotics *in vitro* and *in vivo*', in Waterson, A. P. (ed.), *Recent Advances in Medical Microbiology*, J. & A. Churchill Ltd., p. 254.

Rosenblatt, J. E., Kind, A. C., Brodie, J. L. and Kirby, W. M. M. (1968), 'Mechanisms responsible for the blood level differences of isoxazolyl penicillins, oxacillin, cloxacillin and dicloxacillin', *Arch. Intern. Med.*, **121**, 345.

Sabath, L. D., McCall, C. E., Steigbigel, N. H. and Finland, M. (1967a), 'Synergistic penicillin combinations for treatment of human urinary-tract infections', *Antimicrob. Agents Chemother.*—1966, p. 149.

Sabath, L. D., Elder, H. A., McCall, C. E. and Finland, M. (1967b), 'Synergistic combinations of penicillins in the treatment of bacteriuria', *New Engl. J. Med.*, **277**, 232.

Sabath, L. D., Garner, C., Wilcox, C. and Finland, M. (1975), 'Effect of inoculum and of beta-lactamase on the anti-staphylococcal activity of thirteen penicillins and cephalosporins', *Antimicrob. Ag. Chemother.*, **8**, 344.

Sabath, L. D., Wheeler, N., Laverdiere, M., Blazevic, D. and Wilkinson, B. J. (1977), 'A new type of penicillin resistance of Staphylococcus aureus', *Lancet*, **1**, 443.

Scalley, R. D. and Roark, R. D. (1977), 'Oxacillin-induced agranulocytosis', *Drug. Intellig. Clin. Pharm.*, **2**, 420.

Schwartz, G. J., Hegyi, T. and Spitzer, A. (1976), 'Subtherapeutic dicloxacillin levels in a neonate: possible mechanisms', *J. Pediatrics*, **89**, 310.

Selwyn, S. (1976), 'Rational choice of penicillins and cephalosporins based on parallel *in-vitro* and *in-vivo* tests', *Lancet*, **2**, 616.

Simon, H. J. (1965), 'Current status of methicillin, oxacillin and cloxacillin', *Antimicrob. Agents Chemother.*—1964, p. 280.

Stewart, G. T. (ed.), A Report from Six Hospitals, (1962), 'Clinical and laboratory results with BRL. 1621', *Lancet,* **2,** 634.

Stewart, G. T. (1965), *The Penicillin Group of Drugs,* Elsevier Publishing Company, p. 41.

Sutherland, R. Croydon, E. A. P. and Rolinson, G. N. (1970) 'Flucloxacillin, a new isoxazolyl penicillin, compared with oxacillin, cloxacillin and dicloxacillin', *Brit. med. J.,* **4,** 455.

Tan, J. S., Trott, A., Phair, J. P. and Watanakunakorn, C. (1972), 'A method for measurement of antibiotics in human interstitial fluid', *J. Infect. Dis.,* **126,** 492.

Ten Pas, A. and Quinn, E. L. (1965), 'Cholestatic hepatitis following the administration of sodium oxacillin', *JAMA,* **191,** 674; quoted by Marcy and Klein (1970).

Tetzlaff, T. R., Howard, J. B., McCracken, G. H., Jr., Calderon, E. and Larrondo, J. (1978), 'Antibiotic concentrations in pus and bone of children with osteomyelitis, *J. Pediatrics,* **92,** 135.

Thijssen, H. H. W. and Mattie, H. (1976), 'Active metabolites of isoxazolylpenicillins in humans', *Antimicrob. Ag. Chemother.,* **10,** 441.

Turck, M., Ronald, A. and Petersdorf, R. G. (1965), 'Clinical studies with cloxacillin. A new antibiotic', *JAMA,* **192,** 961.

Turner, G. C. and Cox, P. E. (1967), 'Resistance to cloxacillin among hospital staphylococci', *J. clin. Path.,* **20,** 870.

Walker, S. H. and Standiford, W. E. (1967), 'Treatment of infants with oxacillin sodium', *Amer. J. Dis. Child.,* **114,** 64.

Watanakunakorn, C. and Glotzbecker, C. (1977), 'Comparative *in vitro* activity of nafcillin, oxacillin, and methicillin in combination with gentamicin and tobramycin against enterococci', *Antimicrob. Ag. Chemother.,* **11,** 88.

Westerman, E. L., Bradshaw, M. W. and Williams, T. W., Jr. (1978), 'Agranulocytosis during therapy with orally administered cloxacillin', *Am. J. Clin. Pathol,* **69,** 559.

Wise, R. I. (1973), 'Modern management of severe staphylococcal disease', *Medicine,* **52,** 295.

Yow, M. D., South, M. A. and Hess, C. G. (1964), 'The use of the penicillinase-resistant penicillin in the pneumonias of children', *Postgrad. Med. J.* (Suppl.), **40,** 127.

Nafcillin, Diphenicillin and Quinacillin

Description

In addition to methicillin (page 64) and the isoxazolyl penicillins (page 79), three other penicillinase-resistant penicillins have been derived from the penicillin nucleus (6-aminopenicillanic acid).

1. *Nafcillin*, 6-(2-ethoxy-1-naphthamido) penicillanic acid, described in 1961.
2. *Diphenicillin* (ancillin), 2-biphenylyl penicillin, described in 1961.
3. *Quinacillin*, 3-carboxy-2-quinoxalinyl penicillin, described in 1963.

Nafcillin is the only one of these penicillins which has had wide clinical usage, chiefly in America. Diphenicillin had limited use in America, and compared unfavourably to the other penicillinase-resistant penicillins (Klein *et al.*, 1963). Clinical studies with quinacillin were never pursued.

The following details only apply to nafcillin, which is marketed in America with the trade name of 'Unipen' (Wyeth).

Sensitive Organisms

Nafcillin has a similar antibacterial spectrum to the isoxazolyl penicillins (page 79). It is about as active as oxacillin against both penicillin-sensitive and penicillin-resistant staphylococci (Klein *et al.*, 1963). The stability of nafcillin in the presence of staphylococcal penicillinase, is comparable to that of methicillin (page 64) and greater than that of the isoxazolyl penicillins (page 80) (Sabath *et al.*, 1975). Methicillin-resistant staphylococci (page 64) are resistant to all penicillinase-resistant penicillins, including nafcillin (Barber and Waterworth, 1964; Richmond *et al.*, 1977). Penicillin-tolerant staphylococcal strains (pages 6, 67, 80) are also tolerant to nafcillin. Sabath *et al.* (1977) studied seven such strains; all had low minimum inhibitory concentrations to nafcillin ($0 \cdot 1 - 0 \cdot 4 \, \mu g$ per ml), but their minimum bactericidal concentrations were 128 to 2000 times higher, whereas normally the MBC is only about four-fold higher than the MIC. These staphylococcal strains are deficient in an autolytic enzyme activity, which appears to be necessary for the lethal action of any of the penicillins. Severe staphylococcal infections caused by these tolerant strains, may not respond satisfactorily to nafcillin alone, but may respond if gentamicin is also used (page 80).

There is some evidence that nafcillin may act synergistically with one of the aminoglycosides such as gentamicin (page 325) or rifampicin (page 555), against some strains of *Staph. pyogenes*.

Nafcillin has a higher degree of activity than the isoxazolyl penicillins against a number of strains of pneumococci and haemolytic streptococci (Lane,

1964). *Strep. faecalis* is relatively resistant to nafcillin (Table 6), but the drug may act synergistically with gentamicin against some strains of this organism. Glew *et al.* (1975) found that this combination at clinically achievable concentrations was synergistic against 10 of 14 strains tested. Watanakunakorn and Glotzbecker (1977) also demonstrated enhanced killing of most enterococcal strains by nafcillin/gentamicin and in addition showed that it was superior to combinations of either methicillin/gentamicin or oxacillin/gentamicin (page 79).

In Vitro Sensitivities

TABLE 6

(After Barber and Waterworth, 1964)

ORGANISM	MIC (μg per ml)
Staph. pyogenes (non-penicillinase producer)	0·25–0·5
Staph. pyogenes (penicillinase producer)	0·25–1·0
Strep. pyogenes (Group A)	0·03–0·06
Strep. pneumoniae (Dip. pneumoniae)	0·03–0·06
Strep. faecalis (Enterococcus Group D)	8·0

The minimum inhibitory concentrations of nafcillin against some selected bacteria are shown in Table 6. If the activity of nafcillin against *Staph. pyogenes* is tested in 95 per cent human serum instead of nutrient broth, extensive protein binding occurs and its MIC is increased about ten-fold (Barber and Waterworth, 1964).

Mode of Administration and Dosage

1. *Oral administration.* Nafcillin is poorly and inconsistently absorbed from the gastro-intestinal tract, and it is unreliable if used orally. Therefore its administration by this route is not recommended (Klein *et al.*, 1963; Whitehouse *et al.*, 1963; Watanakunakorn, 1977).

2. *Parenteral administration.* Nafcillin can be given either intramuscularly or intravenously. The usual adult dose is 1 g four-hourly, but this can be doubled for the treatment of severe infections. Doses of up to 18 g intravenously daily have been given to adults with no ill effects (Hamburger, 1964; Eickhoff *et al.*, 1965).

3. *Children.* The usual dose is 100–200 mg per kg per day intramuscularly or intravenously, given in four or six divided doses.

4. *Newborn infants.* As with all penicillins, a smaller dose should be used in this age group (*see* page 82). The suggested dose is 50 mg per kg per day, administered in two divided doses (Wise, 1973).

5. *Patients with renal failure.* Nafcillin is eliminated from the body rapidly by non-renal mechanisms (Kind *et al.*, 1970), so that dosage reduction is not needed in such patients. Anuric patients receiving haemodialysis do not have an altered serum nafcillin half-life either during haemodialysis or in the interval between dialyses. Therefore they can be treated by a nafcillin dosage identical to that used for patients with normal renal function (Diaz *et al.*, 1977).

Availability

1. Vials containing 500 mg, 1 g and 2 g.
2. Capsules: 250 mg and tablets: 500 mg.
3. Oral solution: 250 mg nafcillin per 5 ml.

Serum Levels in Relation to Dosage

1. After an intramuscular injection of 1·0 g nafcillin, a peak serum level of about 8 μg per ml is reached one hour later. The serum concentration thereafter falls and it is about 0·5 μg per ml at six hours (Whitehouse et al., 1963). Concomitant oral administration of probenecid increases and prolongs nafcillin levels similar to other penicillins (Klein et al., 1963).

Nafcillin serum levels are lower than those attained with equal doses of intramuscular oxacillin (page 84), because it is distributed in a larger volume in the body, and also it is more rapidly inactivated by the liver (Kind et al., 1970).

2. Serum levels following orally administered nafcillin are low and quite irregular. If the drug is taken with food, its absorption is even more impaired (Klein et al., 1963; Whitehouse et al., 1963).

Excretion

URINE: About 30 per cent of an intramuscularly administered dose of nafcillin can be recovered from the urine, and urinary concentrations reach as high as 1000 μg per ml. A considerably smaller amount of active nafcillin (about 19 per cent of the administered dose) is recovered from the urine after intramuscular administration if it is given with probenecid (Klein et al., 1963).

BILE: A small amount, probably only about 8 per cent of an intramuscular dose, is eliminated via the bile (Kind et al., 1970).

INACTIVATION IN BODY: The remainder of the administered nafcillin appears to be inactivated in the liver (Kind et al., 1970). This inactivation takes place even more rapidly than in the case of oxacillin (page 85).

Distribution of the Drug in Body

Tissue penetration of nafcillin is probably similar to the isoxazolyl penicillins (page 85), but nafcillin has been reported to reach higher concentrations in the CSF both in patients with normal meninges and in those with meningitis. Fossieck et al. (1977) studied CSF nafcillin levels in seven patients with normal meninges; each received an intravenous nafcillin dose of 40 mg per kg infused over 30 min. The mean nafcillin CSF concentration was 0·05 μg per ml at one hour after the infusion, 0·12 μg per ml at two hours, 0·09 μg per ml at three hours and 0·03 μg per ml at four hours. Ruiz and Warner (1976) treated an adult patient with staphylococcal meningitis using nafcillin in a dose of 200 mg per kg per day. A high CSF nafcillin concentration of 9·5 μg per ml was reached 45 min after a 3 g intravenous nafcillin dose, administered over five minutes. Kane et al. (1977) studied nine patients with severe staphylococcal infections who were treated by intravenous nafcillin. High CSF nafcillin levels (7·5–88·0 μg per ml) were found in three patients with purulent meningitis and in two others with staphylococcal septicaemia who only had a CSF pleocytosis. By contrast lower nafcillin CSF levels (0·13–2·7 μg per ml) were found in the patients without a CSF pleocytosis.

Nafcillin is about 87 per cent serum protein bound (Rolinson and Sutherland, 1965). The significance of protein binding is discussed on page 86).

Mode of Action

The mode of action of nafcillin on bacteria is similar to penicillin G (page 18).

Toxicity

1. *Hypersensitivity reactions*. Nafcillin, like other penicillins, may cause the same hypersensitivity reactions that occur with penicillin G (page 24). The drug is contraindicated in any patient with a history of penicillin sensitivity.

2. *Nephropathy*. Parry *et al.* (1973) described a patient, who developed renal damage due to methicillin, which resolved when lincomycin was substituted. Later when therapy was changed to nafcillin, the 'hypersensitivity nephritis' recurred. Nephropathy has been reported on many occasions with methicillin (page 72), but only rarely with other penicillinase-resistant penicillins. This may partly reflect the less extensive use of these drugs. Parry *et al.* (1973) suggest that if nephropathy develops after the use of one penicillin analogue, it is likely to recur if any other penicillin is subsequently used.

The presence of nafcillin in the urine can cause a false-positive urine reaction for protein, when the sulphasalicylic test is used, but not with the dipstick test. This may lead to unnecessary cessation of the drug and even renal biopsy (Line *et al.*, 1976). Penicillin G and oxacillin can also cause false-positive urine protein determinations, but to a lesser degree.

3. *Neutropenia*. This complication with concomitant fever, occurred in one patient receiving a daily dose of 12 g of nafcillin intravenously. Neutropenia resolved when the drug was stopped (Sandberg *et al.*, 1975). In another patient with right-sided valvular endocarditis, intravenous nafcillin therapy (12 g daily) was associated with the development of agranulocytosis, which only improved after the drug was discontinued (Markowitz *et al.*, 1975). In addition Greene and Cohen (1978) described neutropenia in three children, which developed while they were receiving intravenous nafcillin therapy. The neutropenia again resolved when nafcillin treatment was stopped.

Clinical Uses of the Drug

Parenteral nafcillin has been used successfully for the treatment of severe staphylococcal infections such as septicaemia, endocarditis, osteomyelitis and pneumonia (Martin *et al.*, 1964; Eickhoff *et al.*, 1965). It has also been used for staphylococcal septic arthritis (Goldenberg and Cohen, 1976) and meningitis (Ruiz and Warner, 1976).

The results obtained have been about the same as those with methicillin (page 74) or the parenteral isoxazolyl penicillins, oxacillin, cloxacillin and possibly flucloxacillin (page 88). These drugs therefore can be regarded as equal in their therapeutic efficacy (Waisbren, 1970; Wise, 1973). For this reason each clinician should select the parenteral anti-staphylococcal penicillin with which he is most familiar. Nevertheless many clinicians now prefer cloxacillin to methicillin or, particularly in America, nafcillin to methicillin, mainly because methicillin has a greater propensity to cause nephropathy (page 72). Because of the better penetration of nafcillin into the CSF (page 95), some authors regard it as the drug of choice for staphylococcal meningitis (Ruiz and Warner, 1976; Fossieck *et al.*, 1977). If nafcillin is used for this purpose the parenteral dose should be at least 100–200 mg per kg body weight per day (Kane *et al.*, 1977).

REFERENCES

Barber, M. and Waterworth, P. M. (1964), 'Penicillinase-resistant penicillins and cephalosporins', *Brit. med. J.*, **2**, 344.

Diaz, C. R., Kane, J. G., Parker, R. H. and Pelsor, F. R. (1977), 'Pharmacokinetics of nafcillin in patients with renal failure', *Antimicrob. Ag. Chemother.*, **12**, 98.

Eickhoff, T. C., Kislak, J. W. and Finland, M. (1965), 'Clinical evaluation of nafcillin in patients with severe staphylococcal disease', *New Engl. J. Med.*, **272**, 699.

Fossieck, B. E. Jr., Kane, J. G., Diaz, C. R. and Parker, R. H. (1977), 'Nafcillin entry into human cerebrospinal fluid', *Antimicrob. Ag. Chemother.*, **11**, 965.

Glew, R. H., Moellering, R. C. Jr. and Wennersten, C. (1975), 'Comparative synergistic activity of nafcillin, oxacillin and methicillin in combination with gentamicin against enterococci', *Antimicrob. Ag. Chemother.*, **7**, 828.

Goldenberg, D. L. and Cohen, A. S. (1976), 'Acute infectious arthritis. A review of patients with nongonococcal joint infections (with emphasis on therapy and prognosis)', *Amer. J. Med.*, **60**, 369.

Greene, G. R. and Cohen, E. (1978), 'Nafcillin-induced neutropenia in children', *Pediatrics*, **61**, 94.

Hamburger, M. (1964), 'The new penicillins in endocarditis', *Postgrad. Med. J.* (Suppl.), **40**, 98.

Kane, J. G., Parker, R. H., Jordan, G. W. and Hoeprich, P. D. (1977), 'Nafcillin concentration in cerebrospinal fluid during treatment of staphylococcal infections', *Ann. Intern. Med.*, **87**, 309.

Kind, A. C., Tupasi, T. E., Standiford, H. C. and Kirby, W. M. M. (1970), 'Mechanisms responsible for plasma levels of nafcillin lower than those of oxacillin', *Arch. Intern. Med.*, **125**, 685.

Klein, J. O., Finland, M. and Wilcox, C. (1963), 'Nafcillin. Antibacterial action *in vitro* and absorption and excretion in normal young men', *Amer. J. Med. Sci.*, **246**, 10.

Lane, W. R. (1964), 'Nafcillin: A comparative *in vitro* trial', *Med. J. Aust.*, **2**, 499.

Line, D. E., Adler, S., Fraley, D. S. and Burns, F. J. (1976), 'Massive pseudoproteinuria caused by nafcillin', *JAMA*, **235**, 1259.

Markowitz, S. M., Rothkopf, M., Holden, F. D., Stith, D. M. and Duma, R. J. (1975), 'Nafcillin-induced agranulocytosis', *JAMA*, **232**, 1150.

Martin, C. M., Kushnick, T. H., Nuccio, P. A., Gray, D. F., Bernstein, I. and Webb, N. C. Jr. (1964), 'Controlled double-blind efficacy trial of penicillin, methicillin and nafcillin in 346 adults and children. II. Comparative clinical efficacy', *Antimicrob. Agents Chemother.*—1963, p. 290.

Parry, M. F., Ball, W. D., Conte, J. E. Jr. and Cohen, S. N. (1973), 'Nafcillin nephritis', *JAMA*, **225**, 178.

Ritchmond, A. S., Simberkoff, M. S., Schaefler, S. and Rahal, J. J. Jr. (1977), 'Resistance of Staphylococcus aureus to semisynthetic penicillin and cephalothin', *J. Infect. Dis.*, **135**, 108.

Rolinson, G. N. and Sutherland, R. (1965), 'The binding of antibiotics to serum proteins', *Brit. J. Pharmacol.*, **25**, 638.

Ruiz, D. E. and Warner, J. F. (1976), 'Nafcillin treatment of Staphylococcus aureus meningitis', *Antimicrob. Ag. Chemother.*, **9**, 554.

Sabath, L. D., Garner, C., Wilcox, C. and Finland, M. (1975), 'Effect of inoculum and of beta-lactamase on the anti-staphylococcal activity of thirteen penicillins and cephalosporins', *Antimicrob. Ag. Chemother.*, **8**, 344.

Sabath, L. D., Wheeler, N., Laverdiere, M., Blazevic, D. and Wilkinson, B. J. (1977), 'A new type of penicillin resistance of Staphylococcus aureus', *Lancet*, **1**, 443.

Sandberg, M., Tuazon, C. U. and Sheagren, J. M. (1975), 'Neutropenia probably resulting from nafcillin', *JAMA*, **232**, 1152.

Waisbren, B. A. (1970), 'Antibiotics in the treatment of burns', *Surg. Clin. North Amer.*, **50**, 1311.

Watanakunakorn, C. and Glotzbecker, C. (1977), 'Comparative *in vitro* activity of nafcillin, oxacillin and methicillin in combination with gentamicin and tobramycin against enterococci', *Antimicrob. Ag. Chemother.*, **11**, 88.

Watanakunakorn, C. (1977), 'Absorption of orally administered nafcillin in normal healthy volunteers', *Antimicrob. Ag. Chemother.*, **11**, 1007.

Whitehouse, A. C., Morgan, J. G., Schumacher, J. and Hamburger, M. (1963), 'Blood levels and anti-staphylococcal titers produced in human subjects by a penicillinase-resistant penicillin, nafcillin, compared with similar penicillins', *Antimicrob. Agents Chemother.*—1962, p. 384.

Wise, R. I. (1973), 'Modern management of severe staphylococcal disease', *Medicine*, **52**, 295.

Ampicillin

Description

Ampicillin (BRL 1341) is a semisynthetic penicillin derived from the penicillin nucleus (6-aminopenicillanic acid). The compound is chemically alpha-aminophenylacetamido-penicillanic acid (Rolinson and Stevens, 1961). It was discovered at the Beecham Research Laboratories, which markets it under the trade name of 'Penbritin'.

Sensitive Organisms

Ampicillin is active against most of the bacteria sensitive to penicillin G, but in addition it is active against some Gram-negative bacilli, which are penicillin G-resistant. Ampicillin has thus been referred to loosely as a 'broad spectrum penicillin', but this somewhat misleading term is better avoided.

1. *Gram-positive cocci.* Ampicillin is active against many of these such as Strep. pyogenes, Strep. pneumoniae and the alpha-haemolytic streptococci of the 'viridans' group. The still uncommon pneumococcal strains, which are relatively resistant to penicillin G (page 4), are usually completely sensitive to ampicillin (Hansman, 1976; Howes and Mitchell, 1976). The pneumococcal strains reported from South Africa, which are completely resistant to penicillin G (page 4), are either partially or completely ampicillin-resistant (Center for Disease Control, 1977b). Group B streptococci are always ampicillin-sensitive (Anthony and Concepcion, 1975; Bayer *et al.*, 1976); in addition ampicillin with gentamicin act synergistically against these organisms resulting in accelerated streptococcal killing (Shauf *et al.*, 1976). Anaerobic Gram-positive cocci such as the Peptococcus and Peptostreptococcus spp. and anaerobic streptococci are nearly always ampicillin-sensitive (Sutter and Finegold, 1976). Penicillin G remains the more active agent against all of the above organisms, but its superiority to ampicillin is not great.

Strep. faecalis is usually sensitive to ampicillin and often more so than to penicillin G (page 6). The combination of ampicillin with either streptomycin (page 294) or kanamycin (page 309) is synergistic against approximately 75 per cent of Strep. faecalis strains, whereas ampicillin plus gentamicin (page 329) is synergistic against all such strains. *In vitro* data indicate that ampicillin, combined with some of the newer aminoglycosides such as tobramycin (page 361), will also usually act synergistically against this organism (Iannini *et al.*, 1976).

Ampicillin is destroyed by staphylococcal penicillinase, so that most staphylococcal strains are ampicillin-resistant, just as they are to penicillin G (page 6).

99

2. *Gram-positive bacilli.* C. diphtheriae and B. anthracis are sensitive to ampicillin. Listeria monocytogenes is also usually sensitive, being more consistently sensitive to ampicillin than to penicillin G (Kalis *et al.*, 1976; Wiggins *et al.*, 1978). In addition, gentamicin acts synergistically with ampicillin against this organism (page 329). Most Nocardia asteroides strains are ampicillin-resistant (MIC 25 μg per ml or greater). However ampicillin acts synergistically with either the sulphonamides (Orfanakis *et al.*, 1972) or erythromycin (Bach *et al.*, 1973; Finland *et al.*, 1974) against many of these strains, a finding which may be of clinical importance.

Anaerobic Gram-positive sporing bacilli such as Clostridium tetani, Cl. perfringens (welchii), Cl. botulinum and other Clostridium spp. are nearly always ampicillin-sensitive. Ampicillin is also usually active against the anaerobic Gram-positive asporogenous bacilli such as the Actinomyces, Eubacterium, Arachnia, Propionibacterium, Bifidobacterium and Lactobacillus spp. (Sutter and Finegold, 1976).

3. *Enterobacteriaceae.* By contrast to penicillin G, ampicillin is active against some of these bacteria (Rolinson and Stevens, 1961; Stewart *et al.*, 1961). Esch. coli may be sensitive, but many strains are resistant. This is particularly so in hospitals where more than 50 per cent of Esch. coli strains may be ampicillin-resistant (Nyström, 1971; Yoshioka *et al.*, 1977). Ampicillin-resistant Esch. coli strains also occur in community acquired infections; in one study 18 per cent of patients on admission to hospital already carried these strains in their bowel (Søgaard, 1975). Ampicillin resistance of Esch. coli is always due to beta-lactamase production (Roupas and Pitton, 1974; Konforti and Halperin, 1975), and this may be either R plasmid or chromosomally mediated (*see* pages 104, 422).

Enterobacter, Klebsiella, Serratia, Citrobacter, Hafnia, Edwardsiella and Providencia spp. are nearly always ampicillin-resistant (Eickhoff *et al.*, 1966; Bear *et al.*, 1970). The Arizona spp. which cause human diseases similar to those produced by the salmonellae are usually ampicillin-sensitive (Johnson *et al.*, 1976). Similarly, Proteus mirabilis is usually sensitive unless it is a beta-lactamase producing strain. Other Proteus spp. are resistant. Yersinia enterocolitica is also usually ampicillin-resistant (Raevuori *et al.*, 1978).

The salmonellae are usually ampicillin-sensitive, but resistant strains, particularly of Salm. typhimurium have been reported (Winshell *et al.*, 1970; Bissett *et al.*, 1974; Grant *et al.*, 1976). In one large survey of 718 Salmonella strains isolated from humans, ampicillin resistance was detected in 36·9 per cent of Salm. typhimurium, 30·0 per cent Salm. heidelberg, 31·8 per cent Salm. newport, 13·6 per cent Salm. st. paul, 3·4 per cent Salm. infantis, and 0·9 per cent of Salm. enteritidis strains (Neu *et al.*, 1975a). These authors also tested 688 Salmonella isolations from animal sources and among these ampicillin-resistant Salm. typhimurium was less common (31·0 per cent), but the reverse was true for most of the other Salmonella spp. tested. During the 18 months ending June 1978, 194 Salmonella strains (other than Salm. typhi or paratyphi) were recovered from patients admitted to Fairfield Hospital, Melbourne with infective diarrhoea. Only 21 (10·8 per cent) were ampicillin-resistant, and all resistant strains belonged to Salm. typhimurium serotype. Resistance of salmonellae to ampicillin and other antibiotics is usually due to transferable drug resistance (*see* chloramphenicol, page 421).

Salmonella typhi is usually still susceptible to ampicillin. During the 1972 chloramphenicol-resistant typhoid fever epidemic in Mexico (page 423), when ampicillin was extensively used for treatment of the disease, a few Salm. typhi strains resistant to ampicillin as well as to chloramphenicol were isolated from patients (Olarte and Galindo, 1973). These resistant strains did not become widespread in Mexico at that time (page 423). Since then Salm. typhi strains resistant to both ampicillin and chloramphenicol have been encountered in South-East Asia and India (Lampe et al., 1975; Herzog, 1976), but they seem to be rare elsewhere (Chun et al., 1977; Barros et al., 1977).

Some Shigella spp. strains are sensitive to low ampicillin concentrations in vitro. Soon after the discovery of the drug, Sh. sonnei strains were reported which required at least 10 μg per ml for inhibition (Stewart, 1965). Other strains have shown complete ampicillin resistance. Subsequently in one survey of 1 102 Sh. sonnei strains in London, over 80 per cent were ampicillin-resistant (Davies et al., 1970). Studies in other countries initially showed a lower incidence of ampicillin-resistant Sh. sonnei and Sh. flexneri strains, e.g. 3·7 per cent in North America (Farrar and Eidson, 1971) and 14 per cent in Sweden (Urban, 1972). Thereafter in some areas of the United States ampicillin resistance among shigellae (mainly Sh. sonnei) rose to over 80 per cent (Ross et al., 1972; Tilton et al., 1972). These shigellae were also usually resistant to sulphonamides, streptomycin and tetracycline and this multiple resistance was usually R plasmid mediated. Resistance of Sh. sonnei to ampicillin is due to the production of a number of different beta-lactamases; this is mediated either by a chromosomal mutation, which gives a low level, non-transmissible resistance, or by an R plasmid, which gives high level transmissible resistance (Smith et al., 1974; Prince and Neu, 1976).

Recent surveys indicate that ampicillin resistance is more common with Sh. sonnei than Sh. flexneri. Neu et al. (1975b) investigated 102 Sh. sonnei and 14 Sh. flexneri strains isolated from patients in the New York City hospital. There was no ampicillin resistance among Sh. flexneri strains, but 60 per cent of Sh. sonnei strains were resistant. Byers et al. (1976) studied 113 Sh. sonnei and 56 Sh. flexneri strains isolated from patients in Houston, Texas; 7 per cent of Sh. flexneri and 55 per cent of Sh. sonnei isolates were ampicillin-resistant.

Shigella dysenteriae, type 1 (Shiga bacillus) causes the most severe form of Shigella dysentery. Isolation of ampicillin-resistant strains of this organism was first reported from Bangladesh (Rahaman et al., 1974). Between 1968 and 1970 there was an extensive epidemic of dysentery in Central America and a smaller one in Mexico. The Shiga bacillus strain responsible was resistant to chloramphenicol, tetracyclines, streptomycin and sulphonamides, but consistently sensitive to ampicillin. The first ampicillin-resistant Sh. dysenteriae, type 1 strain from this pandemic, was isolated from a six-year-old girl in Costa Rica (Center for Disease Control, 1974b). Subsequently Olarte et al. (1976) isolated ampicillin-resistant strains from another five children in a Mexico City hospital. As ampicillin has been extensively used for the treatment of Shiga dysentery in Central America and elsewhere, ampicillin-resistant Sh. dysenteriae, type 1 strains may become more widespread in the future. Ampicillin resistance of Sh. dysenteriae type 1 is R plasmid mediated; the ampicillin resistance determinants are carried on one plasmid, and the determinants for resistance to chloramphenicol, tetracycline, sulphonamides and streptomycin on another plasmid (Crosa *et al.*, 1977).

4. *Other Gram-negative aerobic bacteria.* Some of these such as N. meningitidis, B. pertussis and the Brucella spp. are ampicillin-sensitive and resistant strains among these have not been reported. Others such as Pseudomonas aeruginosa and Ps. pseudomallei are always highly ampicillin-resistant. N. gonorrhoeae is usually ampicillin-sensitive, but gonococcal strains relatively resistant to penicillin G (page 7) also show some but less marked resistance to ampicillin (Johnson *et al.*, 1970; Maier *et al.*, 1975; Watts *et al.*, 1977). By contrast penicillinase producing gonococcal strains (page 8), which have emerged more recently, are always completely ampicillin-resistant (Leading article, 1976c).

Haemophilus influenzae type b was considered to be always ampicillin-sensitive until 1974, when the initial reports of highly resistant strains (MIC often higher than 50 μg per ml) came from the United States of America. Resistant strains were isolated from the CSF of children with H. influenzae meningitis (Thomas *et al.*, 1974; Center for Disease Control, 1974a; Tomeh *et al.*, 1974) and also from the nasopharynx of healthy children (Schiffer *et al.*, 1974). In an early American survey of sixty H. influenzae type b strains, isolated from children with various diseases, ten per cent were ampicillin-resistant (Khan *et al.*, 1974). Subsequently these resistant strains were detected in geographically widespread areas in the United States (Nelson, 1974; Katz, 1975; Jacobson *et al.*, 1976). They were also reported from many other countries including Britain (Clymo and Harper, 1974; Kattan *et al.*, 1975; Fallon, 1976; Leading article, 1976a), Sweden (Biörklund *et al.*, 1975) and Australia (Gibbs *et al.*, 1975; Bell and Smith, 1975; Dorman and Kilham, 1976). Ampicillin-resistant H. influenzae type b has been isolated from children with septicaemia, meningitis, epiglottitis, otitis media and other severe childhood infections. Such strains are also isolated from the nasopharynx of healthy carriers of this organism. In addition more recent reports indicate that ampicillin-resistant strains of H. influenzae type b can emerge *in vivo* during a course of ampicillin treatment. Delage *et al.* (1977) described two children, one with septicaemia and the other with meningitis, from whom ampicillin-sensitive H. influenzae type b strains were isolated. Response to ampicillin therapy appeared good, but after cessation of treatment, the infections relapsed and then ampicillin-resistant strains of H. influenzae type b were isolated. Similarly Albritton *et al.* (1977) reported a nine-month-old boy who initially had meningitis due to an ampicillin-sensitive strain; an ampicillin-resistant strain of H. influenzae type b emerged in a subdural empyema following ampicillin treatment. In a 28-month-old boy reported by Granoff *et al.* (1978) osteomyelitis and septic arthritis developed during ampicillin therapy of H. influenzae meningitis. His meningitis was caused by an ampicillin-sensitive strain, but the bone and joint infection responded only after the therapy was changed to chloramphenicol.

Resistance of H. influenzae type b to ampicillin is mediated by an R plasmid (page 422), which codes for the production of beta lactamase (Medeiros and O'Brien, 1975; Catlin, 1975; Vega *et al.*, 1976; Eickhoff *et al.*, 1976). This beta-lactamase is of the TEM-type and it resembles beta-lactamases which are commonly produced by, and widely transferred amongst Gram-negative bacilli (Farrar and O'Dell, 1974; Medeiros and O'Brien, 1975). Transfer of ampicillin resistance from a resistant to a sensitive H. influenzae type b strain apparently by conjugation has been demonstrated *in vitro* (Thorne and Farrar, 1975). Resistance can also be transferred from an ampicillin-resistant H. influenzae type b to other organisms such as H. parainfluenzae, Esch. coli and Ps. aeruginosa (Eickhoff *et al.*, 1976; Saunders and Sykes, 1977).

Ampicillin-resistant H. influenzae type b strains are also highly resistant to penicillin G. They are more sensitive to carbenicillin (page 150) and ticarcillin (page 171) than to any other penicillin (Kattan *et al.*, 1975; Thornsberry *et al.*, 1976), but the MIC's of these drugs are higher against ampicillin-resistant strains (4–32 μg per ml), compared to those against ampicillin-sensitive organisms (0·25–1·0 μg per ml) (Kammer *et al.*, 1975). These strains are nearly always sensitive to chloramphenicol, erythromycin, rifampicin, gentamicin and less consistently to the tetracylines (Emerson *et al.*, 1975). They are also highly sensitive to co-trimoxazole (McGowan *et al.*, 1976). The older cephalosporins are relatively inactive against H. influenzae type b, but three newer compounds, cefamandole (page 269), cefuroxime (page 272) and cefoxitin (page 271) have good *in vitro* activity, comparable to that of chloramphenicol, against both ampicillin-sensitive and ampicillin-resistant strains (Kattan *et al.*, 1975; Kammer *et al.*, 1975; Leading article, 1976a). Ampicillin combined with chloramphenicol acts synergistically against a proportion of both ampicillin-sensitive and ampicillin-resistant H. influenzae strains (*see* page 425).

Non-typable strains of H. influenzae are pathogens in respiratory tract infection in adults. Otitis media in children may be caused either by these strains (Shurin *et al.*, 1976) or by H. influenzae type b (Crosson *et al.*, 1976). Ampicillin-resistant strains of these non-encapsulated H. influenzae have occasionally been isolated from the sputum of patients with chronic bronchitis (Stewart, 1974). They have also been isolated from children with otitis media (Shurin *et al.*, 1976; Syriopoulou *et al.*, 1976; Schwartz *et al.*, 1978). In a recent large survey of non-typable H. influenzae strains in Britain, 10 of 889 isolates were ampicillin-resistant (Howard *et al.*, 1978). These strains, similar to ampicillin-resistant H. influenzae type b, produce beta-lactamase (Syriopoulou *et al.*, 1976; Bysjö and Dornbusch, 1977; Malmvall and Branefors-Helander, 1978). Similarly beta-lactamase producing ampicillin-resistant strains of H. parainfluenzae have been detected (Mayo and McCarthy, 1977).

Most strains of Vibrio parahaemolyticus are ampicillin-resistant because they produce a beta-lactamase (Joseph *et al.*, 1978). The Legionnaires' disease bacterium is sensitive to ampicillin *in vitro* (MIC 0·25–2·0 μg per ml) (Thornsberry *et al.*, 1978). Campylobacter fetus is also usually sensitive (median MIC 1·8 μg per ml) (Chow *et al.*, 1978).

5. *Gram-negative anaerobic bacteria.* Some of these such as Bacteroides melaninogenicus and the Fusobacterium spp. are ampicillin-sensitive, but B. fragilis is usually resistant. Other Bacteroides spp. vary in sensitivity, but about 50 per cent of isolates are inhibited by low ampicillin concentrations (Sutter and Finegold, 1976).

6. Mycobacteria, Mycoplasmas and Rickettsiae are ampicillin-resistant.

7. *Gram-negative bacilli and ampicillin/cloxacillin.* The resistance of Gram-negative bacteria to ampicillin is partly intrinsic (due to a permeability barrier) and partly due to beta-lactamase production (*see* page 10). It was considered

that the beta-lactamase component may be partially overcome in some of these bacteria if cloxacillin is used in combination (Acred and Sutherland, 1967). Cloxacillin has no intrinsic activity against these bacteria but being stable in the presence of their enzymes, it might therefore prevent the destruction of ampicillin by binding some beta-lactamases. An ampicillin/cloxacillin combination did occasionally produce sufficient antibacterial activity in urine to inhibit some Gram-negative bacilli, including Ps. aeruginosa (Sabath *et al.*, 1967), but this effect was difficult to obtain in serum (Sabath *et al.*, 1970). This synergistic combination is now rarely used. It is not synergistic against the majority of Gram-negative bacilli, many of which produce different beta-lactamases, which have no affinity for cloxacillin. In about 80 per cent of ampicillin-resistant Esch. coli strains isolated from patients, enzyme production is R plasmid (page 422) mediated. These strains are highly resistant to ampicillin and carbenicillin, usually sensitive to cephalothin and do not show ampicillin/cloxacillin synergism. In the other 20 per cent of resistant Esch. coli, beta-lactamase production appears to be under the control of a chromosomal gene. These strains are only moderately ampicillin-resistant, they are carbenicillin-sensitive and cephalothin-resistant, and exhibit ampicillin/cloxacillin synergism. On theoretical grounds an ampicillin/cloxacillin combination may be useful for the treatment of urinary tract infections due to Esch. coli strains belonging to the second category (Roupas and Pitton, 1974).

　　8. *Clavulanic acid.* Certain Streptomyces spp. produce substances such as clavulanic acid which inhibit beta-lactamases. Clavulanic acid is a potent inhibitor of many beta-lactamases including those found in Esch. coli (plasmid-mediated), Kl. aerogenes, Pr. mirabilis and Staph. pyogenes. Beta-lactamases found in Ps. aeruginosa and Enterobacter cloacae and the chromosomally-mediated beta-lactamase of Esch. coli are less well inhibited (Reading and Cole, 1977). With most anaerobic bacteria such as Bacteroides spp., it is possible to reduce the MIC's of penicillin G and cephalothin to a susceptible level, by the addition of clavulanic acid in a concentration of 1–5 μg per ml. By contrast the MIC's of cefoxitin (page 271), an antibiotic which is resistant to the beta-lactamases of these bacteria, are not markedly influenced by clavulanic acid (Wüst and Wilkins, 1978). Wise *et al.* (1978) also demonstrated a marked decrease of the MIC's of penicillin G for Bacteroides fragilis strains in the presence of clavulanic acid, and the same effect was noted with beta-lactamase producing strains of N. gonorrhoeae. Beta-lactamase producing strains of Esch. coli, Klebsiella spp. and Pr. mirabilis also showed considerably increased susceptibility to amoxycillin (page 143) in combination with clavulanic acid, but enzyme producing strains of Ps. aeruginosa remained resistant to a carbenicillin/clavulanic acid combination.

　　It is therefore possible to use clavulanic acid with ampicillin or other beta-lactam antibiotics to render some beta-lactamase producing bacteria (Gram-negative and Gram-positive) nearly as sensitive to these antibiotics, as strains which do not produce enzymes (Hamilton-Miller, 1977; Wise, 1977). This only occurs with those bacterial species which produce beta-lactamases readily inhibited by clavulanic acid (*vide supra*). It may be practicable to use clavulanic acid together with beta-lactam antibiotics; clavulanic acid itself is a beta-lactam compound and its oral absorption in man is similar to that of amoxycillin page 136 (Hunter *et al.*, 1978). In a small clinical trial Ninane *et al.* (1978) administered a combination of amoxycillin 500 mg and clavulanic acid 250 mg orally three times a day, for three days to three anthracosilicotic coalminers, presenting with exacerbations of chronic bronchitis. The infecting organism was a beta-lactamase producing Branhamella (Neisseria) catarrhalis, and each patient improved with treatment. No side-effects from clavulanic acid were noted.

In Vitro Sensitivities

The minimum inhibitory concentrations of ampicillin against various bacteria are listed in Table 7.

TABLE 7

Compiled from data published by Rolinson and Stevens (1961), Stewart *et al.* (1961), Bass *et al.* (1969), Bear *et al.* (1970), Smith (1976), Sutter and Finegold (1976) and Schauf *et al.* (1976)

ORGANISM	MIC (μg per ml)
Gram-positive bacteria	
Staph. pyogenes (non-penicillinase producer)	0·05
Staph. pyogenes (pencillinase producer)	125·0
Strep. pyogenes (Group A)	0·05–0·1
Strep. pneumoniae (Dip. pneumoniae)	0·02–0·05
Streptococci, Group B	0·06
Strep. viridans spp.	0·04–1·6
Strep. faecalis (Enterococcus, Group D)	1·0–5·0
Listeria monocytogenes	0·08–0·32
Gram-negative bacteria	
Escherichia coli	5·0
Enterobacter spp.	250·0
Klebsiella pneumoniae	1·25
Proteus mirabilis	1·25
Proteus vulgaris	5·0
Salmonella typhi	0·25
Salmonella typhimurium	1·0–5·0
Shigella sonnei	1·0–10·0
Shigella flexneri	1·25
Neisseria gonorrhoeae	0·02–0·6
Neisseria meningitidis	0·05
H. influenzae (sensitive strains)	0·05
H. influenzae (resistant strains)	3·0–500·0
Bordetella pertussis	0·39–1·56
Brucella spp.	0·25–0·8
Pseudomonas aeruginosa	>250·0
Bacteroides fragilis	4·0–256·0
Bacteroides melaninogenicus	0·5–4·0

Mode of Administration and Dosage

1. *Oral administration.* Ampicillin is acid stable and can be given orally. The usual oral dose for mild to moderate infections is 50–100 mg per kg per day, given in four divided doses. A common adult dose is 500 mg six-hourly, though 250 mg six-hourly may suffice for mild infections due to highly susceptible organisms.

2. *Parenteral administration.* This drug in the form of the sodium salt can also be given either intramuscularly or intravenously. For serious infections high parenteral doses are often necessary. In children a daily dose of 150 mg per kg is commonly used (Mathies *et al.*, 1966), but up to 400 mg per kg per day has been occasionally given (Fleming *et al.*, 1967). In adults a dose as high as 20 g daily intravenously has been used to treat Strep. faecalis endocarditis (Parker and Hoeprich, 1966).

Intramuscularly, ampicillin is usually given every four to six hours, and it can be given intravenously either by intermittent injection or continuous infusion. For intravenous administration, similar to penicillin G (page 13) and methicillin (page 68), intermittent injections or intermittent infusions of high concentration ampicillin solutions via a minibottle or buretrol, are now commonly advocated. In one animal study ampicillin levels in tissue fibrin clots were higher when the drug was injected intermittently, than when the same total dose was given by continuous infusion (Barza *et al.*, 1974). Administration by intermittent injection has not been confirmed to be superior in clinical practice, but it obviates possible inactivation and incompatibilities when ampicillin is added to intravenous flasks for continuous infusion (Brodlie *et al.*, 1974).

Ampicillin is very unstable in concentrated solutions and should not be stored as such. The drug is more stable in dilute solutions (e.g. 500 mg in 500 ml), but this depends on many factors including the type of intravenous fluid used. Sodium ampicillin, an alkaline antibiotic, may raise the pH of the intravenous fluid to 8·0 or higher, and at this level ampicillin is slowly inactivated. For instance, in one study the pH of a Ringers lactate solution rose from 6·23 to 8·20 after the addition of ampicillin, and 70 per cent of the drug was inactivated at 37°C after 12 h (Wyatt *et al.*, 1972). In more acid intravenous fluids such as 5 per cent dextrose in water (pH about 4·7) ampicillin is more stable, but the pH of individual bottles of a particular intravenous solution may vary and other incompatible additives may also be present. Ampicillin is also inactivated at 37°C in amino acid solutions for intravenous use (Feigin *et al.*, 1973). For these reasons it is advisable to avoid adding ampicillin to intravenous flasks whenever possible, unless the above variables can be carefully controlled during the preparation of intravenous solutions containing additives.

3. *Newborn and premature infants.* In these patients a dose as low as 25 mg per kg body weight per day, given in two divided doses, is satisfactory when milder infections are treated (Boe *et al.*, 1967). For severe infections, 50 mg per kg per day in two equal doses is recommended for all infants under one week of age; between the ages of one to four weeks the dose for premature infants is 100 mg per kg per day and for full term infants 150 mg per kg per day, given in three equal doses in both instances (Kaplan *et al.*, 1974; McCracken, 1974).

After the age of one month the dose recommended for older children is used.

4. *Patients with renal failure.* Ampicillin is relatively non-toxic, and is often given in the usual doses to these patients, but if high parenteral doses are used, appropriate dosage reduction is necessary. In anuric patients the average plasma half-life for ampicillin is 8·5 h (*see* page 108), and it has been recommended that in patients with severe renal failure the total daily dose should be halved by giving the usual six-hourly dose every 12 h (Bennett *et al.*, 1970). A nine-fold increase in complications, mainly maculopapular rashes (page 110) has been observed in patients with severe renal failure treated by usual ampicillin doses (Lee and Hill, 1968). These authors suggest that 500 mg ampicillin daily is sufficient for patients with a creatinine clearance of 10 ml per min or less.

5. *Intraperitoneal administration.* Ampicillin can be safely added to peritoneal dialysis fluid; usually a dose of 50 mg is added to each litre of dialysate. A variable amount of the drug is absorbed from the peritoneal cavity and if this dialysate is used continuously, a steady serum ampicillin concentration of around 9 μg per ml is attained (Bulger *et al.*, 1965; Lee and Hill, 1968).

Availability

1. Capsules: 250 and 500 mg.
2. Paediatric tablets: 125 mg.
3. Syrup: 5 ml containing 125 mg or 250 mg.
4. Vials of 100 mg, 250 mg, 500 mg and 1 g suitable for intramuscular and intravenous administration.
5. *Ampiclox:* This is a 2:1 ampicillin/cloxacillin combination advertised for treatment or prophylaxis of neonatal infections. Neonatal oral drops when dispensed contain 60 mg ampicillin and 30 mg cloxacillin per 0·6 ml. Vials for injection contain 50 mg ampicillin and 25 mg cloxacillin. Infections in premature infants and neonates often require treatment before bacteriological data are available, and 'ampiclox' has been advocated for this situation. The addition of a penicillinase-resistant penicillin, cloxacillin, provides therapeutic cover against penicillin-resistant staphylococci for which ampicillin is ineffective. However many neonatal infections, especially serious hospital acquired ones, such as septicaemia are caused by ampicillin-resistant Gram-negative bacilli such as Klebsiella spp. etc. *In vitro* studies (Acred and Sutherland, 1967) have suggested that cloxacillin may render some of these organisms ampicillin-sensitive, but there is little clinical evidence that this synergic combination will be effective in severe systemic infections (page 104). This preparation may therefore be useful for mild neonatal infections, but should not be used for treatment of infections of a more serious nature.

Serum Levels in Relation to Dosage

After oral administration of ampicillin to adults, peak serum concentrations are obtained at about two hours, and the drug is still detectable in the serum at six hours (Fig. 6). Doubling the dose virtually doubles the serum concentration (Knudsen *et al.*, 1961). The oral absorption of this drug, although initially reported to be good even if taken with food (Bear *et al.*, 1970), is significantly impaired when it is administered with meals (*see* page 136). Ampicillin is absorbed normally in patients with coeliac disease (Parsons *et al.*, 1975).

With intramuscular administration, a much higher peak level is achieved within 30 min (Fig. 6). Ampicillin, compared to penicillin G, produces considerably higher serum levels after parenteral administration; this is chiefly due to its slower renal clearance (Tuano *et al.*, 1966; Kirby and Kind, 1967).

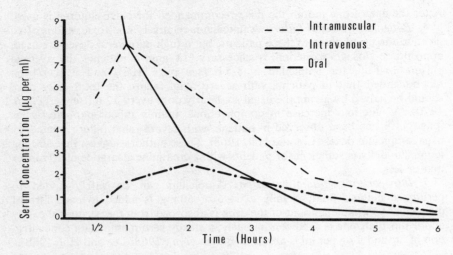

FIG. 6. Comparative serum levels of ampicillin after 0·5 g with three routes of administration. (Redrawn after Kirby and Kind, 1967.)

In newborn and premature infants after an intramuscular dose of 10 mg per kg, a peak serum level of about 20 μg per ml is reached one hour after injection. With a dose of 25 mg per kg, the peak level is approximately 60 μg per ml. Detectable serum levels persist for at least 12 h after injection. The serum half-life of ampicillin in infants declines with increasing postnatal age; it is 4 h in infants aged 2–7 days, 2·8 h in those aged 8–14 days and 1·7 h in infants 15–30 days of age (Axline *et al.*, 1967; McCracken, 1974).

In pregnant women ampicillin serum levels are significantly lower than in the same women after pregnancy. This difference appears to be mainly due to increased volumes of plasma and body water during pregnancy resulting in an increase in the drug's distribution volume. In addition, during pregnancy the renal plasma clearance of ampicillin is increased. It has therefore been suggested that pregnant women may require higher doses of ampicillin per kg body weight compared to non-pregnant patients (Philipson, 1977).

Excretion

URINE: Some 30 per cent of an oral dose of ampicillin is excreted in urine during the first six hours. High concentrations of the active drug are attained in urine; after a 500 mg oral dose urinary concentrations range from 250 to 1000 μg per ml (Knudsen *et al.*, 1961). Ampicillin is excreted partly by glomerular filtration and partly by tubular secretion. Probenecid slows excretion by partial blockage of tubular secretion (*see* penicillin G, page 17). After parenteral administration, about 75 per cent of the dose is excreted in urine. Compared to penicillin G, ampicillin is cleared at a slower rate by the kidney, and its serum half-life in normal adults is 1·5 h, compared to 0·5 h for penicillin G (page 16). Therefore the action of probenecid in lowering renal clearance and elevating serum levels is more marked with penicillin G (Kirby and Kind, 1967; Bennett *et al.*, 1974).

BILE: Ampicillin is also excreted unchanged in bile, and animal studies show that its biliary concentration may be 300 times higher than in blood (Brown and Acred, 1961). However in patients with T-tube drainage after cholecystectomy, only 0·1 per cent of an intravenous or oral dose of ampicillin is excreted via the bile. In these patients biliary concentrations varied from 0·4 to 6·5 μg per ml during a 12 h period after an oral ampicillin dose of 0·5 g (Pinget et al., 1976). These concentrations are higher than the MIC's of ampicillin against highly susceptible pathogens (page 105). Some of the drug excreted in the bile is reabsorbed from the gut, but recycling through the liver is probably only a minor factor in maintaining serum levels (Kirby and Kind, 1967). Data on biliary excretion, obtained from studies on animals and on patients with free biliary drainage, are not wholly applicable to patients with obstructive biliary tract disease. For instance, ampicillin concentrations obtained in a non-functioning gall bladder are low, and therapeutic levels are only present in the common bile duct if it is not obstructed (Mortimer et al., 1969).

INACTIVATION IN BODY: Unexcreted ampicillin appears to be chiefly inactivated in the liver. It is inactivated at a slower rate than penicillin G, and in anuric patients, the average serum half-life for ampicillin is 8·5 h compared to four hours for penicillin G (Kirby and Kind, 1967).

Distribution of the Drug in Body

Ampicillin has been shown to be evenly distributed throughout body tissues by animal studies. With the exception of kidney and liver, tissue concentrations are lower than simultaneous serum levels (Stewart, 1965). In healthy human kidney the intrarenal tissue concentration is about eight-fold higher than the concomitant serum level. By contrast, the ampicillin concentration in chronic glomerulonephritic kidneys is only about half the serum level at the time. In such severe kidney disease, urinary concentration of ampicillin is greatly reduced, and the serum rather than urinary concentration more closely reflects the ampicillin renal tissue level (Whelton et al., 1972).

Adequate ampicillin concentrations are attained in septic joint effusions (Nelson, 1971) and in ascitic fluid of patients with ascites and bacterial peritonitis (Gerding et al., 1977). Ampicillin penetrates poorly into bronchial secretions, though this penetration may be increased two- to three-fold in the presence of inflammation and marked sputum purulence. In bronchial secretions from patients with moderate pulmonary infection, the ampicillin concentration is usually only about 10 per cent of the simultaneous serum level (Wong et al., 1975). Peak interstitial tissue fluid concentrations of ampicillin are lower than those attained in serum, but the drug persists in tissue fluid for a longer period of time. There is no evidence of accumulation of this antibiotic in tissue fluid with repeated doses (Chisholm et al., 1973). Ampicillin is usually undetectable in saliva, sweat and tears (Philipson et al., 1975).

Only minute amounts of ampicillin can be detected in normal CSF, but in patients with bacterial meningitis higher levels occur. In such patients following a parenteral dose of 150 mg per kg per day, a mean CSF ampicillin level of 2·9 μg per ml was detected during the first three days of treatment, but this level fell during convalescence (Thrupp et al., 1966). However these CSF ampicillin levels bore no relation to the clinical outcome.

The drug crosses the placenta. In pregnant women given an oral dose of 500 mg six-hourly, ampicillin levels in amniotic fluid at delivery range from $0 \cdot 42$ to $4 \cdot 1$ μg per ml. Concentrations found in cord blood are lower, being in the range of $0 \cdot 24 - 2 \cdot 0$ μg per ml (Blecher et al., 1966). However the drug does not reach therapeutic concentrations in amniotic fluid during the first trimester (Wasz-Höckert et al., 1970).

The binding of ampicillin to serum proteins (18 per cent) is the lowest of all the penicillins (Rolinson and Sutherland, 1965).

Mode of Action

Ampicillin has an action similar to penicillin G (see page 19). Its differences in antibacterial spectrum compared to penicillin G can probably be explained by its greater ability to penetrate the outer membrane of the cell wall of some Gram-negative bacilli (see page 20). Ampicillin may also be less susceptible to inactivation by some of the beta-lactamases produced by these organisms (see pages 20, 422).

Toxicity

1. *Rashes and allergic reactions*. Ampicillin may be 'cross-allergenic' with other penicillins, and in sensitized patients it may evoke any of the hypersensitivity reactions caused by penicillin G (page 24). Patients allergic to penicillin G do not always react to ampicillin, but because of this possibility ampicillin is contraindicated in such patients. There may be rare exceptions to this, such as when ampicillin is the drug of choice for the treatment of a severe infection. Thus Petheram and Boyce (1976) used intravenous ampicillin plus gentamicin successfully for the treatment of Strep. faecalis endocarditis in a penicillin-allergic patient; prednisolone and an antihistamine were administered concomitantly and full resuscitation facilities were immediately available.

Rashes due to ampicillin are more common than with other penicillins, but most of these may not be due to true penicillin hypersensitivity (*vide infra*). In one large survey the risk of an ampicillin rash was estimated as $7 \cdot 7$ per cent, compared to $2 \cdot 7$ per cent with other penicillins (Shapiro et al., 1969). A multicentre prospective study of 933 patients treated with ampicillin, showed that $7 \cdot 3$ per cent developed rashes (Report, 1973). More recently the Boston Collaborative Drug Surveillance Program detected a somewhat lower occurrence of rashes ($5 \cdot 2$ per cent of 2988 patients), but other possible causes of rashes in ampicillin-treated patients were more carefully excluded (Arndt and Jick, 1976). The frequency of these rashes may be related to the dose of the drug used (Leading article, 1972b; McHardy and Schonell, 1972; Bass et al., 1973; Report, 1973). About 20 per cent of patients developed a rash when large doses of ampicillin were used for treatment of salmonella infections (Sleet et al., 1964). Also rashes are more common in patients with renal failure treated by usual ampicillin doses, which result in high serum concentrations of the drug (Lee and Hill, 1968).

Ampicillin rashes are not always urticarial, but may be macular eruptions resembling measles or rubella. They frequently appear four to five days after starting therapy (Stevenson and Mandal, 1966), usually without other associated signs of allergy, and they may intensify, but often subside if treatment is continued (Stewart, 1969; Kerns et al., 1973). Patients with macular rashes have negative skin tests to ampicillin and to the major and minor penicillin antigenic determinants (Kerns et al., 1973) (see also penicillin G, page 23). These rashes appear to be 'ampicillin-specific' and do not indicate true penicillin hypersensitivity (Annotation, 1969; Leading article, 1975). They may be toxic rather than allergic in nature (Leading article, 1972b; Report, 1973). An allergic mechanism may exist, because some brands of ampicillin appear to cause rashes more often than others (Shapiro et al., 1969). Protein impurities have been reported to exist in commercial ampicillin preparations; the frequency of macular rashes appeared to be reduced in patients treated with a 'purified ampicillin' (Knudsen et al., 1970). However, contrary to these findings by Beecham Research Laboratories, this protein impurity could not be detected in eight different samples of ampicillin produced by Bristol Laboratories in America (Fardig et al., 1970). Most penicillins, especially ampicillin, may readily polymerize in solution to produce complex polymers of high molecular weight (Stewart, 1969; Leading article, 1975). These polymers appear to be responsible for some ampicillin rashes (see also penicillin G, page 24). A polymer-free ampicillin has been prepared; this has been used to treat infections in eight patients with chronic lymphatic leukaemia and in two others with lymphosarcoma. Only one patient developed a rash, whereas the frequency of ampicillin rashes in patients with these underlying diseases is usually much higher (Parker and Richmond, 1976) (vide infra).

Rashes are very common in patients with glandular fever who are given ampicillin. A small percentage of glandular fever patients develop a rash without a history of prior drug therapy, but it has been estimated that 65–95 per cent of them will develop a rash if they are given ampicillin (Pullen et al., 1967; Brown and Kanwar, 1967; Lund and Bergan, 1975). In the eight-year period 1968–1976, 1134 patients with glandular fever were admitted to Fairfield Hospital, Melbourne and 77 (6·8 per cent) had a rash associated with prior ampicillin administration. These figures indicate that ampicillin is frequently prescribed for pharyngitis, a condition for which other forms of penicillin are preferable (page 31). This 'sensitivity' to ampicillin of patients with glandular fever appears to be temporary, because ampicillin skin tests become negative and rashes do not recur if they are given ampicillin when they have recovered from the disease (Nazareth et al., 1972; Lund and Bergan, 1975). The glandular fever-like disease due to cytomegalovirus also predisposes patients to ampicillin rashes (Klemola, 1970). The risk of developing an ampicillin rash is very high (90 per cent) in patients with lymphatic leukaemia (Leading article, 1972b), and it seems to be increased in those with reticulosarcoma and other lymphomas (Potter, 1972). Because of these associations, ampicillin rashes may be due to a 'toxic' mechanism associated with the presence of abnormal lymphocytes, rather than due to hypersensitivity (Leading article, 1972b). Interestingly, these rashes are more common if the drug is given for a viral rather than a bacterial infection, and they are overall more common in females (Report, 1973). An increased rate of ampicillin rashes has been reported in patients with hyperuricaemia receiving concurrent allopurinol therapy (A Report, 1972).

It is clear that ampicillin has a greater predilection to cause rashes than other penicillins, but this is due to a greater prevalence of rashes of the benign macular variety, which are unrelated to true penicillin allergy. Thus the occurrence of an ampicillin rash during or after treatment is not currently considered in itself a contraindication to future treatment with one of the penicillins (Report, 1973).

Ampicillin can cause serious allergic reactions such as anaphylaxis and urticaria, but the frequency of these is probably no higher than with other penicillins (Shapiro *et al.*, 1969; Leading article, 1975).

2. *Gastro-intestinal side-effects*. Oral or less commonly parenteral ampicillin therapy can cause nausea and diarrhoea, but these are usually not serious (Bass *et al.*, 1973). In one study of children, the severity of diarrhoea was such that 8 per cent of all orally and 3 per cent of all intravenously treated patients required discontinuation of ampicillin or the use of anti-diarrhoea drugs (Phillips *et al.*, 1976). Ampicillin-induced diarrhoea appeared to be more common in younger children. In adults, diarrhoea may occur in 5–20 per cent of treated patients and is probably more common in older age groups (Robertson *et al.*, 1977; Gurwith *et al.*, 1977; Lusk *et al.*, 1977).

A more severe complication is pseudomembranous colitis. This occurs more commonly with lincomycin or clindamycin therapy (page 481), but ampicillin can also cause the same illness with the characteristic endoscopic appearance of the rectal mucosa (Keating *et al.*, 1974; Read and Cove-Smith, 1977). In one large co-operative study, diarrhoea was noted in 62 (18 per cent) of 343 clindamycin-treated patients, but only in 16 (5 per cent) of 315 ampicillin-treated patients. Pseudomembranous colitis occurred in 7 (2 per cent) of the clindamycin-treated patients, but only in one (0·3 per cent) of those treated by ampicillin (Gurwith *et al.*, 1977). Similarly in the series reported by Lusk *et al.* (1977), clindamycin therapy was associated with diarrhoea in 30 per cent of patients and pseudomembranous colitis in 1·9 per cent, while ampicillin caused diarrhoea in 17 per cent and pseudomembranous colitis in only 0·7 per cent.

Moniliasis, which sometimes can be a problem, may also be caused by ampicillin therapy, but this complication, as in the case of tetracyclines (page 613), is usually not a causative factor in ampicillin-induced diarrhoea.

3. *Nephropathy*. One case of interstitial nephritis, which immediately followed a small dose of ampicillin, has been reported (Tannenberg *et al.*, 1971). Azotaemia did not occur in this patient, but the other clinical, histological and immunological features were similar to those of methicillin nephritis (page 72). Maxwell *et al.* (1974) reported another patient with ampicillin-induced interstitial nephritis in whom the large dose of the drug used (200 mg per kg per day) was a probable factor. Lee and Hill (1968) observed three patients with renal failure, who, following a severe cutaneous ampicillin reaction, developed further permanent deterioration in renal function. These authors postulated that an ampicillin-induced interstitial nephritis may have occurred as part of an overall hypersensitivity reaction. Two other patients have been described who developed acute renal failure due to interstitial nephritis in association with a hypersensitivity reaction to ampicillin (Ruley and Lisi, 1974; Woodroffe *et al.*, 1975).

Crystalluria has been observed in patients treated with large doses of ampicillin intravenously (Potter *et al.*, 1971). It appears that high urinary ampicillin levels and an acid urine (pH 5) favour crystallization of this drug. The site of crystal formation is unknown, but it may well be intrarenal, as concentration and acidification of urine occurs in the distal tubule. It is uncertain whether nephrotoxicity is associated with ampicillin crystalluria.

4. *Haematological side-effects.* Agranulocytosis with monohistiocytosis has been described in one patient in association with ampicillin therapy (Graf and Tarlov, 1968). The authors noted that ampicillin contains an alpha-aminobenzene, a structure common to many drugs previously implicated as causes of agranulocytosis. If there is a causal relationship between ampicillin and this complication, it must be exceedingly rare. Severe acute thrombocytopenia with bleeding occurred in one patient receiving ampicillin, and no other causal agents could be implicated (Brooks, 1974). With high doses of ampicillin there is also tendency for red cells to become coated with the drug, and it is possible that a Coombs positive haemolytic anaemia may be a sequel as with penicillin G (*see* page 29).

5. *Encephalopathy.* Cerebral irritation with convulsions may be anticipated with very large doses of intravenous ampicillin, particularly if serum levels reach 800 μg per ml (Knudsen, 1970).

6. *Elevated serum aspartate aminotransferase (SGOT) levels.* These have been reported after intramuscular ampicillin. Knirsch and Gralla (1970) consider that this may be due to muscle irritation rather than hepatotoxicity.

7. *Benign intracranial hypertension.* Bhowmick (1972) described one patient with this complication, who had severe headache and papilloedema, which was apparently provoked by ampicillin and then perpetuated by tetracycline therapy (*see also* page 621).

8. *Drug interactions.* Ampicillin can impair the absorption of oral contraceptives; treatment with ampicillin may occasionally result in breakthrough bleeding or pregnancy in patients who are reliable oral contraceptive users. In addition, in pregnant women ampicillin decreases the amount of urinary oestriol excretion, but levels of oestrogens in the blood are largely unaffected. The reason for this is that ampicillin interferes with the normal enterohepatic circulation of oestrogens; oestrogen conjugates normally excreted in the bile are not hydrolysed by intestinal bacteria, reconjugated and absorbed. These changes have no effect on the pregnancy, but are important when interpreting urinary oestriol levels as an index of fetoplacental function (Roberton and Johnson, 1976).

Clinical Uses of the Drug

1. *Urinary tract infections.* Acute and uncomplicated urinary tract infections caused by Esch. coli and in particular by Pr. mirabilis usually respond to ampicillin (Kennedy et al., 1963). The drug is also useful for the treatment of Strep. faecalis infections. High concentrations of ampicillin are attained in urine (page 108), and treatment is sometimes successful despite the demonstration of *in vitro* resistance of the causative organism. Treatment of patients with chronic bacteriuria or underlying renal disease is often unsuccessful, because they either relapse or become re-infected with ampicillin-resistant bacteria such as Klebsiella or Enterobacter spp. (Turck, 1967).

Ampicillin is safe for treatment of urinary tract infections during pregnancy (Kincaid-Smith, 1964). It is also suitable for the treatment of urinary tract infections in patients with renal failure, including those with severely impaired renal function, in whom adequate ampicillin levels are not attained in the urine (Lee and Hill, 1968). In such patients ampicillin serum levels are usually high, and resultant renal parenchymal tissue concentrations may be about half of those existing in the serum (see page 109). Ampicillin may also be used prophylactically for prolonged periods in patients with chronic or recurrent urinary tract infections, but it should be avoided in patients with neurogenic bladders, especially females, because of the likelihood of Monilia infections (Slade, 1977).

2. *Septicaemia due to Gram-negative bacilli*. Some patients with septicaemia due to ampicillin-sensitive strains of Pr. mirabilis or Esch. coli, can be successfully managed by large doses of ampicillin parenterally. However treatment with ampicillin alone, prior to sensitivity testing of the causative organism, is inadvisable (Parker and Hoeprich, 1966; Steigbigel *et al.*, 1967). Ampicillin is commonly used for the treatment of suspected neonatal septicaemia, as it is active against Group B streptococci, Listeria monocytogenes, Strep. faecalis and Pr. mirabilis. In this clinical situation it is usually combined with either kanamycin (page 317), gentamicin (page 343) or one of the newer aminoglycosides (pages 368, 387) to provide cover for ampicillin-resistant Gram-negative bacilli such as Esch. coli, Klebsiella spp. and Ps. aeruginosa (Kaplan *et al.*, 1974; McCracken and Eichenwald, 1974).

3. *Typhoid fever and other salmonella infections*. In recent years strains of Salm. typhi resistant to chloramphenicol and sometimes also to ampicillin have been detected, but this is not yet a world wide problem (pages 101, 423). If sensitive strains are involved, ampicillin is not as effective as chloramphenicol for the treatment of typhoid fever; defervescence is slower and some severe cases even fail to respond to ampicillin whilst response to chloramphenicol is uniformly good (Scioli *et al.*, 1964; Patel, 1964; Sanders, 1965; Manriquez *et al.*, 1965; Snyder *et al.*, 1976). In addition, positive stool cultures persist substantially longer in ampicillin treated patients, compared to those treated by chloramphenicol (Snyder *et al.*, 1976). Chloramphenicol is also superior to ampicillin for the treatment of paratyphoid fever, even when relatively large doses of ampicillin (6 g per day in adults) are used (Sleet *et al.*, 1964). Occasional studies, however, have shown ampicillin to be equally effective to chloramphenicol (Mikhail *et al.*, 1972; Hoffman *et al.*, 1975). In addition, in one study chloramphenicol and ampicillin together were superior to chloramphenicol alone in the treatment of this disease (De Ritis *et al.*, 1972). Nevertheless, in most parts of the world, chloramphenicol (page 440) is preferred to ampicillin for the treatment of typhoid and paratyphoid fevers.

The emergence of Salm. typhi strains relatively or completely resistant to chloramphenicol (page 423) posed new problems. Most patients infected with these strains responded to ampicillin (Overturf *et al.*, 1973) or to a combination of ampicillin and chloramphenicol (page 440). Co-trimoxazole (page 711) is also suitable for such patients, and this combination appears to be the only available treatment if the Salm. typhi strain is resistant to both chloramphenicol and ampicillin (Center for Disease Control, 1973; Herzog, 1976). It is possible that either ampicillin or co-trimoxazole may become increasingly necessary for the treatment of typhoid fever in certain parts of the world.

For the treatment of septicaemia due to other Salmonella spp., chloramphenicol is preferred to ampicillin. Treatment failures with ampicillin have been reported (Parker and Hoeprich, 1966), and ampicillin-resistant salmonellae, particularly Salm. typhimurium, are now common in all parts of the world (page 100). In Salmonella gastro-enteritis, ampicillin (or any other antibiotic) is not of any clinical benefit, either for the treatment of the disease or for the resultant asymptomatic salmonella carrier state (Leading article, 1969; Kazemi et al., 1973). The life-long Salm. typhi carrier state is a different problem, and some success has been reported by using large doses of ampicillin plus probenecid for one to three months or longer (Christie, 1964; Whitby, 1964; Simon and Miller, 1966; Phillips, 1971). In carriers who have gallstones the best results are obtained by a combination of biliary surgery and prolonged ampicillin administration (Dinbar et al., 1969). Short-term chemotherapy with ampicillin or another suitable antibiotic is also advisable in all typhoid or paratyphoid carriers undergoing biliary surgery to prevent possible acute exacerbations of these chronic infections. Despite reported successes, treatment aimed at eradicating the carrier state of Salm. typhi is still unsatisfactory. Some carriers remain refractory to all forms of treatment and results must be critically assessed over a prolonged period, because some subjects are intermittent excretors, and clearance of the faeces may only be temporary. It appears that patients who are regularly followed, and who do not excrete typhoid bacilli within two years after stopping ampicillin, are probably cured of their typhoid carrier state (Johnson et al., 1973).

4. *Shigella infections.* Shigella sonnei dysentery is often an acute self-limiting disease, for which rehydration is the most important measure. Ampicillin treatment in these cases often appears of doubtful value; possibly the clinical status, as well as the social and physical environment of the patient, should be taken into consideration when deciding whether to use this drug (Weissman et al., 1974). Several authors have reported clinical benefit from ampicillin in shigellosis, both in milder cases treated as out-patients (Haltalin et al., 1972), and in severe Shigella flexneri infections in hospitalized children (Howard and Riley, 1965; Haltalin et al., 1967). Another study demonstrated that diarrhoea and fever subsided more rapidly in children treated with ampicillin, compared to a neomycin treated group (Haltalin et al., 1968). Parenteral ampicillin has been recommended for severely ill children with shigellosis (Haltalin et al., 1969). The drug also appears to reduce the duration of faecal excretion of organisms (McCracken and Eichenwald, 1974). Ampicillin has been extensively used for the treatment of dysentery due to Shigella dysenteriae type 1 (Shiga bacillus), especially during a large Central American pandemic (Olarte et al., 1976).

Owing to the emergence of ampicillin-resistant strains among all Shigella spp. in various parts of the world (page 101), this drug may become unsuitable for the treatment of shigellosis. Co-trimoxazole (page 713) is probably the best alternative.

5. *Respiratory tract infections.* Ampicillin is satisfactory for treatment of pneumonia (A Co-operative Controlled Trial, 1966), but should not be used alone for life-threatening forms of this disease, in which the bacteriological aetiology cannot be immediately determined. Ampicillin is also ineffective for mycoplasma pneumonia. In chronic bronchitis, ampicillin appears to be as effective as the tetracyclines (Malone et al., 1968). Ampicillin is frequently

prescribed for children with respiratory tract infections, such as bronchiolitis and croup, which are primarily viral in aetiology. This may be useful in selected severe cases to treat or prevent secondary infection by common bacterial pathogens, such as pneumococci and H. influenzae.

Ampicillin should not be used for acute tonsillitis, which is usually due to Strep. pyogenes infection; penicillin G or one of the phenoxypenicillins are the preferred drugs (Pullen et al., 1967). This is because ampicillin has a greater potential to cause rashes, particularly if the diagnosis of glandular fever is overlooked (page 111).

6. *Otitis media and sinusitis.* For otitis media in adults, penicillin G (page 33) is the drug of choice as pneumococci are the most frequent pathogens. In children, in addition to pneumococci, H. influenzae (mainly non-typable strains) are also frequently involved (Coffey, 1968; Leading article, 1976b), and therefore ampicillin is the drug of choice in this age group (Bosso and Jackman, 1977). If infection by ampicillin-resistant H. influenzae strains is suspected or confirmed, then either co-trimoxazole (page 709) or erythromycin (page 507) may be used (Schwartz et al., 1978). Acute sinusitis in both adults and children is usually caused by pneumococci, so that penicillin G therapy is indicated. Acute ethmoiditis in infants and young children may be caused by H. influenzae, and in these cases ampicillin is recommended (McCracken and Eichenwald, 1974). Ampicillin-resistant H. influenzae strains however may be encountered (page 102).

7. *Pertussis.* Ampicillin may be useful for the treatment and prevention of secondary pulmonary infection in this disease. The main factor in reducing the once large mortality in pertussis has probably been the use of antibiotics to prevent and treat bronchopneumonia, particularly in young babies (Bennett, 1973). Ampicillin, similar to other antibiotics, does not shorten the clinical course of pertussis itself. Erythromycin, oxytetracycline and chloramphenicol eliminate B. pertussis within a few days (presumably rendering patients noninfectious), whereas ampicillin treated patients have positive cultures for periods comparable to those of untreated patients (Bass et al., 1969). For this reason some authors regard erythromycin (page 508) as the drug of choice for treatment of patients with pertussis (Bass, 1973).

8. *Bacterial meningitis.* Haemophilus influenzae type b meningitis in children has been successfully treated by using large doses (150 mg per kg per day) of parenteral ampicillin (Mathies et al., 1966; Barrett et al., 1966). Higher doses of up to 400 mg per kg per day have been used (Fleming et al., 1967), but an intravenous dose of 150–200 mg per day given in six divided doses appeared satisfactory for most patients. The drug has also been given intravenously for the first five days only and then followed by intramuscular administration of the same dose (Wilson and Haltalin, 1975). Some authors have found ampicillin to be equally effective to chloramphenicol (page 441) for the treatment of this disease (Barrett et al., 1972; Feigin et al., 1976; Lindberg et al., 1977). Others have noted that in ampicillin treated patients the duration of fever is prolonged (Schulkind et al., 1971), bacteriological responses are slower and some bacteriological relapses occur, by comparison with the uniformly good results obtained with chloramphenicol (Shackelford et al., 1972). The better penetration of chloramphenicol into the CSF may be a factor responsible for these differences (Smith, 1972). Furthermore, there were single case reports

in which ampicillin treatment for H. influenzae meningitis had failed (Greene, 1968; Gold et al., 1969; Coleman et al., 1969). In one patient relapse occurred following a change from parenteral to oral ampicillin administration (Cherry and Sheenan, 1968).

Since 1974 a more serious doubt has been cast on the role of ampicillin in the treatment of H. influenzae meningitis. Ampicillin-resistant strains of H. influenzae have been isolated in many parts of the world (page 102), and a number of patients with meningitis have been reported in whom ampicillin therapy was ineffective because of this resistance (Khan et al., 1974; Tomeh et al., 1974). In one nine-month-old boy a subdural empyema developed which contained ampicillin-resistant H. influenzae. He had presented initially with an ampicillin-sensitive H. influenzae type b meningitis and was treated by ampicillin (Albritton et al., 1977) (see also page 102).

For the above reasons chloramphenicol is the preferred antibiotic for the treatment of H. influenzae meningitis at Fairfield Hospital and in many other units throughout the world. Other clinicians, particularly in North America, have regarded ampicillin as the drug of choice for this disease. For those who still prefer to use ampicillin for the treatment of H. influenzae meningitis, it has been recommended that initially a combination therapy with either penicillin G/chloramphenicol or ampicillin/chloramphenicol should be used, and only when H. influenzae type b is isolated and its sensitivity to ampicillin confirmed, should ampicillin be continued as a single drug (Nelson, 1974; Committee, 1975; Katz, 1975; Smith, 1976; Barkin et al., 1976).

Ampicillin has also been used for the chemoprophylaxis of H. influenzae meningitis. This may be warranted in special circumstances, for instance if an outbreak of the disease occurs in a crowded institution, and the strain is ampicillin-sensitive. Co-trimoxazole has also been used for this purpose (page 714). Otherwise outbreaks of H. influenzae meningitis are unusual and routine antibiotic prophylaxis for contacts is not advocated (Center for Disease Control, 1977a; Ward et al., 1978). Oral ampicillin therapy also does not always eradicate the carrier state of this organism (Glode et al., 1976; Ginsburg et al., 1977).

Ampicillin is effective against pneumococci and meningococci, the two other major causes of bacterial meningitis; therefore it was advocated as a single agent for the initial treatment of unidentified meningitis in children over two months of age (Yow et al., 1973). Apart from the possibility of ampicillin-resistant strains of H. influenzae, this drug may also not be effective against the small percentage of cases of meningitis due to some other bacteria. Staphylococcal meningitis, although rare, may occur in all age groups (Bennett and Kucers, 1970), and therefore it is unwise to rely on ampicillin alone for initial therapy of bacterial meningitis (see page 441).

Ampicillin, although not the drug of choice, is quite effective for pneumococcal meningitis, provided that large doses are given (Hassan et al., 1976). It may prove of value for cases caused by the still uncommon relatively penicillin G-resistant pneumococcal strains (Howes and Mitchell, 1976) (see also pages 4, 99).

9. *Other severe H. influenzae type b infections.* Ampicillin given in high doses parenterally may be quite effective in epiglottitis, osteomyelitis, septic arthritis, cellulitis, pneumonia or septicaemia (McCracken and Eichenwald,

1974; Nade *et al.*, 1974). Nevertheless, for severe and especially life-threatening infections due to this organism we recommend chloramphenicol (page 442). If ampicillin is selected for severely ill patients, initial treatment with either penicillin G/chloramphenicol or ampicillin/chloramphenicol, as in the case of meningitis (*vide supra*), is necessary, until the sensitivity of the H. influenzae type b strain is determined.

10. *Listeria monocytogenes infections.* Ampicillin is probably the best drug for the treatment of listeria infections, penicillin G (page 33) being less consistently effective (Kalis *et al.*, 1976). It has been used with success to treat listeria meningitis (Macnair *et al.*, 1968; Lavetter *et al.*, 1971), and it also appears valuable for treatment of listeriosis in the neonatal age group (Gordon *et al.*, 1970; McCracken and Eichenwald, 1974; Visintine *et al.*, 1977).

11. *Bacterial endocarditis.* Ampicillin is more active than penicillin G against most strains of Strep. faecalis, and it has been used successfully in large parenteral doses as a single drug for treatment of Strep. faecalis endocarditis (Johnson *et al.*, 1965; Beaty *et al.*, 1966). In one case reported by Parker and Hoeprich (1966), a daily dose of 20 g ampicillin was given intravenously, plus probenecid orally. Although a serum ampicillin level of just over 800 μg per ml was obtained, the patient's serum was only bactericidal to the Strep. faecalis strain at a 1:2 dilution. It is now generally accepted that the use of ampicillin alone is not as reliable as the more commonly used combinations of penicillin G with either streptomycin (page 302), kanamycin (page 318) or gentamicin (page 344), for the treatment of this disease (Mandell *et al.*, 1970). An ampicillin/aminoglycoside combination may be equally effective.

Bacterial endocarditis due to Gram-negative bacilli is uncommon. Ampicillin alone would not be expected to be effective, but ampicillin combined with kanamycin has been used successfully to treat endocarditis due to Esch. coli (Hansing *et al.*, 1967).

12. *Biliary infections.* Ampicillin is useful for the treatment of cholangitis, if the infecting organism is ampicillin-sensitive. Esch. coli is the most frequent cause of biliary infections, but other causes include Strep. faecalis and the Klebsiella, Proteus and Clostridium spp. (Kune and Burdon, 1975). Bacteroides fragilis may be also sometimes involved, especially in elderly patients with bile duct obstruction (Shimada *et al.*, 1977). A combination of ampicillin with either kanamycin or gentamicin is advocated for the treatment of these infections, before the causal organism is identified (*see* pages 317, 341). In very ill patients either chloramphenicol (page 443) or clindamycin (page 484) may be necessary in addition to cover the possibility of B. fragilis infections. It is often stressed that antibiotics which are excreted and concentrated in the bile (including ampicillin) are preferable for treatment of biliary infections. Mortimer *et al.* (1969) demonstrated that therapeutic concentrations of ampicillin are in fact not attained in the bile of patients with obstructive biliary tract disease. In these patients pre-operative control of the associated septicaemia is more important than sterilization of the bile.

In the treatment of patients with acute cholecystitis, unlike cholangitis, chemotherapy is not always indicated. In cholecystitis the administration of an antibiotic such as ampicillin does not decrease the frequency of local septic complications. It does however decrease the number of wound infections and the frequency of septicaemia in high risk patients, such as those over 60 years of age or those with debilitating diseases (Kune and Burdon, 1975).

13. *Other surgical infections.* Parenteral or oral administration of ampicillin may limit the spread of intraperitoneal infection in patients with a perforated appendix, and may reduce the duration of post-operative pyrexia (Magarey *et al.*, 1971). Topical ampicillin may reduce the prevalence of wound infections in such patients (Leading article, 1971).

Ampicillin can also be used for treatment of post-operative sepsis, such as wound infections, pneumonia, etc. (Rutenburg and Greenberg, 1967). In hospital-acquired infections, ampicillin alone is unreliable for severely ill patients without bacteriological investigation, because either ampicillin-resistant strains of staphylococci or Gram-negative bacilli are often involved. The variable activity of ampicillin against Bacteroides spp. (page 103) also makes this drug an unwise choice as the sole agent for treatment of severe peritonitis (Bear *et al.*, 1970).

It has been suggested that ampicillin may be of value in acute pancreatitis, possibly because it may decrease complicating infections. In one controlled trial ampicillin was found to be ineffective in patients with primarily alcohol-related acute pancreatitis (Craig *et al.*, 1975).

14. *Venereal diseases.* Gonorrhoea can be treated by ampicillin (Sullivan, 1970). Ideally it should be given for a period of five to seven days, but it has been extensively used as a 'single-dose' oral treatment. A dose of 3·5 g ampicillin combined with 1 g of probenecid is recommended (Karney *et al.*, 1974; Center for Disease Control, 1975). Results with this treatment schedule have been satisfactory and are approximately the same as with currently recommended 'single-dose' schedules using procaine penicillin (page 37) or spectinomycin (page 588) (Judson *et al.*, 1974; Kaufman *et al.*, 1976). 'Single-dose' ampicillin, although effective in gonorrhoea, rarely eliminates Chlamydia trachomatis (page 626) from the genital tract (Oriel *et al.*, 1976). Single-dose ampicillin is ineffective for treatment of pharyngeal gonorrhoea, but a three-day regimen, consisting of a single oral 3·5 g dose of ampicillin and 1·0 g of probenecid on the first day, followed by 500 mg ampicillin four times a day for next two days, is effective for most cases (Di Caprio *et al.*, 1978). Disseminated gonococcal infections such as the arthritis-dermatitis syndrome, may respond to oral ampicillin in a dose of 2 g daily for 7–10 days (Handsfield *et al.*, 1976). Other systemic or disseminated gonococcal infections such as salpingitis or septicaemia may be treated by intravenous penicillin G in a dose of 20 million units daily until a response is obtained, followed by oral ampicillin 2 g daily to complete a 10–14 day course (Litt *et al.*, 1974; Center for Disease Control, 1975).

Ampicillin may be ineffective in some cases of gonorrhoea because gonococci with increased resistance to penicillin G (page 7) are usually also relatively ampicillin-resistant (page 102), and penicillinase-producing strains (page 8) are completely ampicillin-resistant.

Ampicillin has also been reported as useful for the treatment of granuloma inguinale (Thew *et al.*, 1969), but the tetracyclines are the drugs of choice (page 627).

15. *Brucellosis.* Although all Brucella spp. are sensitive to ampicillin *in vitro*, ampicillin is not clinically useful in Br. abortus and Br. melitensis infections. For infections by Brucella canis, an uncommon human pathogen, am-

picillin has been used in conjunction with other drugs such as tetracycline and streptomycin, but optimal therapy for this infection has not been defined (Blankenship and Sanford, 1975).

REFERENCES

A Co-operative Controlled Trial (1966), 'Ampicillin in the treatment of pneumonia', *Brit. med. J.*, **1**, 1329.

Acred, P. and Sutherland, R. (1967), 'Antibacterial activities of combinations of ampicillin and cloxacillin', *Antimicrob. Agents Chemother.*—1966, p. 53.

Albritton, W. L., Hammond, G., Hoban, S. and Ronald, A. R. (1977), 'Ampicillin-resistant H. influenzae subdural empyema following successful treatment of apparently ampicillin-sensitive H. influenzae meningitis.', *J. Pediatrics*, **90**, 320.

Annotation (1969), 'Ampicillin rashes', *Lancet*, **2**, 993.

Anthony, B. F. and Concepcion, N. F. (1975), 'Group B streptococcus in a general hospital', *J. Infect. Dis.*, **132**, 561.

A Report from the Boston Collaborative Drug Surveillance Program, Boston University Medical Center (1972), 'Excess of ampicillin rashes associated with allopurinol or hyperuricaemia', *New Engl. J. Med.*, **286**, 505.

Arndt, K. A. and Jick, H. (1976), 'Rates of cutaneous reactions to drugs. A report from the Boston Collaborative Drug Surveillance Program', *JAMA*, **235**, 918.

Axline, S. G., Yaffe, S. J. and Simon, H. J. (1967), 'Clinical pharmacology of antimicrobials in premature infants: II. Ampicillin, methicillin, oxacillin, neomycin and colistin', *Pediatrics*, **39**, 97.

Bach, M. C., Sabath, L. D. and Finland, M. (1973), 'Susceptibility of Nocardia asteroides to 45 antimicrobial agents *in vitro*', *Antimicrob. Ag. Chemother.*, **3**, 1.

Barkin, R. M., Greer, C. C., Schumacher, C. J. and McIntosh, K. (1976), 'Haemophilus influenzae meningitis. An evolving therapeutic regimen', *Am. J. Dis. Child.*, **130**, 1318.

Barrett, F. F., Eardley, W. A., Yow, M. D. and Leverett, H. A. (1966), 'Ampicillin in the treatment of acute suppurative meningitis', *J. Pediatrics*, **69**, 343.

Barrett, F. F., Taber, L. H., Morris, C. R., Stephenson, W. B., Clarke, J. and Yow, M. D. (1972), 'A 12 year review of the antibiotic management of Haemophilus influenzae meningitis', *J. Pediatrics*, **81**, 370.

Barros, F., Korzeniowski, O. M., Sande, M. A., Martins, K., Santos, L. C. and Rocha, H. (1977), '*In vitro* antibiotic susceptibility of salmonellae', *Antimicrob. Ag. Chemother.*, **11**, 1071.

Barza, M., Brusch, J., Bergeron, M. G. and Weinstein, L. (1974), 'Penetration of antibiotics into fibrin loci *in vitro*. III. Intermittent vs. continous infusion and the effect of probenecid', *J. Infect. Dis.*, **129**, 73.

Bass, J. W., Klenk, E. L., Kotheimer, J. B., Linnemann, C. C. and Smith, M. H. D. (1969), 'Antimicrobial treatment of pertussis', *J. Pediatrics*, **75**, 768.

Bass, J. W., Crowley, D. M., Steele, R. W., Young, F. S. H. and Harden, L. B. (1973), 'Adverse effects of orally administered ampicillin', *J. Pediatrics*, **83**, 106.

Bass, J. W. (1973), 'The role of antimicrobial agents in the treatment of pertussis', *J. Pediatrics*, **83**, 891.

Bayer, A. S., Chow, A. W., Anthony, B. F. and Guze, L. B. (1976), 'Serious infections in adults due to Group B streptococci. Clinical and serotypic characterization', *Amer. J. Med.*, **61**, 498.

Bear, D. M., Turck, M. and Petersdorf, R. G. (1970), 'Ampicillin', *Med. Clin. North America*, **54**, 1145.

Beaty, H. N., Turck, M. and Petersdorf, R. G. (1966), 'Ampicillin in the treatment of enterococcal endocarditis', *Ann. Intern. Med.*, **65**, 701.

Bell, S. M. and Smith, D. D. (1975), 'Ampicilin-resistant Haemophilus influenzae, type b', *Med. J. Aust.*, **1**, 517.

Bennett, W. M., Singer, I. and Coggins, C. H. (1970), 'A practical guide to drug usage in adult patients with impaired renal function', *JAMA*, **214**, 1468.

Bennett, N. McK. and Kucers, A. (1970), 'Staphylococcal and Gram-negative septicaemia', *Aspects of Infection, Proc. Symp. Auckland, Sydney and Melbourne*, p. 123.

Bennett, N. McK. (1973), 'Whooping cough in Melbourne', *Med. J. Aust.*, **2**, 481.

Bennett, W. M., Singer, I. and Coggins, C. J. (1974), 'A guide to drug therapy in renal failure', *JAMA*, **230**, 1544.

Bhowmick, B. K. (1972), 'Benign intracranial hypertension after antibiotic therapy', *Brit. med. J.*, **3**, 30.

Biörklund, A., Dahlquist, E., Kamme, C. and Nilsson, N. I. (1975), 'Ampicillin-resistant Haemophilus influenzae in otitis media', *Lancet*, **1**, 1135.

Bissett, M. L., Abbot, S. L. and Wood, R. M. (1974), 'Antimicrobial resistance and R factors in salmonella isolated in California (1971–1972)', *Antimicrob. Ag. Chemother.*, **5**, 161.

Blankenship, R. M. and Sanford, J. P. (1975), 'Brucella canis. A cause of undulant fever', *Amer. J. Med.*, **59**, 424.

Blecher, T. E., Edgar, W. M., Melville, H. A. H. and Peel, K. R. (1966), 'Transplacental passage of ampicillin', *Brit. med. J.*, **1**, 137.

Boe, R. W., Williams, C. P. S., Bennett, J. V. and Oliver, T. K. (1967), 'Serum levels of methicillin and ampicillin in newborn and premature infants in relation to postnatal age', *Pediatrics*, **39**, 194.

Bosso, J. A. and Jackman, J. R. (1977), 'Acute otitis media', *Drug. Intel. Clin. Pharm.*, **11**, 665.

Brodlie, P. Henney, C. and Wood, A. J. J. (1974), 'Problems of administering drugs by continuous infusion', *Brit. med. J.*, **1**, 383.

Brooks, A. P. (1974), 'Thrombocytopenia during treatment with ampicillin', *Lancet*, **2**, 723.

Brown, D. M. and Acred, P. (1961), 'Penbritin—a new broad-spectrum antibiotic', *Brit. med. J.*, **2**, 197.

Brown, G. L. and Kanwar, B. S. (1967), 'Drug rashes in glandular fever', *Lancet*, **2**, 1418.

Bulger, R. J., Bennett, J. V. and Boen, S. T. (1965), 'Intraperitoneal administration of broad-spectrum antibiotics in patients with renal failure', *JAMA*, **194**, 1198.

Byers, P. A., Dupont, H. L. and Goldschmidt, M. C. (1976), 'Antimicrobial susceptibilities of shigellae isolated in Houston, Texas, in 1974', *Antimicrob. Ag. Chemother.*, **9**, 288.

Bysjö, E. and Dornbusch, K. (1977), 'Occurrence and transfer of ampicillin resistance associated with ampicillin-resistant Haemophilus influenzae isolated from a case at a day-care centre', *Scand. J. Infect. Dis.*, **9**, 293.

Catlin, B. W. (1975), 'Idometric detection of Haemophilus influenzae beta-lactamase: rapid presumptive test for ampicillin resistance', *Antimicrob. Ag. Chemother.*, **7**, 265.

Center for Disease Control (1973), 'Chloramphenicol-ampicillin resistant salmonella typhi-California', *Morbidity and Mortality Weekly Report*, **22**, 183.

Center for Disease Control (1974a), 'Ampicillin-resistant Hemophilus influenzae meningitis', *Morbidity and Mortality Weekly Report*, **23**, 77 and 259.

Center for Disease Control (1974b), 'Ampicillin-resistant Shigella dysenteriae, type 1—Costa Rica', *Mobidity and Mortality Weekly Report*, **23**, 291.

Center for Disease Control (1975), 'Gonorrhea: Recommended treatment schedules', *Ann. Intern. Med.*, **82**, 230.

Center for Disease Control (1977a), 'Outbreak of Haemophilus influenzae type B disease in a day-care center—Kansas', *Morbidity and Mortality Weekly Report*, **26,** 201.

Center for Disease Control (1977b), 'Multiple-antibiotic resistance of pneumococci —South Africa', *Morbidity and Mortality Weekly Report*, **26,** 285.

Cherry, J. D. and Sheenan, C. P. (1968), 'Bacterologic relapse in Haemophilus influenzae meningitis', *New Engl. J. Med.*, **278,** 1001.

Chisholm, G. D., Waterworth, P. M., Calnan, J. S. and Garrod, L. P. (1973), 'Concentration of antibacterial agents in interstitial tissue fluid', *Brit. med. J.*, **1,** 569.

Chow, A. W., Patten, V. and Bednorz, D. (1978), 'Susceptibility of Campylobacter fetus to twenty-two antimicrobial agents', *Antimicrob. Ag. Chemother.*, **13,** 416.

Christie, A. B. (1964), 'Treatment of typhoid carriers with ampicillin', *Brit. med. J.*, **1,** 1609.

Chun, D., Seol, S. Y., Cho, D. T. and Tak, R. (1977), 'Drug resistance and R plasmids in Salmonella typhi isolated in Korea', *Antimicrob. Ag. Chemother.*, **11,** 209.

Clymo, A. B. and Harper, I. A. (1974), 'Ampicillin-resistant Haemophilus influenzae meningitis', *Lancet*, **1,** 453.

Coffey, J. D. Jr. (1968), 'Concentration of ampicillin in exudate from acute otitis media', *J. Pediatrics*, **72,** 693.

Coleman, S. J., Auld, E. B., Connor, J. D., Rosenman, S. B. and Warren, G. H. (1969), 'Relapse of Haemophilus influenzae type B. meningitis during intravenous therapy with ampicillin', *J. Pediatrics*, **74,** 781.

Committee on Infectious Diseases (1975), 'Ampicillin-resistant strains for Hemophilus influenzae type B', *Pediatrics*, **55,** 145.

Craig, R. M., Dordal, E. and Myles, L. (1975), 'The use of ampicillin in acute pancreatitis., Ann. Intern. Med., **83,** 831.

Crosa, J. H., Olarte, J., Mata, L. J., Luttropp, L. K. and Peñaranda, M. E. (1977), 'Characterization of an R-plasmid associated with ampicillin resistance in Shigella dysenteria type 1 isolated from epidemics', *Antimicrob. Ag. Chemother.*, **11,** 553.

Crosson, F. J. Jr., Watson, C., III, Bailey, D. W. and MacLowry, J. D. (1976), 'Acute otitis media caused by ampicillin-resistant Haemophilus influenzae type B, *JAMA*, **236,** 2778.

Davies, J. R., Farrant, W. N. and Uttley, A. H. C. (1970), 'Antibiotic resistance of Shigella sonnei', *Lancet*, **2,** 1157.

de Ritis, F., Giammanco, G. and Manzillo, G. (1972), 'Chloramphenicol combined with ampicillin in treatment of typhoid', *Brit. med. J.*, **4,** 17.

Delage, G., Declerck, Y., Lescop, J. Déry, P. and Shareck, F. (1977), 'Haemophilus influenzae type B infections: Recurrent disease due to ampicillin-resistant strains', *J. Pediatrics*, **90,** 319.

Di Caprio, J. M., Reynolds, J., Frank, G., Carbone, J. and Nishimura, R. (1978), 'Ampicillin therapy for pharyngeal gonorrhea', *JAMA*, **239,** 1631.

Dinbar, A. Altmann, G. and Tulcinsky, D. B. (1969), 'The treatment of chronic biliary salmonella carriers', *Amer. J. Med.*, **47,** 236.

Dorman, D. C. and Kilham, H. A. (1976), 'Meningitis and ampicillin-resistant Haemophilus influenzae', *Med. J. Aust.*, **2,** 359.

Eickhoff, T. C., Steinhauer, B. W. and Finland, M. (1966), 'The Klebsiella-Enterobacter-Serratia division. Biochemical and serologic characteristics and susceptibility to antibiotics', *Ann. Intern. Med.*, **65,** 1163.

Eickhoff, T. C., Ehret, J. M. and Baines, R. D. (1976), 'Characterization of an ampicillin-resistant Haemophilus influenzae type B', *Antimicrob. Ag. Chemother.*, **9,** 889.

Emerson, B. B., Smith, A. L., Harding, A. L. and Smith, D. H. (1975), 'Hemophilus influenzae type B susceptibility to 17 antibiotics', *J. Pediatrics*, **86,** 617.

Fallon, R. J. (1976), 'Leading article. Haemophilus influenzae meningitis', *J. Antimicrob. Chemother.*, **2,** 3.

Fardig, O. B., Rousche, M. A., Cabana, B. E. and Moyland, D. S. (1970), 'Purification of ampicillin', *Brit. med. J.*, **2**, 735.

Farrar, W. E. Jr. and Eidson, M. (1971), 'Antibiotic resistance in shigella mediated by R factors', *J. Infect. Dis.*, **123**, 477.

Farrar, W. E. Jr. and O'Dell, N. M. (1974), 'Beta-lactamase activity in ampicillin-resistant Haemophilus influenzae', *Antimicrob. Ag. Chemother.*, **6**, 625.

Feigin, R. D., Moss, K. S. and Shackelford, P. G. (1973), 'Antibiotic stability in solutions used for intravenous nutrition and fluid therapy', *Pediatrics*, **51**, 1016.

Feigin, R. D., Stechenberg, B. W., Chang, M. J., Dunkle, L. M., Wong, M. L., Palkes, H., Dodge, P. R. and Davis, H. (1976), 'Prospective evaluation of treatment of Hemophilus influenzae meningitis', *J. Pediatrics*, **88**, 542.

Finland, M., Bach, M. C., Garner, C. and Gold, O. (1974), 'Synergistic action of ampicillin and erythromycin against Nocardia asteroides: Effect of time of incubation', *Antimicrob. Ag. Chemother.*, **5**, 344.

Fleming, P. C., Murray, J. D. M., Fujiwara, M. W., Prichard, J. S. and McNaughton, G. A. (1967), 'Ampicillin in the treatment of bacterial meningitis', *Antimicrob. Agents Chemother.*—1966, p. 47.

Gerding, D. N., Hall, W. H. and Schierl, E. A. (1977), 'Antibiotic concentrations in ascitic fluid of patients with ascites and bacterial peritonitis', *Ann. Intern. Med.*, **86**, 708.

Gibbs, M., Hamdorf, K. and Hansman, D. (1975), 'Ampicillin and amoxycillin resistance in Haemophilus influenzae', *Med. J. Aust.*, **1**, 320.

Ginsburg, C. M., McCracken, G. H. Jr., Rae, S. and Parke, J. C. Jr. (1977), 'Haemophilus influenzae type B disease incidence in a day-care center', *JAMA*, **238**, 604.

Glode, M. P., Schiffer, M. S., Robbins, J. B., Khan, W., Battle, C. U. and Armenta, E. (1976), 'An outbreak of Haemophilus influenzae type B meningitis in an enclosed hospital population', *J. Pediatrics*, **88**, 36.

Gold, A. J., Lieberman, E. and Wright, H. T. Jr. (1969), 'Bacteriologic relapse during ampicillin treatment of Haemophilus influenzae meningitis', *J. Pediatrics*, **74**, 779.

Gordon, R. C., Barrett, F. F. and Yow, M. D. (1970), 'Ampicillin treatment of listeriosis', *J. Pediatrics*, **77**, 1067.

Graf, M. and Tarlov, A. (1968), 'Agranulocytosis with monohistiocytosis associated with ampicillin therapy', *Ann. Intern. Med.*, **69**, 91.

Granoff, D. M., Sargent, E. and Jolivette, D. (1978), 'Haemophilus influenzae type B osteomyelitis', *Am. J. Dis. Child.*, **132**, 488.

Grant, R. B., Bannatyne, R. M. and Shapley, A. J. (1976), 'Resistance to chloramphenicol and ampicillin of Salmonella typhimurium in Ontario, Canada', *J. Infect. Dis.*, **134**, 354.

Greene, H. L. (1968), 'Failure of ampicillin in meningitis', *Lancet*, **1**, 861.

Gurwith, M. J., Rabin, H. R., Love, K. and the Co-operative Antibiotic Diarrhea Study Group (1977), 'Diarrhea associated with clindamycin and ampicillin therapy: preliminary results of a co-operative study', *J. Infect. Dis.* (Suppl.), **135**, 104.

Haltalin, K. C., Nelson, J. D., Hinton, L. V., Kusmiesz, H. T. and Sladoje, M. (1968), 'Comparison of orally absorbable and non-absorbable antibiotics in shigellosis', *J. Pediatrics*, **72**, 708.

Haltalin, K. C., Nelson, J. D., Kusmiesz, H. T. and Hinton, L. V. (1969), 'Optimal dosage of ampicillin for shigellosis', *J. Pediatrics*, **74**, 626.

Haltalin, K. C., Nelson, J. D., Ring, R. Sladoje, M. and Hinton, L. V. (1967), 'Double-blind treatment study of shigellosis comparing ampicillin sulfadiazine and placebo', *J. Pediatrics*, **70**, 970.

Haltalin, K. C., Kusmiesz, H. T., Hinton, L. V. and Nelson, J. D. (1972), 'Treatment of acute diarrhoea in outpatients. Double-blind study comparing ampicillin and placebo', *Amer. J. Dis. Child.*, **124**, 554.

Hamilton-Miller, J. M. T. (1977), 'Inhibition of beta-lactamase: a continuing story', *J. Antimicrob. Chemother.*, **3**, 195.

Handsfield, H. H., Wiesner, P. J. and Holmes, K. K. (1976), 'Treatment of the gonococcal arthritis-dermatitis syndrome', *Ann. Intern. Med.*, **84**, 661.

Hansing, C. E., Allen, V. D. and Cherry, J. D. (1967), 'Escherichia coli endocarditis. A review of the literature and a case study', *Arch. Intern. Med.*, **120**, 472.

Hansman, D. (1976), 'Penicillin-insensitive pneumococci', *Brit. med. J.*, **2**, 1503.

Hassan, A., Yassin, M. W., Girgis, N. I., Sippel, J. E., Miner, W. F., Tadros, S. S. and Abu El Ella, A. H. (1976), 'The value of epicillin and ampicillin in the treatment of meningococcal and pneumococcal meningitis', *Scand. J. Infect. Dis.*, **8**, 181.

Herzog, C. H. (1976), 'Drug treatment of typhoid fever', *Brit. med. J.*, **2**, 941.

Hoffman, T. A., Ruiz, C. J., Counts, G. W., Sachs, J. M. and Nitzkin, J. L. (1975), 'Waterborne typhoid fever in Dade Country, Florida. Clinical and therapeutic evaluation of 105 bacteremic patients', *Amer. J. Med.*, **59**, 481.

Howard, P. Jr. and Riley, H. D. (1965), 'Use of ampicillin in the treatment of shigellosis', *Antimicrob. Agents Chemother.*—1964, p. 233.

Howard, A. J., Hince, C. J. and Williams, J. D. (1978), 'Antibiotic resistance in Streptococcus pneumoniae and Haemophilus influenzae. Report of a study group on bacterial resistance', *Brit. med. J.*, **1**, 1657.

Howes, V. J. and Mitchell, R. G. (1976), 'Meningitis due to relatively penicillin-resistant pneumoccus', *Brit. med. J.*, **1**, 996.

Hunter, P. A., Reading, C. and Witting, D. A. (1978), 'The *in vitro* and *in vivo* properties of BRL 14151. A novel beta-lactam with beta-lactamase inhibitory properties', in Siegenthaler, W. and Lüthy, R. (ed.), *Current Chemotherapy: Proceedings of the 10th International Congress of Chemotherapy*, Zurich/Switzerland, 1977. American Society for Microbiology, Washington, D.C. p. 478.

Iannini, P. B., Ehret, J. and Eickhoff, T. C. (1976), 'Effects of ampicillin-amikacin and ampicillin-rifampin on enterococci., *Antimicrob. Ag. Chemother.*, **9**, 448.

Jacobson, J. A., McCormick, J. B., Hayes, P., Thornsberry, C. and Kirvin, L. (1976), 'Epidemiologic characteristics of infections caused by ampicillin-resistant Haemophilus influenzae', *Pediatrics*, **58**, 388.

Johnson, D. G., Barnes, J. A. and McLeod, E. (1965), 'Subacute bacterial endocarditis caused by Streptococcus faecalis and successfully treated with ampicillin', *Med. J. Aust.*, **2**, 1026.

Johnson, D. W., Kvale, P. A., Afable, V. L., Stewart, S. D., Halverson, C. W. and Holmes, K. K. (1970), 'Single-dose antibiotic treatment of asymptomatic gonorrhea in hospitalized women', *New Engl. J. Med.*, **283**, 1.

Johnson, W. D., Jr., Hook, E. W., Lindsey, E. and Kaye, D. (1973), 'Treatment of chronic typhoid carriers with ampicillin', *Antimicrob. Ag. Chemother.*, **3**, 439.

Johnson, R. H., Lutwick, L. I., Huntley, G. A. and Vosti, K. L. (1976), 'Arizona hinshawii infections. New cases, antimicrobial sensitivities and literature review', *Ann. Intern. Med.*, **85**, 587.

Joseph, S. W., DeBell, R. M. and Brown, W. P. (1978), '*In vitro* response to chloramphenicol, tetracycline, ampicillin, gentamicin, and beta-lactamase production by halophilic vibrios from human and environmental sources', *Antimicrob. Ag. Chemother.*, **13**, 244.

Judson, F. N., Allaman, J. and Dans, P. E. (1974), 'Treatment of gonorrhea. Comparison of penicillin G procaine, doxycycline, spectinomycin, and ampicillin', *JAMA*, **230**, 705.

Kalis, P., Le Frock, J. L., Smith, W. and Keefe, M. (1976), 'Listeriosis', *Amer. J. Med. Sci.*, **271**, 159.

Kammer, R. B., Preston, D. A., Turner, J. R. and Hawley, L. C. (1975), 'Rapid detection of ampicillin-resistant Haemophilus influenzae and their susceptibility to sixteen antibiotics', *Antimicrob. Ag. Chemother.*, **8**, 91.

Kaplan, J. M., McCracken, G. H., Jr., Horton, L. J. Thomas, M. L. and Davis, N. (1974), 'Pharmacologic studies in neonates given large dosages of ampicillin', *J. Pediatrics*, **84**, 571.

Karney, W. W., Turck, M. and Holmes, K. K. (1974), 'Comparative therapeutic and pharmacological evaluation of amoxicillin and ampicillin plus probenecid for the treatment of gonorrhea', *Antimicrob. Ag. Chemother.*, **5**, 114.

Kattan, S., Cavanagh, P. and Williams, J. D. (1975), 'Relationship between β-lactamase production by Haemophilus influenzae and sensitivities to penicillins and cephalosporins', *J. Antimicrob. Chemother.*, **1**, 79.

Katz, S. L. (1975), 'Ampicillin-resistant Haemophilus influenzae type B: a status report', *Pediatrics*, **55**, 6.

Kaufman, R. E., Johnson, R. E., Jaffe, H. W., Thornsberry, C., Reynolds, G. H. and Wiesner, P. J. (1976), 'National gonorrhea therapy monitoring study. Treatment results', *New Engl. J. Med.*, **294**, 1.

Kazemi, M., Gumpert, T. G. and Marks, M. I. (1973), 'A controlled trial comparing sulfamethoxazole-trimethoprim, ampicillin, and no therapy in the treatment of salmonella gastro-enteritis in children', *J. Pediatrics*, **83**, 646.

Keating, J. P., Frank, A. L., Barton, L. L. and Tedesco, F. J. (1974), 'Pseudomembranous colitis associated with ampicillin therapy', *Amer. J. Dis. Child.*, **128**, 369.

Kennedy, W. P. U., Wallace, A. T. and Murdoch, J. McC. (1963), 'Ampicillin in treatment of certain Gram-negative bacterial infections', *Brit. med. J.*, **2**, 962.

Kerns, D. L., Shira, J. E., Go, S., Summers, R. J., Schwab, J. A. and Plunket, D. C. (1973), 'Ampicillin rash in children. Relationship to penicillin allergy and infectious mononucleosis', *Amer. J. Dis. Child.*, **125**, 187.

Khan, W., Ross, S. Rodriguez, W., Controni, G. and Saz, A. K. (1974), 'Haemophilus influenzae type B resistant to ampicillin. A report of two cases', *JAMA*, **229**, 298.

Kincaid-Smith, P. (1964), 'Ampicillin in bacteriuria and pyelonephritis of pregnancy', *Postgrad. Med. J.* (Suppl.), **40**, 74.

Kirby, W. M. M. and Kind, A. C. (1967), 'Clinical pharmacology of ampicillin and hetacillin', *Ann. N.Y. Acad. Sci.*, **145**, 291.

Klemola, E. (1970), 'Hypersensitivity reactions to ampicillin in Cytomegalovirus mononucleosis', *Scand. J. Infect. Dis.*, **2**, 29.

Knirsch, A. K. and Gralla, E. J. (1970), 'Serum transaminase levels after parenteral ampicillin and carbenicillin', *New Engl. J. Med.*, **282**, 1081.

Knudsen, E. T., Rolinson, G. N. and Stevens, S. (1961), 'Absorption and excretion of "Penbritin"', *Brit. med. J.*, **2**, 198.

Knudsen, E. T. (1970), 'Factors influencing penicillin therapy', *Aspects of Infection, Proc. Symp. Auckland, Sydney and Melbourne*, p. 115.

Knudsen, E. T., Dewdney, J. M. and Trafford, J. A. P. (1970), 'Reduction in incidence of ampicillin rash by purification of ampicillin', *Brit. med. J.*, **1**, 469.

Konforti, N. and Halperin, E. (1975), 'Sensitivities of strains of enteropathogenic Escherichia coli to cephalexin and other antibiotics', *Amer. J. Clin, Path.*, **64**, 121.

Kune, G. A. and Burdon, J. G. W. (1975), 'Are antibiotics necessary in acute cholecystitis?', *Med. J. Aust.*, **2**, 627.

Lampe, R. M., Duangmani, C. and Mansuwan, P. (1975), 'Chloramphenicol- and ampicillin-resistant typhoid fever', *JAMA*, **233**, 768.

Lavetter, A., Leedom, J. M., Mathies, A. W., Jr., Ivler, D. and Wehrle, P. F. (1971), 'Meningitis due to Listeria monocytogenes. A review of 25 cases', *New Engl. J. Med.*, **285**, 598.

Leading Article (1969), 'Antibiotics prolong salmonella excretion', *Brit. med. J.*, **4**, 699.

Leading Article (1971), 'Sepsis after appendicectomy', *Lancet*, **2**, 195.

Leading Article (1972a), 'Single-dose treatment of gonorrhoea', *Lancet*, **1**, 885.

Leading Article (1972b), 'Skin reactions to ampicillin', *Brit. med. J.*, **1**, 195.

Leading Article (1975), 'Ampicillin rashes', *Brit. med. J.*, **2**, 708.

Leading Article (1976a), 'Haemophilus influenzae', *Lancet*, **2**, 776.

Leading Article (1976b), 'Antibiotics for otitis media', *Brit. med. J.*, **2**, 1407.

Leading Article (1976c), 'Pencillinase-producing gonococci', *Lancet*, **2**, 725.

Lee, H. A. and Hill, L. F. (1968), 'The use of ampicillin in renal disease', *Brit. J. Clin. Pract.*, **22**, 354.

Lindberg, J., Rosenhall, U., Nylén, O. and Ringnér, Å. (1977), 'Long-term outcome of Haemophilus influenzae meningitis related to antibiotic treatment', *Pediatrics*, **60**, 1.

Litt, I. F., Edberg, S. C. and Finberg, L. (1974), 'Gonorrhea in children and adolescents: a current review', *J. Pediatrics*, **85**, 595.

Lund, B. M. A. and Bergan, T. (1975), 'Temporary skin reactions to penicillins during the acute stage of infectious mononucleosis', *Scand. J. Infect. Dis.*, **7**, 21.

Lusk, R. H., Fekety, F. R., Jr., Silva, J., Jr., Bodendorfer, T., Devine, B. J., Kawanishi, H., Korff, L. Nakauchi, D., Rogers, S. and Siskin, S. B. (1977), 'Gastrointestinal side effects of clindamycin and ampicillin therapy', *J. Infect. Dis.* (Suppl.), **135**, 111.

McCracken, G. H., Jr. (1974), 'Pharmacological basis for antimicrobial therapy in newborn infants', *Am. J. Dis. Child.*, **128**, 407.

McCracken, G. H., Jr. and Eichenwald, H. F. (1974), 'Antimicrobial therapy: therapeutic recommendations and review of newer drugs. Part 1. Therapy of infectious conditions', *J. Pediatrics*, **85**, 297.

McGowan, J. E., Jr., Terry, P. M. and Nahmias, A. J. (1976), 'Susceptibility of Haemophilus influenzae isolates from blood and cerebrospinal fluid to ampicillin, chloramphenicol and trimethoprim-sulfamethoxazole', *Antimicrob. Ag. Chemother.*, **9**, 137.

Macnair, D. R., White, J. E. and Graham, J. M. (1968), 'Ampicillin in the treatment of Listeria monocytogenes meningitis', *Lancet*, **1**, 16.

Magarey, C. J., Chant, A. D. B., Rickford, C. R. K. and Magarey, J. R. (1971), 'Peritoneal drainage and systemic antibiotics after appendicectomy', *Lancet*, **2**, 179.

Maier, T. W., Zubrzycki, L. and Coyle, M. B. (1975), 'Genetic analysis of drug resistance in Neisseria gonorrhoeae: Identification and linkage relationships of loci controlling drug resistance', *Antimicrob. Ag. Chemother.*, **7**, 676.

Malmvall, B.-E. and Branefors-Helander, P. (1978), 'R-factor involvement in a local outbreak of ampicillin-resistant Haemophilus influenzae infections', *Scand. J. Infect. Dis.*, **10**, 53.

Malone, D. N., Gould, J. C. and Grant, I. W. B. (1968), 'A comparative study of ampicillin, tetracycline hydrochloride, and methacycline hydrochloride in acute exacerbations of chronic bronchitis', *Lancet*, **2**, 594.

Mandell, G. L., Kaye, D., Levison, M. E. and Hook, E. W. (1970), 'Enterococcal endocarditis', *Arch. Intern. Med.*, **125**, 258.

Manriquez, L., Salcedo, M., Borgoño, J. M., Marzullo, E., Kraljević, R., Paredes, L. and Valdivieso, R. (1965), 'Clinical trials with ampicillin in typhoid fever and paratyphoid A', *Brit. med. J.*, **2**, 152.

Marks, R. and Ellis, J. (1971), 'Comparative effectiveness of tetracycline and ampicillin in rosacea. A controlled trial', *Lancet*, **2**, 1049.

Mathies, A. W., Jr., Leedom, J. M., Thrupp, L. D., Ivler, D., Portnoy, B. and Wehrle, P. F. (1966), 'Experience with ampicillin in bacterial meningitis', *Antimicrob. Agents Chemother.*—1965, p. 610.

McHardy, V. U. and Schonell, M. E. (1972), 'Ampicillin dosage and use of prednisolone in treatment of pneumonia: Co-operative controlled trial', *Brit. med. J.*, **4**, 569.

Maxwell, D., Szwed, J. J., Wahle, W. and Kleit, S. A. (1974), 'Ampicillin nephropathy', *JAMA*, **230**, 586.

Mayo, J. B. and McCarthy, L. R. (1977), 'Antimicrobial susceptibility of Haemophilus parainfluenzae', *Antimicrob. Ag. Chemother.*, **11**, 844.

Medeiros, A. A. and O'Brien, T. F. (1975), 'Ampicillin-resistant Haemophilus influenzae type B possessing a TEM-type β-lactamase but little permeability barrier to ampicillin', *Lancet*, **1**, 716.

Mero, E. (1976), 'Resistance to antibiotics of shigella strains isolated in Somalia', *Bull. World Health Organ.*, **54**, 473.

Mikhail, I. A., Kent, D. C., Sorensen, K., Sanborn, W. R. and Smith, J. (1972), 'Concentrations of ampicillin and chloramphenicol in the serum of patients with acute salmonella enteric fever', *Antimicrob. Ag. Chemother.*, **2**, 336.

Mortimer, P. R., Mackie, D. B. and Haynes, S. (1969), 'Ampicillin levels in human bile in the presence of biliary tract disease', *Brit. med. J.*, **3**, 88.

Nade, S., Robertson, F. W. and Taylor, T. K. F. (1974), 'Antibiotics in the treatment of acute osteomyelitis and acute septic arthritis in children', *Med. J. Aust.*, **2**, 703.

Nazareth, I., Mortimer, P. and McKendrick, G. D. W. (1972), 'Ampicillin sensitivity in infectious mononucleosis—temporary or permanent?', *Scand. J. Infect. Dis.*, **4**, 229.

Nelson, J. D. (1971), 'Antibiotic concentrations in septic joint effusions', *New Engl. J. Med.*, **284**, 349.

Nelson, J. D. (1974), 'Editorial. Should ampicillin be abandoned for treatment of Haemophilus influenzae disease?', *JAMA*, **229**, 322.

Neu, H. C., Cherubin, C. E., Longo, E. D., Flouton, B. and Winter, J. (1975a), 'Antimicrobial resistance and R-factor transfer among isolates of salmonella in the Northeastern United States: a comparison of human and animal isolates', *J. Infect. Dis.*, **132**, 617.

Neu, H. C., Cherubin, C. E., Longo, E. D. and Winter, J. (1975b), 'Antimicrobial resistance of shigella isolated in New York City in 1973', *Antimicrob. Ag. Chemother.*, **7**, 833.

Ninane, G., Joly, J., Kraytman, M. and Piot, P. (1978), 'Bronchopulmonary infection due to β-lactamase-producing Branhamella catarrhalis treated with amoxycillin/clavulanic-acid', *Lancet*, **2**, 257.

Nyström, B. (1971), 'Patterns of antibiotic sensitivity in bacteria isolated from hospital in-patients', *Scand. J. Infect. Dis.*, **3**, 229.

Olarte, J. and Galindo, E. (1973), 'Salmonella typhi resistant to chloramphenicol, ampicillin, and other antimicrobial agents: Strains isolated during an extensive typhoid fever epidemic in Mexico', *Antimicrob. Ag. Chemother.*, **4**, 597.

Olarte, J., Filloy, L. and Galindo, E. (1976), 'Resistance of Shigella dysenteriae type 1 to ampicillin and other antimicrobial agents: Strains isolated during a dysentery outbreak in a hospital in Mexico City', *J. Infect. Dis.*, **133**, 572.

Orfanakis, M. G., Wilcox, H. G. and Smith, C. B. (1972), '*In vitro* studies of the combined effect of ampicillin and sulfonamides on Nocardia asteroides and results of therapy in four patients', *Antimicrob. Ag. Chemother.*, **1**, 215.

Oriel, J. D., Ridgway, G. L., Reeve, P., Beckingham, D. C. and Owen, J. (1976), 'The lack of effect of ampicillin plus probenecid given for genital infections with Neisseria gonorrhoeae on associated infections with Chlamydia trachomatis', *J. Infect. Dis.*, **133**, 568.

Overturf, G., Marton, K. I. and Mathies, A. W., Jr. (1973), 'Antibiotic resistance in typhoid fever', *New Engl. J. Med.*, **289**, 463.

Parker, R. H. and Hoeprich, P. D. (1966), 'Parenteral sodium ampicillin therapy of endocarditis, salmonellosis, and other bacterial infections', *Antimicrob. Agents Chemother.—1965*, p. 618.

Parker, A. C. and Richmond, J. (1976), 'Reduction in incidence of rash using polymer-free ampicillin', *Brit. med. J.*, **1**, 998.

Parsons, R. L., Hossack, G. and Paddock, G. (1975), 'The absorption of antibiotics in adult patients with coeliac disease', *J. Antimicrob. Chemother.*, **1**, 39.

Patel, K. M. (1964), 'Ampicillin in typhoid fever', *Brit. med. J.*, **1**, 907.

Petheram, I. S. and Boyce, J. M. H. (1976), 'Prosthetic endocarditis treated with ampicillin and gentamicin in a penicillin-hypersensitive patient', *Brit. med. J.*, **2**, 851.

Phillips, W. E. (1971), 'Treatment of chronic typhoid carriers with ampicillin', *JAMA*, **217**, 913.

Phillips, J. A., Lovejoy, F. H., Jr. and Matsumiya, Y. (1976), 'Ampicillin-associated diarrhoea: Effect of dosage and route of administration', *Pediatrics*, **58**, 869.

Philipson, A., Sabath, L. D. and Rosner, B. (1975), 'Sequence effect on ampicillin blood levels noted in an amoxicillin, ampicillin, and epicillin triple crossover study', *Antimicrob. Ag. Chemother.*, **8**, 311.

Philipson, A. (1977), 'Pharmacokinetics of ampicillin during pregnancy', *J. Infect. Dis.*, **136**, 370.

Pinget, M., Brogard, J. M., Dauchel, J. and Lavillaureix, J. (1976), 'Biliary excretion of ampicillin, metampicillin and carbenicillin', *J. Antimicrob. Chemother.*, **2**, 195.

Potter, J. L., Weinberg, A. G. and West, R. (1971), 'Ampicillinuria and ampicillin crystalluria', *Pediatrics*, **48**, 636.

Potter, J. P. L. (1972), 'Skin reactions to ampicillin', *Brit. med. J.*, **1**, 749.

Prince, A. and Neu, H. C. (1976), 'Beta-lactamase activity in Shigella sonnei', *Antimicrob. Ag. Chemother.*, **9**, 776.

Pullen, H., Wright, N. and Murdoch, J. McC. (1967), 'Hypersensitivity reactions to antibacterial drugs in infectious mononucleosis', *Lancet*, **2**, 1176.

Raevuori, M., Harvey, S. M., Pickett, M. J. and Martin, W. J. (1978), 'Yersinia enterocolitica; *in vitro* antimicrobial susceptibility', *Antimicrob. Ag. Chemother.*, **13**, 888.

Rahaman, M. M., Huq, I., Dey, C. R., Kibriya, A. K. M. G. and Curlin, G. (1974), 'Ampicillin-resistant shiga bacillus in Bangladesh, *Lancet*, **1**, 406.

Read, L. and Cove-Smith, J. R. (1977), 'Pseudomembranous enterocolitis complicating ampicillin therapy', *Postgrad. Med. J.*, **53**, 324.

Reading, C. and Cole, M. (1977), 'Clavulanic acid: A beta-lactamase-inhibiting beta-lactam from Streptomyces clavuligerus', *Antimicrob. Ag. Chemother.*, **11**, 852.

Report of a Collaborative Study Group (1973), 'Prospective study of ampicillin rash', *Brit. med. J.*, **1**, 7.

Roberton, Y. R. and Johnson, E. S. (1976), 'Interactions between oral contraceptives and other drugs: a review', *Curr. Med. Res. Opin.*, **3**, 647.

Robertson, M. B., Breen, K. J., Desmond, P. V., Mashford, M. L. and McHugh, A. M. (1977), 'Incidence of antibiotic-related diarrhoea and pseudomembranous colitis: A prospective study of lincomycin, clindamycin and ampicillin', *Med. J. Aust.*, **1**, 243.

Rolinson, G. N. and Stevens, S. (1961), 'Microbiological studies on a new broad-spectrum penicillin, "Penbritin"', *Brit. med. J.*, **2**, 191.

Rolinson, G. N. and Sutherland, R. (1965), 'The binding of antibiotics to serum proteins', *Brit. J. Pharmacol.*, **25**, 638.

Ross, S., Controni, G. and Khan, W. (1972), 'Resistance of shigellae to ampicillin and other antibiotics', *JAMA*, **221**, 45.

Roupas, A. and Pitton, J. S. (1974), 'R factor—mediated and chromosomal resistance to ampicillin in Escherichia coli', *Antimicrob. Ag. Chemother.*, **5**, 186.

Ruley, E. J. and Lisi, L. M. (1974), 'Interstitial nephritis and renal failure due to ampicillin', *J. Pediatrics*, **84**, 878.

Rutenburg, A. M. and Greenberg, H. L. (1967), 'Broad-spectrum penicillins and other antibiotics in the treatment of surgical infections', *Ann. N.Y. Acad. Sci.*, **145**, 451.

Sabath, L. D., McCall, C. F., Steigbigel, N. H. and Finland, M. (1967), 'Synergistic penicillin combinations for treatment of human urinary-tract infections', *Antimicrob. Agents Chemother.*—1966, p. 149.

Sabath, L. D., Gerstein, D. A., Leaf, C. D. and Finland, M. (1970), 'Increasing the usefulness of antibiotics: Treatment of infections by Gram-negative bacilli', *Clin. Pharm. Ther.*, **11**, 161.

Sanders, W. L. (1965), 'Treatment of typhoid fevers: A comparative trial of ampicillin and chloramphenicol', *Brit. med. J.*, **2**, 1226.

Saunders, J. R. and Sykes, R. B. (1977), 'Transfer of a plasmid-specified beta-lactamase gene from Haemophilus influenzae', *Antimicrob. Ag. Chemother.*, **11**, 339.

Schauf, V., Deveikis, A., Riff, L. and Serota, A. (1976), 'Antibiotic-killing kinetics of Group B streptococci', *J. Pediatrics*, **89**, 194.

Schiffer, M. S., MacLowry, J., Schneerson, R. and Robbins, J. B. (1974), 'Clinical bacteriological, and immunological characterisation of ampicillin-resistant Haemophilus influenzae type B', *Lancet*, **2**, 257.

Schulkind, M. L., Altemeier, W. A. and Ayoub, E. M. (1971), 'A comparison of ampicillin and chloramphenicol therapy in Hemophilus influenzae meningitis', *Pediatrics*, **48**, 411.

Schwartz, R., Rodriguez, W., Khan, W. and Ross, S. (1978), 'The increasing incidence of ampicillin-resistant Haemophilus influenzae. A cause of otitis media', *JAMA*, **239**, 320.

Scioli, C. Giusti, G. and Balestrieri, G. (1964), 'Comparison of ampicillin and chloramphenicol in treatment of typhoid fever', *Posgrad. Med. J.* (Suppl.), **40**, 87.

Shackelford, P. G., Bobinski, J. E., Feigin, R. D. and Cherry, J. D. (1972), 'Therapy of Haemophilus influenzae meningitis reconsidered', *New Engl. J. Med.*, **287**, 634.

Shapiro, S., Slone, D., Siskind, V., Lewis, G. P. and Jick, H. (1969), 'Drug rash with ampicillin and other penicillins', *Lancet*, **2**, 969.

Shimada, K., Inamatsu, T. and Yamashiro, M. (1977), 'Anaerobic bacteria in biliary disease in elderly patients', *J. Infect. Dis.*, **135**, 850.

Shurin, P. A., Pelton, S. I., Scheifele, D. and Klein, J. O. (1976), 'Otitis media caused by non-typable, ampicillin-resistant strains of Haemophilus influenzae', *J. Pediatrics*, **88**, 646.

Simon, H. J. and Miller, R. C. (1966), 'Ampicillin in the treatment of chronic typhoid carriers. Report on fifteen treated cases and a review of the literature', *New Engl. J. Med.*, **274**, 808.

Slade, N. (1977), 'Urinary tract infections in neurogenic bladder', *J. Antimicrob. Chemother.*, **3**, 3.

Sleet, R. A., Sangster, G. and Murdoch, J. McC. (1964), 'Comparison of ampicillin and chloramphenicol in treatment of paratyphoid fever', *Brit. med. J.*, **1**, 148.

Smith, A. L. (1972), 'Editorial. Therapy of influenzal meningitis considered', *New Engl. J. Med.*, **287**, 664.

Smith, A. L. (1976), 'Current concepts. Antibiotics and invasive Haemophilus influenzae', *New Engl. J. Med.*, **294**, 1329.

Smith, J. T., Bremner, D. A. and Datta, N. (1974), 'Ampicillin resistance of Shigella sonnei', *Antimicrob. Ag. Chemother.*, **6**, 418.

Snyder, M. J. *et al.* (1976), 'Comparative efficacy of chloramphenicol, ampicillin, and co-trimoxazole in the treatment of typhoid fever', *Lancet*, **2**, 1155.

Søgaard, H. (1975), 'Incidence of antibiotic resistance and transmissible R factors in the Gram-negative bowel flora of hospital patients on admission', *Scand. J. Infect. Dis.*, **7**, 253.

Steigbigel, N. H., McCall, C. E., Read, C. W. and Finland, M. (1967), 'Antibacterial action of "broad spectrum" penicillins, cephalosporins and other antibiotics against Gram-negative bacilli isolated from bacteremic patients', *Ann. N.Y. Acad. Sci.*, **145**, 224.

Stevenson, J. and Mandal, B. K. (1966), 'Ampicillin and the fifth-day rash', *Brit. med. J.*, **1**, 1359.

Stewart, G. T. (1965), *The Penicillin Group of Drugs*, Elsevier Publishing Company.

Stewart, G. T., Coles, H. M. T., Nixon, H. H. and Holt, R. J. (1961), '"Penbritin": An oral penicillin with broad-spectrum activity', *Brit. med. J.*, **2**, 200.

Stewart, G. T. (1969), 'Ampicillin rashes', *Lancet*, **2**, 1356.

Stewart, S. M. (1974), 'Ampicillin-resistant Haemophilus influenzae', *Lancet*, **1**, 1163.

Sullivan, J. F. (1970), 'Ampicillin treatment of gonorrhoea in girls in institutions', *Med. J. Aust.*, **2**, 785.

Sutter, V. L. and Finegold, S. M. (1976), 'Susceptibility of anaerobic bacteria to 23 antimicrobial agents', *Antimicrob. Ag. Chemother.*, **10**, 736.

Syriopoulou, V., Scheifele, D., Howie, V., Ploussard, J., Sloyer, J. and Smith, A. L. (1976), 'Incidence of ampicillin-resistant Hemophilus influenzae in otitis media', *J. Pediatrics*, **89**, 839.

Tannenberg, A. M., Wicher, K. J. and Rose, N. R. (1971), 'Ampicillin nephropathy', *JAMA*, **218**, 449.

Thew, M. A., Swift, J. T. and Heaton, C. L. (1969), 'Ampicillin in the treatment of granuloma inguinale', *JAMA*, **210**, 866.

Thomas, W. J., McReynolds, J. W., Mock, C. R. and Bailey, D. W. (1974), 'Ampicillin-resistant Haemophilus influenzae meningitis', *Lancet*, **1**, 313.

Thorne, G. M. and Farrar, W. E., Jr. (1975), 'Transfer of ampicillin resistance between strains of Haemophilus influenzae type B', *J. Infect. Dis.*, **132**, 276.

Thornsberry, C., Baker, C. N., Kirven, L. A. and Swenson, J. M. (1976), 'Susceptibility of ampicillin-resistant Haemophilus influenzae to seven penicillins', *Antimicrob. Ag. Chemother.*, **9**, 70.

Thornsberry, C., Baker, C. N. and Kirven, L. A. (1978), '*In vitro* activity of antimicrobial agents on Legionnaires' disease bacterium', *Antimicrob. Ag. Chemother.*, **13**, 78.

Thrupp, L. D., Leedom, J. M., Ivler, D., Wehrle, P. F., Portnoy, B. and Mathies, A. W. (1966), 'Ampicillin levels in the cerebro-spinal fluid during treatment of bacterial meningitis', *Antimicrob. Agents Chemother.*—1965, p. 206.

Tilton, R. C., Corcoran, L., Newberg, L. and Sedgwick, A. K. (1972), 'Ampicillin-resistant Shigella sonnei', *JAMA*, **222**, 487.

Tomeh, M. O., Starr, S. E., McGowan, J. E., Jr., Terry, P. M. and Nahmias, A. J. (1974), 'Ampicillin-resistant Haemophilus influenzae type B infection', *JAMA*, **229**, 295.

Tuano, S. B., Johnson, L. D., Brodie, J. L. and Kirby, W. M. M. (1966), 'Comparative blood levels of hetacillin, ampicillin and penicillin G', *New Engl. J. Med.*, **275**, 635.

Turck, M. (1967), 'Broad-spectrum penicillins and other antibiotics in the treatment of urinary tract infections', *Ann. N.Y. Acad. Sci.*, **145**, 344.

Urban, T. (1972), 'Transferable multiple drug resistance of shigella strains isolated in Sweden', *Scand. J. Infect. Dis.*, **4**, 221.

Vega, R., Sadoff, H. L. and Patterson, M. J. (1976), 'Mechanisms of ampicillin resistance in Haemophilus influenzae type B', *Antimicrob. Ag. Chemother.*, **9**, 164.

Visintine, A. M., Oleske, J. M. and Nahmias, A. J. (1977), 'Listeria monocytogenes infection in infants and children', *Am. J. Dis. Child.*, **131**, 393.

Ward, J. I., Gorman, G., Phillips, C. and Fraser, D. W. (1978), 'Hemophilus influenzae type B disease in a day-care center', *J. Pediatrics*, **92**, 713.

Wasz-Höckert, O., Nummi, S., Vuopala, S. and Järvinen, P. A. (1970), 'Transplacental passage of azidocillin, ampicillin and penicillin G during early and late pregnancy', *Scand. J. Infect. Dis.*, **2**, 125.

Watts, B. A., Phillips, I. and Stoate, M. W. (1977), 'The *in vitro* activity of 15 penicillins and mecillinam against Neisseria gonorrhoea', *J. Antimicrob. Chemother.*, **3**, 331.

Weissman, J. B., Gangarosa, E. J., Dupont, H. L., Nelson, J. D. and Haltalin, K. C. (1974), 'Shigellosis. To treat or not to treat?', *JAMA*, **229**, 1215.

Whelton, A., Sapir, D. G., Carter, G. G., Garth, M. A. and Walker, W. G. (1972), 'Intrarenal distribution of ampicillin in the normal and diseased human kidney', *J. Infect. Dis.*, **125**, 466.

Whitby, J. M. F. (1964), 'Ampicillin in treatment of Salmonella typhi carriers', *Lancet*, **2**, 71.

Wiggins, G. L., Albritton, W. L. and Feeley, J. C. (1978), 'Antibiotic susceptibility of clinical isolates of Listeria monocytogenes', *Antimicrob. Ag. Chemother.*, **13**, 854.

Wilson, H. D. and Haltalin, K. C. (1975), 'Ampicillin in Haemophilus influenzae meningitis, *Am. J. Dis. Child.*, **129**, 208.

Winshell, E. B., Cherubin, C., Winter, J. and Neu, H. C. (1970), 'Antibiotic resistance of Salmonella in the eastern United States', *Antimicrob. Agents Chemother.*—1969, p. 86.

Wise, R. (1977), 'Clavulanic acid and susceptibility of Bacteroides fragilis to penicillin', *Lancet*, **2**, 145.

Wise, R., Andrews, J. M. and Bedford, K. A. (1978), '*In vitro* study of clavulanic acid in combination with penicillin, amoxycillin, and carbenicillin', *Antimicrob. Ag. Chemother.*, **13**, 389.

Wong, G. A., Peirce, T. H., Goldstein, E. and Hoeprich, P. D. (1975), 'Penetration of antimicrobial agents into bronchial secretions', *Amer. J. Med.*, **59**, 219.

Woodroffe, A. J., Weldon, M., Meadows, R. and Lawrence, J. R. (1975), 'Acute interstitial nephritis following ampicillin hypersensitivity', *Med. J. Aust.*, **1**, 65.

Wüst, J. and Wilkins, T. D. (1978), 'Effect of clavulanic acid on anaerobic bacteria resistant to beta-lactam antibiotics', *Antimicrob. Ag. Chemother.*, **13**, 130.

Wyatt, R. G., Okamoto, G. A. and Feigin, R. D. (1972), 'Stability of antibiotics in parenteral solutions', *Pediatrics*, **49**, 22.

Yoshioka, H., Rudoy, P., Riley, H. D., Jr. and Yoshida, K. (1977), 'Antimicrobial susceptibility of Escherichia coli isolated at a children's hospital', *Scand. J. Infect. Dis.*, **9**, 207.

Yow, M. D., Baker, C. J., Barrett, F. F. and Ortigoza, C. O. (1973), 'Initial antibiotic management of bacterial meningitis', *Medicine*, **52**, 305.

Amoxycillin, Epicillin, Cyclacillin, Hetacillin, Pivampicillin, Talampicillin, Bacampicillin and Metampicillin

Description

The value of ampicillin as a chemotherapeutic agent is well recognised, and it has been chemically modified in various ways in an attempt to produce an improved compound. Many antibiotics structurally related to ampicillin have been developed and eight of them are described in this chapter. Three, amoxycillin, epicillin and cyclacillin, have intrinsic antibacterial activity. The other five antibiotics are usually completely hydrolysed in the body to ampicillin after administration.

1. *Amoxycillin*. Chemically alpha-amino-p-hydroxybenzyl-penicillin, it is also known as amoxicillin, 'Amoxil', 'Larocin', 'Moxacin' and BRL 2333. This was developed by Beecham Research Laboratories (Sutherland and Rolinson, 1971; Sutherland *et al.*, 1972), and its main advantage over ampicillin is its better absorption from the gastro-intestinal tract (page 136).

2. *Epicillin*. Chemically 6-(D2-amino-2-(1,4-cyclohexadienyl) acetamido)-penicillanic acid (Basch *et al.*, 1971; Gadebusch *et al.*, 1971), it is marketed as 'Dexacillin' (Squibb).

3. *Cyclacillin*. This is a partially penicillinase-resistant penicillin with a chemical formula of 6-(1-aminocyclo-hexanecarboxamide)-penicillanic acid (Gonzaga *et al.*, 1974; Neu, 1975a and b).

4. *Hetacillin*. Developed by Bristol Laboratories in 1965 by reacting ampicillin with acetone, this is also referred to as BL-804, BL-PK-804, phenazacillin or 'Versapen'. Hetacillin hydrolyses in solution to form ampicillin both *in vitro* and *in vivo*, therefore the ultimate active component of this semisynthetic penicillin is mainly ampicillin (Sutherland and Robinson, 1967; Kahrimanis and Pierpaoli, 1971).

5. *Pivampicillin*. This is the hydrochloride salt of pivaloyl-oxymethyl D-alpha-aminobenzyl-penicillinate, which is an ampicillin ester. It is better absorbed from the gastro-intestinal tract than ampicillin, to which after absorption it is rapidly and completely hydrolysed (Daehne *et al.*, 1971).

6. *Talampicillin*. Chemically a thiazolide carboxylic ester of ampicillin, this drug is also known as 'Talpen'. It has no antibacterial activity until it is hydrolysed in the intestine to form ampicillin. Serum levels after administration of this drug, are approximately twice those attained with an equivalent dose of ampicillin (Clayton *et al.*, 1974; Leigh *et al.*, 1976).

7. *Bacampicillin*. Similarly, this is another ester of ampicillin which is chemically 1'-ethoxycarbonyloxy-ethyl 6-(D-alpha-aminophenylacetamido)

penicillinate. After absorption it is rapidly hydrolysed to ampicillin and serum levels achieved are two to three times higher than those after equivalent doses of ampicillin (Bodin *et al.*, 1975; Hallander *et al.*, 1977; Sjövall *et al.*, 1978).

8. *Metampicillin*. This is produced by combining ampicillin with formaldehyde. When administered orally, it is rapidly hydrolysed to ampicillin in the gut and administered in this way it has no advantages over ampicillin (Neu, 1975a and b). After parenteral administration, some of the drug apparently circulates as unchanged metampicillin, because it has a greater stability in serum than in aqueous acid solutions. The sole advantage of this seems that circulating metampicillin is excreted into the bile in a greater concentration than ampicillin (Neu, 1975b; Brogard *et al.*, 1976).

Sensitive Organisms

For practical purposes, the antibacterial activities of these eight compounds are identical to that of ampicillin (page 99).

1. *Hetacillin, pivampicillin, talampicillin, bacampicillin and metampicillin*. Since all of these are hydrolysed to ampicillin *in vivo* before they exert any antibacterial activity, their activity would be expected to be identical to that of ampicillin. With hetacillin there was some controversy about this concept. For example, using fast methods for measuring bacterial inhibition, hetacillin was shown to have an independent antibiotic action prior to its *in vivo* hydrolysis (Faine and Harper, 1973). In such studies, unlike ampicillin, hetacillin was not destroyed by beta-lactamase, and theoretically some ampicillin-resistant bacteria could be susceptible to it. These findings have no practical significance, because all absorbed hetacillin is hydrolysed in the body to ampicillin within 15–30 min. Using conventional microbiological techniques, the *in vitro* activities of hetacillin and ampicillin against various bacteria are identical (Sutherland and Robinson, 1967; Steigbigel *et al.*, 1967).

After parenteral administration, some metampicillin also circulates in the serum in an unhydrolysed form, but *in vitro* activity of metampicillin is identical to that of ampicillin and both drugs are unstable in the presence of beta-lactamase (Neu, 1975b).

2. *Amoxycillin*. This drug's *in vitro* antibacterial activity is virtually identical to that of ampicillin, although it has its own intrinsic activity and it is not converted to ampicillin in the body (Neu and Winshell, 1971a; Sutherland *et al.*, 1972). There are only a few minor differences between the antibacterial activities of these drugs. For instance, amoxycillin is about two-fold more active than ampicillin against Strep. faecalis and Salmonella spp. but two-fold less active against Shigella spp. (Sabto *et al.*, 1973; Neu, 1974). H. influenzae also appears to be slightly less sensitive to amoxycillin than to ampicillin (Kosmidis *et al.*, 1972); the same is true for the anaerobic bacteria, both Gram-positive and Gram-negative (Sutter and Finegold, 1976). Similar to penicillin G and ampicillin, amoxycillin when combined with an aminoglycoside acts synergistically against Strep. faecalis (Russell and Sutherland, 1975; Basker and Sutherland, 1977).

In studies with experimental infections in mice, amoxycillin is more active than ampicillin against infections with both Gram-positive and Gram-negative bacteria (Hunter *et al.*, 1973; Rolinson, 1974). This cannot be explained on the basis of the better absorption of amoxycillin from the gastro-intestinal tract (page 136), but there were differences in the distribution of these two penicillins in the infected animals. Amoxycillin produced better peritoneal concentration after subcutaneous administration and amoxycillin serum levels were also higher after intraperitoneal dosing (Comber *et al.*, 1975). These differences partly explained why amoxycillin was more effective than ampicillin in the experimental infections. The slightly differing mechanisms of action of these two penicillins on bacteria (*see* page 22), may also partly explain the better *in vivo* bactericidal activity of amoxycillin. The clinical significance of these observations remains unknown.

3. *Epicillin*. The antimicrobial spectrum of this compound is also similar to that of ampicillin. It is more active than ampicillin, but usually less active than carbenicillin, against Pseudomonas aeruginosa (Basch *et al.*, 1971). This property has no clinical importance.

4. *Cyclacillin*. This compound has variable but in general an inferior antibacterial activity compared to ampicillin (Gonzaga *et al.*, 1974; Neu, 1975b). It has a slightly greater activity against penicillinase-producing staphylococci, but this is of no therapeutic value. Cyclacillin has greater activity in experimental animal infections than would be predicted from its *in vitro* activity.

5. *Activity against ampicillin-resistant strains*. All these penicillins are inactive against penicillinase-producing Staph. pyogenes strains. There is also no evidence that they are active against any strains of Gram-negative bacilli such as H. influenzae and the Salmonella and Shigella spp., which have developed resistance to ampicillin (*see* page 100).

In Vitro Sensitivities

TABLE 8

Compiled from data published by Basch *et al.* (1971), Sutherland *et al.* (1972) and Sutter and Finegold (1976)

ORGANISM	MIC (μg per ml)	
	Amoxycillin	Epicillin
Gram-positive bacteria		
Staph. pyogenes (non-penicillinase producer)	0·1	0·2
Staph. pyogenes (penicillinase producer)	250·0	50·0
Strep. pyogenes (Group A)	0·01	0·004
Strep. pneumoniae (Dip. pneumoniae)	0·02	0·02
Strep. faecalis (Enterococcus, Group D)	0·5	0·5
Gram-negative bacteria		
Escherichia coli	5·0	1·4
Proteus mirabilis	2·5	1·2
Haemophilus influenzae	0·25	0·3
Pseudomonas aeruginosa	500·0	9·4
Bacteroides fragilis	32·0–64·0	—
Bacteroides melaninogenicus	0·5–1·0	—

The minimum inhibitory concentrations of amoxycillin and epicillin against some selected bacterial species are shown in Table 8. For practical purposes there is no difference between these two drugs and ampicillin (Table 7, page 105).

Mode of Administration and Dosage

Pivampicillin, talampicillin and bacampicillin were introduced to provide compounds with improved oral absorption, and these are not used parenterally. The same is also generally true for amoxycillin, but a parenteral preparation of this has been recently developed. Epicillin, cyclacillin, hetacillin and metampicillin are available for parenteral and oral administration.

1. *Parenteral administration.*

(a)   *Amoxycillin.* Sodium amoxycillin, which is suitable for both intramuscular and intravenous administration, has been developed recently. It produces satisfactory serum levels in adults when it is given intravenously or intramuscularly in single doses of 250 mg, 500 mg and 1·0 g (Spyker *et al.*, 1977) (*see* page 136). This preparation may prove to be satisfactory for parenteral use in doses similar to parenteral ampicillin (page 106).

(b)   *Epicillin.* Sodium epicillin can be administered intramuscularly or intravenously in doses of 250 mg to 1 g six-hourly to adults. As with ampicillin (page 106), even higher doses are probably safe (Limson *et al.*, 1972).

(c)   *Cyclacillin.* This compound can be administered by intravenous route in doses similar to those used orally (*vide infra*).

(d)   *Hetacillin.* Both intramuscular and intravenous administration are satisfactory. Like ampicillin, high parenteral doses are necessary for serious infections; a daily dose of 150 mg per kg, administered in four divided doses has been commonly used.

(e)   *Metampicillin.* This can be administered both intramuscularly and intravenously in an adult dose of 0·5–1·0 g six-hourly (Neu, 1975b; Brogard *et al.*, 1976).

2. *Oral administration.* All eight compounds can be administered by the oral route. The usual oral dose of amoxycillin, epicillin, cyclacillin, hetacillin and metampicillin is 50 to 100 mg per kg body weight per day administered in four divided doses. A common adult dose is 250–500 mg six-hourly.

The adult dose of pivampicillin is 350 to 700 mg six-hourly. On a molar basis, 700 mg of pivampicillin corresponds to 500 mg of ampicillin (Hultberg and Backelin, 1972). Talampicillin is given to adults in a dose of 375 to 750 mg (equivalent to 250 to 500 mg ampicillin) every eight hours (Clayton *et al.*, 1974; Leigh *et al.*, 1976). Bacampicillin has been administered to adults in doses of either 200 mg, 400 mg or 800 mg every eight or twelve hours (Maesen *et al.*, 1976; Hallander *et al.*, 1977).

3. *Newborn and premature infants.* In this age group dosage reduction of these drugs similar to ampicillin (page 106) is advocated. It is preferable at present to use the more familiar ampicillin for the treatment of these patients.

4. *Patients with renal failure.* These drugs are relatively non-toxic and may be given in the usual recommended dosage to patients with mild renal failure. In patients with more severe renal failure, as in the case of ampicillin (page 107), the dose should be reduced (Sabto *et al.*, 1973). In patients undergoing regular

dialysis, a single 250 mg dose of amoyxcillin, given at the end of dialysis, will provide therapeutic serum levels for 24 h (Lawson *et al.*, 1974).

Availability

1. *Amoxycillin*
   (a) Capsules: 125, 250 and 500 mg.
   (b) Oral suspension: 125 mg in 5 ml and 250 mg in 5 ml.
   (c) Sodium amoxycillin: for intramuscular or intravenous use (not yet generally available).
2. *Epicillin*
   (a) Capsules: 250 and 500 mg.
   (b) Paediatric syrup: 125 mg per 5 ml or 250 mg per 5 ml.
   (c) Sodium epicillin for parenteral use: vials of 250 and 500 mg.
3. *Cyclacillin*
   Preparations for both oral and intravenous administration.
4. *Hetacillin*
   (a) Capsules: 250 mg.
   (b) Paediatric suspension: 125 mg per 5 ml.
   (c) Vials: 250 mg for intravenous or intramuscular use.
5. *Pivampicillin*
   (a) Capsules: 178 mg (equimolar to 125 mg ampicillin).
   (b) Capsules: 350 mg (equimolar to 250 mg ampicillin).
   (c) Paediatric suspension of pivampicillin base: 162 mg per 5 ml (equimolar to 125 mg of ampicillin per 5 ml).
6. *Talampicillin*
   (a) Capsules: 375 mg (equimolar to 250 ampicillin).
   (b) Capsules: 750 mg (equimolar to 500 mg ampicillin).
7. *Bacampicillin*
   (a) Capsules: 200 mg (equimolar to 125 mg ampicillin).
   (b) Capsules: 400 mg (equimolar to 250 mg ampicillin).
8. *Metampicillin*
   Preparations suitable for oral and intravenous administration.

Serum Levels in Relation to Dosage

1. *Amoxycillin*. Amoxycillin is well absorbed after oral administration (Neu and Winshell, 1971b; Sutherland *et al.*, 1972; Verbist, 1976). After a 500 mg dose in adults, a peak serum level of 8–10 μg per ml is reached two hours later (Fig. 7). Doubling the dose doubles the peak serum level. Thereafter serum concentrations fall, and reach zero after six to eight hours. These serum levels are about twice as high as those produced by an equivalent dose of oral ampicillin, and about the same as those attained after this dose of ampicillin is given intramuscularly (page 107). Food in the stomach significantly impairs ampicillin absorption, but has little effect on that of amoxycillin (Sabto *et al.*, 1973; Neu, 1974) (*see also* ampicillin, page 107). Amoxycillin absorption is satisfactory in patients with achlorhydria (Lawson *et al.*, 1974), but it is significantly impaired in those with coeliac disease (Parsons *et al.*, 1975).

Intramuscular administration of sodium amoxycillin results in serum concentrations similar to those obtained with intramuscular ampicillin or oral amoxycillin (Spyker *et al.*, 1977). Serum levels of amoxycillin after intravenous administration are the same as those obtained with ampicillin intravenously (page 108).

2. *Epicillin*. This drug is moderately well absorbed from the gastro-intestinal tract and serum levels attained are usually slightly lower than those obtained with oral ampicillin (*see* Fig. 6, page 108). After a 500 mg oral dose to adults, a peak serum level of 2·4 μg per ml is reached two to three hours later. The level

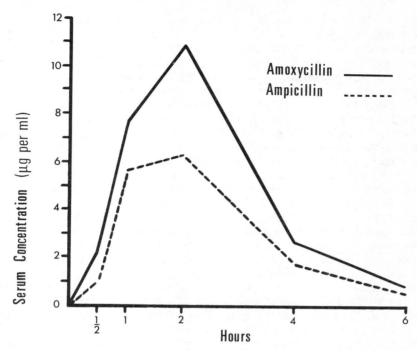

FIG. 7. Mean serum concentrations of amoxycillin and ampicillin after a single 500 mg oral dose in a cross-over study in 12 fasting subjects. (Redrawn after Sutherland *et al.*, 1972.)

is virtually zero eight hours after administration (Philipson *et al.*, 1975). Serum levels attained after parenteral epicillin are probably of the same order as those produced by intramuscular or intravenous ampicillin.

3. *Cyclacillin*. After oral administration it is rapidly absorbed and serum levels reach 10–18 μg per ml 30 min after a 500 mg dose. These serum levels fall rapidly, are low in two hours and usually very low or undetectable at four and six hours (Neu, 1975b).

4. *Hetacillin*. There was controversy about serum levels obtained with this drug compared to those attained with equivalent doses of ampicillin. In practice there is no significant difference, irrespective of the mode of administration. Slightly higher blood levels with oral or intramuscular ampicillin were reported (Sutherland and Robinson, 1967; Ridley, 1967); others showed that although after oral administration hetacillin levels rise more slowly, they are more prolonged (Kirby and Kind, 1967). Hetacillin also produces higher serum levels than ampicillin when these drugs are administered intravenously (Tuano *et al.*, 1966). Therefore it was concluded that hetacillin was only superior to ampicillin if given intravenously (Kahrimanis and Pierpaoli, 1971). Subsequently, Jusko and Lewis (1972) showed that higher serum levels after intravenous hetacillin were due to a technical artefact; during the period taken for microbiological assay all unhydrolysed hetacillin is converted to ampicillin, and they assumed that this unhydrolysed hetacillin is microbiologically inactive. Hetacillin may however have independent activity (page 133), and this

could be significant because the drug exists *in vivo* as ampicillin plus un-hydrolysed hetacillin.

After oral administration the proportion of unchanged hetacillin in the serum is very small at any time (Sutherland and Robinson, 1967). By comparison, there may be a higher proportion of the unchanged drug in the serum when large doses (0.5 g per hour) are given intravenously, as in the study by Tuano *et al.* (1966). Unhydrolysed hetacillin is probably more slowly eliminated from the body (page 139), and this may explain the higher total drug levels achieved with intravenous hetacillin compared to ampicillin. It is still uncertain whether this confers a therapeutic advantage to intravenous hetacillin. Clinically the two drugs seem to be of about the same value (page 143).

5. *Pivampicillin*. The absorption of this ester from the gastro-intestinal tract is superior to that of ampicillin, to which it is immediately hydrolysed, so that it produces higher serum levels than oral ampicillin (Daehne *et al.*, 1971; Jordan *et al.*, 1971; Little and Peddie, 1974). After an oral dose of 700 mg pivam-picillin (equimolar to 500 mg ampicillin), a peak serum level of about 10 μg per ml is reached one to two hours after the dose (Fig. 8). Thereafter the serum concentration gradually falls and at six hours very little drug is detectable.

Serum levels after pivampicillin are at least double those after ampicillin (Fig. 6, page 108) and, although similar, they differ slightly from those attained after an identical oral dose of amoxycillin. During the first one to two hours after dosage, ampicillin levels obtained by pivampicillin administration are slightly higher than amoxycillin levels. According to some investigators, amoxycillin then produces slightly higher serum concentrations than pivam-picillin over the period from two to six hours (Croydon and Sutherland, 1971); others have found that pivampicillin produces slightly higher levels throughout the six-hour period after the dose (Verbist, 1974).

Absorption of pivampicillin is not impaired by food rich in fat and protein (Jordan *et al.*, 1971; Roholt *et al.*, 1974). Serum concentrations of ampicillin after pivampicillin administration, are about the same in patients with acute febrile illnesses and in convalescent patients (Hultberg and Backelin, 1972). Absorption of pivampicillin is reduced in patients with coeliac disease (Parsons *et al.*, 1975), and it is reduced and variable in post-operative, partially mobilized patients (Kunst and Mattie, 1975).

6. *Talampicillin*. Ampicillin serum levels after administration of this ester are about twice as high as those after administration of an equimolar dose of oral ampicillin, and are similar to those attained by amoxycillin (Fig. 7, page 137) Clayton *et al.*, 1974; Verbist, 1976). The presence of food in the stomach reduces and delays the peak serum level, but does not affect the total amount of antibiotic absorbed (Leigh *et al.*, 1976; Jones, 1977).

7. *Bacampicillin*. Serum levels of ampicillin attained after the oral ad-ministration of this ester are also about twice as high as those after oral ad-ministration of an equimolar dose of ampicillin but about the same as attained by intramuscular ampicillin (Bergan, 1978). In one study the mean peak serum level after 800 mg bacampicillin was 11.9 μg per ml, while an equimolar dose of oral ampicillin (500 mg) produced a mean peak serum level of 6.8 μg per ml (Hallander *et al.*, 1977). In young children with a dose of 10 mg per kg body weight, the mean peak serum level reached in 30–60 min, is 7.2 μg per ml (Bergan *et al.*, 1978).

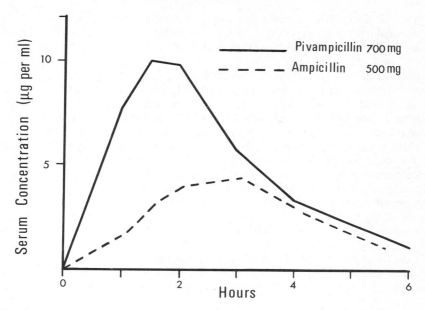

FIG. 8. Mean concentration of ampicillin in serum for 24 patients after oral administration of 700 mg pivampicillin equimolar to 500 mg of ampicillin, and after 500 mg ampicillin. (Redrawn after Hultberg and Backelin, 1972.)

8. *Metampicillin.* Following oral administration, this compound is hydrolysed to ampicillin, and serum levels are approximately the same as after ampicillin administration (Neu, 1975b). With parenteral administration, total serum levels achieved are similar to those attained after ampicillin, but a small proportion of the drug circulates in the body as unhydrolysed metampicillin (page 133).

Excretion

URINE: About 58–68 per cent of an orally administered dose of amoxycillin is excreted in the urine in an unchanged active form, during the first six hours (Sutherland *et al.*, 1972). High amoxycillin urinary levels of 115–1850 μg per ml occur after a 500 mg dose to adults. Like ampicillin (page 108), this drug is excreted by both glomerular filtration and tubular secretion; the latter can be reduced by concomitant administration of probenecid (Bodey and Nance, 1972).

Hetacillin, pivampicillin, talampicillin, bacampicillin and metampicillin are excreted via the kidney as ampicillin (page 108). A small proportion of administered hetacillin and metampicillin may be excreted as such in the urine, but the renal mechanisms involved are not known.

Epicillin is excreted unchanged in the urine in a similar manner to that of ampicillin. Cyclacillin is excreted unchanged in urine more rapidly; at six hours 77 per cent of a 500 mg oral dose can be recovered from urine, but thereafter urinary recovery is negligible (Gonzaga *et al.*, 1974).

BILE: The three drugs which are not hydrolysed to ampicillin in the body (amoxycillin, epicillin and cyclacillin), are probably excreted in the bile, similar to ampicillin (page 109). For instance in animals amoxycillin is concentrated in bile (Acred *et al.*, 1971).

After oral administration of metampicillin biliary concentrations of ampicillin attained are about the same as those obtained after oral administration of ampicillin. Following intravenous administration, some metampicillin circulates in the unhydrolysed form (page 139), and it is claimed that this is excreted in bile in higher concentrations than ampicillin. In patients after cholecystectomy who have T-tube drainage, a 500 mg intravenous metampicillin dose apparently produces a peak biliary drug concentration (probably mainly ampicillin) of approximately 1500 μg per ml in three hours. Overall, 8·3 per cent of an intravenously administered dose, but only 0·16 per cent of a metampicillin dose given orally, is excreted via the bile, probably mainly as ampicillin (Pinget *et al.*, 1976; Brogard *et al.*, 1976). By comparison, only approximately 0·1 per cent of an orally or intravenously administered dose of ampicillin is excreted in the bile (*see* page 109).

INACTIVATION IN BODY: All of these drugs are inactivated in the body to some extent, chiefly in the liver, similar to ampicillin. Unhydrolysed hetacillin may be more resistant to such inactivation than ampicillin (Tuano *et al.*, 1966).

Distribution of the Drugs in Body

All eight drugs, including those which are not converted in the body to ampicillin (amoxycillin, epicillin and cyclacillin) are probably distributed similarly to ampicillin, but some minor differences have been described with amoxycillin.

Amoxycillin penetrates into bronchial secretions better than ampicillin. In purulent sputum similar concentrations of both drugs are attained, but amoxycillin levels are higher in mucoid sputum (May and Ingold, 1974). Amoxycillin is only excreted in small amounts in breast milk. Saliva, sweat and tears also contain very small amounts of amoxycillin, while ampicillin and epicillin are usually undetectable in these secretions (Philipson *et al.*, 1975). Animal studies indicate that amoxycillin may also penetrate into normal CSF to a greater extent than ampicillin or penicillin G (Auvergnat, 1974). Like ampicillin, amoxycillin crosses the placenta and levels in cord blood are about one quarter to a third of those in maternal blood (Furuya *et al.*, 1973). Protein binding of amoxycillin (17 per cent) is similar to that of ampicillin (Sutherland *et al.*, 1972).

Mode of Action

The mode of action of all these penicillins on bacteria is similar to that of penicillin G, but with amoxycillin some differences have been described (*see* penicillin G, page 19).

Toxicity

1. *Hypersensitivity*. These penicillins may be all 'cross-allergenic' with other penicillins, and are therefore contraindicated in penicillin-allergic patients. As

pivampicillin, talampicillin and bacampicillin and nearly all of hetacillin and metampicillin are converted to ampicillin in the body, it is to be expected that the frequency of rashes and other allergic manifestations with these drugs, would be similar to ampicillin (page 110). The overall rate of amoxycillin rashes was reported to be about 3 per cent (Brogden *et al.*, 1975), which is lower than that due to ampicillin (page 110). After more widespread use of the drug, it now appears that amoxycillin rashes are more prevalent and probably as common as those due to ampicillin (Adverse Drug Reactions Advisory Committee, 1978). The maculopapular eruptions produced by amoxycillin are similar to those seen with ampicillin (page 110). Rashes due to amoxycillin have been reported in patients with glandular fever (Mulroy, 1973), and the drug probably has the same predilection to cause rashes in this disease as ampicillin (page 111) (Adverse Drug Reactions Advisory Committee, 1978).

According to the manufacturers, epicillin produces less rashes (2·2 per cent) than ampicillin. Large scale surveys are needed to determine the true frequency of rashes with all of these newer penicillins.

2. *Gastro-intestinal side-effects.* Oral administration of any of these drugs can cause nausea, epigastric discomfort and diarrhoea. As with ampicillin (page 112), these are not usually severe. Amoxycillin, because of its better absorption appears to cause these side-effects less commonly than ampicillin; the reported overall frequency of diarrhoea following amoxycillin treatment is only about 2 per cent (Knudsen, 1977). Pseudomembranous colitis (page 481), with typical clinical and sigmoidoscopic findings, has been described in one ten-year-old boy who received amoxycillin in a dose of 250 mg three times a day for an upper respiratory tract infection (Similä *et al.*, 1976). Oral epicillin (Limson *et al.*, 1972; Guerrero and Groel, 1974) and cyclacillin (Neu, 1975b) have also been relatively free from gastro-intestinal side-effects in clinical trials to date.

Pivampicillin is usually well tolerated (Neu, 1975b; Moe *et al.*, 1977). It produces more upper gastro-intestinal discomfort than ampicillin, whereas the reverse is true for diarrhoea. For example, in one comparative study, nine of 55 pivampicillin treated patients developed upper gastro-intestinal discomfort, which compared unfavourably with ampicillin (Brumfitt *et al.*, 1973). These symptoms are less frequent if pivampicillin is taken with food. Although pivampicillin is an antibacterially inactive ester, it still alters the intestinal bacterial flora (Moe *et al.*, 1977), because some free ampicillin reaches the gut via the bile.

Talampicillin appears to be well tolerated and it has a less profound effect on the faecal bacterial flora than ampicillin (Leigh *et al.*, 1976); the effect that occurs is again presumably the results of biliary excretion of free ampicillin (Symonds and George, 1978). Preliminary evidence from one trial suggests that diarrhoea with talampicillin may be only half as common as that with ampicillin (Knudsen and Harding, 1975; Knudsen, 1977). Gastro-intestinal side-effects have also been infrequent with bacampicillin in clinical trials to date (Maesen *et al.*, 1976; Hallander *et al.*, 1977). In animal studies using high oral doses of the ampicillin esters, gastric ulcerations have been produced. Magnusson *et al.* (1977) studied gastro-intestinal blood loss by a radioisotopic method in 10 male volunteers to whom either pivampicillin or bacampicillin was administered orally. Blood loss was clinically insignificant with both drugs.

3. *Encephalopathy*. This complication which occurs with ampicillin (page 113) may possibly occur if large doses of the parenterally used drugs (amoxycillin, epicillin, cyclacillin, hetacillin and metampicillin) are given intravenously.

Clinical Uses of the Drugs

Since all of these drugs have a similar antibacterial spectrum to ampicillin, their possible indications are the same as those for which ampicillin is advocated (page 113). Some of these drugs are inferior to ampicillin, whilst others in certain clinical situations may have advantages over ampicillin.

1. *Amoxycillin*. Being better absorbed from the gastro-intestinal tract, this drug can be used to treat infections which respond to oral ampicillin. On present evidence it appears that amoxycillin will replace oral ampicillin. Amoxycillin has been used successfully to treat urinary and respiratory tract infections (Handsfield *et al.*, 1973; Sabto *et al.*, 1973), but results of treatment have usually been about the same as with ampicillin. In patients with infections restricted to the bladder, a single amoxycillin dose of 3 g is just as effective as a 10 days course in a dose of 250 mg four times a day (Fang *et al.*, 1978). When amoxycillin is used for urinary tract infections, it significantly alters the normal periurethral flora, most patients acquiring a flora of either resistant aerobic Gram-negative rods or Candida albicans (Ronald *et al.*, 1977). Such alteration of periurethral flora may precede a recurrence of infection with resistant organisms.

For the treatment of chronic bronchial infections amoxycillin may be superior to oral ampicillin (May and Ingold, 1972; 1974), because it penetrates into bronchial secretions to a greater extent (page 140). In streptococcal pharyngitis amoxycillin is about as effective as oral penicillin V (Stillerman *et al.*, 1974). A six weeks course of oral amoxycillin in a dose of 1·0 g every four hours, combined with intramuscular gentamicin, was successful in one patient with Strep. faecalis endocarditis (Seligman, 1974). This treatment was instituted after the patient had relapsed following therapy with intravenous penicillin G plus intramuscular streptomycin and then intravenous vancomycin, and at a time when further intravenous chemotherapy was difficult to maintain.

Amoxycillin in an oral dose of 100 mg per kg per day or 1·0 g (occasionally 1·5 g) six-hourly for adults, is satisfactory treatment for typhoid fever. It was effective for 25 patients with typhoid fever due to chloramphenicol-resistant strains (Calderon, 1974). Gilman *et al.* (1975) also found oral amoxycillin satisfactory for the treatment of chloramphenicol-resistant typhoid fever and about as effective as treatment with co-trimoxazole (page 711). Afifi *et al.* (1976) used amoxycillin for 14 days to treat 30 typhoid fever patients who had haematological contraindications to chloramphenicol; eighteen had gluclose-6-phosphatase dehydrogenase deficiency and 12 a previous history of reversible chloramphenicol bone marrow depression. Their response to treatment was satisfactory and comparable, to that of 30 other patients treated with chloramphenicol. Mild haemolysis occurred in some of the patients with glucose-6-phosphate dehydrogenase deficiency during amoxycillin treatment, but severe life-threatening haemolysis was not observed. In another clinical trial in which the two drugs were given randomly and involving 124 adults with typhoid fever, amoxycillin in a dose of 1·0 g six-hourly for 14 days was as effective as treatment with chloramphenicol (Pillay et al., 1975). A similar trial with 155 African children with typhoid fever showed that oral amoxycillin was slightly superior to chloramphenicol when assessed by clinical response, relapse rate and subsequent carrier state (Scragg, 1976). Patients with Salm. typhi or Salm. paratyphi A bacteriuria and recurrent septicaemia associated with schistosomiasis have responded to amoxycillin in a dose of 250 mg four times a day for four weeks (Farid et al., 1975).

It may be concluded that amoxycillin is effective for the treatment of typhoid fever and it is probably more effective than ampicillin (page 114). The availability of parenteral amoxycillin (page 135) may make its use in typhoid fever even more acceptable. Nevertheless, ampicillin-resistant strains of Salm. typhi occur (page 101), and these are also amoxycillin-resistant.

Amoxycillin in a dose of 2 g three times a day for 28 days has also been successful in the eradication of the chronic typhoid carrier state in a proportion of patients (Nolan and White, 1978) (see also ampicillin, page 115).

Unlike ampicillin (page 115), amoxycillin is ineffective in shigellosis (Nelson and Haltalin, 1974).

Amoxycillin is valuable for the treatment of gonorrhoea, and the un-complicated disease usually responds satisfactorily to a 'single dose' of 3 g given without probenecid (Karney et al., 1974; Roberts, 1974). If gonococcal strains relatively resistant to amoxycillin (MIC 0·05–1·0 μg per ml) are in-volved results of treatment are more satisfactory if this 'single dose' is com-bined with 1·0 g of probenecid (Thin et al., 1977). Gonococcal arthritis usually responds to amoxycillin in a dose of 0·5–1·0 g eight-hourly, for ten days (Neu, 1975b). Gonococcal strains relatively resistant to penicillin G (page 7) are also relatively amoxycillin-resistant, but as in the case of ampicillin (page 102), this resistance is usually lesser in degree than penicillin G resistance (Watts et al., 1977). Penicillinase-producing gonococcal strains (page 8) are completely amoxycillin-resistant.

Certain infections caused by beta-lactamase producing organisms may res-pond to amoxycillin and clavulanic acid used in combination (see page 104).

2. *Epicillin*. This drug also has been used with good results in infections for which ampicillin is commonly indicated, such as urinary tract, respiratory tract, skin and soft tissue infections (Feeney et al., 1972; Limson et al., 1972; Guerrero and Groel, 1974). Meningococcal and pneumococcal meningitis has also been reported to respond to large intravenous doses of the drug (Hassan et al., 1976). There is no evidence to suggest that epicillin is superior to ampicillin.

3. *Cyclacillin*. Although it may be effective in urinary infections (Gonzaga et al., 1974), in most other infections results of treatment with this drug are in-ferior to those obtained with ampicillin (Neu, 1975b). There are no clinical in-dications for the use of cyclacillin.

4. *Hetacillin*. This antibiotic, which can be given orally or parenterally, can be used for all diseases for which ampicillin is advocated (page 113). Results of treatment are about the same as those which would be expected from an iden-tical ampicillin regimen. Louria and Schultz (1967) found that hetacillin was an effective antibiotic for treatment of pneumococcal lung infections, and its side-effects appeared similar to those of ampicillin. Smith et al. (1967) treated seven

children with acute bacterial meningitis (most due to H. influenzae), with hetacillin in an intravenous dose of 100–200 mg per kg body weight per day. Results were satisfactory and comparable to those previously reported with ampicillin (page 116). One trial showed that the response of children with typhoid fever to hetacillin was equal to that obtained with chloramphenicol (Chawla *et al.*, 1970). However, typhoid fever is often a milder disease in children, and contrary to opinion that chloramphenicol is generally superior in this disease (page 114), there have been occasional reports showing that ampicillin is equally effective (Kaye *et al.*, 1967). It appears that hetacillin does not offer any advantages over ampicillin.

5. *Pivampicillin.* Similar to amoxycillin, this has been used for some infections which respond to oral ampicillin. It is effective for treatment of urinary tract infections, but results are not superior to those obtained with ampicillin (Brumfitt *et al.*, 1973; Moe *et al.*, 1977). Patients with purulent bronchial infections and uncomplicated gonorrhoea respond to pivampicillin (Neu, 1975b).

6. *Talampicillin.* This ester, like amoxycillin, can probably be used for some diseases which respond to oral ampicillin, such as urinary tract infections (Leigh *et al.*, 1976) and uncomplicated gonorrhoea (Price *et al.*, 1977). The drug may be preferable to oral ampicillin because of its improved absorption and lesser frequency of gastro-intestinal side-effects (page 141). However it is unlikely to be superior to oral amoxycillin (page 142).

7. *Bacampicillin.* Exacerbations of chronic bronchitis (Maesen *et al.*, 1976) and acute tonsillitis (Hallander *et al.*, 1977) have been treated by this drug. Bacampicillin may be preferable to oral ampicillin because of its better absorption from the gastro-intestinal tract, but it is unlikely to be more effective than oral amoxycillin.

8. *Metampicillin.* Oral metampicillin has no advantages over ampicillin. Some authors consider that parenteral metampicillin is the penicillin of choice for the treatment of biliary infections, because by this mode of administration high concentrations of the antibiotic are attained in bile (Pinget *et al.*, 1976; Brogard *et al.*, 1976) (*see also* page 140). However in patients with biliary infections such as cholangitis, the common bile duct is often obstructed, and under these conditions the antibiotic level in the bile is unlikely to be high (pages 118, 623). In addition, it is often more important to control the associated septicaemia in such patients, than to sterilize the bile.

REFERENCES

Acred, P., Hunter, P. A., Mizen, L. and Rolinson, G. N. (1971), 'α-Amino-p-hydroxybenzylpenicillin (BRL 2333), a new broad-spectrum semisynthetic penicillin: *In vivo* evaluation', *Antimicrobial Agents Chemother.*—1970, p. 416.

Adverse Drug Reactions Advisory Committee (1978), 'Ampicillin and amoxycillin-identical twins', *Australian Prescriber,* **2,** 81.

Afifi, A. M., Adnan, M. and El Garf, A. A. (1976), 'Amoxycillin in treatment of typhoid fever in patients with haematological contraindications to chloramphenicol', *Brit. med. J.,* **2,** 1033.

Auvergnat, J. C. (1947), 'A comparative experimental study of the circulation of amoxycillin and penicillin G in the cerebro-spinal fluid of dogs as function of the type of intravenous administration', *J. Int. Med. Res.,* **2,** 189.

Basch, H., Erickson, R. and Gadebusch, H. (1971), 'Epicillin: *In vitro* laboratory studies', *Infec. Immun.*, **4**, 44.

Basker, M. J. and Sutherland, R. (1977), 'Activity of amoxycillin, alone, and in combination with aminoglycoside antibiotics against streptococci associated with bacterial endocarditis', *J. Antimicrob. Chemother.*, **3**, 273.

Bergan, T. (1978), 'Pharmacokinetic comparison of oral bacampicillin and parenteral ampicillin', *Antimicrob. Ag. Chemother.*, **13**, 971.

Bergan, T., Bratlid, D. and Brøndbo, A. (1978), 'Pharmacokinetics of bacampicillin in infants', *J. Antimicrob. Chemother.*, **4**, 79.

Bodey, G. P. and Nance, J. (1972), 'Amoxicillin: *In vitro* and pharmacological studies', *Antimicrob. Ag. Chemother.*, **1**, 358.

Bodin, N.-O., Ekström, B., Forsgren, U., Jalar, L.-P., Magni, L., Ramsay, C.-H. and Sjöberg, B. (1975), 'Bacampicillin: a new orally well-absorbed derivative of ampicillin', *Antimicrob. Ag. Chemother.*, **8**, 518.

Brogard, J. M., Pinget, M., Adloff, M., Dorner, M. and Lavillaureix, J. (1976), 'Experimental and clinical pharmacology of metampicillin in the biliary tract', *J. Antimicrob. Chemother.*, **2**, 363.

Brogden, R. N., Speight, T. M. and Avery, G. S. (1975), 'Amoxycillin: a review of its antibacterial pharmacokinetic properties and therapeutic use', *Drugs*, **9**, 88.

Brumfitt, W., Franklin, I., Hayek, L. and Pursell, R. (1973), 'Treatment of urinary tract infections with pivampicillin', *Scand. J. Infect. Dis.*, **5**, 59.

Calderon, E. (1974), 'Amoxicillin in the treatment of typhoid fever due to chloramphenicol-resistant Salmonella typhi', *J. Infect. Dis.* (Suppl.), **129**, 219.

Chawla, V., Chandra, R. K., Bhujwala, R. A. and Ghai, O. P. (1970), 'A comparative trial of hetacillin and chloramphenicol in typhoid fever', *J. Pediatrics*, **77**, 471.

Clayton, J. P., Cole, M., Elson, S. W. and Ferres, H. (1974), 'BRL 8988 (Talampicillin), a well-absorbed oral form of ampicillin', *Antimicrob. Ag. Chemother.*, **5**, 670.

Comber, K. R., Osborne, C. D. and Sutherland, R. (1975), 'Comparative effects of amoxycillin and ampicillin in the treatment of experimental mouse infections', *Antimicrob. Ag. Chemother.*, **7**, 179.

Croydon, E. A. P. and Sutherland, R. (1971), 'α-Amino-p-hydroxybenzylpenicillin (BRL 2333), a new semisynthetic penicillin: Absorption and excretion in man', *Antimicrob. Agents Chemother.*—1970, p. 427.

Daehne, W. von, Godtfredsen, W. O., Roholt, K. and Tybring, L. (1971), 'Pivampicillin, a new orally active ampicillin ester', *Antimicrob. Agents Chemother.*—1970, p. 431.

Faine, S. and Harper, M. (1973), 'Independent antibiotic actions of hetacillin and ampicillin revealed by fast methods', *Antimicrob. Ag. Chemother.*, **3**, 15.

Fang, L. S. T., Tolkoff-Rubin, N. E. and Rubin, R. H. (1978), 'Efficacy of single-dose and conventional amoxicillin therapy in urinary-tract infection localized by the antibody-coated bacteria technic', *New Engl. J. Med.*, **298**, 413.

Farid, Z., Bassily, S., Mikhail, I. A., Edman, D. C., Hassan, A. and Miner, W. F. (1975), 'Treatment of chronic enteric fever with amoxicillin', *J. Infect. Dis.*, **132**, 698.

Feeney, D. W., Surynt, J. L., Mason, D. and Stringer, H. C. W. (1972), 'Epicillin (dexacillin): A new semisynthetic penicillin: Report of clinical experience', *N.Z. Med. J.*, **75**, 77.

Furuya, H., Matsuda, S., Mori, S., Tanno, M. and Kobayashi, T. (1973), 'Clinical application of amoxycillin in the field of obstetrics and gynaecology', *Chemotherapy* (Tokyo), **21**, 1752; quoted by Brogden *et al.* (1975).

Gadebusch, H., Miraglia, G., Pansy, F. and Renz, K. (1971), 'Epicillin: Experimental chemotherapy, pharmacodynamics, and susceptibility testing', *Infec. Immun.*, **4**, 50.

Gilman, R. H., Terminel, M., Levine, M. M., Hernandez-Mendosa, P., Calderone, E., Vasquez, V., Martinez, E., Snyder, M. J. and Hornick, R. B. (1975), 'Comparison of trimethoprim-sulfamethoxazole and amoxicillin in therapy of chloramphenicol-resistant and chloramphenicol-sensitive typhoid fever', *J. Infect. Dis.,* **132,** 630.

Gonzaga, A. J., Antonio-Velmonte, M. and Tupasi, T. E. (1974), 'Cyclacillin: A clinical and *in vitro* profile', *J. Infect. Dis.,* **129,** 545.

Guerrero, J. R. and Groel, J. T. (1974), 'Successful clinical experience with twice daily oral epicillin', *Curr. Med. Res. Opin.,* **2,** 366.

Hallander, H. O., Flodström, A. and Sjövall, J. (1977), 'Pharmacological and clinical study of bacampicillin in acute peritonsillitis—a comparison with ampicillin', *Antimicrob. Ag. Chemother.,* **11,** 185.

Handsfield, H. H., Clark, H., Wallace, J. F., Holmes, K. K. and Turck, M. (1973), 'Amoxicillin, a new penicillin antibiotic', *Antimicrob. Ag. Chemother.,* **3,** 262.

Hassan, A., Yassin, M. W., Girgis, N. J., Sippel, J. E., Miner, W. F., Tadros, S. S. and Abu el Ella, H. A. (1976), 'The value of epicillin and ampicillin in the treatment of meningococcal and pneumococcal meningitis', *Scand. J. Infect. Dis.,* **8,** 181.

Hultberg, E. R. and Backelin, B. (1972), 'Studies on the absorption of pivampicillin and ampicillin', *Scand. J. Infect. Dis.,* **4,** 149.

Hunter, P. A., Rolinson, G. N. and Witting, D. A. (1973), 'Comparative activity of amoxycillin and ampicillin in an experimental bacterial infection in mice', *Antimicrob. Ag. Chemother.,* **4,** 285.

Jones, K. H. (1977), 'Bioavailability of talampicillin', *Brit. med. J.,* **2,** 232.

Jordan, M. C., de Maine, J. B. and Kirby, W. M. M. (1971), 'Clinical pharmacology of pivampicillin as compared with ampicillin', *Antimicrob. Agents Chemother.—*1970, p. 438.

Jusko, W. J. and Lewis, G. P. (1972), 'Precaution in pharmacokinetic evaluation of ampicillin precursors', *Lancet,* **1,** 690.

Kahrimanis, R. and Pierpaoli, P. (1971), 'Hetacillin vs. ampicillin', *New Engl. J. Med.,* **285,** 236.

Karney, W. W., Turck, M. and Holmes, K. K. (1974), 'Comparative therapeutic and pharmacological evaluation of amoxicillin and ampicillin plus probenecid for the treatment of gonorrhea', *Antimicrob. Ag. Chemother.,* **5,** 114.

Kaye, D., Rocha, H., Eyckmans, L., Prata, A. and Hook, E. W. (1967), 'Comparison of parenteral ampicillin and parenteral chloramphenicol in the treatment of typhoid fever'. *Ann. N.Y. Acad. Sci.,* **145,** 423.

Kirby, W. M. M. and Kind, A. C. (1967), 'Clinical pharmacology of ampicillin and hetacillin', *Ann. N.Y. Acad. Sci.,* **145,** 291.

Knudsen, E. T. and Harding, J. W. (1975), 'Multicentre comparative trial of talampicillin and ampicillin in general practice', *Brit. J. Clin. Pract.,* **29,** 255.

Knudsen, E. T. (1977), 'Amoxil and talpen', *Brit. med. J.,* **1,** 442.

Kosmidis, J., Williams, J. D., Andrews, J., Goodall, J. A. D. and Geddes, A. M. (1972), 'Amoxycillin—pharmacology, bacteriology and clinical studies', *Brit. J. Clin. Pract.,* **26,** 341.

Kunst, M. W. and Mattie, H. (1975), 'Absorption of pivampicillin in postoperative patients', *Antimicrob. Ag. Chemother.,* **8,** 11.

Lawson, D. H., Henderson, A. K. and McGeachy, R. R. (1974), 'Amoxycillin: Pharmacokinetic studies in normal subjects, patients with pernicious anaemia and those with renal failure', *Postgrad. Med. J.,* **50,** 500.

Leigh, D. A., Reeves, D. S., Simmons, K., Thomas, A. L. and Wilkinson, P. J. (1976), 'Talampicillin: A new derivative of ampicillin', *Brit. med. J.,* **1,** 1378.

Limson, B. M., Siasoco, R. E. and Dial, F. P. (1972), 'The effect of combined sodium epicillin injection and orally administered epicillin in the treatment of acute infective illness', *Med. J. Aust.,* **2,** 1348.

Little, P. J. and Peddie, B. A. (1974), 'Absorption and excretion of amoxycillin and pivampicillin, two new semisynthetic penicillins', *Med. J. Aust.,* **2,** 598.

Louria, D. B. and Schultz, M. (1967), 'Treatment of pneumonia in adults with hetacillin', *Ann. N.Y. Acad. Sci.*, **145**, 387.

Maesen, F. P. V., Beeuwkes, H., Davies, B. I., Buytendijk, H. J., Brombacher, P. J. and Wessman, J. (1976), 'Bacampicillin in acute exacerbations of chronic bronchitis—a dose range study', *J. Antimicrob. Chemother.*, **2**, 279.

Magnusson, B., Sölvell, L. and Wessman, J. (1977), 'Gastrointestinal blood loss in man during administration of two ampicillin esters', *Scand. J. Infect. Dis.*, **9**, 218.

May, J. R. and Ingold, A. (1972), 'Amoxycillin in the treatment of chronic non-tuberculous bronchial infections', *Brit. J. Dis. Chest*, **66**, 185.

May, J. R. and Ingold, A. (1974), 'Amoxicillin in the treatment of infections of the lower respiratory tract., *J. Infect. Dis.* (Suppl.), **129**, 189.

Moe, O. J., Meberg, A. and Eng, J. (1977), 'Ampicillin and pivampicillin in the treatment of urinary tract infection in children', *Scand. J. Infect. Dis.*, **9**, 31.

Mulroy, R. (1973), 'Amoxicillin rash in infectious mononucleosis', *Brit. med. J.*, **1**, 554.

Nelson, J. D. and Haltalin, K. C. (1974), 'Amoxicillin less effective than ampicillin against Shigella *in vitro* and *in vivo*: Relationship of efficacy to activity in serum', *J. Infect. Dis.* (Suppl.), **129**, 222.

Neu, H. C. and Winshell, E. B. (1971a), '*In vitro* antimicrobial activity of 6[D(—)a-amino-p-hydroxyphenylacetamidol] penicillanic acid, a new semisynthetic penicillin', *Antimicrob. Agents Chemother.*—1970, p. 407.

Neu, H. C. and Winshell, E. B. (1971b), 'Pharmacological studies of 6 [D(—)a-amino-p-hydroxyphenylacetamidol] penicillanic acid in humans', *Antimicrob. Agents Chemother.*—1970, p. 423.

Neu, H. C. (1974), 'Antimicrobial activity and human pharmacology of amoxicillin', *J. Infect. Dis.* (Suppl.), **129**, 123.

Neu, H. C. (1975a), 'Editorial. New broad-spectrum penicillins', *Drugs*, **9**, 81.

Neu, H. C. (1975b), 'Aminopenicillins-clinical pharmacology and use in disease states', *Int. J. Clin. Pharmacol.*, **11**, 132.

Nolan, C. M. and White, P. C., Jr. (1978), 'Treatment of typhoid carriers with amoxicillin correlates of successful therapy', *JAMA*, **239**, 2352.

Parsons, R. L., Hossack, G. and Paddock, G. (1975), 'The absorption of antibiotics in adult patients with coeliac disease', *J. Antimicrob. Chemother.*, **1**, 39.

Philipson, A., Sabath, L. D. and Rosner, B. (1975), 'Sequence effect on ampicillin blood levels noted in an amoxicillin, ampicillin, and epicillin triple crossover study', *Antimicrob. Ag. Chemother.*, **8**, 311.

Pillay, N., Adams, E. B. and North-Coombes, D. (1975), 'Comparative trial of amoxycillin and chloramphenicol in treatment of typhoid fever in adults', *Lancet*, **2**, 333.

Pinget, M., Brogard, J. M., Dauchel, J. and Lavillaureix, J. (1976), 'Biliary excretion of ampicillin, metampicillin and carbenicillin', *J. Antimicrob. Chemother.*, **2**, 195.

Price, J. D., Fluker, J. L. and Giles, A. J. H. (1977), 'Oral talampicillin in the treatment of gonorrhoea', *Brit. J. Vener. Dis.*, **53**, 113.

Ridley, M. (1967), 'Hetacillin and ampicillin', *Brit. med. J.*, **3**, 305.

Roberts, F. L. (1974), 'Treatment of uncomplicated gonorrhea with amoxicillin', *J. Infect. Dis.* (Suppl.), **129**, 262.

Roholt, K., Nielsen, B. and Kristensen, E. (1974), 'Clinical pharmacology of pivam-picillin', *Antimicrob. Ag. Chemother.*, **6**, 563.

Rolinson, G. N. (1974), 'Laboratory evaluation of amoxicillin', *J. Infect. Dis.* (Suppl.), **129**, 139.

Ronald, A. R., Jagdis, F. A., Harding, G. K. M., Hoban, S. A., Muir, P. L. and Gurwith, M. J., (1977), 'Amoxicillin therapy of acute urinary tract infections in adults', *Antimicrob. Ag. Chemother.*, **11**, 780.

Russell, E. J. and Sutherland, R. (1975), 'Activity of amoxycillin against enterococci and synergism with aminoglycoside antibiotics', *J. Med. Microbiol.*, **8**, 1.

Sabto, J., Carson, P. and Morgan, T. (1973), 'Evaluation of amoxycillin—a new semisynthetic penicillin', *Med. J. Aust.*, **2**, 537.

Scragg, J. N. (1976), 'Further experience with amoxycillin in typhoid fever in children', *Brit. med. J.*, **2**, 1031.

Seligman, S. J. (1974), 'Treatment of enterococcal endocarditis with oral amoxicillin and intramuscular gentamicin', *J. Infect. Dis.* (Suppl.), **129**, 213.

Similä, S., Kouvalainen, K. and Mäkelä, P. (1976), 'Pseudomembranous colitis after amoxycillin', *Lancet*, **2**, 317.

Sjövall, J., Magni, L. and Bergan, T. (1978), 'Pharmacokinetics of bacampicillin compared with those of ampicillin, pivampicillin and amoxycillin', *Antimicrob. Ag. Chemother.*, **13**, 90.

Smith, M. H. D., Sandstrom, S. M. and Hoffpauir, C. W. (1967), 'Preliminary evaluation of hetacillin in the treatment of acute bacterial meningitis', *Ann. N.Y. Acad. Sci.*, **145**, 502.

Spyker, D. A., Rugloski, R. J., Vann, R. L. and O'Brien, W. M. (1977), 'Pharmacokinetics of amoxicillin: dose dependence after intravenous, oral and intramuscular administration', *Antimicrob. Ag. Chemother.*, **11**, 132.

Steigbigel, N. H., McCall, C. E., Reed, C. W. and Finland, M. (1967), 'Antibacterial action of "broad-spectrum" penicillins, cephalosporins and other antibiotics against Gram-negative bacilli isolated from bacteremic patients', *Ann. N.Y. Acad. SCI.*, **145**, 224.

Stillerman, M., Isenberg, H. D. and Facklam, R. R. (1974), 'Treatment of pharyngitis associated with Group A streptococcus: Comparison of amoxicillin and potassium phenoxymethyl penicillin', *J. Infect. Dis.* (Suppl.), **129**, 169.

Sutherland, R. and Robinson, O. P. W. (1967), 'Laboratory and pharmacological studies in man with hetacillin and ampicillin', *Brit. med. J.*, **2**, 804.

Sutherland, R. and Rolinson, G. N. (1971), 'α-Amino-p-hydroxybenzyl-penicillin (BRL 2333), a new semisynthetic penicillin: *In vitro* evaluation', *Antimicrob. Agents Chemother.*—1970, p. 411.

Sutherland, R., Croydon, E. A. P. and Rolinson, G. N. (1972), 'Amoxycillin: A new semi-synthetic penicillin', *Brit. med. J.*, **3**, 13.

Sutter, V. L. and Finegold, S. M. (1976), 'Susceptibility of anaerobic bacteria to 23 Antimicrobial Agents', *Antimicrob. Ag. Chemother.*, **10**, 736.

Symonds, J. and George, R. H. (1978), 'The effect of talampicillin on faecal flora', *J. Antimicrob. Chemother.*, **4**, 92.

Thin, R. N., Symonds, M. A. E., Shaw, E. J., Wong, J., Hopper, P. K. and Slocombe, B. (1977), 'A double blind trial of amoxycillin in the treatment of gonorrhoea', *Brit. J. Vener. Dis.*, **53**, 118.

Tuano, S. B., Johnson, L. D., Brodie, J. L. and Kirby, W. M. M. (1966), 'Comparative blood levels of hetacillin, ampicillin and penicillin G', *New Engl. J. Med.*, **275**, 635.

Verbist, L. (1974), 'Triple crossover study on absorption and excretion of ampicillin, pivampicillin, and amoxycillin', *Antimicrob. Ag. Chemother.*, **6**, 588.

Verbist, L. (1976). 'Triple crossover study on absorption and excretion of ampicillin, talampicillin and amoxycillin', *Antimicrob. Ag. Chemother.*, **10**, 173.

Watts, B. A., Phillips, I. and Stoate, M. W. (1977), 'The *in vitro* activity of fifteen penicillins and mecillinam against Neisseria gonorrhoeae', *J. Antimicrob. Chemother.*, **3**, 331.

Carbenicillin, Indanyl Carbenicillin and Carfecillin

Description

Carbenicillin (disodium alpha-carboxybenzylpenicillin, 'BRL 2064') is a semisynthetic penicillin derived from the penicillin nucleus (6-aminopenicillanic acid), which was first introduced for clinical use by Beecham Research Laboratories (Knudsen et al., 1967). This drug can only be administered parenterally. It is marketed with the trade names of 'Pyopen' (Beecham), 'Geopen' (Pfizer) and 'Carbapen' (CSL, Australia). Subsequently two carbenicillin esters, carbenicillin indanyl sodium and a phenyl ester of carbenicillin (carfecillin) have been developed, which are absorbed after oral administration. After absorption, both of these esters are rapidly hydrolysed in the body to produce carbenicillin (page 155). Oral indanyl carbenicillin is marketed in North America ('Geocillin', Pfizer) and carfecillin in Britain with the trade name of 'Uticillin' (Beecham).

Sensitive Organisms

1. *Pseudomonas aeruginosa*. Activity against this organism, although of a relatively low order, is the most important feature of carbenicillin. Parenteral carbenicillin can be administered in sufficient dosage to obtain serum concentrations exceeding 50–60 μg per ml, which inhibits most Ps. aeruginosa strains. Unfortunately, a proportion of strains are not inhibited by concentrations as high as 200 μg per ml. Since the introduction of this drug, it has become evident that Ps. aeruginosa strains with increased resistance can develop in patients treated with carbenicillin (Jones and Lowbury, 1967; Darrell and Waterworth, 1969; Holmes et al., 1970). A progressive increase in the incidence of carbenicillin-resistant Ps. aeruginosa was reported in a British burns unit between 1966 and 1969. In 1969 highly resistant strains appeared suddenly and displaced all other Ps. aeruginosa strains from this unit (Lowbury et al., 1969). Carbenicillin-resistant variants can also be induced *in vitro* by culturing Ps. aeruginosa in the presence of the drug (Bell and Smith, 1969). Resistance can be either chromosomally or R plasmid-mediated (*see* page 422), and transfer of plasmids from certain strains of Enterobacteriaceae to Ps. aeruginosa and *vice versa*, can occur (Roe et al., 1971; Roe and Jones, 1972). Resistance of some Ps. aeruginosa strains to carbenicillin is 'intrinsic' (page 10), but many produce a beta-lactamase (carbenicillinase), which destroys carbenicillin (Sykes and Richmond, 1971; Wretlind et al., 1974; Labia et al., 1977). Transferable (R plasmid-mediated) resistance appears to be usually associated with carbenicillinase production (Lowbury et al., 1972; Hewitt and Winters, 1973).

149

Despite these observations, highly resistant Ps. aeruginosa strains have not yet displaced sensitive strains from most general hospitals. Duncan (1974) tested 1500 strains collected from a variety of sources in North America, and found that over 99 per cent of them were inhibited by a carbenicillin concentration of 256 μg per ml or less. Gaman et al. (1976) isolated Ps. aeruginosa from 238 patients during a six month period in one hospital. Carbenicillin-resistant strains emerged in four of 14 patients treated with this drug, and on admission to hospital 17 of the 238 patients were already infected with carbenicillin-resistant organisms. These resistant variants did not spread in the hospital environment. Similarly, Baird et al. (1976) isolated Ps. aeruginosa from 535 hospital patients during an eleven month period; 85 of these patients were colonized or infected with strains resistant to both carbenicillin and gentamicin (page 326). Resistant strains were mainly isolated from the urinary tract of patients who had recently received gentamicin and other antibiotics; they did not appear to have an altered pathogenicity; they did not spread rapidly and only rarely caused infections in the general hospital population, where only a minority of patients were highly vulnerable e.g. immunosuppressed. Of 650 Ps. aeruginosa strains isolated from Australian hospital patients, only 16 were carbenicillin-resistant (Dean et al., 1977). From all these studies, it appears that carbenicillin-resistant Ps. aeruginosa strains are still relatively uncommon in hospitals, except in special areas, such as intensive care and burns units, where carbenicillin is used extensively (Gaman et al., 1976).

A carbenicillin and gentamicin combination may exhibit in vitro synergism against strains of Ps. aeruginosa sensitive to both drugs and also against strains which are carbenicillin-sensitive and only have a low level of gentamicin resistance (MIC lower than 40 μg per ml) (Kluge et al., 1974a) (see also page 161). With gentamicin-resistant and carbenicillin-sensitive strains, there may sometimes be in vitro synergism between carbenicillin and one of the newer aminoglycosides such as tobramycin (page 360), sisomicin (page 395) or amikacin (page 379), even if the strain is not susceptible to a clinically attainable concentration of the aminoglycoside (Kluge et al., 1974b; Marks et al., 1976). The aminoglycoside which will be synergistic is not always predictable from its MIC against the Pseudomonas strain (Anderson et al., 1975; Marks et al., 1976).

2. *Other Gram-negative aerobic bacteria.* Compared to ampicillin, carbenicillin has a relatively high activity against indole-positive Proteus spp. (Pr. vulgaris, rettgeri and morganii). Its range of activity against other Gram-negative bacteria is comparable to that of ampicillin (page 100); it is effective to a degree against Esch. coli, Pr. mirabilis, salmonellae, shigellae and also H. influenzae, N. meningitidis and N. gonorrhoeae. Ampicillin is preferred for treatment of infections due to these bacteria because it is the more active drug. Carbenicillin and ticarcillin (page 171) are the only two penicillins active against ampicillin-resistant H. influenzae strains (page 102). However the activity of carbenicillin against these strains is less (MIC 4–32 μg per ml) than against ampicillin-sensitive strains (MIC 0·25–1·0 μg per ml) (Kammer et al., 1975; Thornsberry et al., 1976). The Klebsiella spp. are almost invariably resistant to carbenicillin, but some strains of Enterobacter spp. are relatively sensitive (Standiford et al., 1969). Up to 50 per cent of strains of Serratia marcescens are susceptible to 25 μg per ml or less (Hewitt and Winters, 1973);

others are either highly carbenicillin-resistant (MIC >8000 μg per ml) or show a moderate degree of resistance (MIC ⩽2000 μg per ml). Carbenicillin in inhibitory or subinhibitory concentrations potentiates the action of the aminoglycosides gentamicin (page 325), amikacin (page 379) and netilmicin (page 396), against Serratia marcescens strains which are either carbenicillin-sensitive or only moderately resistant to this drug (Pogwizd and Lerner, 1976). Most Acinetobacter calcoaceticus var. anitratus strains are inhibited by 62·5 μg per ml of carbenicillin and this drug often acts synergistically with one of the aminoglycosides such as kanamycin, gentamicin or tobramycin against this organism. Such synergy is unlikely if the Acinetobacter strain is highly resistant to the aminoglycoside concerned (Glew et al., 1977). Campylobacter fetus is usually carbenicillin-sensitive (median MIC 4·6 μg per ml) (Chow et al., 1978).

3. *Gram-negative anaerobic bacteria.* Some of these such as Bacteroides melaninogenicus and Fusobacterium spp. are highly sensitive, the MIC's ranging from 0·1 to 8·0 μg per ml. B. fragilis is more resistant, but 80 per cent of strains can be inhibited by 64·0 μg per ml and 95 per cent by 128 μg per ml, both of which are clinically attainable concentrations (page 155). Other Bacteroides spp. vary in sensitivity, but 96 per cent of isolates are inhibited by 64·0 μg per ml. Carbenicillin has a slightly higher activity than penicillin G (page 10) against Bacteroides spp., but otherwise these two penicillins have a similar activity against Gram-negative anaerobic bacteria (Sutter and Finegold, 1975; 1976; Sutter, 1977).

4. *Gram-positive bacteria.* Carbenicillin is active against Staph. pyogenes (non-penicillinase producers), Strep. pyogenes and Strep. pneumoniae, but Listeria monocytogenes is usually not quite as sensitive with an MIC of 10 μg per ml (McCracken et al., 1973). Ampicillin and penicillin G have a higher degree of activity against all of these organisms. Penicillinase-producing staphylococci are resistant and Strep. faecalis needs moderately high carbenicillin concentrations for inhibition (Table 9).

Anaerobic Gram-positive bacteria such as Peptococcus and Peptostreptococcus spp., anaerobic streptococci, Clostridium, Lactobacillus and Actinomyces spp. and Arachnia propionica are all usually sensitive to low carbenicillin concentrations (Sutter and Finegold, 1976).

In Vitro Sensitivities

Table 9 shows the *in vitro* activity of carbenicillin and oral indanyl carbenicillin, compared to that of ampicillin, against some bacterial species. The minimum inhibitory concentrations of carbenicillin are lower than those of ampicillin for Ps. aeruginosa, Serratia marcescens and Proteus spp. other than Pr. mirabilis. Although the MIC's of sensitive Ps. aeruginosa strains are usually about 50–60 μg per ml, some strains have been isolated from the sputum of patients with chronic respiratory infections with an MIC of 0·7–6·0 μg per ml (May and Ingold, 1973; Duncan, 1974).

Oral indanyl carbenicillin itself can be tested *in vitro* against bacteria because it does not hydrolyse to carbenicillin during testing procedures. Its antibacterial activity in general is similar to that of carbenicillin, but it is more active against sensitive Gram-positive bacteria (Table 9). This higher activity is of academic interest only because *in vivo* the drug is rapidly hydrolysed to carbenicillin. Therefore in assessing the value of indanyl carbenicillin for the treatment of patients, MIC's for carbenicillin should only be considered (English *et al.*, 1972).

TABLE 9

Compiled from data published by Knudsen *et al.* (1967), Butler *et al.* (1970), Smith *et al.* (1970), English *et al.* (1972), Kammer *et al.* (1975) and Sutter and Finegold (1976).

ORGANISM	MIC (μg per ml)		
	Carbenicillin	Indanyl Carbenicillin*	Ampicillin
Gram-positive bacteria			
Staph. pyogenes (non-penicillinase producer)	1·25	0·19	0·06
Staph. pyogenes (penicillinase producer)	50·0	12·5	100·0
Strep. pyogenes (Group A)	0·15	0·003	0·008
Strep. pneumoniae (Dip. pneumoniae)	0·15	0·02	0·008
Strep. faecalis	25·0	3·12	—
Clostridium tetani	0·25	—	—
Clostridium perfringens	0·25	—	—
Actinomyces spp.	0·1–0·5	—	—
Gram-negative bacteria			
Escherichia coli	12·5	3·12	6·25
Enterobacter spp.	50·0	3·12	100·0
Klebsiella pneumoniae	>250·0	50·0	1·56
Serratia marcescens	12·5	12·5	200·0
Proteus mirabilis	3·12	1·56	3·12
Proteus vulgaris	25·0	3·12	100·0
Proteus morganii	6·25	—	200·0
Proteus rettgeri	0·78	—	25·0
Salmonella typhi	25·0	12·5	3·12
Neisseria gonorrhoeae	0·3	—	—
Neisseria meningitidis	0·1	—	—
Haemophilus influenzae	0·5	1·0	0·05
Haemophilus influenzae (ampicillin-resistant)	4·0–32·0	—	3·0–500
Pseudomonas aeruginosa	50·0	50·0	500·0
Bacteroides melaninogenicus	0·1–4·0	—	0·1–4·0
Bacteroides fragilis	4·0–128·0	—	4·0–256

* See comments under '*In vitro* sensitivities'

Mode of Administration and Dosage

1. Carbenicillin is not absorbed from the gastro-intestinal tract and must be administered either intramuscularly or intravenously. The dosage used can be varied widely, depending on the nature of the infection and the sensitivity of the organism.

Indanyl carbenicillin and carfecillin are well absorbed from the gastro-intestinal tract, but they are not suitable for the treatment of systemic infections because therapeutic serum levels are not attained. They are useful for the oral treatment of certain urinary tract infections, because adequate urine concentrations of carbenicillin are achieved.

2. *Parenteral carbenicillin for systemic Pseudomonas infections*. An adult dose of 24–40 g per day, given intravenously is necessary for the treatment of these infections. The corresponding high dose schedule for children is 400–600 mg per kg per day. Probenecid in a daily dose of 1–2 g orally should also be administered to delay excretion of the drug. Carbenicillin or any other systemically administered antibiotic is not indicated for the treatment of mild or superficial Ps. aeruginosa infections, unless other factors suggest that the infection is potentially dangerous, in which case full carbenicillin dosage as for a septicaemia should be given. The mere isolation of Ps. aeruginosa from the trachea or a wound may only indicate colonization and in itself is not sufficient reason for treatment (Leading article, 1969). Furthermore, treatment of such infections by small doses of carbenicillin will not benefit the patient, and will enhance emergence of more resistant Ps. aeruginosa strains.

3. *Parenteral carbenicillin for Pseudomonas urinary tract infections*. An adult dose as low as 1 g intramuscularly every six hours may suffice for these, because urine concentrations attained after this dose are usually higher than the MIC's for relatively sensitive Ps. aeruginosa strains. The corresponding low dosage schedule for children is 50–100 mg per kg per day (Turck *et al.*, 1970). When treating infections confined to the urinary tract probenecid should not be administered.

4. *Septicaemia and other systemic infections due to more sensitive organisms such as Proteus species (MIC 5 μg per ml or less)*. Intramuscular carbenicillin in a dose of 2 g every four to six hours may be adequate, but if the organism is less sensitive, higher doses given intravenously, as for Ps. aeruginosa septicaemia, may be necessary. In treating infections other than those of the urinary tract it is usually advantageous to combine probenecid with carbenicillin.

5. *Pseudomonas infections in patients with anuria or severe renal failure*. The mean half-life of carbenicillin in such patients is approximately thirteen hours, and serum levels of around 100 μg per ml can be maintained by giving an intravenous dose of 2 g every eight to twelve hours. During haemodialysis carbenicillin is removed from the body, and a dose of 2 g intravenously every four hours is recommended. During peritoneal dialysis much less carbenicillin is removed, and a dose of 2 g six-hourly is appropriate (Eastwood and Curtis, 1968). It may be necessary to maintain serum levels higher than 100 μg per ml for the treatment of Ps. aeruginosa septicaemia in some patients with renal failure, and in these higher doses may be given than those recommended by Eastwood and Curtis (1968). For such patients Johny *et al.* (1969) suggest an intravenous loading dose of 4 g followed by 2 to 4 g six-hourly. Further reduction of dosage to 2 g per day is recommended in patients with combined hepatic and renal failure (Hoffman *et al.*, 1970).

6. *Parenteral carbenicillin for systemic Pseudomonas infections in neo-nates*. In older children and adults the serum half-life of carbenicillin is one hour. During the first week or life this is prolonged to 2·7 h in normal birth

weight infants, and to 4 h in low birth weight infants. The initial dose of carbenicillin for these infections in the newborn is 100 mg per kg body weight. Neonates with a birth weight higher than 2000 g should then receive 75 mg per kg every six hours until four days of age, followed by 100 mg per kg six-hourly. For neonates with a birth weight lower than 2000 g, the maintenance dose is 75 mg per kg every eight hours until seven days of age, and thereafter a dose of 100 mg per kg six-hourly (the normal dose for older children). Either intramuscular or intravenous carbenicillin administration is suitable for neonates. Therapeutic non-toxic serum levels of 150–200 μg per ml are achieved with these dosage schedules (Morehead et al., 1972; Nelson and McCracken, 1973; McCracken, 1974).

7. *Methods of intravenous carbenicillin administration.* As with other penicillins, carbenicillin can be administered by continuous infusion or intermittently by either injection or rapid infusion. If the former method is used and the intravenous fluid is acid (commonly used fluids have a pH 5·5), the drug may be slowly inactivated. However, carbenicillin usually retains 90 per cent of its activity for 24 h in all commonly used glucose-saline solutions at 37°C (Wyatt et al., 1972), provided there are no incompatible additives (page 106). Carbenicillin should not be added to parenteral amino acid hyperalimentation mixtures, because in these it is more rapidly inactivated (Feigin et al., 1973). If carbenicillin must be administered by continuous infusion, a fresh carbenicillin-gluclose-saline solution should be used every three to four hours.

Most clinicians administer carbenicillin by either intermittent intravenous injection or intermittent intravenous infusion of a concentrated solution of the drug. For example, if a total daily dose of 30 g is needed, 5 g is dissolved in 10 ml of sterile water, and injected into the drip tubing over a period of five minutes, every four hours. Alternatively, this four-hourly dose may be already dispensed in a separate parallel intravenous bottle, or be dissolved in 25–50 ml of intravenous fluid in a paediatric buretrol; in either case the resultant concentrated solution is infused over a period of 15 to 30 m (*see also* methicillin, page 68).

8. *Oral indanyl carbenicillin.* This drug is used in an adult dose of 0·5 or 1·0 g orally every six hours (Knirsch et al., 1973; Turck, 1973). The corresponding dose for children is 50–100 mg per kg per day, administered in four divided doses. The same doses can be used to treat certain urinary tract infections in patients with mild to moderate degrees of renal insufficiency (Cox, 1973). Bailey et al. (1972) found that even in patients with severe renal failure, therapeutically adequate urinary levels were obtained. They suggested that in patients with a creatinine clearance of 20 ml per min or less, the dose of indanyl carbenicillin should be reduced to 1·0–1·5 g daily, as higher doses may lead to accumulation of carbenicillin in the serum. It is not known whether the indanol moiety of this drug accumulates in such patients and whether this would result in toxicity. By contrast, Cox (1973) considers that oral indanyl carbenicillin is not suitable for patients with severe renal failure. He administered the drug in 1·0 g doses to patients with various degrees of renal insufficiency; no measurable carbenicillin was present in the urine of those with severe renal failure (creatinine clearance less than 14 ml per min); usual doses of the drug were satisfactory for patients with mild to moderate renal failure.

9. *Oral carfecillin.* The usual adult dose of this drug is 0·5 g eight-hourly

(Borowski *et al.*, 1976; Leigh and Simmons, 1976). This dosage is also satisfactory for the treatment of urinary tract infections in patients with mild to moderate degrees of renal failure, because adequate urinary levels of active carbenicillin are attained. Serum levels resulting from an increased oral dose of 1·0 g four-hourly are still inadequate for the treatment of systemic infections, even in patients with severe renal failure (Wilkinson *et al.*, 1975).

Availability

1. *Carbenicillin*, vials containing 1·0 g and 5·0 g of powder for intramuscular or intravenous use. This powder is readily soluble in water, giving a clear neutral solution, which shows no significant loss of activity after 24 h at room temperature.

2. *Indanyl carbenicillin*, 0·5 g tablets (each equivalent to 382 mg of active carbenicillin).

3. *Carfecillin*, 0·5 g tablets (each equivalent to 397 mg of active carbenicillin).

Serum Levels in Relation to Dosage

1. After intramuscular administration of carbenicillin a peak serum concentration is obtained about one hour after injection (Fig. 9). Doubling the dose doubles the serum level.

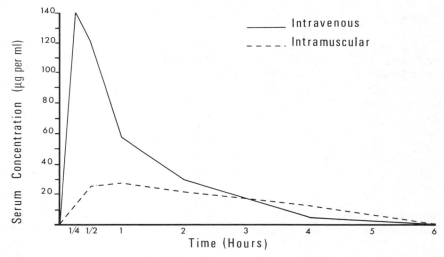

FIG. 9. Serum concentrations in human volunteers after intramuscular and intravenous administration of 1 g of carbenicillin. (Redrawn after Knudsen *et al.*, 1967.)

Figure 10 shows the serum levels achieved with the usual large doses of carbenicillin given intravenously. Intravenous administration of the drug at the rate of 1 g per hour would just achieve adequate serum levels (> 100 μg per ml) for treatment of systemic Ps. aeruginosa infections. The enhancement of serum levels with concomitant oral probenecid is also demonstrated in this figure.

2. The indanyl ester of carbenicillin being acid stable is well absorbed after oral administration. After absorption it is rapidly hydrolysed to carbenicillin plus indanol, probably either in the intestinal mucosa or in the liver (Butler *et al.*, 1973).

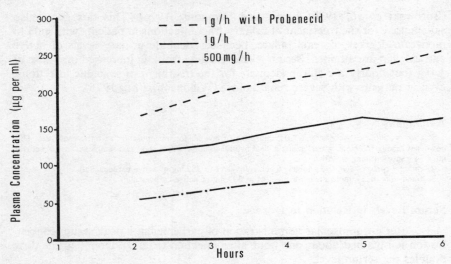

Fig. 10. Average serum concentrations of carbenicillin in four healthy volunteers given a continuous intravenous infusion. (Redrawn after Standiford *et al.*, 1970.)

After an oral dose of 0·5 g of indanyl carbenicillin to adults, a peak serum level of about 10 μg per ml of carbenicillin is reached in 1–1½ h. Thereafter the serum level progressively falls and usually reaches zero six hours later. Doubling the dose to 1·0 g only raises the peak serum level to 15–17 μg per ml. As with other penicillins, simultaneous administration of probenecid results in higher serum levels (Knirsch *et al.*, 1973). These serum levels are inadequate for treatment of systemic Ps. aeruginosa infections. With doses higher than 1·0 g six-hourly, higher serum levels can be obtained, but doubling the dose does not double the serum concentrations. In addition, diarrhoea commonly occurs in patients treated with doses higher than 4 g per day because a large proportion of the dose is unabsorbed (Knirsch *et al.*, 1973).

3. Carfecillin also being acid stable is well absorbed after oral adminstration. After absorption this ester is rapidly hydrolysed to carbenicillin and phenol, the phenol moiety being quickly detoxicated by conjugation (Wilkinson *et al.*, 1975; Wise, 1975). After a 0·5 g dose a mean peak serum level of approximately 3·0 μg per ml is attained in one to two hours, and at six hours the drug is undetectable in serum (Wilkinson *et al.*, 1975; Leigh and Simmons, 1976). Levels after a 1·0 g dose are higher, but not doubled (Wilkinson *et al.*, 1975). However serum levels attained by different individuals are very variable.

Excretion

URINE: Carbenicillin is excreted via the kidney mainly in an unchanged form. During the first six hours after an intramuscular dose of 1·0 g about 80 per cent of the dose is excreted producing urine concentrations of 2000 to 4000 μg per ml (Knudsen *et al.*, 1967). In the first three hours after an oral dose of 1·0 g indanyl carbenicillin, urine carbenicillin concentrations exceed 1000 μg per ml (Knirsch *et al.*, 1973). After a 1·0 g dose of carfecillin, maximal urinary carbenicillin excretion occurs during the first four hours, with a concentration ranging from 52 to 1120 μg per ml (mean 434 μg per ml) (Wilkinson *et al.*, 1975).

Carbenicillin, like penicillin G (page 17) is excreted by both glomerular filtration and renal tubular secretion. Animal studies have shown that like penicillin G it is secreted in the proximal tubule, but at comparable serum levels only 38 per cent of carbenicillin is excreted by tubular secretion, compared to 60 per cent for penicillin G (Bergeron *et al.*, 1975). This is the reason why the renal clearance of carbenicillin is slower than that of other penicillins, being only about a half that of ampicillin, and a quarter that of penicillin G (Standiford *et al.*, 1970). The serum carbenicillin half-life is one hour. Administration of probenecid reduces renal tubular secretion of carbenicillin, thereby increasing serum levels and prolonging the half-life.

All the indanol, which is formed when indanyl carbenicillin is hydrolysed *in vivo* is eliminated in the urine as glucuronide and sulphate conjugates (Knirsch *et al.*, 1973). The phenol resulting from carfecillin hydrolysis, is also rapidly excreted in urine as glucuronide and sulphate conjugates (Wilkinson *et al.*, 1975).

BILE: A small amount of carbenicillin is eliminated via the bile; in patients after cholecystectomy with T-tube drainage, about 0·19 per cent of an intravenously administered carbenicillin dose is excreted this way (Pinget *et al.*, 1976).

INACTIVATION IN BODY: A small amount of carbenicillin appears to be inactivated in the liver, but this is slower than with other penicillins. In severely uraemic or anuric patients the serum half-life of carbenicillin is some 13–15 h, compared to about 3 h for penicillin G and 8 h for ampicillin (Standiford *et al.*, 1970).

Distribution of the Drug in Body

Carbenicillin is probably distributed in body fluids similarly to penicillin G (*see* page 18). Only insignificant amounts appear in the cerebrospinal fluid of patients with uninflamed meninges, but moderately high CSF levels are found in patients with meningitis treated by large doses of intravenous carbenicillin (Richardson *et al.*, 1968). The drug penetrates into bronchial secretions, but the concentrations reached are usually lower than those needed for inhibition of Ps. aeruginosa. In one animal experiment the bronchial secretion concentration was only 11 per cent of the simultaneous peak serum level 30 min after a carbenicillin injection, and after two hours it was only 18 per cent of the serum level (Pennington and Reynolds, 1973). Sputum carbenicillin levels are also low in patients with cystic fibrosis (Govan, 1976); in a study of four patients with this disease, the mean peak sputum concentration was only 78 μg per ml (Marks *et al.*, 1971).

Levels of carbenicillin in healthy renal cortical tissue may be three times higher than serum levels at the time. Tissue concentrations in the renal papillae may be 17 times higher than those in the serum if the patient is dehydrated, but this gradient decreases with rehydration. In severe renal disease due to chronic pyelonephritis or glomerulo-nephritis, the penetration of carbenicillin into renal parenchyma is markedly decreased. In such kidneys carbenicillin concentrations in the cortex, medulla and papillae are only about half the serum levels at the time (Whelton *et al.*, 1973).

Carbenicillin is about 50 per cent bound to serum proteins (Standiford *et al.*, 1970).

Mode of Action

Carbenicillin, like penicillin G inhibits the synthesis of bacterial cell walls (*see* page 19). Its increased activity against organisms such as Ps. aeruginosa and Pr. morganii is mainly due to its superior ability to penetrate their outer cell membrane (page 20). Thus these bacteria have a lesser intrinsic resistance (page 10) to carbenicillin, compared to penicillin G (Butler *et al.*, 1970). Carbenicillin may be also less susceptible to beta-lactamases produced by Ps. aeruginosa and some other Gram-negative bacilli.

Toxicity

1. *Hypersensitivity reactions*. Carbenicillins may provoke any of the reactions which occur with penicillin G (page 24) in penicillin-sensitive subjects. Anaphylaxis due to carbenicillin has been reported (Silverblatt and Turck, 1969). These drugs are contraindicated in patients with a history of penicillin hypersensitivity.

2. *Neurotoxicity*. High doses of intravenous carbenicillin, similar to 'massive' doses of penicillin G (page 28) may cause neurotoxicity (Kurtzman *et al.*, 1970). This is more likely to occur in patients with renal failure. Hoffman and Bullock (1970) reported two patients with severe renal failure, who developed convulsions whilst receiving a daily intravenous dosage of only 4 g. In one of these the carbenicillin CSF level was 37 μg per ml during the fits, and the serum level was only about 320 μg per ml. By contrast, Whelton *et al.* (1971) described another patient with moderately severe renal failure who convulsed on the 13th day of carbenicillin therapy (20 g daily), and the serum level was as high as 1860 μg per ml, three hours after the seizure. It is possible that relatively low serum and CSF carbenicillin levels may provoke convulsions in some uraemic patients. Patients with underlying central nervous system disease may also be more prone to convulsions with high serum levels of any of the penicillins.

3. *Hepatotoxicity*. Elevated serum aspartate aminotransferase (SGOT) levels have been observed during carbenicillin therapy. Knirsch and Gralla (1970) noted this only in patients receiving intramuscular carbenicillin, and concluded that elevations of the SGOT were due to muscle irritation. Other authors have observed raised SGOT levels during intravenous carbenicillin administration, suggesting that the source of the enzyme is the liver, though the degree of hepatotoxicity is usually slight and rapidly reversible after cessation of the drug (Boxerbaum *et al.*, 1970; Gump, 1970). Four other patients who collectively had eight episodes of a mild reversible anicteric hepatitis associated with intravenous carbenicillin therapy have been reported (Wilson *et al.*, 1975). This hepatitis was characterized by nausea, vomiting, a tender slightly enlarged liver, raised serum transaminases and alkaline phosphatase, but a normal serum bilirubin level. Liver biopsy specimens showed spotty liver cell necrosis

with no cholestasis. A toxic mechanism was postulated because skin rashes and other hypersensitivity manifestations were usually absent. Other penicillins could be given to these patients without ill effects, but on readministration of carbenicillin the hepatotoxicity recurred.

4. *Electrolyte and acid-base disturbances.* One g of carbenicillin contains 4·7 mEq of sodium. The sodium load could therefore be significant in patients receiving massive doses of carbenicillin intravenously. This could cause hyper-natraemia and pulmonary oedema in some patients, particularly those with congestive cardiac failure or impaired renal function. Furthermore, some patients receiving large doses of intravenous carbenicillin develop hypoka-laemia, sometimes associated with metabolic alkalosis (Klastersky *et al.*, 1973; Cabizuca and Desser, 1976). Hypokalaemia probably occurs because carbenicillin promotes potassium loss via the renal tubules, but it may also cause a redistribution of potassium within the body (*see* penicillin G, page 30). Hypokalaemia usually responds to oral or intravenous potassium chloride ad-ministration, and carbenicillin need not be discontinued.

Carbenicillin being a weak acid can cause acute acidosis if excessively high serum levels are reached, particularly in patients with renal disease and pre-existing acidosis (Whelton *et al.*, 1971). The high carbenicillin urine concen-trations which result when large intravenous doses are given, produce a high urine specific gravity. For instance one adult patient with normal renal function receiving carbenicillin in a dose of 30 g intravenously daily had a sustained high urine specific gravity of 1042 (Deziel *et al.*, 1977). This finding should not be misinterpreted to mean that the patient is dehydrated.

5. *Bleeding disorders.* These have been noted in association with in-travenous carbenicillin therapy. Lurie *et al.* (1970) described three patients in whom carbenicillin appeared to act as an anticoagulant by interfering with the conversion of fibrinogen to fibrin. All of these patients had severe renal failure, and the dosage used (24 g daily) exceeded that recommended for such patients. Waisbren *et al.* (1971) reported another five patients (two with renal failure), who developed excessive bleeding associated with the administration of moderately high carbenicillin doses. The nature of the bleeding disorder in these patients was not elucidated. Yudis *et al.* (1972) reported an anuric patient who was treated by carbenicillin in the recommended dosage of 2 g eight-hourly, who developed malaena and a marked prolongation of the one-stage prothrombin-time. After carbenicillin was discontinued the prothrombin time returned to normal within three days.

McClure *et al.* (1970) first described carbenicillin-induced disturbance of platelet function. They observed purpura and mucosal bleeding in six patients with fibrocystic disease, who were given carbenicillin in a dose of 500–750 mg per kg daily, and whose serum levels were in the range of 200–400 μg per ml. These six patients and 24 others receiving carbenicillin without overt bleeding were shown to have a disturbance of platelet function. Subsequently, Brown *et al.* (1974) performed detailed blood coagulation and platelet function studies on subjects receiving carbenicillin; these included 17 volunteers given doses of either 300, 400 or 600 mg per kg per day, and five patients receiving the drug for Gram-negative infections. Some defect in platelet function was demon-strated in all subjects; in addition, in 14 there was prolongation of the bleeding time, in 7 reduced clot retraction and in 8 decreased prothrombin consumption.

The severity of these disturbances appeared to be dose dependent and abnormal platelet function persisted for as long as 12 days after the drug was stopped. Three volunteers given 600 mg per kg per day, and two patients given 340 and 375 mg per kg respectively, experienced bleeding during carbenicillin administration. There was no evidence of any disturbance of coagulation. Life-threatening haemorrhage, attributable to carbenicillin-induced platelet dysfunction, has been described in a patient receiving the drug in a dose of 500 mg per kg per day (Woodruff et al., 1976).

It appears that carbenicillin usually only affects the platelet component of haemostasis, and other causes for carbenicillin-induced bleeding, although reported (vide supra), must be rare. The mechanism by which the drug causes abnormal platelet function is unknown (Brown et al., 1974).

6. Neutropenia. Reyes et al. (1973) described reversible neutropenia in two patients, which appeared to be dose related. In one who was treated with 50 g of carbenicillin intravenously per day and who had normal renal function, neutropenia was observed which recurred twice on readministration of the drug. Neutropenia appeared after about 16 days of carbenicillin therapy, and on each occasion resolved within about one week after the drug was ceased. The bone marrow showed depression of myeloid precursors. There was no evidence that an immunological mechanism was involved, and it was concluded that this was probably due to a direct toxic effect of carbenicillin.

7. Local effects. Pain on intramuscular injection is often troublesome, particularly when doses exceed 1 g. Intravenous carbenicillin can cause thrombophlebitis, but this is usually not a major problem.

8. Indanyl carbenicillin side-effects. This drug tastes very bitter, and although the tablets have a special coating, many patients complain of an unpleasant after-taste and nausea. It can also cause diarrhoea, especially if the dose of 1 g six-hourly is exceeded (Knirsch et al., 1973).

9. Carfecillin side-effects. Some patients have developed diarrhoea while taking this drug, but the unpleasant after-taste associated with the indanyl ester has not been noted (Wilkinson et al., 1975; Leigh and Simmons, 1976). Nausea and vomiting also appear to be less common with carfecillin than with indanyl carbenicillin (Kahan-Coppens and Klastersky, 1978).

Clinical Uses of the Drugs

A. Parenteral Carbenicillin

1. Pseudomonas infections. The main use of carbenicillin is for the treatment of systemic Ps. aeruginosa infections, provided that the MIC of the strain is not much higher than 120 μg per ml. It has been effective for these infections, despite the fact that they are usually associated with serious underlying diseases. The drug has been useful in Pseudomonas septicaemia (Brumfitt et al., 1967; Eickhoff and Marks, 1970) including that associated with leukaemia (Bodey et al., 1971), and also in Pseudomonas infections complicating severe burns (Curreri et al., 1970). Likewise, it has been used successfully in children for the treatment of meningitis (Richardson et al., 1968), mastoiditis and osteomyelitis (Nelson, 1970) due to Ps. aeruginosa. Carbenicillin can also be employed for the treatment of purulent bronchial infections (Pines et al., 1970)

and respiratory infections in children with cystic fibrosis (Boxerbaum et al., 1970; Phair et al., 1970). During or after carbenicillin treatment of children with cystic fibrosis, the usual relatively sensitive non-mucoid forms of Ps. aeruginosa (MIC 20–60 μg per ml) in their respiratory tract are often replaced by mucoid variants, which are more resistant to carbenicillin (MIC 40–80 μg per ml). As carbenicillin concentrations are relatively low in the sputum (page 157), such mucoid variants with only slightly increased resistance may have a selective advantage during carbenicillin therapy (Govan, 1976). Theoretically, carbenicillin may be preferable to gentamicin (page 341), polymyxin B (page 541) and colistin (page 541) for the treatment of Ps. aeruginosa and other Gram-negative rod infections, in which multiple abscesses are present. The activity of carbenicillin is unaltered by the presence of purulent material, which however markedly decreases the effective concentrations of these other drugs, probably because they can be bound to particulate components of pus (Bryant and Hammond, 1974).

Pseudomonas urinary tract infections are difficult to eradicate as they usually occur in patients with urinary tract abnormalities. Carbenicillin may sterilize the urine during therapy, but relapses or reinfections with other carbenicillin-resistant bacteria, particularly Klebsiella spp. are common (Silverblatt and Turck, 1969; Turck et al., 1970). Carbenicillin may be more active in urine with a pH of 7·2, whilst other penicillins such as penicillin G and ampicillin have their greatest activity at an acid pH of 5 (Miller and Perkins, 1973).

In vitro synergism between carbenicillin and gentamicin against Ps. aeruginosa may occur (page 150), and this combination is often effective clinically (Rodriguez et al., 1970; Smith et al., 1970; Carpenter and Seidel, 1972). It is still not clear whether this combination only prevents emergence of more highly resistant Ps. aeruginosa strains during treatment, or if true in vivo synergism occurs. Klastersky et al. (1972) showed that the bactericidal effect of sera from patients receiving a carbenicillin/gentamicin combination was higher than that of sera obtained when either gentamicin or carbenicillin were given separately. Also this combination was superior to either drug given alone, for the treatment of experimental Pseudomonas infection in non-neutropenic rats, provided chemotherapy was started within six hours of bacterial challenge (Andriole, 1971; 1974). Similarly in two other studies the combination of gentamicin and carbenicillin was superior to either drug alone in the treatment of severe Pseudomonas infection in neutropenic rats (Scott and Robson, 1976; Lumish and Norden, 1976). By contrast, carbenicillin/gentamicin was not superior to either of the drugs used alone for the treatment of monkeys with induced Pseudomonas sepsis (Saslaw et al., 1973b).

There have been relatively few controlled trials to determine whether a carbenicillin/gentamicin combination is more effective for Pseudomonas infections in man (Davis et al., 1971). Bodey et al. (1976) treated 26 neutropenic patients with Pseudomonas and Proteus infections using either carbenicillin or carbenicillin plus gentamicin; the cure rates were 83 and 93 per cent respectively, indicating that the combination therapy was possibly superior. Klastersky et al. (1976) compared the efficacy of amikacin (page 388) combined with either penicillin G or carbenicillin, for the treatment of 50 patients with severe Gram-negative rod infections superimposed on serious underlying diseases. The amikacin/carbenicillin combination was superior and it appeared that the outcome of treatment was more favourable if the pathogen was sensitive to both antibiotics used, and also when together they exhibited *in vitro* synergism.

Carbenicillin in high concentrations can inactivate gentamicin both *in vitro* and *in vivo* (McLaughlin and Reeves, 1971). Inactivation is more likely to occur if the two antibiotics are mixed together in the same intravenous bottle and administered by continuous infusion. Significant gentamicin inactivation is unlikely to occur *in vivo,* provided that the two drugs are given separately by intermittent intravenous injection, or the gentamicin is administered intramuscularly (Eykyn *et al.,* 1971; Riff and Jackson, 1971; Lynn, 1971; Winters *et al.,* 1971). Nevertheless when this combination is used, it is advisable to estimate gentamicin serum levels to ensure that they are adequate. This is particularly important in patients with renal failure, when both drugs are usually administered less frequently. In such patients there is a high sustained concentration of circulating carbenicillin and because gentamicin also persists in the serum for a longer period, there is ample time for significant gentamicin inactivation (Jacoby, 1971). The *in vitro* half-life of gentamicin is approximately 40 h at 35°C (McLaughlin and Reeves, 1971). The *in vivo* serum half-life of gentamicin in patients with end-stage renal failure is also about 40 h; this is nearly halved to 20 h if carbenicillin is also given to such patients (Davies *et al.,* 1975; Ervin *et al.,* 1976). Patients with renal failure therefore require an increased dosage of gentamicin to compensate for this inactivation when carbenicillin is administered concurrently.

A carbenicillin/polymyxin combination is not synergistic against Ps. aeruginosa *in vitro* (Standiford *et al.,* 1969), nor is a carbenicillin/colistin combination synergistic in monkeys with induced Pseudomonas sepsis (Saslaw *et al.,* 1973a).

2. *Proteus infections.* Carbenicillin is satisfactory for treatment of Proteus infections, particularly those caused by ampicillin-resistant species (*see* page 150). Ross *et al.* (1970) reported the successful treatment of four infants with Proteus meningitis (two each of Pr. mirabilis and Pr. morganii) with large doses of carbenicillin intravenously.

3. *Other Gram-negative aerobic bacterial infections.* Carbenicillin may be useful for the treatment of infections due to Esch. coli and Enterobacter spp. on rare occasions if indicated by sensitivity tests (Standiford *et al.,* 1969). The drug is of more importance for the treatment of Serratia marcescens infections, which recently have been detected more frequently, especially in debilitated hospitalized patients and in intravenous drug abusers (Pogwizd and Lerner, 1976). Serratia marcescens infections are hard to treat successfully. Currently the best therapy appears to be gentamicin (page 344) combined with, depending on the sensitivity of the organism, either chloramphenicol (page 444) or carbenicillin (Mills and Drew, 1976).

4. *Gram-negative anaerobic bacterial infections.* This antibiotic is often successful for the treatment of patients with intra-abdominal and female genital tract infections where anaerobic bacteria, especially Bacteroides fragilis, are the main pathogens (Young *et al.,* 1977; Swenson and Lorber, 1976; 1977). Chloramphenicol (page 442), clindamycin (page 484) and metronidazole (page 771) are also very effective for these infections.

5. *Emergency treatment of neonatal infections.* Infections in the newborn often require treatment before bacteriological data are available. Commonly

either penicillin G or ampicillin is combined with an aminoglycoside such as kanamycin or gentamicin for this purpose. It has been suggested that it may be advantageous to use carbenicillin in place of penicillin G or ampicillin in these combinations, because of its efficacy against Ps. aeruginosa. However Strep. faecalis and Listeria monocytogenes, which also cause neonatal infections, are both relatively resistant to carbenicillin (page 151). Although carbenicillin plus gentamicin are often synergistic against these two latter organisms *in vitro*, further clinical experience with this combination is necessary before it can be recommended as the initial therapy for severe neonatal infections (Nelson and McCracken, 1973; McCracken *et al.*, 1973).

6. *Bacterial meningitis.* Carbenicillin has been suggested as a possible alternative to chloramphenicol for the treatment of meningitis due to ampicillin-resistant H. influenzae. A randomized therapeutic trial using either carbenicillin (200–400 mg per kg per day) or ampicillin was performed in 86 paediatric and adult patients with bacterial meningitis; the causative organisms were H. influenzae 41, Strep. pneumoniae 22 and N. meningitidis 13 (Overturf *et al.*, 1977). Clinical responses were equivalent with either regimen, but in this trial there were no cases of meningitis due to resistant H. influenzae strains. As these strains are less sensitive to carbenicillin than ampicillin-sensitive strains (page 150), it remains undetermined whether carbenicillin can be used effectively to treat meningitis caused by ampicillin-resistant H. influenzae strains.

B. *Oral Indanyl Carbenicillin and Carfecillin*

These drugs are mainly indicated for oral therapy of Ps. aeruginosa urinary tract infections. They may occasionally be useful for the treatment of similar infections caused by Enterobacter and indole-positive Proteus species (Turck, 1973; Kayser *et al.*, 1973; Wilkinson *et al.*, 1975; Leigh and Simmons, 1976). Infections by all of these pathogens usually only occur in patients with some underlying urinary tract pathology, and bacteriuria is often recurrent and difficult to eradicate with any drug. Furthermore, suprainfection with carbenicillin-resistant organisms such as Klebsiella spp. may occur (Hodges and Perkins, 1973). Nevertheless these oral carbenicillins have been used with some success, either as short term therapy (Baker and Andriole, 1973; Leigh and Simmons, 1976), or as long term suppressives in patients with chronic bacteriuria (Holloway and Taylor, 1973).

Oral indanyl carbenicillin and carfecillin should not be used for the treatment of urinary tract infections caused by other bacterial species such as Esch. coli, which respond to many other drugs. Their widespread use is unwise, because it may result in the spread of Ps. aeruginosa strains resistant to carbenicillin. These two drugs should only be used in out-patients in whom the use of the more effective parenteral carbenicillin is inconvenient.

REFERENCES

Anderson, E. L., Gramling, P. K., Vestal, P. R. and Farrar, W. E., Jr. (1975), 'Susceptibility of Pseudomonas aeruginosa to tobramycin or gentamicin alone and combined with carbenicillin', *Antimicrob. Ag. Chemother.*, **8**, 300.

Andriole, V. T. (1971), 'Synergy of carbenicillin and gentamicin in experimental infection with Pseudomonas', *J. Infect. Dis.* (Suppl.), **124**, 46.

Andriole, V. T. (1974), 'Antibiotic synergy in experimental infection with Pseudomonas. II. The effect of carbenicillin, cephalothin or cephanone combined with tobramycin or gentamicin', *J. Infect. Dis.*, **129**, 124.

Bailey, R. R., Eastwood, J. B. and Vaughan, R. B. (1972), 'The pharmacokinetics of an oral form of carbenicillin in patients with renal failure', *Postgrad. Med. J.*, **48**, 422.

Baird, I, M., Slepack, J. M., Kauffman, C. A. and Phair, J. P. (1976), 'Nosocomial infection with gentamicin-carbenicillin-resistant Pseudomonas aeruginosa', *Antimicrob. Ag. Chemother.*, **10**, 626.

Baker, D. A. and Andriole, V. T. (1973), 'The treatment of difficult urinary-tract infections with carbenicillin indanyl sodium', *J. Infect. Dis.* (Suppl.), **127**, 136.

Bell, S. M. and Smith, D. D. (1969), 'Resistance of Pseudomonas aeruginosa to carbenicillin', *Lancet*, **1**, 753.

Bergeron, M. G., Gennari, F. J., Barza, M., Weinstein, L. and Cortell, S. (1975), 'Renal tubular transport of penicillin G and carbenicillin in the rat', *J. Infect. Dis.*, **132**, 374.

Bodey, G. P., Whitecar, J. P., Jr., Middleman, E. and Rodriguez, V. (1971), 'Carbenicillin therapy for Pseudomonas infections', *JAMA*, **218**, 62.

Bodey, G. P., Feld, R. and Burgess, H. A. (1976), 'Beta-lactam antibiotics alone or in combination with gentamicin for therapy of Gram-negative bacillary infections in neutropenic patients', *Amer. J. Med. Sci.*, **271**, 179.

Borowski, J., Musierowicz, A., Czerniawski, J., Dzierzanowska, D., Zarebski, M. and Ginel, Z. (1976), 'Laboratory and clinical studies on carfecillin', *J. Antimicrob. Chemother.*, **2**, 175.

Boxerbaum, B., Doershuk, C. F. and Matthews, L. W. (1970), 'Use of carbenicillin in patients with cystic fibrosis', *J. Infect. Dis.* (Suppl.), **122**, 59.

Brown, C. H., III, Natelson, E. A., Bradshaw, M. W., Williams, T. W., Jr., and Alfrey C. P., Jr. (1974), 'The hemostatic defect produced by carbenicillin', *New Engl. J. Med.*, **291**, 265.

Brumfitt, W., Percival, A. and Leigh, D. A. (1967), 'Clinical and laboratory studies with carbenicillin', *Lancet*, **1**, 1289.

Bryant, R. E. and Hammond, D. (1974), 'Interaction of purulent material with antibiotics used to treat Pseudomonas infections', *Antimicrob. Ag. Chemother.*, **6**, 702.

Butler, K., English, A. R., Ray, V. A. and Timreck, A. E. (1970), 'Carbenicillin: Chemistry and mode of action', *J. Infect. Dis.* (Suppl.), **122**, 1.

Butler, K., English, A. R., Briggs, B., Gralla, E., Stebbins, R. B. and Hobbs, D. C. (1973), 'Indanyl carbenicillin: Chemistry and laboratory studies with a new semisynthetic penicillin', *J. Infect. Dis.* (Suppl.), **127**, 97.

Cabizuca, S. V. and Desser, K. G. (1976), 'Carbenicillin-associated hypokalemic alkalosis', *JAMA*, **236**, 956.

Carpenter, A. A. and Seidel, R. A. (1972), 'The treatment of chronic renal infections with carbenicillin-gentamicin, a report of two cases', *J. of Urology*, **108**, 192.

Chow, A. W., Patten, V. and Bednorz, D. (1978), 'Susceptibility of Campylobacter fetus to twenty-two antimicrobial agents', *Antimicrob. Ag. Chemother.*, **13**, 416.

Cox, C. E. (1973), 'Pharmacology of carbenicillin indanyl sodium in renal insufficiency', *J. Infect. Dis.* (Suppl.), **127**, 157.

Curreri, P. W., Lindberg, R. B., Divincenti, F. C. and Pruitt, B. A., Jr. (1970), 'Intravenous administration of carbenicillin for septicaemia due to Pseudomonas aeruginosa following thermal injury', *J. Infect Dis.* (Suppl.), **122**, 40.

Darrell, J. H. and Waterworth, P. M. (1969), 'Carbenicillin resistance in Pseudomonas aeruginosa from clinical material', *Brit. med. J.*, **3**, 141.

Davies, M., Morgan, J. R. and Anand, C. (1975), 'Interactions of carbenicillin and ticarcillin with gentamicin', *Antimicrob. Ag, Chemother.*, **7**, 431.

Davis, S. D., Iannetta, A. and Wedgwood, R. J. (1971), 'Editorial. Antibiotics for Pseudomonas aeruginosa sepsis: Inadequate proof of efficacy', *J. Infect. Dis.*, **124**, 104.

Dean, H. F., Morgan, A. F., Asche, L. V. and Holloway, B. W. (1977), 'Isolates of Pseudomonas aeruginosa from Australian hospitals having R-plasmid determined antibiotic resistance', *Med. J. Aust.*, **2**, 116.

Deziel, C., Daigneault, B., Marc-Aurele, J., Albert, G. and Brodeur, A. (1977), 'High urine specific gravity induced by carbenicillin', *Lancet*, **2**, 980.

Duncan, I. B. R. (1974), 'Susceptibility of 1500 isolates of Pseudomonas aeruginosa to gentamicin, carbenicillin, colistin and polymyxin B', *Antimicrob. Ag. Chemother.*, **5**, 9.

Eastwood, J. B. and Curtis, J. R. (1968), 'Carbenicillin administration in patients with severe renal failure', *Brit. med. J.*, **1**, 486.

Eickhoff, T. C. and Marks, M. I. (1970), 'Carbenicillin in therapy of systemic infections due to Pseudomonas', *J. Infect. Dis.* (Suppl.), **122**, 84.

English, A. R., Retsema, J. A., Ray, V. A. and Lynch, J. E. (1972), 'Carbenicillin indanyl sodium, an orally active derivative of carbenicillin', *Antimicrob. Ag. Chemother.*, **1**, 185.

Ervin, F. R., Bullock, W. E., Jr. and Nuttall, C. E. (1976), 'Inactivation of gentamicin by penicillins in patients with renal failure', *Antimicrob. Ag. Chemother.*, **9**, 1004.

Eykyn, S., Phillips, I. and Ridley, M. (1971), 'Gentamicin plus carbenicillin', *Lancet*, **1**, 545.

Feigin, R. D., Moss, K. S. and Shackelford, P. G. (1973), 'Antibiotic stability in solutions used for intravenous nutrition and fluid therapy', *Pediatrics*, **51**, 1016.

Gaman, W., Cates, C., Snelling, C. F. T., Lank, B., and Ronald, A. R. (1976), 'Emergence of gentamicin- and carbenicillin-resistant Pseudomonas aeruginosa in a hospital environment', *Antimicrob. Ag. Chemother.*, **9**, 474.

Glew, R. H., Moellering, R. C., Jr. and Buettner, K. R. (1977), '*In vitro* synergism between carbenicillin and aminoglycosidic aminocyclitols against Acinetobacter calcoaceticus var. anitratus', *Antimicrob. Ag. Chemother.*, **11**, 1036.

Govan, M. R. W. (1976), 'Antibiotic therapy and cystic fibrosis: Increased resistance of mucoid Pseudomonas aeruginosa to carbenicillin', *J. Antimicrob. Chemother.*, **2**, 215.

Gump, D. W. (1970), 'Elevated S.G.O.T. levels after carbenicillin', *New Engl. J. Med.*, **282**, 1489.

Hewitt, W. L. and Winters, R. E. (1973), 'The current status of parenteral carbenicillin', *J. Infect. Dis.* (Suppl.), **127**, 120.

Hodges, G. R. and Perkins, R. L. (1973), 'Carbenicillin indanyl sodium oral therapy of urinary tract infections', *Arch, Intern. Med.*, **131**, 679.

Hoffman, T. A., Cestero, R. and Bullock, W. E. (1970), 'Pharmacokinetics of carbenicillin in patients with hepatic and renal failure', *J. Infect Dis.* (Suppl.), **122**, 75.

Hoffman, T. A. and Bullock, W. E. (1970), 'Carbenicillin therapy of Pseudomonas and other Gram-negative bacillary infections', *Ann. Intern. Med.*, **73**, 165.

Holloway, W. J. and Taylor, W. A. (1973), 'Long term oral carbenicillin therapy in complicated urinary tract infections', *J. Infect. Dis.* (Suppl.), **127**, 143.

Holmes, K. K., Clark, H., Silverblatt, F. and Turck, M. (1970), 'Emergence of resistance in Pseudomonas during carbenicillin therapy', *Antimicrob. Agents Chemother.*—1969, p. 391.

Jacoby, G. A. (1971), 'Carbenicillin and gentamicin', *New Engl. J. Med.*, **284**, 1096.

Johny, M., Derrington, A. W., Lawrence, J. R. and Clapp, K. H. (1969), 'Carbenicillin therapy in renal failure', *Med. J. Aust.*, **2**, 681.

Jones, R. J. and Lowbury, E. J. L. (1967), 'Prophylaxis and therapy for Pseudomonas aeruginosa infection with carbenicillin and with gentamicin', *Brit. med. J.*, **3**, 78.

Kahan-Coppens, L. and Klastersky, J. (1978), 'Comparative study of carfecillin and indanyl carbenicillin in patients with complicated urinary tract infections', in Siegenthaler, W. and Lüthy, R. (ed.), *Current Chemotherapy: Proceedings of the*

10th International Congress of Chemotherapy, Zurich/Switzerland, 1977. American Society for Microbiology, Washington, D.C., p. 591.

Kammer, R. B., Preston, D. A., Turner, J. R. and Hawley, L. C. (1975), 'Rapid detection of ampicillin-resistant Haemophilus influenzae and their susceptibility to sixteen antibiotics', *Antimicrob. Ag. Chemother.*, **8**, 91.

Kayser, F. H., Hany, A. and Lupi, G. A. (1973), 'Laboratory studies with indanyl carbenicillin', Proc. Symp., Lond., 1973, *Excerpta Medica*, p. 43.

Klastersky, J., Vamecq, G., Cappel, R., Swings, G. and Vandenborre, L. (1972), 'Effects of the combination of gentamicin and carbenicillin on the bactericidal activity of serum', *J. Infect Dis.*, **125**, 183.

Klastersky, J., Vanderkelen, B., Daneau, D. and Mathieu, M. (1973), 'Carbenicillin and hypokalemia', *Ann. Intern. Med.*, **78**, 774.

Klastersky, J., Hensgens, C. and Meunier-Carpentier, F. (1976), 'Comparative effectiveness of combinations of amikacin with penicillin G and amikacin with carbenicillin in Gram-negative septicemia: double-blind clinical trial', *J. Infect. Dis.* (Suppl.), **134**, 433.

Kluge, R. M., Standiford, H. C., Tatem, B., Young, V. M., Schimpff, S. C., Greene, W. H., Calia, F. M. and Hornick, R. B. (1974a), 'The carbenicillin-gentamicin combination against Pseudomonas aeruginosa', *Ann. Intern. Med.*, **81**, 584.

Kluge, R. M., Standiford, H. C., Tatem, B., Young, V. M., Greene, W. H., Schimpff, S. C., Calia, F. M. and Hornick, R. B. (1974b), 'Comparative activity of tobramycin, amikacin and gentamicin alone and with carbenicillin against Pseudomonas aeruginosa', *Antimicrob. Ag. Chemother.*, **6**, 442.

Knirsch, A. K. and Gralla, E. J. (1970), 'Serum transaminase levels after parenteral ampicillin and carbenicillin', *New Engl. J. Med.*, **282**, 1081.

Knirsch, A. K., Hobbs, D. C. and Korst, J. J. (1973), 'Pharmacokinetics, toleration, and safety of indanyl carbenicillin in man', *J. Infect. Dis.* (Suppl.), **127**, 105.

Knudsen, E. T., Rolinson, G. N. and Sutherland, R. (1967), 'Carbenicillin: A new semisynthetic penicillin active against Pseudomonas pyocyanea', *Brit. med. J.*, **3**, 75.

Kurtzman, N. A., Rogers, P. W. and Harter, H. R. (1970), 'Neurotoxic reaction to penicillin and carbenicillin', *JAMA*, **214**, 1320.

Labia, R., Guionie, M., Masson, J.-M., Phillipon, A. and Barthelemy, M. (1977), 'Beta-lactamases produced by a Pseudomonas aeruginosa strain highly resistant to carbenicillin', *Antimicrob. Ag. Chemother.*, **11**, 785.

Leading Article (1969), 'Resistant Pseudomonas', *Lancet*, **2**, 473.

Leigh, D. A. and Simmons, K. (1976), 'The treatment of simple and complicated urinary tract infections with carfecillin, a new oral ester of carbenicillin', *J. Antimicrob. Chemother.*, **2**, 293.

Lowbury, E. J. L., Kidson, A., Lilly, H. A., Ayliffe, G. A. J. and Jones, R. J. (1969), 'Sensitivity of Pseudomonas aeruginosa to antibiotics: Emergence of strains highly resistant to carbenicillin', *Lancet*, **2**, 448.

Lowbury, E. J. L., Babb, J. R. and Roe, E. (1972), 'Clearance from a hospital of Gram-negative bacilli that transfer carbenicillin-resistance to Pseudomonas aeruginosa', *Lancet*, **2**, 941.

Lumish, R. M. and Norden, C. W. (1976), 'Therapy of neutropenic rats infected with Pseudomonas aeruginosa', *J. Infect. Dis.*, **133**, 538.

Lurie, A., Ogilvie, M., Townsend, R., Gold, C., Meyers, A. M. and Goldberg, B. (1970), 'Carbenicillin-induced coagulopathy', *Lancet*, **1**, 1114.

Lynn, B. (1971), 'Carbenicillin plus gentamicin', *Lancet*, **1**, 654.

Marks, M. I., Prentice, R., Swarson, R., Cotton, E. K. and Eickhoff, T. C. (1971), 'Carbenicillin and gentamicin: Pharmacologic studies in patients with cystic fibrosis and Pseudomonas pulmonary infections', *J. Pediatrics*, **79**, 822.

Marks, M. I., Hammerberg, S., Greenstone, G. and Siliver, B. (1976), 'Activity of newer aminoglycosides and carbenicillin, alone and in combination, against gentamicin-resistant Pseudomonas aeruginosa', *Antimicrob. Ag. Chemother.*, **10**, 399.

McCracken, G. H., Jr. (1974), 'Pharmacological basis for antimicrobial therapy in newborn infants', *Am. J. Dis. Child*, **128**, 407.

May, J. R. and Ingold, A, (1973), 'Sensitivity of respiratory strains of Pseudomonas aeruginosa to carbenicillin', *J. Med. Microbiol.*, **6**, 77.

McClure, P. D., Casserly, J. G., Monsier, C. and Crozier, D. (1970), 'Carbenicillin induced bleeding disorder', *Lancet*, **2**, 1307.

McCracken, G. H., Jr., Nelson, J. D. and Thomas, M. L. (1973), 'Discrepancy between carbenicillin and ampicillin activities against enterococci and Listeria', *Antimicrob. Ag. Chemother.*, **3**, 343.

McLaughlin, J. E. and Reeves, D. S. (1971), 'Clinical and laboratory evidence for inactivation of gentamicin by carbenicillin', *Lancet*, **1**, 261.

Miller, M. A. and Perkins, R. L. (1973), 'Effect of pH on *in vitro* activity of carbenicillin against Proteus mirabilis', *J. Infect. Dis.*, **127**, 689.

Mills, J. and Drew, D. (1976), 'Serratia marcescens endocarditis: a regional illness associated with intravenous drug abuse', *Ann. Intern. Med.*, **84**, 29.

Morehead, C. D., Shelton, S., Kusmiesz, H. and Nelson, J. D. (1972), 'Pharmacokinetics of carbenicillin in neonates of normal and low birth weight', *Antimicrob. Ag. Chemother.*, **2**, 267.

Nelson, J. D. (1970), 'Editorial. Carbenicillin—a major new antibiotic', *Amer. J. Dis. Child.*, **120**, 382.

Nelson, J. D. (1970), 'Carbenicillin therapy of infections due to Pseudomonas in children', *J. Infect. Dis.* (Suppl.), **122**, 48.

Nelson, J. D. and McCracken, G. H. (1973), 'Clinical pharmacology of carbenicillin and gentamicin in the neonate and comparative efficacy with ampicillin and gentamicin', *Pediatrics*, **52**, 801.

Overturf, G. D., Steinberg, E. A., Underman, A. E., Wilkins, J., Leedom, J. M., Mathies, A. W., Jr. and Wehrle, P. F. (1977), 'Comparative trial of carbenicillin and ampicillin therapy for purulent meningitis', *Antimicrob. Ag. Chemother.*, **11**, 420.

Pennington, J. E. and Reynolds, H. Y. (1973), 'Concentrations of gentamicin and carbenicillin in bronchial secretions', *J. Infect. Dis.*, **128**, 63.

Phair, J. P., Tan, J. S., Watanakunakorn, C., Schwab, L. and Sanders, L. W. (1970), 'Carbenicillin treatment of Pseudomonas pulmonary infection. Use in children with cystic fibrosis', *Amer. J. Dis. Child.*, **120**, 22.

Pines, A., Raafat, H., Siddiqui, G. M. and Greenfield, J. S. B. (1970), 'Treatment of severe Pseudomonas infections of the bronchi', *Brit. med. J.*, **1**, 663.

Pinget, M., Brogard, J. M., Dauchel, J. and Lavillaureix, J. (1976), 'Biliary excretion of ampicillin, metampicillin and carbenicillin', *J. Antimicrob. Chemother.*, **2**, 195.

Pogwizd, S. M. and Lerner, S. A. (1976), '*In vitro* activity of gentamicin, amikacin, and netilmicin alone and in combination with carbenicillin against Serratia marcescens', *Antimicrob. Ag. Chemother.*, **10**, 878.

Reyes, M. P., Palutke, M. and Lerner, A. M. (1973), 'Granulocytopenia associated with carbenicillin. Five episodes in two patients', *Amer. J. Med.*, **54**, 413.

Richardson, A. E., Spittle, C. R., James, K. W. and Robinson, O. P. W. (1968), 'Experiences with carbenicillin in the treatment of septicaemia and meningitis', *Postgrad. Med. J.*, **44**, 844.

Riff, L. and Jackson, G. G. (1971), 'Gentamicin plus carbenicillin', *Lancet*, **1**, 592.

Rodriguez, V., Whitecar, J. P., Jr. and Bodey, G. P. (1970), 'Therapy of infections with the combination of carbenicillin and gentamicin', *Antimicrob. Agents Chemother.* —1969, p. 386.

Roe, E., Jones, R. J. and Lowbury, E. J. L. (1971), 'Transfer of antibiotic resistance between Pseudomonas aeruginosa, Escherichia coli, and other Gram-negative bacilli in burns', *Lancet*, **1**, 149.

Roe, E. and Jones, R. J. (1972), 'Effects of topical chemoprophylaxis on transferable antibiotic resistance in burns', *Lancet*, **2**, 109.

Ross, S., Kraybill, E. N. and Khan, W. (1970), 'Treatment of Proteus meningitis with carbenicillin: A report of four cases', *J. Infect. Dis.* (Suppl.), **122**, 62.

Saslaw, S., Carlisle, H. N. and Moheimani, M. (1973a), 'Comparison of colistin-carbenicillin, colistin, and carbenicillin in Pseudomonas sepsis in monkeys', *Antimicrob. Ag. Chemother.*, **3**, 118.

Saslaw, S., Carlisle, H. N. and Moheimani, M. (1973b), 'Comparison of gentamicin, carbenicillin and gentamicin, and carbenicillin in Pseudomonas sepsis in monkeys', *Antimicrob. Ag. Chemother.*, **3**, 274.

Scott, R. E. and Robson, H. G. (1976), 'Synergistic Activity of carbenicillin and gentamicin in experimental Pseudomonas bacteremia in neutropenic rats', *Antimicrob. Ag. Chemother.*, **10**, 646.

Silverblatt, F. and Turck, M. (1969), 'Laboratory and clinical evaluation of carbenicillin (carboxybenzyl penicillin)', *Antimicrob. Agents Chemother.*—1968, p. 279.

Smith, C. B., Wilfert, J. N., Dans, P. E., Kurrus, T. A. and Finland, M. (1970), '*In vitro* activity of carbenicillin and results of treatment of infections due to Pseudomonas with carbenicillin singly and in combination with gentamicin', *J. Infect. Dis.* (Suppl.), **122**, 14.

Standiford, H. C., Jordan, M. C., and Kirby, W. M. M., (1970), 'Clinical pharmacology of carbenicillin compared with other penicillins', *J. Infect. Dis.* (Suppl.), **122**, 9.

Standiford, H. C., Kind, A. L. and Kirby, W. M. M. (1969), 'Laboratory and clinical studies of carbenicillin against Gram-negative bacilli', *Antimicrob. Agents Chemother.*—1968, p. 286.

Sutter, V. L. and Finegold, S. M. (1975), 'Susceptibility of anaerobic bacteria to carbenicillin, cefoxitin, and related drugs', *J. Infect. Dis.*, **131**, 417.

Sutter, V. L. and Finegold, S. M. (1976), 'Susceptibility of anaerobic bacteria to 23 antimicrobial agents', *Antimicrob. Ag. Chemother.*, **10**, 736.

Sutter, V. L. (1977), '*In vitro* susceptibility of anaerobes: Comparison of clindamycin and other antimicrobial agents', *J. Infect. Dis.* (Suppl.), **135**, 7

Swenson, R. M. and Lorber, B. (1976), 'Carbenicillin in the treatment of infections involving anaerobic bacteria', *Antimicrob. Ag. Chemother.*, **9**, 1025.

Swenson, R. M. and Lorber, B. (1977), 'Clindamycin and carbenicillin in treatment of patients with intraabdominal and female genital tract infections', *J. Infect. Dis.*, (Suppl.) **135**, 40.

Sykes, R. B. and Richmond, M. H. (1971), 'R factors, beta-lactamase, and carbenicillin-resistant Pseudomonas aeruginosa', *Lancet*, **2**, 342.

Thornsberry, C., Baker, C. N., Kirven, L. A. and Swenson, J. M. (1976), 'Susceptibility of ampicillin-resistant Haemophilus influenzae to seven penicillins', *Antimicrob. Ag. Chemother.*, **9**, 70.

Turck, M., Silverblatt, F., Clark, H. and Holmes, K. (1970), 'The role of carbenicillin in treatment of infections of the urinary tract', *J. Infect. Dis.* (Suppl.), **122**, 29.

Turck, M. (1973), 'The treatment of urinary-tract infections with an oral carbenicillin', *J. Infect. Dis.* (Suppl.), **127**, 133.

Waisbren, B. A., Evani, S. V. and Ziebert, A. P. (1971), 'Carbenicillin and bleeding', *JAMA*, **217**, 1243.

Whelton, A., Carter, G. G., Barth, M. A., Darwish, M. O. and Walker, W. G. (1971), 'Carbenicillin-induced acidosis and seizures', *JAMA*, **218**, 1942.

Whelton, A., Carter, G. G., Bryant, H. H., Porteous, L. A. and Walker, W. G. (1973), 'Carbenicillin concentrations in normal and diseased kidneys. A therapeutic consideration', *Ann. Intern. Med.*, **78**, 659.

Wilkinson, P. J., Reeves, D. S., Wise, R. and Allen, J. T. (1975), 'Volunteer and clinical studies with carfecillin: A new orally administered ester of carbenicillin', *Brit. med. J.*, **2**, 250.

Wilson, F. M., Belamaric, J., Lauter, C. B. and Lerner, A. M. (1975), 'Anticteric carbenicillin hepatitis. Eight episodes in four patients', *JAMA*, **232**, 818.

Winters, R. E., Chow, A. W., Hecht, R. H. and Hewitt, W. L. (1971), 'Combined use of gentamicin and carbenicillin', *Ann. Intern. Med.*, **75**, 925.

Wise, R. (1975), 'Editorial. For and against carfecillin—a matter of resistance?', *J. Antimicrob. Chemother.*, **1**, 4.

Woodruff, R. K., Bell, W. R. and Castaldi, P. A. (1976), 'Carbenicillin danger', *Med. J. Aust.*, **1**, 278.

Wretlind, B., Nord, C. E. and Wadström, T. (1974), '*In vitro* sensitivity of isolates of Pseudomonas aeruginosa to carbenicillin, gentamicin, tobramycin, and some other antibiotics', *Scand. J. Infect. Dis.*, **6**, 49.

Wyatt, R. G., Okamoto, G. A. and Feigin, R. D. (1972), 'Stability of antibiotics in parenteral solutions', *Pediatrics*, **49**, 22.

Young, L. S., Martin, W. J., Meyer, R. D., Weinstein, R. J. and Anderson, E. T. (1977), 'Gram-negative rod bacteremia: microbiologic, immunologic, and therapeutic considerations', *Ann. Intern. Med.*, **86**, 456.

Yudis, M., Mahood, W. H. and Maxwell, R. (1972), 'Bleeding problems with carbenicillin', *Lancet*, **2**, 599.

Ticarcillin, BL-P1654, Pirbenicillin, Mezlocillin, Azlocillin, Piperacillin and Apalcillin (PC-904)

Other semisynthetic penicillins with antibacterial spectra somewhat similar to that of carbenicillin (page 149) have been developed. Seven of these are described in this chapter. With the exception of ticarcillin, these antibiotics are only available for investigational use.

1. *Ticarcillin*. Developed by Beecham Research Laboratories this has the chemical formula of alpha-carboxyl-3-thienylmethyl penicillin (Sutherland *et al.*, 1971; Rodriguez *et al.*, 1973a and b). It is very similar to carbenicillin, but is more active against Ps. aeruginosa (MIC 25 μg per ml). Earlier it was known as BRL-2288 and it is marketed by Beecham in America with the trade name of 'Ticar'.

2. *BL-P1654*. An alpha-substituted ureido-penicillin with the chemical formula of 6(R-alpha-(guanylureido) phenylacetamido)-penicillanic acid, this compound was developed by Bristol Laboratories (Price *et al.*, 1971). Clinical trials with this penicillin have been suspended, because it has an inferior antibacterial activity to carbenicillin (*see* page 171) and it is potentially nephrotoxic (page 180).

3. *Pirbenicillin*. Chemically 6-(D-2-phenyl-2(N-4-pyridyliformimidoylaminoacetamido)-acetamido) penicillanic acid, this drug was developed by Pfizer Laboratories (Retsema *et al.*, 1976). Due to production difficulties further investigation of this compound was stopped (Wise, 1977).

4. *Mezlocillin*. Also known as BAY 1353, this drug, like BL-P1654 (*vide supra*), is an ureido-penicillin. It has the chemical formula of D-alpha(2-oxo-3-mesyl-imidazolidinyl)-carbonyl-aminobenzylpenicillin (Bodey and Pan, 1977).

5. *Azlocillin*. This is another ureido-substituted penicillin with a chemical formula of 6(D-2-(2-oxoimidazolidine-1-carboxamido)-2-phenylacetamido)-penicillanic acid (Stewart and Bodey, 1977).

6. *Piperacillin*. Also known as T-1220, this is an aminobenzyl-penicillin derivative with a chemical formula of sodium 6-(D(-)-alpha-(4-ethyl-2,3-dioxo-1-piperazinylcarbonylamino)-alpha-phenylacetamido)-penicillanate. It has an *in vitro* antimicrobial spectrum qualitatively but not quantitatively similar to that of carbenicillin (Fu and Neu, 1978a and b; Eickhoff and Ehret, 1978). This compound apparently has a different mode of action to other penicillins, in that it only prevents septum formation in dividing cells (Iida *et al.*, 1978) (*see* also page 21).

7. *Apalcillin* (*PC-904*). Chemically this is sodium 6-(D(-)alpha-(4-hydroxy-1,5-naphthyridine-3-carboxamido)-phenylacetamido)-penicillinate. It has been

reported to be active in quite low concentrations against a large proportion of Gram-negative organisms (Noguchi et al., 1976).

Sensitive Organisms

The antibacterial spectra of these compounds are similar to that of carbenicillin (page 149), but there are differences between their degree of activity against various bacterial species.

1. *Ticarcillin*. This drug is consistently at least twice and sometimes four times as active as carbenicillin against Ps. aeruginosa (Sutherland et al., 1971; Neu and Garvey, 1975; Parry and Neu, 1976c; Prior and Fass, 1978) (see also Table 10). Other Gram-negative aerobic bacteria and Gram-positive bacteria exhibit similar susceptibility to both ticarcillin and carbenicillin (Sutherland et al., 1971; Parry and Neu, 1976c). The same is generally true for Gram-negative anaerobic bacteria (Sutter and Finegold, 1976; Henderson et al., 1977). In one study ticarcillin was slightly more active than carbenicillin against Bacteroides fragilis (Roy et al., 1977). Strains of all bacteria, including Ps. aeruginosa, which have become highly resistant to carbenicillin, are also highly ticarcillin-resistant (Neu and Garvey, 1975; Kalkani and Marketos, 1976). As with carbenicillin (page 150), ampicillin-resistant strains of H. influenzae (page 102) are less susceptible (MIC 4-32 μg per ml) to ticarcillin than ampicillin-sensitive organisms (MIC 0·25–1·0 μg per ml) (Kammer et al., 1975; Thornsberry et al., 1976).

Similar to carbenicillin, ticarcillin combined with an aminoglycoside such as gentamicin, tobramycin or amikacin, exhibits *in vitro* synergism against some strains of Ps. aeruginosa and also against some strains of certain other Gram-negative bacilli such as Esch. coli and Enterobacter spp. (Wald et al., 1975; Comber et al., 1977; Yoshikawa and Shibata, 1978). With Ps. aeruginosa the degree of synergy varies from strain to strain and also from one aminoglycoside to another against the same strain. The MIC's of individual drugs are not predicative of the degree of synergism. Therefore testing of these drug combinations routinely may be as important for the choice of combination therapy as individual susceptibility testing is for the choice of individual antibiotics (Heineman and Lofton, 1978).

2. *BL-P1654*. In addition to having an antibacterial spectrum similar to that of carbenicillin (page 149), this drug initially appeared more active than carbenicillin against Ps. aeruginosa (MIC 12·5 μg per ml or less). Most Enterobacteriaceae were also inhibited by similar concentrations, with the exception of Klebsiella spp., which usually required 25–100 μg per ml (Price et al., 1971; Bodey et al., 1974; Watanakunakorn and Bannister, 1974).

Subsequently other investigators, using different culture media, demonstrated that BL-P1654 is only about as active as carbenicillin against Ps. aeruginosa and Serratia marcescens and that it has less activity against indole-positive Proteus spp. (Adler et al., 1971; Weinstein et al., 1975). Furthermore, in tube dilution studies the MBC of BL-P1654 was often 16–64 fold higher than its MIC against Ps. aeruginosa (Overturf et al., 1974; Wald et al., 1975; Kurtz et al., 1975). This appears to be due to a small number of resistant cells in each culture, whose presence can only be detected by special sub-culturing techniques, rather than due to a bacteristatic action of the drug

(Sanders and Sanders, 1975). Strains of Ps. aeruginosa highly resistant to carbenicillin, are usually also BL-P1654-resistant (Watanakunakorn and Bannister, 1974). Similar to carbenicillin, BL-P1654 plus gentamicin exhibit *in vitro* synergism against Ps. aeruginosa (Wald *et al*., 1975).

Because of the above limitations and its potential toxicity (page 180), BL-P1654 appears inferior to carbenicillin, and is unlikely to be used clinically.

3. *Pirbenicillin*. This compound has a similar activity to carbenicillin (page 149), but it has been reported to be four to eight times more active than carbenicillin and approximately twice as active as ticarcillin against Ps. aeruginosa (Retsema *et al*., 1976; Wise *et al*., 1977; Murakawa and Sabath, 1977). However, its *in vitro* activity against Ps. aeruginosa is much less if a large inoculum is used (Bodey *et al*., 1976; Lopez *et al*., 1977). Pirbenicillin is less active than carbenicillin against indole-positive Proteus spp., and against Esch. coli it is slightly more active than carbenicillin, but less active than ampicillin (Greenwood *et al*., 1977). The drug is as active as carbenicillin against Serratia and Enterobacter spp. and it is also marginally active against Klebsiella spp., as some strains are inhibited by 200 μg per ml (Bodey *et al*., 1976).

4. *Mezlocillin*. This newer ureido-penicillin is more active than carbenicillin against all Proteus and Enterobacter strains (Table 10, page 175). Its activity appears about the same as that of carbenicillin against Esch. coli, Serratia marcescens and Ps. aeruginosa. As with BL-P1654 (*vide supra*), the MBC's of mezlocillin against Ps. aeruginosa are very much higher than the inhibitory concentrations, suggesting that each culture contains some highly mezlocillin-resistant Ps. aeruginosa cells (Bodey and Pan, 1977). Mezlocillin is more active than carbenicillin against Klebsiella spp., and more than 50 per cent of strains can be inhibited by clinically achievable concentrations (Fu and Neu, 1978c). The susceptibility of Bacteroides fragilis is variable (Table 10). Sutter and Finegold (1976) reported that the activity of mezlocillin against this organism was in general similar to that of other penicillins such as penicillin G (page 10), ampicillin (page 103) and carbenicillin (page 151). Other authors have found mezlocillin somewhat more active (MIC of most strains 25–50 μg per ml) (Fu and Neu, 1978c).

Mezlocillin is also quite active against H. influenzae and the Neisseria (meningococci and gonococci). Gonococcal strains relatively resistant to penicillin G, are 4 to 16 times more sensitive to mezlocillin (Wise, 1977). Penicillinase-producing gonococci (page 8) are mezlocillin-resistant. Gram-positive bacteria, including Strep. faecalis, but not penicillinase-producing Staph. pyogenes, are also sensitive to low mezlocillin concentrations (Bywater *et al*., 1978).

In combination with an aminoglycoside such as gentamicin, amikacin or netilmicin, mezlocillin acts synergistically against many strains of Ps. aeruginosa, Esch. coli, the Klebsiella, Citrobacter, Enterobacter and Serratia spp. and indole-positive Proteus. Synergy occurs with both mezlocillin-sensitive or -resistant strains of these bacteria (Neu and Fu, 1978).

5. *Azlocillin*. The main advantage of this drug is its superior activity to carbenicillin, ticarcillin and mezlocillin against Ps. aeruginosa. It is also active against many carbenicillin-resistant strains (Stewart and Bodey, 1977; Wise, 1977). In common with BL-P1654, pirbenicillin and mezlocillin, the activity of azlocillin against Ps. aeruginosa is markedly inoculum dependent, suggesting

that each culture contains some highly azlocillin-resistant bacterial cells. Azlocillin has the same activity as mezlocillin against Bacteroides fragilis, but it is somewhat less active against most other Gram-negative bacilli (Stewart and Bodey, 1977; Fu and Neu, 1978c). The drug is as active as mezlocillin against H. influenzae, N. meningitidis, N. gonorrhoeae and the Gram-positive bacteria (Wise, 1977; Bywater et al., 1978; Wise et al., 1978) (see also Table 10, page 175).

Similar to mezlocillin, azlocillin combined with an aminoglycoside such as gentamicin, amikacin or netilmicin acts synergistically against many strains of Ps. aeruginosa, Esch. coli, the Klebsiella, Citrobacter, Enterobacter and Serratia spp. and indole-positive Proteus. Synergy occurs with both azlocillin-sensitive and -resistant strains of these bacteria (Neu and Fu, 1978).

6. *Piperacillin*. This is a new broad spectrum penicillin active against Gram-positive and Gram-negative organisms. It is marginally more active than carbenicillin against Gram-positive cocci such as Staph. pyogenes (non-penicillinase producers), Staph. epidermidis, Strep. pyogenes, pneumococci and Strep. faecalis. Piperacillin has good activity against most Enterobacteriaceae. Most strains of Esch. coli, Proteus mirabilis and the Klebsiella, Enterobacter, Serratia, Citrobacter, Salmonella and Shigella spp. are inhibited by quite low concentrations (Table 10). Only about 50 per cent of indole-positive Proteus, Providencia and Acinetobacter spp. strains are inhibited by low piperacillin concentrations. Against Pr. rettgeri piperacillin is slightly less active than carbenicillin. The drug is also active against a considerable proportion of cephalothin-resistant Enterobacteriaceae (George et al., 1978), but ampicillin- or carbenicillin-resistant isolates of these bacteria are likely to be piperacillin-resistant (Verbist, 1978). Piperacillin also inhibits many aminoglycoside-resistant Gram-negative bacilli (Winston et al., 1978).

Against Ps. aeruginosa piperacillin is more active than carbenicillin (page 149), mezlocillin (page 172) and azlocillin (page 172), its activity being similar to that of gentamicin (page 326) or amikacin (page 377) (Ueo et al., 1977; Kuck and Forbes, 1978; Eickhoff and Ehret, 1978; Fu and Neu, 1978a and b). The drug has also good activity against Bacteroides fragilis, most strains being inhibited by 25 μg per ml; in this respect it is about equally active to mezlocillin (page 172).

Piperacillin is very active against H. influenzae and it is as active as penicillin G (page 7) against N. gonorrhoeae. It is hydrolysed by many different beta-lactamases produced by Gram-negative bacteria. Fu and Neu (1978b) found that penicillinase-producing gonococci (page 8) were sensitive to piperacillin, but Eickhoff and Ehret (1978) reported that they were piperacillin-resistant.

A combination of piperacillin with an aminoglycoside such as gentamicin (page 325) or amikacin (page 377) is synergistic *in vitro* against many strains of Enterobacteriaceae and Ps. aeruginosa (Fu and Neu, 1978b).

7. *Apalcillin* (*PC 904*). In quite low concentrations (0·1–3·13 μg per ml) this drug is active against a large proportion of Gram-positive and Gram-negative organisms, including Ps. aeruginosa (Table 10) (Noguchi et al., 1976). It is also active against other Pseudomonas spp. such as Ps. cepacia, Ps. maltophilia, Ps. fluorescens and Ps. putida (Noguchi et al., 1978).

Apalcillin is more active than ticarcillin, mezlocillin, azlocillin, carbenicillin (page 150) and amoxycillin (page 133) against Esch. coli, Klebsiella spp. and

Ps. aeruginosa (Bodey *et al.*, 1978). It is also active against many ampicillin-resistant Gram-negative bacilli. However, ampicillin-resistant H. influenzae strains (page 102) are also resistant to apalcillin, as this drug is inactivated by TEM-like beta-lactamases (Wretlind *et al.*, 1978). Ps. aeruginosa strains which are only moderately carbenicillin-resistant (MIC 400–1600 μg per ml) are apalcillin-sensitive. Highly carbenicillin-resistant strains (MIC ⩾ 3200 μg per ml) are moderately apalcillin-resistant (MIC 50–1600 μg per ml) (Noguchi *et al.*, 1978).

In Vitro Sensitivities

The minimum inhibitory concentrations of ticarcillin, mezlocillin, azlocillin, piperacillin and apalcillin, compared to those of carbenicillin, are shown in Table 10.

Mode of Administration and Dosage

A. *Ticarcillin*

This drug is not absorbed from the gastro-intestinal tract and must be administered either intramuscularly or intravenously. The dose used can be varied widely, depending on the nature of the infection and the sensitivity of the organism.

1. *Systemic Pseudomonas aeruginosa infections.* An adult dose of 18–24 g per day given intravenously is necessary for the treatment of these infections. The corresponding high dose schedule for children is 300–400 mg per kg per day. Ticarcillin is best given in six to eight divided doses, and each dose infused intravenously as a concentrated solution over 30 to 60 min. For instance, if a total daily dosage of 18 g is to be administered, a dose of 3 g can be given every four hours; this dose can be dissolved in 50 to 100 ml of 5 per cent dextrose in a paediatric buretrol and the resultant solution infused over 30, 60 or 120 min (Neu and Garvey, 1975; Parry and Neu, 1976b). Alternatively, the drug may be already dispensed in a secondary intravenous bottle. The exact rate selected for infusion of this drug does not appear to influence its efficacy. For serious infections or for larger adults, a dose of 3 g administered every three hours may be used (total daily dose 24 g). Occasionally doses as high as 30 g daily (400 mg per kg per day for a large adult) have been used (Ervin and Bullock, 1976). Probenecid given in a dose of 1–2 g orally per day may also be administered to delay excretion of ticarcillin (page 178).

2. *Systemic infections due to more sensitive organisms.* Some Gram-negative bacteria, such as Esch. coli and the Proteus and Enterobacter spp., may be more highly ticarcillin-sensitive (MIC 5 μg per ml or less, *see also* Table 10). Intramuscular ticarcillin in a dose of 1–2 g given every four to six hours may be adequate for the treatment of infections caused by these bacteria (Neu and Garvey, 1975). If the organism is less sensitive or the precise sensitivity is unknown, higher doses given intravenously, as for Ps. aeruginosa septicaemia, are necessary.

3. *Urinary tract infections.* An adult dose as low as 1 g intramuscularly every six hours may suffice for these, because urine concentrations attained

TABLE 10

Compiled from data published by Sutherland et al. (1971), Adler et al. (1971), Sutter and Finegold (1976), Noguchi et al. (1976), Bodey and Pan (1977), Ueo et al. (1977), Stewart and Bodey (1977), Wise et al. (1978), Eickhoff and Ehret (1978) and Fu and Neu (1978b and c).

ORGANISM	MIC (μg per ml)					
	Carbenicillin	Ticarcillin	Mezlocillin	Azlocillin	Piperacillin	Apalcillin
Gram-positive bacteria						
Staph. pyogenes (non-penicillinase producer)	1·25	1·25	0·2	0·2	0·78	0·39
Staph. pyogenes (penicillinase producer)	50·0	12·5–25·0	100·0	Resistant	3·1–400·0	>200·0
Strep. pyogenes	0·15	0·5	0·025	<0·1	0·2	0·1
Strep. pneumoniae	0·15	1·25	0·025	0·1	0·1	0·05
Strep. faecalis	25·0	125·0	—	—	0·4–1·6	12·5
Clostridium perfringens	0·25	0·5	—	—	—	1·56
Gram-negative bacteria						
Escherichia coli	12·5	5·0	12·5	12·5	0·8	0·39
Enterobacter spp.	50·5	5·0	25·0	12·5–100·0	1·6	—
Klebsiella spp.	>250·0	500·0	12·5–100·0	12·5–>100·0	3·1	3·13
Serratia marcescens	12·5	12·5	12·5	12·5	1·6	—
Proteus mirabilis	3·12	1·25	1·56	1·56	0·2	0·76
Proteus vulgaris*	25·0	2·5	1·56	12·5	0·78	0·006
Proteus morganii*	6·25	2·5	1·56	12·5	0·78	—
Proteus rettgeri*	0·78	2·5	1·56	12·5	—	—
Salmonella typhi	25·0	2·5	—	—	0·39	0·39
Neisseria gonorrhoeae	0·3	0·02	0·005	0·005	<0·1	0·1
Hamophilus influenzae	0·5	0·25	0·12	0·06	<0·1	—
Pseudomonas aeruginosa	50·0	25·0	25·0–50·0	25·0–50·0	6·3	0·78
Bacteroides melaninogenicus	0·1–4·0	0·1–4·0	0·5–4·0	—	—	—
Bacteroides fragilis	4·0–128·0	4·0–128·0	1·0–128·0	1·0–128·0	25·0	0·1

* Indole-positive Proteus spp.

after this dose (page 178) are usually higher than the MIC's for most Ps. aeruginosa strains (Parry and Neu, 1976b). The corresponding low dosage schedule for children is 50–100 mg per kg per day.

4. *Pseudomonas infections in patients with renal failure.* The ticarcillin half-life after an intravenous dose is approximately 70 min in patients with normal renal function; this is prolonged to about 14 h in patients with severe renal failure so that dose reduction is necessary (Wise *et al.*, 1974; Parry and Neu, 1976a). A suggested schedule is that in mild renal insufficiency (creatinine clearance 30–60 ml per min), a dose of 2 g is given every four hours, in moderate renal failure (creatinine clearance 10–30) a dose of 2 g every eight hours, and in patients with severe renal failure (creatinine clearance < 10) a dose of 2 g every 12 h (Parry and Neu, 1976a). All patients with any degree of renal failure should be given an initial loading dose of 3 g. Ticarcillin is effectively removed during haemodialysis, so that the dose should be complemented when patients are undergoing this procedure. An additional dose of 1 g four-hourly may be given during dialysis (Wise *et al.*, 1974); alternatively an extra 3 g may be given intravenously after each dialysis, followed by the standard dose for patients with severe renal failure (2 g every 12 h) between dialyses (Parry and Neu, 1976a).

Renal failure patients who are treated with ticarcillin according to these guidelines have not shown significant accumulation of the drug and their serum levels are usually in the therapeutic range (exceeding 100 μg per ml). Further dosage reduction to 2 g of ticarcillin every 24 h is probably appropriate for patients with severe renal failure who have concomitant severe liver disease (Parry and Neu, 1976a).

5. *Pseudomonas infections in newborn and premature infants.* Intramuscular rather than intravenous administration is often preferred in this age group. Based on pharmacokinetic studies, Nelson *et al.* (1975) published tentative dosage recommendations, which aim to maintain ticarcillin serum levels between 50 and 150 μg per ml. An initial dose of 100 mg per kg may be given to all infants; subsequently babies weighing less than 2000 g receive 75 mg per kg eight-hourly (225 mg per kg per day) during their first week of life, whilst for babies weighing more than 2000 g the dose is 75 mg per kg every four or six hours (300 to 450 mg per kg per day). The higher dose is also suitable for the low birth weight infants after one week of age, and it is the same dose as that recommended for older children (page 174).

Availability

Ticarcillin is available in 1, 3 and 6 g vials for intramuscular or intravenous use. It is also available in 3 g 'piggyback bottles', which are convenient to use as parallel infusion sets.

B. *BL-P1654*

In a few limited human studies this drug was administered intravenously by intermittent intravenous infusions or injections, in a dose of 1 g four- or six-hourly (Bodey *et al.*, 1974; Clarke *et al.*, 1974; Williams *et al.*, 1974).

C. *Pirbenicillin*

No data are at present available.

D. *Mezlocillin*

Preliminary pharmacokinetic studies suggest that a suitable dose for adults is 3 g intravenously, given every four hours. The 3 g dose is infused intravenously over a two-hour period (Issell *et al.*, 1978).

E. *Azlocillin*

In preliminary clinical trials this drug has been administered to patients with systemic Pseudomonas infections. A daily adult dose of 12 to 16 g has been given intravenously, usually administered in four divided doses by intermittent intravenous infusions (Daikos *et al.*, 1978; Matthiessen and Kroening, 1978).

F. *Piperacillin*

In one clinical trial piperacillin was used to treat Serratia marcescens urinary tract infections; a daily adult dose of 4, 6 or 8 g was administered intravenously in two or three divided doses (Washida *et al.*, 1978).

G. *Apalcillin*

This drug has been used in clinical trials in Japan in daily doses ranging from 0·5 to 6·0 g, usually administered intravenously (Miki *et al.*, 1978).

Serum Levels in Relation to Dosage

1. *Ticarcillin*. After administration of 1 g of ticarcillin intramuscularly to adults, a mean peak serum level of 35 μg per ml is reached in one hour. Thereafter the serum level falls and six hours after the injection it is only about 6 μg per ml (Sutherland and Wise, 1971; Rodriguez *et al.*, 1973a).

Following a rapid 5 min intravenous infusion of 3 g ticarcillin, the mean serum level 15 min later is 257 μg per ml; this level falls to 218 at 30 min, 119 at one hour, 70 at two hours and after four hours it is 30 μg per ml (Neu and Garvey, 1975). If a 3 g intravenous ticarcillin dose is infused slowly over 90–120 min, and this is repeated every four hours, the mean peak serum level at the end of the infusion is 239 μg per ml and the mean trough level at the end of the four hours is 94 μg per ml (Parry and Neu, 1976b). When ticarcillin is administered by either of these intravenous methods in a dose of 3 g every four hours, serum levels are adequate for the treatment of systemic Pseudomonas infections (Neu and Garvey, 1975).

Ticarcillin serum levels after both intramuscular and intravenous administration are comparable to those of carbenicillin (page 155) and its serum half-life (70 min) is also similar to that of carbenicillin (Rodriguez *et al.*, 1973a; Neu and Garvey, 1975). Probenecid (page 17) increases both serum levels and the half-life of ticarcillin (Sutherland and Wise, 1971; Neu and Garvey, 1975).

2. *BL-P1654*. In adults a dose of 1 g administered by rapid intravenous injection, produces a peak serum level of 80 μg per ml. If this dose is given as a one-hour infusion, the peak serum level is 47 μg per ml. Following either of

these methods of administration, a serum level of 5–6 μg per ml is still present at six hours (Bodey *et al.*, 1974; Clarke *et al.*, 1974). Its serum half-life is approximately two hours, which is longer than that of other penicillins (pages 16, 157). Probenecid does not significantly change the serum levels produced by this drug, indicating that it is not secreted by the renal tubules (Clarke *et al.*, 1974).

3. *Mezlocillin*. After the intravenous administration of a 3 g dose given over a 15 min period, the mean peak serum level at the end of the infusion is 269 μg per ml. Thereafter the serum levels fall, and the half-life of the drug of 66 min is similar to that of ampicillin (page 108) and carbenicillin (page 157). Six hours after the administration of this dose the serum level is less than 10 μg per ml.

When 3 g of mezlocillin is administered intravenously every four hours as a two hour infusion, the peak serum level just after the infusion is over 100 μg per ml, and mean serum levels above 50 μg per ml are maintained at all times (Issell *et al.*, 1978).

4. *Piperacillin*. Evans *et al.* (1978) studied serum levels in eight adult volunteers who received a 15 mg per kg dose intravenously over 3 min. Mean serum levels at 5, 10, 20, 30 and 60 min after commencement of injection were 105, 66, 56, 44 and 34 μg per ml, respectively. At two hours the serum level was down to 12 and at six hours to 1·5 μg per ml. The same piperacillin dose was also given as a two-hour infusion; the serum level steadily rose during the infusion and at the end of the infusion reached a peak of 33 μg per ml. This level fell to 7 μg per ml at three hours, to 3 μg per ml at four hours and at six hours the drug was no longer detectable in serum.

5. *Pirbenicillin, azlocillin and apalcillin*. Data on human pharmacology of these drugs are not yet available.

Excretion

1. *Ticarcillin*. Like carbenicillin (page 156), it is excreted in urine by both glomerular filtration and tubular secretion. Probenecid reduces its rate of excretion by partially blocking renal tubular secretion (Sutherland and Wise, 1971; Neu and Garvey, 1975). Approximately 80 per cent of an intravenously administered dose can be recovered from the urine as the active drug during the six hours after administration. This is less than the comparable figure for carbenicillin (95 per cent), because more ticarcillin than carbenicillin is converted in the liver to the inactive metabolite penicilloic acid before renal excretion. Approximately 10 per cent of the administered dose of ticarcillin is excreted in the urine as penicilloic acid (Neu and Garvey, 1975).

High urinary concentrations of active ticarcillin are obtained after the administration of usual intravenous doses; these reach 650 to 2475 μg per ml during the first three hours after a single 3 g intravenous dose. Urinary concentrations are also high in patients with varying degrees of renal failure, when doses of the drug appropriate to renal function (page 176) are given; even in patients with a creatinine clearance rate of <10 ml per min, urinary ticarcillin concentrations have ranged from 250 to 3900 μg per ml (Parry and Neu, 1976c).

2. *BL-P1654*. About 50–65 per cent of an intravenously administered dose is excreted in urine during the first six hours (Bodey *et al.*, 1974). BL-P1654 is

excreted via the kidney more slowly than other penicillins. Renal excretion is only by glomerular filtration, there is no tubular component, so that its excretion is unaffected by probenecid (Clarke *et al.*, 1974). High concentrations of the active drug are attained in urine (Bodey *et al.*, 1974).

3. *Mezlocillin.* Excreted in the urine in an active unchanged form, only about 45 per cent of a dose can be recovered from the urine during the first six hours after administration. Mezlocillin, like ampicillin, but unlike carbenicillin, is also excreted and concentrated in the bile to some extent (Issell *et al.*, 1978).

4. *Piperacillin.* This drug is also excreted in urine and after intravenous administration approximately 50 per cent of the dose can be recovered from the urine as the active drug during a 12 h period; most of this is excreted in the urine in the first two to four hours (Evans *et al.*, 1978).

Distribution of the Drugs in Body

Ticarcillin is probably distributed in the body in a similar manner to carbenicillin (page 157). Both carbenicillin and ticarcillin diffuse well into human interstitial fluid (Tan and Salstrom, 1977). Ticarcillin cannot be detected in the CSF of patients with uninflamed meninges (Rodriguez *et al.*, 1973a). According to Sutherland *et al.* (1971) ticarcillin is 45 per cent serum protein bound, but Ullmann (1976) could not demonstrate that it had any protein binding.

In a study of one patient with uninflamed meninges the CSF concentration of BL-P1654 was only one per cent of the serum level at the time (Bodey *et al.*, 1974).

Mode of Action

Ticarcillin probably acts on bacteria in a similar manner to penicillin G (page 19) and carbenicillin (page 158).

Toxicity

A. *Ticarcillin*

1. *Hypersensitivity reactions.* Ticarcillin may provoke any of the reactions which occur with penicillin G (page 24) in penicillin-sensitive subjects. The drug is contraindicated in patients with a history of penicillin hypersensitivity.

Eosinophilia has been fairly frequently noted during ticarcillin therapy (Parry and Neu, 1976b; Parry *et al.*, 1977), and occasionally this has been associated with an urticarial rash (Ervin and Bullock, 1976).

2. *Neurotoxicity.* High doses of intravenous ticarcillin, similar to 'massive' doses of penicillin G (page 28) and carbenicillin (page 158) may cause neurotoxicity. This is more likely to occur in patients with renal failure.

3. *Hepatotoxicity.* This is mainly manifested by elevated serum aspartate aminotransferase (SGOT) levels and can probably occur with ticarcillin as with carbenicillin (page 158), but it appears to be rare (Parry and Neu, 1976b).

4. *Electrolyte and acid-base disturbances.* Problems similar to those caused by intravenous carbenicillin (page 159) may occur with ticarcillin therapy.

Hypokalaemia has been observed in several patients treated by high doses intravenously (Klastersky *et al.*, 1975; Schimpff *et al.*, 1976; Parry *et al.*, 1977).

5. *Bleeding disorders*. Since carbenicillin administered in high doses intravenously is known to inhibit platelet function and occasionally cause bleeding (page 159), Brown *et al.* (1975) studied blood coagulation and platelet function in 17 human volunteers who received intravenous ticarcillin for periods of 3–10 days, in doses of 100, 200 or 300 mg per kg per day (7 to 21 g per day). Blood coagulation was unaffected but platelet function was impaired in all subjects. Lower doses produced only mild defects in platelet function, but with a dose of 300 mg per kg per day haemostasis was more seriously impaired, and the defects were similar in degree to those produced by the same dose of carbenicillin. It is possible that bleeding disorders may be less common with ticarcillin because clinically it is used in lower doses than carbenicillin. Ervin and Bullock (1976) described two patients in whom prolongation of the bleeding time appeared to be caused by ticarcillin; one had received a high dose of 400 mg per kg per day, but the other only 275 mg per kg per day. Another patient who had renal failure and inadvertently received a full dosage of ticarcillin, developed a bleeding disorder characterized by petechiae, ecchymoses and epistaxis; the serum ticarcillin level nine hours after the last dose was 1050 μg per ml (Schimpff *et al.*, 1976).

6. *Thrombophlebitis*. This appears to be more common with intravenous ticarcillin that with carbenicillin (Parry and Neu, 1976b; Parry *et al.*, 1977).

B. *BL-P1654*

Animal studies showed that BL-P1654, unlike other pencillins, has potentially serious nephrotoxocity and possibly also hepatotoxicity. The drug has been given to adult humans in a dose of 1·0 g intravenously every four hours for a period of one week without toxicity (Bodey *et al.*, 1974). One patient with Pseudomonas tricuspid valve endocarditis treated by BL-P1654 developed vertigo and rise in serum creatinine to a level of 3·2 mg per 100 ml; treatment consisted of gentamicin plus BL-P1654 given in a dose of 4 g daily for seven days, then 6 g daily for the next three days, followed by 4 g daily for another four days. Nephrotoxicity appeared to be caused by BL-P1654 as the patient had previously received gentamicin plus carbenicillin for 23 days without evidence of toxicity (Williams *et al.*, 1974).

Clinical Uses of the Drugs

Clinical data on pirbenicillin, mezlocillin, azlocillin, piperacillin and apalcillin are not yet available, and further clinical studies with BL-P1654 have not been pursued because of nephrotoxicity (*vide supra*). The following details only apply to ticarcillin.

1. *Systemic Pseudomonas aeruginosa infections*. Ticarcillin may be a useful and possibly preferable alternative to carbenicillin (page 160) for the treatment of these infections. Like carbenicillin it has been used successfully for Ps. aeruginosa infections despite the fact that they are usually associated with serious underlying diseases. The drug is useful in Pseudomonas septicaemia (Parry and Neu, 1976b), including those occurring in patients with neutropenia

and underlying neoplastic disease (Rodriguez *et al.*, 1973b), Pseudomonas pneumonia (Ervin and Bullock, 1976) and pulmonary infections in patients with cystic fibrosis (Parry *et al.*, 1977). Pseudomonas urinary tract infections may also respond to ticarcillin therapy (Parry and Neu, 1976b).

The response of all these diseases to ticarcillin has been comparable to results previously achieved with larger doses of carbenicillin (Parry and Neu, 1976b). If the lower toxicity of standard ticarcillin doses, compared to the higher standard carbenicillin doses is confirmed (page 180), then ticarcillin may replace carbenicillin for the treatment of systemic Pseudomonas infections.

As with carbenicillin (page 161), there may be *in vitro* synergism between ticarcillin and gentamicin (page 325). These two drugs have been used together clinically, but the response has been usually about the same as that obtained by either drug used alone (Parry and Neu, 1976b; Parry *et al.*, 1977). Some authors consider that when serious Pseudomonas infections are treated, ticarcillin should always be combined with a second drug such as gentamicin to prevent emergence of ticarcillin-resistant Ps. aeruginosa strains during treatment (Peterson *et al.*, 1977). A ticarcillin/gentamicin combination has been used with some success as initial emergency chemotherapy for patients with leucopenia and neoplastic disease and a suspected severe infection (Schimpff *et al.*, 1976; Murillo *et al.*, 1978). Ticarcillin combined with the newer aminoglycoside tobramycin (page 369), has also been used similarly (Klastersky *et al.*, 1975).

Ticarcillin in high concentrations, similar to carbenicillin (page 162), can inactivate gentamicin both *in vitro* and *in vivo*. This is of greater clinical significance in patients with renal failure, when both drugs persist for longer periods in the blood allowing more time for gentamicin inactivation. The serum gentamicin half-life in patients with end-stage renal failure is approximately 40 h, and this is reduced to about 20 h if carbenicillin is also given intravenously in sufficient doses to produce therapeutic serum levels (page 162). With concomitant administration of intravenous ticarcillin, resulting in therapeutic serum levels in the range of 56–169 μg per ml, there is considerably less gentamicin inactivation *in vivo* than is observed with the higher levels of carbenicillin which are needed therapeutically. Under these conditions ticarcillin only reduces the gentamicin half-life by a mean of 26 per cent (Davies *et al.*, 1975; Ervin *et al.*, 1976).

2. *Proteus infections.* Similar to carbenicillin (page 162), ticarcillin may be useful for these infections (Rodriguez *et al.*, 1973b).

3. *Other Gram-negative aerobic bacterial infections.* Ticarcillin, like carbenicillin may on occasions be suitable for the treatment of Esch. coli, Enterobacter spp. and Serratia marcescens infections (Parry and Neu, 1976b; Schimpff *et al.*, 1976).

4. *Gram-negative anaerobic bacterial infections.* Ticarcillin appears at least as useful as carbenicillin (page 162) for the treatment of these infections. Harding *et al.* (1978) treated 25 patients with mixed aerobic-anaerobic intraabdominal or female genital tract infections using a ticarcillin/gentamicin combination. Ticarcillin appeared to be effective for these infections, which were often caused by anaerobic bacteria, including Bacteroides fragilis. In another study of 100 patients with similar infections ticarcillin, clindamycin and chloramphenicol were given randomly; cure rates were 91 per cent for ticar-

cillin, 80 per cent for clindamycin and 82 per cent for chloramphenicol (Medical News, 1978).

REFERENCES

Adler, J. L., Burke, J. P., Wilcox, C. and Finland, M. (1971), 'Susceptibility of Proteus species and Pseudomonas aeruginosa to penicillins and cephalosporins', *Antimicrob. Agents Chemother.*—**1970**, p. 63.

Bodey, G. P., Horikoshi, N. and Rodriguez, V. (1974), 'Human Pharmacology of 6-(D-α-(3-Guanylureido)-Phenylacetamido)-Penicillanic Acid (BL-P1654)', *Antimicrob. Ag. Chemother.*, **5**, 366.

Bodey, G. P., Rodriguez, V. and Weaver, S. (1976), 'Pirbenicillin, a new semisynthetic penicillin with broad-spectrum activity', *Antimicrob. Ag. Chemother.*, **9**, 668.

Bodey, G. P. and Pan, T. (1977), 'Mezlocillin: *In vitro* studies of a new broad-spectrum penicillin, *Antimicrob. Ag. Chemother.*, **11**, 74.

Bodey, G. P., Weaver, S. and Pan, T. (1978), 'PC-904, a new semisynthetic penicillin', *Antimicrob. Ag. Chemother.*, **13**, 14.

Brown, C. H. III, Natelson, E. A., Bradshaw, M. W., Alfrey, C. P., Jr. and Williams, T. W., Jr. (1975), 'Study of the effects of ticarcillin on blood coagulation and platelet function', *Antimicrob. Ag. Chemother.*, **7**, 652.

Bywater, M. J., Holt, H. A., Broughall, J. M. and Reeves, D. S. (1978), 'Laboratory study of azlocillin and mezlocillin, including comparison with other agents', in Siegenthaler, W. and Lüthy, R. (ed.), *Current Chemotherapy: Proceedings of the 10th International Congress of Chemotherapy*, Zurich/Switzerland, 1977. American Society for Microbiology, Washington, D.C., p. 624.

Clarke, J. T., Libke, R. D., Ralph, E. D., Luthy, R. P. and Kirby, W. M. M. (1974), 'Human pharmacokinetics of BL-P1654 compared with ampicillin', *Antimicrob. Ag. Chemother.*, **6**, 729.

Comber, K. R., Basker, M. J., Osborne, C. D. and Sutherland, R. (1977), 'Synergy between ticarcillin and tobramycin against Pseudomonas aeruginosa and Enterobacteriaceae *in vitro* and *in vivo*', *Antimicrob. Ag. Chemother.*, **11**, 956.

Daikos, G. K., Giamarellou, H., Hadjipolydorou, K. and Kanellakopoulou, K. (1978), '*In vitro* and *in vivo* activity of azlocillin against Pseudomonas aeruginosa', in Siegenthaler, W. and Lüthy, R. (ed.), *Current Chemotherapy: Proceedings of the 10th International Congress of Chemotherapy*, Zurich/Switzerland, 1977. American Society for Microbiology, Washington, D.C., p. 626.

Davies, M., Morgan, J. R. and Anand, C. (1975), 'Interactions of carbenicillin and ticarcillin with gentamicin', *Antimicrob. Ag. Chemother.*, **7**, 431.

Eickhoff, T. C. and Ehret, J. M. (1978), '*In vitro* studies of piperacillin, a new broad-spectrum penicillin', in Siegenthaler, W. and Lüthy, R. (ed.), *Current Chemotherapy: Proceedings of the 10th International Congress of Chemotherapy*, Zurich/Switzerland, 1977. American Society for Microbiology, Washington, D.C., p. 598.

Ervin, F. R. and Bullock, W. E. (1976), 'Clinical and pharmacological studies of ticarcillin in Gram-negative infections', *Antimicrob. Ag. Chemother.*, **9**, 94.

Ervin, F. R., Bullock, W. E., Jr. and Nuttall, C. E. (1976), 'Inactivation of gentamicin by penicillins in patients with renal failure', *Antimicrob. Ag. Chemother.*, **9**, 1004.

Evans, M. A. L., Wilson, P. and Leung, T. (1978), 'Pharmacokinetics of piperacillin administered by bolus, infusion, and bolus plus infusion', in Siegenthaler, W. and Lüthy, R. (ed.), *Current Chemotherapy: Proceedings of the 10th International Congress of Chemotherapy*, Zurich/Switzerland, 1977. American Society for Microbiology, Washington, D.C., p. 605.

Fu, K. P. and Neu, H. C. (1978a), 'Antimicrobial activity of piperacillin', in

Siegenthaler, W. and Lüthy, R. (ed.), *Current Chemotherapy: Proceedings of the 10th International Congress of Chemotherapy,* Zurich/Switzerland, 1977. American Society for Microbiology, Washington, D.C., p. 596.

Fu, K. P. and Neu, H. C. (1978b), 'Piperacillin, a new penicillin active against many bacteria resistant to other penicillins', *Antimicrob. Ag. Chemother.,* 13, 358.

Fu, K. P. and Neu, H. C. (1978c), 'Azlocillin and mezlocillin: New ureido penicillins', *Antimicrob. Ag. Chemother.,* 13, 930.

George, W. L., Lewis, R. P. and Meyer, R. D. (1978), 'Susceptibility of cephalothin-resistant Gram-negative bacilli to piperacillin, cefuroxime, and other selected antibiotics', *Antimicrob. Ag. Chemother.,* 13, 484.

Greenwood, D., Pearson, N. J., Olivant, J. and O'Grady, F. (1977), 'Laboratory evaluation of pirbenicillin, a new penicillin with antipseudomonal activity', *J. Antimicrob. Chemother.,* 3, 185.

Harding, G. K. M., Marrie, T. J., Buckwold, F. J., Muir, P., Koss, J., Gratton, C., Gurwith, M. J., Stiver, G., Albritton, W. and Ronald, A. R. (1978), 'Ticarcillin therapy for infections involving anaerobic bacteria', in Siegenthaler, W. and Lüthy, R. (ed.), *Current Chemotherapy: Proceedings of the 10th International Congress of Chemotherapy,* Zurich/Switzerland, 1977. American Society for Microbiology, Washington, D.C., p. 585.

Heineman, H. S. and Lofton, W. M. (1978), 'Unpredictable response of Pseudomonas aeruginosa to synergistic antibiotic combinations *in vitro, Antimicrob. Ag. Chemother.,* 13, 827.

Henderson, D. K., Chow, A. W. and Guze, L. B. (1977), 'Comparative susceptibility of anaerobic bacteria to ticarcillin, cefoxitin, metronidazole, and related antimicrobial agents', *Antimicrob. Ag. Chemother.,* 11, 679.

Iida, K., Hirata, S., Nakamuta, S. and Koike, M. (1978), 'Mode of action of synthetic penicillin T-1220', in Siegenthaler, W. and Lüthy, R. (ed.), *Current Chemotherapy: Proceedings of the 10th International Congress of Chemotherapy,* Zurich/Switzerland, 1977. American Society for Microbiology, Washington, D.C., p. 594.

Issell, B. F., Bodey, G. P. and Weaver, S. (1978), 'Clinical pharmacology of mezlocillin', *Antimicrob. Ag. Chemother.,* 13, 180.

Kalkani, E. and Marketos, N. (1976), 'Comparative *in vitro* evaluation of the effects of ticarcillin and carbenicillin upon Pseudomonas aeruginosa', *Antimicrob. Ag. Chemother.,* 9, 89.

Kammer, R. B., Preston, D. A., Turner, J. R. and Hawley, L. C. (1975), 'Rapid detection of ampicillin-resistant Haemophilus influenzae and their susceptibility to sixteen antibiotics', *Antimicrob. Ag. Chemother.,* 8, 91.

Klastersky, J., Hensgens, C. and Debusscher, L. (1975), 'Empiric therapy for cancer patients: Comparative study of ticarcillin-tobramycin, ticarcillin-cephalothin, and cephalothin-tobramycin', *Antimicrob. Ag. Chemother.,* 7, 640.

Kuck, N. A. and Forbes, M. (1978), '*In vitro* evaluation of piperacillin sodium, a new broad-spectrum penicillin', in Siegenthaler, W. and Lüthy, R. (ed.), *Current Chemotherapy: Proceedings of the 10th International Congress of Chemotherapy,* Zurich/Switzerland, 1977. American Society for Microbiology, Washington, D.C., p. 599.

Kurtz, S., Holmes, K. and Turck, M. (1975), 'Disparity between inhibitory and killing effects of BL-P1654', *Antimicrob. Ag. Chemother.,* 7, 215.

Lopez, C. E., Standiford, H. C., Tatem, B. A., Calia, F. M., Schimpff, S. C., Synder, M. J. and Hornick, R. B. (1977), 'Pirbenicillin: Comparison with carbenicillin and BL-P1654, alone and with gentamicin, against Pseudomonas aeruginosa', *Antimicrob. Ag. Chemother.,* 11, 441.

Matthiessen, W. and Kroening, U. (1978), 'Phase II study on azlocillin for bronchopulmonary infections due to Pseudomonas', in Siegenthaler, W. and Lüthy,

R. (ed.), *Current Chemotherapy: Proceedings of the 10th International Congress of Chemotherapy*, Zurich/Switzerland, 1977. American Society for Microbiology, Washington, D.C., p. 628.

Medical News (1978), 'Bacteroides sensitive to IV metronidazole, ticarcillin', *JAMA*, **239**, 2103.

Miki, F., Shiota, K., Hara, K. and Shibata, K. (1978), 'Clinical experience with PC-904, a new semisynthetic penicillin', in Siegenthaler, W. and Lüthy, R. (ed.), *Current Chemotherapy: Proceedings of the 10th International Congress of Chemotherapy*, Zurich/Switzerland, 1977. American Society for Microbiology, Washington, D.C., p. 642.

Murakawa, T. and Sabath, L. D. (1977), 'Comparative *in vitro* activity of pirbenicillin, ticarcillin and carbenicillin against Pseudomonas aeruginosa', *Antimicrob. Ag. Chemother.*, **11**, 1.

Murillo, J., Standiford, H. C., Schimpff, S. C. and Tatem, B. A. (1978), 'Comparison of serum bactericidal activity among three antimicrobial combinations', *Antimicrob. Ag. Chemother.*, **13**, 992.

Nelson, J. D., Shelton, S. and Kusmiesz, H. (1975), 'Clinical pharmacology of ticarcillin in the newborn infant: Relation to age, gestational age, and weight', *J. Pediatrics*, **87**, 474.

Neu, H. C. and Garvey, G. J. (1975), 'Comparative *in vitro* activity and clinical pharmacology of ticarcillin and carbenicillin', *Antimicrob. Ag. Chemother.*, **8**, 457.

Neu, H. C. and Fu, K. P. (1978), 'Synergy of azlocillin and mezlocillin combined with aminoglycoside antibiotics and cephalosporins', *Antimicrob. Ag. Chemother.*, **13**, 813.

Noguchi, H., Eda, Y., Tobiki, H., Nakagome, T. and Komatsu, T. (1976), 'PC-904', a novel broad-spectrum semisynthetic penicillin with marked antipseudomonal activity: Microbiological evaluation', *Antimicrob. Ag. Chemother.*, **9**, 262.

Noguchi, H., Kubo, M., Kurashige, S. and Mitsuhashi, S. (1978), 'Antibacterial activity of apalcillin (PC-904) against Gram-negative bacilli, especially ampicillin-, carbenicillin-, and gentamicin-resistant clinical isolates', *Antimicrob. Ag. Chemother.*, **13**, 745.

Overturf, G. D., Ressler, R. and Wilkins, J. (1974), 'Comparative *in vitro* evaluation of BL-P1654 and carbenicillin against Pseudomonas', *Antimicrob. Ag. Chemother.*, **6**, 643.

Parry, M. F. and Neu, H. C. (1976a), 'Pharmacokinetics of ticarcillin in patients with abnormal renal function', *J. Infect. Dis.*, **133**, 46.

Parry, M. F. and Neu, H. C. (1976b), 'Ticarcillin for treatment of serious infections with Gram-negative bacteria', *J. Infect. Dis.*, **134, 476.**

Parry, M. F. and Neu, H. C. (1976c), 'Comparison and evaluation of ticarcillin and carbenicillin using disc diffusion methods', *Antimicrob. Ag. Chemother.*, **9**, 625.

Parry, M. F., Neu, H. C., Merlino, M., Gaerlan, P. F., Ores, C. N. and Denning, C. R. (1977), 'Treatment of pulmonary infections in patients with cystic fibrosis: A comparative study of ticarcillin and gentamicin', *J. Pediatrics*, **90**, 144.

Peterson, C. D., Kaatz, B. L. and Angaran, D. M. (1977): 'Drug evaluation data. Ticarcillin and carbenicillin. A Comparison', *Drug. Intellig. Clin. Pharm.*, **11**, 482.

Price, K. E., Leitner, F., Misiek, M., Chisholm, D. R. and Pursiano, T. A. (1971), 'BL-P1654, a new broad-spectrum penicillin with marked antipseudomonal activity', *Antimicrob. Agents Chemother.—***1970**, p. 17.

Prior, R. B. and Fass, R. J. (1978), 'Comparison of ticarcillin and carbenicillin activity against random and select populations of Pseudomonas aeruginosa', *Antimicrob. Ag. Chemother.*, **13**, 184.

Retsema, J. A., English, A. R. and Lynch, J. E. (1976), 'Laboratory studies with a new broad-spectrum penicillin, pirbenicillin', *Antimicrob. Ag. Chemother.*, **9**, 975.

Rodriguez, V., Inagaki, J. and Bodey, G. P. (1973a), 'Clinical pharmacology of ticarcillin (α-carboxyl-3-thienylmethyl penicillin, BRL 2288), *Antimicrob. Ag. Chemother.*, **4**, 31.

Rodriguez, V., Bodey, G. P., Horikoshi, N., Inagaki, J. and McCredie, K. B. (1973b), 'Ticarcillin therapy of infections', *Antimicrob. Ag. Chemother.*, **4**, 427.

Roy, I., Bach, V. and Thadepalli, H. (1977), '*In vitro* activity of ticarcillin against anaerobic bacteria compared with that of carbenicillin and penicillin', *Antimicrob. Ag. Chemother.*, **11**, 258.

Sanders, C. C. and Sanders, W. E., Jr. (1975), 'BL-P1654: A bacteriostatic penicillin?', *Antimicrob. Ag. Chemother.*, **7**, 435.

Schimpff, S. C., Landesman, S., Hahn, D. M., Standiford, H. C., Fortner, C. L., Young, V. M. and Wiernik, P. H. (1976), 'Ticarcillin in combination with cephalothin or gentamicin as empiric antibiotic therapy in granulocytopenic cancer patients', *Antimicrob. Ag. Chemother.*, **10**, 837.

Stewart, D. and Bodey, G. P. (1977), 'Azlocillin: *In vitro* studies of a new semisynthetic penicillin', *Antimicrob. Ag. Chemother.*, **11**, 865.

Sutherland, R., Burnett, J. and Rolinson, G. N. (1971), 'α-carboxy-3-thienylmethylpenicillin (BRL 2288), a new semisynthetic penicillin: *In vitro* evaluation', *Antimicrob. Agents Chemother.*—**1970**, p. 390.

Sutherland, R. and Wise, P. J. (1971), 'Alpha-carboxy-3-thienylmethyl-penicillin (BRL 2288) a new semisynthetic penicillin: Absorption and excretion in man', *Antimicrob. Agents Chemother.*—**1970**, p. 402.

Sutter, V. L. and Finegold, S. M. (1976), 'Susceptibility of anaerobic bacteria to 23 antimicrobial agents', *Antimicrob. Ag. Chemother.*, **10**, 736.

Tan, J. S. and Salstrom, S. J. (1977), 'Levels of carbenicillin, ticarcillin, cephalothin, cefazolin, cefamandole, gentamicin, tobramycin and amikacin in human serum and interstitial fluid', *Antimicrob. Ag. Chemother.*, **11**, 698.

Thornsberry, C., Baker, C. N., Kirven, L. A. and Swenson, J. M. (1976), 'Susceptibility of ampicillin-resistant Haemophilus influenzae to seven penicillins', *Antimicrob. Ag. Chemother.*, **9**, 70.

Ueo, K., Fukuoka, Y., Hayashi, T., Yasuda, T., Taki, H., Tai, M., Watanabe, Y., Saikawa, I. and Mitsuhashi, S. (1977), *In vitro* and *in vivo* antibacterial activity of T-1220, a new semisynthetic penicillin', *Antimicrob. Ag. Chemother.*, **12**, 455.

Ullmann, U. (1976), 'The protein binding of ticarcillin and tobramycin', *J. Antimicrob. Chemother.*, **2**, 213.

Verbist, L. (1978), '*In vitro* activity of piperacillin, a new semisynthetic penicillin with an unusually broad spectrum of activity', *Antimicrob. Ag. Chemother.*, **13**, 349.

Wald, E. R., Standiford, H. C., Tatem, B. A., Calia, F. M. and Hornick, R. B. (1975), 'BL-P1654, ticarcillin and carbenicillin: *In vitro* comparison alone and in combination with gentamicin against Pseudomonas aeruginosa', *Antimicrob. Ag. Chemother.*, **7**, 336.

Washida, H., Ueda, K., Watanabe, H. and Shimizu, K. (1978), 'Clinical studies of T-1220, a new semisynthetic penicillin in urinary tract infections caused by Serratia marcescens', in Siegenthaler, W. and Lüthy, R. (ed.), *Current Chemotherapy: Proceedings of the 10th International Congress of Chemotherapy*, Zurich/Switzerland, 1977. American Society for Microbiology, Washington, D.C., p. 607.

Watanakunakorn, C. and Bannister, T. (1974), 'Comparison of the *in vitro* activity of BL-P1654 with gentamicin and carbenicillin against Pseudomonas aeruginosa', *Antimicrob. Ag. Chemother.*, **6**, 471.

Weinstein, R. J., Young, L. S. and Hewitt, W. L. (1975), 'Activity of three aminoglycosides and two penicillins against four species of Gram-negative bacilli', *Antimicrob. Ag. Chemother.*, **7**, 172.

Williams, B. B., Cushing, R. D. and Lerner, A. M. (1974), 'Severe combined nephrotoxicity of BL-P1654 and gentamicin', *J. Infect. Dis.*, **130**, 694.

Winston, D. J., Wang, D., Young, L. S., Martin, W. J. and Hewitt, W. L. (1978), '*In vitro* studies of piperacillin, a new semisynthetic penicillin', *Antimicrob. Ag. Chemother.*, **13**, 944.

Wise, R., Reeves, D. S. and Parker, A. S. (1974), 'Administration of ticarcillin, a new antipseudomonal antibiotic, in patients undergoing dialysis', *Antimicrob. Ag. Chemother.*, **5**, 119.

Wise, R., Andrews, J. M. and Bedford, K. A. (1977), 'Pirbenicillin—a semi-synthetic penicillin with antipseudomonal activity', *J. Antimicrob. Chemother.*, **3**, 175.

Wise, R. (1977), 'Substituted ampicillins', *J. Antimicrob. Chemother.*, **3**, 289.

Wise, R., Gillett, A. P., Andrews, J. M. and Bedford, K. A. (1978), 'Activity of azlocillin and mezlocillin against Gram-negative organisms: Comparison with other penicillins', *Antimicrob. Ag. Chemother.*, **13**, 559.

Wretlind, B., Gezelius, L., Karlsson, I. and Hagberg, R. (1978), '*In vitro* activity of a new semisynthetic penicillin, PC-904, against ampicillin-resistant Gram-negative bacteria', in Siegenthaler, W. and Lüthy, R. (ed.), *Current Chemotherapy: Proceedings of the 10th International Congress of Chemotherapy*, Zurich/Switzerland, 1977. American Society for Microbiology, Washington, D.C., P. 638.

Yoshikawa, T. T. and Shibata, S. A. (1978), '*In vitro* antibacterial activity of amikacin and ticarcillin, alone and in combination, against Pseudomonas aeruginosa', *Antimicrob. Ag. Chemother.*, **13**, 997.

Mecillinam

Description

Mecillinam is a new antibiotic, developed by Leo Pharmaceutical Laboratories (Lund and Tybring, 1972). It has a beta-lactam structure and is derived from the penicillin nucleus, 6-aminopenicillanic acid, but it belongs to a new class of penicillins. The natural and semisynthetic penicillins are acylamino-penicillinates, but these new derivatives are 6-beta-amidinopenicillanic acids, containing a substituted amidino group (Matsuhashi *et al.*, 1974; Leading article, 1976). Mecillinam in the form of hydrochloride dihydrate (FL-1060) is suitable for intramuscular or intravenous administration, but it is not absorbed when given orally. A pivaloyloxymethyl ester of the drug, pivmecillinam hydrochloride (FL-1039) is suitable for oral administration. This is readily absorbed from the gastro-intestinal tract and after absorption it is hydrolysed by enzymes with the liberation of active mecillinam (Roholt *et al.*, 1975). Pivmecillinam hydrochloride is marketed by Leo Laboratories with the trade name of 'Selexid'. Mecillinam and its ester are not yet available in Australia or United States of America.

Sensitive Organisms

1. *Gram-negative bacteria*. Mecillinam differs fundamentally in its antibacterial activity from other penicillins, being much more active against Gram-negative than against Gram-positive organisms (Lund and Tybring, 1972; Tybring, 1975; Reeves *et al.*, 1975; Neu 1976a). It is highly active against most Enterobacteriaceae such as Esch. coli, the Enterobacter, Klebsiella, Salmonella, Shigella, Yersinia and Citrobacter spp. Proteus mirabilis and Pr. vulgaris are usually sensitive, but Pr. morganii, Pr. rettgeri and Providencia spp. are less often so. A paradoxical effect of mecillinam has been observed with Providencia stuartii; most strains are sensitive to drug concentrations of $1-10\,\mu$g per ml, but at high concentrations, usually $50-400\mu$g per ml, mecillinam is inactive against this organism (Kerry *et al.*, 1976).

Serratia marcescens may be mecillinam-sensitive, but most strains are moderately or highly resistant (Neu, 1976a). Pseudomonas aeruginosa, Acinetobacter and the anaerobic Gram-negative bacilli such as Bacteroides fragilis are completely mecillinam-resistant (Leading article, 1976; Neu, 1976a).

Neisseria spp. are much less sensitive to mecillinam than to ampicillin (Table 11, page 190). Haemophilus influenzae is also moderately resistant and ampicillin-resistant strains of this organism (page 102) are highly mecillinam-resistant (Neu, 1976a).

2. *Gram-positive bacteria.* Compared to ampicillin, the activity of mecillinam against these organisms is relatively low (Table 11). All Strep. faecalis strains are highly resistant (Neu, 1976a). Subgroup 3 micrococci (Staph. saprophyticus), which are common causes of urinary tract infections in otherwise healthy young women, are relatively resistant to mecillinam (Table 11), but sufficiently high concentrations of the drug may be attained in the urine to inhibit these bacteria (Anderson *et al.*, 1976a).

3. *In vitro growth conditions and MIC values.* The ion content or conductivity and the osmolality of the testing medium, have a marked influence upon mecillinam's MIC's against many organisms. In media with high osmolality and high conductivity, MIC values for some organisms are markedly increased (Greenwood and O'Grady, 1973; Tybring and Melchior, 1975; Neu, 1976a; Greenwood, 1976). As mecillinam may have a place in the treatment of urinary tract infections, and as urine normally has a high osmolality and conductivity, these findings may have clinical significance.

4. *Inoculum effect and bactericidal action.* If large inocula of bacteria are used for *in vitro* sensitivity testing, mecillinam's MIC's are markedly increased for all bacteria. With many Gram-negative bacteria there is also a marked difference (8–32 fold) between mecillinam's MIC's and its minimum bactericidal concentrations (Neu, 1976a). Instability of mecillinam in the assay medium may account for these differences, and the drug probably has a bactericidal effect *in vivo* similar to other penicillins. According to Tybring and Melchior (1975), the drug has a bactericidal effect, but this effect is evident *in vitro* only after prolonged incubation of the culture. This can be explained in terms of the mode of action of mecillinam which is different from other penicillins (pages 22, 192). Growing cells of Esch. coli respond to the action of mecillinam by first forming swollen and then spherical cells, with lysis only occurring much later.

5. *Acquired resistance and cross-resistance with ampicillin.* Mecillinam-resistant strains of many bacterial species can be readily selected by their *in vitro* passage in the presence of the antibiotic (Greenwood and O'Grady, 1973; Matsuhashi *et al.*, 1974; Tybring, 1975). Resistant strains may also emerge during treatment with mecillinam. Jonsson and Tunewall (1975) treated 12 chronic Salmonella spp. carriers with the drug; eight were apparently cured but in four others mecillinam-resistant salmonellae emerged, in three of whom an R plasmid was implicated (*see* page 422). The emergence of mecillinam-resistant strains so far has not been a problem when the drug was used for the treatment of typhoid fever (Clarke *et al.*, 1976; Geddes and Clarke, 1977) or urinary tract infections (Bentzen *et al.*, 1975; Verrier Jones and Asscher, 1975; Aaraas *et al.*, 1977). Resistance may become more apparent with increased use of this new antibiotic. At present it appears that short courses are unlikely to select resistant faecal organisms or lead to chemotherapy failure due to development of mecillinam-resistant pathogens (Anderson, 1977). Mecillinam-resistant variants can sometimes be demonstrated in urine containing therapeutic concentrations of the drug. The generation time of these resistant strains is 3·0–4·5 times as long as that of susceptible organisms, and this may provide an explanation why such resistant organisms do not usually colonize the urinary tract during chemotherapy (Anderson *et al.*, 1977).

At this time Enterobacteriaceae resistant to mecillinam are much less common than those resistant to ampicillin, as evidenced by isolates from patients both from the community and hospitals (Anderson *et al.*, 1976b; Hassam, 1978). Most ampicillin-resistant Enterobacteriaceae isolated from faecal flora or infected urines are mecillinam-sensitive. However, some ampicillin-resistant Gram-negative bacilli are also mecillinam-resistant (Greenwood *et al.*, 1974; Neu, 1976a). Bacteria exhibiting this cross-resistance are those which produce large amounts of beta-lactamases. Mecillinam can be inactivated by these enzymes, but they have a relatively low affinity for mecillinam, so that it is generally more stable than ampicillin in their presence. The two drugs may also differ in their sensitivity to the various types of beta-lactamases produced by individual organisms (page 20). Another reason why Enterobacteriaceae are more sensitive to mecillinam than to ampicillin is mecillinam's superior ability to penetrate through the outer layers of the bacterial envelope so that it can reach its site of action (Tybring, 1975; Richmond, 1977).

6. *Synergism with other drugs.* Because of their differing mechanisms of action (pages 22, 192), it was anticipated that mecillinam may be synergistic with other beta-lactam antibiotics, such as ampicillin. *In vitro* synergy has indeed been demonstrated between mecillinam and ampicillin under certain conditions (Tybring and Melchior, 1975; Lorian and Atkinson, 1977). It appears that the large spherical forms of bacteria produced by mecillinam (page 192), are more sensitive to ampicillin than normal cells.

The synergistic action of mecillinam with the other beta-lactam antibiotics is rather selective; it depends on the other antibiotic in the combination, the proportions of the two antibiotics used in the test, the species of the organism and also the individual strain within each species. For instance, bacterial isolates which are highly susceptible to mecillinam are not synergistically inhibited by the addition of any beta-lactam antibiotics. Also if media of low osmolality and conductivity are used, the activity of mecillinam may be too great for synergy to be apparent *in vitro* (Neu, 1976b). Otherwise synergy between mecillinam and beta-lactam antibiotics such as ampicillin, amoxycillin, carbenicillin, cephalothin, cephazolin, cephradine, cefamandole and cefoxitin can be demonstrated with selected isolates of most Enterobacteriaceae (Neu, 1976b; Baltimore *et al.*, 1976; Kerry *et al.*, 1977). Animal experiments have also indicated that mecillinam combined with one of the penicillins or cephalosporins, acts synergistically against infections with most Enterobacteriaceae *in vivo* (Grunberg *et al.*, 1976; Grunberg and Cleeland, 1977).

Neu (1976b) was unable to demonstrate synergy between mecillinam and other antibiotics such as the aminoglycosides (kanamycin, gentamicin, tobramycin, amikacin), chloramphenicol, tetracycline or polymyxins. Baltimore *et al.* (1976) had different results; mecillinam/amikacin was synergistic against ten of eleven Pr. mirabilis strains and gentamicin and tobramycin were also each synergistic with mecillinam against four of these strains; mecillinam combined with chloramphenicol or clindamycin acted synergistically against seven of twelve Pr. morganii strains.

Mecillinam does not increase the activity of beta-lactam antibiotics against Gram-positive bacteria (Neu, 1976b) (*see also* mode of action, page 193).

In Vitro Sensitivities

Table 11 shows the comparative activity of mecillinam and ampicillin against various bacteria; with the exception of Micrococcus subgroup 3 and Serratia marcescens, which are given as the usual MIC, all other values are expressed as the IC_{50}. This latter value indicates the concentration of the antibiotic necessary to cause inhibition of 50 per cent of the growth of the bacterium concerned.

TABLE 11

Compiled from data published by Lund and Tybring (1972), Greenwood *et al.* (1974) and Neu (1976a)

ORGANISM	IC_{50} (μg per ml)	
	Mecillinam	Ampicillin
Gram-positive bacteria		
Staph. pyogenes (non-penicillinase producer)	5·0	0·016
Staph. pyogenes (penicillinase producer)	>100·0	50·0
Strep. pyogenes	0·50	0·006
Strep. pneumoniae	1·60	0·016
Strep. faecalis	>100·0	0·20
Micrococcus subgroup 3	16·0–64·0*	—
Gram-negative bacteria		
Neisseria gonorrhoeae	0·16	0·005
Haemophilus influenzae	16·0	0·16
Escherichia coli	0·016	0·50
Enterobacter cloacae	0·16	>100·0
Klebsiella pneumoniae	0·10	>100·0
Proteus mirabilis	0·10	0·50
Proteus vulgaris	0·16	40·0
Proteus morganii	0·13	>100·0
Salmonella typhimurium	0·10	1·0
Salmonella enteritidis	0·079	0·20
Shigella dysenteriae	0·05	1·0
Serratia marcescens	12·5–100·0*	32·0
Pseudomonas aeruginosa	160·0	500·0

* These two values are expressed as the MIC.

Mode of Administration and Dosage

1. *Parenteral administration.* Mecillinam hydrochloride dihydrate is available as a powder, containing 82 per cent anhydrous mecillinam, which when dissolved in sterile water is only suitable for intramuscular or intravenous administration. Clarke *et al.* (1976) gave this drug intramuscularly or intravenously to adult patients with typhoid fever in a dose of 400 mg every six hours; in one patient the dose was increased to 600 mg every six hours. Op-

timal dosage schedules for use in different infections and under different conditions are yet to be determined.

2. *Oral administration.* Pivmecillinam hydrochloride is available in capsules of 150 or 200 mg each containing 68 per cent anhydrous mecillinam, and this preparation is suitable for oral administration. In clinical trials to date pivmecillinam has been given orally to adults in doses of 200 mg four times daily (Aaraas *et al.*, 1977), 300 mg four times daily (Jonsson, 1974; Jonsson and Tunevall, 1975; Bentzen *et al.*, 1975), 400 mg three times daily (Verrier Jones and Asscher, 1975; Clarke *et al.*, 1977) and 400 mg every six hours (Clarke *et al.*, 1976).

Serum Levels in Relation to Dosage

1. *Intramuscular mecillinam.* After intramuscular injection of a 335 mg dose (equivalent to 273 mg anhydrous mecillinam) to adults, a mean peak serum level of $4.5–5.0 \mu g$ per ml (expressed as anhydrous mecillinam) is reached 30–45 min after the injection. This peak level is approximately double that attained after an equivalent dose of oral pivmecillinam (*vide infra*). Thereafter the serum level falls more rapidly than that after oral pivmecillinam and the drug cannot be detected in the serum six hours after the dose (Williams *et al.*, 1976). Somewhat higher serum levels after intramuscular mecillinam have been reported by Roholt (1977), who detected a peak serum concentration of $6.0 \mu g$ per ml after a 200 mg dose. Doubling the dose, doubles both the peak serum concentration and the 'area under the curve' (Roholt, 1977).

2. *Intravenous mecillinam.* Clarke *et al.* (1976) gave a 600 mg intravenous dose to one adult patient (equivalent to 492 mg anhydrous mecillinam); the serum level after 5 min was $46 \mu g$ per ml, which fell to 30 at 20 min, 27 at 30 min, 14.5 at 1 h, 4.6 at 2 h and $3.5 \mu g$ per ml 4 h after administration. These values are all expressed as anhydrous mecillinam.

After rapid intravenous administration of a 200 mg mecillinam dose to adults, an initial high serum level of $6.5 \mu g$ per ml is attained, this falls to about $2.0 \mu g$ per ml within 1 h and to $0.8 \mu g$ per ml at 2 h (Mitchard *et al.*, 1977). As with intramuscular administration (*vide supra*), doubling the dose, doubles both the peak serum concentration and the 'area under the curve'. The latter indicates bioavailability, and after a given dose it is the same irrespective of whether the drug is given intravenously or intramuscularly (Roholt, 1977).

3. *Oral pivmecillinam.* This is well absorbed after oral administration. After a 400 mg dose (equivalent to 273 mg anhydrous mecillinam) to adults, a mean peak serum level of $2.5 \mu g$ per ml (expressed as anhydrous mecillinam) is reached approximately 1.5 h after the dose. Thereafter, the serum level falls, but some mecillinam is still detectable in the serum 6 h after administration. The serum half-life is approximately one hour (Williams *et al.*, 1976; Mitchard *et al.*, 1977). Higher serum levels after oral administration have been reported. Roholt *et al.* (1975) and Roholt (1977) in human volunteer studies, found a mean serum level as high as $5.0 \mu g$ per ml, after a 400 mg dose. In the latter studies older ambulatory subjects were used, while Williams *et al.* (1976) and Mitchard *et al.* (1977) used younger subjects who also remained supine throughout the study. Older patients are likely to have higher serum concentrations as the renal excretion of the drug is slower, and physical activity after

antibiotic administration also tends to produce higher serum levels (Mitchard *et al.*, 1977).

On doubling the oral pivmecillinam dose, peak serum concentrations increase by approximately 50 per cent, but the 'area under the curve' is doubled. If pivmecillinam is given with food, the peak serum level is slightly lower and delayed. As with other penicillins, concurrent administration of probenecid (page 17) produces higher and more prolonged mecillinam serum levels (Roholt, 1977).

Excretion

URINE: Mecillinam is excreted in the urine. Roholt *et al.* (1975) and Roholt (1977) found that approximately 60 per cent of a parenterally administered dose and 40–45 per cent of an oral pivmecillinam dose was recovered from the urine during the 24 h after administration. Most of this is excreted within the first six hours. Somewhat at variance to this, Williams *et al.* (1976) showed that mecillinam was rather unstable in urine; they were only able to recover 25 per cent of a 400 mg oral pivmecillinam dose from a six-hour urine collection, and urine concentrations of mecillinam varied from 92 to 365 μg per ml.

BILE: The drug is excreted in bile, where levels attained are higher than those in the serum, provided that the biliary tract is not obstructed (Sales *et al.*, 1975). In one post-operative patient with a T-tube in the common bile duct, a peak mecillinam bile level of 6·2 μg per ml was obtained two hours after a 400 mg oral pivmecillinam dose (Clarke *et al.*, 1976). Animal experiments show that biliary secretion accounts for approximately 3·0 per cent of an injected dose (Roholt, 1977).

Distribution of the Drug in Body

In animals mecillinam is evenly distributed in body fluids and tissues with high concentrations in the kidneys, liver and lungs, but low concentrations in animal fetuses. The secretion of mecillinam in animal breast milk is very low (Roholt, 1977).

Mode of Action

Mecillinam acts on bacteria in a different way to other beta-lactam antibiotics (Greenwood and O'Grady, 1973; Matsuhashi *et al.*, 1974; Braun and Wall, 1975; Spratt, 1977a and b). Esch. coli exposed to low mecillinam concentrations, forms large spherical bodies and not the spheroplasts associated with exposure to penicillin G (page 21). Cell division is eventually inhibited and cell lysis occurs after several hours of growth in the presence of mecillinam (*see also* page 188); this is very different from the rapid lysis caused by other beta-lactam antibiotics (Matsuhashi *et al.*, 1974; Tybring and Melchior, 1975; Spratt, 1977a). Enzymes known to be inhibited by other penicillins are not inhibited by a lethal mecillinam concentration, and the drug does not affect proteins which are implicated in cell elongation and septum formation (*see* page 21).

With high affinity, mecillinam appears to compete for one of six penicillin-binding proteins (PBP's) in the cytoplasmic membrane of Esch. coli. It exerts its effect on Esch. coli by binding to PBP2, but a specific corresponding mecillinam-susceptible enzyme has not been identified. By contrast all other beta-lactam antibiotics have a low affinity for PBP2, they bind to most other PBP's, and bacterial lysis is caused by their specific binding to PBP1 (Spratt, 1977a). The mechanism of action of mecillinam appears to be identical in a wide variety of Gram-negative bacilli including Salm. typhimurium, Kl. aerogenes and Serratia marcescens. Some mecillinam-resistant mutants have been isolated which fail to bind mecillinam to PBP2 (Spratt, 1977b).

The morphological effects produced by mecillinam on Bacillus subtilis are similar to those produced by penicillin G (page 21). This organism has five PBP's, and mecillinam binds to all of these proteins. Against B. subtilis the drug acts as a typical but weak beta-lactam antibiotic. It may have the same mode of action on other Gram-positive bacteria. The identical modes of action against Gram-positive bacteria seems to explain the lack of synergy between mecillinam and beta-lactam antibiotics against these organisms (Spratt, 1977b) (see also page 189).

A new amidinopenicillanic acid derivative, referred to as morpholino compound, acts like mecillinam against Gram-negative bacilli in low concentrations, binding only to PBP2. However, in high concentrations this compound, unlike mecillinam, binds extensively also to PBP1 and PBP4. It is therefore possible that modification of the mecillinam side-chain may result in new drugs, which whilst retaining a mecillinam-like mode of action may also act on bacteria in a manner similar to other beta-lactam antibiotics (Spratt, 1977a).

Toxicity

From the results of clinical trials published to date, mecillinam appears to have few toxic effects.

1. *Gastro-intestinal side-effects.* Nausea, vomiting, upper gastro-intestinal discomfort and diarrhoea have been reported in a few patients treated with oral pivmecillinam (Bentzen et al., 1975; Jonsson and Tunevall, 1975; Clarke et al., 1977; Bresky, 1977; Pines et al., 1977).

2. *Hypersensitivity reactions.* Maculopapular or urticarial skin rashes appear to be uncommon side-effects. One patient reported by Verrier Jones and Asscher (1975) and another reported by Bresky (1977) developed erythematous rashes whilst receiving pivmecillinam, which subsided within a few days after cessation of treatment. One patient developed mouth ulcers and vaginitis apparently due to pivmecillinam (Guttmann, 1977). No rashes have been encountered in several other clinical trials (Bentzen et al., 1975; Jonsson and Tunevall, 1975; Clarke et al., 1976; 1977). One patient who developed a skin rash after pivampicillin treatment, was treated two weeks later by pivmecillinam for seven days without recurrence of the rash (Aaraas et al., 1977). Nevertheless, at present it is wise to assume that mecillinam may be cross-allergenic with other penicillins, and only after widespread clinical usage will the types and prevalence of hypersensitivity reactions be defined (Leading article, 1976).

Clinical Uses of the Drug

1. *Urinary tract infections*. Mecillinam has been fairly extensively used for the treatment of these infections. Esch. coli infections respond very well, and infections caused by other Enterobacteriaceae such as the Klebsiella, Proteus and Enterobacter spp. also usually respond satisfactorily (Verrier Jones and Asscher, 1975; Bentzen *et al.*, 1975). As with other drugs, the results of mecillinam treatment are superior in patients with uncomplicated infections, compared to those in patients with recurrent infections and structural abnormalities of the urinary tract (Clarke *et al.*, 1977). The efficacy of mecillinam in both uncomplicated and complicated infections is comparable to that of either ampicillin or co-trimoxazole (Verrier Jones and Asscher, 1975; Bentzen *et al.*, 1975; Wise *et al.*, 1977; Leading article, 1978). Pivmecillinam has been compared to pivampicillin (page 144) in a double blind study. Gynaecological patients with bacteriuria at the time of removal of an indwelling catheter three to four days after surgery were treated. These infections were caused by either Esch. coli, Klebsiella or Proteus spp. After treatment all 17 patients in the pivmecillinam group, but only 6 of 14 patients in the pivampicillin group were cured (Aaraas *et al.*, 1977).

Laboratory experiments with urine containing mecillinam suggest that uncomplicated urinary tract infections caused by subgroup 3 micrococci (a common cause of acute urinary tract infections in healthy young women) may respond to pivmecillinam treatment, but the drug is unlikely to be effective in infections caused by Strep. faecalis (Anderson *et al.*, 1976a). In one trial in which pivmecillinam and co-trimoxazole were compared for the treatment of simple cystitis, both drugs were equally effective, and cystitis attributed to micrococci responded to pivmecillinam as readily as infections caused by highly sensitive bacteria (Guttmann, 1977).

The markedly enhanced effect obtained when Esch. coli is exposed to mecillinam in conditions of low osmolality (page 188), suggests that it may be advisable to reduce urine osmolality by increased fluid intake, when mecillinam is used for the treatment of urinary tract infections (Greenwood, 1976; Reeves, 1977).

2. *Systemic infections caused by Gram-negative bacilli*. Parenterally administered, mecillinam may be suitable for the treatment of septicaemias and other systemic infections caused by Esch. coli and other sensitive Enterobacteriaceae, but clinical data are not yet available. A combination of mecillinam and cephradine (page 256) has been reported to be synergistic against Serratia marcescens (Hamilton-Miller *et al.*, 1977). This combination may be useful if other drugs (pages 162, 344) cannot be used, either because of bacterial resistance or drug toxicity.

3. *Salmonella infections*. Mecillinam, usually in a dose of 400 mg every six hours has been used to treat 13 patients with typhoid and two with paratyphoid fever (Clarke *et al.*, 1976; Geddes and Clarke, 1977). It was initially given parenterally, but when a clinical response was obtained, oral pivmecillinam was substituted in the same dosage. Twelve patients with typhoid fever responded satisfactorily, becoming afebrile in a mean period of five days from the commencement of treatment. The other patient with typhoid remained febrile for 10 days, and blood cultures continued to grow Salm. typhi for six

days after the treatment was started; this patient subsequently responded to chloramphenicol (page 440). One patient with paratyphoid fever responded satisfactorily to mecillinam; the other developed persistent vomiting associated with oral pivmecillinam therapy, and as the parenteral drug was temporarily unavailable, treatment was changed to intravenous co-trimoxazole (page 711) with satisfactory recovery.

The efficacy of mecillinam in typhoid fever is yet to be confirmed by more large scale studies. Better results may be obtained if the drug is combined with probenecid (pages 17, 192), thus ensuring more sustained serum levels (Geddes, 1977).

Mecillinam may also be suitable for the treatment of septicaemias caused by other Salmonella spp. Shanson *et al.* (1977) used a mecillinam/ampicillin combination successfully to control septicaemia in a patient with Salm. enteritidis endocarditis associated with a prosthetic heart valve.

Jonsson and Tunevall (1975) treated twelve chronic salmonella carriers (two Salm. typhi, two Salm. paratyphi B and eight other Salmonella spp.), with oral pivmecillinam in a dosage of 300 mg four times a day for 28 days. The salmonella carrier state appeared to be eradicated in eight patients by this therapy, but in three of these a cholecystectomy was also performed. The carrier state was not eradicated in the remaining four patients; in all of these mecillinam-resistant salmonellae emerged during treatment and in three the resistance was R plasmid-mediated.

4. *Chronic bronchitis.* In one trial an amoxycillin/mecillinam combination (either amoxycillin 250 mg and pivmecillinam 200 mg or double the dose of both drugs, three times daily for 10 days) was compared with amoxycillin alone in a dose of 500 mg three times daily for 10 days, for the treatment of purulent exacerbations of chronic bronchitis (Pines *et al.*, 1977). By the seventh day of treatment a greater improvement was noted in patients receiving the combination chemotherapy, and at the end of treatment, results in patients given the higher doses of the combination were still superior to amoxycillin treatment alone. Also patients who were treated by amoxycillin alone later relapsed more frequently.

A combination of amoxycillin and pivmecillinam may be superior to amoxycillin alone in chronic bronchitis. This may be due to synergy of the combination (page 189) against H. influenzae and against organisms such as Esch. coli, which are sometimes respiratory tract pathogens in debilitated patients (page 710). Further trials are necessary to fully assess the place of mecillinam combinations in the management of patients with chronic bronchitis (Gray, 1977).

REFERENCES

Aarass, I., Skarsten, K. W. and Nees, H. C. (1977), 'Pivmecillinam in the treatment of post-operative bacteriuria in gynecological patients. A double-blind comparison with pivmecillin and pivampicillin', *J. Antimicrob. Chemother.*, **3**, 227.

Anderson, J. D., Adams, M. A., Wilson, L. C. and Shepherd, C. A. (1976a), 'Studies on the effect of mecillinam upon micrococcaceae and faecal streptococci under conditions simulating urinary tract infection', *J. Antimicrob. Chemother.*, **2**, 351.

Anderson, J. D., Adams, M. A., Barrington, J. C., Spence, W. N. and Shepherd, C. A.

(1976b), 'Comparison of the epidemiology of bacterial resistance to mecillinam and ampicillin', *Antimicrob. Ag. Chemother.*, **10**, 872.

Anderson, J. D. (1977), 'Mecillinam resistance in clinical practice—a review', *J. Antimicrob. Chemother.*, **3** (Suppl. B), 89.

Anderson, J. D., Adams, M. A., Webster, H. M. and Smith, L. (1977), 'Growth properties of mecillinam-resistant bacterial variants in urine', *Antimicrob. Ag. Chemother.*, **12**, 559.

Baltimore, R. S., Klein, J. D., Wilcox, C. and Finland, M. (1976), 'Synergy of mecillinam (FL 1060) with penicillins and cephalosporins against proteus and klebsiella, with observations on combinations with other antibiotics and against other bacterial species', *Antimicrob. Ag. Chemother.*, **9**, 701.

Bentzen, A. J., Vejlsgaard, R., Jacobsen, J. and Tybring, L. (1975), 'Clinical evaluation of a novel beta-lactam antibiotic: Pivmecillinam (FL 1039)', *Infection,* **3**, 154.

Braun, V. and Wolff, H. (1975), 'Attachment of lipoprotein to murein (peptidoglycan) of Escherichia coli in the presence and absence of penicillin FL 1060', *J. Bacteriol,* **123**, 888.

Bresky, B. (1977), 'Controlled randomized study comparing amoxycillin and pivmecillinam in adult out-patients presenting with symptoms of acute urinary tract infection', *J. Antimicrob. Chemother.*, **3** (Suppl. B), 121.

Clarke, P. D., Geddes, A. M., McGhie, D. and Wall, J. C. (1976), 'Mecillinam: A new antibiotic for enteric fever', *Brit. med. J.*, **2**, 14.

Clarke, P. D., Geddes, A. M., McGhie, D. and Wall, J. C. (1977), 'Pivmecillinam in urinary tract infections: A correlation of urinary bactericidal activity with clinical efficacy', *J. Antimicrob. Chemother.*, **3**, 169.

Geddes, A. M. (1977), 'Leading article. The antibiotic treatment of typhoid fever', *J. Antimicrob. Chemother.*, **3**, 382.

Geddes, A. M. and Clarke, P. D. (1977), 'The treatment of enteric fever with mecillinam', *J. Antimicrob. Chemother.*, **3** (Suppl. B), 1011.

Gray, J. (1977), 'Leading article. Synergy and mecillinam', *J. Antimicrob. Chemother.*, **3**, 531.

Greenwood, D. and O'Grady, F. (1973), 'FL 1060: A new beta-lactam antibiotic with novel properties', *J. clin. Path.*, **26**, 1.

Greenwood, D., Brooks, H. L., Gargan, R. and O'Grady, F. (1974), 'Activity of FL 1060, a new beta-lactam antibiotic, against urinary tract pathogens', *J. clin. Path.*, **27**, 192.

Greenwood, D. (1976), 'Effect of osmolality on the response of Escherichia coli to mecillinam', *Antimicrob. Ag. Chemother.*, **10**, 824.

Grunberg, E., Cleeland, R., Beskid, G. and De Lorenzo, W. F. (1976), '*In vivo* synergy between 6-beta-amidinopenicillanic acid derivatives and other antibiotics', *Antimicrob. Ag. Chemother.*, **9**, 589.

Grunberg, E. and Cleeland, R. (1977), '*In vivo* activity of the 6-beta-amidinopenicillanic acid derivative, mecillinam, chemically linked or combined in varying ratios with 6-aminopenicillanic acid derivatives', *J. Antimicrob. Chemother.*, **3** (Suppl. B.), 59.

Guttmann, D. (1977), 'A comparison of pivmecillinam and cotrimoxazole in the treatment of simple cystitis in general practice', *J. Antimicrob. Chemother.*, **3** (Suppl. B), 137.

Hamilton-Miller, J. M. T., Kerry, D. W. and Brumfitt, W. (1977), 'The use of antibiotic combinations in the treatment of Serratia marcescens infections', *J. Antimicrob. Chemother.*, **3**, 193.

Hassam, Z. (1978), 'Sensitivity of urinary-tract isolates to mecillinam and amoxycillin', *Lancet*, **1**, 445.

Jonsson, M. and Tunevall, G. (1975), 'FL 1039: A new beta-lactam derivative for the treatment of infections with Gram-negative bacteria', *Infection*, **3**, 31.

Jonsson, M. (1974), 'Is chloramphenicol the drug of choice for the treatment of enteric fever?', *Infection*, **2**, 145.

Kerry, D. W., Hamilton-Miller, J. M. T. and Brumfitt, W. (1976), 'Paradoxical effect of mecillinam on Providencia stuartii', *J. Antimicrob. Chemother.*, **2**, 386.

Kerry, D. W., Hamilton-Miller, J. M. T. and Brumfitt, W. (1977), 'Laboratory studies on mecillinam: Activity alone and combined with cephradine', *J. Antimicrob. Chemother.*, **3** (Suppl. B), 53.

Leading Article (1976), 'Mecillinam', *Lancet*, **2**, 503.

Leading Article (1978), 'Mecillinam', *Lancet*, **1**, 252.

Lorian, V. and Atkinson, B. (1977), 'Comparison of the effects of mecillinam and 6-aminopenicillanic acid on Proteus mirabilis, Escherichia coli, and Staphylococcus aureus', *Antimicrob. Ag. Chemother.*, **11**, 541.

Lund, F. and Tybring, L. (1972), '6-beta-amidinopenicillanic acids—a new group of antibiotics', *Nature New Biol.*, **236**, 135.

Matsuhashi, S., Kamiryo, T., Blumberg, P. M., Linnett, P., Willoughby, E. and Strominger, J. L. (1974), 'Mechanism of action and development of resistance to a new amidino penicillin', *J. Bacteriol.*, **117**, 578.

Mitchard, M., Andrews, J., Kendall, M. J. and Wise, R. (1977), 'Mecillinam serum levels following intravenous injection: A comparison with pivmecillinam', *J. Antimicrob. Chemother.*, **3** (Suppl. B), 83.

Neu, H. C. (1976a), 'Mecillinam, a novel penicillanic acid derivative with unusual activity against Gram-negative bacteria', *Antimicrob. Ag. Chemother.*, **9**, 793.

Neu, H. C. (1976b), 'Synergy of mecillinam, a beta-amidinopenicillanic acid derivative, combined with beta-lactam antibiotics', *Antimicrob. Ag. Chemother.*, **10**, 535.

Pines, A., Nandi, A. R., Raafat, H. and Rahman, M. (1977), 'Pivmecillinam and amoxycillin as combined treatment in purulent exacerbations of chronic bronchitis', *J. Antimicrob. Chemother.*, **3** (Suppl. B), 141.

Reeves, D. S., Wise, R. and Bywater, M. J. (1975), 'A laboratory evaluation of a novel beta-lactam antibiotic mecillinam', *J. Antimicrob. Chemother.*, **1**, 337.

Reeves, D. S. (1977), 'Antibacterial activity of mecillinam', *J. Antimicrob. Chemother.*, **3** (Suppl. B), 5.

Richmond, M. H. (1977), '*In vitro* studies with mecillinam on Escherichia coli and Pseudomonas aeruginosa', *J. Antimicrob. Chemother.*, **3** (Suppl. B), 29.

Roholt, K. (1977), 'Parmacokinetic studies with mecillinam and pivmecillinam', *J. Antimicrob. Chemother.*, **3** (Suppl. B). 71.

Roholt, K., Nielsen, B. and Kristensen, E. (1975), 'Pharmacokinetic studies with mecillinam and pivmecillinam', *Chemother.*, **21**, 146; quoted by Aaraas *et al.* (1977).

Sales, J. E. L., Wilson, A. and Rimmer, D. (1975), 'Excretion of pivmecillinam in the bile of patients with biliary tract disease', *Abstracts* 9th International Congress of Chemotherapy, M-397.

Shanson, D. C., Brigden, W. and Weaver, E. J. M. (1977), 'Salmonella enteritidis endocarditis', *Brit. Med. J.*, **1**, 612.

Spratt, B. G. (1977a), 'Comparison of the binding properties of two 6-beta-amidinopenicillanic acid derivatives that differ in their physiological effects on Escherichia coli', *Antimicrob. Ag. Chemother.*, **11**, 161.

Spratt, B. G. (1977b), 'The mechanism of action of mecillinam', *J. Antimicrob. Chemother.*, **3** (Suppl. B), 13.

Tybring, L. (1975), 'Mecillinam (FL 1060), a 6-beta-amidinopenicillanic acid derivative: *In vitro* evaluation', *Antimicrob. Ag. Chemother.*, **8**, 266.

Tybring, L. and Melchior, N. H. (1975), 'Mecillinam (FL 1060), a 6-beta-amidinopenicillanic acid derivative: Bactericidal action and synergy *in vitro*', *Antimicrob. Ag. Chemother.*, **8**, 271.

Verrier Jones, E. R. and Asscher, A. W. (1975), 'Treatment of recurrent bacteriuria with pivmecillinam (FL 1039)', *J. Antimicrob. Chemother.*, **1,** 193.

Williams, J. D., Andrews, J., Mitchard, M. and Kendall, M. J. (1976). 'Bacteriology and pharmacokinetics of the new amidinopenicillin-mecillinam', *J. Antimicrob. Chemother.*, **2,** 61.

Wise, R., Pippard, M. and Reeves, D. S. (1977), 'A laboratory and clinical investigation of mecillinam and its ester pivmecillinam in the treatment of urinary tract infections', *J. Antimicrob. Chemother.*, **3** (Suppl. B), 113.

Cephalothin and Cephaloridine

Description

Cephalothin and cephaloridine are semisynthetic antibiotics derived from cephalosporin C, a natural antibiotic produced by a strain of the mould Cephalosporium acremonium. The nucleus of cephalosporin C is closely related but not identical to the penicillin nucleus, 6-aminopenicillanic acid (Barber and Waterworth, 1964).

1. *Cephalothin*. This drug is chemically, 7-(thiophene-2-acetamido)-cephalosporanic acid (Griffith and Black, 1964). It is marketed as the sodium salt with the trade name of 'Keflin' (Eli Lilly).

2. *Cephaloridine*. This was derived by adding two side chains to the nucleus, and has a formula of 7-[(2-thienyl) acetamido]-3-(1-pyridylmethyl)-3-cephem-4-carboxylic acid betaine (Muggleton *et al.*, 1964). It is marketed with the trade names of 'Ceporan' (Glaxo) and 'Loridine' (Eli Lilly).

Sensitive Organisms

Cephalothin and cephaloridine have similar but not identical spectra of activity.

1. *Staphylococcus pyogenes*. Cephalothin and cephaloridine are highly active against non-penicillinase producing staphylococci. Both drugs also appear highly active against penicillinase producing strains, if sensitivity is tested by either disc diffusion methods or by dilution tests with low inocula (Bell, 1974). When large inocula are used, resistance of the strain to cephalothin is only increased approximately four-fold whilst it is 60–80 fold with cephaloridine (Bell, 1974; Sabath *et al.*, 1975; Laverdiere *et al.*, 1978b) (*see also* Table 12, page 202). The reason for this is that cephalothin is very resistant to hydrolysis by staphylococcal beta-lactamase, whilst cephaloridine is much more easily hydrolysed (Benner *et al.*, 1966; Regamey *et al.*, 1975; Lacey and Stokes, 1977). This is in accord with clinical findings that cephalothin is a reliable anti-staphylococcal drug, whereas cephaloridine is of doubtful efficacy, particularly for treatment of severe infections caused by beta-lactamase-producing staphylococci (page 213). It has even been suggested that cephaloridine may not be significantly different from penicillin G for the treatment of staphylococcal infections (Bell, 1974; Comments, 1974).

Methicillin-resistant staphylococci (page 64) are usually also resistant to cephalothin and cephaloridine, and this resistance, as in the case of methicillin, is both heterogeneous and temperature-dependent (Richmond *et al.*, 1977; Laverdiere *et al.*, 1978b).

Penicillin-tolerant Staph. pyogenes strains (pages 6, 67, 80) also show

199

similar tolerance to cephalothin and cephaloridine. MIC's of cephalothin against these strains are in the usual low (sensitive) range, but minimum bactericidal concentrations are high. Severe infections caused by these staphylococci, such as septicaemia, may not respond to these cephalosporins (Mayhall *et al.*, 1976; Sabath *et al.*, 1977).

2. *Other Gram-positive cocci.* Most of these such as Staph. epidermidis, Strep. pyogenes, Strep. pneumoniae, Group B streptococci, and the alpha-haemolytic streptococci of the 'viridans' group (page 6) are usually sensitive to both cephalothin and cephaloridine (Muggleton *et al.*, 1964; Bayer *et al.*, 1976; Phillips *et al.*, 1976). By contrast to methicillin-resistant Staph. pyogenes strains (*vide supra*), methicillin-resistant Staph. epidermidis strains are usually sensitive to these cephalosporins (Speller and Mitchell, 1973). However cephalothin usually exhibits poor bactericidal activity against these isolates, and a cephalothin/gentamicin combination may be necessary for the treatment of severe methicillin-resistant Staph. epidermidis infections such as endocarditis (Laverdiere *et al.*, 1978a).

Strep. faecalis is usually both cephalothin- and cephaloridine-resistant (Stewart and Holt, 1964), but the non-enterococcal Group D streptococci such as Strep. bovis are usually quite sensitive (Moellering *et al.*, 1974). A cephalosporin antibiotic combined with an aminoglycoside such as gentamicin may act synergistically against Strep. faecalis, but these combinations are not useful clinically for the treatment of Strep. faecalis endocarditis. It appears that a synergistic and possibly therapeutic effect can only be achieved when very high cephalosporin doses are used which result in serum levels several times in excess of the MIC of the Strep. faecalis strain (Weinstein and Moellering, 1975; Weinstein and Lentnek, 1976). Such levels are difficult to achieve clinically.

Anaerobic Gram-positive cocci such as Peptostreptococcus spp. and anaerobic streptococci are also usually sensitive to both cephalothin and cephaloridine (Tally *et al.*, 1975; Sutter and Finegold, 1976).

3. *Gram-positive bacilli.* B. anthracis, Cl. perfringens (welchii), Cl. tetani, Actinomyces spp. and C. diphtheriae are highly susceptible, but Listeria monocytogenes is usually somewhat less sensitive (Kayser, 1971; Tally *et al.*, 1975; Sutter and Finegold, 1976). The Nocardia spp. are resistant.

4. *Gram-negative aerobic bacteria.* The Neisseria spp. (meningococci and gonococci), Salmonella and Shigella spp., Pasteurella multocida (septica) and Vibrio cholerae are usually sensitive. H. influenzae, B. pertussis and Brucella abortus are only sensitive to a degree, and moderately high cephalosporin concentrations are usually needed for their inhibition (Waterworth, 1971; Williams and Andrews, 1974). Esch. coli is usually sensitive, but resistant strains are not uncommon, especially in hospitals (Yoshioka *et al.*, 1977). Proteus mirabilis, irrespective of beta-lactamase production, is usually sensitive. Indole-positive Proteus spp. and Providencia spp. are resistant, but cephalothin and aminoglycosides, such as gentamicin (page 326) or tobramycin (page 359), act synergistically against these organisms. Even if isolates of these species are resistant to both cephalothin and the aminoglycoside, the MIC and MBC of either gentamicin or tobramycin may be significantly reduced by the addition of cephalothin. These combinations may be useful clinically (Hyams *et al.*, 1974).

The susceptibility of the Klebsiella spp. varies; Kl. pneumoniae is usually sensitive, but Kl. aerogenes less often so. Klebsiella spp. strains which are only slightly sensitive to ampicillin (MIC 32-500 μg per ml), are usually fully sensitive to these cephalosporins, but those strains that are completely ampicillin-resistant, are also cephalosporin-resistant (Greenwood and O'Grady, 1975). In vitro synergy can be demonstrated against most Klebsiella strains by using cephalothin in combination with one of the aminoglycosides such as kanamycin (page 308), gentamicin (page 326) or amikacin (page 379) (D'Alessandri et al., 1976).

All strains of Serratia marcescens (Farrar and O'Dell, 1976), the Enterobacter spp. and most strains of Citrobacter, Edwardsiella and Arizona spp. are highly resistant to these cephalosporins. Pseudomonas aeruginosa and Ps. pseudomallei are always resistant (Barber and Waterworth, 1964; Waterworth, 1971). Campylobacter fetus is relatively resistant to cephalothin (median MIC 11.2 μg per ml) and also to all other cephalosporins (Chow et al., 1978).

The resistance of many Gram-negative bacilli, including Ps. aeruginosa, is partly due to the production of various beta-lactamases, which destroy cephalosporins (Sykes and Matthew, 1976). Laboratory studies have suggested that this enzyme effect may at times be overcome by the simultaneous use of cloxacillin and cephaloridine (Muggleton and O'Callaghan, 1967). Cloxacillin, although ineffective against Gram-negative bacilli, may bind some of these beta-lactamases (page 103). Such combinations have not proved to be of value clinically in the treatment of cephaloridine-resistant Gram-negative infections.

5. *Gram-negative anaerobic bacteria*. Bacteroides fragilis is resistant to both cephalothin and cephaloridine. Bacteroides melaninogenicus and some strains of other Bacteroides spp. may be inhibited by therapeutically achievable concentrations of these drugs (Tally et al., 1975; Sutter and Finegold, 1976). Cephaloridine is more active than cephalothin against these anaerobic bacilli (Table 12).

6. *Treponema pallidum and Leptospirae* are sensitive to these cephalosporins.

7. Both cephalothin and cephaloridine are inactive against the Mycoplasmas, Fungi and Protozoa, and have only an insignificant activity against M. tuberculosis (Murdoch et al., 1964).

8. *Penicillin inactivating enzymes of host origin*. These enzymes which have been found in purulent accumulations such as empyema, and which are presumed to be of host and not bacterial origin, can inactivate cephalothin and cephaloridine in a manner similar to penicillin G (see page 11).

In Vitro Sensitivities

The minimum inhibitory concentrations of cephalothin and cephaloridine against some bacterial species are shown in Table 12. Cephaloridine has a greater activity than cephalothin against some bacteria, particularly Gram-positive organisms (except penicillinase producing Staph. pyogenes). These antibiotics only have high activity against Gram-positive cocci. The Gram-negative bacilli vary greatly in sensitivity; only 50–60 per cent of both Esch.

coli and Proteus mirabilis can be inhibited by relatively low concentrations (Stewart and Holt, 1964).

TABLE 12

Compiled from data published by Barber and Waterworth (1964), Sabath et al. (1975), Tally et al. (1975), Sutter and Finegold (1976) and Lacey and Stokes (1977).

ORGANISM	MIC (μg per ml)	
	Cephalothin	Cephaloridine
Gram-positive bacteria		
Staph. pyogenes (non-penicillinase producer)	0·2	0·04
Staph. pyogenes (penicillinase producer, using light inoculum)	0·25–0·5	0·05–0·1
Staph. pyogenes (penicillinase producer, using heavy inoculum)	0·8	3·1
Strep. pyogenes (Group A)	0·06	0·007
Strep. pneumoniae (Dip. pneumoniae)	0·06–0·12	0·015–0·03
Strep. faecalis (Enterococcus, Group D)	32·0	16·0
Bacillus anthracis	0·25–0·5	0·06–0·12
Clostridium perfringens	1·0	0·5–2·0
Gram-negative bacteria		
Esch. coli	2·0–8·0	2·0–4·0
Enterobacter spp.	128·0–256·0	128·0–256·0
Klebsiella aerogenes	2·0–32·0	2·0–8·0
Proteus mirabilis	4·0–8·0	8·0
Proteus vulgaris	64·0–>256·0	128·0–>256·0
Salmonella typhi	0·5–2·0	2·0
Shigella sonnei	4·0–8·0	1·0–2·0
Neisseria gonorrhoeae	0·25–0·5	4·0
Neisseria meningitidis	0·12–0·5	0·5–1·0
Haemophilus influenzae	2·0–8·0	4·0–16·0
Pseudomonas aeruginosa	Resistant	Resistant
Bacteroides fragilis	64·0–>512·0	4·0–64·0
Bacteroides melaninogenicus	0·5–32·0	—
Other Bacteroides spp.	0·5–256·0	0·1–1·0

Mode of Administration and Dosage

Cephalothin and cephaloridine can only be given parenterally, as absorption after oral administration is negligible. Intramuscular cephaloridine is notably painless, but intramuscular cephalothin is quite painful.

A. *Cephaloridine*

1. *Intramuscular administration*. The dosage by this route is 25–50 mg per kg body weight per day, given in three or four divided doses. The usual adult dose is 500 mg six- or eight-hourly, but this may be increased to 1 g six-hourly for serious infections. A total dose of 6 g daily (or 100 mg per kg body weight

in children) should not be exceeded, because of the danger of renal toxicity (page 210).

2. *Intravenous administration.* The intravenous dose is the same as the intramuscular dose. Cephaloridine is stable in all commonly used intravenous solutions for at least 12 h at room temperature. It may therefore be administered by continuous infusion over this period without loss of activity. Cephaloridine can also be given by intermittent intravenous injection; 0·5 or 1·0 g of the drug is dissolved in 20 ml of 0·9 per cent saline, which can be injected intravenously over a period of five minutes (Curtis and Marhsall, 1970).

3. *Patients with renal failure.* Cephaloridine accumulates in these patients, and a modified dose schedule monitored with serum level estimations should be used. A rapid (three to four hour) method for serum cephalosporin assay has been described (Noone, 1973). An approximate dosage schedule for adults with renal impairment recommended by Gower (1967a), is shown in Table 13.

TABLE 13

Approximate cephaloridine dosage schedule for adults with renal impairment (After Gower, 1967a).

Serum creatinine		Creatinine clearance ml/min	Dose (g)	Intervals between doses (h)
mg/100 ml	mmol/l			
<1·1	<0·09	>70	1·0	6–8
1·1–2	0·09–0·17	70–30	1·0	12
2–6	0·17–0·50	30–10	0·5	12
>6·0	>0·50	<10	0·5	24

Curtis and Marshall (1970) recommended higher doses than those shown in Table 13 for anephric patients maintained by haemodialysis. The half-life of cephaloridine is shorter in these patients, compared to other patients with severe renal failure (page 206), and in addition the drug is removed during haemodialysis. These authors suggested that haemodialysis patients requiring treatment for Gram-positive infections, should be given 1 g intravenously daily, when not being dialysed, but this should be increased to 1 g intravenously six-hourly during haemodialysis. For infections due to Gram-negative bacilli a dosage schedule of 1 g twelve-hourly when not dialysed, and 1 g four-hourly during haemodialysis was recommended. These doses are high, but nephrotoxicity is obviously not a consideration. Cephaloridine is also removed during peritoneal dialysis, and in patients with end-stage renal disease undergoing this procedure, a cephaloridine dose of 1 g at 12 to 24 h intervals is recommended (Perkins *et al.*, 1969).

4. *Newborn and premature infants.* Smaller doses of cephaloridine will suffice, since glomerular filtration is reduced at this age resulting in higher and more prolonged serum levels. For instance, in neonates a single dose of 15 mg per kg produces a higher and more prolonged serum level than is obtained after a 1 g dose in adults. No toxic effects were noted when a total of 30 mg per kg per day was given to newborns (Burland and Simpson, 1967), but pharmacokinetic data indicate that a dose of 12·5 mg per kg administered every

12 h, is suitable for most patients of this age group (McCracken and Nelson, 1977).

B. *Cephalothin*

1. *Intramuscular and intravenous administration*. The dosage by both of these routes is 50–100 mg per kg body weight per day for children, and 0·5–1·0 g every four or six hours for adults. For serious infections adult doses as high as 12 g daily have been used (Rahal *et al.*, 1968; Wise, 1973), but with these doses a serum sickness-like reaction (page 209) may occur. When large doses are used, intravenous administration is preferable because intramuscular injections are painful. Similar to cephaloridine, cephalothin can be given intravenously by either continuous infusion or intermittent injections and also by intermittent intravenous infusion of a concentrated drug solution via a buretrol (*see* methicillin, page 68). Cephalothin is stable in all commonly used glucose-saline intravenous fluids, for at least six hours at 37°C (Wyatt *et al.*, 1972). Thrombophlebitis can sometimes be a problem when the drug is used intravenously (Kabins and Cohen, 1965), and this is probably reduced if the acid pH of the cephalothin solution is buffered by sodium bicarbonate (Carrizosa *et al.*, 1974; Bergeron *et al.*, 1976). Preparations of cephalothin sodium suitably buffered to produce a pH ranging between 6 and 8·5 are now available commercially for clinical use.

2. *Patients with renal failure*. By contrast to cephaloridine, cephalothin has usually been administered to patients with mild to moderate renal impairment with only minor modification of dosage. Venuto and Plaut (1971), studying haemodialysis patients, found that an intravenous dose of 1 g of cephalothin at the beginning of haemodialysis provided an adequate level throughout dialysis; the same dose after dialysis provided adequate serum levels for at least 48 h, indicating that prolonged cephalothin retention did occur in severely uraemic patients. However, the drug itself does not accumulate to any great extent in such patients, but its breakdown product desacetylcephalothin does (page 207). This metabolite also has antibacterial activity, but this is two- to four-fold less than that of cephalothin against Gram-positive bacteria and eight- to sixteen-fold less against Gram-negative bacteria (Kirby *et al.*, 1971). Therefore cephalothin dosage cannot be greatly reduced for the treatment of Gram-negative infections in uraemic patients, because such therapy may be ineffective. In this situation accumulation of therapeutically relatively inactive desacetylcephalothin in the serum must be accepted. The toxicity of this metabolite is probably not great (Kirby *et al.*, 1971), but it is possible that this together with high serum levels of cephalothin may aggravate pre-existing renal failure (Benner, 1970b) and cause a Coombs positive haemolytic anaemia (page 211). For these reasons, it is best not to use cephalothin for the treatment of severe Gram-negative infections in anephric patients or in those with severe renal failure (Venuto and Plaut, 1971). However, it is practicable to reduce the dose of cephalothin for the treatment of Gram-positive infections in such patients (Weinstein and Kaplan, 1970), and a dosage reduction almost as extensive as that suggested for cephaloridine (page 203) may be indicated (Perkins *et al.*, 1969).

Cephalothin is removed during peritoneal dialysis, and during this procedure a dose of 1 g six- to twelve-hourly is usually needed (Perkins *et al.*, 1969).

Cephaloridine is preferable to cephalothin for the treatment of patients with end-stage failure in whom nephrotoxicity is not a consideration. Cephaloridine does not produce metabolites in the body and therefore it has a more sustained and predictable antibacterial activity in the serum. In patients with some remaining renal function, cephalothin has the advantage of lesser nephrotoxicity (Perkins *et al.*, 1969).

3. *Newborn and premature infants.* A dose of 20 mg per kg body weight, administered every twelve hours is recommended for infants aged less than seven days. Those older than seven days can be given 20 mg per kg every eight hours (McCracken and Nelson, 1977).

4. *Intraperitoneal administration.* Cephalothin can be added to peritoneal dialysis fluid and a concentration of 50 μg per ml is usually used. If this is used continuously during dialysis, some cephalothin is absorbed, and serum levels of about 10 μg per ml may be attained in patients with renal failure (Bulger *et al.*, 1965).

Availability

1. *Cephaloridine*, a white crystalline powder, is supplied in 250 mg, 500 mg and 1 g vials for reconstitution with water for intramuscular or intravenous use.

2. *Cephalothin sodium (neutral)* is available in 1 g, 2 g, 4 g and 20 g rubber-stoppered ampoules.

Serum Levels in Relation to Dosage

After intramuscular injection, the peak serum level of cephaloridine is attained after half an hour (Fig. 11), and is about twice that obtained after a similar dose of cephalothin. Doubling these usual doses of both drugs, doubles their respective peak serum concentrations. After a 500 mg intramuscular dose of cephaloridine, the serum level at six hours is still at least 2 μg per ml, but the

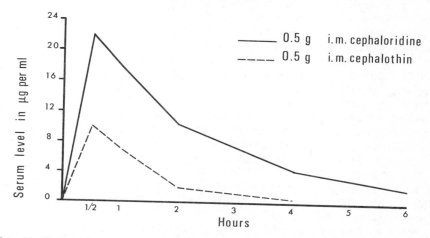

FIG. 11. Comparison of serum levels of cephaloridine and cephalothin in healthy male volunteers. (Redrawn after Benner *et al.*, 1966.)

cephalothin level with a similar dose falls below 2 μg per ml after four hours, and at six hours there is no detectable cephalothin activity (Benner *et al.*, 1966).

When a large dose of 12 g cephalothin is administered every 24 h by continuous intravenous infusion, serum levels fluctuate between 10 and 30 μg per ml. If the same daily dose is given by intermittent intravenous injections (3 g every 6 h), peak levels of 150–200 μg per ml are attained but these fall to zero before the next dose (Griffith and Black, 1971).

If a 1 g dose of cephaloridine, diluted in 20 ml of 0·9 per cent saline, is given by rapid intravenous injection, the mean serum level at 15 min after the injection is 60 μg per ml, this falls to 40 at 30 min, 30 at 1 h, 15 at 2 h, and 2–3 μg per ml at 6 h (Mathews, 1975). A 2 g dose of cephaloridine given intravenously over 10 min produces a serum level of about 100 μg per ml half an hour after the injection, and detectable serum concentrations remain for at least eight hours (Griffith and Black, 1971).

Excretion

URINE:

1. *Cephaloridine*. This drug is rapidly excreted in urine, and very high urinary concentrations (400–1000 μg per ml) of the active drug are obtained with normal dosage (Muggleton *et al.*, 1964). Some 80 per cent of a parenterally administered dose appears unchanged in urine during the first twenty-four hours, most excretion occurring during the first six hours. Cephaloridine is excreted mainly by glomerular filtration. Some investigators have been unable to detect any renal tubular secretion (Currie, 1967), but Foley *et al.* (1967) demonstrated that in man tubular secretion also plays a minor role, but probenecid did not influence the exretion rate. Others have found that probenecid can cause slight elevation of cephaloridine serum levels (Saslaw, 1970).

If a single dose of cephaloridine is given to an anuric patient, the serum level as measured by a microbiological method decreases slowly during a 54-h period, but if a chemical method of assay is used, the rate of loss is much slower. When a cephaloridine solution is incubated *in vitro* at 37°C, the rates at which the concentrations of the drug decline, when measured by the two methods, are the same as observed *in vivo* (Currie, 1967). Thus the slow loss of activity from the serum of an anuric patient is probably mainly due to chemical breakdown, and there is no evidence for a significant non-renal mechanism for removal of cephaloridine from the body. The drug therefore accumulates in patients with renal failure. The serum cephaloridine half-life in patients with normal renal function is approximately 1·5 h, but in patients with severe renal failure (creatinine clearance less than 3 ml per min), the half-life is prolonged to 20–23 h (Kabins and Cohen, 1966; Kunin and Atuk, 1966). Surprisingly, in anephric patients receiving maintenance haemodialysis for some time, the half-life of this drug becomes shorter (Pryor *et al.*, 1967). For instance a mean cephaloridine half-life of only 10·4 h was found in patients who had been treated by haemodialysis for over two years (Curtis and Marshall, 1970). Presumably extrarenal mechanisms of cephaloridine degradation (e.g. inactivation in liver), which are normally insignificant, may become increasingly important with increasing duration of maintenance haemodialysis.

2. *Cephalothin*. This cephalosporin is also excreted in large amounts in the urine of healthy persons. It is primarily excreted by tubular secretion, and its elimination is diminished by probenecid (Saslaw, 1970). Cephalothin is also rapidly deacetylated in the body, presumably mainly in the liver, producing the metabolite, desacetylcephalothin. Some cephalothin may be inactivated in the blood because *in vitro* the drug is destroyed when incubated with human serum at body temperature (Pitkin *et al.*, 1977). About 65 per cent of cephalothin is excreted unchanged and the remainder as its metabolite (Griffith and Black, 1971). Desacetylcephalothin also has antibacterial activity, but this is of a lower order than that of cephalothin (page 204). This metabolite is only about one-fifth as active as cephalothin against B. subtilis, one of the organisms often used for estimation of cephalothin serum levels. This explains some of the discrepancies which have been observed in the estimation of cephalothin serum half-lives in uraemic patients. Some studies showed that renal functional impairment only caused a slight decrease in the rate of disappearance of cephalothin from the serum; the normal half-life of 0·85 h, was increased only to 2·9 h in patients with severe renal failure (Kunin and Atuk, 1966). Other investigators confirmed that in uraemic patients there was an early rapid decline in cephalothin serum levels with an apparent half-life of only about 2·8 h, but there was also subsequently a slower decline over the next 8 h resulting in a half-life of about 12 h (Kabins and Cohen, 1965). An equivalent prolongation of serum concentrations for both cephalothin and cephaloridine after 1 g doses in uraemic patients, was observed by Perkins *et al.* (1969). They also showed that during the slow decline phase, cephaloridine serum levels were higher than those of cephalothin. Blood levels also decline slowly (half-life of 18 h) when multiple doses of cephalothin are given to uraemic patients (Kabins and Cohen, 1965). By using methods which measure cephalothin and desacetylcephalothin serum levels separately, the secondary slow decline in serum levels has been shown to be chiefly due to the metabolite. For instance when a 1 g cephalothin dose was given to a uraemic patient, the cephalothin level fell rapidly (half-life 2 h), but the desacetylcephalothin concentrations increased over the first 12 h, and then declined slowly with a half-life of 8 h (Kirby *et al.*, 1971). A high desacetylcephalothin serum level (177 μg per ml) has also been recorded in one uraemic patient treated by cephalothin 1 g every 4 h, confirming that this metabolite, which is normally rapidly excreted via the kidney, accumulates in patients with renal failure (Kirby *et al.*, 1971).

BILE: Both cephalothin and cephaloridine are excreted in the bile and measurable concentrations of each drug can usually be detected in both gall bladder and common duct bile, provided that the biliary tract is not obstructed. These drugs are not concentrated in the bile to any extent, and bile concentrations are usually lower than serum levels at the time (Ratzan *et al.*, 1974; Mendelson *et al.*, 1974).

Distribution of the Drugs in Body

1. *Cephaloridine*. This drug penetrates well into body fluids and tissues. High levels are found in renal tissue and inflamed muscle. Therapeutic concentrations of cephaloridine are achieved in bone, synovial capsule and synovial

fluid after usual doses (Hughes *et al.*, 1975). The concentration in inflammatory exudate is about the same as that in the serum, and it peaks simultaneously with the serum (Ellis *et al.*, 1975). The usual cephaloridine dose of 2 g intramuscularly daily, yields levels of 30–36 µg per ml in pleural fluid (Murdoch *et al.*, 1964). In normal CSF levels of only 0·03–0·25 µg per ml have been detected after a 0·5 g intramuscular dose (Murdoch *et al.*, 1964). In patients with inflamed meninges receiving parenteral doses of 4 g per day, the CSF concentrations range from 0·4 to 5·6 µg per ml (Lerner, 1971). Considerably higher CSF levels (up to 20 µg per ml) may be achieved when parenteral cephaloridine is accompanied by intrathecal administration (Fisher *et al.*, 1975). A concentration of 0·9 µg per g was found in brain biopsy tissue two to four hours after a single 2 g dose of cephaloridine (Griffith and Black, 1971). Levels in cord and fetal blood are approximately 60 per cent of that in the maternal circulation (Arthur and Burland, 1969).

Cephaloridine is only 20 per cent bound to serum proteins (Kunin, 1967).

2. *Cephalothin*. This antibiotic penetrates very poorly into normal cerebrospinal fluid. Even in patients with meningitis CSF concentrations only approximate 1 per cent of serum levels at the time; one hour after a 2 g intravenous cephalothin dose to these patients, CSF levels were only 0·16 to 0·31 µg per ml (Vianna and Kaye, 1967).

Perkins and Saslaw (1966) studied tissue levels of cephalothin after death in a patient who had received the drug in a dosage of 2 g four-hourly. High levels were found in the renal cortex, pleural fluid, myocardium, striated muscle, skin and stomach wall. Cephalothin also penetrates well into ascitic fluid and into the peritoneal fluid in patients with bacterial peritonitis (Gerding *et al.*, 1977).

A measurable amount (1·6 µg per g) of cephalothin has been found in brain tissue of a patient who received 2 g of the drug two to four hours previously (Griffith and Black, 1971). The concentration in bronchial secretions is usually about 25 per cent of the serum level at the time (Wong *et al.*, 1975). Cephalothin concentrations are very low in both normal and infected bone (Hierholzer *et al.*, 1974; Smilack *et al.*, 1976). The drug can be detected in prostatic tissue in a concentration approximately 25 per cent of the simultaneous serum level (Adam *et al.*, 1975). It is also transferred across the placenta (Morrow *et al.*, 1968).

Cephalothin is about 50–60 per cent serum protein bound (Kunin, 1967).

Mode of Action

Cephalosporin antibiotics, like the penicillins (page 19) inhibit bacterial cell wall synthesis (Chang and Weinstein, 1964; Izaki and Strominger, 1968; Curtis *et al.*, 1976). It has been presumed that these two groups of antibiotics have identical modes of action, but the observation of different morphologic responses of Gram-negative bacilli to penicillins and cephalosporins (Lorian and Sabath, 1972), suggests that there may be some differences (*see also* page 21).

Toxicity

1. *Hypersensitivity reactions*. On the assumption that they are not cross-allergenic with the penicillins, cephalothin and cephaloridine are frequently

recommended for the treatment of severe infections in penicillin-allergic patients. Stewart (1962) using skin-tests in patients sensitized to penicillin G, obtained positive reactions with the semisynthetic penicillins but not with cephalosporin C. Since then in many clinical studies allergic reactions have not been observed in penicillin-allergic patients treated with cephalothin (Weinstein *et al.*, 1964; Perkins and Saslaw, 1966; Rahal *et al.*, 1968) or cephaloridine (Apicella *et al.*, 1966; Cohen *et al.*, 1966; Steigbigel *et al.*, 1968). However, occasionally penicillin-sensitive patients have reacted to cephalosporin C derivatives (Editorial, 1967). For instance, immediate severe reactions to cephalothin in penicillin-allergic patients have been described (Rothschild and Doty, 1966; Scholand *et al.*, 1968; Spruill *et al.*, 1974). A skin-sensitizing antibody to cephalothin, cephaloridine and 7-amino-cephalosporanic acid was demonstrated in one patient who had suffered an anaphylactic reaction to penicillin G five months previously (Grieco, 1967). This author suggested that cross-reactivity between penicillins and cephalosporins may be more common than is apparent from clinical data, as only 10 per cent of patients with a past history of penicillin allergy exhibit recurrent reactions on readministration of penicillin. It is still not clear whether 'true cross-reactivity' between the penicillins and cephalosporins exists, because penicillin-allergic patients often have an allergic diathesis and therefore have an increased tendency to allergic reactions from many drugs (Petz, 1971). It appears from large surveys, that 91–94 per cent of patients with a history of penicillin allergy do not react to cephalosporins (Dash, 1975). Therefore the risk seems small, and cephalosporins may be used in patients with a past history of penicillin hypersensitivity, but special precautions should be taken in those who have had a previous severe penicillin reaction. It is best to avoid the use of cephalosporins in patients with a past history of anaphylaxis or other immediate-type penicillin hypersensitivity reaction (Petz, 1978).

Allergic manifestations due to cephalothin and cephaloridine occur in the absence of a history of penicillin allergy, indicating that these drugs themselves are allergenic. Kaplan and Weinstein (1967) described a severe immediate allergic reaction in a nurse who received 1 g of cephaloridine intravenously. It was subsequently shown that she was not allergic to penicillin G, but for the previous six months she had frequently prepared injections of cephalothin and cephaloridine. Saleh and Tischler (1974) described a severe anaphylactic reaction, following intravenous cephaloridine administration to a pregnant patient; she also had no previous history of any drug reactions and had never been treated with penicillin.

When cephalothin was administered to 15 volunteers in increasing doses up to a maximum of 2 g four times daily by intermittent rapid infusions, surprisingly, after two to four weeks' therapy, they all developed a serum sickness-like illness consisting of malaise, weakness, arthralgia, myalgia, fever, lymphadenopathy and skin rashes. These symptoms appeared to be due to a hypersensitivity reaction (Sanders *et al.*, 1974). Similar reactions were also noted in volunteers treated with the newer cephalosporin cephapirin (page 247). The authors postulated that the use of large doses of these drugs by rapid intravenous infusion for prolonged periods, may have been responsible for the high rate of reactions. It is possible that similar reactions have occurred in patients treated by cephalosporins in this way, but they may have been attributed to other causes.

As with penicillin G (page 25) routine testing for possible cephalosporin hypersensitivity, is not yet practicable.

2. *Nephrotoxicity*. This may occur with cephaloridine therapy, and appears to be dose related (Benner, 1970a). Daily doses of 4 g or even 6 g are quite safe for adults with normal renal function (Foord, 1971; Winchester and Kennedy, 1972). With higher doses the renal tubules can be affected. Animal studies show that the middle portion of the proximal tubule is the site of the damage (Silverblatt *et al.*, 1970). Initially there are alterations in the proximal tubular brush border and then progression to massive proximal tubular necrosis (Mitchell *et al.*, 1977). Although there is little or no active tubular secretion of cephaloridine (page 206), this drug is taken up into the proximal tubular cells of the renal cortex to a greater extent than other cephalosporins, where it reaches high intracellular concentrations (Tune, 1975). This probably explains its greater nephrotoxicity (Tune, 1975; Appel and Neu, 1977). By contrast, cephalothin is actively secreted into the renal tubules (page 207) so that there is a lesser tendency for it to accumulate in possible toxic concentrations inside the proximal tubular cells (Foord, 1975).

When high cephaloridine doses are used in humans, frank renal damage may be preceded by a massive excretion of hyaline casts (Annotation, 1967a; Appel and Neu, 1977). Severe renal failure with oliguria has been described in at least one hundred patients (Ballingall and Turpie, 1967; Hinman and Wolinsky, 1967; Foord, 1975). Diuretics such as frusemide, which cause potassium loss, and which by some unexplained mechanism prolong the cephaloridine half-life in the body, potentiate its nephrotoxicity (Lawson *et al.*, 1970; 1972; Norrby *et al.*, 1976). Cephaloridine nephrotoxicity appears more likely if other potentially nephrotoxic antibiotics such as kanamycin or gentamicin are given at the same time (Busuttil *et al.*, 1973; Foord, 1975). Surprisingly, some animal experiments show that cephaloridine actually protects kidneys from gentamicin toxicity (Luft *et al.*, 1976). Probenecid has some protective effect against cephaloridine nephrotoxicity in certain experimental animals. This is presumably because it prevents cephaloridine uptake in proximal tubular cells, thereby reducing the high intracellular concentration of the drug (Tune and Kempson, 1973; Tune, 1975). However, there is no evidence that probenecid decreases cephaloridine nephrotoxicity in humans (Appel and Neu, 1977).

In patients with pre-existing renal impairment cephaloridine may be used safely if the dose is adjusted (page 203). Dillon and Postlewait (1971) administered cephaloridine in appropriately reduced doses to 81 patients with varying degrees of renal functional impairment, and there was no apparent aggravation of their renal disease. In patients aged more than 50 years suitable dose reduction is also indicated to avoid nephrotoxicity, because these patients have a decreased capacity to excrete cephaloridine (Foord, 1971). Nephrotoxicity does not seem to occur if serum cephaloridine levels are maintained between 20 and 80 μg per ml (Winchester and Kennedy, 1972). Serum levels greater than 100 μg per ml are unsafe and should be avoided, and severe renal failure or anuria usually develops if they exceed 150 μg per ml (Gower, 1967; Foord, 1975). In the majority of reported cases of cephaloridine nephrotoxicity, it has been associated with either excessive dosage or doses inappropriately high for patients with impaired renal function. Other possible aggravating factors have been the associated use of other nephrotoxic antibiotics or frusemide, as well as conditions which may lead to a temporary reduction in renal clearance such as operations, shock and dehydration (Foord, 1975).

The nephrotoxicity of cephalothin is much less than that of cephaloridine. Cephalothin or its metabolite, desacetylcephalothin (pages 204, 207), or both, may be responsible for this side-effect. There are reports indicating that cephalothin may occasionally aggravate pre-existing renal failure (Rahal et al., 1968; Benner, 1970b). In the other reports of this complication there was either some evidence of pre-existing renal damage or the cephalothin dose was unusually large, such as 8–24 g daily for 8 to 35 days (Hansten, 1973; Kleinknecht et al., 1973; Engle et al., 1975; Barrientos et al., 1976). While the renal lesion produced by cephaloridine is primarily due to intrinsic toxicity of this drug for the cells of the proximal renal tubule (vide supra), the renal injury due to cephalothin somewhat resembles that of the penicillins. Some instances of cephalothin nephropathy appear to be toxic in nature with the histological picture of acute tubular necrosis, but others resemble hypersensitivity interstitial nephritis (Barza, 1978) (see also pages 29, 72).

Acute, usually reversible renal failure, has also occurred in patients receiving high doses of cephalothin in combination with gentamicin (Bobrow et al., 1972; Fillastre et al., 1973; Kleinknecht et al., 1973). Gentamicin alone can cause renal damage (page 339), but it has been suggested that this drug combination is more nephrotoxic than either agent acting alone. Nephrotoxicity may also occur if cephalothin is combined with one of the other aminoglycosides or with one of the polymyxins (Hansten, 1973; Appel and Neu, 1977). The Boston Collaborative Drug Surveillance Program analysed data from over 22 000 consecutive patients admitted to hospital. This showed that after standardization of the figures, a rise in the blood urea was attributed to antibiotic therapy in 8·6 per cent of patients receiving gentamicin alone, 2·9 per cent of those receiving cephalothin alone and 9·3 per cent of those receiving the two drugs together. These data therefore did not demonstrate that cephalothin potentiates gentamicin nephrotoxicity (Fanning et al., 1976). Animal experiments, as with cephaloridine (vide supra), show that the nephrotoxicity of gentamicin is actually significantly reduced by the simultaneous administration of cephalothin (Dellinger et al., 1976a and b).

In animals, similarly to cephaloridine, diuretics such as frusemide may potentiate cephalothin nephrotoxicity (Lawson et al., 1972; Foord, 1975). By contrast to cephaloridine, these diuretics do not have a significant effect on the renal clearance of cephalothin in humans (Tice et al., 1975).

3. *Encephalopathy.* Neurological disturbances similar to those associated with large doses of penicillin G (page 28), can also occur when high cephaloridine serum levels are reached. Myoclonus, twitchings and rapid onset of coma have been observed in a few patients (Steigbigel et al., 1968; Gabriel et al., 1970). Two other patients developed hallucinations and nystagmus following a 100 mg dose of cephaloridine given intrathecally, but these effects were not observed when daily intrathecal doses were reduced to 50 mg (Murdoch et al., 1964).

4. *Haematological side-effects.* A positive direct Coombs test occurs in

many patients receiving cephalothin (Molthan *et al.*, 1967) and in some patients receiving cephaloridine (Fass *et al.*, 1970). This may interfere with blood cross-matching procedures, but otherwise usually there are no ill effects. Only a few cases of Coombs positive haemolytic anaemia due to cephalothin have been reported; antibodies of the IgG class against cephalothin were present in the serum (Gralnick *et al.*, 1971; Rubin and Burka, 1977). In another patient with haemolytic anaemia due to penicillin G, the disease worsened when cephalothin was substituted, but full recovery occurred twelve days after cephalothin was stopped (Medical News, 1968). Circulating antibodies in this patient were identical to those of another patient who had haemolysis caused by penicillin G only, in that the sera of both patients were equally reactive with penicillin and cephalothin coated red cells (*see* penicillin G, page 29). A severe cephalothin-induced haemolytic anaemia has been described in another patient following aortic valve replacement (Lemole *et al.*, 1972).

Cephalothin usually causes an aggregation type haemolytic anaemia; it binds to the red cells, but during this process serum proteins are also aggregated. In this condition either the IgG Coombs test, or C3 Coombs test, or both, may be positive (Abramson and Lee, 1974; Garratty and Petz, 1975).

Other haematological effects due to these cephalosporins are rare. An unusual coagulopathy occurred in two patients possibly related to cephaloridine therapy (Steigbigel *et al.*, 1968). Both patients had severe renal failure and very high cephaloridine serum levels were attained. The coagulopathy was due to an inhibitor of thromboplastin generation and was accompanied by a true deficiency of prothrombin and antithrombin activity. Prolongation of the prothrombin time had been observed previously during cephaloridine therapy (Hermans *et al.*, 1966). Natelson *et al.* (1976) demonstrated combined defects of platelet function and blood coagulation in volunteers receiving cephalothin in a very high dose of 300 mg per kg per day. The platelet defect was similar to that seen with carbenicillin (page 159). When the dose of cephalothin was reduced to 200 mg per kg per day, platelet and coagulation defects disappeared. This suggests that patients with normal renal function are unlikely to develop bleeding problems due to the cephalosporins, even when maximum dosages are used. Bleeding may occur in those with impaired renal function or possibly if a cephalothin/carbenicillin combination is used.

Thrombocytopenia caused by cephalothin apparently due to the binding of a specific antibody to cephalothin-coated platelets, has been described (Gralnick *et al.*, 1972). There are reports of leucopenia due to cephaloridine (Stewart and Holt, 1964) and cephalothin (Martin and Wellman, 1967; Di Cato and Ellman, 1975). Eosinophilia can also be associated with the administration of both of these drugs.

5. *Other side-effects*. Raised serum aspartate aminotransferase (SGOT) levels have been occasionally noted during therapy with cephalothin (Martin and Wellman, 1967) and cephaloridine (Kabins and Cohen, 1966). No other evidence of hepatotoxicity has been observed. Diarrhoea and pseudomembranous colitis (page 481) developed in one patient who had been treated successively over a month with oral cephalexin, parenteral cephalothin and parenteral cephazolin. The colitis responded to cholestyramine (page 483) therapy (Tures *et al.*, 1976).

The development of bacterial meningitis in five patients receiving cephalothin for other severe infections has been described (Mangi et al., 1973). Two patients had pneumococcal meningitis and the other three were due to meningococcus, a Klebsiella spp. and Listeria monocytogenes, respectively. Freij et al. (1975) reported another patient who developed pneumococcal meningitis during cephalothin treatment for pneumococcal septicaemia. The occurrence of meningitis in these circumstances was erroneously described as a specific complication of cephalothin therapy (Leading article, 1973). However, meningitis is not an uncommon association of any septicaemia. Furthermore it may develop during treatment, particularly if the antibiotic used, such as cephalothin, does not easily pass into the CSF (page 208) and the bacterial species involved is not highly susceptible (Shedden, 1973).

Teratogenicity in humans due to cephalothin and cephaloridine has not been described (Williams and Smith, 1973). Similar to penicillins, cephalosporins can probably be safely used during the first trimester of pregnancy. No adverse effects, such as haemolytic anaemia in the newborn, have been detected due to cephalosporin administration to mothers near term (Hirsch, 1971).

Clinical Uses of the Drugs

1. *Streptococcal and pneumococcal infections.* Cephalothin and cephaloridine are useful alternatives to penicillin G for the treatment of these infections, but being less effective and more expensive, they are mainly indicated in penicillin-allergic patients (page 208). Strep. pyogenes infections such as scarlet fever, and pneumococcal pneumonia (Tempest and Austrian, 1967) respond well to these antibiotics. Pneumococcal meningitis has also been successfully treated by a combination of parenteral and intrathecal cephaloridine (Murdoch et al., 1964; Love et al., 1970), but chloramphenicol (page 441) is the preferred and more reliable alternative for penicillin-allergic patients (Fisher et al., 1975). Cephalothin appears quite unsatisfactory for the treatment of pneumococcal and all other types of meningitis (Leading article, 1973; Fisher et al., 1975). These cephalosporins are effective for the treatment of Strep. viridans or Strep. bovis endocarditis, but ineffective, even in combination with aminoglycosides, for the treatment of Strep. faecalis endocarditis (Rahal et al., 1968; Abrutyn et al., 1978).

2. *Staphylococcal infections.* Cephalothin is a satisfactory antistaphylococcal agent, but cephaloridine, being easily hydrolysed by penicillinase (page 199), is of doubtful value for the treatment of severe infections caused by penicillin G-resistant staphylococci. The clinical efficacy of cephalothin in severe staphylococcal sepsis appears to be about the same as that of the parenteral penicillinase-resistant penicillins (Wise, 1973), such as methicillin (page 74), oxacillin, cloxacillin and flucloxacillin (page 88) and nafcillin (page 96). This cephalosporin can therefore be regarded as another satisfactory drug for the treatment of staphylococcal infections resistant to penicillin G.

In some reports good results have been obtained using cephaloridine for staphylococcal infections of moderate severity (Apicella et al., 1966; Steigbigel et al., 1968). Other reports describe failure of cephaloridine in the treatment of staphylococcal endocarditis (Burgess and Evans, 1966; Rountree and Bullen,

1967). Relative *in vivo* resistance to cephaloridine probably only occurs when the staphylococcal strain produces large amounts of penicillinase. These strains which are not detected by ordinary disc tests, can be differentiated by tube dilution tests using both small and large inocula (Leading article, 1967) (*see also* (page 199).

For hospital acquired methicillin-resistant Staph. pyogenes infections, cephalothin and especially cephaloridine are usually ineffective. Cephalothin may be useful if combined with another antibiotic such as kanamycin (Bulger, 1967).

Staph. epidermidis strains acquired in hospitals are usually penicillin G-resistant and may also be methicillin-resistant, but are often sensitive to the cephalosporins (Speller and Mitchell, 1973). These cephalosporins may, therefore, be useful for some infections due to these strains, but when severe infections such as endocarditis are treated, a cephalothin/gentamicin combination is preferable (page 200).

3. *Urinary tract infections*. These drugs are effective in eradicating sensitive strains of Esch. coli and Pr. mirabilis from urine (Steigbigel *et al.*, 1968), but results are less satisfactory with infections due to Klebsiella and Enterobacter spp. In severe urinary tract infections, a two weeks' course of cephaloridine appears to be superior to a one week course (Burgess *et al.*, 1968). In chronic infections, associated with urinary tract abnormalities, results of treatment with cephalosporins, as with other antibiotics, are unsatisfactory.

4. *Septicaemias due to Gram-negative bacilli*. These diseases may be treated by either cephaloridine or cephalothin provided the organism is sensitive to a concentration of the drug which is easily attainable *in vivo* (Cohen *et al.*, 1966; Benner *et al.*, 1966). Cephalosporins are not reliable as single agents for initial emergency treatment of severe unidentified Gram-negative infections, but a combination of cephalothin and gentamicin has been often used successfully (Leading article, 1973). However, this regimen is not effective against all common septicaemias, because infections due to N. meningitidis, H. influenzae type b, and Salmonella and Bacteroides spp. will not respond. Furthermore, this combination may cause nephrotoxicity (page 211). For suspected severe Gram-negative organism sepsis, combinations of either chloramphenicol plus gentamicin (pages 342, 443), carbenicillin plus gentamicin (pages 161, 341) or clindamycin plus gentamicin (pages 342, 485) may be more suitable for initial emergency chemotherapy. A cephalothin/gentamicin regimen may only be advantageous for the treatment of Klebsiella spp. infections (Young *et al.*, 1977).

5. *Haemophilus influenzae infections*. Compared to chloramphenicol and ampicillin, these cephalosporins are unsatisfactory for the treatment of severe H. influenzae type b infections. For example, Walker and Collins (1968) treated three infants with meningitis due to this organism by high doses of cephaloridine, but without clinical improvement. These drugs may be useful in adult respiratory tract infections, which are caused by non-typable H. influenzae strains. However in one study, these strains of H. influenzae relatively resistant to cephaloridine were detected in about 50 per cent of patients, who responded poorly to treatment with this drug (Howard, 1967). Cephaloridine was regarded as a somewhat satisfactory drug for treatment of acute or chronic bronchitis (Annotation, 1967b; Pines, 1974), but other drugs such as

ampicillin (page 115), amoxycillin (page 142) or co-trimoxazole (page 709) are superior.

6. *Klebsiella pneumonia*. This disease has been successfully treated by either cephaloridine or cephalothin (Perkins and Saslaw, 1966), but resistant strains of Kl. pneumoniae exist or may emerge during treatment with each drug. For severe cases one of these cephalosporins combined with gentamicin or chloramphenicol is more reliable.

7. *Listeria monocytogenes meningitis*. Satisfactory results have been obtained by using cephaloridine for this disease (Cohen *et al.*, 1966), but alternative drugs are available (pages 33, 118), with ampicillin (page 118) being the drug of choice.

8. *Chemoprophylaxis and treatment of Clostridium perfringens infections.* It was suggested that cephalothin, administered intravenously in large doses, may be the best alternative drug to penicillin G for treatment of this infection in penicillin-allergic patients (Schwartzman *et al.*, 1977). However Mohr *et al.* (1978) described four cases of clostridial myonecrosis that developed in patients with open fractures who had received intravenous cephalothin prophylactically. Subsequently these authors, on testing seven human isolates of Cl. perfringens, found four to be cephalothin-resistant. This experience indicates that cephalothin should not be used for the prophylaxis or treatment of gas gangrene. Erythromycin (page 508), clindamycin (page 470) and chloramphenicol (page 420) are effective for this infection.

9. *Venereal diseases*. A course of cephaloridine appears to be an effective alternative to penicillin G for the treatment of gonorrhoea (Oller, 1967a). If 'single-dose' treatment is used (usually 2 to 2·5 g) results are unsatisfactory (Duncan and Knox, 1971). Cephaloridine is not widely used for this disease, because penicillin G (page 36) still remains the drug of choice, and cheaper alternatives are available for penicillin-allergic patients. Cephaloridine is ineffective for infections caused by penicillinase-producing gonococci (page 8).

Cephaloridine is an effective alternative to penicillin G for the treatment of primary and secondary stages of syphilis (Oller, 1967b; Glicksman *et al.*, 1968), but erythromycin (page 509) and the tetracyclines (page 627) are also effective. A dosage of 0·5 g daily, given for 10 days, has proved satisfactory. Cephaloridine may be a satisfactory alternative to penicillin G in penicillin-allergic patients for the treatment of syphilis in pregnancy (Holder and Knox, 1972), but currently in the United States erythromycin (pages 39, 509) is recommended for this purpose. Cephaloridine may also be useful for treatment of lymphogranuloma venereum (Oller *et al.*, 1970).

10. *Chemoprophylaxis in surgical patients*. Cephaloridine in a dose of 1·0 g has been instilled into potentially contaminated surgical wounds just before skin closure, in an attempt to reduce the wound sepsis rate (Roy, 1976). In one study involving 2491 operations, the primary wound sepsis rate with cephaloridine used in this manner was less than half the rate in controls (Pollock and Evans, 1975). Parenteral cephaloridine also may be a useful chemoprophylaxis for patients undergoing total hip replacement, because after usual therapeutic doses, adequate levels of the drug are achieved in bone and associated tissues (Hughes *et al.*, 1975).

Bain *et al.* (1977) used cephalothin as a prophylactic antibiotic in 100 consecutive patients undergoing open heart surgery. It was given intravenously in a high dose of 28 g which was administered by continuous infusion over 48 h. The frequency of post-operative infections was low and drug toxicity was not encountered.

11. *Meningococcal infections.* Cephalothin and cephaloridine are not suitable alternatives to penicillin G for treatment of meningococcal meningitis. McKenzie *et al.* (1967) treated ten patients with meningococcal meningitis by cephaloridine. These patients recovered, but response to cephaloridine was slower than in comparable cases treated by penicillin G and sulphonamides. Other authors have also described unsatisfactory results following the use of cephalothin for meningococcal meningitis (Almond, 1969; Southern and Sanford, 1969; Brown *et al.*, 1970).

12. *Typhoid fever.* Although Salm. typhi is sensitive to cephaloridine *in vitro*, the drug is ineffective clinically (Walker, 1964).

13. *Actinomycosis.* A few patients with this disease have been successfully treated by cephalothin (Caldwell, 1971).

14. *Choice between cephalothin and cephaloridine.* In some diseases only one of these drugs is suitable and not the other (*vide supra*). However in several instances either drug may be satisfactory, and the clinician should select the drug with which he is more familiar. Cephalothin, being less toxic, but more painful on intramuscular injection, is often the better choice for the seriously ill patient in hospital, in whom intravenous chemotherapy is necessary. In other situations cephaloridine may be more suitable, because intramuscular injections need not be given as frequently and they are less painful.

REFERENCES

Abramson, N. and Lee, D. P. (April 1974), 'Immune hemolytic anemias', *Disease-a-Month,* Year Book Medical Publishers inc. Chicago.

Abrutyn, E., Lincoln, L., Gallagher, M. and Weinstein, A. J. (1978), 'Cephalothin-gentamicin synergism in experimental entercoccal endocarditis', *J. Antimicrob. Chemother.*, **4**, 153.

Adam, D., Hofstetter, A. G., Jacoby, W. and Reichardt, B. (1975), 'Studies on the diffusion of cephradine and cephalothin into human tissue', *Proceedings of 9th International Congress of Chemotherapy*, Abstract M-69.

Almond, H. R. (1969), 'Meningococcal infection unresponsive to cephalothin', *New Engl. J. Med.*, **281**, 218.

Annotation (1967a), 'Cephalosporins', *Lancet*, **1**, 1264.

Annotation (1967b), 'Cephaloridine in chronic bronchitis', *Lancet*, **2**, 603.

Apicella, M. A., Perkins, R. L. and Saslaw, S. (1966), 'Treatment of bacterial endocarditis with cephalosporin derivatives in penicillin-allergic patients', *New Engl. J. Med.*, **274**, 1002.

Appel, G. B. and Neu, H. C. (1977), 'The nephrotoxicity of antimicrobial agents (First of three parts)', *New Engl. J. Med.*, **296**, 663.

Arthur, L. J. H. and Burland, W. L. (1969), 'Transfer of cephaloridine from mother to fetus', *Arch. Dis. Child.*, **44**, 82; quoted by Holder and Knox (1972).

Azimi, P. H. and Cramblett, H. G. (1968), 'Cephaloridine; clinical and laboratory studies in children', *J. Pediatrics*, **73**, 255.

Bain, W. H., McGeachie, J., Lindsay, G. and Underwood, J. (1977), 'The use of cephalothin sodium (Keflin) as the prophylactic antibiotic for open heart surgery', *J. Antimicrob. Chemother.*, **3**, 339.

Ballingall, D. L. K. and Turpie, A. G. G. (1967), 'Cephaloridine toxicity', *Lancet*, **2**, 835.

Barber, M. and Waterworth, P. M. (1964), 'Penicillinase-resistant penicillins and cephalosporins', *Brit. Med., J.*, **2**, 344.

Barrientos, A., Bello, I., Gutierrez-Millet, V., Ruilope, L. and Rodicio, J. (1976), 'Renal failure and cephalothin', *Ann. Intern. Med.*, **84**, 612.

Barza, M. (1978), 'The nephrotoxicity of cephalosporins: An overview', *J. Infect. Dis.* (Suppl.), **137**, 60.

Bayer, A. S., Chow, A. W., Anthony, B. F. and Guze, L. B. (1976), 'Serious infections in adults due to Group B streptococci. Clinical and serotypic characterization', *Amer. J. Med.*, **61**, 498.

Bell, S. M. (1974), 'The significance of sensitivity tests of Staphylococcus aureus to cephaloridine', *Med. J. Aust.*, **2**, 902.

Benner, E. J., Brodie, J. S. and Kirby, W. M. M. (1966), 'Laboratory and clinical comparison of cephaloridine and cephalothin', *Antimicrob. Agents Chemother.—1965*, p. 888.

Benner, E. J. (1970a), 'Editorial. Cephaloridine and the kidneys', *J. Infect. Dis.*, **122**, 104.

Benner, E. J. (1970b), 'Renal damage associated with prolonged administration of ampicillin, cephaloridine and cephalothin', *Antimicrob. Agents Chemother.—1969*, p. 417.

Bergeron, M. G., Brusch, J. L., Barza, M. and Weinstein, L. (1976), 'Significant reduction in the incidence of phlebitis with buffered versus unbuffered cephalothin', *Antimicrob. Ag. Chemother.*, **9**, 646.

Bobrow, S. N., Jaffe, E. and Young, R. C. (1972), 'Anuria and acute tubular necrosis associated with gentamicin and cephalothin', *JAMA*, **222**, 1546.

Brewer, N. S., Spencer, R. J. and Nichols, D. R. (1974), 'Primary anorectal actinomycosis', *JAMA*, **228**, 1397.

Brown, J. D., Mathies, A. W., Jr., Ivler, D., Warren, W. S. and Leedom, J. M. (1970), 'Variable results of cephalothin therapy for meningococcal meningitis', *Antimicrob. Agents Chemother.—1969*, p. 432.

Bulger, R. J., Bennett, J. V. and Boen, S. T. (1965), 'Intraperitoneal administration of broad-spectrum antibiotics in patients with renal failure', *JAMA*, **194**, 1198.

Bulger, R. J. (1967), '*In vitro* activity of cephalothin/kanamycin and methicillin/kanamycin combinations against methicillin-resistant Staphylococcus aureus', *Lancet*, **1**, 17.

Burgess, H. A. and Evans, R. J. (1966), 'Failure of cephaloridine in a case of staphylococcal endocarditis', *Brit. med. J.*, **2**, 1244.

Burgess, M. A., Fairley, K. F. and Habersberger, P. (1968), 'Cephaloridine in urinary tract infections', *Med. J., Aust.*, **1**, 947.

Burland, W. L. and Simpson, K. (1967), 'Administration of cephaloridine to the newborn infant', *Postgrad. Med. J.* (Suppl.), **43**, 112.

Busuttil, A. A. Gibson, A. A. and Kerr, M. M. (1973), 'Possible cephaloridine nephrotoxicity in a neonate', *Lancet*, **1**, 264.

Caldwell, J. L. (1971), 'Actinomycosis treated with cephalothin', *South Med. J.*, **64**, 987; quoted by Brewer *et al.* (1974).

Carrizosa, J., Levison, M. E. and Kaye, D. (1974), 'Double-blind comparison of phlebitis produced by cephalothin infusions with buffered and unbuffered diluents', *Antimicrob. Ag. Chemother.*, **5**, 192.

Center for Disease Control (1977), 'Multiple-antibiotic resistance of pneumococci—South Africa', *Morbidity and Mortality Weekly Report*, **26**, 285.

Chang, T. and Weinstein, L. (1964), 'Inhibition of synthesis of cell wall of Staphylococcus aureus by cephalothin', *Science*, **143**, 807; quoted by Grieco, M. H. (1967).

Chow, A. W., Patten, V. and Bednorz, D. (1978), 'Susceptibility of Campylobacter fetus to twenty-two antimicrobial agents', *Antimicrob. Ag. Chemother.*, **13**, 416.

Cohen, P. G., Romansky, M. J. and Johnson, A. C. (1966), 'Laboratory and clinical evaluation of cephaloridine in 78 patients', *Antimicrob. Agents Chemother.*—1965, p. 894.

Comments (1974), 'Cephaloridine and staphylococci', *Med. J. Aust.*, **2**, 891.

Currie, J. P. (1967), 'Cephaloridine: Pharmacology and Toxicology', *Postgrad. Med. J.* (Suppl.), **43**, 22.

Curtis, J. R. and Marshall, M. J. (1970), 'Cephaloridine serum levels in patients on maintenance haemodialysis', *Brit. med. J.*, **2**, 149.

Curtis, N. A. C., Hughes, J. M. and Ross, G. W. (1976), 'Inhibition of peptidoglycan cross-linking in growing cells of Escherichia coli by penicillins and cephalosporins, and its prevention by R factor—mediated beta-lactamase', *Antimicrob. Ag. Chemother.*, **9**, 208.

D'Alessandri, R. M., McNeely, D. J. and Kluge, R. M. (1976), 'Antibiotic synergy and antagonism against clinical isolates of Klebsiella species', *Antimicrob. Ag. Chemother.*, **10**, 889.

Dash, C. H. (1975), 'Penicillin allergy and the cephalosporins', *J. Antimicrob. Chemother.* (Suppl.), **1**, 107.

Dellinger, P., Murphy, T., Barza, M., Pinn, V. and Weinstein, L. (1976a), 'Effect of cephalothin on renal cortical concentrations of gentamicin in rats', *Antimicrob. Ag. Chemother.*, **9**, 587.

Dellinger, P., Murphy, T., Pinn, V., Barza, M. and Weinstein, L. (1976b), 'Protective effect of cephalothin against gentamicin-induced nephrotoxocity in rats', *Antimicrob. Ag. Chemother.*, **9**, 172.

Di Cato, M.-A. and Ellman, L. (1975), 'Cephalothin-induced granylocytopenia', *Ann. Intern. Med.*, **83**, 671.

Dillon, M. L. and Postlewait, R. W. (1971), 'Cephaloridine in patients with impaired renal function', *JAMA*, **218**, 250.

Duncan, W. C. and Knox, J. M. (1971), 'Cephalosporin antibiotics in venereal disease', *Postgrad. Med. J.* (Suppl.), **47**, 119.

Editorial (1967), 'Cross-allergenicity of penicillins and cephalosporins', *JAMA*, **199**, 495.

Ellis, B. W., Stanbridge, R. DeL., Sikorski, J. M., Dudley, H. A. F. and Spencer, R. C. (1975), 'Pentration into inflammatory exudate and wounds of two cephalosporins for the prevention of surgical infections', *J. Antimicrob. Chemother.*, **1**, 291.

Engle, J. E., Drago, J., Carlin, B. and Schoolwerth, A. C. (1975), 'Reversible acute renal failure after cephalothin', *Ann. Intern. Med.*, **83**, 232.

Fanning, W. L., Gump, D. and Jick, H. (1976), 'Gentamicin- and cephalothin-associated rises in blood urea nitrogen', *Antimicrob. Ag. Chemother.*, **10**, 80.

Farrar, W. E., Jr. and O'Dell, N. M. (1976), 'Beta-lactamases and resistance to penicillins and cephalosporins in Serratia marcescens', *J. Infect. Dis.*, **134**, 245.

Fass, R. J., Perkins, R. L. and Saslaw, S. (1970), 'Positive direct Coombs test associated with cephaloridine therapy', *JAMA*, **213**, 121.

Fillastre, J. P., Laumonier, R., Humbert, G., Dubois, D., Metayer, J., Delpech, A., Leroy, J. and Robert, M. (1973), 'Acute renal failure associated with combined gentamicin and cephalothin therapy', *Brit. med. J.*, **2**, 396.

Fisher, L. S., Chow, A. W., Yoshikawa, T. A. and Guze, L. B. (1975), 'Cephalothin and cephaloridine therapy for bacterial meningitis. An evaluation', *Ann. Intern. Med.*, **82**, 689.

Foley, T. H., Jones, N. F., Barraclough, M. A., Cranston, W. I. and Hunt, A. P. (1967), 'The renal excretion of cephaloridine in man', *Postgrad. Med. J.* (Suppl.), **43**, 85.

Foord, R. D. (1971), 'Nephrotoxocity of cephaloridine', *Brit. med. J.*, **4**, 493.

Foord, R. D. (1975), 'Cephaloridine, cephalothin and the kidney', *J. Antimicrob.*

Chemother. (Suppl.), **1**, 119.

Freij, L., Hebelka, M. and Seeberg, S. (1975), 'Meningitis developing during cephalothin therapy of septicaemia', *Scand. J. Infect. Dis.*, **7**, 153.

Gabriel, R., Foord, R. D. and Joekes, A. M. (1970), 'Reversible encephalopathy and acute renal failure after cephaloridine', *Brit. med. J.*, **4**, 283.

Garratty, G. and Petz, L. D. (1975), 'Drug-induced immune hemolytic anemia', *Amer. J. Med.*, **58**, 398.

Gerding, D. N., Hall, W. H. and Schierl, E. A. (1977), 'Antibiotic concentrations in ascitic fluid of patients with ascites and bacterial peritonitis', *Ann. Intern. Med.*, **86**, 708.

Glicksman, J. M., Short, D. H. and Knox, J. M. (1968), 'Parenteral cephaloridine treatment of patients with early syphilis', *Arch. Intern. Med.*, **121**, 342.

Gower, P. E. (1967a), 'The effect of cephaloridine on renal function in patients with renal failure', *Postgrad. Med. J.* (Suppl.), **43**, 92.

Gower, P. E. (1967b), 'Cephaloridine toxicity', *Lancet, **2**, 1086.

Gralnick H. R., McGinniss, M., Elton, W. and McCurdy, P. (1971), 'Hemolytic anemia associated with cephalothin', *JAMA*, **217**, 1193.

Gralnick, H. R., McGinniss, M. and Halterman, R. (1972), 'Thrombocytopenia with sodium cephalothin therapy', *Ann. Intern. Med.*, **77**, 401.

Greenwood, D. and O'Grady, F. (1975), 'Resistance categories of enterobacteria to beta-lactam antibiotics', *J. Infect. Dis.*, **132**, 233.

Grieco, M. H. (1967), 'Cross-allergenicity of the penicillins and the cephalosporins', *Arch. Intern. Med.*, **119**, 141.

Griffith, R. S. and Black, H. R. (1964), 'Cephalothin—a new antibiotic', *JAMA*, **189**, 823.

Griffith, R. S. and Black, H. R. (1971), 'Blood, urine and tissue concentrations of the cephalosporin antibiotics in normal subjects', *Postgrad. Med. J.* (Suppl.), **47**, 32.

Hansten, P. D. (1973), 'Cephalothin, gentamicin, colistin hazards', *JAMA*, **223**, 1158.

Hermans, P. E., Martin, J. K., Needham, G. M. and Nichols, D. R. (1966), 'Laboratory and clinical evaluation of cephaloridine, a cephalosporin derivative', *Antimicrob. Agents Chemother.*—1965, p. 879.

Hierholzer, G., Lienzenmeier, G., Kleining, R. and Hoerster, G. (1974), 'Study of the diffusion of various cephalosporins in the bone tissue', *Aktuelle Traumatologie*, **4**, 191.

Hinman, A. R. and Wolinsky, E. (1967), 'Nephrotoxicity associated with the use of cephaloridine', *JAMA*, **200**, 724.

Hirsch, H. A. (1971), 'The use of cephalosporin antibiotics in pregnant women', *Postgrad. Med. J.* (Suppl), **47**, 90.

Holder, W. R. and Knox, J. M. (1972), 'Syphilis in pregnancy', *Med. Clin. North Amer.*, **56**, 1151.

Howard, P. (1967), 'Cephaloridine in acute pulmonary infections', *Brit. med. J.*, **2**, 573.

Hughes, S. P. F., Benson, M. K. D., Dash, C. H. and Field, C. A. (1975), 'Cephaloridine penetration into bone and synovial capsule of patients undergoing hip joint replacement', *J. Antimicrob. Chemother.* (Suppl.), **1**, 41.

Hyams, P. J., Simberkoff, M. S. and Rahal, J. J., Jr. (1974), 'Synergy between cephalosporin and aminoglycoside antibiotics against Providencia and Proteus', *Antimicrob. Ag. Chemother.*, **5**, 571.

Izaki, K. and Strominger, J. L. (1968), 'Biosynthesis of the peptidoglycan of bacterial cell walls', *J. Biol. Chem.*, **243**, 3193.

Kabins, S. A. and Cohen, S. (1965), 'Cephalothin serum levels in the azotemic patient', *Antimicrob. Agents Chemother.*—1964, p. 207.

Kabins, S. A. and Cohen, S. (1966), 'Cephaloridine therapy as related to renal function', *Antimicrob. Agents Chemother.*—1965, p. 922.

Kaplan, K. and Weinstein, L. (1967), 'Anaphylaxis to cephaloridine in a nurse', *JAMA*,

200, 75.

Kayser, F. H. (1971), '*In vitro* activity of cephalosporin antibiotics against Gram-positive bacteria', *Postgrad. Med. J.* (Suppl.), **47,** 14.

Kirby, W. M. M., de Maine, J. B. and Serrill, W. S. (1971), 'Pharmacokinetics of the cephalosporins in healthy volunteers and uremic patients', *Postgrad. Med. J.* (Suppl.), **47,** 41.

Kleinknecht, D., Ganeval, D. and Droz, D. (1973), 'Acute renal failure after high doses of gentamicin and cephalothin', *Lancet,* **1,** 1129.

Kunin, C. M. (1967), 'A guide to use of antibiotics in patients with renal disease', *Ann. Intern. Med.,* **67,** 151.

Kunin, C. M. and Atuk, N. (1966), 'Excretion of cephaloridine and cephalothin in patients with renal impairment', *New Engl. J. Med.,* **274,** 654.

Lacey, R. W. and Stokes, A. (1977), 'Susceptibility of the "penicillinase-resistant" penicillins and cephalosporins to penicillinase of Staphylococcus aureus', *J. clin. Path.,* **30,** 35.

Laverdiere, M., Peterson, P. K., Verhoef, J., Williams, D. N. and Sabath, L. D. (1978a), '*In vitro* activity of cephalosporins against methicillin-resistant, coagulase-negative staphylococci', *J. Infect. Dis.,* **137,** 245.

Laverdiere, M., Welter, D. and Sabath, L. D. (1978b), 'Use of a heavy inoculum in the *in vitro* evaluation of the anti-staphylococcal activity of 19 cephalosporins', *Antimicrob. Ag. Chemother.,* **13,** 669.

Lawson, D. H., Macadam, R. F., Singh, H., Gavras, H. and Linton, A. L. (1970), 'The nephrotoxicity of cephaloridine', *Postgrad. Med. J.* (Suppl.), **46,** 36.

Lawson, D. H., Macadam, R. F., Singh, H., Gavras, H., Hartz, S., Turnbull, D. and Linton, A. L. (1972), 'Effect of furosemide on antibiotic-induced renal damage in rats', *J. Infect. Dis.,* **126,** 593.

Leading Article (1967), 'Treatment of staphylococcal endocarditis', *Brit. med. J.,* **1,** 515.

Leading Article (1973), 'Antibiotic-induced meningitis', *Brit. med. J.,* **3,** 366.

Lemole, G. M., Fadali, A. M. A. and Molthan, L. (1972), 'Cephalothin-induced tachycardia following aortic valve replacement', *JAMA,* **221,** 593.

Lerner, P. I. (1971), 'Penetration of cephaloridine into cerebrospinal fluid', *Amer. J. Med. Sci.,* **262,** 321; *quoted* by Fisher *et al.* (1975).

Lorian, V. and Sabath, L. D. (1972), 'Penicillins and cephalosporins: Differences in morphologic effects on Proteus mirabilis', *J. Infect Dis.,* **125,** 560.

Love, W. C., McKenzie, P., Lawson, J. H., Pinkerton, I. W., Jamieson, W. M., Stevenson, J., Roberts, W. and Christie, A. B. (1970), 'Treatment of pneumococcal meningitis with cephaloridine', *Postgrad. Med. J.* (Suppl.), **46,** 155.

Luft, F. C., Patel, V., Nahm Yum, M. and Kleit, S. A. (1976), Nephrotoxicity of cephalosporin-gentamicin combinations in rats, *Antimicrob. Ag. Chemother.,* **9,** 831.

Mangi, R. J., Kundargi, R. S., Quintiliani, R. and Andriole, V. T. (1973), 'Development of meningitis during cephalothin therapy', *Ann. Intern. Med.,* **78,** 347.

Martin, W. J. and Wellman, W. E. (1967), 'Clinically useful antimicrobial agents', *Postgrad. Medicine,* **42,** 350.

Mathews, D. D. (1975), 'Cephaloridine serum levels after intravenous injection', *J. Antimicrob. Chemother.* (Suppl.), **1,** 37.

McCracken, G. H., Jr. and Nelson, J. D. (1977), *Antimicrobial Therapy for Newborns: Practical Application of Pharmacology to Clinical Usage,* Grune & Stratton, New York, San Francisco, London, p. 27.

McKenzie, P., Love, W. C., Lawson, J. H., Pinkerton, I. W., Jamieson, W. M. and Stevenson, J. (1967), 'Cephaloridine in pneumococcal and other forms of pyogenic meningitis', *Postgrad. Med. J.* (Suppl.), **43,** 142.

Mayhall, C. G., Medoff, G. and Marr, J. J. (1976), 'Variation in the susceptibility of strains of Staphylococcus aureus to oxacillin, cephalothin, and gentamicin', *Antimicrob. Ag. Chemother.*, **10**, 707.

Medical News (1968), 'Reactions to cephalothin', *JAMA*, **206**, 1701.

Mendelson, J., Portnoy, J., Sigman, H. and Dick, V. (1974), 'Pharmacology of cephalothin in the biliary tract of humans', *Antimicrob. Ag. Chemother.*, **6**, 659.

Mitchell, J. R., McMurtry, R. J., Statham, C. N. and Nelson, S. D. (1977), 'Molecular basis for several drug-induced nephropathies', *Amer. J. Med.*, **62**, 518.

Moellering, R. C., Jr., Watson, B. K. and Kunz, L. J. (1974), 'Endocarditis due to Group D streptococci. Comparison of disease caused by Streptococcus bovis with that produced by the Enterococci', *Amer. J. Med.*, **57**, 239.

Mohr, J. A., Griffiths, W., Holm, R., Garcia-Moral, C. and Flournoy, D. J. (1978), 'Clostridial myonecrosis ("Gas Gangrene") during cephalosporin prophylaxis', *JAMA*, **239**, 847.

Molthan, L., Reidenberg, M. M. and Eichman, M. F. (1967), 'Positive direct Coombs tests due to cephalothin', *New Engl. J. Med.*, **277**, 123.

Morrow, S., Palmisano, P. and Cassady, G. (1968), 'The placental transfer of cephalothin', *J. Pediatrics*, **73**, 262.

Muggleton, P. W., O'Callaghan, C. H. and Stevens, W. K. (1964), 'Laboratory evaluation of a new antibiotic—cephaloridine (ceporan)', *Brit. med. J.*, **2**, 1234.

Muggleton, P. W. and O'Callaghan, C. H. (1967), 'The antibacterial activities of cephaloridine: Laboratory investigations', *Postgrad. Med. J.* (Suppl.), **43**, 17.

Murdoch, J. McC., Speirs, C. F., Geddes, A. M. and Wallace, E. T. (1964), 'Clinical trial of cephaloridine (ceporan), a new broad-spectrum antibiotic derived from cephalosporin C', *Brit. med. J.*, **2**, 1238.

Natelson, E. A., Brown, C. H. III., Bradshaw, M. W., Alfrey, C. P., Jr. and Williams, T. W., Jr. (1976), 'Influence of cephalosporin antibiotics on blood coagulation and platelet function', *Antimicrob. Ag. Chemother.*, **9**, 91.

Noone, P. (1973), 'A rapid assay method for cephalosporins', *J. clin. Path.*, **26**, 506.

Norrby, R., Stenquist, K. and Elgefors, B. (1976), 'Interaction between cephaloridine and furosemide in man', *Scand. J. Infect. Dis.*, **8**, 209.

Oller, L. Z. (1967a), 'Further experience with cephaloridine in gonorrhoea', *Postgrad. Med. J.* (Suppl.), **43**, 124.

Oller, L. Z. (1967b), 'Cephaloridine in early syphilis', *Postgrad. Med. J.* (Suppl.), **43**, 128.

Oller, L. Z., Smith, H. G. and Marshall, M. J. (1970), 'Cephaloridine and cephalexin in venereological practice', *Postgrad. Med. J.* (Suppl.), **46**, 99.

Perkins, R. L. and Saslaw, S. (1966), 'Experience with cephalothin', *Ann. Intern. Med.*, **64**, 13.

Perkins, R. L., Smith, E. J. and Saslaw, S. (1969), 'Cephalothin and cephaloridine: Comparative pharmacodynamics in chronic uremia', *Amer. J. Med. Sci.*, **257**, 116.

Petz, L. D. (1971), 'Immunologic reactions of humans to cephalosporins', *Postgrad. Med. J.* (Suppl.), **47**, 64.

Petz, L. D. (1978), 'Immunologic cross-reactivity between penicillins and cephalosporins: A review', *J. Infect. Dis.* (Suppl.), **137**, 74.

Phillips, I., Warren, C., Harrison, J. M., Sharples, P., Ball, L. C. and Parker, M. T. (1976), 'Antibiotic susceptibilities of streptococci from the mouth and blood of patients treated with penicillin or lincomycin and clindamycin', *J. Med. Microbiol.*, **9**, 393.

Pines, A. (1974), 'Cephalosporins in bronchitis', *Brit. Med. J.*, **2**, 440.

Pitkin, D., Actor, P., Filan, J. J., White, R. and Weisbach, J. A. (1977), 'Comparative stability of cephalothin and cefazolin in buffer in human serum', *Antimicrob. Ag. Chemother.*, **12**, 284.

Pollock, A. V. and Evans, M. (1975), 'The prophylaxis of surgical wound sepsis with cephaloridine-experiences in 2491 general surgical operations and reporting a controlled clinical trial against framycetin', *J. Antimicrob. Chemother.* (Suppl.), **1**, 71.

Pryor, J. S., Joekes, A. M. and Foord, R. D. (1967), 'Cephaloridine excretion in patients with normal and impaired renal function', *Postgrad. Med. J.* (Suppl.), **43**, 82.

Rahal, J. J., Jr., Meyers, B. R. and Weinstein, L. (1968), 'Treatment of bacterial endocarditis with cephalothin', *New Engl. J. Med.*, **279**, 1305.

Ratzan, K. R., Ruiz, C. and Irvin, G. L. III (1974), 'Biliary tract excretion of cefazolin, cephalothin, and cephaloridine in the presence of biliary tract disease', *Antimicrob. Ag. Chemother.*, **6**, 426.

Regamey, C., Libke, R. D., Engelking, E. R., Clarke, J. T. and Kirby, W. M. M. (1975), 'Inactivation of cefazolin, cephaloridine and cephalothin by methicillin-sensitive and methicillin-resistant strains of Staphylococcus aureus', *J. Infect. Dis.*, **131**, 291.

Richmond, A. S., Simberkoff, M. S., Schaefler, S. and Rahal, J. J., Jr. (1977), 'Resistance of Staphylococcus aureus to semisynthetic penicillins and cephalothin', *J. Infect. Dis.*, **135**, 108.

Rothschild, P. D. and Doty, D. B. (1966), 'Cephalothin reaction after penicillin sensitization', *JAMA*, **196**, 372.

Rountree, P. M. and Bullen, M. M. (1967), 'Cephaloridine and staphylococcal endocarditis', *Brit. med. J.*, **2**, 373.

Roy, A. D. (1976), 'The prophylactic use of antimicrobial agents in the surgery of the intestine', *J. Antimicrob. Chemother.*, **2**, 233.

Rubin, R. N. and Burka, E. R. (1977), 'Anti-cephalothin antibody and Coombs-positive hemolytic anemia', *Ann. Intern. Med.*, **86**, 64.

Sabath, L. D., Garner, C., Wilcox, C. and Finland, M. (1975), 'Effect of inoculum and of beta-lactamase on the anti-Staphylococcal activity of thirteen penicillins and cephalosporins', *Antimicrob. Ag. Chemother.*, **8**, 344.

Sabath, L. D., Wheeler, N., Laverdiere, M., Blazevic, D. and Wilkinson, B. J. (1977), 'A new type of penicillin resistance of Staphylococcus aureus', *Lancet*, **1**, 443.

Saleh, Y. and Tischler, E. (1974), 'Severe anaphylactic reaction to intravenous cephaloridine in a pregnant patient', *Med. J. Aust.*, **2**, 490.

Sanders, W. E., Jr., Johnson, J. E., III and Taggart, J. G. (1974), 'Adverse reactions to cephalothin and cephapirin. Uniform occurrence on prolonged intravenous administration of high doses', *New Engl. J. Med.*, **290**, 424.

Saslaw, S. (1970), 'Cephalosporins', *Med. Clin. North America*, **54**, 1217.

Scholand, J. F., Tennenbaum, J. I. and Cerilli, G. J. (1968), 'Anaphylaxis to cephalothin in a patient allergic to penicillin', *JAMA*, **206**, 130.

Schwartzman, J. D., Reller, L. B. and Wang, W.-L. L. (1977), 'Susceptibility of Clostridium perfringens isolated from human infections to twenty antibiotics', *Antimicrob. Ag. Chemother.*, **11**, 695.

Shedden, W. I. H. (1973), 'Antibiotic-induced meningitis', *Brit. med. J.*, **3**, 638.

Silverblatt, F., Turck, M. and Bulger, R. (1970), 'Nephro-toxicity due to cephaloridine: A light and electron-microscopic study in rabbits', *J. Infect. Dis.*, **122**, 33.

Smilack, J. D., Flittie, W. H. and Williams, T. W., Jr. (1976), 'Bone concentrations of antimicrobial agents after parenteral administration', *Antimicrob. Ag. Chemother.*, **9**, 169.

Southern, P. M., Jr. and Sanford, J. P. (1969), 'Meningococcal meningitis—suboptimal response to cephalothin therapy', *New Engl. J. Med.*, **280**, 1163.

Speller, D. C. E. and Mitchell, R. G. (1973), 'Coagulase-negative staphylococci causing endocarditis after cardiac surgery', *J. clin. Path.*, **26**, 517.

Spruill, F. G., Minette, L. J. and Sturner, W. Q. (1974), 'Two surgical deaths associated with cephalothin', *JAMA*, **229**, 440.

Steigbigel, N. H., Kislak, J. W., Tilles, J. G. and Finland, M. (1968)', 'Clinical evaluation of cephaloridine', *Arch. Intern. Med.*, **121**, 24.

Stewart, G. T. (1962), 'Cross-allergenicity of penicillin G and related substances', *Lancet*, **1**, 509.

Stewart, G. T. and Holt, R. J. (1964), 'Laboratory and clinical results with cephaloridine', *Lancet*, **2**, 1305.

Sutter, V. L. and Finegold, S. M. (1976), 'Susceptibility of anaerobic bacteria to 23 antimicrobial agents', *Antimicrob. Ag. Chemother.*, **10**, 736.

Sykes, R. B. and Matthew, M. (1976), 'The beta-lactamases of Gram-negative bacteria and their role in resistance to beta-lactam antibiotics', *J. Antimicrob. Chemother.*, **2**, 115.

Tally, F. P., Jacobus, N. V., Bartlett, J. G. and Gorbach, S. L. (1975), 'Susceptibility of anaerobes to cefoxitin and other cephalosporins', *Antimicrob. Ag. Chemother.*, **7**, 128.

Tempest, B. and Austrian, R. (1967), 'Cephaloridine and penicillin G in the treatment of pneumococcal pneumonia; A comparative study', *Ann. Intern. Med.*, **66**, 1109.

Tice, A. D., Barza, M., Bergeron, M. G., Brusch, J. L. and Weinstein, L. (1975), 'Effect of diuretics on urinary excretion of cephalothin in humans', *Antimicrob. Ag. Chemother.*, **7**, 168.

Tune, B. M. and Kempson, R. L. (1973), 'Nephrotoxic drugs', *Brit. med. J.*, **3**, 635.

Tune, B. M. (1975), 'Relationship between the transport and toxocity of cephalosporins in the kidney', *J. Infect. Dis.*, **132**, 189.

Tures, J. F., Townsend, W. F. and Rose, H. D. (1976), 'Cephalosporin-associated pseudomembranous colitis', *JAMA*, **236**, 948.

Venuto, R. C. and Plaut, M. E. (1971), 'Cephalothin handling in patients undergoing hemodialysis', *Antimicrob. Agents Chemother.—*1970, p. 50.

Vianna, N. J. and Kaye, D. (1967), 'Penetration of cephalothin into the spinal fluid', *Amer. J. Med. Sci.*, **254**, 216; *quoted* by Fisher *et al.* (1975).

Walker, S. H. and Collins, C. C., Jr. (1968), 'Failure of cephaloridine in Hemophilus influenzae meningitis', *Amer. J. Dis. Child.*, **116**, 285.

Walker, W. (1964), 'Cephaloridine in typhoid', *Brit. med. J.*, **2**, 1529.

Waterworth, P. M. (1971), 'The susceptibility of pathogenic Gram-negative bacilli to cephalosporins', *Postgrad. Med. J.* (Suppl.), **47**, 25.

Weinstein, L. Kaplan, K. and Chang, T. (1964), 'Treatment of infections in man with cephalothin', *JAMA*, **189**, 829.

Weinstein, L. and Kaplan, K. (1970), 'The cephalosporins. Microbiological, chemical and pharmacological properties and use in chemotherapy of infection', *Ann. Intern. Med.*, **72**, 729.

Weinstein, A. J. and Moellering, R. C., Jr. (1975), 'Studies of cephalothin: Aminoglycoside synergism against Enterococci', *Antimicrob. Ag. Chemother.*, **7**, 522.

Weinstein, A. J. and Lentnek, A. L. (1976), 'Cephalosporin-aminoglycoside synergism in experimental enterococcal endocarditis', *Antimicrob. Ag. Chemother.*, **9**, 983.

Williams, J. D. and Smith, E. K. (1973), 'Antibiotic use in obstetric patients', in Geddes, A. M. and Williams, J. D. (ed.) *Current Antibiotic Therapy*, Churchill Livingstone, Edinburgh and London, p. 71.

Williams, J. D. and Andrews, J. (1974), 'Sensitivity of Haemophilus influenzae to antibiotics', *Brit. med. J.*, **1**, 134.

Winchester, J. F. and Kennedy, A. C. (1972), 'Absence of nephrotoxicity during cephaloridine therapy for urinary-tract infection', *Lancet*, **2**, 514.

Wise, R. I. (1973), 'Modern management of severe staphylococcal disease', *Medicine*, **52**, 295.

Wong, G. A., Peirce, T. H., Goldstein, E. and Hoeprich, P. D. (1975), 'Penetration of antimicrobial agents into bronchial secretions', *Amer. J. Med.*, **59**, 219.

Wyatt, R. G., Okamoto, G. A. and Feigin, R. D. (1972), 'Stability of antibiotics in parenteral solutions', *Pediatrics*, **49**, 22.

Yoshioka, H., Rudoy, P., Riley, H. D., Jr. and Yoshida, K. (1977), 'Antimicrobial susceptibility of Escherichia coli isolated at a children's hospital', *Scand. J. Infect. Dis.*, **9,** 207.
Young, L. S., Martin, W. J., Meyer, R. D., Weinstein, R. J. and Anderson, E. T. (1977), Gram-negative rod bacteremia: Microbiologic, immunologic, and therapeutic considerations', *Ann. Intern. Med.*, **86,** 456.

Cephalexin and Cephaloglycin

Description

Cephalexin and cephaloglycin are semisynthetic antibiotics derived from cephalosporin C, but unlike cephalothin and cephaloridine (page 199) they are absorbed after oral administration.

1. *Cephalexin* or 7-(D-alpha-amino-alpha-phenylacetamido)-3-methyl-3-cephem-4-carboxylic acid (Wick, 1967) is marketed with the trade name of 'Keflex' (Eli Lilly) and 'Ceporex' (Glaxo).

2. *Cephaloglycin* or 7-(D-alpha-aminophenyl acetamido)-cephalosporanic acid was the first available 'oral' cephalosporin (Pitt *et al.*, 1968; Johnson *et al.*, 1968). It is marketed in America with the trade name of 'Kafocin' (Eli Lilly).

Cephalexin is the more useful of these two 'oral' cephalosporins, because of its much better absorption (Braun *et al.*, 1968), so that cephaloglycin now has very little clinical application. The data given below only apply to cephalexin.

Sensitive Organisms

The antibacterial spectrum of cephalexin resembles that of cephalothin and cephaloridine (page 199), but in general its activity is of a lower order against most bacterial species (Muggleton *et al.*, 1969).

1. *Gram-positive cocci*. Staph. pyogenes, including most penicillin-resistant strains, is cephalexin-sensitive. Similar to cephalothin (page 199), cephalexin is relatively resistant to inactivation by staphylococcal penicillinase (Sabath *et al.*, 1975; Lacey and Stokes, 1977). Nevertheless, only penicillin-sensitive Staph. pyogenes strains are uniformly cephalexin-sensitive; penicillinase-producing strains vary in their degree of susceptibility and their MIC's are generally higher than those of penicillin-sensitive strains (Braun *et al.*, 1968) (*see* Table 14, page 227). Methicillin-resistant staphylococcal strains (page 64) are also resistant to cephalexin (Griffith and Black, 1970; Kayser, 1971). Penicillin-tolerant staphylococci (page 6) presumably also show similar tolerance to cephalexin.

Most other aerobic Gram-positive cocci such as Staph. epidermidis (albus), Strep. pyogenes, Strep. pneumoniae and the alpha-haemolytic streptococci of the 'viridans' group are cephalexin-sensitive. Strep. faecalis is always resistant (Braun *et al.*, 1968).

Anaerobic Gram-positive cocci such as the Peptococcus and Peptostreptococcus spp. are usually moderately sensitive. Most strains recovered from airway associated infections are inhibited by 8·16 μg per ml. Other strains are

225

resistant, needing 64 μg per ml or higher for inhibition (Tally *et al.*, 1975; Busch *et al.*, 1976).

2. *Gram-positive bacilli*. C.diphtheriae is cephalexin-sensitive, but Listeria monocytogenes is relatively resistant (Wick, 1967; Kayser, 1971). Anaerobic Gram-positive rods such as C1. perfringens (welchii), C1. tetani and other Clostridium spp. are relatively resistant. Some strains may be inhibited by 8–16 μg per ml of cephalexin, but others need 32 or 64 μg per ml or even higher for inhibition (Tally *et al.*, 1975).

3. *Gram-negative aerobic bacteria*. The Neisseria spp. (meningococci and gonococci) are sensitive. Cephalexin, unlike cephaloridine (page 8), retains moderate *in vitro* activity against penicillinase-producing gonococci (page 8); it inhibits large inocula of these strains at a concentration of 2·5 μg per ml (Selwyn and Bakhtiar, 1977).

Other Gram-negative bacteria vary in their sensitivity. Some strains of Esch. coli, Proteus mirabilis and the Klebsiella, Salmonella and Shigella spp. may be inhibited by concentrations of cephalexin that can be easily attained *in vivo*, but other strains require much higher concentrations (Braun *et al.*, 1968; Konforti and Halperin, 1975). Such high concentrations of cephalexin can be attained in the urine. Bordetella pertussis and H. influenzae are both moderately resistant to cephalexin (Waterworth, 1971). Proteus spp., other than mirabilis, Enterobacter spp. and especially Pseudomonas aeruginosa are always cephalexin-resistant. Serratia marcescens and the Providencia, Hafnia, Citrobacter, Edwardsiella and Arizona spp. are also usually resistant. Drug inactivation by beta-lactamases is a major reason for the resistance of some of these Gram-negative bacilli, but as with other beta-lactam antibiotics (page 10), other mechanisms are also involved (O'Callaghan and Kirby, 1970; Sykes and Matthew, 1976).

4. *Gram-negative anaerobic bacteria*. Bacteroides fragilis is cephalexin-resistant, but other Bacteroides spp., especially those that populate the oropharynx, are quite sensitive. Similarly Fusobacterium and Veillonella spp. are usually sensitive to cephalexin, especially strains recovered from airway-related infections as opposed to those isolated from intra-abdominal infections (Tally *et al.*, 1975; Busch *et al.*, 1976).

5. *Mycoplasmas and Mycobacteria* are resistant to cephalexin.

6. *Cephalexin sensitivity testing*. The antibacterial spectra of cephalexin and the older parenteral cephalosporins, cephalothin and cephaloridine (page 199) are similar, so that the use of only one of these cephalosporins for sensitivity tests is usually satisfactory. However, some strains of Gram-negative bacteria produce enzymes that destroy cephaloridine, but not cephalexin; in such instances sensitivity testing with individual cephalosporins may be important (Guttmann, 1970; Selwyn and Bakhtiar, 1977).

In Vitro Sensitivities

TABLE 14

Compiled from data published by Braun *et al.* (1968) and Tally *et al.* (1975)

ORGANISM	MIC (μg per ml)	
	Range	Median
Gram-positive bacteria		
Staph. pyogenes (non-penicillinase producer)	1·6–12·5	3·1
Staph. pyogenes (penicillinase producer)	1·6–>100	12·5
Strep. pyogenes (Group A)	0·2–6·3	0·4
Strep. pneumoniae (Dip. pneumoniae)	1·6–6·3	3·1
Strep. viridans spp.	0·8–12·5	6·3
Strep. faecalis (Enterococcus, Group D)	100–>100	100
Peptostreptococcus spp.	0·5–64·0	—
Clostridium perfringens	8·0–64·0	—
Gram-negative bacteria		
Escherichia coli	25–>100	>100
Enterobacter spp.	50–>100	50
Klebsiella pneumoniae	50–>100	>100
Serratia marcescens	50–>100	100
Proteus mirabilis	>100	>100
Proteus (other than mirabilis)	25–>100	>100
Neisseria gonorrhoeae	0·1–6·3	3·1
Neisseria meningitidis	1·6–6·3	3·1
Haemophilus influenzae	12·5–>100	>100
Pseudomonas aeruginosa	>100	>100
Bacteroides fragilis	>64·0	—
Other Bacteroides spp.	0·5–32·0	—

The minimum inhibitory concentrations of cephalexin against some bacterial species are shown in Table 14. Braun *et al.* (1968) found that most strains of Gram-negative aerobic bacilli were resistant to cephalexin at 100 μg per ml. More sensitive strains of Esch. coli, Proteus mirabilis and Klebsiella spp. have been reported by others as shown in Table 15.

TABLE 15

(After Muggleton *et al.*, 1969)

ORGANISM	MIC (μg per ml)
Escherichia coli	16·0
Proteus mirabilis	31·0
Klebsiella pneumoniae	16·0

Mode of Administration and Dosage

1. *Mild to moderate infections.* The usual adult dose of cephalexin for these infections is 250 to 500 mg four times a day, and for children 25 to 50 mg per kg body weight per day.

2. *Severe systemic infections.* Cephalexin has been tried in moderately severe systemic infections, in a higher dosage of 3–4 g daily (Bailey *et al.*, 1970). The corresponding dose for children has been up to 100 mg per kg per day. In endocarditis, an adult dose of 6 g daily has been given, sometimes with probenecid (Zabransky *et al.*, 1969; Stratford, 1970).

3. *Patients with renal failure.* Cephalexin accumulates in these patients, so that dosage modification with serum level estimations is necessary. Table 16 shows a proposed dose regimen for treatment of moderately severe systemic infections, in patients with various degrees of renal impairment (Kabins *et al.*, 1970). The oral cephalexin dosage schedules in this table are designed to produce sustained serum levels of 12 or 30 μg per ml. The former level is sufficient to inhibit staphylococci, the latter, the most susceptible Gram-negative bacilli. The drug is removed by haemodialysis, and an additional dose is needed on the day when this procedure is performed.

TABLE 16

Proposed oral dose schedule of cephalexin
(After Kabins *et al.*, 1970)

Group	Creatinine clearance (ml per min)	For sustained levels of:				Loading Dose (mg)
		12 μg per ml		30 μg per ml		
		Dose (mg)	Interval (hours)	Dose (mg)	Interval (hours)	
1.	58–124	1000	4	—	—	—
2.	33–48	250	12	250	8	1000
3.	3–10	250	24	250	12	500
4.	0–2·5	250	48	250	24	500
4. (on day of dialysis)	0–2·5	500	—	750	—	—

Cephalexin is suitable for treatment of urinary tract infections in azotaemic patients, because it produces satisfactory and prolonged concentrations in the urine, even in the presence of severe renal functional impairment (Bailey *et al.*, 1970; Butcher *et al.*, 1972). Suitable dosage adjustments for this situation are shown in Table 17. Alternatively the appropriate daily dose of cephalexin may be calculated by dividing the usual dose of 2 g per day by the patient's serum creatinine level in mg per cent (Butcher *et al.*, 1972). For conversion from SI units to mg per cent, *see* gentamicin, page 333.

4. *Newborn infants.* The dose as for older children i.e. 25–50 mg per kg of body weight per day, given in two or three divided doses, is usually recommended, but up to 100 mg per kg per day has been well tolerated (Marget, 1971).

5. *Parenteral cephalexin.* This is not generally available, but the clinical pharmacology of intravenous and intramuscular cephalexin has been studied (deMaine and Kirby, 1971; Davies and Holt, 1972; Gower *et al.*, 1973; Hughes *et al.*, 1974). It appears that in patients with normal renal function an

intramuscular or intravenous dose of 1 g every four to six hours may be suitable, but for severe infections an intravenous dose of up to 12 g per day can probably be used. In patients with severe renal failure a dose of 1 g every eight to twelve hours seems satisfactory. Cephalexin is removed from the blood during haemodialysis, but an intravenous dose of 1 g maintains an adequate serum level for up to eight hours during this procedure (Davies and Holt, 1972).

TABLE 17

Recommended dosage of cephalexin for urinary tract infections in patients with impaired renal function. (After Bailey et al., 1970)

Creatinine clearance or Glomerular filtration rate in ml per min	Intervals for 500 mg dose
<20	daily
20–50	twelve-hourly
>50	eight-hourly
Intermittent haemodialysis	daily plus 500 mg at end of each dialysis

Availability

Cephalexin is available in both 250 and 500 mg capsules and 500 mg tablets. Cephalexin elixir is available for children. Parenteral cephalexin is not currently available for general use.

Serum Levels in Relation to Dosage

1. *Oral cephalexin.* Cephalexin is almost completely absorbed after oral administration, and doubling the usual dose doubles the serum concentration (Fig. 12). These serum levels are about the same as those attained after equivalent intramuscular doses of cephaloridine, and are higher than those after intramuscular cephalothin (page 205) (Perkins et al., 1968; Meyers et al., 1969). Food delays absorption, resulting in lower peak but more prolonged serum levels; the total amount of the drug absorbed is only slightly less when given with food (Tetzlaff et al., 1978). In fasting patients 82 per cent of orally administered cephalexin is found in urine, compared to 73 per cent in those given food simultaneously (Griffith and Black, 1968). Probenecid prolongs and enhances serum levels (Braun et al., 1968; Griffith and Black, 1968).

Cephalexin absorption and serum levels attained are unimpaired in patients with obstructive jaundice, gastric achlorhydria, partial gastrectomy and congestive cardiac failure. The absorption of the drug is also not impaired in elderly patients, who develop more sustained serum levels due to slower cephalexin excretion (Davies and Holt, 1975).

Improved absorption of cephalexin occurs in patients with coeliac disease, small bowel diverticulosis and fibrocystic disease, but absorption is slightly impaired in those with Crohn's disease. Concomitant administration of cholestyramine significantly reduces cephalexin absorption and therefore these two drugs should not be administered simultaneously (Parsons *et al.*, 1975; Parsons and Paddock, 1975).

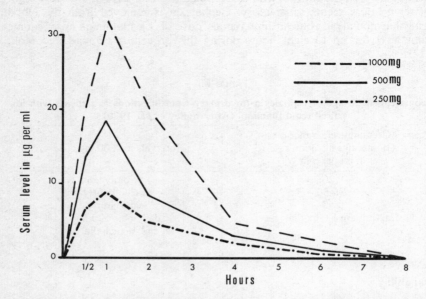

FIG. 12. Cephalexin blood levels with increasing dosage in fasting adults. (Redrawn after Griffith and Black, 1968.)

2. *Parenteral cephalexin.* After an intravenous dose of 1 g administered over a period of 5 min, a serum level of about 60 μg per ml is attained 15 min later. Thereafter the serum concentration rapidly falls to 5–10 μg per ml at 2 h and to 1–4 μg per ml at 4 h. The mean serum half-life of intravenous cephalexin is 1·1 h, but this can be nearly doubled by the concomitant administration of probenecid (Davies and Holt, 1972). Following an intramuscular injection of 1·0 g cephalexin, an average peak serum level of 10·6 μg per ml is reached 2 h later. At 6 h the cephalexin level is down to 2·5 μg per ml and at 12 h it is undetectable in serum (Nicholas *et al.*, 1973). These serum levels are lower than those obtained after equivalent doses of oral cephalexin (*vide supra*). It is possible that a local depot effect occurs after the intramuscular injection (Gower *et al.*, 1973).

Excretion

URINE: Cephalexin is excreted in urine in an active unchanged form by glomerular filtration and tubular secretion. Eighty per cent or more of an oral dose can be recovered from urine and high urinary concentrations are attained. Probenecid delays its excretion by partially blocking renal tubular secretion (Braun *et al.*, 1968; Griffith and Black, 1971).

Cephalexin accumulates in patients with impaired renal function. In normal subjects the mean serum half-life of cephalexin is 0·9 h (Bennett *et al.*, 1977), but in patients with severe renal functional impairment it increases to 20–30 h (Kabins *et al.*, 1970; Linquist *et al.*, 1970).

BILE: Some cephalexin is excreted in bile. After repeated doses, moderately high cephalexin levels (15–90 μg per ml) are attained in gallbladder bile, provided that the gall bladder is functioning normally. Biliary levels are much lower in patients with non-functioning gall bladders, and in the presence of complete biliary obstruction no cephalexin is excreted in the bile (Sales *et al.*, 1972).

INACTIVATION IN BODY: Cephalexin is not metabolized in the body (Griffith and Black, 1971).

Distribution of the Drug in Body

Griffith and Black (1971) studied post mortem tissue levels of cephalexin, in a patient who had received 2 g every 6 h, and the last dose was 5·5 h prior to death. The level in heart blood was 1·9 μg per ml, and tissue levels in lung, spleen, liver, adrenals, pancreas, heart muscle and stomach ranged from 0·12 μg to 0·6 μg per g. A higher concentration of 4·05 μg per g was found in kidney tissue. Moderately high cephalexin concentrations are reached in purulent sputum of patients with inflamed bronchi, but this decreases as the bronchial inflammation resolves (Halprin and McMahon, 1973). Therapeutic levels of cephalexin are achieved in amniotic fluid and cord blood if the drug is given in late pregnancy (Goodspeed 1975). Cephalexin is about 15 per cent serum protein bound (Kind *et al.*, 1969).

Mode of Action

Cephalexin, similar to penicillin G (page 19) and other cephalosporins (page 208), inhibits the synthesis of bacterial cell walls (Russell and Fountain, 1971).

Toxicity

1. *Gastro-intestinal side-effects.* Diarrhoea, vomiting and abdominal cramps occur in some patients receiving oral cephalexin therapy. Pruritus and moniliasis have also been observed (Griffith and Black, 1970). One patient who was treated successively over one month with oral cephalexin, parenteral cephalothin and cefazolin, developed pseudomembranous colitis, which responded to cholestyramine therapy (*see* page 481).

2. *Hypersensitivity reactions.* Skin rashes and eosinophilia have been observed in cephalexin-treated patients. It has been assumed that cephalexin is not 'cross-allergenic' with the penicillins, but as with cephalothin and cephaloridine (page 208), 'cross-allergy' may occasionally be encountered. Published data indicate that 91 to 94 per cent of patients with a history of penicillin-allergy have not reacted to cephalexin, cephalothin or cephaloridine (page 209); therefore the risk appears to be small (Dash, 1975).

3. *Nephrotoxicity.* In view of the known nephrotoxicity of cephaloridine (page 210), renal function has been studied carefully in many patients receiving cephalexin, but evidence of renal impairment is rare (Kabins *et al.*, 1970). In addition, the drug does not appear to aggravate pre-existing renal disease

(Kunin and Finkelberg, 1970). Haematuria and eosinophilia occurred in two patients with bacterial endocarditis who were treated with very high oral cephalexin doses (20 or 24 g per day plus probenecid); one patient also developed a transient elevation of serum creatinine. All abnormalities disappeared when cephalexin was ceased (Verma and Kieff, 1975).

4. *Haematological side-effects*. A positive Coombs test has been reported with cephalexin therapy (Erikssen *et al.*, 1970). As with other cephalosporins (page 211) the clinical significance of this is not clear. Coombs positive haemolytic anaemia is rare. Forbes *et al.* (1972) described a 14-year-old haemophiliac patient who developed severe intravascular haemolysis nine days after starting cephalexin in a dose of 2 g daily. Haemolysis ceased after cephalexin was stopped.

5. *Neurotoxicity*. Like cephaloridine (page 211), cephalexin may occasionally cause central nervous system disturbances. Diplopia, headache, tinnitus and an unstable gait occurred in one patient, and these symptoms gradually disappeared within two weeks after cessation of the drug (Erikssen *et al.*, 1970). Similar symptoms were observed in another patient by Kind *et al.* (1969). If very high serum levels of cephalexin are reached, convulsions and coma may result. Saker *et al.* (1973) described a patient with severe renal disease treated by cephalexin, who developed a grand mal seizure which was followed by disorientation lasting for over a week. The drug was given in a dose of 2 g daily and its serum level prior to the seizure was 120 μg per ml.

6. *Changes in gut flora*. Gaya *et al.* (1970) reported that some hospital patients treated with cephalexin had high concentrations of Ps. aeruginosa in the faeces. However all antibiotics in the gastro-intestinal tract alter the gut flora, and such changes are likely to be more profound with tetracyclines than cephalexin (Dash and Gower, 1970). In addition, colonization of the gut with environmental strains of Ps. aeruginosa and other Gram-negative bacilli is a common occurrence in hospitalized patients.

7. *Side-effects from parenteral cephalexin*. This preparation has been well tolerated in clinical trials to date. Intramuscular injections are painful, and this can be avoided by dissolving cephalexin in lignocaine hydrochloride (Hughes *et al.*, 1974; Svensson and Seeberg, 1974).

8. *Effects on fetus*. Cephalexin has been administered as early as the second month of pregnancy without evidence of fetal damage (Goodspeed, 1975).

Clinical Uses of the Drug

A. *Oral Cephalexin*

Extensive clinical trials have shown that this drug is satisfactory for some conditions in which parenteral cephalosporins (page 213) are used, provided that the use of an oral antibiotic is not contraindicated. However, compared to cephalothin, cephalexin has an inferior antibacterial activity against most bacterial species (page 225).

1. *Streptococcal and pneumococcal infections*. Cephalexin is an alternative to the oral phenoxypenicillins (page 60) for the treatment of relatively mild infections due to these organisms, particularly in penicillin-allergic patients. It has been used successfully for Strep. pyogenes throat and soft tissue infections (Azimi *et al.*, 1972; Stillerman *et al.*, 1972; Solberg *et al.*, 1972; Matsen *et al.*,

1974) and pneumococcal pneumonia (Rosenthal *et al.*, 1971). Two patients with bacterial endocarditis (one Strep. pyogenes and the other Strep. viridans), in whom oral cephalexin was successful, have been reported (Stratford, 1970). In these more severe infections parenteral chemotherapy is indicated and if penicillin G cannot be used, cephaloridine or cephalothin may be suitable (page 213).

2. *Other respiratory tract infections.* Cephalexin has been used for bronchitis, bronchopneumonia and otitis media (Nassar and Allen, 1974). The bacterial aetiology of these infections cannot always be easily determined, especially in children (Donnison and Davison, 1970), and poor results with cephalexin may be expected especially if H. influenzae is the pathogen. For instance, cephalexin is not suitable for the treatment of otitis media due to H. influenzae (Stechenberg *et al.*, 1977). In general, antibiotics other than cephalexin (page 115) are preferable for the treatment of all of these infections.

3. *Staphylococcal infections.* Minor staphylococcal infections such as skin and soft tissue sepsis can be satisfactorily treated by cephalexin (Kind *et al.*, 1969; Henning *et al.*, 1970). Chronic staphylococcal osteomyelitis has been managed by administering large doses of oral cephalexin for a prolonged period (Hedlund, 1970). One patient with endocarditis due to Staph. epidermidis was cured by oral cephalexin, given in a dose of 6 g daily for one month (Zabransky *et al.*, 1969). Despite this success parenteral antibiotics are preferable for bacterial endocarditis.

4. *Urinary tract infections.* The drug has been used extensively for these infections (Kind *et al.*, 1969; Fairley, 1970; Glass, 1973). It is reasonably effective in eradicating relatively sensitive strains of Esch. coli, Pr. mirabilis and Klebsiella spp. (Clark and Turck, 1969). Cephalexin appears to be about as effective as ampicillin for the treatment of these infections (Davies *et al.*, 1971). In a study of 100 women with urinary tract infections, cephalexin in a dose of 1 g twice daily was found to be significantly inferior to co-trimoxazole (page 706), administered in a dose of two standard tablets twice a day, both regimens given for one week (Gower and Tasker, 1976). Cephalexin is more slowly bactericidal to Enterobacteriaceae than other beta-lactam antibiotics, and it is also somewhat susceptible to beta-lactamases produced by Gram-negative bacilli. These and other factors (page 706) may explain the superior performance of co-trimoxazole compared to cephalexin in urinary tract infections (Greenwood and O'Grady, 1976).

Relatively resistant strains of Esch. coli, Pr. mirabilis and Klebisella spp. are often encountered in urinary tract infections, but urine levels inhibitory to the majority of these strains can be attained with usual oral doses of cephalexin (Levison *et al.*, 1969). Similar to the use of other chemotherapeutic agents, in patients with predisposition to urinary tract infections, relapses or reinfections are common after cephalexin treatment (Guttmann, 1970). Some selected patients with relapsing urinary tract infections may benefit from long-term, low dose cephalexin administration (Cox and Montgomery, 1971; Fairley *et al.*, 1971). A dose as low as 125 mg nightly appears to be efficient in preventing recurrent urinary tract infections (Gower, 1975).

5. *Venereal diseases.* Cephalexin is reasonably satisfactory for the treatment of uncomplicated gonorrhoea (Willcox and Woodcock, 1970) and even

for some cases of gonococcal septicaemia (Henning *et al.*, 1970). Nevertheless parenteral cephaloridine appears to be superior for this disease (Oller *et al.*, 1970). The use of either cephaloridine or cephalexin will probably be limited in this disease as penicillin G remains the drug of choice (page 36). The penicillinase-producing gonococci (page 8) are somewhat sensitive to cephalexin *in vitro* (page 226), but other drugs are preferred for the treatment of infections due to these strains (pages 319, 589).

Unlike intramuscular cephaloridine (page 215), oral cephalexin is unsatisfactory for the treatment of primary and secondary syphilis (Duncan and Knox, 1971).

6. *Shigella infections*. Cephalexin has been tried in patients with Shigella dysentery, caused by ampicillin-resistant organisms. Results were unsatisfactory, and cephalexin cannot be recommended for shigellosis (Nelson and Haltalin, 1975).

B. *Parenteral Cephalexin*

Hughes *et al.* (1974) treated 20 patients, the majority of whom had either urinary tract infections following prostatectomy or pulmonary infections, by intramuscular or intravenous cephalexin in a dose of 1·0 g every six hours. Results of treatment were satisfactory in most patients. Svensson and Seeberg (1974) used parenteral cephalexin to treat staphylococcal infections such as chronic osteomyelitis, soft tissue and wound infections and septicaemia. Satisfactory clinical improvement occurred in most patients and side-effects of treatment were minimal.

REFERENCES

Azimi, P. H., Cramblett, H. G., Del Rosario, A. J., Kronfol, H., Haynes, R. E. and Hilty, M. D. (1972), 'Cephalexin: Treatment of streptococcal pharyngitis', *J. Pediatrics*, **80**, 1042.

Bailey, R. R., Gower, P. E. and Dash, C. H. (1970), 'The effect of impairment of renal function and haemodialysis on serum and urine levels of cephalexin', *Postgrad. Med. J.* (Suppl.), **46**, 60.

Bennett, W. M., Singer, I., Golper, T., Feig, P. and Coggins, C. J. (1977), 'Guidelines for drug therapy in renal failure', *Ann. Intern. Med.*, **86**, 754.

Braun, P., Tillotson, J. R., Wilcox, C. and Finland, M. (1968), 'Cephalexin and cephaloglycin activity *in vitro* and absorption and urinary excretion of single oral doses in normal young adults', *Appl. Microbiol.*, **16**, 1684.

Busch, D. F., Kureshi, L. A., Sutter, V. L. and Finegold, S. M. (1976), 'Susceptibility of respiratory tract anaerobes to orally administered penicillins and cephalosporins', *Antimicrob. Ag. Chemother.*, **10**, 713.

Butcher, R. H., Dawborn, J. K. and Pattison, G. (1972), 'Blood and urine levels of cephalexin in patients with impaired renal function', *Med. J. Aust.*, **2**, 1282.

Clark, H. and Turck, M. (1969), '*In vitro* and *in vivo* evaluation of cephalexin', *Antimicrob. Agents Chemother.*—1968. p. 296.

Cox, C. E. and Montgomery, W. G. (1971), 'Cephalosporin therapy of urinary tract infections', *Postgrad. Med. J.* (Suppl.), **47**, 107.

Dash, C. H. and Gower, P. E. (1970), 'Gut flora after cephalexin', *Brit. med. J.*, **4**, 181.

Dash, C. H. (1975), 'Penicillin allergy and the cephalosporins', *J. Antimicrob. Chemother.*, **1** (Suppl.), 107.

Davies, J. A., Strangeways, J. E. M., Mitchell, R. G., Beilin, L. J., Ledingham, J. G. G. and Holt, J. M. (1971), 'Comparative double-blind trial of cephalexin and ampicillin in treatment of urinary infections', *Brit. med. J.*, **3**. 215.

Davies, J. A. and Holt, J. M. (1972), 'Clinical pharmacology of cephalexin administered by intravenous injection', *J. clin. Path.*, **25**, 518.

Davies, J. A. and Holt, J. M. (1975), 'Absorption of cephalexin in diseased and aged subjects', *J. Antimicrob. Chemother.*, **1**, (Suppl.) 69.

Donnison, A. B. and Davison, C. E. (1970), 'Cephalexin in paediatric infections', *Postgrad. Med. J.* (Suppl.), **46**, 93.

Duncan, W. C. and Knox, J. M. (1971, 'Cephalosporin antibiotics in venereal disease', *Postgrad. Med. J.* (Suppl.), **47**, 119.

Erikssen, J., Midtvedt, T. and Bergan, T. (1970), 'Treatment of urinary tract infections with cephalexin', *Scand. J. Infect. Dis.*, **2**, 53.

Fairley, K. F. (1970), 'Cephalexin in recurrent urinary tract infection', *Postgrad. Med. J.* (Suppl.), **46**, 24.

Fairley, K. F., Hubbard, M. and Whitworth, J. A. (1974), 'Prophylactic long-term cephalexin in recurrent urinary infection', *Med. J. Aust.*, **1**, 318.

Forbes, C. D., Craig, J. A., Mitchell, R. and McNicol, G. P. (1972), 'Acute intravascular haemolysis associated with cephalexin therapy', *Postgrad. Med. J.*, **48**, 186.

Gaya, H., Adnitt, P. I. and Turner, P. (1970), 'Changes in gut flora after cephalexin treatment', *Brit. med. J.*, **3**, 624.

Glass, R. D. (1973), 'Cephalexin in the treatment of urinary infection in childhood', *Med. J. Aust.*, **1**, 793.

Goodspeed, A. H. (1975), 'Cephalexin in special cases', *J. Antimicrob. Chemother.*, **1**, (Suppl.) 105.

Gower, P. E., Dash, C. H. and O'Callaghan, C. H. (1973), 'Serum and blood concentration of sodium cephalexin in man given single intramuscular and intravenous injections', *J. Pharm. Pharmac.*, **25**, 376.

Gower, P. E. (1975), 'The use of small doses of cephalexin (125 mg) in the management of recurrent urinary tract infection in women', *J. Antimicrob. Chemother.*, **1**, (Suppl.) 93.

Gower, P. E. and Tasker, P. R. W. (1976), 'Comparative double-blind study of cephalexin and co-trimoxazole in urinary tract infections', *Brit. med. J.*, **1**, 684.

Greenwood, D. and O'Grady, F. (1976), 'Co-trimoxazole and cephalexin in urinary tract infection', *Brit. med. J.*, **1**, 1073.

Griffith, R. S. and Black, H. R. (1968), 'Cephalexin: A new antibiotic', *Clinical Medicine*, **75**, 14.

Griffith, R. S. and Black, H. R. (1970), 'Cephalexin', *Med. Clin. North America*, **54**, 1229.

Griffith, R. S. and Black, H. R. (1971), 'Blood, urine and tissue concentrations of the cephalosporin antibiotics in normal subjects', *Postgrad. Med. J.* (Suppl.), **47**, 32.

Guttmann, D. (1970), 'Cephalexin in chronic and recurrent urinary infections: Laboratory and clinical studies', *Postgrad. Med. J.* (Suppl.), **46**, 75.

Halprin, G. M. and McMahon, S. M. (1973), 'Cephalexin concentrations in sputum during acute respiratory infections', *Antimicrob. Ag. Chemother.*, **3**, 703.

Hedlund, P. (1970), 'Clinical evaluation of cephalexin in staphylococcal infections', *Postgrad. Med. J.* (Suppl.), **46**, 152.

Henning, C., Kallings, L. O., Lidman, K. and Sterner, G. (1970), 'Studies of absorption, excretion, antibacterial and clini al effect of cephalexin', *Scand. J. Infect. Dis.*, **2**, 131.

Hughes, S. P. F., Hurst, L. and Dash, C. H. (1974), 'Parenteral cephalexin in a general surgical unit', *Brit. J. Clin. Pract.*, **28**, 51.

Johnson, W. D., Applestein, J. M. and Kaye, D. (1968), 'Cephaloglycin. Clinical and laboratory experience with an orally administered cephalosporin', *JAMA*, **206**, 2698.

Kabins, S. A., Kelner, B., Waltone, E. and Goldstein, E. (1970), 'Cephalexin therapy as related to renal function', *Amer. J. Med. Sci.*, **259**, 133.

Kayser, F. H. (1971), '*In vitro* activity of cephalosporin antibiotics against Gram-positive bacteria', *Postgrad. Med. J.* (Suppl.), **47**, 14.

Kind, A. C., Kestle, D. G., Standiford, H. C. and Kirby, W. M. M. (1969), 'Laboratory and clinical experience with cephalexin', *Antimicrob. Agents Chemother.*—1968, p. 361.

Konforti, N. and Halperin, E. (1975), 'Sensitivities of strains of enteropathogenic Escherichia coli to cephalexin and other antibiotics', *Amer. J. Clin. Path.*, **64**, 121.

Kunin, C. M. and Finkelberg, Z. (1970), 'Oral cephalexin and ampicillin: Antimicrobial activity, recovery in urine, and persistence in blood of uremic patients', *Ann. Intern. Med.*, **72**, 349.

Lacey, R. W. and Stokes, A. (1977), 'Susceptibility of the 'penicillinase-resistant' penicillins and cephalosporins to penicillinase of Staphylococcus aureus', *J. clin. Path.*, **30**, 35.

Levision, M. E., Johnson, W. D., Thornhill, T. S. and Kaye, D. (1969), 'Clinical and *in vitro* evaluation of cephalexin', *JAMA*, **209**, 1331.

Linquist, J. A., Siddiqui, J. Y. and Smith, I. M. (1970), 'Cephalexin in patients with renal disease', *New Engl. J. Med.*, **283**, 720.

De Maine, J. B. and Kirby, W. M. M. (1971), 'Clinical pharmacology of cephalexin administered intravenously', *Antimicrob. Agents Chemother.*—1970, p. 190.

Marget, W. (1971), 'Special aspects of cephalosporin therapy in infants and children', *Postgrad. Med. J.* (Suppl.), **47**, 54.

Matsen, J. M., Torstenson, O., Siegel, S. E. and Bacaner, H. (1974), 'Use of available dosage forms of cephalexin in clinical comparison with phenoxymethyl penicillin and benzathine penicillin in the treatment of streptococcal pharyngitis in children', *Antimicrob. Ag. Chemother.*, **6**, 501.

Meyers, B. R., Kaplan, K. and Weinstein, L. (1969), 'Cephalexin: Microbiological effects and pharmacologic parameters in man', *Clin. Pharm. Ther.*, **10**, 810.

Muggleton, P. W., O'Callaghan, C. H., Foord, R. D., Kirby, S. M. and Ryan, D. M. (1969), 'Laboratory appraisal of cephalexin', *Antimicrob. Agents Chemother.*—1968, p. 353.

Nassar, W. Y. and Allen, B. M. (1974), 'A double-blind comparative clinical trial of cephalexin and ampicillin in the treatment of childhood acute otitis media', *Curr. Med. Res. Opin.*, **2**, 198.

Nelson, J. D. and Haltalin, K. C. (1975), 'Comparative efficacy of cephalexin and ampicillin for shigellosis and other types of acute diarrhoea in infants and children', *Antimicrob. Ag. Chemother.*, **7**, 415.

Nicholas, P., Meyers, B. R. and Hirschman, S. Z. (1973), 'Cephalexin: Pharmacologic evaluation following oral and parenteral administration', *J. Clin. Pharmicol.*, **13**, 463.

O'Callaghan, C. H. and Kirby, S. M. (1970), 'Some cephalosporins in clinical use and their structure-activity relationship', *Postgrad. Med. J.* (Suppl.), **46**, 9.

Oller, L. Z., Smith, H. G. and Marshall, M. J. (1970), 'Cephaloridine and cephalexin in venereological practice', *Postgrad. Med. J.* (Suppl.), **46**, 99.

Parsons, R. L., Hossack, G. and Paddock, G. (1975), 'The absorption of antibiotics in adult patients with coeliac disease', *J. Antimicrob. Chemother.*, **1**, 39.

Parsons, R. L. and Paddock, G. M. (1975), 'Absorption of two antibacterial drugs, cephalexin and co-trimoxazole, in malabsorption syndromes', *J. Antimicrob. Chemother.*, **1**, (Suppl.) 59.

Perkins, R. L., Carlisle, H. N. and Saslaw, S. (1968), 'Cephalexin: *In vitro* bacterial susceptibility, absorption in volunteers, and antibacterial activity of sera and urine',

CEPHALEXIN AND CEPHALOGLYCIN

Amer. J. Med. Sci., **256,** 122.

Pitt, J., Siasoco, R., Kaplan, K. and Weinstein, L. (1968), 'Antimicrobial activity and pharmacological behaviour of cephaloglycin', *Antimicrob. Agents Chemother.*—1967, p. 630.

Rosenthal, I. M., Metzger, W. A. and Laxminarayana, M. S. (1971), 'Treatment of pneumonia in childhood with cephalexin', *Postgrad. Med. J.* (Suppl.), **47,** 51.

Russell, A. D. and Fountain, R. H. (1971), 'Aspects of the mechanism of action of some cephalosporins', *J. Bacteriol.*, **106,** 65.

Sabath, L. D., Garner, C., Wilcox, C. and Finland, M. (1975), 'Effect of inoculum and of beta-lactamase on the anti-staphylococcal activity of thirteen penicillins and cephalosporins', *Antimicrob. Ag. Chemother.*, **8,** 344.

Saker, B. M., Musk, A. W., Haywood, E. F. and Hurst, P. E. (1973), 'Reversible toxic psychosis after cephalexin', *Med. J. Aust.*, **1,** 497.

Sales, J. E. L., Sutcliffe, M. and O'Grady, F. (1972), 'Cephalexin levels in human bile in presence of biliary tract disease', *Brit. med. J.*, **3,** 441.

Selwyn, S. and Bakhtiar, M. (1977), 'Penicillin-resistant gonococci', *Brit. med. J.*, **2,** 118.

Solberg, C. O., Schreiner, A. and Digranes, A. (1972), 'Cephalexin therapy of lower respiratory tract, soft tissue and bone infections', *Scand. J. Infect. Dis.*, **4,** 241.

Stechenberg, B. W., Anderson, D., Chang, M. J., Dunkle, L., Wong, M., Van Reken, D., Pickering, L. K., and Feigin, R. D. (1977), 'Cephalexin compared to ampicillin treatment of otitis media', *Pediatrics*, **58,** 532.

Stillerman, M., Isenberg, H. D. and Moody, M. (1972), 'Streptococcal pharyngitis therapy. Comparison of cephalexin, phenoxymethyl-penicillin, and ampicillin', *Amer. J. Dis. Child.*, **123,** 457.

Stratford, B. C. (1970), 'Clinicolaboratory experience with cephalexin', *Postgrad. Med. J.* (Suppl.), **46,** 138.

Svensson, R. and Seeberg, S. (1974), 'Clinical evaluation of parenteral cephalexin sodium', *Scand. J. Infect. Dis.*, **6,** 279.

Sykes, R. B. and Matthew, M. (1976), 'The beta-lactamases of Gram-negative bacteria and their role in resistance to beta-lactam antibiotics', *J. Antimicrob. Chemother.*, **2,** 115.

Tally, F. P., Jacobus, N. V., Bartlett, J. G. and Gorbach, S. L. (1975), 'Susceptibility of anaerobes to cefoxitin and other cephalosporins', *Antimicrob. Ag. Chemother.*, **7,** 128.

Tetzlaff, T. R., McCracken, G. H., Jr. and Thomas, M. L. (1978), 'Bioavailability of cephalexin in children: Relationship to drug formulations and meals', *J. Pediatrics*, **92,** 292.

Verma, S. and Kieff, E. (1975), 'Cephalexin-related nephropathy', *JAMA*, **234,** 618.

Waterworth, P. M. (1971), 'The susceptibility of pathogenic Gram-negative bacilli to cephalosporins', *Postgrad. Med. J.* (Suppl.), **47,** 25.

Wick, W. E. (1967), 'Cephalexin, a new orally absorbed cephalosporin antibiotic', *Appl. Microbiol.*, **15,** 765.

Willcox, R. R. and Woodcock, K. S. (1970), 'Cephalexin in the oral treatment of gonorrhoea by a double-dose method', *Postgrad. Med. J.* (Suppl.), **46,** 103.

Zabransky, R. J., Gardner, M. A. and Geraci, J. E. (1969), 'Cephalexin: Preliminary *in vitro* studies of a new orally administered cephalosporin and report of a case of en-docarditis cured with cephalexin', *Mayo Clin. Proc.*, **44,** 876.

Cephazolin, Cephacetrile, Cephapirin, Cephanone, Ceftezole, BL-S786 and FR 10024

Description

Many compounds have been derived from the cephalosporin C nucleus in an attempt to produce antibiotics with significant advantages over the older parenteral cephalosporins, cephalothin and cephaloridine (page 199) or over oral cephalexin (page 225). Some of these newer cephalosporins are already in clinical use, others are still undergoing clinical trials, while for some only *in vitro* data are available.

The new cephalosporins described in this chapter are grouped together because they can only be administered parenterally and their antibacterial spectrum is rather similar to that of cephalothin (page 199).

1. *Cephazolin*. This has many similarities to both cephalothin and cephaloridine (Wick and Preston, 1972), but it produces higher serum levels than both of these drugs, and its intramuscular administration is less painful than that of cephalothin (Ishiyama *et al.*, 1971; Ries *et al.*, 1973; Kirby and Regamey, 1973). It is marketed with the trade names of 'Ancef' (Smith, Kline and French) and 'Kefzol' (Lilly).

2. *Cephacetrile (Ciba 36278-Ba)*. Chemically this is 7-cyanacetamido-cephalosporanic acid. It is rather similar to cephalothin, but after intravenous administration higher peak serum levels are attained, and its plasma half-life is more prolonged (Brogard *et al.*, 1973a and b; Hodges *et al.*, 1973). Cephacetrile is marketed as 'Celospor' (Ciba).

3. *Cephapirin*. The chemical formula of this drug is 7-(pyrid-4-yl-thioacetamido) cephalosporonate. It is also very similar to cephalothin, and the pain produced by intramuscular injection of both of these drugs is the same (Bran *et al.*, 1972). The initial impression that intravenous administration of cephapirin may cause less thrombophlebitis than cephalothin (Lane *et al.*, 1972), has not been confirmed (Carrizosa *et al.*, 1973; Robson and Bowmer, 1974). Cephapirin is marketed by Bristol with the trade names of 'Cefadyl' and 'Cefatrexyl'.

4. *Cephanone*. It has similarities to cephalothin, but after both intravenous and intramuscular administration, cephanone produces serum levels which are about four times higher and more prolonged (Meyers *et al.*, 1972; Regamey and Kirby, 1973; Fare *et al.*, 1974).

5. *Ceftezole*. This has an antimicrobial activity similar to that of cephazolin. It differs from cephazolin in that its binding to serum proteins is less, and it is more rapidly excreted via the kidney so that lower serum levels are produced which are less sustained (Nishida *et al.*, 1976). Data from clinical trials are not yet available.

238

6. *BL-S786*. Similar to ceftezole, clinical information about this new drug is not yet available. It is more active than cephalothin against most Gram-negative bacteria, but is somewhat less active against Gram-positive pathogens. After intramuscular administration to mice, high serum levels are attained and its half-life is longer than that of cephalothin, cephaloridine and cephazolin (Leitner *et al.*, 1976).

7. *FR 10024*. Apparently this is more active than cephalothin against certain Gram-negative bacteria and its serum levels after intramuscular injection are twice as high as those attained by cephalothin. It has been reported to be excreted in high concentrations in the bile of experimental animals (Nishida *et al.*, 1977). Data from clinical trials are not yet available.

The following details only apply to cephazolin, cephacetrile, cephapirin and cephanone.

Sensitive Organisms

The antibacterial spectra of these antibiotics are similar, and in general resemble that of cephalothin (page 199).

1. *Gram-positive cocci*. These cephalosporins are active against Staph. pyogenes, including penicillin-resistant, but not methicillin-resistant strains. Stability of cephacetrile to staphylococcal penicillinase is similar to that of cephalothin (page 199) but cephapirin is somewhat more easily hydrolysed; cephazolin is even more vulnerable to the enzyme but not to the same degree as cephaloridine (page 199) (Sabath *et al.*, 1975; Regamey *et al.*, 1975; Farrar and Gramling, 1976; Fong *et al.*, 1976; Lacey and Stokes, 1977).

Most other Gram-positive cocci such as Staph. epidermidis, Strep. pyogenes, Strep. pneumoniae and the alpha-haemolytic streptococci of the 'viridans' group are sensitive, but Strep. faecalis is usually moderately resistant (Axelrod *et al.*, 1971; Knüsel *et al.*, 1971; Wick and Preston, 1972; Meyers *et al.*, 1972; Brogard *et al.*, 1973a; Motley and Shadomy, 1974; Shadomy *et al.*, 1974; Hamilton-Miller, 1974). At clinically achievable concentrations cephazolin and gentamicin act synergistically against Strep. faecalis *in vitro*, and it has been suggested that in penicillin-allergic patients this combination may be considered for treatment of Strep. faecalis infections (Bourque *et al.*, 1976).

Anaerobic Gram-positive cocci such as Peptococcus and Peptostreptococcus spp. are usually sensitive to these cephalosporins (Tally *et al.*, 1975; Sutter and Finegold, 1975).

2. *Gram-positive bacilli*. B. anthracis, C. diphtheriae and Listeria monocytogenes are usually sensitive. Anaerobes such as Cl. perfringens, Cl. tetani and other Clostridium spp. are also sensitive (Tally *et al.*, 1975; Sutter and Finegold, 1975).

3. *Gram-negative aerobic bacteria*. The Neisseria spp. (meningococci and gonococci) are usually sensitive. Cephazolin may be quite active against gonococcal strains which are relatively resistant to penicillin G (page 7) (Phillips *et al.*, 1976), but this drug and cephacetrile, cephapirin and cephanone are all inactive against penicillinase-producing gonococci (page 8). The latter organisms, however, are inhibited by some other cephalosporins such as cefuroxime (page 272), which possess an increased resistance to beta-lactamases produced by Gram-negative bacteria.

Salmonella and Shigella spp., H. influenzae and B. pertussis are usually sensitive. Esch. coli, Kl. pneumoniae and Proteus mirabilis are commonly sensitive unless they are derived from a hospital environment. Other species of Klebsiella, such as Kl. aerogenes are frequently resistant. Species of Proteus other than mirabilis, Enterobacter and Providencia spp., Serratia marcescens and Pseudomonas aeruginosa are always resistant (Axelrod et al., 1971; Ries et al., 1973; Brogard et al., 1973a; Motley and Shadomy, 1974; Shadomy et al., 1974; Yourassowsky et al., 1976; Verbist, 1976). Cephazolin and amikacin (page 379) often show in vitro synergism against Klebsiella spp. strains (Klastersky et al., 1976).

4. *Gram-negative anaerobic bacteria*. Bacteroides fragilis is highly resistant, but other Bacteroides spp., especially B. melaninogenicus, and the Fusobacterium and Veillonella spp. are usually sensitive to these cephalosporins (Tally et al., 1975).

5. *Differences in antibacterial activity*. Cephacetrile has been reported to be slightly less active against most bacteria than cephalothin (Leading article, 1973), but other investigators have found the two drugs virtually identical (Isenberg et al., 1973). Cephacetrile may be more active than cephalothin against Strep. faecalis (Edselius, 1976). The activities of cephapirin (Axelrod et al., 1971; Bran et al., 1972) and cephanone (Meyers et al., 1972) are almost identical to that of cephalothin. Cephazolin has much the same activity as cephalothin against Gram-positive cocci and Proteus mirabilis, but it is more active against Esch. coli, Kl. pneumoniae and the salmonellae (Ries et al., 1973; Sabath et al., 1973; Bergeron et al., 1973; Greenwood et al., 1975; Strausbaugh et al., 1978).

6. *Acquired resistance*. There is almost complete cross-resistance between these four drugs and cephalothin (Verbist, 1976). Of a hundred cephalothin-resistant strains of Gram-negative bacilli studied by Phair et al. (1972), with the exception of some Esch. coli strains, all were resistant to cephazolin. Occasionally cephalothin-resistant Esch. coli, Klebsiella and Enterobacter strains may be sensitive to cephazolin or to cephapirin (Kisch and Bartholomew, 1976; Jones and Fuchs, 1976).

In Vitro Sensitivities

The minimum inhibitory concentrations of cephazolin, cephacetrile and cephapirin against some selected bacterial species, are compared to those of cephalothin in Table 18.

Mode of Administration and Dosage

These four cephalosporins can only be administered parenterally and each can be given either intramuscularly or intravenously in the same dosage.

1. *Cephazolin*. This is commonly administered intramuscularly, and the usual adult dosage is 0·5 g every eight hours (Reller et al., 1973). The total daily dose can be varied widely according to the nature and severity of infection. Daily doses ranging from 1·0 to 4·0 g (occasionally up to 6·0 g), administered in two, three or four divided doses have been used (Ries et al., 1973; Reinarz et al., 1973). Like cephaloridine (page 202), cephazolin causes less

TABLE 18

Compiled from data published by Axelrod *et al.* (1971), Knüsel *et al.* (1971), Wick and Preston (1972), Brogard *et al.* (1973a), Hamilton-Miller (1974) and Tally *et al.* (1975).

ORGANISM	MIC (μg per ml)			
	Cephalothin	Cephazolin	Cephacetrile	Cephapirin
Gram-positive bacteria				
Staph. pyogenes (non-penicillinase producer)	0.25	0.5	0.4–3.0	0.18
Staph. pyogenes (penicillinase producer)	0.5	0.5	0.4–3.0	0.37
Staph. epidermidis	0.12–0.5	0.25–0.5	—	0.135
Strep. pyogenes (Group A)	0.06–0.12	0.12	0.1–0.3	0.09
Strep. pneumoniae (Dip. pneumoniae)	0.12–0.25	0.12–0.25	<0.1	<0.045
Strep. viridans	0.5	0.5–1.0	—	0.135
Strep. faecalis (Enterococcus, Group D)	16.0–32.0	32.0	4.0–25.0	25.0
Gram-negative bacteria				
Escherichia coli	4.0–32.0	2.0–4.0	5.0	12.5
Klebsiella spp.	1.0–2.0	1.0–2.0	4.0–7.0	6.2
Proteus mirabilis	4.0–8.0	8.0	10.0	12.5
Proteus vulgaris	>100.0	>100.0	>100.0	>100.0
Bacteroides fragilis	64.0	64.0	—	—

pain on intramuscular injection than cephalothin, and also thrombophlebitis is not a major problem when the drug is used intravenously (Reller *et al.*, 1973; Shemonsky *et al.*, 1975).

Cephazolin can be administered intravenously by either continuous infusion, intermittent infusions (via a paediatric buretrol or separate secondary intravenous bottles), or by direct intravenous injections. The continuous infusion method may have some pharmacological advantages; when resultant serum levels are graphed, the area under the curve is greater with continuous infusion and also biliary levels are more sustained (Thys *et al.*, 1976). However incompatibility and drug inactivation problems may arise if cephazolin is added to intravenous solution bottles (*see* pages 13, 106), and in general the intermittent infusion method, as with methicillin (page 68) is preferable.

The dosage for children is 25–50 mg per kg body weight per day, divided into three or four divided doses (Pickering *et al.*, 1973). Total daily dosage may be increased to 100 mg per kg per day for the treatment of severe infections. For newborn and premature infants a dose of 20 mg per kg every 12 h is recommended (McCracken and Nelson, 1977).

Patients with renal failure require dosage reduction and serum level monitoring (Levison *et al.*, 1973; Benner *et al.*, 1975; Madhavan *et al.*, 1975). All adults with renal failure should receive an initial loading dose of 0·5 g. Thereafter those with mild to moderate renal failure (creatinine clearance 40–60 ml per min) may be given 60 per cent of the normal daily dose in two divided doses. The dose for patients with moderate renal failure (creatinine clearance 20–40 ml per min) is 25–35 per cent of the normal daily dose, given in two divided doses. In severe renal failure (creatinine clearance 5–20 ml per min), a dose of approximately 10 per cent of the normal daily one administered as a single dose every 24 h is recommended. For patients with essentially no renal function (creatinine clearance <5 ml per min) only 5 per cent of the normal daily dose should be given, as a single dose once every 24 h.

Cephazolin is removed relatively slowly by haemodialysis and over four hours about 46 per cent of an administered dose is removed (Madhavan *et al.*, 1976). Therefore for anephric patients undergoing twice-weekly haemodialysis, an extra dose of 250 mg at end of each dialysis is recommended (Levison *et al.*, 1973; McCloskey *et al.*, 1973). Cephazolin is not removed by peritoneal dialysis so that additional dosing is not needed during this procedure (Levison *et al.*, 1973; Madhavan *et al.*, 1976).

2. *Cephacetrile.* Intramuscular or intravenous administration is suitable for this drug, but like cephalothin it causes pain and induration when injected intramuscularly (Hodges *et al.*, 1973). Thrombophlebitis with intravenous use also can be a problem. The adult dose is 3–6 g daily in three or four divided doses. The dosage for children is 50–100 mg per kg body weight per day (Di Nola and Soranzo, 1976).

For patients with renal failure the following dosage schedules have been recommended (Brogard *et al.*, 1973a); in moderate renal failure (creatinine clearance 30–80 ml per min) a dose of 1·0 g every 12 h; in severe renal failure (creatinine clearance <30 ml per min) a dose of 1·0–1·5 g every 24 h. In anephric patients treated by haemodialysis a dose of 1·0 g at the beginning and again at the end of dialysis, and 1·0 g every 30 h between dialyses, should be used.

3. *Cephapirin*. This has been used in adults in doses varying from 2·0 to 8·0 g per day, administered in four or six divided doses, either intravenously or intramuscularly (Bran *et al.*, 1972). Occasionally, doses as high as 18 g daily intravenously, have been given (Robson and Bowmer, 1974). A commonly used adult dose is 0·5–1·0 g administered every six hours (Wiesner *et al.*, 1972). Cephapirin causes pain on intramuscular injection. It was reported by some authors to cause less pain and thrombophlebitis than cephalothin, when administered by the intravenous route (Bran *et al.*, 1972; Lane *et al.*, 1972; Siebert *et al.*, 1976), but others have found no difference between these two drugs (Carrizosa *et al.*, 1973; Robson and Bowmer, 1974). Buffered cephalothin (page 204) may even cause less phlebitis than cephapirin (Berger *et al.*, 1976).

Similar to cephalothin (page 204), the dose reduction of cephapirin for patients with renal failure is less than that needed with the other cephalosporins. A dose of 1·0 g (15–18 mg per kg body weight) every 12 h, has been recommended for patients with severe renal failure (serum creatinine higher than 6 mg per cent or 0·5 mmol/l). In patients undergoing chronic haemodialysis the same dose can be given just prior to dialysis and every 12 h thereafter (McCloskey *et al.*, 1972).

However when Gram-positive infections are treated, adequate serum levels of cephapirin (combined unchanged and deacetylated drug) can be maintained for 48 h between dialyses without further drug administration. Therefore it is satisfactory and convenient to treat dialysis patients by doses of cephapirin (50 mg per kg body weight), administered only during the first and last half hours of haemodialysis (Berman *et al.*, 1978). As with cephalothin (page 204), the deacetylated drug has satisfactory activity against Gram-positive, but not against Gram-negative organisms. Cephapirin, like cephalothin (page 204), is removed from the serum by haemodialysis.

4. *Cephanone*. Intramuscular or intravenous administration may be used with this cephalosporin, but the best dosage schedules have not been determined. Pharmacological studies in humans indicate that a dose of 0·5 g (7 mg per kg body weight), administered either eight- or twelve-hourly may be suitable (Meyers *et al.*, 1972; Regamey and Kirby, 1973).

Serum Levels in Relation to Dosage

1. *Cephazolin*. A peak level as high as 34 μg per ml is attained one hour after a 0·5 g intramuscular dose, and six hours later the level is about 6·0 μg per ml (Ishiyama *et al.*, 1971). These levels are about twice as high as those after cephaloridine and four times as high as those after cephalothin (page 205). In addition, measurable levels of cephazolin may still be present 12 h after this dose (Ries *et al.*, 1973). Doubling the dose usually doubles the serum concentrations (Cahn *et al.*, 1974). After intravenous infusion of 0·5 g cephazolin over a 20 min period, a peak serum level of 118 μg per ml is obtained, and a detectable level is still present eight hours later (Kirby and Regamey, 1973). When a 1·5 g dose of cephazolin is injected intravenously over a three minute period, the peak serum level five minutes after the injection is 206 μg per ml. If 6 g of cephazolin is administered by a continuous infusion over 24 h (using a constant infusion device), a stable serum level of 52 μg per

ml is maintained. In one study the area under the curve (graph of serum levels against time) associated with such continuous infusion, was 24 per cent greater than that associated with rapid injections of 1·5 g doses every six hours (Thys et al., 1976). The serum half-life of cephazolin is 1·8 h.

2. *Cephacetrile.* Following an intramuscular injection of 1·0 g, the peak serum level attained one hour later is about 15 μg per ml. Thereafter the serum level falls to 6–7 μg per ml at three hours and to 4–5 μg per ml at four hours. After nine hours the drug is usually undetectable in the serum (Brogard et al., 1973a). Serum cephacetrile levels are higher if the drug is injected into the thigh compared to levels obtained after buttock injections; with cephaloridine no such differences are observed (Reeves et al., 1974).

After a rapid intravenous injection of 1·0 g cephacetrile, a high serum level of about 60 μg per ml is reached in 15 min. This falls rapidly to 20 μg per ml in one hour, to 8·0 μg per ml after two hours, to only about 2·0 μg per ml in four hours and to zero in six hours (Brogard et al., 1973a). Serum levels of cephacetrile after both intramuscular and intravenous administration, are therefore slightly more sustained than those of cephalothin (page 205). The serum half-life of this drug is approximately 1·0 h (Meyer-Brunot et al., 1976).

3. *Cephapirin.* Serum levels attained with this cephalosporin are similar to those of cephalothin (page 205). After an intramuscular dose of 1·0 g to adults, a peak serum concentration of about 15 μg per ml is reached one hour later (Bran et al., 1972). Levels then decline rather rapidly and after four hours no therapeutic serum levels are detectable (Gordon et al., 1971; Bodner and Koenig, 1972). If 2·0 g of cephapirin is infused intravenously over 30 min, the serum level soon after the infusion is over 100 μg per ml; this then falls rapidly and at four hours is less than 1·0 μg per ml (Barza et al., 1976). The serum half-life of cephapirin is only 0·36 h.

4. *Cephanone.* After intravenous or intramuscular administration serum concentrations attained with this drug are about twice as high as those after a similar dose of cephalothin, and are also more prolonged. When a 0·5 g dose is given intramuscularly to adults, an average peak serum level of 36 μg per ml is attained one hour later. Six and eight hours after this dose, the average serum concentrations are 11·2 and 6·6 μg per ml, respectively (Regamey and Kirby, 1973).

Excretion

1. *Cephazolin.* Like cephaloridine this drug is rapidly excreted via the kidney in an unchanged form. High urinary concentrations (4000 μg per ml) of the active drug are attained, and about 60 per cent of an intramuscularly administered dose is excreted in the urine during the first six hours (Ishiyama et al., 1971). Its renal clearance is about 80 per cent of the simultaneous creatinine clearance, and nearly all of a given dose can be recovered from the urine in 24 h (Reller et al., 1973; Rattie and Ravin, 1975). Cephazolin is excreted primarily by glomerular filtration and to a lesser degree by tubular secretion; its excretion can be reduced and serum levels elevated by concomitant administration of probenecid (Kirby and Regamey, 1973). The renal clearance of cephazolin is slower than that of cephalothin and cephaloridine,

and this explains its higher and more prolonged serum levels (page 243).

In the presence of impaired renal function, excretion is delayed and serum concentrations are even more sustained (Ries et al., 1973; Bergan et al., 1977). Nevertheless in uraemic patients with a creatinine clearance in excess of 10 ml per min, high cephazolin concentrations are still attained in the urine (Craig et al., 1973; Brodwall et al., 1977). The serum half-life of cephazolin in anephric patients is approximately 42 h (Rein et al., 1973).

Only small quantities are excreted via the bile, where the concentration is about the same or slightly in excess of the simultaneous serum level, provided that the biliary tract is not obstructed (Ram and Watanatittan, 1973; Brogard et al., 1975; Thys et al., 1976). In patients with cystic duct obstruction, cephazolin, like other antibiotics (pages 109, 623), cannot be detected in gall bladder bile. Cephazolin concentrations attained in bile after usual therapeutic doses are higher (17–31 μg per ml) and more sustained than those attained by cephalothin and cephaloridine (page 207); this is entirely due to the higher serum levels which are attained with cephazolin (Ratzan et al., 1974).

Cephazolin does not appear to be inactivated in the body.

2. *Cephacetrile.* Urinary excretion in an unchanged form is the main method by which this drug is eliminated from the body. It is excreted by both glomerular filtration and tubular secretion (Edselius, 1976). About 70 per cent of an administered dose can be recovered from the urine as the active drug within six hours, and about 75 per cent of the dose within 24 h (Brogard et al., 1973a; Meyer-Brunot et al., 1976). Very high urine levels of the active drug are attained. Cephacetrile accumulates in the serum of patients with impaired renal function if usual doses are given.

Biliary excretion of cephacetrile is very low. The drug is metabolized in the liver to some extent, to produce a desacetyl metabolite as in the case of cephalothin (page 207). Approximately 20 per cent of an administered dose of cephacetrile is excreted in the urine as the desacetyl metabolite (Meyer-Brunot et al., 1976; Dörhöfer and Faigle, 1976).

3. *Cephapirin.* This is rapidly excreted by the normal kidney; about 60 per cent of a dose can be recovered from the urine as the active drug within eight hours (Gordon et al., 1971; McCloskey et al., 1972). Cephapirin, like cephalothin (page 207) is also inactivated in the body by deacetylation in the liver. In healthy individuals, the desacetyl metabolite only comprises 5–15 per cent of the serum concentration of the parent substance, but in urine some 40 per cent of the administered dose is excreted as the metabolite (Barza et al., 1976).

As cephapirin in inactivated in the body, it has a lesser tendency to accumulate in patients with renal failure. The serum half-life of cephapirin is only about 1·5 h in patients with moderate renal insufficiency (McCloskey et al., 1972).

4. *Cephanone.* About 90 per cent of an administered dose is excreted unchanged via the kidney; after an intramuscular dose of 0·5 g the urinary concentration may reach 900 μg per ml. Cephanone is cleared by the kidney more slowly than cephalothin and cephaloridine, and this may largely account for its higher and more sustained serum levels. This drug is mainly eliminated by tubular secretion and only a small amount is filtered through glomeruli (Regamey and Kirby, 1973).

Distribution of the Drugs in Body

1. *Cephazolin*. This drug is highly bound to serum proteins (approximately 80 per cent) and apparently the volume in which it is distributed in the body is the smallest among the cephalosporins; this apparent volume of distribution has been estimated as 10 litres per $1 \cdot 73M^2$ body surface area (Kirby and Regamey, 1973). This together with its low renal clearance (page 244) is partly responsible for its high serum levels (page 243). Therefore despite high cephazolin serum levels, concentrations of this drug may be low at the site of infection, at least in some tissues.

Cephazolin does not penetrate into the cerebrospinal fluid in the absence of meningeal inflammation (Thys *et al.*, 1976). It readily crosses inflamed synovial membranes, and penetrates into bone reaching considerably higher concentrations in acutely inflamed compared to normal bone tissue (Reller *et al.*, 1973; Parsons, 1976; Fass, 1978). The drug is present in the ascitic fluid of patients with ascites and bacterial peritonitis (Gerding *et al.*, 1977). It also penetrates into pleural fluid in adequate concentrations, which however are lower than the serum levels at the time (Cole and Pung, 1977). Concentrations of cephazolin in inflammatory exudate are almost identical to concomitant serum levels, but its levels are lower in fluid aspirated from surgical wounds (Ellis *et al.*, 1975). Cephazolin crosses the placenta, but its concentrations are lower in fetal than in maternal serum; in one study the drug, while present in fetal body fluids, was undetectable in fetal tissues (Bernard *et al.*, 1977).

In animals cephazolin penetrates well into interstitial fluid (Waterman *et al.*, 1976) and peritoneal tissue fluid (Gerding *et al.*, 1976). It also reaches satisfactory concentrations in lung, heart, liver and kidney, but tissue concentrations in animals are somewhat lower in the spleen and much lower in the brain (Ishiyama *et al.*, 1971).

2. *Cephacetrile*. Protein binding of this compound is only 38 per cent (Brogard *et al.*, 1973a), and its apparent volume of distribution ($22 \cdot 5$ litres per $1 \cdot 73M^2$) is much greater than that of cephazolin (*vide supra*). Therefore it is possible that despite lower serum levels (page 244), higher concentrations of this drug may reach various tissues (Meyer-Brunot *et al.*, 1976).

When a high cephacetrile dose of 3 g intravenously every six hours is administered to patients with acute bacterial meningitis, a peak CSF concentration of approximately 20 μg per ml is attained on the first day of treatment. As the meningitis resolves, CSF concentrations fall and may only be 2–3 μg per ml on the fifth day of treatment. The drug is detectable in only very low concentrations in normal CSF (Dettli *et al.*, 1976).

Significant concentrations of cephacetrile are detectable in amniotic, peritoneal and ascitic fluid, umbilical cord blood and bone (Edselius, 1976). The drug also diffuses well into pericardial and pleural fluid (Regamey *et al.*, 1976) and into myocardial tissue (Adam *et al.*, 1976). In liver tissue the cephacetrile concentration is usually only 25 per cent of the serum level at the time (Maroske *et al.*, 1976).

3. *Cephapirin*. The distribution of this drug in the body is probably similar to cephalothin (page 208), and its protein binding is also about the same (50–60 per cent).

4. *Cephanone*. This drug is 88 per cent bound to serum proteins and phar-

macokinetic studies suggest that it is distributed poorly outside the vascular compartment (Regamey and Kirby, 1973).

Mode of Action

These drugs inhibit bacterial cell wall synthesis similar to penicillin G (page 19) and other cephalosporins (page 208).

Toxicity

These cephalosporins appear to have low toxicity, but only cephazolin and to a lesser extent cephacetrile and cephapirin have had wide clinical usage. During volunteer pharmacokinetic studies cephanone has been well tolerated with no untoward side-effects (Meyers et al., 1972).

1. *Hypersensitivity reactions.* Eosinophilia commonly occurs in association with cephazolin (Ries et al., 1973), cephacetrile (Hodges et al., 1973) and cephapirin (Wiesner et al., 1972) therapy. Allergic rashes have been uncommon. Primary allergic reactions occur in approximately 5 per cent of patients treated with the older cephalosporins (Moellering and Swartz, 1976), so that a higher prevalence of these reactions may become apparent with increased clinical use of these newer drugs. A serum sickness-like illness has been ascribed to cephapirin hypersensitivity (Sanders et al., 1974). Volunteers given the drug in a dose of 2 g four times a day by rapid intravenous infusion, all developed fever, malaise, headache, joint and muscle pains, and a rash, after two to four weeks treatment (*see also* cephalothin, page 209). Drug fever alone has been occasionally observed during cephazolin (Ries et al., 1973), cephapirin (Wiesner et al., 1972) and cephacetrile (Edselius, 1976) administration.

These cephalosporins, like cephalothin and cephaloridine (page 209), are probably only occasionally cross-allergenic with the penicillins (Levine, 1973). Ideally, they should never be given to patients with a past history of anaphylaxis or other immediate-type hypersensitivity to any of the penicillins, but their use may be considered in patients with a history of less severe penicillin reactions (Moellering and Swartz, 1976).

2. *Nephrotoxicity.* This appears to be rare, mild and reversible with these cephalosporins (Moellering and Swartz, 1976). Cephazolin, cephapirin and cephacetrile have each been given to humans in doses as high as 12 g daily, without any evidence of nephrotoxicity (Reinarz et al., 1973; Robson and Bowmer, 1974; Dettli et al., 1976). Abnormalities of the proximal renal tubules which occur with cephaloridine (page 210), have not been observed in experimental animals given large doses of cephapirin (Wiesner et al., 1972). Both cephazolin and cephacetrile produce renal tubular damage in experimental animals, but the lesions are much less marked than those caused by cephaloridine (Silverblatt et al., 1973; Luscombe and Nicholls, 1975). Renal effects caused by cephacetrile are not increased by the concomitant administration of frusemide.

It is not yet known whether any of these cephalosporins enhance nephrotoxicity of the aminoglycoside antibiotics (Moellering and Swartz, 1976).

3. *Haematological side-effects*. Marked neutropenia has been described in one patient after a six day course of cephapirin, but this returned to normal after the drug was stopped. Bone marrow examination showed maturation arrest of the white cell series at the metamyelocyte stage (Levison *et al.*, 1973). Leucopenia has also been observed in one patient during cephacetrile therapy (Hodges *et al.*, 1973). Elevated platelet counts have been noted in several patients receiving cephacetrile, but this may have resulted from the infection being treated (Hodges *et al.*, 1973). These authors also detected a positive direct Coombs test during the second week of treatment with cephacetrile in four of 27 patients. Haemolytic anaemia has not been reported. A bleeding disorder developed in one uraemic patient who was treated with cephazolin, and in whom high serum levels of the drug were attained (Lerner and Lubin, 1974).

4. *Hepatotoxicity*. Transient elevations of serum aspartate aminotransferase (SGOT) or alkaline phosphatase have been noted in association with cephapirin (Wiesner *et al.*, 1972), cephacetrile (Hodges *et al.*, 1973) and cephazolin (Ries *et al.*, 1973) therapy. No cases of serious hepatotoxity have been reported.

5. *Encephalopathy*. As with the penicillins (pages 28, 158) and other cephalosporins (page 211), this complication may occur if very high serum levels of these drugs are reached. A patient reported by Gardner *et al.* (1978), who had renal functional impairment, and who was initially treated by inappropriately high doses of cephazolin (12 g per day), developed repeated convulsions while undergoing haemodialysis. A post-dialysis serum cephazolin level was greater than 512 μg per ml.

6. *Other side-effects*. Lorber *et al.* (1975) described one patient who developed Listeria meningitis, in whom treatment with cephazolin for five days for Listeria septicaemia had been initially successful. Meningitis has also developed during cephalothin therapy (page 212). Therefore drugs like cephalothin and cephazolin, which penetrate poorly into the CSF, should be used with caution in infections such as a septicaemia, which may be complicated by meningitis.

Clinical Uses of the Drugs

1. *Cephazolin*. This drug may have some clinical advantages over cephaloridine and cephalothin because it produces higher serum levels and is well tolerated. It has been used with success in streptococcal cellulitis, pneumococcal pneumonia and staphylococcal infections such as septicaemia, pneumonia, osteomyelitis, septic arthritis and endocarditis (Reller *et al.*, 1973; Reinarz *et al.*, 1973; Turck *et al.*, 1973; Fass, 1978), As cephazolin is somewhat less stable to staphylococcal beta-lactamase than cephalothin (page 239), it may not be the ideal drug for the treatment of severe staphylococcal infections such as endocarditis. Although cephazolin appeared to be as effective as cephalothin in experimental staphylococcal endocarditis in animals (Carrizosa *et al.*, 1978), similar to cephaloridine (page 213), there are several case reports of its failure in the treatment of human staphylococcal endocarditis (Quinn *et al.*, 1973; Bryant and Alford, 1977). Others however have obtained satisfactory results with cephazolin in this disease, and the role of this drug for staphylococcal endocarditis remains controversial (Bryant and

Alford, 1978; Kaye *et al.*, 1978). In common with other cephalosporins, cephazolin is ineffective for the treatment of Strep. faecalis endocarditis.

The efficacy of cephazolin for the treatment of urinary tract infections is comparable with that of cephalothin and cephaloridine (Ries *et al.*, 1973; Reller *et al.*, 1973) or ampicillin (Benner *et al.*, 1975). Uncomplicated gonorrhoea and gonococcal arthritis also respond well to a course of cephazolin (Karney *et al.*, 1973; Reller *et al.*, 1973). However 'single-dose' treatment for uncomplicated gonorrhoea, using an intramuscular dose of 2 g, with or without probenecid, is quite unsatisfactory and it cannot be recommended (Duncan, 1974).

Children with soft tissue infections, pneumonia and osteomyelitis have been treated with cephazolin. Clinical response was satisfactory in most patients and similar to that obtained with cephalothin (Pickering *et al.*, 1974).

Cephazolin has been used prophylactically in patients undergoing routine cholecystectomy. In one trial it appeared that wound sepsis rate was reduced by this treatment (Strachan *et al.*, 1977), but the results of such chemoprophylaxis are very difficult to assess. Uwaydah (1976) used cephazolin in daily doses of 3–6 g to treat seven patients with typhoid and two patients with paratyphoid fever. The acute infection was controlled in all patients, but one of the typhoid fever patients relapsed when treatment was stopped. More extensive clinical data are necessary before it can be concluded that this drug is satisfactory for the treatment of enteric fevers.

2. *Cephacetrile.* This has been used effectively to treat staphylococcal and streptococcal soft tissue infections, staphylococcal osteomyelitis, pneumococcal pneumonia and urinary tract infections (Hodges *et al.*, 1973; Edselius, 1976). It is unsatisfactory for the treatment of gonorrhoea (Edselius, 1976). Cephacetrile probably has no definite advantages over cephalothin for the treatment of most infections (page 213). In one comparative trial these two drugs were found to be about equally effective and their side-effects were also about the same (Jackson *et al.*, 1974). However, unlike cephalothin, cephacetrile has been claimed to be effective for the treatment of both pneumococcal and meningococcal meningitis, provided that a large intravenous dose (3 g every six hours) is given (Dettli *et al.*, 1976). In view of the poor results obtained with other cephalosporins in meningitis (pages 216, 285), this claim requires confirmation.

3. *Cephapirin.* Clinical studies show that this drug is satisfactory for those infections which normally respond to cephalothin (page 213). For example, it has been effective for treatment of staphylococcal and streptococcal soft tissue infections, pneumococcal and staphylococcal pneumonia and urinary tract infections (Bran *et al.*, 1972; Wiesner *et al.*, 1972; Robson and Bowmer, 1974). Used as a single 4·0 g intramuscular dose it is ineffective for gonorrhoea, but a course of 1·0 g six-hourly for eight days is satisfactory (Wiesner *et al.*, 1972). Cephapirin does not appear to have any definite advantages over cephalothin.

4. *Cephanone.* Clinical studies with this drug have not been pursued.

REFERENCES

Adam, D., Pätzold, J. and Reichardt, B. (1976), 'Concentration of cephacetrile in myocardial tissue', Cephacetrile—a review of progress to date. *Proceedings of an*

International Symposium on Cephalosporins, Munich 1976, p. 97.

Axelrod, J., Meyers, B. R. and Hirschman, S. Z. (1971), 'Cephapirin: *In vitro* antibacterial spectrum', *Appl. Microbial.,* **22,** 904.

Barza, M., Melethil, S., Berger, S. and Ernst, E. C. (1976), 'Comparative pharmacokinetics of cefamandole, cephapirin, and cephalothin in healthy subjects and effect of repeated dosing', *Antimicrob. Ag. Chemother.,* **10,** 421.

Benner, E. J., Kranhold, J. F. and Bush, W. G. (1975), 'Cephazolin: A comparison to ampicillin in respiratory and urinary infections with dosage regulation by a nomogram', *Scot. med. J.,* **20,** 244.

Bergan, T., Brodwall, E. K. and Ørjavik, O. (1977), 'Pharmacokinetics of cefazolin in patients with normal and impaired renal function', *J. Antimicrob. Chemother.,* **3,** 435.

Berger, S., Ernst, E. C. and Barza, M. (1976), 'Comparative incidence of phlebitis due to buffered cephalothin, cephapirin, and cefamandole', *Antimicrob. Ag. Chemother.,* **9,** 575.

Bergeron, M. G., Brusch, J. L., Barza, M. and Weinstein, L. (1973), 'Bactericidal activity and pharmacology of cefazolin', *Antimicrob. Ag. Chemother.,* **4,** 396.

Berman, S. J., Boughton, W. H., Sugihara, J. G., Wong, E. G. C. and Siemsen, A. W. (1978), 'Hemodialysis-associated infections: Treatment with cephapirin', *Antimicrob. Ag. Chemother.,* **13,** 4.

Bernard, B., Barton, L., Abate, M. and Ballard, C. A. (1977), 'Maternal-fetal transfer of cefazolin in the first twenty weeks of pregnancy', *J. Infect. Dis.,* **136,** 377.

Bodner, S. J. and Koenig, M. G. (1972), 'Clinical and *in vitro* evaluation of cephapirin: A new parenteral cephalosporin', *Amer. J. Med. Sci.,* **263,** 43.

Bourque, M., Quintiliani, R. and Tilton, R. C. (1976), 'Synergism of cefazolin-gentamicin against enterococci', *Antimicrob. Ag. Chemother.,* **10,** 157.

Bran, J. L., Levison, M. E. and Kaye, D. (1972), 'Clinical and *in vitro* evaluation of cephapirin, a new cephalosporin antibiotic', *Antimicrob. Ag. Chemother.,* **1,** 35.

Brodwall, E. K., Bergan, T. and Ørjavik, O. (1977), 'Kidney transport of cefazolin in normal and impaired renal function', *J. Antimicrob. Chemother.,* **3,** 585.

Brogard, J. M., Kuntzmann, F. and Lavillaureix, J. (1973a), 'Blood levels, renal and biliary excretions of a new cephalosporin, cephacetrile (Ciba 36278 Ba)', *Schweiz, med. Wschr.,* **103,** 110.

Brogard, J. M., Haegele, P., Dorner, M. and Lavillaureix, J. (1973b), 'Biliary excretion of a new semisynthetic cephalosporin cephacetrile', *Antimicrob. Ag. Chemother.,* **3,** 19.

Brogard, J. M., Dorner, M., Pinget, M., Adloff, M. and Lavillaureix, J. (1975), 'The biliary excretion of cefazolin', *J. Infect. Dis.,* **131,** 625.

Bryant, R. E. and Alford, R. H. (1977), 'Unsuccessful treatment of staphylococcal endocarditis with cefazolin', *JAMA,* **237,** 569.

Bryant, R. E. and Alford, R. H. (1978), 'Treatment of staphylococcal endocarditis', *JAMA,* **239,** 1130.

Cahn, M. M., Levy, E. J., Actor, P. and Pauls, J. F. (1974), 'Comparative serum levels and urinary recovery of cefazolin, cephaloridine and cephalothin in man', *J. Clin. Pharmacol.,* **14,** 61.

Carrizosa, J., Levison, M. E. and Kaye, D. (1973), 'Double-blind controlled comparison of phlebitis produced by cephapirin and cephalothin', *Antimicrob. Ag. Chemother.,* **3,** 306.

Carrizosa, J., Santoro, J. and Kaye, D. (1978), 'Treatment of experimental Staphylococcus aureus endocarditis: Comparison of cephalothin, cefazolin, and methicillin', *Antimicrob. Ag. Chemother.,* **13,** 74.

Cole, D. R. and Pung, J. (1977), 'Penetration of cefazolin into pleural fluid', *Antimicrob. Ag. Chemother.,* **11,** 1033.

Craig, W. A., Welling, P. G., Jackson, T. C. and Kunin, C. M. (1973), 'Pharmacology of cefazolin and other cephalosporins in patients with renal insufficiency', *J. Infect. Dis.* (Suppl.), **128**, 347.

Dettli, L., Spring, P. and Lomar, A. V. (1976), 'Pharmacokinetics of cephalosporins in the cerebrospinal fluid', Cephacetrile—a review of progress to date. *Proceedings of an International Symposium on Cephalosporins*, Munich, 1976, p. 61.

Di Nola, F. and Soranzo, M. L. (1976), 'Clinical trials with cephacetrile in the treatment of secondary respiratory infections in childhood pertussis', Cephacetrile—a review of progress to date. *Proceedings of an International Symposium on Cephalosporins*, Munich, 1976, p. 109.

Dörhöfer, G. and Faigle, J. W. (1976), 'Biotransformation of cephacetrile in man', Cephacetrile—a review of progress to date. *Proceedings of an International Symposium on Cephalosporins*, Munich, 1976, p. 46.

Duncan, W. C. (1974), 'Treatment of gonorrhea with cefazolin plus probenecid', *J. Infect. Dis.*, **130**, 398.

Edselius, B. R. (1976), 'Introductory remarks on cephacetrile', Cephacetrile—a review of progress to date. *Proceedings of an International Symposium on Cephalosporins*, Munich, 1976, p. 17.

Ellis, B. W., Stanbridge, R. DeL., Sikorski, J. M., Dudley, H. A. F. and Spencer, R. C. (1975), 'Penetration into inflammatory exudate and wounds of two cephalosporins for the prevention of surgical infections', *J. Antimicrob. Chemother.*, **1**, 291.

Fare, L. R., Actor, P., Sachs, C., Phillips, L., Joloza, McD., Pauls, J. F. and Weisbach, J. A. (1974), 'Comparative serum levels and protective activity of parenterally administered cephalosporins in experimental animals', *Antimicrob. Ag. Chemother.*, **6**, 150.

Farrar, W. E., Jr. and Gramling, P. K. (1976), 'Antistaphylococcal activity and beta-lactamase resistance of newer cephalosporins', *J. Infect. Dis.*, **133**, 691.

Fass, R. J. (1978), 'Treatment of osteomyelitis and septic arthritis with cefazolin', *Antimicrob. Ag. Chemother.*, **13**, 405.

Fong, I. W., Engelking, E. R. and Kirby, W. M. M. (1976), 'Relative inactivation by Staphylococcus aureus of eight cephalosporin antibiotics', *Antimicrob. Ag. Chemother.*, **9**, 939.

Gardner, M. E., Fritz, W. L. and Hyland, R. N. (1978), 'Antibiotic-induced seizures. A case attributed to cefazolin', *Drug Intelligence and Clinical Pharmacy*, **12**, 268.

Gerding, D. N., Hall, W. H., Schierl, E. A. and Manion, R. E. (1976), 'Cephalosporin and aminoglycoside concentrations in peritoneal capsular fluid in rabbits', *Antimicrob. Ag. Chemother.*, **10**, 902.

Gerding, D. N., Hall, W. H. and Schierl, E. A. (1977), 'Antibiotic concentrations in ascitic fluid of patients with ascites and bacterial peritonitis', *Ann. Intern. Med.*, **86**, 708.

Gordon, R. C., Barrett, F. F., Clark, D. J. and Yow, M. D. (1971), 'Laboratory and pharmacologic studies of BL-P-1322 (Cephapirin sodium) in children', *Curr. Ther. Res.*, **13**, 398.

Greenwood, D., Chan-Teoh, C. H. and O'Grady, F. (1975), 'Activity of cefazolin against dense populations of Enterobacteria', *Antimicrob. Ag. Chemother.*, **7**, 191.

Hamilton-Miller, J. M. T. (1974), 'Comparative activity of ampicillin and seven cephalosporins against Group D streptococci', *J. clin. Path.*, **27**, 828.

Hodges, G. R., Scholand, J. F. and Perkins, R. L. (1973), 'Cephacetrile: Clinical evaluation in 27 patients', *Antimicrob. Ag. Chemother.*, **3**, 228.

Isenberg, H. D., Painter, B. G., Sampson-Scherer, J. and Siegel, M. (1973), 'Clinical laboratory study of cephacetrile and cephalothin against bacteria recently isolated from clinical specimens', *Amer. J. Clin. Path.*, **59**, 700.

Ishiyama, S., Nakayama, I., Iwamoto, H., Iwai, S., Okui, M. and Matsubara, T. (1971), 'Absorption, tissue concentration, and organ distribution of cefazolin', *Antimicrob. Agents. Chemother.*—1970, p. 476.

Jackson, G. G., Riff, L. J., Zimelis, V. M., Daood, M. and Youssuf, M. (1974), 'Double-blind comparison of cephacetrile with cephalothin/cephaloridine', *Antimicrob. Ag. Chemother.*, **5**, 247.

Jones, R. N. and Fuchs, P. C. (1976), 'Comparison of *in vitro* antimicrobial activity of cefamandole and cefazolin with cephalothin against over 8000 clinical bacterial isolates', *Antimicrob. Ag. Chemother.*, **9**, 1066.

Karney, W. W., Turck, M. and Holmes, K. K. (1973), 'Cefazolin in the treatment of gonorrhoea', *J. Infect. Dis.* (Suppl.), **128**, 399.

Kaye, D., Hewitt, W., Remington, J. S. and Turck, M. (1978), 'Treatment of Staphylococcal endocarditis', *JAMA*, **239**, 1130.

Kirby, W. M. M. and Regamey, C. (1973), 'Pharmacokinetics of cefazolin compared with four other cephalosporins', *J. Infect. Dis.* (Suppl.), **128**, 341.

Kisch, A. L. and Bartholomew, L. (1976), 'Comparison of the *in vitro* activity of several cephalosporin antibiotics against Gram-negative and Gram-positive bacteria resistant to cephaloridine', *Antimicrob. Ag. Chemother.*, **10**, 507.

Klastersky, J., Meunier-Carpentier, F., Prevost, J. M. and Staquet, M. (1976), 'Synergism between amikacin and cefazolin against Klebsiella: *In vitro* studies and effect on the bactericidal activity of serum', *J. Infect. Dis.*, **134**, 271.

Knüsel, F., Konopka, E. A., Gelzer, J. and Rosselet, A. (1971), 'Antimicrobial studies *in vitro* with CIBA 36278-Ba, a new cephalosporin derivative', *Antimicrob. Agents Chemother.*—1970, p. 140.

Lacey, R. W. and Stokes, A. (1977), 'Susceptiblity of the 'penicillinase-resistant' penicillins and cephalosporins to pencillinase of Staphylococcus aureus', *J. clin. Path.*, **30**, 35.

Lane, A. Z., Taggart, J. G. and Iles, R. L. (1972), 'Relative incidence of phlebitis caused by continuous intravenous infusion of cephapirin and cephalothin', *Antimicrob. Ag. Chemother.*, **2**, 234.

Leading Article (1973), 'Cephalosporins, present and future', *Lancet*, **2**, 364.

Leitner, F., Misiek, M., Pursiano, T. A., Buck, R. E., Chisholm, D. R., De Regis, R. G., Tsai, Y. H. and Price, K. E. (1976), 'Laboratory evaluation of BL-S786 a cephalosporin with broad-spectrum antibacterial activity', *Antimicrob. Ag. Chemother.*, **10**, 426.

Lerner, P. I. and Lubin, A. (1974), 'Coagulopathy with cefazolin in uremia', *New Engl. J. Med.*, **290**, 1324.

Levine, B. B. (1973), 'Antigenicity and cross-reactivity of penicillins and cephalosporins', *J. Infect. Dis.* (Suppl.), **128**, 364.

Levison, M. E., Levison, S. P., Ries, K. and Kaye, D. (1973), 'Pharmacology of cefazolin in patients with normal and abnormal renal function', *J. Infect. Dis.* (Suppl.), **128**, 354.

Lorber, B., Santoro, J. and Swenson, R. M. (1975), 'Listeria meningitis during cefazolin therapy', *Ann. Intern. Med.*, **82**, 226.

Luscombe, D. K. and Nicholls, P. J. (1975), 'Possible interaction between cephacetrile and frusemide in rabbits and rats', *J. Antimicrob. Chemother.*, **1**, 67.

Madhavan, T., Yaremchuk, K., Levin, N., Fisher, E., Cox, F., Burch, K., Haas, E., Pohlod, D. and Quinn, E. L. (1975), 'Effects of renal failure and dialysis on cefazolin pharmacokinetics', *Antimicrob. Ag. Chemother.*, **8**, 63.

Maroske, D., Knothe, H. and Rox, A. (1976), 'Liver tissue concentration of cephradine and cephacetril and their excretion in bile', *Infection*, **4**, 159.

McCloskey, R. V., Terry, E. E., McCracken, A. W., Sweeney, M. J. and Forland, M. F. (1972), 'Effect of hemodialysis and renal failure on serum and urine concentrations of cephapirin sodium', *Antimicrob. Ag. Chemother.*, **1**, 90.

McCloskey, R. V., Forland, M. F., Sweeney, M. J. and Lawrence, D. N. (1973), 'Hemodialysis of cefazolin', *J. Infect. Dis.* (Suppl.), **128**, 358.

McCracken, G. H., Jr. and Nelson, J. D. (1977), '*Antimicrobial Therapy for Newborns:*

Practical Application of Pharmacology to Clinical Usage', Grune and Stratton, Inc., New York, San Francisco, London, p. 28.

Meyer-Brunot, H. G., Randazzo, D., Spring, P. and Theobald, W. (1976), 'Pharmacokinetic characteristics of cephalosporins', Cephacetrile—a review of progress to date. *Proceedings of an International Symposium on Cephalosporins, Munich*, 1976, p. 31.

Meyers, B. R., Hirschman, S. Z. and Nicholas, P. (1972), 'Cephanone: *In vitro* antibacterial activity and pharmacology in normal human volunteers', *Antimicrob. Ag. Chemother.*, **2**, 250.

Moellering, R. C., Jr. and Swartz, M. N. (1976), 'Drug therapy: The newer cephalosporins', *New Engl. J. Med.*, **294**, 24.

Motley, M. and Shadomy, S. (1974), *'In vitro* studies with cefazolin', *Antimicrob. Ag. Chemother.*, **6**, 856.

Nishida, M., Murakawa, T., Kamimura, T., Okada, N., Sakamoto, H., Fukada, S., Nakamoto, S., Yokota, Y. and Miki, K. (1976), *'In vitro* and *in vivo* evaluation of ceftezole, a new cephalosporin derivative', *Antimicrob. Ag. Chemother.*, **10**, 1.

Nishida, M., Murakawa, T., Kamimura, T., Okada, N., Fukada, S., Sakamoto, H., Nakamoto, S., Yokota, Y. and Kono, Y. (1977), 'Laboratory evaluation of FR 10024, a new cephalosporin derivative', *Antimicrob. Ag. Chemother.*, **11**, 51.

O'Callaghan, C. H. (1975), 'Classification of cephalosporins by their antibacterial activity and pharmacokinetic properties', *J. Antimicrob. Chemother.*, **1** (Suppl.), 1.

Parsons, R. L. (1976), Leading Article. 'Antibiotics in bone', *J. Antimicrob. Chemother.*, **2**, 228.

Phair, J. P., Carleton, J. and Tan, J. S. (1972), 'Comparison of cefazolin, a new cephalosporin antibiotic, with cephalothin', *Antimicrob. Ag. Chemother.*, **2**, 329.

Phillips, I., King, A., Warren, C., Watts, B. and Stoate, M. W. (1976), 'The activity of penicillin and eight cephalosporins on Neisseria gonorrhoeae', *J. Antimicrob. Chemother.*, **2**, 31.

Pickering, L. K., O'Connor, D. M., Anderson, D., Bairan, A. C., Feigin, R. D. and Cherry, J. D. (1973), 'Clinical and pharmacologic evaluation of cefazolin in children', *J. Infect. Dis.* (Suppl.), **128**, 407.

Pickering, L. K., O'Connor, D. M., Anderson, D., Bairan, A. C., Feigin, R. D. and Cherry, J. D. (1974), 'Comparative evaluation of cefazolin and cephalothin in children', *J. Pediatrics*, **85**, 842.

Quinn, E. L., Pohlod, D., Madhavan, T., Burch, K., Fisher, E. and Cox, F. (1973), 'Clinical experiences with cefazolin and other cephalosporins in bacterial endocarditis', *J. Infect. Dis.* (Suppl.), **128**, 386.

Ram, M. D. and Watanatittan, S. (1973), 'Levels of cefazolin in human bile', *J. Infect. Dis.* (Suppl.), **128**, 361.

Rattie, E. S. and Ravin, L. J. (1975), 'Pharmacokinetic interpretation of blood levels and urinary excretion data for cefazolin and cephalothin after intravenous and intramuscular administration in humans', *Antimicrob. Ag. Chemother.*, **7**, 606.

Ratzan, K. R., Ruiz, C. and Irvin, G. L. III (1974), 'Biliary tract excretion of cefazolin, cephalothin, and cephaloridine in the presence of biliary tract disease', *Antimicrob. Ag. Chemother.*, **6**, 426.

Reeves, D. S., Bywater, M. J. and Wise, R. (1974), 'Availability of three antibiotics after intramuscular injection into thigh and buttock', *Lancet*, **2**, 1421.

Regamey, C. and Kirby, W. M. M. (1973), 'Pharmacokinetics of cephanone in healthy adult volunteers', *Antimicrob. Ag. Chemother.*, **4**, 589.

Regamey, C., Libke, R. D., Engelking, E. R., Clarke, J. T. and Kirby, W. M. M. (1975), 'Inactivation of cefazolin, cephaloridine and cephalothin by methicillin-sensitive and methicillin-resistant strains of Staphylococcus aureus', *J. Infect. Dis.*, **131**, 291.

Regamey, C., Vicquerat, C., Sutter, P. M. and Waldvogel, F. A. (1976), 'Concen-

trations of cephacetrile in pericardial effusions following cardiac surgery',
Cephacetrile—a review of progress to date. *Proceedings of an International Symposium on Cephalosporins,* Munich, 1976, p. 86.

Rein, M. F., Westervelt, F. B. and Sande, M. A. (1973), 'Pharmacodynamics of cefazolin in the presence of normal and impaired renal function', *Antimicrob. Ag. Chemother.*, **4,** 366.

Reinarz, J. A., Kier, C. M. and Guckian, J. C. (1973), 'Evaluation of cefazolin in the treatment of bacterial endocarditis and bacteremia', *J. Infect. Dis.* (Suppl.), **128,** 392.

Reller, L. B., Karney, W. W., Beaty, H. N., Holmes, K. K. and Turck, M. (1973), 'Evaluation of cefazolin, a new cephalosporin antibiotic', *Antimicrob. Ag. Chemother.*, **3,** 488.

Ries, K., Levison, M. E. and Kaye, D. (1973), 'Clinical and *in vitro* evaluation of cefazolin, a new cephalosporin antibiotic', *Antimicrob. Ag. Chemother.*, **3,** 168.

Robson, H. G. and Bowmer, M. I. (1974), 'Treatment of pneumonia and other serious bacterial infections with cephapirin', *Antimicrob. Ag. Chemother.*, **6,** 274.

Sabath, L. D., Wilcox, C. Garner, C. and Finland, M. (1973), '*In vitro* activity of cefazolin against recent clinical bacterial isolates', *J. Infect. Dis.* (Suppl.), **128,** 320.

Sabath, L. D., Garner, C., Wilcox, C. and Finland, M. (1975), 'Effect of inoculum and of beta-lactamase on the anti-staphylococcal activity of thirteen penicillins and cephalosporins', *Antimicrob. Ag. Chemother.*, **8,** 344.

Sanders, W. E., Jr., Johnson, J. E. III and Taggart, J. G. (1974), 'Adverse reactions to cephalothin and cephapirin. Uniform occurrence on prolonged intravenous administration of high doses', *New Engl. J. Med.*, **290,** 424.

Shadomy, S., Kirchoff, C. and Wagner, G. (1974), '*In vitro* studies with cephanone', *Antimicrob. Ag. Chemother.*, **6,** 862.

Shemonsky, N. K., Carrizosa, J., Kaye, D. and Levison, M. E. (1975), 'Double-blind comparison of phlebitis produced by cefazolin versus cephalothin', *Antimicrob. Ag. Chemother.*, **7,** 481.

Siebert, W. T., Westerman, E. L., Smilack, J. D., Bradshaw, M. W. and Williams, T. W., Jr. (1976), 'Comparison of thrombophlebitis associated with three cephalosporin antibiotics', *Antimicrob. Ag. Chemother.*, **10,** 467.

Silverblatt, F., Harrison, W. O. and Turck, M. (1973), 'Nephrotoxicity of cephalosporin antibiotics in experimental animals', *J. Infect. Dis.* (Suppl.), **128,** 367.

Strachan, C. J. L., Black, J., Powis, S. J. A., Waterworth, T. A., Wise, R., Wilkinson, A. R., Burdon, D. W., Severn, M., Mitra, B. and Norcott, H. (1977), 'Prophylactic use of cephazolin against wound sepsis after cholecystectomy', *Brit. med. J.,* **1,** 1254.

Strausbaugh, L. J., Mikhail, I. A. and Edman, D. C. (1978), 'Comparative *in vitro* activity of five cephalosporin antibiotics against salmonellae', *Antimicrob. Ag. Chemother.*, **13,** 134.

Sutter, V. L. and Finegold, S. M. (1975), 'Susceptibility of anaerobic bacteria to carbenicillin, cefoxitin, and related drugs', *J. Infect. Dis.,* **131,** 417.

Tally, F. P., Jacobus, N. V., Bartlett, J. G. and Gorbach, S. L. (1975), 'Susceptibility of anaerobes to cefoxitin and other cephalosporins', *Antimicrob. Ag. Chemother.*, **7,** 128.

Thys, J. P., Vanderkelen, B. and Klastersky, J. (1976), 'Pharmacological study of cefazolin during intermittent and continuous infusion: A crossover investigation in humans', *Antimicrob. Ag. Chemother.*, **10,** 395.

Turck, M., Clark, R. A., Beaty, H. N., Holmes, K. K., Karney, W. W. and Reller, L. B. (1973), 'Cefazolin in the treatment of bacterial pneumonia', *J. Infect. Dis.* (Suppl.), **128,** 382.

Uwaydah, H. (1976), 'Cefazolin in the treatment of acute enteric fever', *Antimicrob. Ag. Chemother.*, **10,** 52.

Verbist, L. (1976), 'Comparison of the antibacterial activity of nine cephalosporins against Enterobacteriaeceae and nonfermentative Gram-negative bacilli', *Antimicrob. Ag. Chemother.*, **10,** 657.

Waterman, N. G., Raff, M. J., Scharfenberger, L. and Barnwell, P. A. (1976), 'Protein binding and concentrations of cephaloridine and cefazolin in serum and interstitial fluid of dogs', *J. Infect. Dis.*, **133,** 642.

Wick, W. E. and Preston, D. A. (1972), 'Biological properties of three 3-heterocyclic-thiomethyl cephalosporin antibiotics', *Antimicrob. Ag. Chemother.*, **1,** 221.

Wiesner, P., MacGregor, R., Bear, D., Berman, S., Holmes, K. and Turck, M. (1972), 'Evaluation of a new cephalosporin antibiotic, cephapirin', *Antimicrob. Ag. Chemother.*, **1,** 303.

Yourassowsky, E., Schoutens, E. and Vanderlinden, M. P. (1976), 'Antibacterial activity of eight cephalosporins against Haemophilus influenzae and Streptococcus pneumoniae', *J. Antimicrob. Chemother.*, **2,** 55.

Cephradine, Cefatrizine, Cefadroxil and Cefaclor

Description

These four newer cephalosporins, similar to cephalexin (page 225), are all suitable for oral administration. Cephradine and cefatrizine can also be administered parenterally.

1. *Cephradine*. This semisynthetic cephalosporin was developed at the Squibb Institute for Medical Research (Dolfini *et al.*, 1971; Miraglia *et al.*, 1973; Hubsher *et al.*, 1973). It is very similar to cephalexin (page 225) in its antimicrobial activity and in most other respects (Leading article, 1973; Moellering and Swartz, 1976). Unlike cephalexin, for which a parenteral preparation is not generally available (page 229), cephradine is marketed for both oral and parenteral use with the trade names of 'Velosef' (Squibb) and 'Anspor' (Smith Kline and French).

2. *Cefatrizine*. In initial studies this was known at Bristol Laboratories as 'BL-S640' (Leitner *et al.*, 1975a and b) and at Smith Kline and French Laboratories as 'SK-F60771' (Actor *et al.*, 1976). Cefatrizine is slightly more active than cephalexin against most Gram-negative and Gram-positive bacteria (Leitner *et al.*, 1975a; Overturf *et al.*, 1975). Peak serum levels obtained after oral cefatrizine are lower than those after cephalexin, but they decline at a slower rate (Del Busto *et al.*, 1976; Actor *et al.*, 1976). This drug can also be administered parenterally.

3. *Cefadroxil*. This cephalosporin has been investigated by Bristol-Meyers Company (Buck and Price, 1977; Pfeffer *et al.*, 1977). Its antibacterial activity is similar to that of cephalexin and cephradine. After oral administration of cefadroxil its peak serum level is slightly lower than that of cephalexin, but it is excreted more slowly and so it has a longer serum half-life. It may therefore be possible to use this drug for oral administration at eight- or twelve-hourly intervals.

4. *Cefaclor*. Although this drug is similar in many aspects to cephalexin and cephradine, it differs by being more active *in vitro* against a number of both Gram-positive and Gram-negative bacteria (Bill and Washington, 1977).

Sensitive Organisms

1. *Cephradine*. The antimicrobial spectrum of this drug (Table 19, page 259) is similar to that of cephalexin (page 225) with only minor differences (O'Callaghan, 1975; Moellering and Swartz, 1976). Like cephalexin, cephradine is less active against most bacterial species, compared to cephalothin and cephaloridine (page 225).

Gram-positive bacteria are usually sensitive to cephradine. Staph. pyogenes, including most penicillin-resistant, but not methicillin-resistant strains, is sensitive. Cephradine is about as resistant as cephalothin (page 199) to inactivation by staphylococcal beta-lactamase (Fong *et al.*, 1976; Selwyn, 1976; 1977; Lacey and Stokes, 1977). Most other aerobic Gram-positive cocci such as Staph. epidermidis, Strep. pyogenes, Strep. pneumoniae and alpha-haemolytic streptococci are cephradine-sensitive. Cephradine (MIC 100 μg per ml) is slightly more active than cephalexin (MIC 200 μg per ml) against Strep. faecalis, but from a practical point of view this organism is resistant to both drugs (Hamilton-Miller, 1974).

Anaerobic Gram-positive cocci such as the Peptococcus and Peptostreptococcus spp. are usually cephradine-sensitive. Most strains recovered from airway associated infections are relatively sensitive (MIC 8–16 μg per ml), but other strains are less sensitive (Busch *et al.*, 1976). The activity of cephradine against Gram-positive bacilli is similar to that of cephalexin (page 226).

Cephradine's activity against Gram-negative bacteria is like that of cephalexin (Klastersky *et al.*, 1973; Scholand *et al.*, 1974). Some authors have found that cephradine is less active against Esch. coli, Proteus mirabilis and Klebsiella spp. (McGowan *et al.*, 1974; O'Callaghan, 1975; Bill and Washington, 1977). Both cephalexin (page 226) and cephradine are only moderately active against N. gonorrhoeae (Phillips *et al.*, 1976), but they retain this activity against penicillinase-producing gonococci (page 8) (Selwyn and Bakhtiar, 1977). Like cephalexin (page 226), cephradine is relatively inactive against H. influenzae, many strains of which are completely resistant to these drugs (Yourassowsky *et al.*, 1976; Sinai *et al.*, 1978).

2. *Cefatrizine.* This cephalosporin has a somewhat similar antibacterial spectrum to both cephalexin and cephradine (Table 19). However this newer drug is more active against H. influenzae and some strains of both Esch. coli and Klebsiella spp. In addition, cefatrizine is active against some strains of Enterobacter and Providencia spp. and of Proteus morganii and Pr. rettgeri, all of which are generally completely resistant to cephalexin and cephradine (Leitner *et al.*, 1975a; Overturf *et al.*, 1975; Stillwell *et al.*, 1975; Vuye *et al.*, 1976; Kisch and Bartholomew, 1976; Verbist, 1976; Shadomy *et al.*, 1977).

Against most Gram-positive bacteria, cefatrizine is more active than cephalexin and cephradine (Table 19), but not as active as the older parenteral cephalosporins, cephalothin (page 199) and cephazolin (page 239) (Del Busto *et al.*, 1976; Vuye *et al.*, 1976).

3. *Cefadroxil.* For practical purposes, the antibacterial activity of cefadroxil against both Gram-positive and Gram-negative bacteria is identical to that of cephalexin (page 225) and cephradine (Buck and Price, 1977) (Table 19).

4. *Cefaclor.* This drug is substantially more active than cephalexin and cephradine against Gram-positive bacteria such as staphylococci and streptococci, but against Staph. pyogenes it is not as active as cephalothin. Cefaclor is also more active than cephalexin against many Gram-negative bacteria such as meningococci, gonococci, H. influenzae, Esch. coli, Kl. pneumoniae, Pr. mirabilis and the salmonellae and shigellae (Bill and Washington, 1977; Scheld *et al.*, 1977; Sanders, 1977; Gray *et al.*, 1978) (*see also* Table 19). Cefaclor at a concentration of 6·25 μg per ml consistently inhibits beta-lactamase-producing Haemophilus influenzae (Neu and Fu, 1978; Sinai *et al.*, 1978). The

drug is somewhat less resistant to staphylococcal penicillinase than cephalexin (page 225), and so it may not be a reliable anti-staphyl coccal agent (Bill and Washington, 1977). It is inactive against Serratia and Acinetobacter spp. and also against most strains of indole-positive Proteus spp. (Neu and Fu, 1978).

Anaerobic Gram-positive cocci and most strains of Bacteroides spp. other than B. fragilis are also usually cefaclor-sensitive. The Clostridium spp. and B. fragilis are usually resistant (Bach *et al.*, 1978).

In Vitro Sensitivities

The minimum inhibitory concentrations of cephradine, cefatrizine, cefadroxil and cefaclor against some selected bacteria are shown in Table 19. Those for cephalexin (Table 14, page 227) are included for comparison.

Mode of Administration and Dosage

1. *Cephradine*. The usual oral adult dose is 0·5 g every six hours. For mild infections 250 mg six-hourly may suffice, and up to 1·0 g every four hours may be given for severe or chronic infections (Whitworth *et al.*, 1973; Klastersky *et al.*, 1973; Scholand *et al.*, 1974). The oral dose for children is 25–50 mg per kg body weight per day, given in four divided doses, but up to 100 mg per kg per day may be given for severe infections.

The parenteral dose for adults is 2·0 to 4·0 g daily, given in four divided doses intramuscularly or intravenously. For treatment of severe infections a daily dose of up to 8·0 g can be used. The usual parenteral dose for children is 50–100 mg per kg per day, given in four divided doses. For serious infections, up to 300 mg per kg has been given intravenously to children without toxicity (Hubsher *et al.*, 1973; Macias and Eller, 1975; Mogabgab, 1976).

In patients with renal failure, cephradine accumulates if the usual doses are given, so that dosage reduction is necessary. The recommendations are for moderate renal failure (creatinine clearance 10–50 ml per min), 50 per cent of the usual daily dose, and for severe renal failure (creatinine clearance less than 10 ml per min), 25 per cent of the usual daily dose. The drug is removed by both peritoneal and haemodialysis, so that dosage supplements are necessary during or after these procedures (Bennett *et al.*, 1977).

2. *Cefatrizine*. In preliminary clinical trials this has been given orally to adult patients in daily doses of 1·0 g or 2·0 g, administered in four divided doses (Del Busto *et al.*, 1976). In pharmacological studies using volunteers, cefatrizine has also been given in single 0·5 g intramuscular doses, which have been well tolerated (Actor *et al.*, 1976).

3. *Cefadroxil*. Pharmacological studies indicate that this can be administered orally at less frequent intervals than cephalexin (page 227), and either eight-hourly or twelve-hourly administration may be satisfactory (Pfeffer *et al.*, 1977; Hartstein *et al.*, 1977). A dose of 0·5 g either two or three times a day may prove to be suitable for most mild to moderate infections for which an oral cephalosporin is indicated. For children a dosage of 15 mg of cefadroxil per kg, given three or four times daily is advocated (Ginsburg *et al.*, 1978).

4. *Cefaclor*. The properties of this cephalosporin indicate that oral doses for adults of 250 to 500 mg six-hourly may be suitable (Korzeniowski *et al.*, 1978).

TABLE 19

Compiled from data published by Hamilton-Miller (1974), Overturf *et al.* (1975), Leitner *et al.* (1975a), Selwyn (1976), Buck and Price (1977) and Bill and Washington (1977)

ORGANISM	MIC (µg per ml)				
	Cephalexin	Cephradine	Cefatrizine	Cefadroxil	Cefaclor
Gram-positive bacteria					
Staph. pyogenes (non-penicillinase producer)	1.6–12.5	2.0	—	2.0	4.0
Staph. pyogenes (penicillinase producer)	1.6–>100	8.0	0.8–6.25	8.0	8.0
Strep. pyogenes (Group A)	0.2–6.3	1.0	0.025–0.1	0.63	0.25
Strep. faecalis (Enterococcus Group D)	200.0	100.0	25.0	57.0	64.0
Gram-negative bacteria					
Escherichia coli	25.0–>100.0	16.0–>125.0	1.6–>100.0	16.0–>125.0	8.0
Enterobacter spp.	50.0–>100.0	>125.0	1.6–>100.0	>125.0	>128.0
Klebsiella spp.	50.0–>100.0	4.0–125.0	0.8–50.0	4.0–125.0	8.0
Proteus mirabilis	25.0–>100.0	4.0–63.0	1.6–50.0	4.0–63.0	>128.0
Proteus (other than mirabilis)	>100.0	>125.0	1.6–50.0	>125.0	>128.0
Providencia spp.	>125.0	>125.0	12.5–>100.0	>125.0	>128.0
Serratia spp.	>125.0	>125.0	>100.0	>125.0	>128.0
Haemophilus influenzae	12.5–>100.0	4.0–63.0	1.6–3.13	8.0–63.0	2.0
Pseudomonas aeruginosa	>100.0	>125.0	>100.0	>125.0	>128.0

These doses are similar to those of oral cephalexin (page 227). The cefaclor half-life in normal subjects is 40–60 min, and this increases to 3 h in patients with essentially no renal function. Patients with severe renal failure should receive one quarter of the usual dose, and those with moderate renal failure (creatinine clearance < 40 ml per min) one half of the usual dose. In patients with mild renal failure (creatinine clearance > 40 ml per min), modification of cefaclor dose is probably unnecessary (Bloch *et al.*, 1977; Santore *et al.*, 1978).

Availability

1. *Cephradine*
    (a) *For oral administration:*
        Capsules: 250 and 500 mg.
        For children a powder for reconstitution, 125 or 250 mg in 5 ml.
    (b) *For parenteral administration:*
        Vials: 250 mg, 500 mg, 1·0 g, 2 g and 4 g.
2. *Cefadroxil* (oral administration only)
    Cefadroxil monohydrate capsules: 300 and 500 mg.
    Cefadroxil trihydrate capsules: 300 mg.
3. *Cefaclor* (oral administration only)
    Capsules: 250 mg.

Serum Levels in Relation to Dosage

1. *Cephradine.* Serum levels after oral administration of this drug are similar to those after cephalexin (Fig. 12, page 230). After a 0·5 g oral dose to adults, a peak serum level of approximately 15·0 μg per ml is reached in 1 h, which falls to 6·5 μg per ml at 2 h, 1·0 μg per ml at 4 h and 0·10 μg per ml at 6 h. Doubling the dose to 1·0 g increases the peak serum level by over 50 per cent, but usually does not double it. (Scholand *et al.*, 1974; Pfeffer *et al.*, 1977).

Following intravenous or intramuscular administration, serum levels attained are identical to those after cephalexin (page 230). As with cephalexin, intramuscular cephradine produces lower serum levels than equivalent oral doses.

2. *Cefatrizine.* Serum levels after oral administration are lower than those after cephalexin and cephradine (*vide supra*). With a 0·5 g oral dose, the peak serum level attained 1–2 h after dosing, is only about 6·0 μg per ml (Actor *et al.*, 1976; Del Busto *et al.*, 1976). Four hours after this dose the serum level is slightly higher than that of cephalexin, and in some subjects it can still be detected at 8 h, whereas cephalexin is always undetectable at this time. Thus oral cefatrizine has a more prolonged serum half-life than cephalexin (page 230). In a study in pregnant patients Bernard *et al.* (1977) estimated its half-life to be 2·4 h.

After intramuscular injection of 0·5 g of cefatrizine, an average peak serum level of 12·0 μg per ml is reached in 30 min. This peak is reached earlier and it is higher than that after intramuscular cephalexin and cephradine (page 230). Thereafter, the serum concentration falls, being 9·0 μg per ml at 1 h, 5·7 μg per ml at 2 h, 2·0 μg per ml at 4 h and 0·2 μg per ml at 8 h. The serum half-life after intramuscular injection has been estimated to be 86 min (Actor *et al.*, 1976).

3. *Cefadroxil.* The peak serum level, attained 1 h after an oral dose of this drug is about the same or slightly lower than that after cephalexin (page 230).

Cefadroxil differs from cephalexin and cephradine by having a longer serum half-life, and a slower urinary excretion rate as demonstrated by a greater area under the serum level against time curve. Thus cephadroxil's serum levels are more sustained. Doubling its dose results in doubling its serum concentrations (Hartstein et al., 1977; Pfeffer et al., 1977). After a 0·5 g oral dose to adults, the peak serum level in 1 h is approximately 15·0 μg per ml, which falls to 12·5 μg per ml at 2 h, 4·5 μg per ml at 4 h, 1·8 μg per ml at 6 h, 0·65 μg per ml at 8 h and the level at 12 h is still 1·1 μg per ml (Pfeffer et al., 1977). These authors estimated the serum half-life of cefadroxil to be 1·2 h and that of cephalexin to be 0·6 h, and the 'area under the curve' for cephadroxil was 1·6 times greater than that for cephalexin. Other authors have reported a somewhat longer half-life (0·9 h) for cephalexin (Bennett et al., 1977) (see also page 230).

Cefadroxil absorption is not impaired by food in the stomach. There is no difference in the serum levels produced by the two cefadroxil preparations, the monohydrate and trihydrate (Pfeffer et al., 1977).

4. *Cefaclor*. This drug is rapidly absorbed from the gastro-intestinal tract, but the peak level is lower than that after cephalexin (page 230) and subsequent serum levels also decline more rapidly. After a 200 mg oral cefaclor dose, the mean peak serum level at about 1 h is 6·0 μg per ml (comparable level for cephalexin 9·4), and this level falls to 0·33 μg per ml at 4 h (comparable level for cephalexin 0·68). Cefaclor is more rapidly excreted than cephalexin and their half-lives have been estimated to be 0·58 and 0·8 h, respectively (Korzeniowski et al., 1977). Concomitant administration of probenecid prolongs cefaclor's serum levels. Food intake significantly reduces its absorption. The serum half-life of cefaclor in patients with severe renal failure is only about 3 h, which suggests that the drug may also be eliminated by non-renal mechanisms (Santoro et al., 1978).

Excretion

1. *Cephradine*. Similar to cephalexin (page 230) this drug is excreted unchanged in urine. Up to 30 per cent of an orally administered dose is excreted during the first 6 h, resulting in high urine concentrations (Scholand et al., 1974). Probenecid delays its excretion by partially blocking renal tubular secretion. Cephradine accumulates in patients with impaired renal function. The serum half-life of cephradine is 1·3 h in normal subjects, but this rises to 15 h in patients with end-stage renal disease (Bennett et al., 1977).

Like cephalexin, some cephradine is also excreted in bile, where its concentration may be about four times higher than the serum level at the time. This biliary excretion is reduced if there is biliary tract obstruction and also if jaundice is present (Maroske et al., 1976).

2. *Cefatrizine*. Only about 35 per cent of an orally administered dose and 45 per cent of one given intramuscularly can be recovered from the urine as the active drug during the first 12 h. Urine concentrations during this time after a 0·5 g dose, vary from 50 to 400 μg per ml after oral administration and from 50–1650 μg per ml after intramuscular administration (Actor et al., 1976).

Some orally administered cefatrizine is probably unabsorbed, but the relatively low urine recovery of the active drug after intramuscular dosing raises the possibility that some if it may be metabolized in the body.

3. *Cefadroxil*. This cephalosporin is excreted in the urine in the active form by both glomerular filtration and tubular secretion (Pfeffer *et al.*, 1977). Approximately 93 per cent of a 0·5 g oral dose can be recovered from the urine as active drug during the first 24 h; most of this excretion occurs during the first 6 h, when urine concentrations are in the range 400–2400 μg per ml (Hartstein *et al.*, 1977). The tubular secretion rate of cefadroxil is less than that of cephalexin so that the urinary excretion of cephadroxil is of longer duration. This explains its more prolonged serum levels (page 261). Initial urine concentrations of cefadroxil are lower than those of cephalexin, but during the period 3–12 h after a dose, they are higher (Pfeffer *et al.*, 1977).

4. *Cefaclor*. Approximately 70 per cent of an orally administered dose can be recovered from urine as the active drug during the first 6 h. During this period, after a 250 mg oral dose urine concentrations range from 50 to 1000 μg per ml. The urinary levels of cefaclor are adequate to inhibit susceptible pathogens even in patients with moderately severe renal failure (Santoro *et al.*, 1978). Some of the drug may be metabolized in the body, but no metabolites have been identified (Korzeniowski *et al.*, 1977).

Distribution of the Drugs in Body

1. *Cephradine*. This drug has been reported to distribute well into various body fluids and tissues. It does not penetrate into the CSF of patients with uninflamed meninges, but some cephradine can be found in human brain tissue after usual therapeutic doses (Adam *et al.*, 1975). Its concentration in liver tissue approximates to the serum level at the time (Maroske *et al.*, 1976), and satisfactory concentrations are also reached in heart muscle, uterine muscle, lung and prostatic tissue (Adam *et al.*, 1975; Michel *et al.*, 1975; Kiss *et al.*, 1976). Cephradine also penetrates well into both normal and infected bone (Hierholzer *et al.*, 1974; Parsons *et al.*, 1976; Parsons, 1976), and crosses the placenta so that it is detectable in amniotic fluid.

The serum protein binding of cephradine is only 10 per cent (Bennett *et al.*, 1977).

2. *Cefatrizine*. Detailed data on the distribution of this drug are not yet available. It crosses the placenta readily, thereby achieving a wide distribution in various fetal tissues in the first half of gestation (Bernard *et al.*, 1977).

3. *Cefadroxil*. This is probably distributed in a similar manner to cephalexin (page 231), but as it is eliminated more slowly, it remains in body tissues for longer after single doses. It is 20 per cent serum protein bound (Pfeffer *et al.*, 1977).

4. *Cefaclor*. No body distribution data about this drug are available.

Mode of Action

These cephalosporins probably act on bacteria in a manner similar to cephalothin and cephaloridine (page 208) and cephalexin (page 231).

Toxicity

1. *Cephradine*. In general this drug is well tolerated. Gastro-intestinal symp-

toms after oral administration are probably similar and as frequent as those after oral cephalexin (page 231). Candida vaginitis can occur. Other side-effects include urticarial skin rashes, joint pains, headache and dizziness, all of which are uncommon (Klastersky *et al.*, 1973; Hubsher *et al.*, 1973; Scholand *et al.*, 1974; Mogabgab, 1976). Intramuscular cephradine can cause pain, but this is usually not severe. Thrombophlebitis can follow its intravenous use, but it is relatively infrequent. Mild elevations of blood urea have been noted during cephradine therapy, but serious nephrotoxicity has not been reported (Hubsher *et al.*, 1973; Macias and Eller, 1975; Mogabgab, 1976).

2. *Cefatrizine.* In one clinical trial involving 33 patients oral cefatrizine was well tolerated and, except for mild diarrhoea in five patients, no adverse effects were noted (Del Busto *et al.*, 1976).

3. *Cefadroxil.* During a pharmacological study in 20 healthy men it was well tolerated and no side-effects occurred (Hartstein *et al.*, 1977).

4. *Cefaclor.* In one pharmacological study this was administered orally to 20 healthy volunteers in a dose of 250 mg six-hourly; four developed mild gastro-intestinal symptoms, but there were no serious toxic effects (Korzeniowski *et al.*, 1977).

Clinical Uses of the Drugs

1. *Cephradine.* The oral preparation of this drug is suitable for the same indications as those for oral cephalexin (page 232). It has been used with success in pharyngeal, skin, soft tissue, respiratory and urinary tract infections (Whitworth *et al.*, 1973; Klastersky *et al.*, 1973; Scholand *et al.*, 1974; Mogabgab, 1976; Davies, 1977). Overall results with cephradine are similar to those obtained with cephalexin (page 232).

Parenteral cephradine has been advocated for some infections which would usually be treated by older parenteral cephalosporins such as cephaloridine and in particular cephalothin (page 213). However, the place of parenteral cephradine in severe infections such as pneumococcal pneumonia, Strep. viridans endocarditis and staphylococcal septicaemia in penicillin-allergic patients is not yet well defined. Some authors have obtained good results by using intravenous cephradine for severe infections of this type (Hubsher *et al.*, 1973; Macias and Eller, 1975).

It has been suggested that parenteral cephradine could completely replace cephalothin and cephaloridine for reasons such as its lesser toxicity, low serum protein binding and good stability to staphylococcal beta-lactamase; the drug can be also administered orally, intramuscularly and intravenously (Selwyn, 1976). This view is not justified. Cephradine and cephalexin (Table 19, page 259) have a lesser intrinsic antibacterial activity than cephalothin and cephaloridine (Table 12, page 202). In addition, compared to cephalothin (page 213), experience with parenteral cephradine for serious infections is still limited. Daggett and Nathan (1975) reported a case of Strep. viridans endocarditis which failed to respond to intravenous cephradine in a dose of 0·5 g every 3 h; the MIC of cephradine for this organism was 0·312 μg per ml.

2. *Cefatrizine.* Thirty-three patients with urinary tract or soft tissue infections or bacterial pneumonia have been treated by oral cefatrizine in a daily dose of 1·0–2·0 g. Most patients responded satisfactorily to this treatment (Del

Busto *et al.*, 1976), similar to the response previously reported with cephalexin (page 232).

3. *Cefadroxil and cefaclor.* These oral cephalosporins may be suitable for some of the indications for which cephalexin (page 232) is used. In one randomized controlled study of 50 children with impetigo, cefadroxil was as effective as penicillin G in curing existing lesions and in preventing the development of new lesions (Ginsburg *et al.*, 1978). Cefaclor has also been used successfully for the treatment of staphylococcal bullous impetigo (Gray *et al.*, 1978). Because of its antimicrobial spectrum (page 257), cefaclor may prove more effective than cephalexin (page 233) for some Gram-negative bacterial infections.

REFERENCES

Actor, P., Pitkin, D. H., Lucyszyn, G., Weisbach, J. A. and Bran, J. L. (1976), 'Cefatrizine (SK & F 60771), a new oral cephalosporin: Serum levels and urinary recovery in humans after oral or intramuscular administration—comparative study with cephalexin and cefazolin', *Antimicrob. Ag. Chemother.*, **9**, 800.

Adam, D., Hofstetter, A. G., Jacoby, W. and Reichardt, B. (1975), *Studies on the Diffusion of Cephradine and Cephalothin into Human Tissue*, 9th International Congress of Chemotherapy, London, 1975, Abstract M69.

Bach, V. T., Khurana, M. M. and Thadepalli, H. (1978), *In vitro* activity of cefaclor against aerobic and anaerobic bacteria, *Antimicrob. Ag. Chemother.*, **13**, 210.

Bennett, W. M., Singer, I., Golper, T., Feig, P. and Coggins, C. J. (1977), 'Guidelines for drug therapy in renal failure', *Ann. Intern. Med.*, **86**, 754.

Bernard, B., Thielen, P., Garcia-Cázares, S. J. and Ballard, C. A. (1977), 'Maternal-fetal pharmacology of cefatrizine in the first 20 weeks of pregnancy', *Antimicrob. Ag. Chemother.*, **12**, 231.

Bill, N. J. and Washington, J. A. II (1977), 'Comparison of *in vitro* activity of cephalexin, cephradine and cefaclor', *Antimicrob. Ag. Chemother.*, **11**, 470.

Bloch, R., Szwed, J. J., Sloan, R. S. and Luft, F. C. (1977), 'Pharmacokinetics of cefaclor in normal subjects and patients with chronic renal failure', *Antimicrob. Ag. Chemother.*, **12**, 730.

Buck, R. E. and Price, K. E. (1977), 'Cefadroxil, a new broad-spectrum cephalosporin', *Antimicrob. Ag. Chemother.*, **11**, 324.

Busch, D. F., Kureshi, L. A., Sutter, V. L. and Finegold, S. M. (1976), 'Susceptibility of respiratory tract anaerobes to orally administered penicillins and cephalosporins', *Antimicrob. Ag. Chemother.*, **10**, 713.

Daggett, P. R. and Nathan, A. W. (1975), 'Failure of cephradine in infective endocarditis', *Lancet*, **2**, 877.

Davies, B. I. (1977), 'Cephradine and ampicillin in urinary infection', *J. Antimicrob. Chemother.*, **3**, 219.

Del Busto, R., Haas, E., Madhavan, T., Burch, K., Cox, F., Fisher, E., Quinn, E. and Pohlod, D. (1976), '*In vitro* and clinical studies of cefatrizine, a new semisynthetic cephalosporin', *Antimicrob. Ag. Chemother.*, **9**, 397.

Dolfini, J. E., Applegate, H. E., Bach, G., Basch, H., Bernstein, J., Schwartz, J. and Weisenborn, F. L. (1971), 'A new class of semisynthetic penicillins and cephalosporins derived from D-2-(1, 4-Cyclohexadienyl) glycine', *J. Med. Chem.*, **14**, 117.

Fong, I. W., Engelking, E. R. and Kirby, W. M. M. (1976), 'Relative inactivation by Staphylococcus aureus of eight cephalosporin antibiotics', *Antimicrob. Ag. Chemother.*, **9**, 939.

Ginsburg, C. M., McCracken, G. H. Jr., Clahsen, J. C. and Thomas, M. L. (1978), 'Clinical pharmacology of cefadroxil in infants and children', *Antimicrob. Ag. Chemother.*, **13**, 845.

Gray, B. M., Hubbell, C. A. and Dillon, H. C., Jr. (1978), 'Susceptibility of Staphylococcus aureus to cefaclor and cephalothin: Laboratory and clinical studies', *Antimicrob. Ag. Chemother.*, **13**, 988.

Hamilton-Miller, J. M. T. (1974), 'Comparative activity of ampicillin and seven cephalosporins against Group D streptococci', *J. clin. Path.*, **27**, 828.

Hartstein, A. I., Patrick, K. E., Jones, S. R., Miller, M. J. and Bryant, R. E. (1977), 'Comparison of pharmacological and antimicrobial properties of cefadroxil and cephalexin', *Antimicrob. Ag. Chemother.*, **12**, 93.

Hierholzer, G., Lienzenmeier, G., Kleining, R. and Hoerster, G. (1974), 'Study of the diffusion of various cephalosporins in the bone tissue', *Aktuelle Traumatologie*, **4**, 191.

Hubsher, J. A., Calóza, D. L. and Bernfeld, G. E. (1973), *Worldwide Clinical Experience with Cephradine for Injection*, Proceedings of 8th International Congress of Chemotherapy, Athens, Sept. 1973, p. 17.

Kisch, A. L. and Bartholomew, L. (1976), 'Comparison of the *in vitro* activity of several cephalosporin antibiotics against Gram-negative and Gram-positive bacteria resistant to cephaloridine', *Antimicrob. Ag. Chemother.*, **10**, 507.

Kiss, I. J., Faragó, E. and Pintér, J. (1976), 'Serum and lung tissue levels of cephradine in thoracic surgery', *Br. J. clin.Pharmac.*, **3**, 891.

Klastersky, J., Daneau, D. and Weerts, D. (1973), 'Cephradine Antibacterial activity and clinical effectiveness', *Chemotherapy*, **18**, 191.

Korzeniowski, O. M., Scheld, W. M. and Sande, M. A. (1977), 'Comparative pharmacology of cefaclor and cephalexin', *Antimicrob. Ag. Chemother.*, **12**, 157.

Lacey, R. W. and Stokes, A. (1977), 'Susceptibility of the "penicillinase-resistant" penicillins and cephalosporins to penicillinase of Staphylococcus aureus', *J. clin. Path.*, **30**, 35.

Leading Article (1973), 'Cephalosporins, present and future', *Lancet*, **2**, 364.

Leitner, F., Buck, R. E., Misiek, M., Pursiano, T. A. and Price, K. E. (1975a), BL-S 640, a cephalosporin with a broad spectrum of antibacterial activity: Properties *in vitro*', *Antimicrob. Ag. Chemother.*, **7**, 298.

Leitner, F., Chisholm, D. R., Tsai, Y. H., Wright, G. E., Deregis, R. G. and Price, K. E. (1975b), 'BL-S640, a cephalosporin with a broad spectrum of antibacterial activity: Bioavailability and therapeutic properties in rodents', *Antimicrob. Ag. Chemother.*, **7**, 306.

Macias, E. G. and Eller, J. J. (1975), 'Intravenous cephradine in serious paediatric infections', *Lancet*, **1**, 38.

Maroske, D., Knothe, H. and Rox, A. (1976), 'Liver tissue concentration of cephradine and cephacetrile and their excretion in bile', *Infection*, **4**, 159.

McGowan, J. E., Jr., Garner, C., Wilcox, C. and Finland, M. (1974), 'Antibiotic susceptibility of Gram-negative bacilli isolated from blood cultures: Results of tests with 35 agents and strains from 169 patients at Boston City Hospital during 1972' *Amer. J. Med.*, **57**, 225; *quoted by* Bill and Washington (1977).

Michel, C. F., Knothe, H., Lauer, B. and Werner, E. (1975), 'Concentration of cephradine and cephalothin in the serum and uterus musculature', *Geburtsh u. Frauenheilk.*, **35**, 24.

Miraglia, G. J., Renz, K. J. and Gadebusch, H. H. (1973), 'Comparison of the chemotherapeutic and pharmacodynamic activities of cephradine, cephalothin and cephaloridine in mice', *Antimicrob. Ag. Chemother.*, **3**, 270.

Moellering, R. C., Jr. and Swartz, M. N. (1976), 'Drug therapy. The newer cephalosporins', *New Engl. J. Med.*, **294**, 24.

Mogabgab, W. J. (1976), 'Treatment of urinary tract infections with cephradine',

Curr.Ther. Res., **19**, 520.

Neu, H. C. and Fu, K. P. (1978), 'Cefaclor: *In vitro* spectrum of activity and beta-lactamase stability', *Antimicrob. Ag. Chemother.*, **13**, 584.

O'Callaghan, C. H. (1975), 'Classification of cephalosporins by their antibacterial activity and pharmacokinetic properties', *J. Antimicrob. Chemother.* **1** (Suppl.), 1.

Overturf, G. D., Ressler, R. L., Marengo, P. B. and Wilkins, J. (1975), '*In vitro* evaluation of BL-S640, a new oral cephalosporin antibiotic', *Antimicrob. Ag. Chemother.*, **8**, 305.

Parsons, R. L. (1976), Leading article. 'Antibiotics in bone', *J. Antimicrob. Chemother.*, **2**, 228.

Parsons, R. L., Beavis, J. P., Paddock, G. M. and Hossack, G. M. (1976), 'Cephradine bone concentrations during total hip replacement', *Chemotherapy* (Ed. Williams J. D. and Geddes, A. M.), *Plenum Press*, **1**, 201.

Pfeffer, M., Jackson, A., Ximenes, J. and De Menezes, J. P. (1977), 'Comparative human oral clinical pharmacology of cefadroxil, cephalexin, and cephradine', *Antimicrob. Ag. Chemother.*, **11**, 331.

Phillips, I., King, A., Warren, C., Watts, B. and Stoate, M. W. (1976), 'The activity of penicillin and eight cephalosporins on Neisseria gonorrhoeae', *J. Antimicrob. Chemother.*, **2**, 31.

Sanders, C. C. (1977), '*In vitro* studies with cefaclor, a new oral cephalosporin', *Antimicrob. Ag. Chemother.*, **12**, 490.

Santoro, J., Agarwal, B. N., Martinelli, R., Wenger, N. and Levison, M. E. (1978), 'Pharmacology of cefaclor in normal volunteers and patients with renal failure', *Antimicrob. Ag. Chemother.*, **13**, 951.

Scheld, W. M., Korzeniowski, O. M. and Sande, M. A. (1977), '*In vitro* susceptibility studies with cefaclor and cephalexin', *Antimicrob. Ag. Chemother.*, **12**, 290.

Scholand, J. F., Hodges, G. R., Fass, R. J. and Saslaw, S. (1974), 'Clinical evaluation of cephradine, a new oral cephalosporin', *Amer. J. Med. Sci.*, **267**, 111.

Selwyn, S. (1976), 'Rational choice of penicillins and cephalosporins based on parallel *in-vitro* and *in-vivo* tests', *Lancet*, **2**, 616.

Selwyn, S. (1977), 'Susceptibility of penicillins and cephalosporins to beta-lactamases assessed by a new test', *J. Antimicrob. Chemother.*, **3**, 161.

Selwyn, S. and Bakhtiar, M. (1977), 'Penicillin-resistant gonococci', *Brit. med. J.*, **2**, 118.

Shadomy, S., Wagner, G. and Carver, M. (1977), '*In Vitro* activities of five oral cephalosporins against aerobic pathogenic bacteria', *Antimicrob. Ag. Chemother.*, **12**, 609.

Sinai, R., Hammerberg, S., Marks, M. I. and Pai, C. H. (1978), '*In vitro* susceptibility of Haemophilus influenzae to sulfamethoxazole-trimethoprim and cefaclor, cephalexin, and cephradine', *Antimicrob. Ag. Chemother.*, **13**, 861.

Stilwell, G. A., Adams, H. G. and Turck, M. (1975), '*In vitro* evaluation of a new oral cephalosporin, cefatrizine (BL-S640)', *Antimicrob. Ag. Chemother.*, **8**, 751.

Verbist, L. (1976), 'Comparison of the antibacterial activity of nine cephalosporins against Enterobacteriaceae and nonfermentative Gram-negative bacilli', *Antimicrob. Ag. Chemother.*, **10**, 657.

Vuye, A., Pijck, J. and Soep, H. (1976), '*In vitro* activity of BL-S640 against Gram-negative bacilli and Staphylococcus aureus compared with activity of four other semisynthetic cephalosporins', *Antimicrob. Ag. Chemother.*, **9**, 422.

Whitworth, J. A., Fairley, K. F. and McIvor, M. M. (1973), 'Cephradine in recurrent urinary tract infection', *Med. J. Aust.*, **2**, 742.

Yourassowsky, E., Schoutens, E. and Vanderlinden, M. P. (1976), 'Antibacterial activity of eight cephalosporins against Haemophilus influenzae and Streptococcus pneumoniae', *J. Antimicrob. Chemother.*, **2**, 55.

Cefamandole, Cefoxitin, Cefuroxime, Cefazaflur, Cefotaxime, SK & F75073 and Cefsulodin

Description

These seven compounds are described collectively, because compared to all other cephalosporins, they possess an increased resistance to beta-lactamases produced by Gram-negative bacteria. Therefore they are active against many Gram-negative bacteria which are resistant to other cephalosporins. However, there are important differences in their antimicrobial activities.

1. *Cefamandole*. Developed at Lilly Research Laboratories, this drug was first shown by Wick and Preston (1972) to have a very good activity against Gram-negative bacteria, including beta-lactamase producing strains of Proteus and Enterobacter spp. It also has a higher *in vitro* activity than cephalothin (page 200) against H. influenzae and other cephalosporin-sensitive Gram-negative bacilli (Eykyn *et al.*, 1973; Ernst *et al.*, 1976). Cefamandole is used clinically as the sodium salt of the O-formyl ester which is called cefamandole nafate. The independent antibacterial activity of cefamandole nafate is about 10 times less than that of cefamandole itself, but after administration this ester is rapidly converted to cefamandole *in vivo*, so that cefamandole is the predominant circulating antibiotic (Turner *et al.*, 1977; Wold *et al.*, 1978a).

2. *Cefoxitin*. This drug is a cephamycin. Cephamycins A, B and C are naturally occurring antibiotics which were obtained from several Streptomyces spp. at Merck Sharp and Dohme Research Laboratories (Stapley *et al.*, 197'). Elthough they are not cephalosporin antibiotics, they are structurally related to cephalosporin C (page 199), and are therefore included in this chapter. Cephamycin C has the greatest activity, particularly against Gram-negative bacteria. It is more stable to beta-lactamases than most cephalosporins, and it is active *in vitro* against many cephalothin-resistant strains of Gram-negative bacilli (Miller *et al.*, 1972a; Daoust *et al.*, 1973). Cephamycin C is non-toxic to animals (Miller *et al.*, 1972b). Chemically modified semisynthetic cephamycins have been produced from cephamycin C, and one of these is cefoxitin, a parenterally administered antibiotic, which is now marketed as 'Mefoxin'.

3. *Cefuroxime*. Research at the Glaxo Laboratories led to the development of this new cephalosporin with increased stability to beta-lactamases (O'Callaghan *et al.*, 1976; Ryan *et al.*, 1976). In addition to its activity against non-beta-lactamase producing Gram-negative bacteria, cefuroxime is active against many beta-lactamase producing strains of Enterobacter, Klebsiella and indole-positive Proteus spp. It is also highly active against N. gonorrhoeae 'including penicillinase producing strains), N. meningitidis and H. influenzae,

including ampicillin-resistant strains (O'Callaghan *et al.*, 1976; Norrby *et al.*, 1976).

4. *Cefazaflur*. This is another new cephalosporin with increased stability to beta-lactamases, and an antibacterial spectrum apparently similar to that of cefuroxime (Verbist, 1976). It is effective *in vitro* against Staph. pyogenes and the Enterobacteriaceae, but has relatively poor activity against Bacteroides fragilis and no useful activity against Ps. aeruginosa (Sutter and Finegold, 1976; Counts *et al.*, 1977). Marked differences in the *in vitro* activity of this antibiotic against many bacteria occur with different media, inocula and methods of testing, so that an evaluation of its usefulness will depend on *in vivo* studies (Counts *et al.*, 1977).

5. *Cefotaxime*. This compound which has been investigated by Hoechst/Roussel is also stable to many beta-lactamases produced by Gram-negative becitli. It has about the same *in vitro* activity against Staph. pyogenes as cephazolin (page 239). However, it is much more active then cephazolin against all Enterobacteriaceae, having good *in vitro* activity also against those which are always cephalothin- and cephazolin-res stant such as Enterobacter and Serratia species. Cefotaxime is also significantly more active against H. influenzae and N. gonorrhoeae than cephazotin, including beta-lactamase producing strains of these organisms. Pseudomonas spp. (MIC > 16 μg per ml) is usually resistent, but Bacteroides fragilis shows a wide range of susceptibility with an MIC range of 0·2–100 μg per ml (Leading article, 1978; Vanhoof *et al.*, 19   8). This compound is also known as HR 756.

6. *SK & F 75073*. A new parenteral cephalosporin, this is also more active than cephalothin against Gram-negative bacteria. It is quite active against Esch. coli, Klebsiella and Enterobacter spp., all Proteus spp. and some Serratia isolates. Neisseria spp. and H. influenzae, including ampicillin-resistant strains, are also susceptible. Ps. aeruginosa and B. fragilis are resistant. SK & F 75073 is some two- to eight-fold less active than cephalothin against Gram-positive bacteria such as staphylococci and streptococci (Actor *et al.*, 1978).

7. *Cefsulodin*. High activity against Ps. aeruginosa (MIC 3–6 μg per ml) is the important property of this new cephalosporin. Against other Gram-negetive bacilli it is not as active as carbenicillin (page 150), and against Gram-positive bacteria such as Staph. pyogenes, cephalothin (page 199) is more active than cefsulodin (Tsuchiya *et al.*, 1978). This drug is also known as SCE-129.

The following details apply only to cefamandole, cefoxitin and cefuroxime.

Sensitive Organisms

A. *Cefamandole*

1. *Gram-positive bacteria*. Cefamandole is quite active against Staph. pyogenes (non-penicillinase and penicillinase producing strains), Staph. epidermidis, Strep. pyogenes, Strep. pneumoniae and alpha-haemolytic streptococci (Strep. viridans). Strep. faecalis requires high cefamandole concentrations for its inhibition. This activity against Gram-positive cocci is comparable to that of cephalothin (Table 20, page 273), although some authors have found cefamandole to be marginally less active, particularly against Staph. pyogenes (Wick and Preston, 1972; Neu, 1974b; Bodey and Weaver, 1976). Cefamandole

appears to be as resistant to inactivation by staphylococcal beta-lactamase as cephalothin (page 199), and therefore it is a reliable anti-staphylococcal druo (Fong *et al.*, 1976a; Farrar and Gramling, 1976).

Gram-positive bacilli such as Clostridium tetani, Cl. perfringens and C. diphtheriae are also cefamandole-sensitive (Wick and Preston, 1972).

2. *Gram-negative cocci.* Cefamandole is quite active against the Neisseria (Table 20). It is more active than cephalothin and cefoxitin and about equally active to cefuroxime against meningococci. The activity of cefamandole against gonococci is greater than that of cephalothin and cefoxitin but less than that of cefuroxime (Wick and Preston, 1972; Eykyn *et al.*, 1976; O'Callaghan *et al.*, 1976). Cefamandole also remains quite active against penicillinase-producing gonococci (Sparling *et al.*, 1977) (*see also* page 8).

3. *Gram-negative aerobic bacilli.* As cefamandole is more stable to many beta-lactamases produced by these bacilli, it is more active against them than cephalothin, and it is also active against some cephalothin-resistant species (O'Callaghan, 1975). Thus bacteria which are normally cephalothin-sensitive such as Esch. coli, Proteus mirabilis and the Klebsiella spp. are even more sensitive to cefamandole (Wick and Preston, 1972; Neu, 1974b). Cefamandole is active against most cephalothin-resistant isolates of Esch. coli, but not against those of Kl. pneumoniae (Bodey and Weaver, 1976; Jackson *et al.*, 1977).

Among bacteria which are normally cephalothin-resistant, cefamandole exhibits good activity against indole-positive Proteus spp., with the exception of Pr. vulgaris which is usually moderately resistant. In addition, most Enterobacter strains and a proportion of those of Providencia and Citrobacter spp. are cefamandole-sensitive (Wick and Preston, 1972; Neu, 1974b; Shemonsky *et al.*, 1975; Meyers *et al.*, 1975; Russell, 1975; Meyers and Hirschman, 1978). Strains of Enterobacter spp. can be readily made resistant to cefamandole *in vitro*, by repeated passage in cultures containing the drug. Some of these resistant variants inactivate cefamandole enzymatically, others appear to possess intrinsic resistance (Findell and Sherris, 1976). Some strains of Yersinia enterocolitica are also sensitive to cefamandole (Simon *et al.*, 1978).

Cefamandole is active, and considerably more so than cephalothin, against all salmonellae, including Salm. typhi (Hirschman *et al.*, 1977; Barros *et al.*, 1977; Strausbaugh *et al.*, 1978). Ampicillin-resistant strains of Salm. typhi (page 101) are also cefamandole-sensitive (Hirschman *et al.*, 1977). The Shigella spp. are moderately sensitive (Wick and Preston, 1972; Neu, 1974b).

The drug is highly active against H. influenzae, an activity which is greater than that of cephalothin and cefoxitin, but about equal to that of cefuroxime (Table 20). Ampicillin-resistant strains of H. influenzae remain cefamandole-sensitive (Kammer *et al.*, 1975; Yourassowsky *et al.*, 1976; Meyers and Hirschman, 1978).

About 25 per cent of Serratia marcescens isolates are inhibited by cefamandole concentrations of 12 to 50 μg per ml; others require higher concentrations or are completely resistant. Acinetobacter spp. also need high concentrations (100–400 μg per ml) for inhibition or are completely resistant. Pseudomonas aeruginosa is always completely resistant (Neu, 1974b; Verbist, 1976; Griffith *et al.*, 1976; Fu and Neu, 1978).

4. *Gram-negative anaerobic bacilli.* B. melaninogenicus, some other

Bacteroides spp. and Fusobacterium spp. are sensitive to cefamandole, but Bacteroides fragilis is usually resistant (Ernst *et al.*, 1976; Sutter and Finegold, 1976). Erythromycin and cefamandole act synergistically against B. fragilis; in one study 0·25–0·5 μg per ml of erythromycin plus 0·4 μg per ml of cefamandole inhibited all strains tested, erythromycin increasing the potency of cefamandole by more than a hundred-fold (Griffith *et al.*, 1977b).

B. *Cefoxitin*

1. *Gram-positive bacteria*. Most pyogenic cocci such as Staph. pyogenes both sensitive and resistant to penicillin G, Staph. epidermidis, Strep. pyogenes, Strep. pneumoniae and the alpha-haemolytic streptococci (Strep. viridans) are cefoxitin-sensitive (Kosmidis *et al.*, 1973; Wallick and Hendlin, 1974; Neu, 1974a). However, cefoxitin's activity against these cocci is five to ten times less than that of cephalothin or cefamandole (Table 20, page 273), and is comparable to that of cephalexin (Table 14, page 227). Strep. faecalis (MIC 800 μg per ml) is more resistant to cefoxitin than to most cephalosporins (Hamilton-Miller, 1974). Cefoxitin is as resistant as cephalothin (page 199) to inactivation by staphylococcal beta-lactamase (Fong *et al.*, 1976a; Farrar and Grambling, 1976), so that except for its lesser intrinsic activity, it can be regarded as a reliable anti-staphylococcal agent.

Anaerobic Gram-positive cocci such as the Peptococcus and Peptostreptococcus spp. and anaerobic streptococci are nearly always cefoxitin-sensitive (Sutter and Finegold, 1976; Bach *et al.*, 1977).

Gram-positive bacilli such as Clostridium perfringens, other Clostridium spp. and Actinomyces spp. are also moderately cefoxitin-sensitive (Sutter and Finegold, 1976). Three strains of Listeria monocytogenes tested by Moellering *et al.* (1974) were sensitive to cephalothin, but resistant to cefoxitin.

2. *Gram-negative cocci*. Cefoxitin is active against meningococci, but to a lesser extent than cefuroxime (page 272) or cefamandole (page 269). It also has a slightly lesser activity than cephalothin against these organisms (Eickhoff and Ehret, 1976; Norrby *et al.*, 1976) (Table 20). Cefoxitin's activity against gonococci is marginally greater than that of cephalothin, but less than that of cefamandole (page 269) or especially cefuroxime (page 272) (Eickhoff and Ehret, 1976; Phillips *et al.*, 1976). Similar to cefamandole and cefuroxime, cefoxitin retains good activity against penicillinase-producing gonococci (Sparling *et al.*, 1977).

3. *Gram-negative aerobic bacteria*. A feature of cefoxitin is its high resistance to hydrolysis by various types of beta-lactamanses produced by Gram-negative organisms (Onishi *et al.*, 1974). Therefore it is active against many of these bacteria which are normally cephalothin-resistant or which have acquired resistance to this drug and other cephalosporins (Kosmidis *et al.*, 1973; Neu, 1974a). Against cephalothin-sensitive strains of Esch. coli, Proteus mirabilis and Klebsiella spp., cefoxitin is only slightly more active than cephalothin (Kosmidis *et al.*, 1973; Neu, 1974a; Brumfitt *et al.*, 1974) (*see also* Table 20). However, cefoxitin usually remains highly active against ampicillin-resistant Esch. coli strains (Norrby *et al.*, 1976) and also against strains of Esch. coli, Pr. mirabilis and Kl. pneumoniae which have become cephalothin-resistant. Cephalothin and gentamicin-resistant Kl. pneumoniae isolates are

also usually cefoxitin-sensitive (Wallick and Hendlin, 1974; Jackson *et al.*, 1977). Nevertheless, Kl. pneumoniae can become resistant if it is exposed to subinhibitory concentrations of cefoxitin *in vitro*; this resistance appears to be intrinsic in type because beta-lactamase activity was not demonstrated (Hoeprich and Huston, 1976).

Among bacterial species normally resistant to cephalothin, cefoxitin has good *in vitro* activity against all indole-positive Proteus spp. and Providencia spp. It is more active than both cefamandole and cefuroxime against Serratia marcescens, about 50 per cent or more of all isolates being inhibited by low cefoxitin concentrations. Cefoxitin is not as active as cefamandole against Enterobacter spp., and approximately one half of all strains are either completely resistant or need high concentrations for inhibition. Some strains of Citrobacter and Acinetobacter spp. are also sensitive to cefoxitin (Kosmidis *et al.*, 1973; Neu, 1974a; Wallick and Hendlin, 1974; Brumfitt *et al.*, 1974; Lewis *et al.*, 1976; Verbist, 1976; Adams *et al.*, 1976).

Cefoxitin's activity against salmonellae and shigellae is comparable to that of cephalothin, but inferior to that of cefamandole (Neu, 1974a; Moellering *et al.*, 1974) (*see also* Table 20). It is considerably less active against H. influenzae than cefamandole and cefuroxime, and also slightly less active than cephalothin (Yourassowsky *et al.*, 1976; Norrby *et al.*, 1976). Cefoxitin is also active against ampicillin-resistant strains of H. influenzae (page 102) (Kammer *et al.*, 1975). Similar to cefamandole and cefuroxime, Ps. aeruginosa is always highly cefoxitin-resistant (Kosmidis *et al.*, 1973; Wallick and Hendlin, 1974). The Legionnaires' disease bacterium is sensitive to cefoxitin *in vitro* (MIC 0·06–0·25 μg per ml) (Thornsberry *et al.*, 1978).

4. *Gram-negative anaerobic bacilli.* An important property of cefoxitin is that, unlike cefamandole and cefuroxime, it has good activity against Bacteroides fragilis, approximately 80 per cent of isolates being inhibited by a concentration of 16 μg per ml or less (Tally *et al.*, 1975; Sutter and Finegold, 1975; 1976; Norrby *et al.*, 1976; Henderson *et al.*, 1977; Bach *et al.*, 1977). Cefoxitin is also quite active against other Gram-negative anaerobes such as B. melaninogenicus and other Bacteroides and Fusobacterium spp. (Sutter and Finegold, 1976; Bach *et al.*, 1977). Resistance to beta-lactamase hydrolysis is the main reason for cefoxitin's action against B. fragilis. Darland and Birnbaum (1977) examined 79 strains of this organism; several isolates were resistant to cefuroxime because they produced enzymes capable of hydrolysing it, but cefoxitin was active against over 90 per cent of strains, and no strains produced an enzyme capable of hydrolysing it.

C. *Cefuroxime*

1. *Gram-positive bacteria.* Staph. pyogenes irrespective of penicillinase production is cefuroxime-sensitive, but 'methicillin-resistant' staphylococci (page 64) are relatively resistant (O'Callaghan *et al.*, 1976). Staph. epidermidis is usually sensitive (Eykyn *et al.*, 1976) and Strep. pyogenes, Strep. pneumoniae and the alpha-haemolytic streptococci (Strep. viridans) are sensitive. Strep. faecalis is usually resistant (O'Callaghan *et al.*, 1976). The activity of cefuroxime against all of these organisms is rather similar to that of cephalothin, but Staph. pyogenes and Staph. epidermidis are slightly less

susceptible to cefuroxime than cephalothin, and the reverse is true for Strep. viridans (Eykyn *et al.*, 1976; Jones *et al.*, 1977).

The Clostridium spp. is also usually cefuroxime-sensitive (O'Callaghan *et al.*, 1976).

2. *Gram-negative cocci.* Cefuroxime is quite active against N. meningitidis. It is especially active against N. gonorrhoeae, being more active than cefamandole, cefoxitin and cephalothin (O'Callaghan *et al.*, 1976; Phillips *et al.*, 1976). It is also fully active against penicillinase producing strains (Sparling *et al.*, 1977) (*see also* page 8).

3. *Gram-negative bacilli.* Activity of cefuroxime against these bacteria is rather similar to that of defamandole (page 269). Cefuroxime, like cefamandole and cefoxitin, is also very stable to most enterobacterial beta-lactamases (Hamilton-Miller, 1977; Greenwood, 1977). Enterobacteriaceae which are usually cephalothin-susceptible, such as Esch. coli, Pr. mirabilis and Kl. pneumoniae, are even more sensitive to cefuroxime (Eykyn *et al.*, 1976). However, the drug is not as active as cefoxitin against ampicillin-resistant Esch. coli (Norrby *et al.*, 1976).

In low concentrations cefuroxime inhibits approximately 60 per cent of Gram-negative bacilli which are normally cephalothin-resistant; these include indole-positive Proteus, Enterobacter, Providencia, Citrobacter and Hafnia spp. (O'Callaghan *et al.*, 1976; Eykyn *et al.*, 1976; Greenwood *et al.*, 1976; George *et al.*, 1978). A few Serratia marcescens strains are inhibited by cefuroxime in low concentrations, but the majority require either high concentrations or are completely resistant (O'Callaghan *et al.*, 1976; Verbist, 1976; Neu and Fu, 1978) (*see also* Table 20).

Cefuroxime is as active as cephalothin against the Salmonella spp., but slightly more active than cephalothin against Shigella spp. (O'Callaghan *et al.*, 1976).

Cefuroxime is very active against H. influenzae, being more active than cephalothin and cefoxitin, but having about the same activity as cefamandole (Table 20). This activity is also maintained against ampicillin-resistant strains, because cefuroxime is resistant to their specific beta-lactamase (page 102) (O'Callaghan *et al.*, 1976; Eykyn *et al.*, 1976; Norrby *et al.*, 1976; Sykes *et al.*, 1977).

Most strains of Acinetobacter spp. and all strains of Pseudomonas aeruginosa are completely cefuroxime-resistant. Some strains of other Pseudomonas spp. such as Ps. cepacia may be sensitive to cefuroxime. Certain Gram-negative anaerobic bacilli such as B. melaninogenicus are sensitive to cefuroxime, but Bacteroides fragilis usually needs high concentrations for inhibition or is completely resistant (O'Callaghan *et al.*, 1976; Eykyn *et al.*, 1976; Jones *et al.*, 1977).

In Vitro Sensitivities

The minimum inhibitory concentrations of cefamandole, cefoxitin and cefuroxime compared to those of cephalothin, against some selected bacterial species are shown in Table 20.

Compiled from data published by **Wick and Preston (1972), Wallick and Hendlin (1974), Neu (1974a and b), Brumfitt et al. (1974), Kammer et al. (1975), O'Callaghan et al. (1976), Norrby et al. (1976), Phillips et al. (1976), Sutter and Finegold (1976), Verbist (1976) and Report (1978).**

ORGANISM	MIC (µg per ml)			
	Cephalothin	Cefamandole	Cefoxitin	Cefuroxime
Gram-positive bacteria				
Staph. pyogenes (non-penicillinase producer)	0.25	0.25–1.0	1.6–6.4	0.25
Staph. pyogenes (penicillinase-producer)	0.5	0.5–1.0	1.6–6.4	0.25
Strep. pyogenes (Group A)	0.06–0.12	0.03–0.06	<0.8–1.6	≤0.125
Strep. pneumoniae (Dip. pneumoniae)	0.12–0.25	0.12–0.25	1.6–6.4	≤0.125
Strep. 'viridans'	0.5–1.0	0.5	<0.8–1.6	≤0.125
Strep. faecalis (Enterococcus, Group D)	16.0–32.0	32.0	200.0–800.0	>125.0
Clostridium perfringens	0.25–0.5	0.03–0.5	0.5–16.0	0.23
Gram-negative bacteria				
Esch. coli	4.0–32.0	0.5–1.0	0.78–25.0	2.9
Enterobacter spp.	16.0–>128.0	1.0–8.0	1.56–100.0	10.2
Klebsiella spp.	2.0–32.0	0.5–1.0	0.78–50.0	8.2
Proteus mirabilis	4.0–8.0	1.0–2.0	0.25–4.0	2.2
Proteus morganii	>128.0	1.0	0.25–8.0	16.0
Proteus rettgeri	>128.0	0.5–2.0	0.25–8.0	—
Proteus vulgaris	>128.0	8.0–32.0	0.25–8.0	39.0
Providencia spp.	50.0–>100.0	1.63–100.0	3.1	11.5
Salmonella spp.	4.0	1.0	0.8–3.12	3.6
Shigella spp.	8.0	2.0	0.8–6.25	4.6
Serratia marcescens	>128.0	4.0–>100.0	12.5–>100.0	116.0
Neisseria gonorrhoeae	0.15	0.02	0.12	0.005
N. gonorrhoeae (beta-lactamase producer)	—	0.25–2.0	—	0.25–1.0
N. meningitidis	0.5	0.125	0.25–4.0	0.125
H. influenzae	2.0–8.0	0.5	2.0–8.0	0.5
H. influenzae (ampicillin-resistant)	2.0–8.0	0.5–2.0	2.0–8.0	0.5
Pseudomonas aeruginosa	>128.0	>128.0	640.0–>1,000	>125.0
Bacteroides fragilis	64.0–>512.0	32.0–>512.0	0.5–32.0	53.0
Bacteroides melaninogenicus	0.5–32.0	0.1–8.0	0.1–8.0	0.5–8.0
Other Bacteroides spp.	0.5–256.0	0.1–100.0	0.5–32.0	—

Mode of Administration and Dosage

1. *Cefamandole*. Cefamandole nafate can only be given parenterally and it is suitable for both intramuscular and intravenous administration. In clinical trials to date, the total daily adult dose has ranged from 1·5 g to 8·0 g (22·5–120 mg per kg per day). Common dosage schedules employed have been 0·5 g eight- or six-hourly, 1·0 g every six, four or three hours and 2·0 g every six hours (Short *et al.*, 1976; Minor *et al.*, 1976). The higher doses have usually been administered intravenously, and it is possible that even higher doses of 12·0–16·0 g per day may be safe and suitable for use in severe infections (Griffith *et al.*, 1976).

Intravenously, cefamandole has usually been given by intermittent rapid infusions. Some have administered the intravenous dose, suitably diluted, over a period of 5 min (Appel *et al.*, 1976), others over periods of 10, 15 or 30 min (Griffith *et al.*, 1976; Minor *et al.*, 1976; Short *et al.*, 1976). All these methods appear equally satisfactory. Intravenous cefamandole can cause thrombophlebitis, and one study suggested that this may be slightly more common with cefamandole than buffered cephalothin (Berger *et al.*, 1976) (*see also* page 204).

Patients with impaired renal function need a suitably reduced dosage, because cefamandole is excreted almost exclusively by the kidneys. Mellin *et al.* (1977) suggest a simple dosage schedule for such patients making two assumptions. The half-life of the drug can be calculated by adding 1·0 to the patient's serum creatinine measured in mg per 100 ml. (For conversion of serum creatinine values expressed in SI units, *see* page 333.) Secondly the normal six-hourly dose should be given once every third half-life. For example, a patient with normal renal function (creatinine 1·0 mg per 100 ml) should receive a usual cefamandole dose such as 1·0 g every $(1 + 1) \times 3 = 6$ h. A patient with a serum creatinine of 3·0 mg per 100 ml should receive this cefamandole dose every $(3 + 1) \times 3 = 12$ h; alternatively in such patients to avoid long intervals between doses, one-third of the usual dose could be administered once every half-life. In patients with end-stage renal failure the cefamandole half-life has been estimated to be 7·0–8·0 h (Appel *et al.*, 1976; Ahern *et al.*, 1976), but Meyers and Hirschman (1977) found it to be 12–18 h. According to the above schedule these patients could be given a 1·0 g dose once every third half-life (approximately 24 h), or alternatively after a loading dose of 1·0 g, one-half or one-third of this dose could be given once every half-life (7·0–8·0 h).

Very little cefamandole is removed during peritoneal dialysis, so that additional dosing is not necessary during this procedure. For patients treated with haemodialysis, which removes more cefamandole, several dosage regimens have been advocated. Appel *et al.* (1976) suggest that no extra dosage of cefamandole is necessary, provided that the patient has received a dose just before dialysis. Meyers and Hirschman (1977) agree that no change of dosage is necessary during haemodialysis, but recommend that an extra one-third to one-half of the loading dose should be given at the end of dialysis. However, Ahern *et al.* (1976) found that the cefamandole half-life was shorter during haemodialysis (6·6 h), and advised that reduced cefamandole doses (1/3–1/2 of the loading dose) should be administered at this shorter 6–7 h interval, during dialysis. All these recommendations appear satisfactory and would achieve about the same result.

2. *Cefoxitin*. This cephamycin, like cefamandole (page 274) can only be administered parenterally. It can be given either intramuscularly or intravenously, but the latter is usually preferred because intramuscular injections are only slightly less painful than those of cephalothin (Kosmidis *et al.*, 1973; Brumfitt *et al.*, 1974) (*see also* page 202). The adult dose used so far has ranged from 1·0 g eight-hourly to 2·0 g six-hourly. Occasionally a dose as high as 2·0 g every four hours has been used (Geddes *et al.*, 1977; Haseltine *et al.*, 1977). On this basis, the corresponding doses for children would be from 15 mg per kg eight-hourly to 30 mg per kg six- to four-hourly. Cefoxitin has not been used in children to any extent so far.

The drug is usually administered intravenously by intermittent intravenous injections or by intermittent infusions, over a period of 3–30 min or even as long as 120 min (Goodwin *et al.*, 1974; Geddes *et al.*, 1977; Haseltine *et al.*, 1977). All these rates of infusion appear to be satisfactory.

As cefoxitin is excreted almost entirely via the kidney (page 281), it accumulates in patients with impaired renal function if usual doses are given. Its serum half-life in patients with normal renal function is 45 min (Kosmidis *et al.*, 1973). This is prolonged to 2 h in patients with a creatinine clearance of 30–80 ml per min, and to approximately 6 h in those with a creatinine clearance of 10–30 ml per min. In patients with virtually no renal function (creatinine clearance <10 ml per min) the cefoxitin serum half-life is approximately 12 h (Leroy *et al.*, 1978). All patients, irrespective of the degree of renal failure, may be given one loading dose of 1·0–2·0 g cefoxitin. Thereafter the dose is adjusted according to the severity of the patient's renal failure; with a creatinine clearance of 30–80 ml per min the usual daily dose is halved, with a clearance value of 10–30 ml per min one-sixth of the usual daily dose is given and for patients with virtually no renal function, a twelfth of the usual daily dose is recommended. These dosage reductions may be achieved by lengthening the intervals between doses, reducing the individual doses or combining the two approaches.

During haemodialysis approximately 85 per cent of the circulating antibiotic is removed, so that patients treated in this way should receive an extra loading dose of the drug after dialysis (Leroy *et al.*, 1978).

3. *Cefuroxime*. This drug like cefamandole (page 274) and cefoxitin (*vide supra*) is only suitable for intramuscular or intravenous administration. In clinical trials to date, the adult cefuroxime dose used has been in the range 0·5–2·0 g eight-hourly (Norrby *et al.*, 1977). For intravenous administration each dose is dissolved in 100 ml of saline and infused over 30 min, but more concentrated solutions have been used and injected over a period of 3 or 5 min (Foord, 1976; Norrby *et al.*, 1977; Goodwin *et al.*, 1977).

Cefuroxime is excreted almost entirely by the kidney (page 282), and patients with renal failure require a modified dosage schedule. The normal cefuroxime serum half-life of 75 min is prolonged to 24 h in anephric patients (Kosmidis *et al.*, 1978). Patients with a creatinine clearance of less than 10 ml per min may receive 0·5 g cefuroxime daily, those with a clearance of 10–20 ml per min, 0·5 g twice a day, and those with a clearance of 20–50 ml per min 0·5 g three times daily. When the creatinine clearance is greater than

50 ml per min, normal dosage may be used (Gower *et al.*, 1978).

Haemodialysis removes cefuroxime and patients treated this way should receive 0·5 g before and again after dialysis (Gower *et al.*, 1978). A variable amount of cefuroxime is removed during peritoneal dialysis, and this shortens the drug's half-life in anephric patients to approximately 14 h. During peritoneal dialysis these patients may be given 1·0 g once every 24 h (Kosmidis *et al.*, 1978).

Serum Levels in Relation to Dosage

1. *Cefamandole*. After an intramuscular injection of 1·0 g to adults, a peak serum level of approximately 20 μg per ml is reached 45 min after the dose (Fig. 13). This peak level is similar to that attained after a 1·0 g intramuscular cephalothin dose, but with cephalothin the peak occurs 30 min after the injection (page 205).

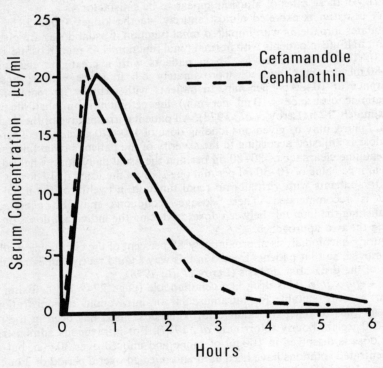

FIG. 13. Average serum levels after a 1 g intramuscular injection showing consistently higher levels for cefamandole beginning at 45 min, and an area under the curve about 25 per cent greater than for cephalothin (Redrawn after Fong *et al.*, 1976b).

Beginning at 45 min after intramuscular administration, cefamandole serum levels are consistently higher than those of cephalothin, and its area under the serum level curve is about 25 per cent larger (Fong *et al.*, 1976b). After a 1·0 g intramuscular dose, cephalothin can be detected in the serum for only 5–6 h (Fig. 13), but cefamandole activity is detectable for 6–8 h (Griffith *et al.*, 1976; Meyers *et al.*, 1976; Mellin *et al.*, 1977). The serum half-life of cefamandole after intramuscular injection is approximately one hour (Fong *et al.*, 1976b).

Immediately following a 1·0 g intravenous infusion of cefamandole over 20 min, the mean peak serum level is 88·0 μg per ml, the comparable figure for cephalothin being 64·0 μg per ml (Fig. 14). In addition, successive cefamandole levels are higher than those of cephalothin at all time intervals; at 2·5 h the cefamandole level is 3·0 μg per ml and that of cephalothin less than 1·0 μg per ml. Higher peaks are obtained if the dose is infused over a period of 3 or 5 min.

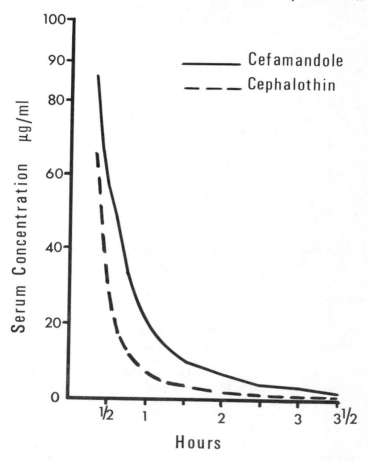

FIG. 14. Average serum cefamandole and cephalothin concentrations after a 1 g intravenous infusion given in 20 min (Redrawn after Fong *et al.*, 1976b).

Repeated intravenous dosing with 2·0 g of cefamandole every 6 h has no effect on peak serum levels, half-life, serum clearance or apparent volume of distribution of the drug (Barza *et al.*, 1976). The serum half-life of cefamandole after intravenous administration is only 34 min (Fong *et al.*, 1976b).

With both intramuscular and intravenous administration, doubling the dose of cefamandole approximately doubles peak serum levels, and prolongs, but does not double, the period during which the drug is detectable in the serum (Griffith *et al.*, 1976). Concomitant administration of probenecid (page 17) increases and prolongs serum levels of cefamandole (Griffith *et al.*, 1977a).

2. *Cefoxitin*. Serum levels of cefoxitin after both intramuscular and intravenous administration, like those of cefamandole, are higher than those of cephalothin (Kosmidis *et al.*, 1973; Brumfitt *et al.*, 1974). After a 1·0 g intramuscular dose to adults, a mean peak serum level of 22·5 μg per ml is reached 20 min later (Fig. 15). Thereafter the level falls, but cefoxitin can be detected in the serum for at least four hours.

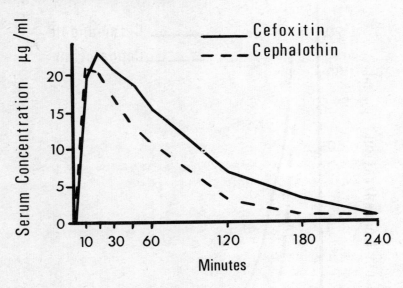

FIG. 15. Serum concentrations of cefoxitin and cephalothin after intramuscular administration of 1 g (Redrawn after Brumfitt *et al.*, 1974).

If 2·0 g of cefoxitin is administered intravenously over 3 min to adults, the mean peak serum level attained at approximately 5 min, is 222·6 μg per ml (Fig. 16). Thereafter this level falls more slowly than that of cephalothin, and a concentration of 3·4 μg per ml is still detectable at 3 h. When the same dose of cefoxitin is given as a 30 min intravenous infusion, the peak serum level (immediately after the infusion) is lower, but subsequent serum concentrations are slightly more sustained (Goodwin *et al.*, 1974). It is doubtful whether the rate of infusion influences clinical efficacy, as experience with the penicillins and other cephalosporins shows that within a given dose range, all methods of giving multiple intravenous doses are equally effective.

Doubling the intramuscular or intravenous dose of cefoxitin, virtually doubles serum concentrations (Brumfitt *et al.*, 1974; Geddes *et al.*, 1977). The mean cefoxitin serum half-life after either intramuscular or intravenous ad-

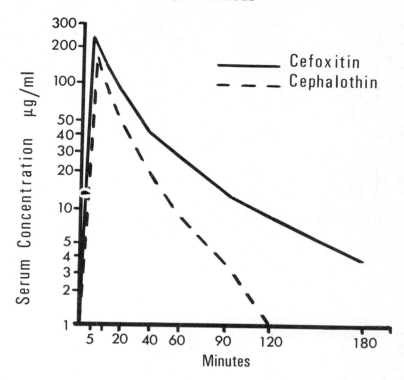

FIG. 16. Serum concentrations of cefoxitin and cephalothin after intravenous administration of 2 g (Redrawn after Brumfitt *et al.*, 1974).

ministration is 45 min. Concomitant administration of probenecid greatly enhances and prolongs cefoxitin serum levels, so that its half-life is then 83 min (Goodwin *et al.*, 1974).

3. *Cefuroxime*. After 0·5 g intramuscular dose to adults, a mean peak serum level of 25·3 μg per ml is reached in 30 min. Following a 1·0 g intramuscular dose the peak is higher (39·1 μg per ml), but not doubled, and it is reached in 45–60 min (Fig. 17). Serum levels after both doses are prolonged, and measurable concentrations of cefuroxime are still present eight hours after the injection. The area under the concentration time curve increases, but does not double with the higher dose.

If a 0·5 g dose of cefuroxime is infused intravenously over 30 min into adults, the mean peak serum level immediately after the infusion is 37·8 μg per ml; this level falls to 5·1 μg per ml at 3 h and the drug is still detectable in serum for 5–6 h (Fig. 18). If the same dose is given by rapid intravenous injection (over 3 min), the peak serum level is much higher (82·7 μg per ml), but at 3 h and thereafter the levels are slightly lower than after the 30 min infusion (Foord, 1976; Goodwin *et al.*, 1977).

The cefuroxime serum half-life after intramuscular or intravenous administration has been variously estimated as 1·16 h (Foord, 1976), 1·4 h (Norrby *et al.*, 1977) and 2 h (Goodwin *et al.*, 1977). Concomitant administra-

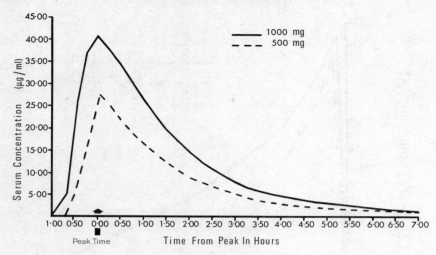

Fɪɢ. 17. Serum concentrations of cefuroxime after intramuscular injections (Redrawn after Foord, 1976).

tion of probenecid increases cefuroxime's serum concentrations, the total area under the curve, and its serum half-life (Foord, 1976). The pharmacokinetics of cefuroxime are rather similar to that of cephaloridine (page 205), but after intramuscular administration, the mean peak serum concentration and the mean area under the curve are significantly greater with cefuroxime, while the serum half-life and mean apparent volume of distribution are greater with cephaloridine (Foord, 1976).

Excretion

1. *Cefamandole*. Unlike cephalothin (page 207) cefamandole is not metabolized in the body (Barza *et al.*, 1976), and nearly all of a parenterally administered dose is excreted via the kidney in an unchanged active form (Meyers *et al.*, 1976; Griffiths *et al.*, 1976). High concentrations are attained in the urine; in one study during the first eight-hour period, the mean urinary concentration was 1633 μg per ml after a 0·5 g intramuscular dose and 3458 μg per ml after a 1·0 g dose (Meyers *et al.*, 1976).

The renal clearance of cefamandole is approximately 234 ml per min per 1·72 M^2, of body surface area; this exceeds the creatinine clearance of patients with normal renal function (82 ml per min per 1·72 M^2). Therefore cefamandole is not only excreted by glomerular filtration, but also by active tubular secretion (Mellin *et al.*, 1977). Probenecid (page 17) delays the drug's excretion by partly blocking tubular secretion (Griffith *et al.*, 1977a). The mean serum clearance of cefamandole (272 ml per min per 1·72 M^2) is similar to its renal clearance (*vide supra*), indicating that it is excreted mainly by the kidneys (Fong *et al.*, 1976b; Mellin *et al.*, 1977). This concept is also supported by animal experiments (Sullivan *et al.*, 1977).

A small amount of cefamandole is also eliminated via the bile. In one animal study biliary concentrations were approximately 30 times higher than the serum

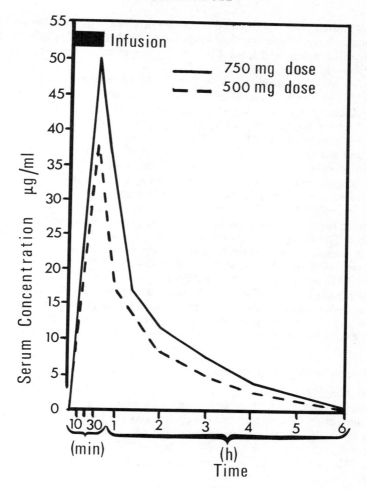

FIG. 18. Serum concentrations of cefuroxime: mean values during a six-hour period after the commencement of a 30 min infusion (Redrawn after Goodwin *et al.*, 1977).

levels at the time (Waterman *et al.*, 1976). In patients with a T-tube in the common bile duct peak biliary levels after 1 g intravenously average 352 μg per ml. After the same dose of cephazolin and cephalothin, comparative biliary levels were only 46 and 12 μg per ml, respectively. It therefore has been suggested that if a cephalosporin is indicated in biliary sepsis, cefamandole may be the drug of choice (Ratzan *et al.*, 1978).

2. *Cefoxitin*. Excretion in the urine in an unchanged form is virtually the only way this cephamycin is eliminated from the body. It is excreted by both glomerular filtration and active tubular secretion, so that probenecid (page 17) delays its excretion (Goodwin *et al.*, 1974). About 90 per cent or more of a parenterally administered dose can be recovered from the urine as the active unchanged drug during the following 12 h (Kosmidis *et al.*, 1973; Brumfitt *et*

al., 1974). High cefoxitin concentrations are attained in urine; after a 0·5 g intramuscular dose, concentrations range from 1000 to 3500 μg per ml during the first three hours, and from 22·0 to 350 μg per ml in the succeeding nine hours (Kosmidis *et al.*, 1973).

In a few subjects cefoxitin is deacylated in the body to detectable amounts of antibacterially inactive descarbamyl-cefoxitin. This does not appear to occur to any significant extent, as the metabolite can only be found in the urine after a delay of several hours, and it always accounts for less than 2 per cent of the administered dose (Goodwin *et al.*, 1974).

A small amount of cefoxitin may also be excreted in the bile. Cefoxitin bile levels in two patients with T-tube drainage after cholecystectomy were four to twelve times higher than simultaneous serum levels (Geddes *et al.*, 1977).

3. *Cefuroxime*. This drug also is not inactivated in the body, and virtually all of a parenterally administered dose is excreted via the kidney in an active unchanged form. It is excreted by both glomerular filtration and active tubular secretion. The latter accounts for 43–54 per cent of the total drug excreted, so that concomitant administration of probenecid (page 17) decreases cefuroxime clearance by about 40 per cent (Foord, 1976).

Over 95 per cent of intramuscularly or intravenously administered cefuroxime can be recovered from the urine during the first 24 h (Foord, 1976; Goodwin *et al.*, 1977). High concentrations of the drug are attained in urine; after a 0·5 g intramuscular dose, urinary concentrations are in the range 300–3000 μg per ml during the first six hours (Goodwin *et al.*, 1977).

Distribution of the Drugs in Body

1. *Cefamandole*. This drug, like other cephalosporins, probably does not penetrate into normal CSF to any extent. In animals with induced pneumococcal meningitis, CSF cefamandole concentrations are 3 per cent of simultaneous serum levels. When serum levels were achieved in these animals which were considered therapeutic for humans, the mean CSF cefamandole concentration was 0·98 μg per ml, which is higher than the MIC for pneumococci. The drug also penetrates into the brain tissue in therapeutic concentrations in such animals (Beam and Allen, 1977). In humans cefamandole also reaches inflamed meninges in significant concentrations. Steinberg *et al.* (1977) studied CSF cefamandole levels in twelve patients with bacterial meningitis, all of whom had received a single intravenous cefamandole dose (33 mg per kg), 75–140 min before lumbar puncture. Most of these patients had a detectable CSF level which correlated with the CSF protein; in six with a CSF protein less than 100 mg per 100 ml (1000 mmol/l), the concentration was zero to 0·62 μg per ml, and in the other six with a CSF protein greater than 100 mg per 100 ml, the range was 0·57–7·4 μg per ml (*see also* penicillin G, page 18).

Cefamandole also diffuses well into human interstitial fluid (Tan and Salstrom, 1977). Four adult patients with pneumonia caused by Gram-negative organisms receiving a cefamandole dose of 6·0 to 8·0 g daily had sputum cefamandole levels ranging from 0·27 to 2·5 μg per ml (Minor *et al.*, 1976).

It probably penetrates into other body fluids and tissues in a manner similar to cephalothin (page 208). The drug is approximately 70 per cent serum protein bound (Fong *et al.*, 1976b; Neu, 1978).

2. *Cefoxitin.* Like penicillins (pages 18, 109) and cephalosporins (pages 208, 246), this cephamycin does not penetrate into normal CSF (Haseltine *et al.*, 1977; Geddes *et al.*, 1977). It penetrates well into normal human interstitial fluid, where concentrations of the drug are very similar to serum levels (Gillett and Wise, 1978). The cefoxitin concentration in the breast milk of one patient, collected two hours after an intravenous dose of 1·0 g, was 5·6 µg per ml (Geddes *et al.*, 1977).

In animals cefoxitin penetrates into brain, heart, kidney, liver, lung, muscle and spleen, where its concentration is greater than that of cephalothin and approaches cephaloridine tissue levels (Miller *et al.*, 1974). Binding of cefoxitin to serum proteins is approximately 20 per cent (O'Callaghan, 1975).

3. *Cefuroxime.* This drug also penetrates well into the normal human interstitial fluid, reaching concentrations there similar to the serum levels at the time (Gillett and Wise, 1978). It is approximately 33 per cent bound to serum proteins (Foord, 1976).

Mode of Action

These cephalosporins and cefoxitin probably act on bacteria in a manner similar to cephalothin and cephaloridine (page 208).

Toxicity

All three compounds appear to have low toxicity to humans, but none have had wide clinical usage.

1. *Cefamandole.* Only a few side-effects have been reported with this drug. An allergic urticarial rash was observed in a few patients which rapidly subsided when the drug was ceased (Short *et al.*, 1976; Minor *et al.*, 1976; Steinberg *et al.*, 1977; Azimi, 1978). Eosinophilia has also been occasionally noted (Shemonsky *et al.*, 1975; Perkins *et al.*, 1978). Cefamandole, like cephalothin and cephaloridine (page 209), is probably only occasionally cross-allergenic with the penicillins. A positive Coombs test without haemolysis can occur with cefamandole as with other cephalosporins (Rodriguez *et al.*, 1978) (*see also* page 211).

One child developed what appeared to be drug fever due to cefamandole, occurring nearly two hours after its administration (Steinberg *et al.*, 1977). Elevated serum aspartate aminotransferase (SGOT) levels, and in a few patients also elevated creatinine phosphokinase levels, have occurred during cefamandole administration, usually when it has been given intramuscularly (Shemonsky *et al.*, 1975; Minor *et al.*, 1976). In one patient diarrhoea was attributed to parenteral cefamandole (Shemonsky *et al.*, 1975).

Nephrotoxicity due to cefamandole appears to be an uncommon complication. In a survey of 2000 treated patients, two sustained reversible nephropathy which might have been related to the drug therapy, and a third died of infection when renal damage was present, possibly due to cefamandole (Barza, 1978). In animals nephrotoxicity due to cefamandole is considerably less than that of cephazolin (page 247) (Wold *et al.*, 1978b). Also in animals high cefamandole doses do not increase tobramycin nephrotoxicity, but actually protect against aminoglycoside-induced renal injury, presumably by enhancing tobramycin excretion (Wold et al., 1977; Barza et al., 1978).

Severe pain after intramuscular cefamandole has only been recorded in a small number of patients (Shemonsky et al., 1975; Short et al., 1976). Thrombophlebitis can occur when it is used intravenously, and severe phlebitis is probably more likely with cefamandole than with buffered cephalothin (Berger et al., 1976) (see also page 204).

2. *Cefoxitin*. Eosinophilia (Haseltine et al., 1977) and a rash (McCloskey, 1977) have been reported in a few patients treated by cefoxitin. Two patients developed a positive Coombs test during therapy (Haseltine et al., 1977). Eight of 31 patients treated by Geddes et al. (1977) developed transient slight rises in serum aspartate aminotransferase (SGOT) levels.

During pharmacological studies in human volunteers cefoxitin appeared free from nephrotoxicity (Kosmidis et al., 1973; Brumfitt et al., 1974). Proteinuria without a rise in blood urea was observed in two of 31 patients treated by Geddes et al. (1977). Haseltine et al. (1977) treated 38 patients and four developed deterioration of renal function. Two of these had pre-existing renal functional impairment, and in the other two, factors such as hepatic failure and septicaemia may have contributed to renal failure. These reports suggest that cefoxitin may have nephrotoxic potential.

Intramuscular cefoxitin is only slightly less painful than intramuscular cephalothin (Kosmidis et al., 1973; Brumfitt et al., 1974). Thrombophlebitis due to intravenous administration was noted in 12 of 38 patients in one clinical study (Haseltine et al., 1977).

3. *Cefuroxime*. This drug has been well tolerated during human volunteer studies. Intramuscular injections appeared only slightly more painful than those of cephaloridine (page 202), and single intravenous infusions were administered without thrombophlebitis (Foord, 1976; Goodwin et al., 1977).

In one clinical study some minor side-effects were observed (Norrby et al., 1977). Eighteen of 60 patients developed slight reversible rises in SGOT levels and two a positive direct Coombs test without any signs of haemolysis. Nephrotoxicity or allergic reactions were not observed.

Clinical Uses of the Drugs

These three drugs may prove useful for the treatment of infections caused by Gram-negative bacteria, especially those which are resistant to cephalothin and other cephalosporins. All three, under certain conditions, may be suitable for the treatment of infections such as pyelonephritis and septicaemia caused by Gram-negative rods. Cefoxitin may be especially valuable for the treatment of sepsis following abdominal surgery, because it alone is active against both aerobic and anaerobic Gram-negative bacteria. Both cefamandole and cefuroxime may be suitable for H. influenzae infections, especially those due to ampicillin-resistant strains. There is also some evidence that cefamandole may be useful in systemic salmonella infections, and cefuroxime appears very promising for gonococcal infections due to penicillinase-producing strains.

None of these drugs is preferable to cephalothin for the treatment of infections caused by Gram-positive bacteria such as staphylococcal septicaemia or Strep. viridans endocarditis. Cefamandole and cefuroxime would probably be equally effective to cephalothin in this respect, but cefoxitin, being five to ten times less active *in vitro* than cephalothin against these bacteria (page 270), is likely to be inferior.

1. *Cefamandole*. This has been used with success for the treatment of urinary tract infections, mainly caused by cephalothin-sensitive Esch. coli and Klebsiella and Proteus spp. (Short *et al.*, 1976; Hoyme and Madsen, 1978). Complicated urinary tract and some systemic infections caused by cephalothin-resistant Enterobacter and indole-positive Proteus spp. also respond to cefamandole. Levine and McCain (1978a) reviewed patients treated by cefamandole for infections due to these two organisms; of 45 patients with Enterobacter infections, 41 had a satisfactory clinical response, and of 37 patients with indole-positive Proteus infection, 28 responded to treatment.

Satisfactory clinical results were obtained in 13 of 17 patients in whom cefamandole was used to treat pulmonary infections caused by Gram-negative bacilli. Organisms isolated included H. influenzae, Pr. mirabilis, Kl. pneumoniae, Serratia marcescens and some had infections with mixed Gram-negative rods (Minor *et al.*, 1976). Cefamandole has also been used with success for treatment of other infections in which a mixture of Gram-negative rods, mainly aerobic, were involved. Examples are the use of the drug in bacterial peritonitis (Stone *et al.*, 1978) and its use with carbenicillin for the treatment of infections in patients with cancer (Bodey *et al.*, 1978).

Results of cefamandole treatment of staphylococcal and streptococcal infections appear to be about the same as those obtained with cephalothin (page 213). Cefamandole is satisfactory for the treatment of respiratory tract, skin and soft tissue infections (Perkins *et al.*, 1978), pneumococcal pneumonia (Plaut and Perlino, 1978) and infections of bones and joints (Levine and McCain, 1978b). Similar infections in children including those due to H. influenzae such as sinusitis, cellulitis and pneumonia, also usually respond well to cefamandole (Azimi, 1978; Rodriguez *et al.*, 1978). However, one infant reported by Rodriguez *et al.* (1978) who had both periorbital cellulitis and H. influenzae septicaemia developed bacterial meningitis while receiving cefamandole treatment (*see also* cephalothin, page 212 and cephazolin, page 248).

The drugs *in vitro* activity against H. influenzae (page 269), and satisfactory penetration into the CSF of patients with bacterial meningitis (page 282), suggested that cefamandole may be satisfactory for the treatment of meningitis caused by ampicillin-resistant H. influenzae strains (Sherertz *et al.*, 1976; Steinberg *et al.*, 1977). Furthermore, it was found to be as effective as ampicillin in the therapy of experimental H. influenzae meningitis in rabbits (Sande *et al.*, 1978). In one clinical trial 24 of 25 adult patients with bacterial meningitis were cured by cefamandole used in a dose of 175–200 mg per kg per day. Most of these patients had meningococcal meningitis and only three, all of whom were cured, had H. influenzae type b meningitis (Korzeniowski *et al.*, 1978). By contrast, Steinberg *et al.* (1978) reported unsatisfactory results with cefamandole in children with H. influenzae type b meningitis. They treated three children with cefamandole (200 mg per kg per day), including one child with meningitis due to an ampicillin-resistant strain. All patients showed initial improvement, but in two patients the organism could still be cultured from the CSF during the first 72–96 h of therapy. The third patient relapsed with a recurrence of positive cultures during the seventh day of treatment. Cefamandole, therefore, appears unsatisfactory for the treatment of this disease, but further cautious trials with higher doses may be justified.

Hirschman *et al.* (1977) treated one adult patient with typhoid fever, using 2 g cefamandole intravenously every 6 h, for 14 days. Defervescence occurred within 24 h and the patient was subjectively well after 48 h. Recovery was uneventful and stool cultures remained negative during a six-month follow-up period.

2. *Cefoxitin.* Geddes and Wilcox (1978) used intravenous cefoxitin to treat successfully 30 of 34 patients with abdominal sepsis. All were seriously ill, 12 were septicaemic, including 5 due to Bacteroides fragilis. In two other studies, cefoxitin was used to treat soft tissue infections and pneumonia (both mainly due to Gram-negative bacilli), urinary tract infections, Gram-negative organism septicaemias and intra-abdominal infections such as peritonitis (Geddes *et al.*, 1977; Haseltine *et al.*, 1977). The majority of patients responded well.

McCloskey (1977) treated 143 patients with intravenous cefoxitin; 62 had Gram-positive infections (streptococcal or staphylococcal), 67 aerobic Gram-negative infections and 14 either anaerobic or mixed anaerobic and aerobic infections. Most patients responded satisfactorily, and the author suggested that cefoxitin may be suitable for staphylococcal and other Gram-positive coccal infections despite its inferior *in vitro* antibacterial activity against these organisms (page 270). Christophidis *et al.* (1978) found that the drug was useful for the treatment of nine patients with lung or urinary tract infections caused by cefoxitin-sensitive either Gram-negative or Gram-positive organisms. Cefoxitin was also equally effective to cephazolin (page 248) for the treatment of infections caused by organisms, mainly Gram-positive, which were sensitive to both antibiotics (Gurwith *et al.*, 1978).

3. *Cefuroxime.* In one trial cefuroxime was used to treat 60 patients with various types of sepsis, including soft tissue and lower respiratory tract infections, septicaemia and urinary tract infections (Norrby *et al.*, 1977). Most of the soft tissue infections were caused by Gram-positive bacteria such as Staph. pyogenes or Strep. pyogenes, and overall Gram-positive organisms predominated in the patients treated. Results of this trial were generally satisfactory. Daikos *et al.* (1977) treated 41 patients who had either urinary tract, respiratory tract, or bone and soft tissue infections, mainly due to Gram-negative aerobic bacilli. Twenty-nine of the 41 patients were cured, 9 improved and in 3 treatment failed. These results were regarded as satisfactory, as many patients were suffering from serious infections often due to multi-resistant Gram-negative bacilli.

Present evidence suggests that cefuroxime may be very useful for the treatment of gonorrhoea caused by penicillinase-producing gonococci (Willcox, 1977; McCormack, 1977). In preliminary clinical trials, when given as a single intramuscular dose of 1·5 g (750 mg in each buttock) together with 1·0 g probenecid orally, it was quite effective for both men and women with uncomplicated gonorrhoea (Medical News, 1977). A single 1 g dose of intramuscular cefuroxime plus 1 g probenecid orally also appears effective for men with uncomplicated gonorrhoea (Price and Fluker, 1978).

REFERENCES

Actor, P., Uri, J. V., Zajac, I., Guarini, J. R., Phillips, L., Pitkin, D. H., Berges, D. A., Dunn, G. L., Hoover, J. R. E. and Weisbach, J. A. (1978), 'SK & F 75073, new parenteral broad-spectrum cephalosporin with high and prolonged serum levels', *Antimicrob. Ag. Chemother.*, **13**, 784.

Adams, H. G., Stilwell, G. A. and Turck, M. (1976), '*In vitro* evaluation of cefoxitin and cefamandole', *Antimicrob. Ag. Chemother.*, **9**, 1019.

Ahern, M. J., Finkelstein, F. O. and Andriole, V. T. (1976), 'Pharmacokinetics of cefamandole in patients undergoing hemodialysis and peritoneal dialysis', *Antimicrob. Ag. Chemother.*, **10**, 457.

Appel, G. B., Neu, H. C., Parry, M. F., Goldberger, M. J. and Jacob, G. B. (1976), 'Pharmacokinetics of cefamandole in the presence of renal failure and in patients undergoing hemodialysis', *Antimicrob. Ag. Chemother.*, **10**, 623.

Azimi, P. H. (1978), 'Clinical and laboratory investigation of cefamandole therapy of infections in infants and children', *J. Infect. Dis.* (Suppl.), **137**, 155.

Bach, V. T., Roy, I. and Thadepalli, H. (1977), 'Susceptibility of anaerobic bacteria to cefoxitin and related compounds', *Antimicrob. Ag. Chemother.*, **11**, 912.

Barros, F., Korzeniowski, O. M., Sande, M. A., Martins, K., Santos, L. C. and Rocha, H. (1977), '*In vitro* antibiotic susceptibility of salmonellae', *Antimicrob. Ag. Chemother.*, **11**, 1071.

Barza, M., Melethil, S., Berger, S. and Ernst, E. C. (1976), 'Comparative pharmacokinetics of cefamandole, cephapirin and cephalothin in healthy subjects and effect of repeated dosing', *Antimicrob. Ag. Chemother.*, **10**, 421.

Barza, M. (1978), 'The nephrotoxicity of cephalosporins: An overview', *J. Infect. Dis.* (Suppl.), **137**, 60.

Barza, M., Pinn, V., Tanguay, P. and Murray, T. (1978), 'Nephrotoxicity of newer cephalosporins and aminoglycosides alone and in combination in a rat model', *J. Antimicrob. Chemother.* (Suppl.), **4**, 59.

Beam, T. R., Jr. and Allen, J. C. (1977), 'Blood, brain and cerebrospinal fluid concentrations of several antibiotics in rabbits with intact and inflamed meninges', *Antimicrob. Ag. Chemother.*, **12**, 710.

Berger, S., Ernst, E. C. and Barza, M. (1976), 'Comparative incidence of phlebitis due to buffered cephalothin, cephapirin, and cefamandole', *Antimicrob. Ag. Chemother.*, **9**, 575.

Bodey, G. P. and Weaver, S. (1976), '*In vitro* studies of cefamandole', *Antimicrob. Ag. Chemother.*, **9**, 452.

Bodey, G. P., Ketchel, S. and Rodriguez, V. (1978), 'Carbenicillin plus cefamandole in the treatment of infections in patients with cancer', *J. Infect. Dis.* (Suppl.), **137**, 139.

Brumfitt, W., Kosmidis, J., Hamilton-Miller, J. M. T. and Gilchrist, J. N. G. (1974), 'Cefoxitin and cephalothin: antimicrobial activity, human pharmacokinetics, and toxicology', *Antimicrob. Ag. Chemother.*, **6**, 290.

Christophidis, N., Dawborn, J. K. and Vajda, F. J. E. (1978), 'Studies of intravenous cefoxitin (MK 306)', *Med. J. Aust.*, **1**, 512.

Counts, G. W., Gregory, D. Zeleznik, D. and Turck, M. (1977), 'Cefazaflur, a new parenteral cephalosporin: *In vitro* studies', *Antimicrob. Ag. Chemother.*, **11**, 708.

Daikos, G. K., Kosmidis, J. C., Stathakis, Ch. and Giamarellou, H. (1977), 'Cefuroxime: antimicrobial activity, human pharmacokinetics and therapeutic efficacy', *J. Antimicrob. Chemother.*, **3**, 555.

Daoust, D. R., Onishi, H. R., Wallick, H., Hendlin, D. and Stapley, E. O. (1973), 'Cephamycins, a new family of β-lactam antibiotics: Antibacterial activity and resistance to β-lactamase degradation', *Antimicrob. Ag. Chemother.*, **3**, 254.

Darlano, G. and Birnbaum, J. (1977), 'Cefoxitin resistance to β-lactamase: A major

288   THE USE OF ANTIBIOTICS

factor for susceptibility of Bacteroides fragilis to the antibiotic', *Antimicrob. Ag. Chemother.*, **11**, 725.

Eickhoff, T. C. and Ehret, J. M. (1976), '*In vitro* comparison of cefoxitin, cefamandole, cephalexin and cephalothin', *Antimicrob. Ag. Chemother.*, **9**, 994.

Ernst, E. C., Berger, S., Barza, M., Jacobus, N. V. and Tally, F. P. (1976), 'Activity of cefamandole and other cephalosporins against aerobic and anaerobic bacteria', *Antimicrob. Ag. Chemother.*, **9**, 852.

Eykyn, S., Jenkins, C., King, A. and Phillips, I. (1973), 'Antibacterial activity of cefamandole, a new cephalosporin antibiotic, compared with that of cephaloridine, cephalothin and cephalexin', *Antimicrob. Ag. Chemother.*, **3**, 657.

Eykyn, S., Jenkins, C., King, A. and Phillips, I. (1976), 'Antibacterial activity of cefuroxime, a new cephalosporin antibiotic, compared with that of cephaloridine, cephalothin and cefamandole', *Antimicrob. Ag. Chemother.*, **9**, 690.

Farrar, W. E., Jr. and Gramling, P. K. (1976), 'Anti-staphylococcal activity and β-lactamase resistance of newer cephalosporins', *J. Infect. Dis.*, **133**, 691.

Findell, C. M. and Sherris, J. C. (1976), 'Susceptibility of Enterobacter to cefamandole: evidence for a high mutation rate to resistance', *Antimicrob. Ag. Chemother.*, **9**, 970.

Fong, I. W., Engelking, E. R. and Kirby, W. M. M. (1976a), 'Relative inactivation by Staphylococcus aureus of eight cephalosporin antibiotics', *Antimicrob. Ag. Chemother.*, **9**, 939.

Fong, I. W., Ralph, E. D., Engelking, E. R. and Kirby, W. M. M. (1976b), 'Clinical pharmacology of cefamandole as compared with cephalothin', *Antimicrob. Ag. Chemother.*, **9**, 65.

Foord, R. D. (1976), 'Cefuroxime: Human pharmacokinetics', *Antimicrob. Ag. Chemother.*, **9**, 741.

Fu, K. P. and Neu, H. C. (1978), 'A comparative study of the activity of cefamandole and other cephalosporins and analysis of the β-lactamase stability and synergy of cefamandole with aminoglycosides', *J. Infect. Dis.* (Suppl.), **137**, 38.

Geddes, A. M., Schnurr, L. P., Ball, A. P., McGhie, D., Brookes, G. R., Wise, R. and Andrews, J. (1977), 'Cefoxitin: a hospital study', *Brit. med. J.*, **1**, 1126.

Geddes, A. M. and Wilcox, R. M. L. (1978), 'Treatment of abdominal sepsis with cefoxitin', in Siegenthaler, W. and Lüthy, R. (Ed.), *Current Chemotherapy: Proceedings of the 10th International Congress of Chemotherapy*, Zurich/Switzerland, 1977. American Society for Microbiology, Washington, D.C., p. 299.

George, W. L., Lewis, R. P. and Meyer, R. D. (1978), 'Susceptibility of cephalothin—resistant Gram-negative bacilli to piperacillin, cefuroxime and other selected antibiotics', *Antimicrob. Ag. Chemother.*, **13**, 484.

Gillett, A. P. and Wise, R. (1978), 'Penetration of four cephalosporins into tissue fluid in man', *Lancet*, **1**, 962.

Goodwin, C. S., Raftery, E. B., Goldberg, A. D., Skeggs, H., Till, A. E. and Martin, C. M. (1974), 'Effects of rate of infusion and probenecid on serum levels, renal excretion, and tolerance of intravenous doses of cefoxitin in humans: comparison with cephalothin', *Antimicrob. Ag. Chemother.*, **6**, 338.

Goodwin, C. S., Dash, C. H., Hill, J. P. and Goldberg, A. D. (1977), 'Cefuroxime: pharmacokinetics after a short infusion, and *in vitro* activity against hospital pathogens', *J. Antimicrob. Chemother.*, **3**, 253.

Gower, P. E., Dash, C. H. and Kennedy, M. R. K. (1978), 'Pharmacokinetics of cefuroxime in the presence of renal failure and dialysis', in Siegenthaler, W. and Lüthy, R. (Ed.), *Current Chemotherapy: Proceedings of the 10th International Congress of Chemotherapy*, Zurich/Switzerland, 1977. American Society for Microbiology, Washington, D.C., p. 877.

Greenwood, D., Pearson, N. J. and O'Grady, F. (1976), 'Cefuroxime: a new cephalosporin antibiotic with enhanced stability to enterobacterial β-lactamases', *J. Antimicrob. Chemother.*, **2**, 337.

Greenwood, D. (1977), 'Enterobacterial β-lactamases', *J. Antimicrob. Chemother.*, **3**, 7.

Griffith, R. S., Black, H. R., Brier, G. L. and Wolny, J. D. (1976), 'Cefamandole: *in vitro* and clinical pharmacokinetics', *Antimicrob. Ag. Chemother.*, **10**, 814.

Griffith, R. S., Black, H. R., Brier, G. L. and Wolny, J. D. (1977a), 'Effect of probenecid on the blood levels and urinary excretion of cefamandole', *Antimicrob. Ag. Chemother.*, **11**, 809.

Griffith, R. S., Brier, G. L. and Wolny, J. D. (1977b), 'Synergistic action of erythromycin and cefamandole against Bacteroides fragilis Subsp. fragilis., *Antimicrob. Ag. Chemother.*, **11**, 813.

Gurwith, M., Albritton, W., Lank, B., Harding, G. and Ronald, A. (1978), 'Prospective comparison of cefoxitin and cefazolin in infections caused by aerobic bacteria', *Antimicrob. Ag. Chemother.*, **13**, 255.

Hamilton-Miller, J. M. T. (1974), 'Comparative activity of ampicillin and seven cephalosporins against Group D streptococci', *J. clin. Path.*, **27**, 828.

Hamilton-Miller, J. M. T. (1977), 'Leading article. Inhibition of β-lactamase: a continuing story', *J. Antimicrob. Chemother.*, **3**, 195.

Henderson, D. K., Chow, A. W. and Guze, L. B. (1977), 'Comparative susceptibility of anaerobic bacteria to ticarcillin, cefoxitin, metronidazole, and related antimicrobial agents', *Antimicrob. Ag. Chemother.*, **11**, 679.

Heseltine, P. N. R., Busch, D. F., Meyer, R. D. and Finegold, S. M. (1977), 'Cefoxitin: clinical evaluation in thirty-eight patients', *Antimicrob. Ag. Chemother.*, **11**, 427.

Hirschman, S. Z., Meyers, B. R. and Miller, A. (1977), 'Antimicrobial activity of cefamandole against Salmonella typhi', *Antimicrob. Ag. Chemother.*, **11**, 369.

Hoeprich, P. D. and Huston, A. C. (1976), 'Induction of resistance in Staphylococcus aureus and Klebsiella pneumoniae by exposure to cephalothin and cefoxitin', *J. Infect. Dis.*, **133**, 681.

Hoyme, U. and Madsen, P. O. (1978), 'Cefamandole and cefazolin in the therapy of complicated urinary tract infections', *J. Infect. Dis.* (Suppl.), **137**, 100.

Jackson, R. T., Thomas, F. E. and Alford, R. H. (1977), 'Cefoxitin activity against multiple antibiotic-resistant Klebsiella pneumoniae *in vitro*', *Antimicrob. Ag. Chemother.*, **11**, 84.

Jones, R. N., Fuchs, P. C., Gavan, T. L., Gerlach, E. H., Barry, A. L. and Thornsberry, C. (1977), 'Cefuroxime, a new parenteral cephalosporin: collaborative *in vitro* susceptibility comparison with cephalothin against 5,887 clinical bacterial isolates', *Antimicrob. Ag. Chemother.*, **12**, 47.

Kammer, R. B., Preston, D. A., Turner, J. R. and Hawley, L. C. (1975), 'Rapid detection of ampicillin-resistant Haemophilus influenzae and their susceptibility to sixteen antibiotics', *Antimicrob. Ag. Chemother.*, **8**, 91.

Korzeniowski, O. M., Carvalho, E. M., Jr., Rocha, H. and Sande, M. A. (1978), 'Evaluation of cefamandole therapy of patients with bacterial meningitis', *J. Infect. Dis.* (Suppl.), **137**, 169.

Kosmidis, J., Hamilton-Miller, J. M. T., Gilchrist, J. N. G., Kerry, D. W. and Brumfitt, W. (1973), 'Cefoxitin, a new semi-synthetic cephamycin: an *in vitro* and *in vivo* comparison with cephalothin', *Brit. med. J.*, **4**, 653.

Kosmidis, J., Stathakis, C. and Anyfantis, A. (1978), 'Cefuroxime kinetics in renal failure', in Siegenthaler, W. and Lüthy, R. (Ed.), *Current Chemotherapy: Proceedings of the 10th International Congress of Chemotherapy*, Zurich/Switzerland, 1977. American Society for Microbiology, Washington, D.C., p. 875.

Leading Article (1978), 'Cephalosporins compared', *Lancet*, **1**, 863.

Leroy, A., Fillastre, J. P., Oksenhendler, G. and Humbert, G. (1978), 'Pharmacokinetics of cefoxitin in normal subjects and in uremic patients', in Siegenthaler, W. and Lüthy, R. (Ed.), *Current Chemotherapy: Proceedings of the 10th International Congress of Chemotherapy*, Zurich/Switzerland, 1977. American Society for Microbiology, Washington, D.C., p. 763.

Levine, L. R. and McCain, E. (1978a), 'Cefamandole in the treatment of infections due to Enterobacter and indole-positive Proteus', *J. Infect. Dis.* (Suppl.), **137**, 125.

Levine, L. R. and McCain, E. (1978b), 'Clinical experience with cefamandole for treatment of serious bone and joint infections', *J. Infect. Dis.* (Suppl.), **137**, 119.

Lewis, R. P., Meyer, R. D. and Kraus, L. L. (1976), 'Antibacterial activity of selected β-lactam and aminoglycoside antibiotics against cephalothin-resistant enterobacteriaceae', *Antimicrob. Ag. Chemother.*, **9**, 780.

McCloskey, R. V. (1977), 'Results of a clinical trial of cefoxitin, a new cephamycin antibiotic', *Antimicrob. Ag. Chemother.*, **12**, 636.

McCormack, W. M. (1977), 'Treatment of gonorrhea – is penicillin passé?', *New Engl. J. Med.*, **296**, 934.

Medical News (1977), 'Classification and therapy challenging in penicillin-resistant gonorrhea', *JAMA*, **238**, 2339.

Mellin, H.-E., Welling, P. G. and Madsen, P. O. (1977), 'Pharmacokinetics of cefamandole in patients with normal and impaired renal function', *Antimicrob. Ag. Chemother.*, **11**, 262.

Meyers, B. R., Leng, B. and Hirschman, S. Z. (1975), 'Cefamandole: antimicrobial activity *in vitro* of a new cephalosporin', *Antimicrob. Ag. Chemother.*, **8**, 737.

Meyers, B. R., Ribner, B., Yancovitz, S. and Hirschman, S. Z. (1976), 'Pharmacological studies with cefamandole in human volunteers', *Antimicrob. Ag. Chemother.*, **9**, 140.

Meyers, B. R. and Hirschman, S. Z. (1977), 'Pharmacokinetics of cefamandole in patients with renal failure', *Antimicrob. Ag. Chemother.*, **11**, 248.

Meyers, B. R. and Hirschman, S. Z. (1978), 'Antibacterial activity of cefamandole *in vitro*', *J. Infect. Dis.* (Suppl.), **137**, 25.

Miller, A. K., Celozzi, E., Pelak, B. A., Stapley, E. O. and Hendlin, D. (1972a), 'Cephamycins, a new family of β-lactam antibiotics. III. *In vitro* studies', *Antimicrob. Ag. Chemother.*, **2**, 281.

Miller, A. K., Celozzi, E., Kong, Y., Pelak, B. A., Kropp, H., Stapley, E. O. and Hendlin, D. (1972b), 'Cephamycins, a new family of β-lactam antibiotics. IV. *In vivo* studies', *Antimicrob. Ag. Chemother.*, **2**, 287.

Miller, A. K., Celozzi, E., Kong, Y., Pelak, B. A., Hendlin, D. and Stapley, E. O. (1974), 'Cefoxitin, a semisynthetic cephamycin antibiotic: *in vivo* evaluation', *Antimicrob. Ag. Chemother.*, **5**, 33.

Minor, M. R., Sande, M. A., Dilworth, J. A. and Mandell, G. L. (1976), 'Cefamandole treatment of pulmonary infection caused by Gram-negative rods', *J. Antimicrob. Chemother.*, **2**, 49.

Moellering, R. C., Jr., Dray, M. and Kunz, L. J. (1974), 'Susceptibility of clinical isolates of bacteria to cefoxitin and cephalothin', *Antimicrob. Ag. Chemother.*, **6**, 320.

Neu, H. C. (1974a), 'Cefoxitin, a semisynthetic cephamycin antibiotic: antibacterial spectrum and resistance to hydrolysis by Gram-negative β-lactamases', *Antimicrob. Ag. Chemother.*, **6**, 170.

Neu, H. C. (1974b), 'Cefamandole, a cephalosporin antibiotic with an unusually wide spectrum of activity', *Antimicrob. Ag. Chemother.*, **6**, 177.

Neu, H. C. (1978), 'Comparison of the pharmacokinetics of cefamandole and other cephalosporin compounds', *J. Infect. Dis.* (Suppl.), **137**, 80.

Neu, H. C. and Fu, K. P. (1978), 'Cefuroxime, a β-lactamase-resistant cephalosporin with a broad spectrum of Gram-positive and -negative activity', *Antimicrob. Ag. Chemother.*, **13**, 657.

Norrby, R., Brorsson, J.-E. and Seeberg, S. (1976), 'Comparative study of the *in vitro* antibacterial activity of cefoxitin, cefuroxime, and cephaloridine', *Antimicrob. Ag. Chemother.*, **9**, 506.

Norrby, R., Foord, R. D. and Hedlund, P. (1977), 'Clinical and pharmacokinetic studies on cefuroxime', *J. Antimicrob. Chemother.*, **3**, 355.

O'Callaghan, C. H. (1975), 'Classification of cephalosporins by their antibacterial activity and pharmacokinetic properties', *J. Antimicrob. Chemother.* (Suppl.), **1**, 1.

O'Callaghan, C. H., Sykes, R. B., Griffiths, A. and Thornton, J. E. (1976), 'Cefuroxime, a new cephalosporin antibiotic: Activity *in vitro*', *Antimicrob. Ag. Chemother.*, **9**, 511.

Onishi, H. R., Daoust, D. R., Zimmerman, S. B., Hendlin, D. and Stapley, E. O. (1974), 'Cefoxitin, a semisynthetic cephamycin antibiotic: Resistance to β-lactamase inactivation', *Antimicrob. Ag. Chemother.*, **5**, 38.

Perkins, R. L., Fass, R. J., Warner, J. F., Prior, R. B., File, T. H., Tight, R. R., Gardner, W. G., Ruiz, D. E. and Slama, T. B. (1978), 'Cefamandole nafate therapy of respiratory tract, skin, and soft tissue infections in 74 patients', *J. Infect. Dis.* (Suppl.), **137**, 110.

Phillips, I., King, A., Warren, C., Watts, B. and Stoate, M. W. (1976), 'The activity of penicillin and eight cephalosporins of Neisseria gonorrhoeae', *J. Antimicrob. Chemother.*, **2**, 31.

Plaut, M. E. and Perlino, C. A. (1978), 'Cefamandole vs. procaine penicillin for treatment of pneumonia due to Streptococcus pneumoniae: A random trial', *J.Infect. Dis.* (Suppl.), **137**, 133.

Price, J. D. and Fluker, J. L. (1978), 'The efficacy of cefuroxime for the treatment of acute gonorrhoea in men', *Brit. J. vener. Dis.*, **54**, 165.

Ratzan, K. R., Baker, H. B. and Lauredo, I. (1978), 'Excretion of cefamandole, cefazolin, and cephalothin into T-tube bile', *Antimicrob. Ag. Chemother.*, **13**, 985.

Report of a WHO Scientific Group (1978), 'Neisseria gonorrhoeae and gonococcal infections', *Wld. Hlth. Org. techn. Rep. Ser.*, No. **616**, p. 130.

Rodriguez, W. J., Ross, S., Khan, W. N. and Goldenberg, R. (1978), 'Clinical and laboratory evaluation of cefamandole in infants and children', *J. Infect. Dis.* (Suppl.), **137**, 150.

Russell, A. D. (1975), 'The antibacterial activity of a new cephalosporin, cefamandole', *J. Antimicrob. Chemother.*, **1**, 97.

Ryan, D. M., O'Callaghan, C. H. and Muggleton, P. W. (1976), 'Cefuroxime, a new cephalosporin antibiotic: Activity *in vivo*', *Antimicrob. Ag. Chemother.*, **9**, 520.

Sande, M. A., Sherertz, R. J., Zak, O. and Strausbaugh, L. J. (1978), 'Cephalosporin antibiotics in therapy of experimental Streptococcus pneumoniae and Haemophilus influenzae meningitis in rabbits', *J. Infect. Dis.* (Suppl.), **137**, 161.

Shemonsky, N. K., Carrizosa, J. and Levison, M. (1975), '*In vitro* activity and pharmacokinetics in patients of cefamandole, a new cephalosporin antibiotic', *Antimicrob. Ag. Chemother.*, **8**, 679.

Sherertz, R. J., Dacey, R. and Sande, M. A. (1976), 'Cefamandole in the therapy of experimental pneumococcal meningitis', *J. Antimicrob. Chemother.*, **2**, 159.

Short, H. D., Gentry, I. O. and Sessoms, S. (1976), 'Cefamandole nafate therapy in the treatment of acute urinary tract infections', *J. Antimicrob. Chemother.*, **2**, 345.

Simon, V. C., Malerczyk, V. and Noxdorf, F. (1978), '*In vitro* activity and clinical pharmacology of cefamandole in comparison to cephalothin', *J. Antimicrob. Chemother.*, **4**, 85.

Sparling, P. F., Holmes, K. K., Wiesner, P. J. and Puziss, M. (1977), 'Summary on the conference on the problem of penicillin-resistant gonococci', *J. Infect. Dis.*, **135**, 865.

Stapley, E. O., Jackson, M., Hernandez, S., Zimmerman, S. B., Currie, S. A., Mochales, S., Mata, J. M., Woodruff, H. B. and Hendlin, D. (1972), 'Cephamycins, a new family of β-lactam antibiotics', *Antimicrob. Ag. Chemother.*, **2**, 122.

Steinberg, E. A., Overturf, G. D., Baraff, L. J. and Wilkins, J. (1977), 'Penetration of cefamandole into spinal fluid', *Antimicrob. Ag. Chemother.*, **11**, 933.

Steinberg, E. A., Overturf, G. D., Wilkins, J., Baraff, L. J., Streng, J. M. and Leedom, J. M. (1978), 'Failure of cefamandole in treatment of meningitis due to Haemophilus influenzae type b', *J. Infect. Dis.* (Suppl.), **157**, 180.

Stone, H. H., Guest, B. S., Geheber, C. E. and Kolb, L. D. (1978), 'Cefamandole in treatment of peritonitis', *J. Infect. Dis.* (Suppl.), **137**, 103.

Strausbaugh, L. J., Mikhail, I. A. and Edman, D. C. (1978), 'Comparative *in vitro* activity of five cephalosporin antibiotics against salmonellae', *Antimicrob. Ag. Chemother.*, **13**, 134.

Sullivan, H. R., Due, S. L., Kau, D. L. K., Quay, J. F. and Miller, W. M. (1977), 'Metabolic fate of [^{14}C] cefamandole, a parenteral cephalosporin antibiotic, in rats and dogs', *Antimicrob. Ag. Chemother.*, **12**, 73.

Sutter, V. L. and Finegold, S. M. (1975), 'Susceptibility of anaerobic bacteria to carbenicillin, cefoxitin, and related drugs', *J. Infect. Dis.*, **131**, 417.

Sutter, V. L. and Finegold, S. M. (1976), 'Susceptibility of anaerobic bacteria to 23 antimicrobial agents', *Antimicrob. Ag. Chemother.*, **10**, 736.

Sykes, R. B., Griffiths, A. and Ryan, D. M. (1977), 'Comparative activity of ampicillin and cefuroxime against three types of Haemophilus influenzae', *Antimicrob. Ag. Chemother.*, **11**, 599.

Tally, F. P., Jacobus, N. V., Bartlett, J. G. and Gorbach, S. L. (1975), 'Susceptibility of anaerobes to cefoxitin and other cephalosporins', *Antimicrob. Ag. Chemother.*, **7**, 128.

Tan, J. S. and Salstrom, S. J. (1977), 'Levels of carbenicillin, ticarcillin, cephalothin, cefazolin, cefamandole, gentamicin, tobramycin, and amikacin in human serum and interstitial fluid', *Antimicrob. Ag. Chemother.*, **11**, 698.

Thornsberry, C., Baker, C. N. and Kirven, L. A. (1978), '*In vitro* activity of antimicrobial agents on Legionnaires' disease bacterium', *Antimicrob. Ag. Chemother.*, **13**, 78.

Tsuchiya, K., Kondo, M. and Nagatomo, H. (1978), 'SCE-129, antipseudomonal cephalosporin: *In vitro* and *in vivo* antibacterial activities', *Antimicrob. Ag. Chemother.*, **13**, 137.

Turner, J. R., Preston, D. A. and Wold, J. S. (1977), 'Delineation of the relative antibacterial activity of cefamandole and cefamandole nafate', *Antimicrob. Ag. Chemother.*, **12**, 67.

Vanhoof, R., Butzler, J. P. and Yourassowsky, E. (1978), '*In vitro* activity of new cephalosporin (HR 756) and cefazolin', *Lancet*, **2**, 209.

Verbist, L. (1976), 'Comparison of the antibacterial activity of nine cephalosporins against enterobacteriacea and nonfermentative Gram-negative bacilli', *Antimicrob. Ag. Chemother.*, **10**, 657.

Wallick, H. and Hendlin, D. (1974), 'Cefoxitin, a semisynthetic cephamycin antibiotic: susceptibility studies', *Antimicrob. Ag. Chemother.*, **5**, 25.

Waterman, N. G., Eickenberg, H. U. and Scharfenberger, L. (1976), 'Concentration of cefamandole in serum, interstitial fluid, bile and urine', *Antimicrob. Ag. Chemother.*, **10**, 733.

Wick, W. E. and Preston, D. A. (1972), 'Biological properties of three 3-heterocyclic-thiomethyl cephalosporin antibiotics', *Antimicrob. Ag. Chemother.*, **1**, 221.

Willcox, R. R. (1977), 'How suitable are available pharmaceuticals for the treatment of sexually transmitted diseases? 1: Conditions presenting as genital discharges', *Brit. J. vener. Dis.*, **53**, 314.

Wold, J. S., Turnipseed, S. A., Broddle, W. D. and Owen, N. V. (1977), 'Effect of cefamandole nafate on the toxicity of tobramycin', *Antimicrob. Ag. Chemother.*, **12**, 465.

Wold, J. S., Joost, R. R., Black, H. R. and Griffith, R. S. (1978a), 'Hydrolysis of cefamandole nafate to cefamandole *in vivo*', *J. Infect. Dis.* (Suppl.), **137**, 17.

Wold, J. S., Welles, J. S., Owen, N. V., Gibson, W. R. and Morton, D. M. (1978b),

'Toxicologic evaluation of cefamandole nafate in laboratory animals', *J. Infect. Dis.* (Suppl.), **137**, 51.

Yourassowsky, E., Schoutens, E. and Vanderlinden, M. P. (1976), 'Antibacterial activity of eight cephalosporins against Haemophilus influenzae and Streptococcus pneumoniae', *J. Antimicrob. Chemother.*, **2**, 55.

Streptomycin

Description

Streptomycin was isolated from Streptomyces griseus in 1944 by Schatz, Bugie and Waksman. This drug belongs to the group of antibiotics known as the aminoglycosides or aminohexoses, which are basic compounds containing amino sugars. They also have an aminocyclitol structure and are more correctly called aminoglycoside aminocyclitols. Many streptomycin salts have been prepared, but the sulphate, being the least painful and irritative on intramuscular injection, is the only one used clinically.

Dihydrostreptomycin is a closely related compound produced by catalytic reduction of streptomycin trihydrochloride. Its antibacterial activity is similar to that of streptomycin, but it is not used because of its greater toxicity.

Sensitive Organisms

1. *Mycobacteria*. Streptomycin is particularly active against both human and bovine strains of M. tuberculosis. By contrast, in general the 'anonymous mycobacteria' (page 832) are nearly always streptomycin-resistant (Barter and Camens, 1968). Harris *et al.* (1975) however found that 76 per cent of patients with pulmonary infection due to M. kansasii in Texas, between 1971 and 1974, had strains sensitive to streptomycin. Although Mycobacterium ulcerans is usually sensitive to streptomycin *in vitro*, this disease does not usually respond to treatment with any chemotherapeutic agents (*see* page 833).

2. *Gram-negative bacteria*. Streptomycin is active against a large number of Gram-negative bacteria such as Esch. coli, the Enterobacter, Klebsiella, Salmonella, Shigella and Brucella spp., N. meningitidis, N. gonorrhoeae, H. influenzae, Pasteurella multocida, Francisella tularensis and Yersinia spp., which includes Y. pestis, Y. pseudotuberculosis and Y. enterocolitica. Some strains of Proteus spp. and less commonly even Pseudomonas aeruginosa are sensitive, but Bacteroides spp. are always resistant (Kislak, 1972).

3. *Gram-positive bacteria*. Some strains of Staph. pyogenes are sensitive, but most other Gram-positive cocci and bacilli are resistant. Strep. faecalis is always resistant to concentrations of streptomycin which can be attained *in vivo*, but penicillin G and streptomycin act synergistically against many strains of Strep. faecalis in both *vitro* and *vivo* (Sapico *et al.*, 1972). Strains of Strep. faecalis unaffected by this combination are highly streptomycin-resistant, often requiring 6000 μg per ml of streptomycin alone for inhibition. By contrast, strains against which the two drugs act synergistically, require only 250 μg per ml or less of streptomycin alone for inhibition (Kirby, 1970; Ruhen and Darrell, 1973). In a study of clinical isolates collected in Britain in 1975, 23 per

cent of Strep. faecalis strains had a high level of resistance to streptomycin. These strains were either sensitive or had a low level of resistance to gentamicin, tobramycin and amikacin, and each of these aminoglycosides when combined with penicillin G or amoxycillin showed synergism against the organism (Basker et al., 1977). Of 203 strains of Strep. faecalis isolated at the Massachusetts General Hospital during the period 1973–1976, depending on the source of the isolate, 36–54 per cent had high-level resistance to streptomycin, 16–49 per cent to kanamycin and 0–14 per cent to amikacin. A combination of penicillin G and amikacin failed to show synergism against a number of strains (Calderwood et al., 1977). Despite extensive use of gentamicin during the period, there were no Strep. faecalis strains which were highly resistant to it, and penicillin G plus gentamicin or tobramycin were synergistic against all strains tested. Combinations of penicillin G and sisomicin (Gutschik et al., 1977; Calderwood et al., 1977) or penicillin G and netilmicin (Sanders, 1977) are also synergistic against Strep. faecalis strains highly resistant to streptomycin. Vancomycin and streptomycin in combination are also often synergistic against Strep. faecalis (Westenfelder et al., 1973).

Some of the actinomycetes (see page 303) such as S. somaliensis may be sensitive to streptomycin (Mahgoub, 1976).

4. *Acquired resistance.* Practically all of the bacteria usually sensitive to streptomycin, including M. tuberculosis, can readily become resistant to this drug. Patients who have not received previous treatment, but who have tubercle bacilli resistant to streptomycin or other antituberculosis drugs, are described as having primary drug resistance. This is relatively rare in developed countries such as Britain, North America and Australia. The percentage of resistant strains in some areas, such as Hong Kong is as high as thirty (Leading article, 1972). In a co-operative study involving twenty-two hospitals in the United States during an eight-year period 1961 through 1968, the overall average resistance to streptomycin was 2·3 per cent and there was no clear trend of any change (Doster et al., 1976). In a continuing study of drug resistance of M. tuberculosis in veterans in the United States from 1969 to 1973, primary resistance to streptomycin has remained less than 5·6 per cent and has not increased (Hobby et al., 1971; 1974). Studies in Massachusetts in 1972 and 1975/76 showed incidences of primary resistance to streptomycin of 1·65 and 2·05 per cent respectively (Stottmeier and Burkes, 1974; Stottmeier and Baker, 1977). Primary drug resistance is also still relatively rare in Australia; in the five-year period 1972–1976, the incidence has remained less than 4·6 per cent (Commonwealth Dept. Health, 1973–1977). Acquired (secondary) drug resistance in tuberculosis occurs as a result of previous chemotherapy.

Streptomycin-resistant Gram-negative bacilli have been common for years. Sabath (1969) reported that 50 per cent of Esch. coli, and 73 per cent of Klebsiella, 58 per cent of Enterobacter and 44 per cent of Proteus spp. isolated in a Boston hospital during 1967 were resistant to streptomycin. In a survey in London from 1967 to 1969, more than half of the Shigella sonnei strains isolated were also resistant to this drug (Davies et al., 1970).

There is partial cross-resistance between streptomycin, kanamycin and neomycin. Strains of M. tuberculosis and other bacteria resistant to kanamycin or neomycin are nearly always resistant to streptomycin, but the reverse is not always true and streptomycin-resistant bacteria are frequently still sensitive to the other two drugs (*Today's Drugs,* 1963). Strep faecalis strains highly resistant to streptomycin now not uncommonly show the same degree of resistance to kanamycin (Basker *et al.*, 1977; Gutschick *et al.*, 1977). Streptomycin-resistant strains of M. tuberculosis are usually sensitive to capreomycin (page 849).

In Vitro Sensitivities

The minimum inhibitory concentrations of sensitive strains of Staph. pyogenes and Gram-negative bacteria are usually in the range of $1-8\,\mu g$ per ml. Organisms with an MIC greater than $16\,\mu g$ per ml can be considered, from a practical point of view, resistant. The usual MIC of streptomycin for M. tuberculosis is $8\cdot0\,\mu g$ per ml. The 'resistance ratio' is often used as a convenient method for reporting sensitivities of M. tuberculosis. The MIC of the strain isolated from the patient is compared with the MIC of a standard H 37 R V strain of M. tuberculosis. Resistance ratio is the MIC of patient's strain divided by the MIC of the standard strain. A ratio lower than four indicates a sensitive organism, but ratios of four or higher for practical purposes indicate resistance.

Mode of Administration and Dosage

1. Streptomycin is given by the intramuscular route for the treatment of systemic infections because it is not significantly absorbed from the intestinal tract, The usual adult dose is 1 g daily given either once a day or in two divided doses. For serious infections such as miliary tuberculosis this dose can be doubled for short periods, preferably for no longer than one week. Doses higher than 2 g daily should not be given under any circumstances.

2. *In patients over the age of 40 years,* if prolonged treatment is indicated as for tuberculosis, a lower dosage such as $0\cdot75$ g or even $0\cdot5$ g daily is recommended to avoid toxicity, even if the patient's renal function appears normal.

3. *In children* the intramuscular dose is 20–40 mg per kg body weight per day, given once a day or in two divided doses. For short-term treatment of serious infections the higher dosage may be used, but for long-term treatment of tuberculosis the lower dose is advisable.

4. *Newborn and premature infants.* The dosage in these patients should be lower, and 10–20 mg per kg body weight per day is recommended (Yaffe, 1965; Yaffe and Back, 1966). A streptomycin dosage of $7\cdot5$ mg per kg given every 12 h is satisfactory for most infants (Herngren *et al.*, 1977).

5. *Patients with renal failure.* Streptomycin accumulates in these patients, so a modified dosage schedule depending on streptomycin serum levels is necessary. A peak serum level of $40-50\,\mu g$ per ml attained one hour after intramuscular injection should not be exceeded. Persistent levels over $20\,\mu g$ per ml are undesirable and levels estimated 24 h after injection should not exceed $3\,\mu g$ per ml (Commonwealth Dept. Health Australia, 1977). The streptomycin half-life in patients with normal renal function is $2\cdot4-2\cdot7$ h but in patients with severe oliguria or anuria, this may be prolonged to 50–100 h. These patients may be treated by using a loading dose of 1 g of streptomycin, followed by half

this dose every three to four days. Patients who have a creatinine clearance of less than 10 ml per min should be treated in the same way as anuric patients. Uraemic patients whose creatinine clearance is in excess of 10 ml per min excrete the drug more rapidly. It is difficult to formulate exact dosage schedules for these, but a loading dose of 1 g, followed by half this dose every one or two days is usually satisfactory (Kunin, 1967).

Streptomycin is removed slowly from the body by haemodialysis, and this is the treatment of choice for acute streptomycin poisoning (Edwards and Whyte, 1959). A safe effective dose for patients undergoing dialysis is 10 mg per kg per day, every five to seven days (Usuda and Sekine, 1978).

6. *Oral administration.* If oral streptomycin is selected for treatment of bacillary dysentery, the adult dose is 2 g every six hours, and for young babies 0·5 g six-hourly (Christie, 1968).

7. *Intravenous streptomycin* is rarely used.

8. *Intrathecal streptomycin.* This was once used in a daily adult dose of 25–50 mg to treat tuberculous meningitis. Meningeal irrigation occurred in a number of patients and nowadays administration of streptomycin by this route is unnecessary for this infection (*see* page 814). Meade (1978) gave intrathecal streptomycin to children with Haemophilus influenzae meningitis; the dose was 2 mg per kg which amounted to 10–15 mg for children aged three to six months to a maximum of 40 mg for children aged six years. This dose was given intrathecally two or three times over the first 24 h (*see* page 303).

Serum Levels in Relation to Dosage

Streptomycin is rapidly absorbed after intramuscular administration, and the peak serum level is reached within one hour (Fig. 19). Doubling the dose,

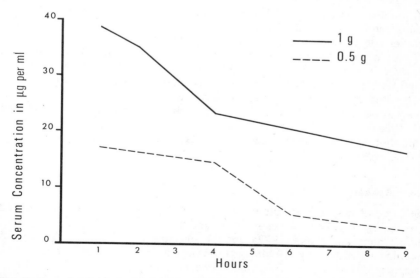

FIG. 19. Serum levels of streptomycin after intramuscular administration of 0·5 and 1·0 g doses. (Redrawn after Welch, 1954.)

doubles the serum concentration. A measurable level is usually maintained for approximately 12 h following a 0·5 g dose in an adult, and for up to 24 h after a 1·0 g dose.

Excretion

URINE: Streptomycin is rapidly excreted by glomerular filtration. In patients with normal renal function, most excretion occurs during the first twelve hours after intramuscular injection, but the amount may vary from 40 to 90 per cent of the administered dose in different individuals (Adcock and Hettig, 1946; Buggs *et al.*, 1946). High concentrations of the active drug are attained in urine, e.g. 200–400 μg per ml after an intramuscular dose of 0·5 g.

BILE: Small amounts of streptomycin, probably only 1 per cent of the total dose, are excreted unchanged in bile. Streptomycin concentrations in bile of 10–20 μg per ml have been recorded after the administration of the usual doses.

INACTIVATION IN BODY: From 10 to 30 per cent of parenterally administered streptomycin does not appear to be excreted, and is presumably inactivated in the body, but no streptomycin metabolites have been identified.

FAECES: Large amounts of active streptomycin appear in faeces, if the drug is administered orally (Adcock and Hettig, 1946).

Distribution of the Drug in Body

Streptomycin diffuses fairly rapidly into body fluids and tissues. It also enters ascitic and pleural fluids. After a single intramuscular injection, the concentration in these is initially much lower than that in the serum, but some four to six hours later, as the serum level falls, the level in the aberrant fluid may equal that found in the serum at the time (Adcock and Hettig, 1946). Streptomycin when given in normal doses penetrates the walls of tuberculous abscesses and achieves adequate levels even in caseous tissue (Fellander *et al.*, 1952).

Streptomycin does not enter the CSF, unless the meninges are inflamed. However the CSF streptomycin concentration is usually much lower than the serum level even in patients with acute meningitis (Buggs *et al.*, 1946).

The drug crosses the 'placental barrier', and simultaneous fetal blood levels are usually at least 50 per cent of maternal serum concentrations (Conway and Birt, 1965).

Streptomycin is approximately 34 per cent serum protein bound (Kunin, 1967; Gordon *et al.*, 1972).

Mode of Action

The mode of action of streptomycin on bacteria has been extensively studied (Cox *et al.*, 1964; Davies, 1964; Gorini and Kataja, 1964; Sparling and Davis, 1972; Chang and Flaks, 1972a and b). Informative reviews on this subject have been written by Goldberg (1965), Carter and McCarthy (1966), Kaempfer and Meselson (1969), and Gale *et al.* (1972).

Streptomycin and other aminoglycoside antibiotics interfere with bacterial protein synthesis (*see* page 433 for a descrption of the basic mechanisms involved). This action of streptomycin is dependent on its ability to bind to a particular protein or proteins of the 30 S subunit of bacterial ribosomes. As with some other aminoglycoside antibiotics (neomycin, kanamycin and gentamicin), this binding of streptomycin to the subunit results in a misreading (or miscoding) of m-RNA codons. Consequently, wrong amino acids are incorporated into growing peptide chains and faulty bacterial proteins are produced. The resultant alteration in the protein molecule may be small and it does not necessarily affect all bacterial proteins. It therefore is difficult to accept that this effect alone would be lethal to bacteria, yet streptomycin and other aminoglycosides are rapidly 'bactericidal'. It is postulated that streptomycin is bactericidal because it also causes detachment of ribosomes from m-RNA; two hypotheses have been put forward to explain this effect. Modolell and Davis (1970) suggest that streptomycin prevents binding of aminoacyl-t RNA to the ribosomal acceptor site, peptidyl-t RNA is subsequently released from the ribosome which then detaches from m-RNA. Luzzatto et al., (1968; 1969) propose that 30 S and 50 S subunits are released from m-RNA by completion of peptide chains in the presence of streptomycin, and then reassociate with m-RNA to form abnormal initiation complexes. Cell death occurs because of accumulation of these abnormal initiation complexes. More recently Kogut and Prizant (1975) have tried to explain most of the known *in vivo* actions of streptomycin. The gradual combination of intracellular streptomycin with specific proteins of 30 S ribosomes leads to faulty alignment or recognition with respect to messenger RNA and perhaps t-RNA during initiation; these affected ribosomes are released and may be able to re-initiate and repeat the process and increasing proportions of nonfunctional, shortened peptide chains are synthetized. This postulated selective misreading caused by streptomycin, therefore, would effect protein synthesis and growth before effects on the ribosome cycle are observable. *In vitro* studies, however, have demonstrated that streptomycin can have many effects on the protein synthesizing system of bacteria (Gale et al., 1972), and the exact mechanism of the drug's lethal effect on bacterial cells remains unclear.

In electron microscopic studies, streptomycin (and other aminoglycosides) cause the formation of blebs on the outer layer of the cell walls of Esch. coli and Ps. aeruginosa; chloramphenicol, tetracycline and erythromycin block the bactericidal action and bleb formation caused by streptomycin and kanamycin; the cell wall alteration caused by the bacteristatic drug spectinomycin is also blocked by chloramphenicol. It is suggested that this action of aminoglycoside antibiotics on the cell wall is an indirect effect due to dependence on ribosomal function for cell envelope biosynthesis (Iida and Koike, 1974).

Streptomycin resistance of bacteria may be due to drug inactivating enzymes, which are usually R plasmid-mediated (Kawabe et al., 1978), or due to genetic mutation causing a change in a particular protein of the 30 S ribosome subunit. Mutant strains may also occur which are streptomycin dependent, i.e. the ribosomes of such bacteria require streptomycin for 'normal' protein synthesis.

The processes by which streptomycin (and gentamicin) are taken up by bacteria have been recently investigated further (Bryan and Van Den Elzen, 1977). They postulate that these antibiotics initially associate with the cell wall and external surface of the cytoplasmic membrane on an electrostatic basis which is energy-independent. The next phase is energy-dependent and involves the binding of the antibiotics to membranous structures and respiratory quinones to form complexes, for their transport into the cell. There is a good correlation between susceptibility of bacteria to aminoglycosides and their possession of respiratory quinones. For instance quinones are not present in obligate anaerobes such as the Clostridia, which are resistant to aminoglycosides. The third phase is also energy-dependent, and involves membrane-bound aminoglycoside becoming bound to higher-affinity binding sites on membrane-associated ribosomes, which carry out protein synthesis. The latter phase results in a more rapid transport rate of the drugs into the cell. This hypothesis suggests that uptake of aminoglycosides is dependent on energy derived from aerobic metabolism (Saunders and Saunders, 1977).

Toxicity

1. *Ototoxicity*. This is the most serious toxic effect of streptomycin, usually resulting in vestibular disturbance with vertigo, but deafness can also occur (Cawthorne and Ranger, 1957). The risk of vestibular disturbance is related to total dosage, and also to excessive serum levels maintained for short periods. Peak serum levels of 40–50 μg per ml should probably not be exceeded and persistent levels greater than 20 μg per ml should be avoided. In patients aged more than 40 years, the risk of damage is higher despite apparently normal renal function. In addition, patients in this age group cannot compensate for vestibular damage as well as younger people. There appears to be also considerable individual variation in susceptibility to the drug.

If streptomycin is given in the usual doses for prolonged periods during pregnancy, the fetus may suffer ear damage, but severe effects appear to be uncommon. Robinson and Cambon (1964) reported two cases of congenital hearing loss that were probably caused by streptomycin administered to mothers during pregnancy. Conway and Birt (1965) examined seventeen children aged 6–13 years, whose mothers had received streptomycin during pregnancy. None of these children had any obvious disability, but detailed examination revealed minor abnormalities of 8th nerve function in eight; abnormalities in the caloric tests were present in six and in the audiograms in four. The authors suggest that such children may be very liable to ototoxicity if streptomycin or other related drugs were administered to them subsequently.

Dihydrostreptomycin, although less liable to cause vestibular disturbance is much more liable to cause deafness, which is often complete and almost always permanent. The onset of dihydrostreptomycin deafness may be delayed, so it is not possible to prevent continuing damage by stopping treatment at the first sign of ototoxicity. For this reason dihydrostreptomycin is no longer used.

2. *Hypersensitivity*. The most common manifestations of this complication are rash and fever. The rash is usually morbilliform or urticarial, but occasionally severe or even fatal exfoliative dermatitis may develop. Contact dermatitis may occur in persons handling the drug. Other manifestations include joint pains, lymphadenopathy or occasionally hepatitis (Thompson, 1969). Anaphylaxis is exceedingly rare. Streptomycin antibodies can be detected in serum of some sensitized individuals (Cronin, 1969). In most patients allergic

manifestations subside when streptomycin is stopped, but treatment with corticosteroids may be required for severe reactions. In the past, when streptomycin hypersensitivity developed in patients treated for tuberculosis, desensitization was often attempted. Nowadays, when more first-line antituberculosis drugs are available (ethambutol, page 832 and rifampicin, page 552) one of these is usually substituted for streptomycin if it causes hypersensitivity.

3. *Neuromuscular blockade*. This may occur with streptomycin and related drugs, especially if large amounts are introduced into the peritoneal cavity during surgery (Emery, 1963; McQuillen *et al.*, 1968). Fisk (1961) described neuromuscular blockade in an adult patient after 5 g of streptomycin was placed into the peritoneal, and another 5 g into the pleural cavity. Busch (1961) reported the case of a baby aged six months, who also developed this complication after instillation of 1 g of streptomycin in the peritoneal cavity. Another baby of the same age, reported by Pinkerton and Munro (1965) developed total paralysis necessitating mechanical ventilation for five hours, after 2 g of streptomycin was similarly administered. It appears that streptomycin can be just as completely absorbed from the peritoneum, especially if it is inflamed, as from intramuscular sites. Therefore if streptomycin is given intraperitoneally, a dose higher than that recommended for intramuscular use should not be given. Neuromuscular blockade in these patients is enhanced by prior use of muscle relaxants and other anaesthetic agents, but is antagonized by calcium and neostigmine. Similarly, patients suffering from myasthenia gravis may be more susceptible to this toxic effect (*see* also kanamycin, page 317 and neomycin, page 411).

4. *Other toxic effects*. Agranulocytosis and aplastic anaemia have been rarely reported following streptomycin therapy. A bleeding disorder due to the development of transient factor V inhibitor, possibly related to streptomycin treatment has also been reported (Feinstein *et al.*, 1973). Some patients develop circumoral paraesthesiae, and some others rarely develop a temporary lack of mental concentration after streptomycin injections.

5. *Nephrotoxicity*. In animals streptomycin is the least nephrotoxic of the aminoglycoside antibiotics, and human nephrotoxicity is very rare (Appell and Neu, 1977). Monitoring of renal function in ill patients is advisable to detect deterioration due to any cause because this may lead to accumulation of the drug and ototoxicity.

6. *Pain and irritation* at the site of intramuscular injection is fairly common, but the pain can be relieved by injecting the antibiotic together with procaine.

Clinical Uses of the Drug

1. *Tuberculosis*. Streptomycin is one of the standard 'first-line' drugs for this disease, and it should be used initially in combination with two other 'first-line' drugs. In such regimens isoniazid (page 810) is always included but either rifampicin (page 568), ethambutol (page 836) or less commonly para-amino salicyclic acid (page 825) may be chosen as the third drug. Nowadays streptomycin is not always included in initial regimens; in many situations, isoniazid in combination with two of the above other oral drugs may be used satisfactorily. Initial triple therapy should be continued for two to four months, or at least until results of sensitivity tests of the organism are available. At this stage the

injectable antibiotic, streptomycin, is usually stopped, and oral chemotherapy is continued with isoniazid combined with either rifampicin, ethambutol or PAS (*see* isoniazid, page 810).

Initial treatment with three antituberculosis drugs is used for pulmonary disease and for other forms of tuberculosis. Streptomycin is also often included in the initial phase of treatment in the short-course chemotherapy of pulmonary tuberculosis (page 812).

Streptomycin in a dose of 1 g two or three times weekly is also suitable for the fully supervised intermittent chemotherapy of pulmonary tuberculosis (*see* isoniazid, page 811).

2. *Brucellosis*. Streptomycin in combination with one of the tetracyclines is regarded as the best treatment for brucellosis (Martin, 1970) (*see also* page 623). *In vitro* studies suggest that kanamycin or gentamicin combined with tetracycline may be more effective than the classical streptomycin/tetracycline regimen (Robertson *et al.*, 1973). However clinical data regarding the efficacy of kanamycin and gentamicin regimens are not available.

3. *Bacterial endocarditis*. Streptomycin combined with either penicillin G or ampicillin has been considered for many years as the treatment of choice for Strep. faecalis endocarditis (Kirby, 1970; Mandell *et al.*, 1970). Penicillin G and streptomycin do not show synergism *in vitro* against every strain of Strep. faecalis (page 294), but a penicillin G/gentamicin combination is usually synergistic against all strains (Ruhen and Darrell, 1973). In addition, Strep. faecalis strains with a high level of resistance to streptomycin are frequently encountered in some areas (page 294). It has therefore been suggested that a penicillin G/gentamicin (page 344) or a penicillin G/tobramycin combination may be the best initial regimen for the treatment of Strep. faecalis endocarditis (Gutschik *et al.*, 1977). The efficacy of such regimens have not yet been confirmed by clinical studies. Also strains of Strep. faecalis relatively resistant to gentamicin have been detected which show variable responses in amoxycillin/gentamicin tests for bactericidal synergy (Basker *et al.*, 1977). These authors therefore emphasized the importance of appropriate laboratory tests in selecting the most suitable penicillin/aminoglycoside combination for these infections.

A penicillin G/streptomycin combination may also on rare occasions be necessary for the treatment of Strep. viridans endocarditis, if an uncommon strain relatively resistant to penicillin G is involved. Carey *et al.* (1977) used these drugs to treat two patients successfully with Vitamin B6-dependent Strep. mitior endocarditis; these organisms were resistant to penicillin G and relatively sensitive to streptomycin, but these two antibiotics demonstrated synergism against them *in vitro* and in experimental endocarditis. Antibiotic synergism between penicillin and streptomycin has also been demonstrated against many penicillin-sensitive Strep. viridans strains, both *in vitro* and in experimental animal endocarditis (Sande and Irvin, 1974). A combination of either penicillin G or V with streptomycin, has been used for the treatment of endocarditis caused by Strep. viridans strains highly sensitive to penicillin. Results obtained using such combinations for only two weeks compared favourably with the results after the usual six weeks' course of penicillin G (Tan *et al.*, 1971). Wolfe and Johnson (1974) also reported the successful use of a penicillin G/streptomycin combination; over 100 patients with endocarditis caused by penicillin-sensitive strains of Strep. viridans were treated parenterally with this combination for two weeks, followed by parenteral penicillin G for another two weeks. They had no relapses and because of the almost universal *in vitro* synergism of this combination against Strep. viridans, they recommended it as the optimal therapy for penicillin-sensitive viridans streptococcal endocarditis. Nevertheless, many clinicians still prefer prolonged treatment for this disease with penicillin G alone (*see* page 34). A vancomycin/streptomycin combination (page 295) may be used on rare occasions for the treatment of Strep. faecalis endocarditis, if the penicillins are contraindicated (Westenfelder *et al.*, 1973) (*see* page 650). A penicillin G/streptomycin combination is also recommended for the prevention of endocarditis in certain circumstances (*see* page 35).

4. *Haemophilus influenzae meningitis.* Streptomycin (30 mg per kg per day) administered intramuscularly in four divided doses (plus intrathecal streptomycin, page 297), together with intravenous and then oral sulfisoxazole (150 mg per kg per day) for 14 days, has been used successfully to treat H. influenzae meningitis (Meade, 1978). This regimen was suggested as an effective alternative to chloramphenicol (page 441) for the treatment of this disease caused by ampicillin-resistant strains (page 102).

5. *Plague and Tularaemia.* Streptomycin is probably the best drug for the treatment of plague but the tetracyclines are also effective (page 625). For tularaemia the tetracyclines are the drugs of choice, but streptomycin is also effective.

6. *Infections due to Gram-negative bacilli.* Streptomycin is rarely indicated for the treatment of septicaemias or simple urinary tract infections due to organisms such as Esch. coli and the Klebsiella and Proteus species. Its use may be rarely justified if other drugs are contraindicated and the organism is sensitive to streptomycin. If streptomycin is used for urinary tract infections, the urine should be made alkaline (*see* gentamicin, page 343).

7. *Intestinal infections.* Streptomycin administered orally, which is not absorbed from the intestinal tract, was previously considered of some value for Shigella sonnei infections (Christie, 1968). However it was always doubtful whether any antibiotics were of benefit in this disease (Smith and Young, 1966), and nowadays since most Shigella sonnei strains are streptomycin-resistant (page 295) the drug is of no value (Christie, 1973). Similarly oral streptomycin is ineffective for salmonella infections.

8. *Treatment of mycetoma.* This infection is caused either by actinomycetes (actinomycetoma) or fungi (eumycetoma), but only those caused by actinomycetes may respond to chemotherapy (Annotation, 1977). The actinomycetes include Nocardia asteroides, N. brasiliensis, Actinomadura madurae, Streptomyces somaliensis, Actinomadura pelletierii and Actinomyces israelii. Mahgoub (1976) treated 144 patients with a mycetoma caused by one of the actinomycetes (S. somaliensis, A. pelletierii, A. madurae and N. brasiliensis) with various drug regimens. He obtained a 63·2 per cent cure rate and another 21·5 per cent of patients showed great clinical improvement; the most effective treatments were dapsone plus streptomycin or co-trimoxazole plus streptomycin; sulfadoxine-pyrimethamine plus streptomycin, and rifampicin plus streptomycin also gave good results.

9. *Mycobacterium kansasii infections.* Streptomycin in combination with

isoniazid and ethambutol has been used to treat pulmonary infections due to this organism successfully (*see* page 838).

10. *Venereal diseases*. Streptomycin is effective for the treatment of chancroid and granuloma inguinale, but not for lymphogranuloma venereum; tetracyclines are usually preferred for all of these infections (Willcox, 1977). Because of the high prevalence of streptomycin-resistant gonococcal strains still present in many parts of the world (Report, 1978), streptomycin is not recommended for the treatment of gonorrhoea. Streptomycin is effective for non-specific urethritis caused by Ureaplasma urealyticum but not that caused by Chlamydia trachomatis (*see* pages 626, 627).

REFERENCES

Adcock, J. D. and Hettig, R. A. (1946), 'Absorption, distribution and excretion of streptomycin', *Arch. Intern. Med.*, **77**, 179.

Annotation (1977), 'Treatment of mycetoma', *Lancet*, **2**, 23.

Appel, G. B. and Neu, H. C. (1977), 'The nephrotoxicity of antimicrobial agents (second of three parts)', *New Engl. J. Med.*, **296**, 722.

Barter, C. E. and Camens, I. M. H. (1968), 'Lung infection with anonymous mycobacteria', *Med. J. Aust.*, **1**, 408.

Basker, M. J., Slocombe, B. and Sutherland, R. (1977), 'Aminoglycoside-resistant enterococci', *J. clin. Path.*, **30**, 375.

Bryan, L. E. and Van Den Elzen, H. M. (1977), 'Effects of membrane-energy mutations and cations on streptomycin and gentamicin accumulation by bacteria: A model for entry of streptomycin in susceptible and resistant bacteria', *Antimicrob. Ag. Chemother.*, **12**, 163.

Buggs, C. W., Pilling, M. A., Bronstein, B. and Hirshfeld, J. W. (1946), 'The absorption, distribution, and excretion of streptomycin in man', *J. Clin. Investig.*, **25**, 94.

Bush, G. H. (1961), 'Prolonged neuromuscular block due to intraperitoneal streptomycin', *Brit. med. J.*, **1**, 557.

Calderwood, S. A., Wennersten, C., Moellering, R. C. Jr., Kunz, L. J. and Krogstad, D. J. (1977), 'Resistance to six aminoglycosidic aminocyclitol antibiotics among enterococci: prevalence, evolution, and relationship to synergism with penicillin', *Antimicrob. Ag. Chemother.*, **12**, 401.

Carey, R. B., Brause, B. D. and Roberts, R. B. (1977), 'Antimicrobial therapy of vitamin B_6-dependent streptococcal endocarditis', *Ann. Intern. Med.*, **87**, 150.

Carter, W. and McCarthy, K. S. (1966), 'Molecular mechanisms of antibiotic action', *Ann. Intern. Med.*, **64**, 1087.

Cawthorne, T. and Ranger, D. (1957), 'Toxic effect of streptomycin upon balance and hearing', *Brit. med. J.*, **1**, 1444.

Chang, F. N. and Flaks, J. G. (1972a) 'Binding of dihydrostreptomycin to Escherichia coli ribosomes: Characteristics and equilibrium of the reaction', *Antimicrob. Ag. Chemother.*, **2**, 294.

Chang, F. N. and Flaks, J. G. (1972b), 'Binding of dihydrostreptomycin to Escherichia coli ribosomes: Kinetics of the reaction', *Antimicrob. Ag. Chemother.*, **2**, 308.

Christie, A. B. (1968), 'Bacillary dysentery', *Brit. med. J.*, **2**, 285.

Christie, A. B. (1973), 'Treatment of gastro-intestinal infections: A clinician's viewpoint', in Geddes, A. M. and Williams, J. D. (ed.), *Current Antibiotic Therapy*, Churchill Livingstone, Edinburgh and London, p. 183.

Commonwealth Department of Health Australia (1973–1977), Tuberculosis Statistics, Canberra.

Commonwealth Department of Health Australia (1977), *Treatment of Tuberculosis with Particular Reference to Chemotherapy*, 4th Edn., Australian Government Publishing Service, Canberra.

Conway, N. and Birt, B. D. (1965), 'Streptomycin in pregnancy: Effect on the foetal ear', *Brit. med. J.,* **2**, 260.

Cox, E. C., White, J. R. and Flaks, J. G. (1964), 'Streptomycin action and the ribosome', *Proc. Nat. Acad. Sci. U.S.A.,* **51**, 703.

Cronin, A. E. (1969), 'Antibodies to streptomycin in rabbits and man', *Suppl. Bulletin of the Post-Graduate Committee in Medicine, the University of Sydney,* **25**, lxxviii.

Davies, J. E. (1964), 'Studies on the ribosomes of streptomycin-sensitive and resistant strains of Escherichia coli', *Proc. Nat. Acad. Sci. U.S.A.,* **51**, 659.

Davies, J. R., Farrant, W. N. and Uttley, A. H. C. (1970), 'Antibiotic resistance of Shigella sonnei', *Lancet,* **2**, 1157.

Doster, B., Caras, G. J. and Snider, D. E. Jr. (1976), 'A continuing survey of primary drug resistance in tuberculosis, 1961 to 1968', *Amer. Rev. Resp. Dis.,* **113**, 419.

Edwards, K. D. G. and Whyte, H. M. (1959), 'Streptomycin poisoning in renal failure: an indication for treatment with an artificial kidney', *Brit. med. J.,* **1**, 752.

Emery, E. R. J. (1963), 'Neuromuscular blocking properties of antibiotics as a cause of post-operative apnoea', *Anaesthesia,* **18**, 57.

Feinstein, D. I., Rapaport, S. I. and Chong, M. M. Y. (1973), 'Factor V inhibitor: Report of a case, with comments on a possible effect of streptomycin', *Ann. Intern. Med.,* **78**, 385.

Fellander, M., Hiertonn, T. and Wallmark, G. (1952), 'Studies on the concentration of streptomycin in the treatment of bone and joint tuberculosis', *Acta Tuberculosea Scandinavica,* **27**, 176.

Fisk, G. C. (1961), 'Respiratory paralysis after a large dose of streptomycin', *Brit. med. J.,* **1**, 556.

Gale, E. F., Cundliffe, E., Reynolds, P. E., Richmond, M. H. and Waring, M. J. (1972), *The Molecular Basis of Antibiotic Action,* John Wiley and Sons Ltd., p. 300.

Goldberg, I. H. (1965), 'Mode of action of antibiotics II, drugs affecting nucleic acid and protein synthesis', *Amer. J. Med.,* **39**, 722.

Gordon, R. C., Regamey, C. and Kirby, W. M. M. (1972), 'Serum protein binding of the aminoglycoside antibiotics', *Antimicrob. Ag. Chemother.,* **2**, 214.

Gorini, L. and Kataja, E. (1964), 'Streptomycin-induced oversuppression in E. coli', *Proc. Nat. Acad. Sci. U.S.A.,* **51**, 995.

Gutschik, E., Jepsen, O. B. and Mortensen, I. (1977), 'Effect of combinations of penicillin and aminoglycosides on Streptococcus faecalis: A comparative study of seven aminoglycoside antibiotics', *J. Infect. Dis.,* **135**, 832.

Harris, G. D., Johanson, W. G. Jr. and Nicholson, D. P. (1975), 'Response to chemotherapy of pulmonary infection due to Mycobacterium kansasii', *Amer. Rev. Resp. Dis.,* **112**, 31.

Herngren, L., Boréus, L. O., Jalling, B. and Lagercrantz, R. (1977), 'Pharmacokinetic aspects of streptomycin treatment of neonatal septicaemia', *Scand. J. Infect. Dis.,* **9**, 301.

Hobby, G. L., Johnson, P. M. and Boytar-Papirnyik, V. (1971), 'Primary drug resistance: A continuing study of drug resistance in tuberculosis in a veteran population within the United States IX. September 1969—September 1970', *Amer. Rev. Resp. Dis.,* **103**, 842.

Hobby, G. L., Johnson, P. M. and Boytar-Papirnyik, V. (1974), 'Primary drug resistance: a continuing study of drug resistance in tuberculosis in a veteran population within the United States. X. September 1970 to September 1973', *Amer. Rev. Resp. Dis.,* **110**, 95.

Hussar, A. E. and Holley, H. L. (1954), *Antibiotics and Antibiotic Therapy,* The Macmillan Company, New York.

Iida, K. and Koike, M. (1974), 'Cell wall alterations of Gram-negative bacteria by aminoglycoside antibiotics', *Antimicrob. Ag. Chemother.*, **5**, 95.

Kaempfer, R. and Meselson, M. (1969), 'Studies of ribosomal subunit exchange', *Cold. Spr. Harb. Symp. quart. Biol.*, **34**, 209.

Kawabe, H., Tanaka, T. and Mitsuhashi, S. (1978), 'Streptomycin and spectinomycin resistance mediated by plasmids', *Antimicrob. Ag. Chemother.*, **13**, 1031.

Kirby, W. M. M. (1970), 'Editorial. Antibiotic synergism against enterococci', *J. Infect. Dis.*, **122**, 462.

Kislak, J. W. (1972), 'The susceptibility of Bacteroides fragilis to 24 antibiotics', *J. Infect. Dis.*, **125**, 295.

Kogut, M. and Prizant, E. (1975), 'Effects of dihydrostreptomycin on ribosome function *in vivo*: lack of correlation between changes in ribosome patterns and growth', *Antimicrob. Ag. Chemother.*, **7**, 341.

Kunin, C. M. (1967), 'A guide to use of antibiotics in patients with renal disease', *Ann. Intern. Med.*, **67**, 151.

Leading Article (1972), 'Resistant tubercle bacilli', *Lancet*, **2**, 412.

Lorian, V. (1971), 'The mode of action of antibiotics on Gram-negative bacilli', *Ach. Intern. Med.*, **128**, 623.

Luzzatto, L., Apirion, D. and Schlessinger, D. (1968), 'Mechanism of action of streptomycin in E. coli: Interruption of the robosome cycle at the initiation of protein synthesis', *Proc. Nat. Acad. Sci. USA.*, **60**, 873.

Luzzatto, L., Apirion, D. and Schlessinger, D. (1969), 'Polyribosome depletion and blockage of the ribosome cycle by streptomycin in Escherichia coli', *J. Mol. Biol.*, **42**, 315.

McQuillen, M. P., Cantor, H. E. and O'Rourke, J. R. (1968), 'Myasthenic syndrome associated with antibiotics', *Arch. Neurol.*, **18**, 402.

Mahgoub, E. L. (1976), 'Medical management of mycetoma', *Bull. Wld. Hlth. Org.*, **54**, 303.

Mandell, G. L., Kaye, D., Levison, M. E. and Hook, E. W. (1970), 'Enterococcal endocarditis', *Arch. Intern. Med.*, **125**, 258.

Martin, W. J. (1970), 'The present status of streptomycin in antimicrobial therapy', *Med. Clin. North America*, **54**, 1161.

Meade, R. H. III (1978), 'Streptomycin and sulfisoxazole for treatment of Haemophilus influenzae meningitis', *JAMA*, **239**, 324.

Modolell, J. and Davis, B. D. (1970), 'Breakdown by streptomycin of initiation complexes formed on ribosomes of Escherichia coli.' *Proc. Nat. Acad. Sci.*, **67**, 1148.

Pinkerton, H. H. and Munro, J. R. (1965), 'Respiratory insufficiency associated with streptomycin', *Scottish med. J.*, **9**, 256.

Report of a WHO Scientific Group (1978), 'Neisseria gonorrhoeae and gonococcal infections', *Wld. Hlth. Org. techn. Rep. Ser.*, No. **616.**

Robertson, L., Farrell, I. D. and Hinchliffe, P. M. (1973), 'The sensitivity of Brucella abortus to chemotherapeutic agents', *J. Med. Microbiol.*, **6**, 549.

Robinson, G. C. and Cambon, K. G. (1964), 'Hearing loss in infants of tuberculous mothers treated with streptomycin during pregnancy', *New Engl. J. Med.*, **271**, 949.

Ruhen, R. W. and Darrell, J. H. (1973), 'Antibiotic synergism against Group D streptococci in the treatment of endocarditis', *Med. J. Aust.*, **2**, 114.

Sabath, L. D. (1969), 'Current concepts: Drug resistance of bacteria', *New Engl. J. Med.*, **280**, 91.

Sande, M. A. and Irvin, R. G. (1974), 'Penicillin-aminoglycoside synergy in experimental Streptococcus viridans endocarditis', *J. Infect. Dis.*, **129**, 572.

Sanders, C. C. (1977), 'Synergy of penicillin-netilmicin combinations against enterococci including strains highly resistant to streptomycin or kanamycin', *Antimicrob. Ag. Chemother.*, **12**, 195.

Sapico, F. L., Keys, T. F. and Hewitt, W. L. (1972), 'Experimental enterococcal endocarditis. II: Study of *in vivo* synergism of penicillin and streptomycin', *Amer. J.*

Med. Sci., **263,** 128.

Saunders, J. R. and Saunders, V. A. (1977), 'Energetics and antibiotic uptake', *Nature,* **270,** 475.

Schatz, A., Bugie, E. and Waksman, S. A. (1944), 'Streptomycin, a substance exhibiting antibiotic activity against Gram-positive and Gram-negative bacteria', *Proc. Soc. Exper. Biol. and Med.,* **55,** 66; quoted by Hussar and Holley (1954).

Smith, H. G. and Young, S. E. J. (1966), 'Sonne dysentery', *Brit. med. J.,* **1,** 481.

Sparling, P. F. and Davis, B. D. (1972), 'Bactericidal action of streptomycin and comparison with spectinomycin in heterozygotes of Escherichia coli', *Antimicrob. Ag. Chemother.,* **1,** 252.

Stottmeier, K. D. and Burkes, J. (1974), 'Primary drug-resistant Mycobacterium tuberculosis isolated in Massachusetts in 1972', *J. Infect. Dis.,* **130,** 293.

Stottmeier, K. D. and Baker, S. (1977), 'Primary drug-resistant tuberculosis in Massachusetts, 1975/76', *New Engl. J. Med.,* **296,** 823.

Tan, J. S., Terhune, C. A. Jr., Kaplan, S. and Hamburger, M. (1971), 'Successful two-week treatment schedule for penicillin-susceptible Streptococcus viridans endocarditis', *Lancet,* **2,** 1340.

Thompson, J. E. (1969), 'The management of hypersensitivity reactions to antituberculosis drugs', *Med. J. Aust.,* **2,** 1058.

Today's Drugs (1963), 'Streptomycin. neomycin, kanamycin and paromomycin', *Brit. med. J.,* **1,** 1393.

Usuda, Y. and Sekine, O. (1978), 'Chemotherapy of tuberculosis in patients on dialysis', in Siegenthaler, W. and Lüthy, R. (Ed.), *Current Chemotherapy: Proceedings of the 10th International Congress of Chemotherapy,* Zurich/Switzerland, 1977. American Society for Microbiology, Washington, D. C., p. 241.

Welch, H. (1954), *Principles and Practice of Antibiotic Therapy,* Med. Encyc. Inc., New York, p. 103.

Westenfelder, G. O., Paterson, P. Y., Reisberg, B. E. and Carlson, G. M. (1973), 'Vancomycin-streptomycin synergism in enterococcal endocarditis'. *JAMA,* **223,** 37.

Willcox, R. R. (1977), 'How suitable are available pharmaceuticals for the treatment of sexually transmitted diseases? (2) Conditions presenting as sores or tumours'. *Brit. J. vener. Dis.,* **53,** 340.

Wolfe, J. C. and Johnson, W. D., Jr. (1974), 'Penicillin-sensitive streptococcal endocarditis. *In-vitro* and clinical observations on penicillin-streptomycin therapy', *Ann. Intern. Med.,* **81,** 178.

Yaffe, S. J. (1965), 'Antibiotic dosage in newborn and premature infants', *JAMA,* **193,** 818.

Yaffe, S. J. and Back, N. (1966), 'Pediatric pharmacology', *Postgraduate Medicine,* **40,** 193.

Kanamycin

Description

Kanamycin was isolated in Japan from Streptomyces kanamyceticus (Umezawa *et al.*, 1957). The drug is an aminoglycoside, chemically similar to streptomycin and neomycin. Clinically it is used as the sulphate, which is water soluble. Trade names include 'Kantrex' (Bristol) and 'Kanasig' (Sigma).

Sensitive Organisms

1. *Gram-negative aerobic bacteria.* Kanamycin is active against most of the Enterobacteriaceae such as Esch. coli, Enterobacter and Klebsiella spp., all Proteus spp. and Salmonella, Shigella, Providencia, Serratia, Citrobacter, Hafnia, Edwardsiella and Arizona species. Yersinia pestis (Butler *et al.*, 1974), Y. enterocolitica (Hammerberg *et al.*, 1977) and Y. pseudotuberculosis (Brodie *et al.*, 1973) are also kanamycin-sensitive. Resistance to kanamycin of those Enterobacteriaceae which are normal inhabitants of the human bowel first became a significant problem 8–10 years after its discovery. During 1967 in one Boston hospital, 11 per cent Esch. coli and 33 per cent Klebsiella, 26 per cent Enterobacter, 16 per cent Proteus and 47 per cent of Serratia spp. were kanamycin-resistant (Sabath, 1969). Between 1969 and 1971, 16·2 per cent of Esch. coli, 70·9 per cent of Pr. mirabilis and 55·8 per cent of Kl. aerogenes isolates were resistant to kanamycin in a British burns unit (Roe and Lowbury, 1972). In some hospitals resistant Klebsiella spp. were even more common (Adler *et al.*, 1970; Terman *et al.*, 1972). Other authors at that time confirmed that resistant Klebsiella spp. strains (Eickhoff *et al.*, 1966; Dans *et al.*, 1970), and Esch. coli strains (Baker *et al.*, 1974) were more frequent in hospital acquired infections. In a study of septicaemic patients in Melbourne, kanamycin-resistant Gram-negative bacilli were not encountered in patients who acquired infection in their home environment (Bennett and Kucers, 1970). As with neomycin (page 406), kanamycin-resistant variants of Salmonella and Shigella spp. were also encountered with increasing frequency. Many streptomycin-resistant strains of all the Enterobacteriaceae may be sensitive to kanamycin, but there is usually complete cross-resistance between kanamycin and neomycin with these organisms (Murdoch *et al.*, 1962).

Recently, presumably because kanamycin has been largely replaced by gentamicin (page 341) in many hospitals, kanamycin-resistant strains are no longer increasing and their prevalence has actually decreased in some areas. In seven North American nurseries the percentage of Esch. coli strains resistant to kanamycin obtained from neonates decreased from a high of 71 per cent in 1971 to 12 per cent in 1974; this coincided with the substitution of gentamicin for kanamycin for the treatment of neonatal infections (Howard and McCracken, 1975). In a large contemporary survey in a London hospital, only about 10 per cent of all Enterobacteriaceae isolates were kanamycin-resistant (Phillips *et al.*, 1977). Similarly only 6 per cent of 97 strains of Esch. coli recently isolated in an Oklahoma City children's hospital were resistant (Yoshioka *et al.*, 1977). In both of these surveys gentamicin-resistant strains, however, were even less common. This contrasts with the report of Keane *et al.* (1975) on the sensitivities of 98 isolates of Providencia stuartii; 76·5 per cent of these were kanamycin-sensitive, but only 16·4 per cent were gentamicin-sensitive (*see also* page 325). This organism in contrast to most other aerobic Gram-negative rods isolated from hospital patients is usually more likely to be sensitive to kanamycin than to gentamicin. However in one laboratory, serving six hospitals, increasing numbers of high-level kanamycin-resistant Providencia stuartii strains have been isolated during the five-year period January, 1972 to December, 1976. The resistance of these isolates was R plasmid-mediated (McHale *et al.*, 1978).

The combination of cephalothin (page 201) and kanamycin usually exhibits *in vitro* synergism against Klebsiella spp., while a kanamycin-chloramphenicol (page 421) combination may show *in vitro* antagonism (D'Alessandri *et al.*, 1976).

Among other Gram-negative bacteria, the Neisseria spp. (meningococci and gonococci), H. influenzae, and the Brucella spp. are kanamycin-sensitive, but Pseudomonas aeruginosa is almost invariably resistant (Finegold, 1959). Gonococci relatively resistant to kanamycin have been reported (Fischnallen *et al.*, 1968), but penicillinase-producing strains (page 8) are usually kanamycin-sensitive. Acinetobacter calcoaceticus var. anitratus is usually sensitive to kanamycin, but resistant strains occur. Carbenicillin (page 151) plus kanamycin exhibit *in vitro* synergism against this organism, provided that the strain is kanamycin-sensitive or only moderately resistant. If the MIC of the strain for kanamycin is 62·5 μg per ml or higher, synergism is usually not demonstrable (Glew *et al.*, 1977). The Legionnaires' disease bacterium is sensitive to kanamycin *in vitro* (MIC 0·5–2·0 μg per ml) (Thornsberry *et al.*, 1978). Campylobacter fetus is also sensitive to the aminoglycosides, including kanamycin (median MIC 2·0 μg per ml) (*see also* gentamicin, page 328).

2. *Gram-negative anaerobic bacteria.* Most of these are resistant to kanamycin. The drug has moderate activity against some strains of Fusobacterium spp. and Bacteroides melaninogenicus, but all others and in particular Bacteroides fragilis are always resistant (Martin *et al.*, 1972; Kislak, 1972).

3. *Gram-positive bacteria.* Staph. pyogenes (irrespective of penicillinase production) and Staph. epidermidis are kanamycin-sensitive, but all other Gram-positive bacteria such as Strep. pyogenes, Strep. pneumoniae, alpha-haemolytic streptococci, Strep. faecalis and the Nocardia, Actinomyces and Clostridium spp. are resistant. Kanamycin-resistant staphylococci, which are nearly always also neomycin-resistant (page 406), have been detected in some hospitals (Barber and Waterworth, 1966), and resistance to both of these drugs appears to be mediated by an R plasmid (Stiffler *et al.*, 1974).

Strep. faecalis is usually resistant to ordinary kanamycin concentrations. However the combination of penicillin G and kanamycin, similar to penicillin

G/streptomycin (page 294), often acts synergistically against this organism. A penicillin/kanamycin combination is synergistic against occasional Strep. faecalis strains, against which penicillin/streptomycin is not synergistic. Kanamycin combined with penicillin G was found to be more effective for treatment of endocarditis caused by such Strep. faecalis strains (Garrod and Waterworth, 1962). Such Strep. faecalis strains are uncommon, because most strains showing high-level resistance to streptomycin (page 294) also show similar resistance to kanamycin (MIC > 5000 μg per ml). With these strains (20–50 per cent of Strep. faecalis isolates) there is no *in vitro* synergism with penicillin G/streptomycin or penicillin G/kanamycin. By contrast, penicillin G combined with either gentamicin (page 329), tobramycin (page 361), sisomicin (page 395) or netilmicin (page 397) shows synergy with all Strep. faecalis strains (Ruhen and Darrell, 1973; Basker *et al.*, 1977; Gutschik *et al.*, 1977; Calderwood *et al.*, 1977).

4. *Mycobacterium tuberculosis* is kanamycin-sensitive, but resistant strains can emerge.

5. *Treponema pallidum*, Leptospirae, Mycoplasmas and Fungi are insensitive.

In Vitro Sensitivities

Table 21 shows the minimum inhibitory concentrations of kanamycin against some selected bacterial species.

TABLE 21

(After Barber and Waterworth, 1966)

ORGANISM	(μg per ml)
Gram-positive bacteria	
Staph. pyogenes	0·5–2·0
Staph. pyogenes (kanamycin-resistant)	64–>512
Strep. pyogenes (Group A)	64–256
Strep. pneumoniae (Dip. pneumoniae)	64–128
Strep. faecalis (Enterococcus, Group D)	8–32
Gram-negative bacteria	
Esch. coli	2–8
Klebsiella aerogenes	1–4
Klebsiella (other spp.)	0·12–2
Proteus mirabilis	2–8
Proteus vulgaris	2–8
Proteus morganii	2–8
Proteus rettgeri	2–4
Salmonella spp.	1–4
Shigella spp.	4–8
Pseudomonas aeruginosa	8–128

Mode of Administration and Dosage

1. *Intramuscular administration.* Kanamycin is poorly absorbed from the gastro-intestinal tract, and it is usually administered by the intramuscular route. The adult dose is 15 mg per kg per day, most commonly administered in two divided doses, but it can be given in three or four divided doses. A common dose for adults is 0·5 g twelve-hourly or 250 mg six-hourly. Occasionally this dose may be increased to 0·5 g eight-hourly for severe infections, but only for short periods. Usually adult doses higher than 1·0 g per day are unnecessary even for very severe infections, and kanamycin should not be used for periods longer than 14 days (Murdoch *et al.*, 1962; 1966).

It was assumed for many years that the adult dose of 15 mg per kg of body weight should also be used for children. Hieber and Nelson (1976) have demonstrated that this dose fails to produce serum concentrations in the therapeutic range in many children aged two months to 12 years. Accordingly they made a preliminary recommendation that kanamycin dosage for this age group should be increased to 30 mg per kg given in three divided doses. In infants and children (page 316) the total dose for a course of treatment should not exceed 500 mg per kg body weight (Yow, 1966).

2. *Intravenous administration.* The drug may be administered intravenously using the same dosage schedule as used for intramuscular therapy. The best method is to dissolve each dose in 20–50 ml of intravenous solution in a paediatric buretrol or a secondary intravenous bottle for infusion over 20 to 30 min. Kanamycin doses well diluted can also be given by intermittent injection into the intravenous tubing. This is less satisfactory, as following such injections, serum kanamycin levels temporarily exceed the safe maximum of 30 μg per ml (page 316) (McCracken *et al.*, 1977). Concentrated kanamycin solutions also readily cause thrombophlebitis. Kanamycin administration by continuous intravenous infusion is not generally advocated. The drug is incompatible with many additives to intravenous fluids. Nevertheless it is stable for at least 12 h in all commonly used glucose-saline intravenous fluids (Wyatt *et al.*, 1972), so that under special circumstances it may be added to intravenous bottles and administered by continuous infusion.

3. *Patients with renal failure.* These require a modified dosage schedule. A loading dose of 0·5–1·0 g can be safely administered to any uraemic patient. The peak serum kanamycin concentration attained after the first dose is higher in patients with renal failure, as the peak is determined not only by the distribution volume, but also by excretion which commences as soon as there is absorption (Mawer *et al.*, 1972a). However with a single dose there is usually no danger of toxicity, and the first dose often has to be given before the patient's renal function is known. Thereafter the frequency with which the standard 0·5 g dose can be repeated depends on the severity of the renal failure (Kunin, 1966).

A linear relationship between the serum kanamycin half-life and the serum creatinine concentration has been demonstrated (Cutler and Orme, 1969). Kanamycin in a dose of 0·5 g given every third half-life will result in therapeutic non-toxic levels in patients with renal failure. The serum kanamycin half-life in hours is approximately equal to the patient's serum creatinine in mg per cent, multiplied by four. (For conversion of creatinine

values from SI units to mg per cent *see* page 333). Table 22 exemplifies the use
of this formula. This calculation may be simplified further; the interval between
kanamycin doses is obtained by multiplying the serum creatinine (in mg per
cent) by 12, which is the usual period in hours between doses for patients with

TABLE 22

Renal function	Kanamycin half-life	Frequency of administration of adult dose of 0·5 g
Normal	4 hours	$4 \times 3 = $ 12-hourly
Renal failure with serum creatinine of 6 mg per cent	$6 \times 4 = $ 24 hours	$24 \times 3 = $ 72-hourly

N.B. (a) Serum kanamycin half-life in hours = serum creatinine in mg per cent × 4.
     (b) The dose of kanamycin should be administered once every 3rd half-life of the
         drug.

normal renal function (McCloskey and Becker, 1971). Alternatively, the time
intervals between doses may be left unchanged, but individual doses are
suitably reduced; the maintenance dose can be calculated by dividing the ordinary dose by the patient's creatinine in mg per cent. Methods using a combination of individual dose reduction and extension of the intervals between
doses are also useful (Healy *et al.*, 1973). Computer-assisted prescribing of
kanamycin has been used for patients with renal failure and a nomogram for
kanamycin dosage has been published (Mawer *et al.*, 1972a and b). With these
methods, which aim for more precision, the loading dose, maintenance dose
and intervals between doses are all altered in an attempt to maintain serum
kanamycin levels within the range of 10–30 μg per ml, for two hours after each
dose.
    All these dose schedules are useful guides, but when possible dosage should
be governed by serum kanamycin estimations (Reeves, 1977). In many patients
renal function varies from day to day, and often improves when infection is
controlled. Suitable times to collect blood for kanamycin assays are one hour
after an intramuscular dose, and just before the next dose. The first or peak
level should not exceed 30 μg per ml and the second or trough level should approach zero and should never exceed 10 μg per ml (*see also* amikacin, page
381). Most of the commonly used microbiological methods for antibiotic serum
level estimation require overnight incubation, but nowadays, as with gentamicin (page 334), several rapid methods are also available.
    Kanamycin is removed from the body by haemodialysis. In anephric
patients undergoing this procedure, the kanamycin half-life is approximately
4·9 h. During a 6–8 h haemodialysis some 50 per cent of kanamycin is
removed from the body, while about 7–80 per cent of the drug is removed
during a 12 h dialysis (Ory *et al.*, 1966; Danish *et al.*, 1974). Therapeutic non-
toxic levels of kanamycin will usually be maintained in anephric patients
managed by twice-weekly haemodialysis, if a dose of 7 mg per kg is given after
each dialysis. Haemodialysis is the best way to treat kanamycin poisoning.

This drug is also removed by peritoneal dialysis. In anuric patients treated by peritoneal dialysis (two litre exchanges every 2·5 h), after a dose of 0·5 g kanamycin intramuscularly, serum levels decrease promptly during the first 6–12 h and the half-life of the drug during this time is approximately 5 h, a figure similar to the normal one. As dialysis continues, removal of the drug is slower and the half-life is prolonged to 48 h. The average rate of removal of kanamycin is 4·4 mg per hour during peritoneal dialysis (about 100 mg per day). This suggests that a daily dose of 250 mg during peritoneal dialysis would suffice for anuric patients (Greenberg and Sanford, 1967). Alternatively, these patients may be treated by intramuscular kanamycin in doses appropriate to their renal function, and the kanamycin lost via dialysis compensated for by adding the drug to the peritoneal dialysate, usually in a concentration of 15–20 µg per ml (Atkins et al., 1973).

A significant amount of kanamycin is absorbed if the drug is added to peritoneal dialysis fluid. If 0·5 g of kanamycin is introduced into the peritoneal cavity, blood levels are reached which are approximately 30 per cent of those obtained with the same intramuscular dose (Sanford, 1966). More commonly 20 mg of the drug is added to each litre of peritoneal dialysis fluid (concentration 20 µg per ml) to prevent or treat intraperitoneal infections (Atkins et al., 1973). In such patients, who are not receiving kanamycin by other routes, after 16 h of dialysis the serum kanamycin concentration stabilizes at approximately 45 per cent of the dialysis inflow level.

Peritoneal lavage, using a solution containing 40 µg per ml kanamycin, has been used for the management of peritonitis in patients with normal renal function (Atkins et al., 1976). The rate of kanamycin absorption from the inflamed peritoneum of these patients may be greater than that from normal peritoneum.

4. *Patients aged more than fifty years.* Compared to younger adults the half-life of kanamycin and many other drugs may be prolonged or even doubled in these patients, despite normal creatinine values. For this reason the dose may require suitable reduction in this age group (Hansen et al., 1970).

5. *Newborn and premature infants.* Many of these, similar to children (page 311), need a higher kanamycin dosage than adults. In infants who weigh more than 2000 g at birth, peak serum levels of kanamycin after intramuscular doses of 7·5 mg per kg, are below the desired therapeutic range of 15–25 µg per ml. The same also applies to all babies aged more than seven days (Howard and McCracken, 1975). It is now recommended that babies whose birth weight is less than 2000 g should receive 7·5 mg of kanamycin per kg every 12 h, until seven days of age, and thereafter 10 mg per kg every 12 h. Infants weighing more than 2000 g at birth should receive 10 mg per kg every 12 h until seven days of age, and thereafter 10 mg per kg every eight hours (McCracken and Threlkeld, 1976; McCracken and Nelson, 1977).

Kanamycin can also be safely administered to neonates by the intravenous route, provided that each dose is dissolved in a suitable volume of intravenous fluid and then given as a constant infusion over 20 min. With this method of administration serum levels attained are similar to those after intramuscular administration. The intravenous kanamycin dosage for infants is the same as that recommended for intramuscular use (McCracken et al., 1977).

6. *Pulmonary tuberculosis.* A dose of 15 mg per kg per day for five days a week only, continued for several months, has been used for patients with nor-

mal renal function (Kass, 1966). Kanamycin should be administered in conjunction with at least two other (preferably oral) antituberculosis drugs.

7. *Intrathecal administration.* This is usually unnecessary for the treatment
of meningitis. However in infants with meningitis, who have associated
anatomical abnormalities such as meningomyelocoeles or who have shunts inserted because of hydrocephalus, intrathecal and intraventricular kanamycin
has been used in addition to systemic treatment. Intrathecal doses of
kanamycin used for infants have ranged from 5–25 mg daily (Lorber, 1967).

8. *Oral administration.* Kanamycin has been used orally as an 'intestinal
antiseptic' in a dose of 4–8 g per day (1–2 g six-hourly). Some of this
kanamycin is absorbed, and in patients with impaired renal function, after
several days treatment serum levels can approach those usually attained after
intramuscular injection.

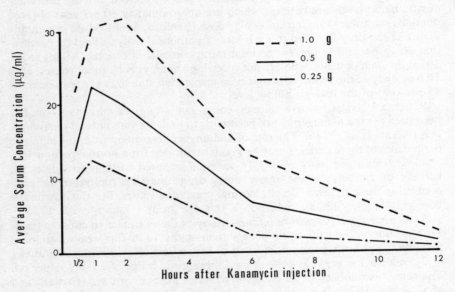

FIG. 20. Average serum concentrations following single intramuscular injections of kanamycin
at three dose levels: 0·25, 0·5 and 1·0 g. (Redrawn after Welch *et al.*, 1958.)

Availability

Kanamycin sulphate is available in vials as a stable aqueous solution containing 0·25 g or 0·5 g
in 2 ml and 1 g in 3 ml. Ampoules are also available e.g. each containing 30 mg per ml.
    The drug is also available in capsules (250 mg) and suspensions for oral administration.

Serum Levels in Relation to Dosage

After intramuscular injection, kanamycin may be detected in the blood in
15–30 min, and a peak level is reached in about one hour. At two hours the
level is usually slightly lower, and then falls rapidly, the kanamycin half-life in

serum being about four hours (Fig. 20). Kanamycin levels are usually low 6–8 h after injection, and negligible at twelve hours. This drug does not accumulate with repeated doses of 0·5 g twelve-hourly, unless the patient has impaired renal function. The serum half-life of kanamycin in severely uraemic patients may be prolonged to 70–80 h.

Excretion

URINE: 50–80 per cent of intramuscularly administered kanamycin is excreted in the urine in an active unchanged form, and most of this is excreted in six hours. High concentrations of the active drug are attained in urine, and with normal doses urine levels are in the range 100–600 μg per ml (Welch et al., 1958; Kunin, 1966). The mechanism for renal excretion of kanamycin is glomerular filtration. Probenecid does not delay kanamycin excretion (Berger et al., 1959). The kanamycin clearance is slightly less than simultaneously determined creatinine clearance, indicating that some of the antibiotic undergoes tubular reabsorption after glomerular filtration (see amikacin, page 384). Boger and Gavin (1959) found that the clearance rate in an adult patient was about 80 per cent of simultaneous creatinine clearance, but Berger et al. (1959) reported that kanamycin was cleared at a somewhat higher rate in children.

BILE: After intramuscular administration only about 1 per cent of the administered dose is excreted in the bile. The concentration of kanamycin in bile is similar to that obtained in serum, but the peak is only reached about six hours after injection (Kunin, 1966).

INACTIVATION OF THE DRUG IN BODY: This probably does occur to a minor extent, but nothing definite is known about the fate of the small fraction of kanamycin that cannot be recovered in the free form in urine and bile (Kunin, 1966).

Distribution of the Drug in Body

Kanamycin serum protein binding, if any, is very low (Berger et al., 1959; Gordon et al., 1972).

Kanamycin diffuses into pleural and ascitic fluids, where it may reach concentrations similar to those obtained in serum at the time (Finegold, 1959). Only traces of kanamycin can be detected in the spinal fluid of patients with uninflamed meninges, in saliva (Boger and Gavin, 1959), and in bronchial secretions (Finegold, 1959). Animal experiments have shown that kanamycin accumulates in the renal cortex, probably intracellularly (Luft and Kleit, 1974).

Mode of Action

In vitro kanamycin has a bactericidal action which is more apparent against bacteria in their multiplication phase. It primarily affects bacterial protein synthesis, but also alters the permeability of the bacterial cell membrane. The mode of action of kanamycin and other aminoglycosides on bacteria is similar to that of streptomycin (page 298).

Toxicity

1. *Ototoxicity*. This is the most important toxic effect of kanamycin, causing deafness through irreversible cochlear damage. Vestibular function may also be affected, but this is less common than with streptomycin (Finegold, 1959; 1966). The following factors predispose to kanamycin ototoxicity:

(a) pre-existing renal impairment
(b) high serum levels
(c) prolonged use of the drug
(d) increasing age of patient
(e) pre-existing hearing loss and possibly also previous treatment with ototoxic drugs.

Kanamycin is potentially more toxic for cochlear function than streptomycin or even dihydrostreptomycin, but less than neomycin (Frost *et al.*, 1959). 'Acute ototoxicity' most commonly occurs when there are sustained kanamycin serum levels higher than 30 μg per ml. 'Chronic ototoxicity' may occur when a large total dose is administered over a long period, even if the daily dose is small. For this reason, if possible, the total adult dose for a course of treatment should not exceed 14 g. Children with normal renal function usually tolerate treatment well if the total dose administered does not exceed 500 mg per kg (Yow, 1966). Ototoxicity was frequent (6 to 39 per cent in different series), when kanamycin was used for prolonged periods in pulmonary tuberculosis (Kass, 1966). By contrast a survey in Boston showed that only four (1·6 per cent) of 243 medical in-patients receiving kanamycin developed deafness (A Co-operative Study, 1973). Patients receiving kanamycin should be questioned daily for tinnitus and for a sensation of 'pressure or fullness in the ears', which indicate that the drug should be stopped. Serial weekly audiograms should be performed, where feasible, during therapy (Finegold, 1966).

The use of other ototoxic drugs together with kanamycin should be avoided, whenever possible. Sudden deafness has been reported in association with the intravenous use of the diuretic, ethacrynic acid in a few patients (A Cooperative Study, 1973). In some of these patients aminoglycosides such as kanamycin or gentamicin had been used concurrently, so it is possible that their combination with this diuretic may be more liable to cause ototoxicity (Meriwether *et al.*, 1971).

Kanamycin ototoxicity appears to be rare in newborn and premature infants. Many children aged 4–5 years who have had kanamycin in the recommended dosage in infancy have been studied by audiograms, and their hearing did not significantly differ from that of controls (Eichenwald, 1966). There is also little evidence of ototoxicity in children whose mothers have been treated with kanamycin during pregnancy.

2. *Nephrotoxicity*. Similar to other aminoglycosides such as neomycin (page 410) and gentamicin (page 339), kanamycin may cause renal damage. Kanamycin is not as nephrotoxic as neomycin, but it is more toxic than streptomycin, which is the least nephrotoxic aminoglycoside (Appel and Neu, 1977). Although kanamycin is only excreted by glomerular filtration and not by tubular secretion, the drug accumulates in renal cortical tissue (page 315) and can cause changes in the proximal tubules that range from cloudy swelling

to acute necrosis. Mild renal toxicity with the appearance of casts, red and white cells and protein in the urine is relatively common. Increasing azotaemia is infrequent, except perhaps in older patients. Oliguric renal failure with features of acute tubular necrosis may occasionally develop. Recovery from these more severe nephrotoxic effects is usually slow and may only be partial (Appel and Neu, 1977; Bennett *et al.*, 1977). Early recognition of kanamycin nephrotoxicity is also important because it may predispose patients to otoxicity (Finegold *et al.*, 1959; Finegold, 1966).

3. *Neuromuscular blockade.* Similar to streptomycin (page 301) and neomycin (page 411), kanamycin can cause paralysis which may affect respiration, especially if a large dose is introduced intraperitoneally in an anaesthetized patient (Finegold, 1966; Pindell, 1966). Neuromuscular blockade due to streptomycin and neomycin appears to be competitive in type and may be reversed by neostigmine (Finegold, 1966). Calcium gluconate has been helpful in some patients with kanamycin paralysis. Finegold (1966) considered that the blockade with kanamycin is usually noncompetitive and similar to that caused by succinylcholine. Patients with myasthenia gravis may be particularly sensitive to this effect of the drug.

4. *Other neurotoxicity.* Many other infrequent neurotoxic side-effects have been attributed to kanamycin. These include circumoral and other paraesthesiae, headaches, restlessness, nervousness, tachycardia, and an acute brain syndrome with hysterical features and blurring of vision (Finegold, 1966).

5. *Hypersensitivity.* Pruritus, rash, drug fever and even anaphylaxis have been reported, but these are rare (Finegold, 1966). Eosinophilia without clinical manifestations is more common.

6. *Pain* of moderate intensity may be experienced at the site of intramuscular injection.

7. *Side-effects due to oral administration.* Vomiting and diarrhoea can be caused by oral kanamycin. The severe but rare complication of staphylococcal enterocolitis may occur as with neomycin (page 411), if staphylococci resistant to this group of drugs are present. Prolonged oral kanamycin administration can also induce a state of malabsorption with steatorrhoea, but neomycin (page 411) appears to be more potent in this regard (Faloon *et al.*, 1966).

Clinical Uses of the Drug

1. *Septicaemia due to Gram-negative enteric bacilli.* These septicaemias are usually associated with some predisposing disease state such as pyelonephritis, cholangitis, agranulocytosis, immunosuppression or they may be associated with operative procedures. Prior to the advent of gentamicin (page 325) and at the time when kanamycin-resistant Gram-negative bacilli were still rare, kanamycin was regarded as the antibiotic of first choice for the treatment of these infections (Murdoch *et al.*, 1962; 1966; Bunn and Lunn, 1966). Kanamycin was also very suitable for treatment of severe Gram-negative bacterial infections in newborn and premature infants, such as Esch. coli meningitis (Eichenwald, 1966). It is still a very useful drug for the treatment of these infections when the bacterial strain involved is kanamycin-sensitive. Compared to gentamicin, it has the advantage of a wider safety margin

between therapeutically effective and toxic doses. In addition its use in place of gentamicin would minimize the emergence of gentamicin-resistant bacilli. Since the late 1960's kanamycin has often not been considered to be sufficiently reliable for the emergency treatment of these infections. Gentamicin was usually selected, particularly if the infection was acquired in a hospital known to harbour kanamycin-resistant Gram-negative bacilli, such as Klebsiella spp. Nevertheless, kanamycin may still be quite useful for the initial treatment of Gram-negative septicaemias in some hospitals where kanamycin resistance to these bacilli has again become uncommon (page 308), or if the infection is not hospital acquired (Bennett and Kucers, 1970). It has also been demonstrated that neonates who develop sepsis within the first five days after birth are less likely to be infected with kanamycin-resistant Gram-negative enteric bacteria than are neonates who develop sepsis later (Crosson and Moxon, 1978).

2. *Urinary tract infections*. Although kanamycin is very effective, other less toxic drugs are usually preferred for the treatment of acute uncomplicated cases. It may be indicated for the treatment of seriously ill patients with known chronic bacteriuria, and possibly in relatively young patients with asymptomatic bacteriuria, which has remained refractory to other drugs (Petersdorf and Turck, 1966). Women in whom the infection is confined to the bladder can be usually cured with a single intramuscular injection of 0·5 g kanamycin, whereas those with infection originating from the kidneys almost always relapse after such 'single-dose' therapy (Ronald *et al.*, 1976). If kanamycin is used for urinary tract infections, the urine should be made alkaline (Sabath *et al.*, 1970) (*see also* gentamicin, page 343).

3. *Klebsiella pneumonia*. Kanamycin is effective for this disease, provided the Kl. pneumoniae strain is sensitive. Alternative drugs are available, such as gentamicin (page 342), the cephalosporins (page 215), chloramphenicol (page 444) and co-trimoxazole (page 710).

4. *Staphylococcal infections*. These respond to kanamycin, but usually other drugs are preferred. In special situations kanamycin in combination with other drugs has been recommended. Cephalothin/kanamycin or methicillin/kanamycin combinations may be effective for treatment of infections caused by methicillin-resistant staphylococci (Bulger, 1967) (page 67). Occasionally in staphylococcal endocarditis, despite sensitivity of the strain to the penicillinase-resistant penicillins and cephalosporins, the disease may not respond, unless a synergistic drug combination is used. In these cases special *in vitro* sensitivity studies may predict the drug combination which may be most beneficial (Garrod and Waterworth, 1962). If facilities for testing drug combinations are not available, the combination of a penicillinase-resistant penicillin or cephalosporin with an aminoglycoside such as kanamycin or gentamicin (page 344) is most likely to be effective for this disease (Leading article, 1967).

5. *Bacterial endocarditis*. Kanamycin, usually in combination with other drugs, may be useful for treatment of endocarditis due to organisms other than staphylococci. In the past, sometimes kanamycin, rather than streptomycin, was combined with penicillin G or ampicillin for treatment of Strep. faecalis endocarditis (page 310). Nowadays if a penicillin G/streptomycin combination is not synergistic against the Strep. faecalis strain, a penicillin G/gentamicin regimen is usually selected (page 344).

It is difficult to cure the uncommon endocarditis due to Gram-negative enteric bacilli with kanamycin alone, as the drug cannot be used in high doses over a prolonged period. Drug combinations are likely to be more successful. A combination of ampicillin and kanamycin has been reported to be effective in Esch. coli endocarditis (Hansing et al., 1967). Sabath et al. (1970) used ampicillin, cloxacillin and kanamycin together for an unusual case of endocarditis due to Enterobacter cloacae, but in spite of initial improvement, the patient did not survive (see page 103 re-ampicillin/cloxacillin synergism).

6. *Peritonitis and other surgical infections.* Good results have been obtained in treating peritonitis in adults by introducing kanamycin into the peritoneal cavity in a solution of 1·0 g in 50 ml (Cohn, 1966). Gross generalized peritonitis can also be managed by prolonged peritoneal lavage, using a kanamycin solution in a concentration of 40 μg per ml with added cephalothin 100 μg per ml (Atkins et al., 1976). In such cases systemic antibiotics are usually also necessary.

Intramuscular kanamycin is useful for other surgical infections, such as infected wounds, provided that the organism concerned is kanamycin-sensitive, and treatment is supplemented by appropriate surgical measures (Rutenburg, 1966). A disadvantage is that kanamycin is inactive against Bacteroides fragilis.

7. *Bowel sterilization.* Orally administered kanamycin is poorly absorbed, and therefore it has been used as an 'intestinal antiseptic' for the preparation of patients for bowel surgery (Cohn, 1966). The use of pre-operative bowel sterilization however is controversial (page 413). Kanamycin is ineffective against most Bacteroides spp. and nowadays if such chemoprophylaxis is given at all, it should be combined with an agent effective against anaerobes such as metronidazole (page 774).

Oral kanamycin is also sometimes preferred to neomycin (page 413) for bowel sterilization in patients with liver failure, especially if they also have renal failure (Kunin, 1966). Both of these drugs are slightly absorbed from the gastro-intestinal tract, but kanamycin has a lower ototoxic and nephrotoxic potential. Kanamycin is also less liable to cause changes in the intestinal mucosa and a consequent malabsorption syndrome (Faloon et al., 1966).

8. *Intestinal infections.* Oral neomycin was regarded as a useful drug for treatment of infantile gastro-enteritis caused by enteropathogenic strains of Esch. coli (page 412). Oral kanamycin did not have extensive trials in this disease, but was considered of much the same value as neomycin (Nelson and Haltalin, 1966). Nowadays it is considered very doubtful whether any antibiotics are beneficial in this infection (Christie, 1973). Orally administered kanamycin is of no value for the treatment of salmonella infections or the salmonella carrier state, and the same is true for shigellosis.

9. *Gonorrhoea.* Kanamycin has been advocated as an alternative to penicillin G for treatment of this disease (Wilkinson et al., 1967). Satisfactory results in acute uncomplicated gonorrhoea have been obtained using single 2·0 g intramuscular doses (Fischnallen et al., 1968; Report, 1978). The drug is probably also effective for gonorrhoea caused by penicillinase-producing strains (page 8). Another possible advantage of kanamycin is that it does not interfere with the diagnosis of coexistent syphilis.

10. *Tuberculosis.* Kanamycin is not a 'first-line' drug for the treatment of

this disease. In the past it was often of value for the treatment of patients with M. tuberculosis resistant to streptomycin, isoniazid and para-amino salicylic acid (Kass, 1966). Kanamycin will now be used rarely, if at all, because of the availability of relatively safer and effective drugs such as ethambutol (page 832) and rifampicin (page 552).

11. *Necrotizing enterocolitis.* This is a disease predominantly affecting infants of low birth weight who have received intensive care treatment. It is characterized by abdominal distension, ileus, passage of blood in stools, intestinal perforation and a high mortality (30–70 per cent). It has been claimed that kanamycin at twice the normal parenteral dose, given through a nasogastric tube, improves survival rate of necrotizing enterocolitis (Leading article, 1977). Prevention of this disease has also been reported when kanamycin is administered via nasogastric tube prophylactically, in a dose of 15 mg per kg per day to low birth weight infants believed to be at risk (Egan *et al.*, 1976; 1977). The aetiology of necrotizing enterocolitis is not known and the mechanism of action of kanamycin in this disease is not understood.

REFERENCES

A Co-operative Study (1973), 'Drug-induced deafness', *JAMA*, **224,** 515.

Adler, J. L., Shulman, J. A., Terry, P. M., Feldman, D. B. and Skality, P. (1970), 'Nosocomial colonization with kanamycin-resistant Klebsiella pneumoniae, types 2 and 11, in a premature nursery', *J. Pediatrics*, **77,** 376.

Appel, G. B. and Neu, H. C. (1977), 'The nephrotoxicity of antimicrobial agents (second of three parts)', *New Engl. J. Med.*, **296,** 722.

Atkins, R. C., Mion, C., Despaux, E., Van-Hai, N., Julien, C. and Mion, H. (1973), 'Peritoneal transfer of kanamycin and its use in peritoneal dialysis', *Kidney International*, **3,** 391.

Atkins, R. C., Scott, D. F., Holdsworth, S. R. and Davidson, A. J. (1976), 'Prolonged antibiotic peritoneal lavage in the management of gross generalized peritonitis', *Med. J. Aust.*, **1,** 954.

Baker, C. J., Barrett, F. F. and Clark, D. J. (1974), 'Incidence of kanamycin resistance among Escherichia coli isolates from neonates', *J. Pediatrics*, **84,** 126.

Barber, M. and Waterworth, P. M. (1966), 'Activity of gentamicin against Pseudomonas and hospital staphylococci', *Brit. med. J.*, **1,** 203.

Basker, M. J., Slocombe, B. and Sutherland, R. (1977), 'Aminoglycoside-resistant enterococci', *J. clin. Path.*, **30,** 375.

Bennett, M. McK. and Kucers, A. (1970), 'Staphylococcal and Gram-negative septicaemia', *Aspects of Infection, Proc. Symp. Auckland, Sydney and Melbourne*, p. 123.

Bennett, W. M., Plamp, C. and Porter, G. A. (1977), 'Drug-related syndromes in clinical nephrology', *Ann. Intern. Med.*, **87,** 582.

Berger, S. H., Bergstrom, W. H. and Wehrle, P. F. (1959), 'Renal clearance of kanamycin in children', *Antibiot. Annual*—1958–1959, p. 684.

Boger, W. P. and Gavin, J. J. (1959), 'Kanamycin: Its cerebrospinal fluid diffusion, renal clearance, and comparison with streptomycin', *Antibiot, Annual*—1958–1959, p. 677.

Brodie, M. J., Boot, P. A. and Girdwood, R. W. A. (1973), 'Severe Yersinia pseudotuberculosis infection diagnosed at laparoscopy', *Brit. med. J.*, **4,** 88.

Bulger, R. J. (1967), '*In vitro* activity of cephalothin/kanamycin and methicillin/kanamycin combinations against methicillin-resistant Staphylococcus aureus', *Lancet*, **1,** 17.

Bunn, P. A. and Lunn, J. S. (1966), 'Status of kanamycin in therapy of infections', *Ann. N.Y. Acad. Sci.*, **132**, 819.

Butler, T., Bell, W. R., Linh, N. N., Tiep, N. D. and Arnold, K. (1974), 'Yersinia pestis infection in Vietnam I. clinical and hematological aspects', *J. Infect. Dis.* (May Suppl.), **129**, 78.

Calderwood, S. A., Wennersten, C., Moellering, R. C., Jr., Kunz, L. J. and Krogstad, D. J. (1977), 'Resistance to six aminoglycosidic aminocyclitol antibiotics among enterococci: prevalence, evolution, and relationship to synergism with penicillin', *Antimicrob. Ag. Chemother.*, **12**, 401.

Christie, A. B. (1973), 'Treatment of gastro-intestinal infections: A clinician's viewpoint', in Geddes, A. M. and Williams, J. D. (ed.), *Current Antibiotic Therapy*, Churchill Livingstone, p. 183.

Cohn, I., Jr. (1966), 'Kanamycin as an intestinal antiseptic and in the treatment of peritonitis: Resume of clinical experience', *Ann. N.Y. Acad. Sci.*, **132**, 860.

Crosson, F. J., Jr. and Moxon, E. R. (1978), 'Factors influencing kanamycin resistance of Gram-negative enteric neonatal sepsis', *Pediatrics*, **61**, 488.

Cutler, R. E. and Orme, B. M. (1969), 'Correlation of serum creatinine concentration and kanamycin half-life. Therapeutic implications', *JAMA*, **209**, 539.

D'Alessandri, R. M., McNeely, D. J. and Kluge, R. M. (1976), 'Antibiotic synergy and antagonism against clinical isolates of Klebsiella species', *Antimicrob. Ag. Chemother.*, **10**, 889.

Danish, M., Schultz, R. and Jusko, W. J. (1974), 'Pharmacokinetics of gentamicin and kanamycin during hemodialysis', *Antimicrob. Ag. Chemother.*, **6**, 841.

Dans, P. E., Barrett, F. F., Casey, J. I. and Finland, M. (1970), 'Klebsiella-Enterobacter at Boston City Hospital, 1967', *Arch. Intern. Med.*, **125**, 94.

Egan, E. A., Mantilla, G., Nelson, R. M. and Eitzman, D. V. (1976), 'A prospective controlled trial of oral kanamycin in the prevention of neonatal necrotizing enterocolitis', *J. Pediatrics*, **89**, 467.

Egan, E. A., Nelson, R. M., Mantilla, G. and Eitzman, D. V. (1977), 'Additional experience with routine use of oral kanamycin prophylaxis for necrotizing enterocolitis in infants under 1500 grams', *J. Pediatrics*, **90**, 331.

Eichenwald, H. F. (1966), 'Some observations on dosage and toxicity of kanamycin in premature and full-term infants', *Ann. N.Y. Acad. Sci.*, **132**, 984.

Eickhoff, T. C., Steinhauer, B. W. and Finland, M. (1966), 'The Klebsiella-Enterobacter-Serratia division. Biochemical and serological characteristics and susceptibility to antibiotics', *Ann. Intern. Med.*, **65**, 1163.

Faloon, W. W., Paes, I. C., Woolfolk, D., Nankin, H., Wallace, K. and Haro, E. N. (1966), 'Effect of neomycin and kanamycin upon intestinal absorption', *Ann. N.Y. Acad. Sci.*, **132**, 879.

Finegold, S. M., Winfield, M. E., Nishizawa, A., Kantor, E. A., Kvinge, V. E. and Hewitt, W. L. (1959), 'Clinical evaluation of kanamycin', *Antibiot. Annual*—1958–1959, p. 606.

Finegold, S. M. (1959), 'Kanamycin', *Arch. Intern. Med.*, **104**, 15.

Finegold, S. M. (1966), 'Toxicity of kanamycin in adults', *Ann. N.Y. Acad. Sci.*, **132**, 942.

Frost, J. O., Daly, J. F. and Hawkins, J. E., Jr. (1959), 'The ototoxicity of kanamycin in man', *Antibiot. Annual*—1958–1959, p. 700.

Fischnallen, J. E., Pedersen, A. H. B., Ronald, A. B., Bonin, P. and Tronca, E. L. (1968), 'Kanamycin sulfate in the treatment of acute gonorrheic urethritis in man', *JAMA*, **203**, 909.

Garrod, L. P. and Waterworth, P. M. (1962), 'Methods of testing combined antibiotic bactericidal action and the significance of the results', *J. clin. Path.*, **15**, 328.

Glew, R. H., Moellering, R. C., Jr. and Buettner, K. R. (1977), '*In vitro* synergism between carbenicillin and aminoglycosidic aminocyclitols against Acinetobacter calcoaceticus var. anitratus', *Antimicrob. Ag. Chemother.*, **11**, 1036.

Gordon, R. C., Regamey, C. and Kirby, W. M. M. (1972), 'Serum protein binding of the aminoglycoside antibiotics', *Antimicrob. Ag. Chemother.*, **2**, 214.

Greenberg, P. A. and Sanford, J. P. (1967), 'Removal and absorption of antibiotics in patients with renal failure undergoing peritoneal dialysis', *Ann. Intern. Med.*, **66**, 465.

Gutschik, E., Jepsen, O. B. and Mortensen, I. (1977), 'Effect of combinations of penicillin and aminoglycosides on Streptococcus faecalis: a comparative study of seven aminoglycoside antibiotics', *J. Infect. Dis.*, **135**, 832.

Hammerberg, S., Sorger, S. and Marks, M. I. (1977), 'Antimicrobial susceptibilities of Yersinia enterocolitica Biotype 4, Serotype 0:3', *Antimicrob. Ag. Chemother.*, **11**, 566.

Hansen, J. M., Kampmann, J. and Laursen, H. (1970), 'Renal excretion of drugs in the elderly', *Lancet*, **1**, 1170.

Hansing, C. E., Allen, V. D. and Cherry, J. D. (1967), 'Escherichia coli endocarditis. A review of the literature and a case study', *Arch. Intern. Med.*, **120**, 472.

Healy, J. K., Drum, P. J. and Elliott, A. J. (1973), 'Kanamycin dosage in renal failure', *Aust. N. Z. J. Med.*, **3**, 474.

Hieber, J. P. and Nelson, J. D. (1976), 'Re-evaluation of kanamycin dosage in infants and children', *Antimicrob. Ag. Chemother.*, **9**, 899.

Howard, J. B. and McCracken, G. H., Jr. (1975), 'Reappraisal of kanamycin usage in neonates', *J. Pediatrics*, **86**, 949.

Kass, I. (1966), 'Kanamycin in the therapy of pulmonary tuberculosis in the United States', *Ann. N. Y. Acad. Sci.*, **132**, 892.

Keane, C. T., English, L. F. and Wise, R. (1975), 'Providencia stuartii infections', *Lancet*, **2**, 1045.

Kislak, J. W. (1972), 'The susceptibility of Bacteroides fragilis to 24 antibiotics', *J. Infect. Dis.*, **125**, 295.

Kunin, C. M. (1966), 'Absorption, distribution, excretion and fate of kanamycin', *Ann. N.Y. Acad. Sci.*, **132**, 811.

Leading Article (1967), 'Treatment of staphylococcal endocarditis', *Brit. med. J.*, **1**, 515.

Leading Article (1977), 'Necrotising enterocolitis', *Lancet*, **1**, 459.

Lorber, J. (1967), 'Intrathecal and intraventricular kanamycin in the treatment of meningitis and ventriculitis in infants', *Postgrad. Med. J.* (May Suppl.), p. 52.

Luft, F. C. and Kleit, S. A. (1974), 'Renal parenchymal accumulation of aminoglycoside antibiotics in rats', *J. Infect. Dis.*, **130**, 656.

Martin, W. J., Gardner, M. and Washington, J. A. II (1972), '*In vitro* antimicrobial susceptibility of anaerobic bacteria isolated from clinical specimens', *Antimicrob. Ag. Chemother.*, **1**, 148.

Mawer, G. E., Knowles, B. R., Lucas, S. B., Stirland, R. M. and Tooth, J. A. (1972a), 'Computer-assisted prescribing of kanamycin for patients with renal insufficiency', *Lancet*, **1**, 12.

Mawer, G. E., Lucas, S. B. and McGough, J. G. (1972b), 'Nomogram for kanamycin dosage', *Lancet*, **2**, 45.

McCloskey, R. V. and Becker, G. G. (1971), 'Evaluation of the Cutler-Orme method for administration of kanamycin during renal failure', *Antimicrob. Agents Chemother.*—1970, p. 161.

McCracken, G. H., Jr. and Threlkeld, N. (1976), 'Kanamycin dosage in newborn infants', *J. Pediatrics*, **89**, 313.

McCracken, G. H., Jr. and Nelson, J. D. (1977), *Antimicrobial Therapy for Newborns: Practical Application of Pharmacology to Clinical Usage*, Grune and Stratton, Inc., New York, San Francisco, London, p. 31.

McCracken, G. H., Jr., Threlkeld, N. and Thomas, M. L. (1977), 'Intravenous administration of kanamycin and gentamicin in newborn infants', *Pediatrics*, **60**, 463.

McHale, P., English, L., Speekenbrink, A., Keane, C. and Wise, R. (1978), 'Kanamycin resistance in Providencia stuartii', *J. Antimicrob. Chemother.*, **4**, 273.

Meriwether, W. D., Mangi, R. J. and Serpick, A. A. (1971), 'Deafness following standard intravenous dose of ethacrynic acid', *JAMA*, **216**, 795.

Murdoch, J. McC., Geddes, A. M. and Syme, J. (1962), 'Studies with kanamycin sulphate', *Lancet*, **1**, 457.

Murdoch, J. McC., Gray, J. A., Geddes, A. M. and Wallace, E. T. (1966), 'Clinical experiences with kanamycin in septicemia caused by Gram-negative organisms', *Ann. N. Y. Acad. Sci.*, **132**, 842.

Nelson, J. D. and Haltalin, K. C. (1966), '*In-vitro* susceptibility of E. coli, shigellae and salmonellae to kanamycin and therapeutic implications', *Ann. N.Y. Acad. Sci.*, **132**, 1006.

Ory, E. M., Williams, T. W., Jr., Camp, F. A., Register, R. F. and Morgen, R. O. (1966), 'Kanamycin in the treatment of patients with diminished kidney function', *Ann. N.Y. Acad. Sci.*, **132**, 933.

Petersdorf, R. G. and Turck, M. (1966), 'Kanamycin in urinary tract infections', *Ann. N.Y. Acad. Sci.*, **132**, 834.

Phillips, I., Eykyn, S., King, B. A., Jenkins, C., Warren, C. A. and Shannon, K. P. (1977), 'The *in vitro* antibacterial activity of nine aminoglycosides and spectinomycin on clinical isolates of common Gram-negative bacteria', *J. Antimicrob. Chemother.*, **3**, 403.

Pindell, M. H. (1966), 'The pharmacology of kanamycin—A review and new developments', *Ann. N.Y. Acad. Sci.*, **132**, 805.

Reeves, D. S. (1977), 'Prescription of aminoglycosides by nomogram', *J. Antimicrob. Chemother.*, **3**, 533.

Report of a WHO Scientific Group (1978), 'Neisseria gonorrhoeae and gonococcal infections', *Wld. Hlth. Org. Techn. Rep. Ser.*, No. **616**, p. 96.

Roe, E. and Lowbury, E. J. L. (1972), 'Changes in antibiotic sensitivity patterns of gram-negative bacilli in burns', *J. clin. Path.*, **25**, 176.

Ronald, A. R., Boutros, P. and Mourtada, H. (1976), 'Bacteriuria localization and response to single-dose therapy in women', *JAMA*, **235**, 1854.

Ruhen, R. W. and Darrell, J. H. (1973), 'Antibiotic synergism against Group D Streptococci in the treatment of endocarditis', *Med. J. Aust.*, **2**, 114.

Rutenburg, A. M. (1966), 'Status of kanamycin in the treatment of surgical infections', *Ann. N.Y. Acad. Sci.*, **132**, 824.

Sabath, L. D. (1969), 'Current concepts: Drug resistance of bacteria', *New Engl. J. Med.*, **280**, 91.

Sabath, L. D., Gerstein, D. A., Leaf, C. D. and Finland, M. (1970), 'Increasing the usefulness of antibiotics: Treatment of infections caused by Gram-negative bacilli', *Clin. Pharm. Ther.*, **11**, 161.

Sanford, J. (1966), 'Panel discussion: Toxicity of kanamycin in adults', *Ann. N.Y. Acad. Sci.*, **132**, 970.

Stiffler, P. W., Sweeney, H. M., Schneider, M. and Cohen, S. (1974), 'Isolation and characterization of a kanamycin resistance plasmid from Staphylococcus aureus', *Antimicrob. Ag. Chemother.*, **6**, 516.

Terman, J. W., Alford, R. H. and Bryant, R. E. (1972), 'Hospital-acquired Klebsiella bacteremia', *Amer. J. Med. Sci.*, **264**, 191.

Thornsberry, C., Baker, C. N. and Kirven, L. A. (1978), '*In vitro* activity of antimicrobial agents on Legionnaires' disease bacterium', *Antimicrob. Ag. Chemother.*, **13**, 78.

Umezawa, H., Ueda, M., Maeda, K., Yagishita, K., Kondo, S., Okami, Y., Utahara, R., Osato, Y., Nitta, K. and Takeuchi, T. (1957), 'Production and isolation of a new antibiotic, kanamycin', *J. Antibiotics Japan*, Ser. A., **10**, 181; quoted by Finegold (1959).

Welch, H., Wright, W. W., Weinstein, H. I. and Ataffa, A. W. (1958), 'In vitro and pharmacological studies with kanamycin', Ann. N.Y. Acad. Sci., 76, 66.

Wilkinson, A. E., Race, J. W. and Curtis, F. R. (1967), 'Kanamycin in the treatment of gonorrhoea in males', Postgrad. Med. J. (May Suppl.), p. 65.

Wyatt, R. G., Okamoto, G. A. and Feigin, R. D. (1972), 'Stability of antibiotics in parenteral solutions', Pediatrics, 49, 22.

Yoshioka, H., Rudoy, P., Riley, H. D., Jr. and Yoshida, K. (1977), 'Antimicrobial susceptibility of Escherichia coli isolated at a children's hospital', Scand. J. Infect. Dis., 9, 207.

Yow, M. (1966), 'Kanamycin in pediatric practice with special reference observations on ototoxicity', Ann. N.Y. Acad. Sci., 132, 1037.

Gentamicin

Description

Gentamicin is produced by a species of bacteria of the genus Micromonospora and was discovered in the Schering Research Laboratories (Weinstein *et al.*, 1964; Black *et al.*, 1964). It is structurally related to the other aminoglycosides, streptomycin, kanamycin, neomycin, amikacin, tobramycin, sisomicin and netilmicin. Gentamicin is marketed as gentamicin sulphate and trade names include 'Garamycin' (Schering) and 'Cidomycin' (Roussel).

Sensitive Organisms

1. *Gram-negative aerobic bacteria*. Gentamicin is active against nearly all the Enterobacteriaceae such as Esch. coli, the Enterobacter, Klebsiella, Proteus, Salmonella, Shigella, Providencia, Serratia, Citrobacter, Hafnia, Edwardsiella and Arizona spp. (Weinstein *et al.*, 1964; Jao and Jackson, 1964; Waitz and Weinstein, 1969). Yersinia pestis (Butler *et al.*, 1974), Y. pseudotuberculosis (Gurry, 1974) and Y. enterocolitica (Chessum *et al.*, 1971; Hammerberg *et al.*, 1977) are also usually gentamicin-sensitive.

For a number of years after this drug was introduced for use in hospitals, gentamicin-resistant strains of even those Enterobacteriaceae which are normal inhabitants of the human bowel were uncommon. This contrasted with the higher prevalence of kanamycin-resistant organisms at the time (page 308). During a two-month survey in a Boston hospital in 1967 only 2 per cent of Esch. coli and 4 per cent of Klebsiella spp. isolates were gentamicin-resistant, and no resistant strains of Enterobacter, Proteus and Serratia spp. were encountered (Sabath, 1969). Since then gentamicin has been extensively used in hospital practice and the prevalence of Enterobacteriaceae resistant to gentamicin has gradually increased in many hospitals or special hospital areas, such as burns or intensive-care units. Thus in a survey in a burns unit, 0·9 per cent of Esch. coli, 4·7 per cent of Kl. aerogenes, 0·37 per cent of Pr. mirabilis, 14·3 per cent of Pr. morganii and 41·2 per cent of Providencia spp. were found to be resistant (Roe and Lowbury, 1972). Hospital infections and outbreaks caused by gentamicin-resistant Klebsiella spp. have been especially prevalent (Martin *et al.*, 1971; Richmond *et al.*, 1975; Noriega *et al.*, 1975; Casewell *et al.*, 1977; Rennie and Duncan 1977; Forbes *et al.*, 1977). The frequency of gentamicin-resistant Klebsiella spp. in a hospital often declines rapidly when the use of this antibiotic is restricted, and increases again several months after restrictions are removed (Noriega *et al.*, 1975).

Resistant strains of Serratia marcescens whilst rare in Great Britain (Annotation, 1977; Phillips *et al.*, 1977) have been a problem in several North

American hospitals. Cooksey *et al.* (1975) in a survey of 102 isolates of Serratia marcescens from three American medical centres found that approximately 20 per cent were gentamicin-resistant. Similarly Meyer *et al.* (1976) reported 50 per cent resistance amongst Serratia isolates from one American general hospital. Schaberg *et al.* (1976) described a large epidemic of infections due to a strain of Serratia marcescens resistant to gentamicin and all then available parenteral antibiotics; 210 patients in four separate hospitals were affected, and there was evidence of inter-hospital spread. In a survey of a large Australian general hospital, 7 of 34 Serratia isolates were gentamicin-resistant (Kwitko *et al.*, 1977).

Gentamicin-resistant strains of many other Enterobacteriaceae, particularly those which are normal inhabitants of human bowel, have also been isolated from hospital patients. Reports include resistant Esch. coli (Drasar *et al.*, 1976; Phillips *et al.*, 1977; Minshew *et al.*, 1977), Enterobacter spp. (Poston *et al.*, 1976; Drasar *et al.*, 1976; Phillips *et al.*, 1977), Proteus spp. (Shafi and Datta, 1975; Drasar *et al.*, 1976), Providencia spp. (Hamilton-Miller *et al.*, 1974; Drasar *et al.*, 1976) and Citrobacter spp. (Richmond *et al.*, 1975; Drasar *et al.*, 1976). Resistance of Enterobacteriaceae may arise by a mutation or be R plasmid-mediated (page 422). R plasmids code for the production of gentamicin-modifying enzymes, and this seems to be the predominant mechanism of resistance of Enterobacteriaceae to gentamicin (Shannon *et al.*, 1978). These plasmids coding resistance to gentamicin have been identified in several bacterial species. They have also been implicated in many hospital outbreaks of infections caused by resistant Enterobacteriaceae, in which gentamicin resistance is often associated with resistance to other antibiotics (Richmond *et al.*, 1975; Shafi and Datta, 1975; Poston *et al.*, 1976; Davey and Pittard, 1977).

Gentamicin-resistant strains of Esch. coli, produced *in vitro* by passage in a gentamicin containing medium, show complete cross-resistance with streptomycin, neomycin, kanamycin and tobramycin. By contrast, naturally occurring gentamicin-resistant strains are not necessarily resistant to the three older drugs, but are usually resistant to tobramycin (page 359) (Houang and Greenwood, 1977).

The MIC's and MBC's of Proteus and Providencia spp. strains, which are only moderately gentamicin-resistant, can be significantly reduced by the simultaneous use of either cephalothin (page 200) or cephazolin (page 239). However with gentamicin strains with a MBC of 25 μg per ml or greater, this synergy is unlikely to result from clinically attainable concentrations of the two antibiotics (Hyams *et al.*, 1974). A cephalothin/gentamicin combination also acts synergistically against many Klebsiella spp. strains (D'Alessandri *et al.*, 1976).

Many strains of Enterobacteriaceae, which are resistant to gentamicin, are sensitive to either amikacin (page 378) or netilmicin (page 396), but they are usually resistant to tobramycin (page 359) and sisomicin (page 395).

Pseudomonas aeruginosa is quite sensitive and activity against this organism is one of the most important features of gentamicin. Resistant strains have been noted in many hospitals ever since the advent of this drug. With increased clinical use of gentamicin both parenterally and topically, the prevalence of such strains has gradually increased. Nevertheless in general medical and surgical wards of most hospitals, gentamicin-resistant Ps. aeruginosa isolates are still relatively uncommon (Duncan, 1974; Holmes et al., 1974a and b; Gaman et al., 1976; Phillips et al., 1977; Dean et al., 1977). In special hospital areas (or occasionally throughout a hospital), usually following the widespread use of this drug, outbreaks of infections or colonizations of patients by gentamicin-resistant Ps. aeruginosa have occurred. For example, such outbreaks have been described in burns units (Shulman et al., 1971; Minshew et al., 1977). In one cancer research centre, the percentage of gentamicin-resistant Ps. aeruginosa isolates increased over a period from 1971 (Greene et al., 1973). Similarly an outbreak of gentamicin- and tobramycin-resistant Ps. aeruginosa infection occurred in a surgical ward over a three-month period (Falkiner et al., 1977). A 12 months' survey in 1974–1975 at one hospital in the United States showed that 19·1 per cent of Ps. aeruginosa isolates were gentamicin-resistant (Meyer et al., 1976), and in another American hospital the percentage of resistant isolates increased from 13·9 per cent in 1969 to 38·9 per cent in 1972 (Maliwan et al., 1975). These resistant strains are frequently isolated from urine (Baird et al., 1976; Meyer et al., 1976; Falkiner et al., 1977). In special hospital areas, where the emergence and spread of gentamicin-resistant Pseudomonas has been clearly related to excessive use of both parenteral and topical gentamicin, the percentage of resistant strains has decreased when the clinical use of this drug was restricted (Holder, 1976; Roberts and Douglas, 1978).

Resistant strains of Ps. aeruginosa appear to be as virulent as sensitive strains (Meyer et al., 1976). Low-level resistance of this organism to gentamicin appears to be chromosomal due to a genetic mutation (Seal and Strangeways, 1976; Phillips et al., 1978). High-level resistance is due to the acquisition of R plasmids, which code for the production of enzymes, which modify gentamicin by either acetylation or adenylylation (Bryan et al., 1974; Kabins et al., 1974). These R plasmids are readily transmissible to other Ps. aeruginosa, but not to Esch. coli strains (Jacoby, 1974). They may also determine multiple drug resistance including that to both gentamicin and carbenicillin (Korfhagen et al., 1975; 1976).

Similar to gentamicin-resistant Enterobacteriaceae (page 326), gentamicin-resistant Ps. aeruginosa strains are often sensitives to amikacin (page 378) and may be sometimes sensitive to netilmicin (page 396). Unlike the Enterobacteriaceae, a proportion of these strains have remained sensitive to tobramycin (page 360) (Meyer et al., 1976; Drasar et al., 1976; Kauffman et al., 1978).

Occasionally other Pseudomonas spp. may cause infections in debilitated patients, such as Ps. maltophilia, Ps. cepacia and Ps. multivorans. These are usually resistant to gentamicin (Moody et al., 1972; Phillips et al., 1977). Ps. pseudomallei is also resistant to gentamicin at concentrations attainable in vivo (Franklin, 1971). Ps. stutzeri may be gentamicin-sensitive, but resistant strains occur (Uwaydah and Taqi-Eddin, 1976).

Among other Gram-negative bacteria, the Neisseria spp. (meningococci and gonococci) are only moderately sensitive to gentamicin, the degree varying with individual strains. H. influenzae is also only moderately sensitive. The Brucella and Moraxella spp., Pasteurella multocida (Waitz and Weinstein, 1969) and Francisella tularensis (Alford et al., 1972) are usually sensitive.

Acinetobacter calcoaceticus var. anitratus (Herellea vaginicola) is usually sensitive to gentamicin, but moderately or highly resistant strains occur. Gentamicin similar to kanamycin (page 309), when combined with carbenicillin (page 151) exhibits *in vitro* synergism against this organism, provided that the strains is gentamicin-sensitive or only moderately resistant (MIC < 31 µg per ml) (Glew *et al.*, 1977). Acinetobacter calcoaceticus var. lwoffi (Mima polymorpha) is also usually gentamicin-sensitive. The Alcaligenes spp. is commonly resistant to gentamicin and other aminoglycosides (Uwaydah and Taqi-Eddin, 1976). The Flavobacterium spp. which may be sensitive to rifampicin (page 552), erythromycin (page 498) and novobiocin (page 525), is always resistant to aminoglycosides including gentamicin (Drasar *et al.*, 1976; Lee *et al.*, 1977). The Legionnaires' disease bacterium is sensitive to gentamicin *in vitro* (MIC 0·12–0·5 µg per ml) (Thornsberry *et al.*, 1978). The drug, administered prophylactically or up to 48 h after infection, can prevent the death of embryonated eggs infected with this organism (Lewis *et al.*, 1978), but it does not prevent the death of infected guinea pigs (Fraser *et al.*, 1978). Campylobacter fetus is sensitive to gentamicin and also to other aminoglycosides such as kanamycin (page 309) and amikacin (page 378) (Chow *et al.*, 1978).

2. *Gram-negative anaerobic bacteria.* Fusobacterium spp. and some strains of Bacteroides melaninogenicus may be moderately sensitive, but all other Gram-negative anaerobic bacteria, in particular Bacteroides fragilis, are gentamicin-resistant (Martin *et al.*, 1972). Gentamicin does not interfere with the *in vitro* activity of clindamycin (page 472) or chloramphenicol (page 421) against B. fragilis (Klastersky and Husson, 1977), and gentamicin plus clindamycin may act synergistically against B. fragilis (Okubadejo and Allen, 1975). Chloramphenicol, however, may interfere with the action of gentamicin on aerobic Gram-negative bacilli such as Esch. coli, but this antagonism, although observed *in vitro*, probably is of little significance *in vivo* (page 443).

3. *Gram-positive bacteria.* Staph. pyogenes is highly sensitive to gentamicin. Barber and Waterworth (1966) tested 102 strains which were sensitive to kanamycin (MIC usually 1 µg per ml), and showed that gentamicin was four times more active. They also tested 57 strains which were resistant to both kanamycin and neomycin, and found that, with only a few exceptions, these were also gentamicin-sensitive. Naturally acquired neomycin and kanamycin resistance does not seem to be accompanied by resistance to gentamicin. Hoeprich (1969) observed that 20 strains of Staph. pyogenes resistant to methicillin and the cephalosporins were all inhibited by 0·4 µg per ml of gentamicin. In addition, Jordan and Hoeprich (1977) tested 22 penicillin G-susceptible, 51 penicillin G-resistant and 47 methicillin-resistant strains of Staph. pyogenes, and these were all gentamicin-sensitive.

By the mid-seventies, almost a decade after the introduction of gentamicin, several reports of outbreaks of infection in hospitals caused by gentamicin-resistant strains of Staph. pyogenes appeared (Speller *et al.*, 1976; Bint *et al.*, 1977; Wyatt *et al.*, 1977; Lewis and Altemeier, 1978). These staphylococci were often resistant to many other antibiotics such as penicillin G, tetracycline, streptomycin, neomycin, kanamycin, tobramycin, erythromycin and clindamycin. Shanson *et al.* (1976) reported an outbreak of hospital infection with a Staph. pyogenes strain resistant to gentamicin and methicillin, as well as to other antibiotics. In some of these outbreaks there was evidence that prior excess use of gentamicin, particularly topically, was associated with the appearance and spread of these strains. Such outbreaks may be prevented or contained by rational prescribing of parenteral gentamicin, and severe restriction or prohibition of its topical use (Bint, 1976).

Resistance of Staph. pyogenes to gentamicin appears to be mediated by R plasmids (page 422). Genes or determinants for gentamicin resistance reside on a 50 S plasmid, which codes for gentamicin-inactivating enzymes; two of these have been identified, an aminoglycoside 6′-N-acetyltransferase and a gentamicin phosphotransferase (Porthouse et al., 1976; Wood et al., 1977; Dowding, 1977; Scott et al., 1978).

Staph. epidermidis, including penicillin G–and methicillin-resistant strains, is also gentamicin-sensitive (Laverdiere et al., 1978). Other Gram-positive cocci such as Strep. pyogenes, Group B streptococci, Strep. pneumoniae, and the alpha-haemolytic streptococci (Strep. viridans) have only a low degree of sensitivity to gentamicin or are completely resistant. Ampicillin (or penicillin G), combined with gentamicin acts synergistically against Group B streptococci (Schauf et al., 1976; Deveikis et al., 1977). Similar to streptomycin (page 302), gentamicin combined with penicillin G acts synergistically against most Strep. viridans strains (Sande and Irvin, 1974).

Strep. faecalis is moderately resistant, but gentamicin combined with penicillin G (or ampicillin) is synergistic against this organism. This effect occurs with nearly all Strep. faecalis strains, whereas penicillin/streptomycin (page 294) and penicillin/kanamycin (page 310) combinations are not synergistic against a proportion of strains (Ruhen and Darrell, 1973; Gutschik et al., 1977; Calderwood et al., 1977). Basker et al. (1977) reported the isolation of two Strep. faecalis strains from patients who had been treated with topical gentamicin; these had MIC's of 250 and 500 μg per ml and were 50 to 100 times less sensitive to gentamicin than control sensitive strains. In addition, they were less sensitive to a penicillin/gentamicin combination than typical strains of Strep. faecalis, and showed variable responses to this combination in tests for bactericidal synergy. The combination of gentamicin with vancomycin is also nearly always synergistic against Strep. faecalis (Watanakunakorn and Bakie, 1973).

The Gram-positive bacilli such as the Bacillus, Clostridium. Actinomyces and Corynebacterium spp. and Listeria monocytogenes are sensitive to gentamicin to a degree (Waitz and Weinstein, 1969). Nocardia asteroides is relatively resistant (Bach et al., 1973). As with Strep. faecalis, a gentamicin/penicillin G or a gentamicin/ampicillin combination acts synergistically against Listeria monocytogenes (Moellering et al., 1972; Mohan et al., 1977).

4. *Mycobacteria.* Gentamicin has no activity against M. tuberculosis at clinically attainable concentrations, most strains having an MIC of 64 μg per ml or higher. It also has no activity against other mycobacteria (Gangadharam and Candler, 1977). The administration of this drug is unlikely to impede the bacteriological diagnosis of tuberculosis.

5. *Other microorganisms.* Mycoplasma pneumoniae and Mycoplasma hominis are sensitive to gentamicin. Yeasts, other fungi and Entamoeba histolytica are resistant (Waitz and Weinstein, 1969; Brenciaglia et al., 1975).

In Vitro Sensitivities

Table 23 shows the minimum inhibitory concentrations of gentamicin against some selected bacterial species. The main clinical importance of gentamicin is its activity against all the Gram-negative bacilli that are normal inhabitants of the human bowel. By comparison to the polymyxins and kanamycin, gentamicin is active against both the Proteus spp. and Ps. aeruginosa. The activity of gentamicin is equal or greater than that of the polymyxins (page 534) against Ps. aeruginosa and it has a similar activity to kanamycin (page 310) against Proteus spp. (Jao and Jackson, 1964).

TABLE 23

(After Barber and Waterworth, 1966)

ORGANISM	MIC (μg per ml)
Gram-positive bacteria	
Staph. pyogenes	0·12– 1·0
Staph. pyogenes (kanamycin-resistant)	0·12– 4·0
Strep. pyogenes (Group A)	16·0
Strep. pneumoniae (Dip. pneumoniae)	16·0–32·0
Strep. faecalis (Enterococcus, Group D)	8·0 –16·0
Gram-negative bacteria	
Esch. coli	1·0 – 4·0
Klebsiella aerogenes	1·0 – 2·0
Klebsiella (other spp.)	0·06– 1·0
Proteus mirabilis	2·0 – 8·0
Proteus vulgaris	1·0 – 4·0
Proteus morganii	1·0 – 4·0
Proteus rettgeri	1·0 – 8·0
Salmonella spp.	0·25– 1·0
Shigella spp.	1·0 – 2·0
Pseudomonas aeruginosa	1·0 – 8·0

Mode of Administration and Dosage

Gentamicin is not absorbed after oral administration, and it is usually administered by the intramuscular or intravenous routes.

1. *Intramuscular administration to adults.* Relatively high gentamicin doses are necessary for treatment of systemic infections caused by Ps. aeruginosa and other Gram-negative rods. A commonly recommended dose is 80 mg eight-hourly or 4·5 mg per kg body weight per day given in three divided doses (Darrell and Waterworth, 1967; Gingell and Waterworth, 1968). This dosage produces mean peak serum levels of 4–6 μg per ml in most adults (Siber *et al.*, 1975.

For seriously ill patients larger doses may be needed to obtain higher peak serum levels and satisfactory therapeutic results. As there is only a narrow safety margin between therapeutically effective and toxic serum levels with gentamicin, near toxic doses are often required for the successful treatment of these patients. In these circumstances it is preferable to calculate each patient's dose according to body weight, rather than rely on a single 'standard' adult dose. During the first day of treatment of critically ill patients, a dose ranging from 5 mg per kg body weight per day (Noone et al., 1974a) to 7–8 mg per kg body weight per day (Riff and Jackson, 1971), given in three divided doses may be used. Subsequent gentamicin dosage is then determined according to results of gentamicin serum level estimations (page 334), a gentamicin dosage nomogram (page 333), or both.

After the first day of therapy the dose can usually be reduced. The maintenance dose will vary in different patients, because there is individual variation in the absorption of gentamicin from intramuscular sites, and also possibly because of other reasons. Serum concentrations achieved with identical doses vary a great deal between patients. For instance serum gentamicin levels are lower in febrile compared to non-febrile patients (Pennington et al., 1975). Therefore, if the drug is used in high dosage for serious infections, serum level estimations are advisable, even in patients with normal renal function (Noone et al., 1974b; Reeves, 1977). The dose should be adjusted to produce peak serum levels of about 6–10 μg per ml, which occur about one hour after intramuscular injection. Serum levels just before the next dose (trough levels) should probably not exceed 1·5–2·0 μg per ml (Annotation, 1974; McGhie et al., 1974) (see page 340). In some patients the commonly used adult dose of 80 mg eight-hourly may produce toxic serum levels (page 338), but in others it may be inadequate. Some adults require a maintenance dose of 120 mg or even 160 mg every eight hours (up to 7 mg per kg per day), to achieve adequate serum levels and a satisfactory therapeutic result.

2. *Intramuscular administration to children.* As with kanamycin (page 311), children need relatively higher doses of gentamicin than adults to achieve similar serum levels. For children less than five years of age a dose of 7·5 mg per kg per day is recommended, while for those aged 5–10 years a dose of 6 mg per kg per day is appropriate, both given in three divided doses. These regimens produce serum levels similar to those attained in adults with the commonly used dose of 4·5 mg per kg per day (*vide supra*). Therefore in some children with severe infections, doses higher than those recommended will be needed, particularly for initiation of therapy (Echeverria et al., 1975; Siber et al., 1975).

3. *Newborn and premature infants.* The serum gentamicin half-life is prolonged in babies during the first week of life. Such patients should only be given 5 mg per kg per day, administered in two divided doses; all other infants may be given 7·5 mg per kg per day in three divided doses, the dose recommended for older children (Nelson and McCracken, 1972; Ingham and Emslie, 1972; McCracken and Nelson, 1977).

4. *Intravenous administration.* Gentamicin can be administered intravenously in the same dosage as recommended for intramuscular use. The intravenous route is essential for shocked patients and preferable for those who have a bleeding tendency. Gentamicin in the usual doses should not be administered intravenously by continuous infusion. If an 80 mg dose is added to an intravenous bottle, and this is infused over eight hours to an adult patient with normal renal function, a 'steady-state' serum concentration of about 2·5 μg per ml will only be reached after ten to twelve hours. This relatively low concentration may not be inhibitory to many Gram-negative bacilli (O'Grady, 1971; O'Grady et al., 1971). Higher 'steady state' gentamicin serum levels can

be achieved if larger doses are infused continuously (Bodey *et al.*, 1975), but this may be associated with an increased risk of toxicity (*see* tobramycin, page 363).

A satisfactory method for intravenous administration is to dilute each eight-hourly dose in 50–100 ml of intravenous fluid (a smaller volume for children) for infusion over 20 to 30 min (Hendeles, 1971; Siber *et al.*, 1975; McCracken *et al.*, 1977). Serum levels comparable to those reached after intramuscular injection of the same dose are attained (page 335). It is recommended that this is the only method by which gentamicin should be administered intravenously to neonates (McCracken and Nelson, 1977; McCracken *et al.*, 1977).

In adults and older children, it is often more convenient to inject the undiluted eight-hourly dose directly into the intravenous tubing, over two to three minutes. This produces adequate serum levels, and the half-life and peak serum concentrations are often similar to those reached after intramuscular injection (Stratford *et al.*, 1974). There is, however, a great individual variation in peak serum levels attained after this method of administration; in some patients levels above 12·5 μg per ml are reached 2–4 min after the start of the injection and persist for 5–13 min (Michel *et al.*, 1974). Gentamicin may be administered even more rapidly by the intravenous route; when a standard dose is injected over 10 s, a higher peak level of about 18 μg per ml occurs in 1–3 min, but this falls to levels of about 9 μg per ml at 10 min and 5 μg per ml at 60 min (Bailey and Lynn, 1974). These transiently high serum levels are unlikely to cause vestibular damage (page 338). Furthermore, no local or systemic reactions occur with rapid intravenous gentamicin injections (Curtis *et al.*, 1967; Mendelson *et al.*, 1976). Intravenous gentamicin administration by injection over 2–3 min is used frequently at Fairfield Hospital.

5. *Patients with renal failure.* These require a modified dosage schedule. Gingell and Waterworth (1968) suggested that an initial loading dose of 80 mg intramuscularly can be given to adult patients, and that the subsequent frequency of administration of this dose depends on the degree of renal impairment (Table 24). This schedule is simple to use because only intervals between standard doses are altered. It is feasible to use a smaller dose of 60 or 40 mg at more frequent intervals (after the initial loading dose of 80 mg), to maintain therapeutic serum levels.

TABLE 24

Approximate scheme of dosage for gentamicin
(After Gingell and Waterworth, 1968)

Blood urea		Creatinine clearance	Dosage
mg/100 ml	mmol/l		
< 35	< 5·8	> 70	80 mg every 8 h
50–100	8·4–16·8	30–50	80 mg every 12 h
> 200	> 33·6	5–10	80 mg every 48 h
Twice-weekly intermittent haemodialysis		< 3	80 mg after each dialysis

Since then gentamicin has been widely used in hospitals, and a number of other dosage schedules for patients with renal failure have appeared.

A simple way is to assume that as with kanamycin (page 311), there is a linear relationship between the gentamicin half-life and the patient's serum creatinine concentration. The gentamicin half-life (measured in hours) is roughly equal to the serum creatinine concentration (mg per cent)* multiplied by four. In patients with renal failure the usual gentamicin dose of 80 to 120 mg (or 2·5 mg per kg in children) may be administered intramuscularly once every two half-lives. For example an adult with a normal creatinine of 1·0 mg per cent may be given 80 mg every $(1 \times 4 \times 2) = 8$ hours, whilst a patient with severe renal failure (creatinine 10 mg per cent) should be given this dose once every $(10 \times 4 \times 2) = 80$ hours (McHenry et al., 1971). A simplication is that the time interval in hours between doses can be obtained by multiplying the patient's serum creatinine (mg per cent) by eight (Goodman et al., 1975). This method has the disadvantage that there may be a prolonged period of time during which gentamicin serum levels are non-therapeutic, prior to the next injection.

An alternative approach is to reduce the individual doses of the drug which are administered at constant intervals (Cutler et al., 1972). A full loading dose of 1·5–2·5 mg per kg is given, but the subsequent eight-hourly dose is calculated by dividing the loading dose by the patient's serum creatinine in mg per cent. Regular administration in this way to patients with impaired renal function results in an almost 'steady state therapy'. In patients with severe renal failure serum gentamicin levels should continuously approximate or slightly exceed the MIC's of gentamicin for many aerobic Gram-negative bacilli (Goodman et al., 1975).

As in the case of kanamycin (page 312), nomograms for gentamicin dosage have been published (Chan et al., 1972; Mawer et al., 1974). Loading and maintenance doses and intervals between doses can be derived from these, and nomograms are designed to give serum gentamicin concentrations of 3–10 μg per ml. Calculations by a nomogram are certainly more accurate than the other methods described, particularly when large gentamicin doses are needed for severe infections. In one comparative study in patients with proven bacterial sepsis, the response rate was improved in those in whom gentamicin was prescribed by nomogram (Wilkinson et al., 1977).

Nevertheless, all these methods of calculating dosage, including nomograms, are at the best only useful approximations, so that whenever possible maintenance doses of gentamicin should be governed by serum level estimations (Bell, 1976; Noone et al., 1978). In many patients pharmacokinetic assumptions fail to match individual patient characteristics. For instance, some authors have found that the serum gentamicin half-life often correlates poorly with serum creatinine (Kaye et al., 1974; Barza et al., 1975). Also the apparent distribution volume of gentamicin often may not be a fixed proportion of the body mass, especially in obese or dehydrated patients. Gentamicin doses can be prescribed in terms of mg per kg of lean body weight (calculated from a for-

---

* The serum creatinine in mg per cent may be obtained by multiplying the creatinine value in mmol/l SI units) by a factor of 12. For instance, a serum creatinine of 0·1 mmol/l equals 1·2 mg per cent and a serum creatinine of 1·0 mg per cent equals 0·088 mmol/l.

mula) instead of total body weight. If lean body weight is used in nomogram calculations, predictive values are apparently improved (Hull and Sarubbi, 1976), but other variables remain. In particular the serum creatinine value may be unreliable as it often changes rapidly (Reeves, 1977).

Gentamicin serum levels can be estimated within a period of four hours by many methods. These include microbiological plate diffusion assay (Sabath *et al.*, 1971; Noone *et al.*, 1971; Sabath and Toftegaard, 1974), chemical assay (Smith *et al.*, 1972), enzymatic assay (Holmes and Sanford, 1974), radioimmunoassay (Mahon *et al.*, 1973; Longmore *et al.*, 1976) and haemagglutination inhibition assay (Mahon *et al.*, 1977). The microbiological plate diffusion method is probably still the best for routine use in clinical laboratories (Waterworth, 1977). Contrary to previous beliefs, jaundiced serum does not inactivate gentamicin and it does not interfere with serum gentamicin estimations (McDonald and Waterworth, 1974).

Gentamicin is removed from the body by haemodialysis, and its half-life in anephric patients of approximately 50 h is reduced to about 10 h during dialysis (Halpren *et al.*, 1976). Patients receiving regular haemodialysis two or three times a week can usually be treated satisfactorily by a dosage of 1·5–2·0 mg per kg body weight, given at the end of each 8 h dialysis (Curtis *et al.*, 1967). This regimen results in therapeutic serum levels during most of a 48 h interdialysis period, but they are in an ineffective range for the duration of the next haemodialysis (Halpren *et al.*, 1976). For this reason these authors suggest an alternate approach. After an initial post-dialysis dose of 1·5–2·0 mg per kg, patients undergoing dialysis every 48 h are given one half of the initial dose immediately preceding, and again following, each dialysis. This schedule avoids both ineffective concentrations during dialysis, and potentially toxic peak concentrations after dialysis. If 6 h dialyses are used twice or thrice a week, it is suggested that a loading dose of 1·5–2·0 mg per kg be given after the first dialysis, but thereafter only three quarters of this dose after each subsequent dialysis (Danish *et al.*, 1974).

Peritoneal dialysis also removes gentamicin, but the rate of clearance varies, probably according to the degree of peritoneal inflammation (Smithivas *et al.*, 1971). A single daily dose of 1·5–2·0 mg per kg of intramuscular gentamicin may result in therapeutic non-toxic serum levels in uraemic patients undergoing peritoneal dialysis, but this should be confirmed by serum level estimations. Gentamicin may also be added to peritoneal dialysis fluid in a concentration of 5–10 mg per litre. If this is used to treat peritonitis, results are improved if parenteral gentamicin is also administered (Smithivas *et al.*, 1971; Hyams *et al.*, 1971).

6. *Intrathecal and intraventricular administration.* Gentamicin may be administered by these routes for the treatment of meningitis due to Gram-negative bacilli (Newman and Holt, 1971; Moellering and Fischer, 1972). The dose for newborn babies is 1–2 mg daily (Nelson and McCracken 1972; Lee *et al.*, 1977). For adults the dose is 5–10 mg daily (Rahal, 1972; Kaiser and McGee, 1975), although doses as high as 20 mg daily have been used safely (Smilack and McCloskey, 1972).

The role of intrathecal gentamicin in conjunction with parenteral treatment for neonatal meningitis or meningitis caused by Gram-negative enteric bacilli in other age groups has been controversial (Annotation, 1976; Leading article,

1976a; Lambert, 1977). In one comparative trial, 117 infants with meningitis due to Gram-negative enteric organisms were treated by either ampicillin and gentamicin given parenterally, or by the same parenteral drugs plus intrathecal gentamicin; there was no additional benefit from intrathecal therapy (McCracken and Mize, 1976). Gentamicin administration into the lumbar intrathecal space results in adequate drug concentrations in lumbar CSF, but not in ventricular CSF. Gentamicin administered into the cerebral ventricles produces adequate concentrations in both the ventricle and lumbar CSF (Kaiser and McGee, 1975). Intraventricular administration of gentamicin (or other antibiotics) is therefore preferable to the intrathecal route. As intraventricular administration is not without problems and risks (Lambert, 1977), it should not be used routinely for meningitis caused by Gram-negative bacilli, but it should be reserved for problem patients, not responding or not likely to respond to parenteral therapy alone (Kaiser and McGee, 1975; Kortopoulos and Holm, 1976; Leading article, 1976a; Olsen et al., 1977; Pickering et al., 1978).

Availability

1. *Intramuscular or intravenous administration:*
   (a) 1, 1·5 and 2 ml ampoules or vials containing 40, 60 and 80 mg gentamicin sulphate, respectively, in an aqueous solution.
   (b) 2 ml vials containing 20 mg and ampoules containing 10 mg per ml, for paediatric use.
2. *Topical and ophthalmic preparations:*
   (a) 0·3 per cent ointment in a 4 g tube, for both ophthalmic and cutaneous use.
   (b) 0·3 per cent ophthalmic drops in a 5 ml plastic squeeze bottle.

Serum Levels in Relation to Dosage

The mean peak serum level of gentamicin, after intramuscular injection of 80 mg in an adult is 7 μg per ml (range 4·2 to 12·0 μg per ml). This level is attained in 0·5–2·0 h after the injection (Gingell and Waterworth, 1968). Doubling the dose results in approximately twice the serum concentrations (Jao and Jackson, 1964). The serum half-life of the drug in patients with normal renal function is approximately four hours, and eight hours after injection the serum level falls to about 1 μg per ml (Fig. 21). The serum half-life in patients with severe renal failure may be prolonged to 40–50 h.

In neonates and young children serum levels similar to those shown in Figure 21 are attained after administration of 2·5 mg per kg of gentamicin intramuscularly (McCracken, 1972; Nelson and McCracken, 1972).

Intravenous gentamicin also produces serum levels comparable to those obtained after intramuscular injection, provided that the dose is infused over 20–30 min (McCracken et al., 1977). After an intravenous injection given over 2–3 min, the serum half-life of the drug is also similar to that after intramuscular administration, but the peak serum level is variable (page 332). In some patients this peak transiently exceeds 12·5 μg per ml, and in others measured levels 5–10 min after the injection are no higher than those after intramuscular administration.

Some authors have found that peak serum levels in patients with renal impairment after a single gentamicin dose are comparable to those obtained in normal subjects (Gingell and Waterworth, 1968), but others have noted higher

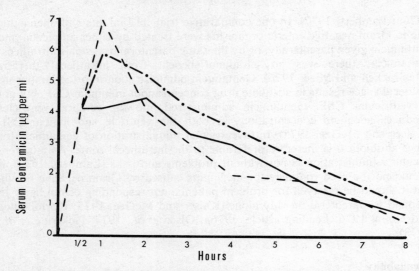

Fig. 21. Serum gentamicin levels in three cases with normal renal function after 80 mg intramuscularly. (Redrawn after Gingell and Waterworth, 1968.)

peak levels in azotaemic patients (Curtis *et al.*, 1967; Riff and Jackson, 1971). In one of these studies 1·6 mg of gentamicin per kg body weight was injected intravenously; in two subjects with normal renal function serum concentrations of 5 and 7·5 μg per ml, respectively, were detected after ten minutes, but in three patients with chronic renal failure, the level at that time was 16 μg per ml (Curtis *et al.*, 1967). Higher peak serum gentamicin levels are expected after the initial dose in patients with renal failure, because this peak is determined not only by the distribution volume, but also by excretion which commences as soon as gentamicin is present in the blood.

Excretion

URINE: Gentamicin is excreted by glomerular filtration almost entirely in the active form (Black *et al.*, 1964). Its renal clearance in normal subjects is about 60 ml per minute (Jao and Jackson, 1964). For the first one or two days of gentamicin therapy, excretion is partly delayed and during this time only about 40 per cent of the administered drug can be recovered from urine. With continued administration, equilibration between the serum and body tissues occurs, the daily urinary excretion increases, and after about one week nearly all of the daily dose is excreted in the urine. After two days treatment with a dose of 2·4 mg per kg per day, the urine concentration is about 40–50 μg per ml (Jao and Jackson, 1964). However the urinary gentamicin concentration varies inversely with urine volume and in oliguric patients concentrations as high as 500–1000 μg per ml of urine have been observed (Riff and Jackson, 1971).

BILE: A small amount of gentamicin is also excreted in bile, but the mean biliary concentration is usually only 30–40 per cent of the mean serum level. Gentamicin is not detected in gall bladder bile in the presence of cystic duct obstruction (Pitt *et al.*, 1973; Mendelson *et al.*, 1973).

Distribution of the Drug in Body

Binding of gentamicin to serum proteins under normal conditions is very low, and estimated values have been in the range 0–25 per cent (Black et al., 1964; Gordon et al., 1972). Serum protein binding of gentamicin and other aminoglycoside antibiotics increases progressively with decreasing concentrations of the divalent cations, calcium and magnesium. In the absence of divalent cations the drug is approximately 70 per cent protein bound. Therefore under normal circumstances the binding of the aminoglycosides to serum proteins is not pharmacologically important, but significant binding may occur in certain pathological conditions (Ramirez-Ronda et al., 1975).

Very low gentamicin concentrations are attained in the CSF of patients with uninflamed meninges (Riff and Jackson, 1971). Levels in pleural, pericardial and ascitic fluids are usually about half of those found in the serum at the time (Cox, 1970; Riff and Jackson, 1971). The drug concentration is usually higher and may reach 90 per cent of the serum level in ascitic fluid of patients with bacterial peritonitis (Gerding et al., 1977). Gentamicin penetrates well into the synovial fluid, even in the absence of bacterial infection, where concentrations consistently exceed 50 per cent of simultaneous serum levels (Dee and Kozin, 1977).

Some gentamicin apparently enters or is absorbed onto red cells, and this is released when the serum level falls (Riff and Jackson, 1971). The drug is detectable in bronchial secretions, but concentrations are only 25–50 per cent of simultaneous serum levels (Pennington and Reynolds, 1973; Wong et al., 1975). Gentamicin depends upon a concentration gradient for passive diffusion into bronchial secretions, and it is cleared from these secretions rather rapidly (Pennington and Reynolds, 1975). It crosses the placenta, where the mean peak level in cord serum is 30–40 per cent of that in maternal serum (Yoshioka et al., 1972).

Incomplete recovery of gentamicin from urine during the first few days of therapy (page 336), and the persistence of measurable concentrations in urine of patients with normal renal function for ten days or more after a final dose, suggest that gentamicin persists in tissues for long periods (Schentag et al., 1977; Schentag and Jusko, 1977; Kahlmeter et al., 1978). Following the final dose of a course of gentamicin, the serum concentration declines in a biphasic fashion; there is an initial rapid decline phase which is similar to that which follows maintenance doses, and then a slow phase, during which low serum concentrations ($< 0.5\,\mu$g per ml) are measurable for ten or more days. The gentamicin half-life of the second phase, when tissue bound drug is excreted, averages 112 h (Schentag et al., 1977). Trough gentamicin serum levels (page 331) may reflect tissue levels, which in turn may be related to nephrotoxicity (page 339).

Studies in humans (Edwards et al., 1976; Schentag and Jusko, 1977) and in experimental animals (Kornguth and Kunin, 1977), indicate that the kidneys are the major site of gentamicin deposition, accounting for 40 per cent of the total antibiotic in the body. The main site of this deposition is the renal cortex, which contains approximately 85 per cent of the total renal drug (Luft and Kleit, 1974). The same is true for other aminoglycosides such as kanamycin (page 315), tobramycin (page 365), amikacin (page 385) and netilmicin (page

400), but the less nephrotoxic streptomycin (page 301) is distributed evenly throughout the kidney. In renal cortical tissue gentamicin levels are often at least 100 times higher than those in the serum (Schentag and Jusko, 1977). Gentamicin is transported into renal cortical cells by an active process, aerobic phosphorylation (Hsu *et al.*, 1977).

Animal experiments show that gentamicin is also distributed in heart, liver and muscle tissue (Black *et al.*, 1964), and concentrations in these tissues and the lymph are about the same as in serum (Chisholm *et al.*, 1968). The drug also penetrates into ascitic fluid of experimental animals, but concentrations are lower than in the serum for the first three to four hours after administration (Gerding *et al.*, 1976a and b). In animals with experimental peritonitis, peritoneal fluid levels are higher, and one hour after administration may exceed serum gentamicin levels (MacGregor, 1977). Interstitial fluid levels have also been studied in animals; the level is lower than that attained in serum, but the drug persists for a longer period of time in this fluid. After usual gentamicin doses interstitial fluid levels are consistently above the MIC's of susceptible organisms (Carbon *et al.*, 1978). With repeated doses gentamicin does not accumulate in tissue fluid (Chisholm *et al.*, 1973; Tan and Salstrom, 1977). Tissue fluid levels are higher during the first two hours when gentamicin is administered by a 2·5 min intravenous injection than by a 30 min infusion. Beyond two hours, levels are the same for both of these methods of administration (Kozak *et al.*, 1977).

Mode of Action

Gentamicin inhibits bacterial growth by inhibiting protein synthesis, and the mechanism of its action appears to be similar to that of streptomycin (page 298). The drug is bactericidal by *in vitro* tests similar to other aminoglycosides (Hahn and Sarre, 1969).

Toxicity

1. *Ototoxicity*. This is an important side-effect of gentamicin, but in the absence of renal insufficiency it only occurs if high doses are used. Animal experiments show that ototoxicity is due to degeneration of vestibular, and to some extent cochlear hair cells (Wërsall *et al.*, 1969). In large scale surveys the frequency of this complication is about 2 per cent (Jackson and Arcieri, 1971). Labyrinthine damage, rather than deafness, usually occurs and this results in symptoms varying from an acute Ménière's syndrome to slight vertigo or tinnitus. The damage is usually permanent and affected patients remain insecure on ambulation, particularly in the dark, but they can usually compensate for this disability (Jao and Jackson, 1964). Ototoxicity is related to high serum levels, and in affected patients these have ranged from 8·0 to 15·6 μg per ml (Jao and Jackson, 1964). Ototoxicity can be avoided in the majority of patients with normal kidney function if peak serum levels are maintained below 10–12 μg per ml, provided treatment is not prolonged (Wersäll *et al.*, 1969). Delayed ototoxicity occuring 10–14 days after stopping gentamicin has been observed, but is exceedingly rare except in patients with markedly impaired renal function (Hewitt, 1974).

By contrast to kanamycin (page 316), deafness due to gentamicin has been uncommon. In one survey of 1327 patients treated with gentamicin, 31 (2·3 per cent) developed ototoxicity (Arcieri et al., 1970). Twenty-seven had vestibular impairment, eight of whom also had high tone hearing loss, and the remaining four had high tone hearing loss alone. Total deafness due to gentamicin was not observed in this survey, but it has been reported occasionally Wersäll et al., 1969; A Co-operative Study, 1973). Deafness may be more likely to occur if gentamicin is administered concurrently with intravenous ethacrynic acid (Meriwether et al., 1971). As deafness is a more serious toxic effect than labyrinthine damage, kanamycin would appear to be more ototoxic than gentamicin. However, kanamycin is easier to use safely, because there is a greater margin between its therapeutically active and toxic serum levels (page 317).

Similar to neomycin (page 410), gentamicin applied topically to the ear as ear drops can cause severe inner ear deafness, especially if a perforation of the ear drum is present. For this reason the use of gentamicin ear drops is not advocated (Jones, 1978).

2. *Nephrotoxicity*. Gentamicin is selectively concentrated in renal cortical cells (page 337), and it can cause functional and structural damage to the proximal tubules. With moderate doses there is cloudy swelling of tubules, but at higher doses acute tubular necrosis results (Appel and Neu, 1977; Bennett et al., 1977). Electron microscopic studies in animals show characteristic vacuolation and lysosomal 'myeloid bodies' in proximal tubules (Appel and Neu, 1977), and similar changes have been observed in human allograft biopsy specimens obtained during gentamicin treatment (Wellwood et al., 1975). Various renal proximal tubular enzymes may be excreted in the urine during gentamicin treatment; this enzymuria appears to be an early manifestation of gentamicin nephrotoxicity, and as it precedes the rise of serum creatinine, it may be of some clinical value in predicting nephron damage before renal function deteriorates (Patel et al., 1975; Wellwood et al., 1975; Beck et al., 1977). There are also reports of hypokalaemia (Young et al., 1973; Mitchell et al., 1977), renal glycosuria (Ginsburg et al., 1976), hypomagnesaemia, hypocalcaemia and alkalosis (Appel and Neu, 1977) induced by gentamicin therapy, but their causative role in nephrotoxicity is not clear.

The most common clinical manifestation is a gradual onset over several days of non-oliguric renal failure with proteinuria and a rising blood urea and serum creatinine; this nephrotoxicity appears dose-related and reversible (Appel and Neu, 1977; Bennett et al., 1977). Some degree of nephrotoxicity has been observed in 5–10 per cent of treated patients (Wilfert et al., 1971; Appel and Neu, 1977). Less commonly an acute oliguric renal failure may occur; the oliguric phase lasts about 10 days, and is followed by a diuretic phase and a slow return to 50 per cent or greater of normal renal function (Kahn and Stein, 1972; Hewitt, 1974). Acute severe renal failure may also occur without oliguria (Gary et al., 1976). Gentamicin nephrotoxicity is likely to be more severe if other aggravating factors such as hypovolaemia are present (Bygbjerg and Møller, 1976). Similar to kanamycin (page 317), renal damage may cause higher serum levels of gentamicin and thus predispose to ototoxicity (page 338).

In man nephrotoxicity is dose related, but there has been controversy as to whether peak or trough serum levels are the best indices for predicting this complication. Although peak drug levels in excess of $12 \mu g$ per ml are associated with an increased frequency of nephrotoxicity (Hewitt, 1974), trough levels appear to be more useful for predicting accumulation of gentamicin, which correlates with early renal impairment. Dahlgren et al. (1975) monitored gentamicin serum levels in 86 patients. Twenty-one had trough levels over $2 \cdot 0 \mu g$ per ml and in 36 per cent of these the serum creatinine rose. Elevated serum creatinine levels were not observed in patients with a trough level less than $2 \cdot 0 \mu g$ per ml, and peak levels of higher than $10 \mu g$ per ml did not correlate with nephrotoxicity.

Several reports have indicated that the risk of gentamicin nephrotoxicity is increased if it is used with cephalothin (page 211) or cephaloridine (page 210). However, data collected by the Boston Collaborative Drug Surveillance Program have not confirmed this role of cephalothin (Fanning et al., 1976) (see also page 211). In animal experiments, cephalosporins such as cephalothin and cephaloridine do not augment, but sometimes protect against gentamicin nephrotoxicity (Harrison et al., 1975; Luft et al., 1976).

Regular monitoring of renal function is advisable for all patients treated by gentamicin (Wilfert et al., 1971). The drug should be used cautiously in patients with pre-existing renal disease and whenever other factors known to impair renal function, such as hypotension or dehydration, are present (Bygbjerg and Møller, 1976).

3. *Hypersensitivity reactions.* Skin rashes due to parenteral gentamicin and skin sensitization due to topical gentamicin are very rare (Cox, 1970). One case of anaphylaxis, presenting within a minute of an intravenous gentamicin injection, has been reported (Hall, 1977).

4. *Neuromuscular blockade.* Gentamicin in common with other aminoglycosides (page 411) can cause this complication. Warner and Sanders (1971) described an adult patient receiving normal doses of gentamicin, who developed respiratory failure two days after an operation. In this patient it appeared that renal impairment and a lowered serum calcium may have been contributory. Another patient with Parkinson's disease reported by Holtzman (1976) developed profound weakness after a short course of gentamicin; this recovered after the drug was stopped but recurred on rechallenge. The symptoms in this patient may have been due to a drug interaction with his anti-Parkinsonian medication. That this side-effect of gentamicin has been uncommon (Arcieri et al., 1970) is presumably due to the later introduction of the drug when the effects of 'overdosages' of the other aminoglycosides (streptomycin, page 301; neomycin, page 411) into the peritoneal cavity were already known.

5. *Kernicterus in infants.* Some reports suggested that gentamicin interferes with the binding of bilirubin to serum albumin (Kapitulnik et al., 1972). This has not been confirmed by subsequent studies, and gentamicin does not predispose to the development of kernicterus in the human neonate (Malaka-Zafiriu et al., 1973; Wennberg and Rusmussen, 1975; Woods et al., 1976).

6. *Other side-effects.* These appear to be rare. A transient leucopenia has been observed occasionally, and one patient has been reported who developed acute agranulocytosis in association with gentamicin therapy (Chang and Reyes, 1975). *In vitro* therapeutic concentrations of gentamicin and other

aminoglycosides inhibit leucocyte migration but do not interfere with phagocytosis (Seklecki *et al.*, 1978). Transient elevations of serum aspartate aminotransferase levels have occurred, but there has been no other evidence of hepatotoxicity (Klein *et al.*, 1964). Two patients have been reported who developed an acute organic brain syndrome, apparently related to gentamicin therapy (Byrd, 1977). Loss of hair, possibly related to gentamicin therapy, has been reported (Yoshioka and Matsuda, 1970).

7. The safety of gentamicin during pregnancy has not been established. The drug crosses the placenta (page 337), but the degree of risk of ototoxicity to the fetus is not known.

Clinical Uses of the Drug

1. *Septicaemia and other severe infections due to aerobic Gram-negative bacilli.* Gentamicin is a useful drug for treatment of these infections, and prior to the development of the newer aminoglycosides such as tobramycin (page 359) and amikacin (page 377), it was often the only antibiotic available to which organisms causing hospital acquired infections were still sensitive. Early studies indicated that gentamicin either alone or sometimes combined with one of the cephalosporins was quite effective for the treatment of Gram-negative septicaemias. The results of treatment were about the same as those obtained with a combination of kanamycin with polymyxin B or colistin (Martin *et al.*, 1969; Cox and Harrison, 1971; McHenry *et al.*, 1971). Since then gentamicin has been widely acknowledged as the drug of first choice for treating life-threatening sepsis caused by aerobic Gram-negative rods in hospital patients (Noone *et al.*, 1974b; Young *et al.*, 1977).

For initial emergency treatment of an unidentified septicaemia, possibly due to Gram-negative aerobes, gentamicin has some advantages. It is active against most commonly encountered aerobic Gram-negative enteric bacilli, and acquired bacterial resistance, although becoming more frequent in recent years (page 325), is still relatively uncommon. Compared to kanamycin (page 317), gentamicin has the disadvantage of having a very narrow safety margin between therapeutically effective and toxic doses (page 330), and there is a tendency to administer low and ineffective doses to seriously ill patients. For this reason kanamycin is often preferred alone or in combination with other drugs for the initial treatment of such life-threatening infections, especially if the infection is community acquired, or if infection by Ps. aeruginosa or other kanamycin-resistant bacteria appears unlikely. If the organism is suspected or confirmed to be not only kanamycin- but also gentamicin-resistant, one of the newer aminoglycosides, tobramycin (page 368), but more commonly amikacin (page 386), is indicated.

When gentamicin is used for initial emergency chemotherapy before the organism is identified, it is often combined with other drugs. For the treatment of suspected septicaemia in cancer patients with neutropenia, combinations such as penicillin G/gentamicin, cephalothin/gentamicin or carbenicillin/gentamicin are often suitable (Bishop *et al.*, 1977; Young *et al.*, 1977). In one large international prospective trial involving such patients, cephalothin/gentamicin was of comparable efficacy to carbenicillin/gentamicin, but the former combination caused more nephrotoxicity (page 211). It was concluded that a combination of carbenicillin (or ticarcillin) with an aminoglycoside such as gentamicin currently appears to be the best initial empiric therapy of infection in neutropenic patients with cancer (EORTC, 1978).

In septicaemias arising from intra-abdominal or female genital tract sepsis, mixed infection with both aerobic and anaerobic Gram-negative bacteria may be involved, and gentamicin combined with either chloramphenicol (page 443) or clindamycin (Fass, 1977; Bartlett *et al.*, 1977 (page 485) are suitable treatment regimens. Chloramphenicol and gentamicin do not appear to be antagonistic clinically (page 443). There is also no antagonism between gentamicin and clindamycin *in vitro* (Fass *et al.*, 1974; Fass, 1977) or in animal experiments (Ekwo and Peter, 1976). Antagonism between gentamicin and minocycline has also not been detected *in vitro* (Fass *et al.*, 1976), but this combination is less commonly used to treat aerobic and anaerobic infections.

For confirmed severe Ps. aeruginosa infections, the combination of gentamicin and carbenicillin has been used with success (Smith *et al.*, 1969; Rodriguez *et al.*, 1970; Klastersky *et al.*, 1972; Bodey *et al.*, 1976). It is still uncertain whether these two drugs always act synergistically against these infections in patients (page 161). Under certain conditions high carbenicillin concentrations may inactivate gentamicin both *in vitro* and *in vivo* (page 162). In patients with normal renal function this can be avoided if the two antibiotics are not mixed together in intravenous infusion fluids (Noone and Pattison, 1971; Winters *et al.*, 1971). High sustained concentration of carbenicillin, which can occur in patients with renal failure, may cause significant gentamicin inactivation; these patients require an increased dosage of gentamicin to compensate for this inactivation (*see* page 162). By contrast, if gentamicin is administered together with 5-fluorocytosine (page 885), the gentamicin serum level may be increased. This may occur with other aminoglycosides and 5-fluorocytosine and a possible mechanism is competition for renal excretion by the drugs. In this situation gentamicin doses may need to be decreased and serum levels monitored (Noone *et al.*, 1978).

Gentamicin alone, used both topically and parenterally, has produced good results in Pseudomonas septicaemia complicating burns (Stone *et al.*, 1965; Stone, 1969). The drug is also useful for the treatment of acute septic arthritis due to Gram-negative bacilli. This form of arthritis commonly occurs in elderly patients with underlying diseases or in patients receiving immunosuppressive drugs (Goldenberg and Cohen, 1976).

Purulent bronchial infections or pneumonia due to either Ps. aeruginosa, Klebsiella spp. or other Gram-negative rods are hard to treat successfully, because they usually occur in patients with chronic lung disease. Satisfactory results with gentamicin therapy have been reported in a considerable proportion of such patients (Louria *et al.*, 1969; Hodges and Saslaw, 1972; Parry *et al.*, 1977), but other authors have found the drug largely ineffective (Pines *et al.*, 1967). Ps. aeruginosa pneumonia associated with septicaemia is nearly always fatal, despite treatment with gentamicin and other appropriate antibiotics, as it is always associated with serious underlying diseases (Iannini *et al.*, 1974). If combined topical (tracheal instillation) and systemic gentamicin is given to patients with pulmonary infection, serum levels should be monitored and the systemic dose reduced if necessary, because some of the topically administered drug is absorbed (Lake *et al.*, 1975).

2. *Severe Gram-negative sepsis in children*. For neonatal meningitis, ampicillin combined with gentamicin is considered to be the best initial chemotherapy before the organism is identified (page 114). Gentamicin alone, only given parenterally or combined with intrathecal therapy, is continued if the causative organism is Esch. coli, Klebsiella spp. or another Gram-negative rod (Mathies *et al*., 1971; Riley *et al*., 1971). It was considered that intrathecal therapy may be of value for the treatment of Gram-negative rod meningitis in infants or adults. This was because gentamicin serum levels are relatively low in relation to the MIC's of these organisms, and the drug does not penetrate well into the CSF even when the meninges are inflamed (Rahal, 1972; Rahal *et al*., 1974). Gentamicin administered into the lumbar intrathecal space results in adequate drug concentrations in the lumbar CSF, but not in ventricular CSF, whereas drug administration into the cerebral ventricles produces adequate concentrations in both ventricular and lumbar CSF (page 335). There is also doubt whether any clinical benefit accrues from intrathecal gentamicin (page 334). Parenteral treatment alone is now recommended for most cases of meningitis caused by Gram-negative rods, but special problem patients may require additional intraventricular therapy (page 335). Combined intramuscular and intrathecal (or intraventricular) gentamicin has been used successfully to treat Esch. coli, Klebsiella and Pseudomonas meningitis and ventriculitis associated with meningomyelocoeles (Newman and Holt, 1967; 1971; van der Waarde and van der Wiel-Korstanje, 1972).

Gentamicin has been effective for the treatment of infants and children with other severe Gram-negative rod infections such as septicaemia, pyelonephritis, pneumonia, septic arthritis and osteomyelitis (Nunnery and Riley, 1969; Klein *et al*., 1971; Pittard *et al*., 1976). Gentamicin (combined with one of the penicillins) is valuable as initial therapy for newborns with life-threatening bacterial infections (Klein, 1969).

3. *Urinary tract infections*. Gentamicin is effective against most organisms causing urinary tract infections, with the notable exception of Strep. faecalis (Cox, 1969). The drug is not indicated for the majority of urinary infections which usually respond to the safer oral drugs. It is valuable for treatment of infections due to Ps. aeruginosa, Klebsiella spp. and other Gram-negative bacilli resistant to commonly used drugs, especially if such infections occur in an abnormal urinary tract (Sweedler *et al*., 1964; Chisholm, 1974). Gentamicin is more effective for urinary tract infections, if the urine is made alkaline (Lindberg *et al*., 1967). It is about a hundred times more active against most strains of Gram-negative bacilli, when tested *in vitro* at a pH of 8·5 than at a pH of 5·0 (Sabath *et al*., 1970). A concentrated urine has an inhibitory effect on the antibacterial activity of gentamicin, the degree of which depends on the total urine osmolality and also on the presence of individual solutes (Minuth *et al*., 1976). Somewhat smaller doses of gentamicin are often recommended for the treatment of uncomplicated urinary tract infections to lessen the risk of toxicity. Under these circumstances alkalinization and dilution of the urine may be important to ensure that optimal conditions for antibacterial activity of gentamicin are present in the urine (Minuth *et al*., 1976). Urine alkalinization can be conveniently achieved by the concomitant administration of bicarbonate or acetazolamide (Sabath *et al*., 1970). Gentamicin treatment may fail to eradicate urinary tract infections in patients with renal failure, because their

urine may be strongly acid and only relatively low urinary gentamicin concentrations are attained (Minuth *et al.*, 1976).

For uncomplicated lower urinary tract infection, low dosage regimens may be effective; a single daily dose of 160 mg of gentamicin intramuscularly appears convenient for the treatment of selected adult out-patients (Labovitz *et al.*, 1974). However, most patients requiring gentamicin have difficult infections with renal tissue involvement, which are often caused by organisms resistant to many drugs, and these should be treated by gentamicin in full dosage (Chisholm, 1974).

4. *Staphylococcal infections*. Gentamicin, used alone, is quite effective for these infections (Richards *et al.*, 1971). It is a valuable 'reserve drug' used singly or in combination with another antibiotic for infections due to Staph. pyogenes strains resistant to methicillin and other drugs (Hoeprich, 1969). Occasionally in staphylococcal endocarditis, despite sensitivity of the strain to penicillinase-resistant penicillins and cephalosporins, the infection may not respond unless a synergistic drug combination is used. Usually a combination of a penicillinase-resistant penicillin or cephalosporin with an aminoglycoside such as kanamycin (page 318) or gentamicin shows *in vitro* synergy against Staph. pyogenes (Watanakunakorn and Glatzbecker, 1974). Animal experiments also indicate that a penicillin/gentamicin combination is more effective than penicillin alone in treatment of experimental peritonitis and endocarditis caused by penicillin-sensitive strains of Staph. pyogenes (Steigbigel *et al.*, 1975; Sande and Johnson, 1975).

5. *Bacterial endocarditis*. A combination of penicillin G and gentamicin is effective for the treatment of Strep. faecalis endocarditis (Weinstein and Moellering, 1973). This combination exhibits synergism against virtually all strains of Strep. faecalis *in vitro* page 329), and it has now largely replaced the formerly used penicillin/streptomycin regimen (page 302).

Endocarditis due to Gram-negative bacilli usually occurs in patients with serious underlying diseases or in intravenous drug abusers. Gentamicin alone is rarely successful in this disease, as the drug cannot be given in large doses for prolonged periods. Drug combinations have therefore been used. Gentamicin combined with either chloramphenicol or carbenicillin (depending on drug sensitivities) has been successful in some cases of Serratia marcescens endocarditis (Mills and Drew, 1976). A gentamicin/carbenicillin combination followed by gentamicin/colistin was successful in one patient with Ps. aeruginosa endocarditis (Bryan *et al.*, 1975). Studies with experimental Ps. aeruginosa endocarditis in animals suggest that a gentamicin/carbenicillin combination is superior to either drug used alone (Archer and Fekety, 1977).

A regimen of two or three drugs is often used before cardiac valve surgery to prevent prosthetic valve endocarditis. These drugs are usually started two days before and then continued for eight days after surgery. Gentamicin is sometimes included in these regimens together with either cloxacillin (page 79), one of the cephalosporins (page 215) or sodium fusidate (Ward *et al.*, 1977).

6. *Gastro-enteritis*. Orally administered gentamicin was used for gastro-enteritis caused by pathogenic Esch. coli (Valman and Wilmers, 1969) and for shigella and salmonella infections (Nunnery and Riley, 1969). This treatment, similar to oral kanamycin (page 319) and neomycin (page 412), is of no value Campylobacter enteritis also usually responds to symptomatic measures only,

but for more severe cases erythromycin (page 510) has been used with apparent success. For Campylobacter septicaemia, parenteral gentamicin is regarded as the treatment of choice (Leading article, 1978).

7. *Suppression of intestinal flora.* Gentamicin in a dose of 50 mg orally every 4 h for 48 h, has been used for pre-operative bowel sterilization (Houghton, 1968). Its large scale use for this purpose cannot be advocated, as this may encourage emergence of gentamicin-resistant Gram-negative bacilli. Oral gentamicin, in combination with oral vancomycin and nystatin has also been used with some success to reduce intestinal flora and consequently the frequency of serious infections such as septicaemia in granulocytopenic patients with leukaemia or other malignancies (Levi *et al.*, 1973; Hahn *et al.*, 1978) (*see also* pages 651, 925).

8. *Chemoprophylaxis in abdominal surgery.* A single intramuscular injection of 80 mg gentamicin, given just before colonic and rectal surgery, appeared ineffective in prevention of post-operative wound infection, intraperitoneal abscess and faecal fistula formation (Burton *et al.*, 1975). If parenteral gentamicin is combined with either parenteral clindamycin (page 485) or rectal or intravenous metronidazole (page 774), and both antibiotics are started just before surgery and then continued for five days, there is a significant reduction of post-operative infections after large bowel surgery (*see* pages 369, 774).

9. *Biliary tract infections.* Gentamicin in combination with ampicillin (page 118) or one of the cephalosporins (pages 214, 249) is often used to treat acute cholangitis. In seriously ill and particularly elderly patients, either chloramphenicol (page 442) or clindamycin (page 484) may also be needed to cover the possibility of Gram-negative anaerobic bacterial infection. Gentamicin and/or cephaloridine have also been given with some success as single doses just before surgery in an attempt to prevent post-operative sepsis after both elective cholecystectomy and that performed during the first week after an attack of acute cholecystitis (Leading article, 1976b; Cunha *et al.*, 1978).

10. *Skin infections.* Local applications containing 0·1–0·3 per cent gentamicin in a cream have been used successfully for infected bed sores, impetigo and for the nasal staphylococcal carrier state. Gentamicin cream has also been used for treatment of infected burns (Stone *et al.*, 1965) and for chemoprophylaxis in this situation (Lowbury and Jackson, 1968). The use of topical gentamicin should be restricted as far as possible, because it encourages emergence of gentamicin-resistant bacilli (page 329) (Leading article, 1977).

11. *Other infections.* Gentamicin can be given by subconjunctival injection in a dose of 20–40 mg to treat or prevent intra-ocular infections (Mathalone, 1974). The drug also appears to be effective in the treatment of tularaemia (Alford *et al.*, 1972), but streptomycin (page 303) remains the drug of choice for this disease. Gentamicin is effective in gonorrhoea (Felarca *et al.*, 1971). Preliminary evidence indicates that uncomplicated gonorrhoea responds to a single intramuscular injection of 240–280 mg of gentamicin and that this dose is non-toxic to adults with normal renal function (Thuillier *et al.*, 1977; Report, 1978). Gentamicin is not currently recommended for the treatment of gonorrhoea, but it may have to be considered in the future for disease produced by penicillinase-producing gonococci. One case report suggested that gentamicin in high doses may be useful for the acute septicaemic form of

melioidosis (Zimmerman, 1970), although the causative organism (Pseudomonas pseudomallei) is usually resistant to this drug *in vitro* (page 327). Similar to kanamycin (page 320), oral gentamicin in a dose of 2·5 mg per kg body weight every six hours for one week, seems to protect high risk babies from necrotizing enterocolitis (Grylack and Scanlon, 1977).

REFERENCES

A Co-operative Study (1973), 'Drug-induced deafness', *JAMA*, **224**, 515.

Alford, R. H., John, J. T. and Bryant, R. E. (1972), 'Tularemia treated successfully with gentamicin', *Amer. Rev. Resp. Dis.,* **106**, 265.

Annotation (1974), 'Serum gentamicin', *Lancet*, **2**, 1185.

Annotation (1976), 'Intrathecal antibiotics in purulent meningitis', *Lancet*, **2**, 1068.

Annotation (1977), 'The importance of S. marcescens', *Lancet*, **1**, 636.

Appel, G. B. and Neu, H. C. (1977), 'The nephrotoxicity of antimicrobial agents (second of three parts)', *New Engl. J. Med.*, **296**, 722.

Archer, G. and Fekety, F. R., Jr. (1977), 'Experimental endocarditis due to Pseudomonas aeruginosa. II. Therapy with carbenicillin and gentamicin'. *J. Infect. Dis.* **136**, 327.

Arcieri, G. M., Falco, F. G., Smith, H. M. and Hobson, L. B. (1970), 'Clinical research experience with gentamicin: Incidence of adverse reactions', *Med. J. Aust.* (Spec. Suppl.), **1**, 30.

Bach, M. C., Sabath, L. D. and Finland, M. (1973), 'Susceptibility of Nocardia asteroides to 45 antimicrobial agents *in vitro*', *Antimicrob. Ag. Chemother.*, **3**, 1.

Bailey, R. R. and Lynn, K. L. (1974), 'Serum levels of gentamicin after intravenous bolus injection', *Lancet*, **1**, 730.

Baird, I,. M., Slepack, J. M., Kauffman, C. A. and Phair, J. P. (1976), 'Nosocomial infection with gentamicin-carbenicillin-resistant Pseudomonas aeruginosa', *Antimicrob. Ag. Chemother.*, **10**, 626.

Barber, M. and Waterworth, P. M. (1966), 'Activity of gentamicin against Pseudomonas, and hospital staphylococci', *Brit. med. J.*, **1**, 203.

Bartlett, J. G., Miao, P. V. W. and Gorbach, S. L. (1977), 'Empiric treatment with clindamycin and gentamicin of suspected septis due to anaerobic and aerobic bacteria', *J. Infect. Dis.* (Suppl.), **135**, 80.

Barza, M., Brown, R. B., Shen, D., Gibaldi, M. and Weinstein, L. (1975), 'Predictability of blood levels of gentamicin in man', *J. Infect. Dis.,* **132**, 165.

Basker, M. J., Slocombe, B. and Sutherland, R. (1977), 'Aminoglycoside-resistant enterococci', *J. clin. Path.*, **30**, 375.

Beck, P. R., Thomson, R. B. and Chaudhuri, A. K. R. (1977), 'Aminoglycoside antibiotics and renal function: changes in urinary gamma-glutamyltransferase excretion', *J. clin. Path.* **30**, 432.

Bell, S. M. (1976), 'Treatment with gentamicin monitored by serum antibiotic assay', *Med. J. Aust.*, **2**, 481.

Bennett, W. M., Plamp, C. and Porter, G. A. (1977), 'Drug-related syndromes in clinical nephrology', *Ann. Intern. Med.*, **87**, 582.

Bint, A. J. (1976), 'Gentamicin-resistant Staphylococcus aureus', *J. Antimicrob. Chemother.*, **2**, 225.

Bint, A. J., George, R. H., Healing, D. E., Wise, R. and Davies, M. (1977), 'An outbreak of infection caused by a gentamicin-resistant Staphylococcus aureus', *J. clin. Path.*, **30**, 165.

Bishop, J. F., McLennan, R. and Whiteside, M. G. (1977), 'The management of febrile episodes in neutropenic cancer patients', *Med. J. Aust.*, **1**, 473.

Black, J. Calesnick, B., Williams, D. and Weinstein, M. J. (1964), 'Pharmacology of gentamicin, a new broad-spectrum antibiotic', *Antimicrob. Agents Chemother.*—1963, p. 138.

Bodey, G. P., Chang, H.-Y., Rodriguez, V. and Stewart, D. (1975), 'Feasibility of administering aminoglycoside antibiotics by continuous intravenous infusion', *Antimicrob. Ag. Chemother.*, **8**, 328.

Bodey, G. P., Feld, R. and Burgess, M. A. (1976), 'Beta-lactam antibiotics alone or in combination with gentamicin for therapy of Gram-negative bacillary infections in neutropenic patients', *Amer. J. Med. Sci.*, **271**, 179.

Brenciaglia, M. I., Cipriani, P. and Mancini, C. (1975), 'Antimicrobial activity of aminoglycosides against clinical strains of Mycoplasma hominis', *J. Antimicrob. Chemother.*, **1**, 333.

Bryan, L. E., Shahrabadi, M. S. and Van Den Elzen, H. M., (1974), 'Gentamicin resistance in Pseudomonas aeruginosa: R-factor-mediated resistance', *Antimicrob. Ag. Chemother.*, **6**, 191.

Bryan, C. S., Marney, S. R., Jr., Alford, R. H. and Bryant, R. E. (1975), 'Gram-negative bacillary endocarditis. Interpretation of the serum bactericidal test', *Amer. J. Med.*, **58**, 209.

Burton, R. C., Hughes, E. S. R. and Cuthbertson, A. M. (1975), 'Prophylactic use of gentamicin in colonic and rectal surgery', *Med. J. Aust.*, **2**, 597.

Butler, T., Bell, W. R., Linh, N. N., Tiep, N. D. and Arnold, K. (1974), 'Yersinia pestis infection in Vietnam. I. Clinical and hematological aspects, *J. Infect. Dis.* (Suppl.), **129**, 78.

Bygbjerg, I. C. and Møller, R. (1976), 'Gentamicin-induced nephropathy', *Scand. J. Infect. Dis.*, **8**, 203.

Byrd, G. J. (1977), 'Acute organic brain syndrome associated with gentamicin therapy', *JAMA*, **238**, 53.

Calderwood, S. A., Wennersten, C., Moellering, R. C., Jr., Kunz, L. J. and Krogstad, D. J. (1977), 'Resistance to six aminoglycosidic aminocyclitol antibiotics among enterococci: prevalence, evolution, and relationship to synergism with penicillin', *Antimicrob. Ag. Chemother.*, **12**, 401.

Carbon, C., Contrepois, A. and Lamotte-Barrillon, S. (1978), 'Comparative distribution of gentamicin, tobramycin, sisomicin, netilmicin, and amikacin in interstitial fluid in rabbits', *Antimicrob. Ag. Chemother.*, **13**, 368.

Casewell, M. W., Dalton, M. T., Webster, M. and Phillips, I. (1977), 'Gentamicin-resistant Klebsiella aerogenes in a urological ward', *Lancet*, **2**, 444.

Chan, R. A., Benner, E. J. and Hoeprich, P. D. (1972), 'Gentamicin therapy in renal failure: A nomogram for dosage', *Ann. Intern. Med.*, **76**, 773.

Chang, J. C. and Reyes, B. (1975), 'Agranulocytosis associated with gentamicin', *JAMA*, **232**, 1154.

Chessum, B., Frengley, J. D., Fleck, D. G. and Mair, N. S. (1971), 'Case of septicaemia due to Yersinia enterocolitica', *Brit. med. J.*, **3**, 466.

Chisholm, G. D., Calnan, J. S., Waterworth, P. M. and Reis, N. D. (1968), 'Distribution of gentamicin in body fluids', *Brit. med. J.*, **2**, 22.

Chisholm, G. D., Waterworth, P. M., Calnan, J. S. and Garrod, L. P. (1973), 'Concentration of antibacterial agents in interstitial tissue fluid', *Brit. med. J.*, **1**, 569.

Chisholm, G. D. (1974), 'The use of gentamicin in urinary tract infections with special reference to drug levels in complicated (urological) infections', *Postgrad. Med. J.* (Suppl. 7), **50**, 23.

Chow, A. W., Patten, V. and Bednorz, D. (1978), 'Susceptibility of Campylobacter fetus to twenty-two antimicrobial agents', *Antimicrob. Ag. Chemother.*, **13**, 416.

Cooksey, R. C., Bannister, E. R. and Farrar, W. E., Jr. (1975), 'Antibiotic resistance patterns of clinical isolates of Serratia marcescens', *Antimicrob. Ag. Chemother.*, **7**, 396.

Cox, C. E. (1969), 'Gentamicin, a new aminoglycoside antibiotic: Clinical and laboratory studies in urinary tract infection', *J. Infect. Dis.*, **119,** 486.

Cox, C. E. (1970), 'Gentamicin', *Med. Clin. North America,* **54,** 1305.

Cox, C. E. and Harrison, L. H. (1971), 'Comparison of gentamicin and polymyxin B-kanamycin in therapy of bacteremia due to Gram-negative bacilli', *J. Infect. Dis.* (Suppl.), **124,** 156.

Cunha, B. A., Pyrtek, L. J. and Quintiliani, R. (1978), 'Prophylactic antibiotics in cholecystectomy', *Lancet,* **1,** 207.

Curtis, J. R., McDonald, S. J. and Weston, J. H. (1967), 'Parenteral administration of gentamicin in renal failure: Patients undergoing intermittent haemodialysis', *Brit. med. J.,* **2,** 537.

Cutler, R. E., Gyselynck, A., Fleet, W. P. and Forrey, A. W. (1972), 'Correlation of serum creatinine concentration and gentamicin half-life', *JAMA*, **29,** 1037.

Dahlgren, J. G., Anderson, E. T. and Hewitt, W. L. (1975), 'Gentamicin blood levels: A guide to nephrotoxicity', *Antimicrob. Ag. Chemother.*, **8,** 58.

Danish, M., Schultz, R. and Jusko, W. J. (1974), 'Pharmacokinetics of gentamicin and kanamycin during hemodialysis', *Antimicrob. Ag. Chemother.*, **6,** 841.

D'Alessandri, R. M., McNeely, D. J. and Kluge, R. M. (1976), 'Antibiotic synergy and antagonism against clinical isolates of Klebsiella species', *Antimicrob. Ag. Chemother.*, **10,** 889.

Darrell, J. H. and Waterworth, P. M. (1967), 'Dosage of gentamicin for Pseudomonas infections', *Brit. med. J.,* **2,** 535.

Davey, R. B. and Pittard, J. (1977), 'Plasmids mediating resistance to gentamicin and other antibiotics in Enterobacteriaceae from four hospitals in Melbourne', *Aust. J. Exper. Biol. Med. Sci.,* **55,** 299.

Dean, H. F., Morgan, A. F., Asche, L. V. and Holloway, B. W. (1977), 'Isolates of Pseudomonas aeruginosa from Australian hospitals having R-plasmid determined antibiotic resistance', *Med. J. Aust.,* **2,** 116.

Dee, T. H. and Kozin, F. (1977), 'Gentamicin and tobramycin penetration into synovial fluid', *Antimicrob. Ag. Chemother.*, **12,** 548.

Deveikis, A., Schauf, V., Mizen, M. and Riff, L. (1977), 'Antimicrobial therapy of experimental Group B streptococcal infection in mice', *Antimicrob. Ag. Chemother.*, **11,** 817.

Dowding, J. E. (1977), 'Mechanisms of gentamicin resistance in Staphylococcus aureus', *Antimicrob. Ag. Chemother.*, **11,** 47.

Drasar, F. A., Farrell, W., Maskell, J. and Williams, J. D. (1976), 'Tobramycin, amikacin, sisomicin, and gentamicin-resistant Gram-negative rods', *Brit. med. J.,* **2,** 1284.

Duncan, I. B. R. (1974), 'Susceptibility of 1500 isolates of Pseudomonas aeruginosa to gentamicin, carbenicillin, colistin and polymyxin B', *Antimicrob. Ag. Chemother.*, **5,** 9.

Echeverria, P., Siber, G. R., Paisley, J., Smith, A. L., Smith, D. H. and Jaffe, N. (1975), 'Age-dependent dose response to gentamicin', *J. Pediatrics,* **87,** 805.

Edwards, C. Q., Smith, C. R., Baughman, K. L., Rogers, J. F. and Lietman, P. S. (1976), 'Concentrations of gentamicin and amikacin in human kidneys', *Antimicrob. Ag. Chemother.*, **9,** 925.

Ekwo, E. and Peter, G. (1976), 'Effect of clindamycin on aminoglycoside activity in a murine model of invasive Escherichia coli infection', *Antimicrob. Ag. Chemother.*, **10,** 893.

EORTC International Antimicrobial Therapy Project Group (1978), 'Three antibiotic regimens in the treatment of infection in febrile granulocytopenic patients with cancer', *J. Infect. Dis.,* **137,** 14.

Falkiner, F. R., Keane, C. T., Dalton, M., Clancy, M. T. and Jacoby, G. A. (1977), 'Cross infection in a surgical ward caused by Pseudomonas aeruginosa with transferable resistance to gentamicin and tobramycin', *J. clin. Path.,* **30,** 731.

Fanning, W. L., Gump, D. and Jick, H. (1976), 'Gentamicin-and cephalothin-associated rises in blood urea nitrogen', *Antimicrob. Ag. Chemother.*, **10**, 80.

Fass, R. J., Rotilie, C. A. and Prior, R. B. (1974), 'Interaction of clindamycin and gentamicin *in vitro*', *Antimicrob. Ag. Chemother.*, **6**, 582.

Fass, R. J., Ruiz, D. E., Prior, R. B. and Perkins, R. L. (1976), '*In vitro* activity of gentamicin and minocycline alone and in combination against bacteria associated with intra-abdominal sepsis', *Antimicrob. Ag. Chemother.*, **10**, 34.

Fass, R. J. (1977), 'Treatment of mixed bacterial infections with clindamycin and gentamicin', *J. Infect. Dis.* (Suppl.), **135**, 74.

Felarca, A. B., Laqui, E. M. and Ibarra, L. M. (1971), 'Gentamicin in gonococcal urethritis in Filipino males: Dosage and response', *J. Infect. Dis.* (Suppl.). **124**, 287.

Forbes, I., Gray, A., Hurse, A. and Pavillard, R. (1977), 'The emergence of gentamicin-resistant Klebsiellae in a large general hospital', *Med. J. Aust.*, **1**, 14.

Franklin, M. (1971), 'Effect of gentamicin on Pseudomonas pseudomallei', *J. Infect. Dis.* (Suppl.), **124**, 30.

Fraser, D. W., Wachsmuth, I. K., Bopp, C., Feeley, J. C. and Tsai, T. F. (1978), 'Antibiotic treatment of guinea-pigs infected with agent of Legionnaires' disease'. *Lancet*, **1**, 175.

Gaman, W., Cates, C., Snelling, C. F. T., Lank, B. and Ronald, A. R. (1976), 'Emergence of gentamicin-and carbenicillin-resistant Pseudomonas aeruginosa in a hospital environment', *Antimicrob. Ag. Chemother.*, **9**, 474.

Gangadharam, P. R. J. and Candler, E. R. (1977), '*In vitro* anti-mycobacterial activity of some new aminoglycoside antibiotics', *Tubercle*, **58**, 35.

Gary, N. E., Buzzeo, L., Salaki, J. and Eisinger, R. P. (1976), 'Gentamicin-associated acute renal failure', *Arch. Intern. Med.,* **136**, 1101.

Gerding, D. N., Kromhout, J. P., Sullivan, J. J. and Hall, W. H. (1976a), 'Antibiotic penetrance of ascitic fluid in dogs', *Antimicrob. Ag. Chemother.*, **10**, 850.

Gerding, D. N., Hall, W. H., Schierl, E. A. and Manion, R. E. (1976b), 'Cephalosporin and aminoglycoside concentrations in peritoneal capsular fluid in rabbits', *Antimicrob. Ag. Chemother.*, **10**, 902.

Gerding, D. N., Hall, W. H. and Schierl, E. A. (1977), 'Antibiotic concentrations in ascitic fluid of patients with ascites and bacterial peritonitis', *Ann. Intern. Med.*, **86**, 708.

Gingell, J. C. and Waterworth, P. M. (1968), 'Dose of gentamicin in patients with normal renal function and renal impairment', *Brit. med. J.*, **2**, 19.

Ginsburg, D. S.,Quintanilla, A. P. and Levin, M. (1976), 'Renal glycosuria due to gentamicin in rabbits', *Infect. Dis.*, **134**, 119.

Glew, R. H., Moellering, R. C., Jr. and Buettner, K. R. (1977), '*In vitro* synergism between carbenicillin and aminoglycosidic aminocyclitols against Acinetobacter calcoaceticus var. anitratus', *Antimicrob. Ag. Chemother.*, **11**, 1036.

Goldenberg, D. L. and Cohen, A. S. (1976), 'Acute infectious arthritis. A review of patients with nongonococcal joint infections (with emphasis on therapy and prognosis), *Amer. J. Med.,* **60**, 369.

Goodman, E. L., Van Gelder, J., Holmes, R., Hull, A. R. and Sanford, J. P. (1975), 'Prospective comparative study of variable dosage and variable frequency regimens for administration of gentamicin', *Antimicrob. Ag. Chemother.*, **8**, 434.

Gordon, R. C., Regamey, C. and Kirby, W. M. M. (1972), 'Serum protein binding of the aminoglycoside antibiotics', *Antimicrob. Ag. Chemother.,* **2**, 214.

Greene, W. H., Moody, M., Schimpff, S., Young, V. M. and Wiernik, P. H. (1973), 'Pseudomonas aeruginosa resistant to carbenicillin and gentamicin'. *Ann. Intern. Med.*, **79**, 684.

Grylack, L. and Scanlon, J. W. (1977), 'Prevention of necrotising enterocolitis with gentamicin', *Lancet*, **2**, 506.

Gurry, J. F. (1974), 'Acute terminal ileitis and Yersinia infection', *Brit. med. J.*, **2**, 264.

Gutschik, E., Jepsen, O. B. and Mortensen, I. (1977), 'Effect of combinations of penicillin and aminoglycosides on Streptococcus faecalis: A comparative study of seven aminoglycoside antibiotics', *J. Infect. Dis.*, **135**, 832.

Hahn, F. E. and Sarre, S. G. (1969), 'Mechanism of action of gentamicin', *J. Infect. Dis.,* **119**, 364.

Hahn, D. M., Schimpff, S. C., Fortner, C. L., Smyth, A. C., Young, V. M. and Wiernik, P. H. (1978), 'Infection in acute leukemia patients receiving oral nonabsorbable antibiotics', *Antimicrob. Ag. Chemother.*, **13**, 958.

Hall, F. J. (1977), 'Anaphylaxis after gentamicin', *Lancet*, **2**, 455.

Halpren, B. A., Axline, S. G., Coplon, N. S. and Brown, D. M. (1976), 'Clearance of gentamicin during hemodialysis: Comparison of four artificial kidneys', *J. Infect. Dis.,* **133**, 627.

Hamilton-Miller, J. M. T., Reynolds, A. V. and Brumfitt, W. (1974), 'Apparent emergence of gentamicin-resistant Providencia stuartii during therapy with gentamicin', *Lancet*, **2**, 527.

Hammerberg, S., Sorger, S. and Marks, M. I., (1977), 'Antimicrobial susceptibilities of Yersinia enterocolitica biotype 4, serotype 0:3', *Antimicrob. Ag. Chemother.*, **11**, 566.

Harrison, W. O., Silverblatt, F. J. and Turck, M. (1975), 'Gentamicin nephrotoxicity: Failure of three cephalosporins to potentiate injury in rats', *Antimicrob. Ag. Chemother.*, **8**, 209.

Hendeles, L. (1971), 'A guide to gentamicin therapy', *Drug Intelligence and Clinical Pharmacy*, **5**, 393.

Hewitt, W. L. (1974), 'Gentamicin: Toxicity in perspective', *Postgrad. Med. J.* (Suppl. 7), **50**, 55.

Hodges, G. R. and Saslaw, S. (1972), 'Gentamicin in the treatment of respiratory tract infections', *The Ohio State Medical Journal*, **68**, 475.

Hoeprich, P. D. (1969), 'Gentamicin versus Staphylococcus aureus', *J. Infect. Dis.,* **119**, 391.

Holder, I. A. (1976), 'Gentamicin-resistant Pseudomonas aeruginosa in a burns unit', *J. Antimicrob. Chemother.*, **2**, 309.

Holmes, R. K. and Sanford, J. P. (1974), 'Enzymatic assay for gentamicin and related aminoglycoside antibiotics', *J. Infect. Dis.,* **129**, 519.

Holmes, R. K., Minshew, B. H., Gould, K. and Sanford, J. P. (1974a), 'Resistance of Pseudomonas aeruginosa to gentamicin and related aminoglycoside antibiotics', *Antimicrob. Ag. Chemother.*, **6**, 253.

Holmes, R. K., Minshew, B. H. and Sanford, J. P. (1974b), 'Resistance of Pseudomonas aeruginosa to aminoglycoside antibiotics', *J. Infect. Dis.,* (Suppl.), **130**, 163.

Holtzman, J. L. (1976), 'Gentamicin and neuromuscular blockade', *Ann. Intern. Med.,* **84**, 55.

Houang, E. T. and Greenwood, D. (1977), 'Aminoglycoside cross-resistance patterns of gentamicin-resistant bacteria', *J. clin. Path.*, **30**, 738.

Houghton, G. W. (1968), 'Gentamicin for preoperative preparation of the large bowel', *Med. J. Aust.*, **1**, 796.

Hsu, C. H., Kurtz, T. W. and Weller, J. M. (1977), '*In vitro* uptake of gentamicin by rat renal cortical tissue', *Antimicrob. Ag. Chemother.*, **12**, 192.

Hull, J. H. and Sarubbi, F. A., Jr. (1976), 'Gentamicin serum concentrations: Pharmacokinetic predictions', *Ann. Intern. Med.,* **85**, 183.

Hyams, P. J., Smithivas, T., Matalon, R., Katz, L., Simberkoff, M. S. and Rahal, J. J. Jr. (1971), 'The use of gentamicin in peritoneal dialysis. II. Microbiologic and clinical results', *J. Infect. Dis.* (Suppl.), **124**, 84.

Hyams, P. J., Simberkoff, M. S. and Rahal, J., Jr. (1974), 'Synergy between cephalosporin and aminoglycoside antibiotics against Providencia and Proteus', *Antimicrob. Ag. Chemother.*, **5**, 571.

Iannini, P. B., Claffey, T. and Quintiliani, R. (1974), 'Bacteremic Pseudomonas pneumonia', *JAMA*, **230**, 558.

Ingham, H. R. and Emslie, J. A. N. (1972), 'Gentamicin dosage', *Brit. med. J.*, **4**, 732.

Jackson, G. G. and Arcieri, G. (1971), 'Ototoxicity of gentamicin in man: A survey and controlled analysis of clinical experience in the United States', *J. Infect. Dis.* (Suppl.), **124**, 130.

Jacoby, G. A. (1974), 'Properties of R plasmids determining gentamicin resistance by acetylation in Pseudomonas aeruginosa', *Antimicrob. Ag. Chemother.*, **6**, 239.

Jao, R. L. and Jackson, G. G. (1964), 'Gentamicin sulphate, new antibiotic against Gram-negative bacilli', *JAMA*, **189**, 817.

Jones, R. J. and Lowbury, E. J. L. (1967), 'Prophylaxis and therapy for Pseudomonas aeruginosa infection with carbenicillin and with gentamicin', *Brit. med. J.*, **3**, 78.

Jones, R. A. K. (1978), 'Ototoxicity of gentamicin ear-drops', *Lancet*, **1**, 1161.

Jordan, G. W. and Hoeprich, P. D. (1977), 'Susceptibility of three groups of Staphylococcus aureus to newer antimicrobial agents', *Antimicrob. Ag. Chemother.*, **11**, 7.

Kabins, S., Nathan, C. and Cohen, S. (1974), 'Gentamicin adenylytransferase activity as a cause of gentamicin resistance in clinical isolates of Pseudomonas aeruginosa', *Antimicrob. Ag. Chemother.*, **6**, 565.

Kahlmeter, G., Jonsson, S. and Kamme, C. (1978), 'Longstanding post-therapeutic gentamicin serum and urine concentrations in patients with unimpaired renal function. A pharmacokinetic evaluation', *J. Antimicrob. Chemother.*, **4**, 143.

Kahn, T. and Stein, R. M. (1972), 'Gentamicin and renal failure', *Lancet*, **1**, 498.

Kaiser, A. B. and McGee, Z. A. (1975), 'Aminoglycoside therapy of Gram-negative bacillary meningitis', *New. Engl. J. Med.*, **293**, 1215.

Kapitulnik, J., Eyal, F. and Simcha, A. J. (1972), 'Gentamicin and bilirubin-binding by plasma', *Lancet*, **2**, 1195.

Kauffman, C. A., Ramundo, N. C., Williams, S. G., Dey, C. R., Phair, J. P. and Watanakunakorn, C. (1978), 'Surveillance of gentamicin-resistant Gram-negative bacilli in a general hospital', *Antimicrob. Ag. Chemother.*, **13**, 918.

Kaye, D., Levison, M. E. and Labovitz, E. D. (1974), 'The unpredictability of serum concentrations of gentamicin: pharmacokinetics of gentamicin in patients with normal and abnormal renal function', *J. Infect. Dis.*, **130**, 150.

Klastersky, J., Cappel, R. and Daneau, D. (1972), 'Clinical significance of *in vitro* synergism between antibiotics in Gram-negative infections', *Antimicrob. Ag. Chemother.*, **2**, 470.

Klastersky, J. and Husson, M. (1977), 'Bactericidal activity of the combinations of gentamicin with clindamycin or chloramphenicol against species of Escherichia coli and Bacteroides fragilis', *Antimicrob. Ag. Chemother.*, **12**, 135.

Klein, J. O., Eickhoff, T. C. and Finland, M. (1964), 'Gentamicin: activity *in vitro* and observations in 26 patients', *Amer. J. Med., Sci.*, **248**, 528; quoted by Curtis *et al.* (1967).

Klein, J. O. (1969), 'Consideration of gentamicin for therapy of neonatal sepsis', *J. Infect. Dis.*, **119**, 457.

Klein, J. O., Herschel, M., Therakan, R. M. and Ingall, D. (1971), 'Gentamicin in serious neonatal infections: absorption, excretion and clinical results in 25 cases', *J. Infect. Dis.* (Suppl.), **124**, 224.

Korfhagen, T. R., Loper, J. C. and Ferrel, J. A. (1975), 'Pseudomonas aeruginosa R factors determining gentamicin plus carbenicillin resistance from patients with urinary tract colonizations', *Antimicrob. Ag. Chemother.*, **7**, 64.

Korfhagen, T. R., Ferrel, J. A., Menefee, C. L. and Loper, J. C. (1976). 'Resistance plasmids of Pseudomonas aeruginosa: change from conjugative to non conjugative in a hospital population', *Antimicrob. Ag. Chemother.*, **9**, 810.

Kornguth, M. L. and Kunin, C. M. (1977), 'Distribution of gentamicin and amikacin in rabbit tissues', *Antimicrob. Ag. Chemother.*, **11**, 974.

Kourtopoulos, H. and Holm, S. E. (1976), 'Intraventricular treatment of Serratia marcescens meningitis with gentamicin', *Scand. J. Infect. Dis.,* **8**, 57,

Kozak, A. J., Gerding, D. N., Peterson, L. R. and Hall, W. H. (1977), 'Gentamicin intravenous infusion rate: Effect on interstitial fluid concentration', *Antimicrob. Ag. Chemother.*, **12**, 606.

Kwitko, A. O., Hamra, L. K. and Atkinson, J. M. (1977), 'Serratia: Opportunistic pathogen of increasing clinical importance', *Med. J. Aust.,* **2**, 119.

Labovitz, E., Levision, M. E. and Kaye, D. (1974), 'Single-dose daily gentamicin therapy in urinary tract infection', *Antimicrob. Ag. Chemother.*, **6**, 465.

Lake, K. B., Van Dyke, J. J. and Rumsfeld, J. A. (1975), 'Combined topical pulmonary and systemic gentamicin: The question of safety', *Chest*, **68**, 62.

Lambert, H. P. (1977), 'Problems with neonatal meningitis', *J. Antimicrob. Chemother.*, **3**, 381.

Laverdiere, M., Peterson, P. K., Verhoef, J., Williams, D. N. and Sabath, L. D. (1978), '*In vitro* activity of cephalsporins against methicillin-resistant, coagulase-negative straphylococci', *J. Infect. Dis.,* **137**, 245.

Leading Article (1976a), 'Chemotherapeutic routes in meningitis', *Brit. med. J.,* **1**, 977.

Leading Article (1976b), 'Treatment of acute cholecystitis', *Lancet*, **1**, 182.

Leading Article (1977), 'Topical antibiotics', *Brit. med. J.,* **1**, 1494.

Leading Article (1978) 'Campylobacter enteritis', *Lancet*, **2**, 135.

Lee, E. L., Robinson, M. J., Thong, M. L., Puthucheary, S. D., Ong, T. H. and Ng, K.K. (1977), 'Intraventricular chemotherapy in neonatal meningitis', *J. Pediatrics*, **91**, 991.

Levi, J. A., Vincent, P. C., Jennis, F., Lind, D. E. and Gunz, F. W. (1973), 'Prophylactic oral antibiotics in the management of acute leukaemia', *Med. J. Aust.,* **1**, 1025.

Lewis, B. R. and Gupta, J. M. (1977), 'Present prognosis in neonatal meningitis', *Med. J. Aust.,* **1**, 695.

Lewis, S. A. and Altemeier, W. A. (1978), 'Emergence of clinical isolates of Staphylococcus aureus resistant to gentamicin and correlation of resistance with bacteriophage type', *J. Infect. Dis.,* **137**, 314.

Lewis, V. J., Thacker, W. L., Shepard, C. C. and McDade, J. E. (1978), '*In vivo* susceptibility of the Legionnaires' disease bacterium to ten antimicrobial agents', *Antimicrob. Ag. Chemother.*, **13**, 419.

Lindberg, A. A., Bucht, H. and Kallings, L. O. (1967), 'Treatment of chronic urinary tract infections with gentamicin', *Proceedings—Gentamicin—First International Symposium, Paris*, p. 75.

Longmore, P., Atkins, R. C., Casley, D. and Johnston, C. I. (1976), 'Radioimmunoassay as an improved method for measurement of serum levels of gentamicin', *Med. J. Aust.,* **1**, 738.

Louria, D. B., Young, L., Armstrong, D. and Smith, J. K. (1969), 'Gentamicin in the treatment of pulmonary infections', *J. Infect Dis.,* **119**, 483.

Lowbury, E. J. L. and Jackson, D. M. (1968), 'Local chemoprophylaxis for burns with gentamicin and other agents', *Lancet*, **1**, 654.

Luft, F. C. and Kleitt, S. A. (1974), 'Renal parenchymal accumulation of aminoglycoside antibiotics in rats', *J. Infect. Dis.,* **130**, 656.

Luft, F. C., Patel, V., Yum, M. N. and Kleit, S. A. (1976), 'Nephrotoxicity of cephalosporin-gentamicin combinations in rats', *Antimicrob. Ag. Chemother.*, **9**, 831.

Mahon, W. A., Ezer, J. and Wilson, T. W. (1973), 'Radioimmunoassay for measurement of gentamicin in blood', *Antimicrob. Ag. Chemother.*, **3**, 585.

Mahon, W. A., Feldman, R. I. and Scherr, G. H. (1977), 'Hemagglutination inhibition assay for gentamicin', *Antimicrob. Ag. Chemother.*, **11**, 359.

Malaka-Zafiriu, K., Tsiouris, I. and Cassimos, C. (1973), 'The effect of gentamicin on liver glucuronyl transferase', *J. Pediatrics*, **82**, 118.

Maliwan, N., Grieble, H. G. and Bird, T. J. (1975), 'Hospital Pseudomonas aeruginosa: Surveillance of resistance to gentamicin and transfer of aminoglycoside R factor', *Antimicrob. Ag. Chemother.*, **8**, 415.

Martin, C. M., Cuomo, A. J., Geraghty, M. J., Zager, J. R. and Mandes, T. C. (1969), 'Gram-negative rod bacteremia', *J. Infect. Dis.*, **119**, 506.

Martin, C. M., Ikari, N. S., Zimmerman, J. and Waitz, J. A. (1971), 'A virulent nosocomial Klebsiella with a transferable R factor for gerˑᵃmicin: Emergence and suppression', *J. Infect. Dis.* (Suppl.), **124**, 24.

Martin, W. J., Gardner, M. and Washington, J. A., II (1972), '*In vitro* antimicrobial susceptibility of anaerobic bacteria isolated from clinical specimens', *Antimicrob. Ag. Chemother.*, **1**, 148.

Mathalone, B. (1974), 'Gentamicin in eye infection', *Postgrad. Med. J.*, (Suppl. 7), **50**, 38.

Mathies, A. W., Jr., Lavetter, A., Leedom, J. M., Ivler, D. and Wehrle, P. F. (1971), 'Gentamicin in the treatment of meningitis', *J. Infect. Dis.* (Suppl.), **124**, 249.

Mawer, G. E., Ahmad, R., Dobbs, S. M., McGough, J. G., Lucas, C. B. and Tooth, J. A. (1974), 'Prescribing aids for gentamicin', *Brit. J. Clin. Pharmacol.*, **1**, 45.

McCracken, G. H., Jr. (1972), 'Clinical pharmacology of gentamicin in infants 2 to 24 months of age', *Amer. J. Dis. Child.*, **124**, 884.

McCracken, G. H., Jr. and Mize, S. G. (1976), 'A controlled study of intrathecal antibiotic therapy in Gram-negative enteric meningitis of infancy', *J. Pediatrics*, **89**, 66.

McCracken, G. H., Jr., Threlkeld, N. and Thomas, M. L. (1977), 'Intravenous administration of kanamycin and gentamicin in newborn infants', *Pediatrics*, **60**, 463.

McCracken, G. H., Jr. and Nelson, J. D. (1977), *Antimicrobial Therapy for Newborns: Practical Application of Pharmacology to Clinical Usage*, Grune and Stratton, New York, San Francisco, London, p. 35.

McDonald, D. R. and Waterworth, P. M. (1974), 'Alleged effect of bile constituents on gentamicin assays', *Antimicrob. Ag. Chemother.*, **5**, 562.

McGhie, D., Hutchison, J. G. P. and Geddes, A. M. (1974), 'Serum gentamicin', *Lancet*, **2**, 1463.

MacGregor, R. R. (1977), 'Comparative penetration of amikacin, gentamicin and penicillin G into exudate fluid in experimental sterile peritonitis', *Antimicrob. Ag. Chemother.*, **11**, 110.

McHenry, M. C., Gavan, T. L., Gifford, R. W., Jr., Geurkink, N. A., Van Ommen, R. A., Town, M. A. and Wagner, J. G. (1971), 'Gentamicin dosages for renal insufficiency', *Ann. Intern. Med.*, **74**, 192.

McHenry, M. C., Gaven, T. L., Van Ommen, R. A. and Hawk, W. A. (1971), 'Therapy with gentamicin for bacteremic infections: results with 53 patients', *J. Infect. Dis.* (Suppl.), **124**, 164.

Mendelson, J., Portnoy, J. and Sigman, H. (1973), 'Pharmacology of gentamicin in the biliary tract of humans', *Antimicrob. Ag. Chemother.*, **4**, 538.

Mendelson, J., Portnoy, J., Dick, V. and Black, M. (1976), 'Safety of the bolus administration of gentamicin', *Antimicrob. Ag. Chemother.*, **9**, 633.

Meriwether, W. F., Mangi, R. J. and Serpick, A. A. (1971), 'Deafness following standard intravenous dose of ethacrynic acid', *JAMA*, **216**, 795.

Meyer, R. D., Lewis, R. P., Halter, J. and White, M. (1976), 'Gentamicin-resistant Pseudomonas aeruginosa and Serratia marcescens in a general hospital', *Lancet*, **1**, 580.

Michel, J., Sacks, T., Stessman, J. and Light, A. (1974), 'Serum-gentamicin levels after intravenous bolus injection', *Lancet*, **2**, 525.

Mills, J. and Drew, D. (1976), 'Serratia marcescens endocarditis: A regional illness associated with intravenous drug abuse', *Ann. Intern. Med.*, **84**, 29.

Minshew, B. H., Pollock, H. M., Schoenknecht, F. D. and Sherris, J. C. (1977), 'Emergence in a burn center of populations of bacteria resistant to gentamicin, tobramycin, and amikacin: Evidence for the need for changes in zone diameter interpretative standards', *Antimicrob. Ag. Chemother.*, **12**, 688.

Minuth, J. N., Musher, D. M. and Thorsteinsson, S. B. (1976), 'Inhibition of the antibacterial activity of gentamicin by urine', *J. Infect. Dis.*, **133**, 14.

Mitchell, C. J., Bullock, S. and Ross, B. D. (1977), 'Renal handling of gentamicin and other antibiotics by the isolated perfused rat kidney: Mechanism of nephrotoxicity', *J. Antimicrob. Chemother.*, **3**, 593.

Moellering, R. C., Jr. and Fischer, E. G. (1972), 'Relationship of intraventricular gentamicin levels to cure of meningitis', *J. Pediatrics*, **81**, 534.

Moellering, R. C., Jr., Medoff, G., Leech, I., Wennersten, C. and Kunz, L. J. (1972), 'Antibiotic synergism against Listeria monocytogenes', *Antimicrob. Ag. Chemother.*, **1**, 30.

Mohan, K., Gordon, R. C., Beaman, T. C., Belding, R. C., Luecke, D., Edmiston, C. and Gerhardt, P. (1977), 'Synergism of penicillin and gentamicin against Listeria monocytogenes in *ex vivo* hemodialysis culture', *J. Infect. Dis.*, **135**, 51.

Moody, M. R., Young, V. M. and Kenton, D. M. (1972), '*In vitro* antibiotic susceptibility of pseudomonads other than Pseudomonas aeruginosa recovered from cancer patients', *Antimicrob. Ag. Chemother.*, **2**, 344.

Nelson, J. D. and McCracken, G. H., Jr. (1972), 'Editorial. The current status of gentamicin for the neonate and young infant', *Amer. J. Dis. Child.*, **124**, 13.

Newman, R. L. and Holt, R. J. (1967), 'Intrathecal gentamicin in treatment of ventriculitis in children', *Brit. med. J.*, **2**, 539.

Newman, R. L. and Holt, R. J. (1971), 'Gentamicin in pediatrics. I. Report on intrathecal gentamicin', *J. Infect. Dis.* (Suppl.), **124**, 254.

Noone, P., Pattison, J. R. and Samson, D. (1971), 'Simple, rapid method for assay of aminoglycoside antibiotics', *Lancet*, **2**, 16.

Noone, P. and Pattison, J. R. (1971), 'Therapeutic implications of interaction of gentamicin and penicillins', *Lancet*, **2**, 575.

Noone, P., Parsons, T. M. C., Pattison, J. R., Slack, R. C. B. Garfield-Davies, D. and Hughes, K. (1974), 'Experience in monitoring gentamicin therapy during treatment of serious Gram-negative sepsis', *Brit. med. J.*, **1**, 477.

Noone, P., Pattison, J. R. and Davies, D. G. (1974b), 'The effective use of gentamicin in life-threatening sepsis', *Postgrad. Med. J.* (Suppl. 7), **50**, 9.

Noone, P., Beale, D. F., Pollock, S. S., Perera, M. R., Amirak, I. D., Fernando, O. N. and Moorhead, J. F. (1978), 'Monitoring aminoglycoside use in patients with severely impaired renal function', *Brit. med. J.*, **2**, 470.

Noriega, E. R., Leibowitz, R. E., Richmond, A. S., Rubinstein, E., Schaefler, S., Simberkoff, M. S. and Rahal, J. J., Jr. (1975) 'Nosocomial infection caused by gentamicin-resistant, streptomycin-sensitive Klebsiella', *J. Infect. Dis.* (Suppl.), **131**, 45.

Nunnery, A. W. and Riley, H. D. Jr. (1969), 'Gentamicin: Clinical and laboratory studies in infants and children', *J. Infect. Dis.*, **119**, 460.

O'Grady, F. (1971), 'Antibiotics in renal failure', *Brit. med. Bull.*, **27**, 142.

O'Grady, F., Brown, W. R. L., Gaya, H., Mackintosh, I. P. (1971), 'Antibiotic levels on continuous intravenous infusion', *Lancet*, **2**, 209.

Okubadejo, O. A. and Allen, J. (1975), 'Combined activity of clindamycin and gentamicin on Bacteroides fragilis and other bacteria', *J. Antimicrob. Chemother.*, **1**, 403.

Olsen, L., Grotte, G. and Nordbring, F. (1977), 'Successful treatment of Pseudomonas aeruginosa-ventriculitis with intraventricular gentamicin in a child with hydrocephalus', *Scand. J. Infect. Dis.*, **9**, 243.

Parry, M. F., Neu, H. C., Merlino, M., Gaerlan, P. F., Ores, C. N. and Denning, C. R.

(1977), 'Treatment of pulmonary infections in patients with cystic fibrosis: a comparative study of ticarcillin and gentamicin', *J. Pediatrics*, **90,** 144.

Patel, V., Luft, F. C., Yum, M. N., Patel, B., Zeman, W. and Kleit, S. A. (1975), 'Enzymuria in gentamicin-induced kidney damage', *Antimicrob. Ag. Chemother.*, **7,** 364.

Pennington, J. E. and Reynolds, H. Y. (1973), 'Concentrations of gentamicin and carbenicillin in bronchial secretions', *J. Infect. Dis.*, **128,** 63.

Pennington, J. E. and Reynolds, H. Y. (1975), 'Pharmacokinetics of gentamicin sulfate in bronchial secretions', *J. Infect. Dis.*, **131,** 158.

Pennington, J. E., Dale, D. C., Reynolds, H. Y. and MacLowry, J. D. (1975), 'Gentamicin sulfate pharmacokinetics: Lower levels of gentamicin in blood during fever, *J. Infect. Dis.*, **132,** 270.

Phillips, I., Eykyn, S., King, B. A., Jenkins, C., Warren, C. A. and Shannon, K. P. (1977), 'The *in vitro* antibacterial activity of nine aminoglycosides and spectinomycin on clinical isolates of common Gram-negative bacteria', *J. Antimicrob. Chemother.*, **3,** 403.

Phillips, I., King, B. A. and Shannon, K. P. (1978), 'The mechanisms of resistance to aminoglycosides in the genus Pseudomonas', *J. Antimicrob. Chemother.*, **4,** 121.

Pickering, L. K., Ericsson, C. D., Ruiz-Palacios, G., Blevins, J. and Miner, M. E. (1978), 'Intraventricular and parenteral gentamicin therapy for ventriculitis in children', *Am. J. Dis. Child.*, **132,** 480.

Pines, A., Raafat, H. and Plucinski, K. (1967), 'Gentamicin and colistin in chronic purulent bronchial infections', *Brit. med. J.*, **2,** 543.

Pitt, H. A., Roberts, R. B. and Johnson, W. D., Jr. (1973), 'Gentamicin levels in the human biliary tract', *J. Infect. Dis.*, **127,** 299.

Pittard, W. B. III, Thullen, J. D. and Fanaroff, A. A. (1976), 'Neonatal septic arthritis', *J. Pediatrics*, **88,** 621.

Pogwizd, S. M. and Lerner, S. A. (1976), '*In vitro* activity of gentamicin, amikacin and netilmicin alone and in combination with carbenicillin against Serratia marcescens', *Antimicrob. Ag. Chemother.*, **10,** 878.

Porthouse, A., Brown, D. F. J., Smith, R. G. and Rogers, T. (1976), 'Gentamicin resistance in Staphylococcus aureus', *Lancet*, **1,** 20.

Poston, S. M., Aubrey, C. and Cameron, J. M. (1976), 'Transferable gentamicin resistance in Enterobacter cloacae', *J. Antimicrob. Chemother.*, **2,** 189.

Rahal, J. J., Jr. (1972), 'Treatment of Gram-negative bacillary meningitis in adults', *Ann. Intern. Med.*, **77,** 295.

Rahal, J. J., Jr., Hyams, P. J., Simberkoff, M. S. and Rubinstein, E. (1974), 'Combined intrathecal and intramuscular gentamicin for Gram-negative meningitis. Pharmacologic study of 21 patients', *New Engl. J. Med.*, **290,** 1394.

Ramirez-Ronda, C. H., Holmes, R. K., and Sanford, J. P. (1975), 'Effects of divalent cations on binding of aminoglycoside antibiotics to human serum proteins and to bacteria', *Antimicrob. Ag. Chemother.*, **7,** 239.

Reeves, D. S. (1977), 'Prescription of aminoglycosides by nomogram', *J. Antimicrob. Chemother.*, **3,** 533.

Rennie, R. P. and Duncan, I. B. R. (1977), 'Emergence of gentamicin-resistant Klebsiella in a general hospital', *Antimicrob. Ag. Chemother.*, **11,** 179.

Report of a Who Scientific Group (1978), 'Neisseria gonorrhoeae and gonococcal infections', *Wld. Hlth. Org. Techn. Rep. Ser.* No. 616, p. 96.

Richards, F., McCall, C. and Cox, C. (1971), 'Gentamicin treatment of staphylococcal infections', *JAMA*, **215,** 1297.

Richmond, A. S., Simberkoff, M. S., Rahal, J. J., Jr. and Schaefler, S. (1975), 'R factors in gentamicin-resistant organisms causing hospital infection', *Lancet*, **2,** 1176.

Riff, L. J. and Jackson, G. G. (1971), 'Pharmacology of gentamicin in man', *J. Infect. Dis.* (Suppl.), **124,** 98.

Riley, H. D. Jr., Rubio, T., Hinz, W., Nunnery, A. W. and Englund, J. (1971), 'Clinical and laboratory evaluation of gentamicin in infants and children', *J. Infect. Dis.* (Suppl.), **124**, 236.

Roberts, N. J., Jr. and Douglas, R. G., Jr. (1978), 'Gentamicin use and Pseudomonas and Serratia resistance: Effect of a surgical prophylaxis regimen', *Antimicrob. Ag. Chemother.*, **13**, 214.

Rodriguez, V., Whitecar, J. P. Jr. and Bodey, G. P. (1970), 'Therapy of infections with the combination of carbenicillin and gentamicin', *Antimicrob. Agents Chemother.*—1969, p. 386.

Roe, E. and Lowbury, E. J. L. (1972), 'Changes in antibiotic sensitivity patterns of Gram-negative bacilli in burns', *J. clin. Path.*, **25**, 176.

Ruhen, R. W. and Darrell, J. H. (1973), 'Antibiotic synergism against group D Streptococci in the treatment of endocarditis', *Med. J. Aust.*, **2**, 114.

Sabath, L. D. (1969), 'Current concepts: Drug resistance of bacteria', *New Engl. J. Med.*, **280**, 91.

Sabath, L. D., Casey, J. I., Ruch, P. A., Stumpf, L. L. and Finland, M. (1971), 'Rapid microassay for circulating nephrotoxic antibiotics', *Antimicrob. Agents Chemother.*—1970, p. 83.

Sabath, L. D., Gerstein, D. A., Leaf, C. D. and Finland, M. (1970), 'Increasing the usefulness of antibiotics: Treatment of infections caused by Gram-negative bacilli', *Clin. Pharm. Ther.*, **11**, 161.

Sabath, L. D., and Toftegaard, I. (1974), 'Rapid microassay for clindamycin and gentamicin when present together and the effect of pH and of each on the antibacterial activity of the other', *Antimicrob. Ag. Chemother.*, **6**, 54.

Sande, M. A. and Irvin, R. G. (1974), 'Penicillin-aminoglycoside synergy in experimental Streptococcus viridans endocarditis', *J. Infect. Dis.*, **129**, 572.

Sande, M. A. and Johnson, M. L. (1975), 'Antimicrobial therapy of experimental endocarditis caused by Staphylococcus aureus', *J. Infect. Dis.*, **131**, 367.

Schaberg, D. R., Alford, R. H., Anderson, R., Farmer, J. J. III, Melly, M. A. and Schaffner, W. (1976), 'An outbreak of nosocomial infection due to multiply resistant Serratia marcescens: Evidence of interhospital spread', *J. Infect. Dis.*, **134**, 181.

Schauf, V., Deveikis, A., Riff, L. and Serota, A. (1976), 'Antibiotic-killing kinetics of Group B streptococci', *J. Pediatrics*, **89**, 194.

Schentag, J. J. and Jusko, W. J. (1977), 'Gentamicin persistence in the body', *Lancet*, **1**, 486.

Schentag, J. J., Jusko, W. J., Plaut, M. E., Cumbo, T. J., Vance, J. W. and Abrutyn, E. (1977), 'Tissue persistence of gentamicin in man', *JAMA*, **238**, 327.

Scott, D. F., Wood, D. O., Brownell, G. H., Carter, M. J. and Best, G. K. (1978), 'Aminoglycoside modification by gentamicin-resistant isolates of Staphylococcus aureus', *Antimicrob. Ag. Chemother.*, **13**, 641.

Seal, D. V. and Strangeways, J. E. M. (1976), 'Gentamicin-resistant Pseudomonas aeruginosa', *Lancet*, **1**, 747.

Seklecki, M. M., Quintiliani, R. and Maderazo, E. G. (1978), 'Aminoglycoside antibiotics moderately impair granulocyte function', *Antimicrob. Ag. Chemother.*, **13**, 552.

Shafi, M. S. and Datta, N. (1975), 'Infection caused by Proteus mirabilis strains with transferable gentamicin-resistance factors', *Lancet*, **1**, 1355.

Shannon, K. P., Phillips, I. and King, B. A. (1978), 'Aminoglycoside resistance among Enterobacteriaceae and Acinetobacter species', *J. Antimicrob. Chemother.*, **4**, 131.

Shanson, D. C., Kensit, J. G. and Duke, R. (1976), 'Outbreak of hospital infection with a strain of Staphylococcus aureus resistant to gentamicin and methicillin', *Lancet*, **2**, 1347.

Shulman, J. A., Terry, P. M. and Hough, C. E. (1971), 'Colonization with gentamicin-resistant Pseudomonas aeruginosa, pyocine type 5, in a burn unit', *J. Infect. Dis.*

(Suppl.), **124**, 18.

Siber, G. R., Echeverria, P., Smith, A. L., Paisley, J. W. and Smith, D. H. (1975), 'Pharmacokinetics of gentamicin in children and adults', *J. Infect. Dis.*, **132**, 637.

Smilack, J. and McCloskey, R. V. (1972), 'Intrathecal gentamicin', *Ann. Intern. Med.*, **77**, 1002.

Smith, C. B., Dans, P. E., Wilfert, J. N. and Finland, M. (1969), 'Use of gentamicin in combinations with other antibiotics', *J. Infect. Dis.*, **119**, 370.

Smith, D. H., Van Otto, B. and Smith, A. L. (1972), 'A rapid chemical assay for gentamicin', *New Engl. J. Med.*, **286**, 583.

Smithivas, T., Hyams, P. J., Matalon, R., Simberkoff, M. S. and Rahal, J. J. Jr. (1971), 'The use of gentamicin in peritoneal dialysis. I. Pharmacologic results', *J. Infect. Dis.* (Suppl.), **124**, 77.

Speller, D. C. E., Raghunath, D., Stephens, N., Viant, A. C., Reeves, D. S., Wilkinson, P. J., Broughall, J. M., and Holt, H. A. (1976), 'Epidemic infection by a gentamicin-resistant Staphylococcus aureus in three hospitals', *Lancet*, **1**, 464.

Steigbigei, R. T., Greenman, R. L. and Remington, J. S. (1975), 'Antibiotic combinations in the treatment of experimental Staphylococcus aureus infection', *J. Infect. Dis.*, **131**, 245.

Stone, H. H., Martin, J. D. and Kolb, L. (1965), 'Experiences in the use of gentamicin sulfate ointment', *Antimicrob. Agents Chemother.*—1964, p. 156.

Stone, H. H. (1969), 'The diagnosis and treatment of Pseudomonas sepsis in major burns', *J. Infect. Dis.*, **119**, 504.

Stratford, B. C., Dixson, S. and Cobcroft, A. J. (1974), 'Serum levels of gentamicin and tobramycin after slow intravenous bolus injection', *Lancet*, **1**, 378.

Sweedler, D. R., Gravenkemper, C. F., Bulger, R. J., Brodie, J. L. and Kirby, W. M. M. (1964), 'Laboratory and clinical studies of gentamicin', *Antimicrob. Agents Chemother.*—1963, p. 157.

Tan, J. S. and Salstrom, S. J. (1977), 'Levels of carbenicillin, ticarcillin, cephalothin, cefazolin, cefamandole, gentamicin, tobramycin, and amikacin in human serum and interstitial fluid', *Antimicrob. Ag. Chemother.*, **11**, 698.

Thornsberry, C., Baker, C. N. and Kirven, L. A. (1978), '*In vitro* activity of antimicrobial agents on Legionnaires' disease bacterium', *Antimicrob. Ag. Chemother.*, **13**, 78.

Thuillier, C., Fillastre, J. P. and Godin, M. (1977), 'Pharmacokinetic data on single dose of 280 mg gentamicin i.m.', *J. Antimicrob. Chemother.*, **3**, 527.

Uwaydah, M. and Taqi-Eddin, A. (1976), 'Susceptibility of non-formentative Gram-negative bacilli to tobramycin', *J. Infect. Dis.*, (Suppl.), **134**, 28.

Valman, H. B. and Wilmers, M. (1969), 'Use of antibiotics in acute gastroenteritis among infants in hospital', *Lancet*, **1**, 1122.

Van der Waarde, K. and van der Wiel-Korstanje, M. (1972), 'Treatment of ventriculitis with gentamicin in an infant born with spina bifida', *Scand. J. Infect. Dis.*, **4**, 165.

Waitz, J. A. and Weinstein, M. J. (1969), 'Recent microbiological studies with gentamicin', *J. Infect. Dis.*, **119**, 355.

Ward, C., Jephcott, A. E. and Hardisty, C. A. (1977), 'Perioperative antibiotic prophylaxis and prosthetic valve endocarditis', *Postgrad. Med. J.*, **53**, 353.

Warner, W. A. and Sanders, E. (1971), 'Neuromuscular blockade associated with gentamicin therapy', *JAMA*, **215**, 1153.

Watanakunakorn, C. and Bakie, C. (1973), 'Synergism of vancomycin-gentamicin and vancomycin-streptomycin against enterococci', *Antimicrob. Ag. Chemother.*, **4**, 120.

Watanakunakorn, C. and Glotzbecker, C. (1974), 'Enhancement of the effects of anti-staphylococcal antibiotics by aminoglycosides', *Antimicrob. Ag. Chemother.*, **6**, 802.

Waterworth, P. M. (1977), 'Which gentamicin assay method is the most practicable?', *J. Antimicrob. Chemother.*, **3**, 1.

Weinstein, M. J., Luedemann, G. M., Oden, E. M. and Wagman, G. H. (1964), 'Gentamicin, A new broad-spectrum antibiotic complex', *Antimicrob. Agents Chemother.*—1963, p. 1.

Weinstein, M. J. and Moellering, R. C., Jr. (1973), 'Penicillin and gentamicin therapy for enterococcal infections', *JAMA*, **223**, 1030.

Wellwood, J. M., Simpson, P. M., Tighe, J. R. and Thompson, A. E. (1975), 'Evidence of gentamicin nephrotoxicity in patients with renal allografts', *Brit. med. J.*, **3**, 278.

Wennberg, R. P. and Rasmussen, L. F. (1975), 'Effects of gentamicin on albumin binding of bilirubin', *J. Pediatrics,* **86**, 611.

Wersäll, J., Lundquist, P. G. and Björkroth, B. (1969), 'Ototoxicity of gentamicin', *J. Infect. Dis.,* **119**, 410.

Wilfert, J. N., Burke, J. P., Bloomer, H. A. and Smith, C. B. (1971), 'Renal insufficiency associated with gentamicin therapy', *J. Infect. Dis.* (Suppl.), **124**, 148.

Wilkinson, P. M., Gorst, D. W., Tooth, J. A. and Delamore, I. W. (1977), 'The management of fever in blood dyscrasias: Results of a prospective controlled trial of a prescribing aid for gentamicin', *J. Antimicrob. Chemother.*, **3**, 297.

Winters, R. E., Chow, A. W., Hecht, R. H. and Hewitt, W. L. (1971), 'Combined use of gentamicin and carbenicillin', *Ann. Intern. med.*, **75**, 925.

Wong, G. A., Peirce, T. H., Goldstein, E. and Hoeprich, P. D. (1975), 'Penetration of antimicrobial agents into bronchial secretions', *Amer. J. Med.,* **59**, 219.

Woods, J. T., Bryan, L. E., Chan, G. and Schiff, D. (1976), 'Gentamicin and albumin-bilirubin binding', *J. Pediatrics*, **89**, 483.

Wood, D. O., Carter, M. J. and Best, G. K. (1977), 'Plasmid-mediated resistance to gentamicin in Staphylococcus aureus', *Antimicrob. Ag. Chemother.*, **12**, 513.

Wyatt, T. D., Ferguson, W. P., Wilson, T. S. and McCormick, E. (1977), 'Gentamicin-resistant Staphylococcus aureus associated with the use of topical gentamicin', *J. Antimicrob. Chemother.*, **3**, 213.

Yoshioka, H. and Matsuda, I. (1970), 'Loss of hair related to gentamicin treatment', *JAMA*, **211**, 123.

Yoshioka, H., Monma, T. and Matsuda, S. (1972), 'Placental transfer of gentamicin', *J. Pediatrics*, **80**, 121.

Young, G. P., Sullivan, J. and Hurley, T. (1973), 'Hypokalaemia due to gentamicin/cephalexin in leukaemia', *Lancet,* **2**, 855.

Young, L. S., Martin, W. J., Meyer, R. D., Weinstein, R. J. and Anderson, E. T. (1977), 'Gram-negative rod bacteremia: microbiologic, immunologic, and therapeutic considerations', *Ann. Intern. Med.,* **86**, 456.

Zimmerman, J. E. (1970), 'Acute septicemic melioidosis. Successful treatment with gentamicin', *JAMA,* **213**, 2266.

Tobramycin

Description

Tobramycin, previously known as nebramycin factor 6, is an aminoglycoside aminocyclitol antibiotic (page 294), which is one of several compounds in an antibiotic complex (nebramycin), produced by Streptomyces tenebrarius (Preston and Wick, 1971). It is a very similar drug to gentamicin (page 325), but its advantages include a greater intrinsic activity against Pseudomonas aeruginosa, activity against a variable proportion of gentamicin-resistant Ps. aeruginosa strains and possibly also lesser toxicity. Tobramycin sulphate is marketed with the trade name of 'Nebcin' (Lilly).

Sensitive Organisms

The antibacterial spectrum of tobramycin is similar to that of gentamicin (page 325).

1. *Gram-negative bacteria.* Tobramycin is active against all the Enterobacteriaceae such as Esch. coli, the Enterobacter, Klebsiella, Proteus, Salmonella, Shigella, Providencia, Serratia, Citrobacter, Hafnia, Edwardsiella, Arizona and Yersinia spp. (Waterworth, 1972; Dienstag and Neu, 1972; Levison *et al.*, 1972; Karney *et al.*, 1973; Neu, 1976; Moellering, 1977; Hammerberg *et al.*, 1977). Against some of these bacteria such as Esch. coli, tobramycin is usually about two-fold less active than gentamicin, and it is at least four-fold less active than gentamicin against Serratia spp. (Waterworth, 1972; Reynolds *et al.*, 1974; Neu, 1976). With the Enterobacteriaceae cross-resistance between tobramycin and gentamicin is almost complete (Neu, 1976; Meyer *et al.*, 1976; Houang and McKay-Ferguson, 1976; Moellering, 1977; Seligman, 1978). Only occasional gentamicin-resistant isolates of this group such as the Klebsiella and Serratia spp. may be tobramycin-sensitive (Drasar *et al.*, 1976; Verbist *et al.*, 1978). Resistance of Enterobacteriaceae to tobramycin and other aminoglycoside antibiotics is R plasmid-mediated (Elwell *et al.*, 1978) (*see also* page 326). Resistant strains contain plasmid-mediated enzymes, which inactivate these drugs by acetylation, adenylylation and phosphorylation. Nine such bacterial enzymes have been characterized (Minshew *et al.*, 1974). Gentamicin and sisomicin (page 395) are susceptible to six of these enzymes and tobramycin to five, but amikacin is only inactivated by one of them (*see* page 378). R plasmid-mediated enzymatic inactivation of tobramycin and other aminoglycosides is probably the most common mechanism for their resistance, but genetic mutation resulting in alterations in ribosomal proteins can also occur (Minshew *et al.*, 1974).

An important feature of tobramycin is that Pseudomonas aeruginosa is quite sensitive, against which it is about two to four times more active than gentamicin (Waterworth, 1972; Meyers and Hirschman, 1972; Bodey and Stewart, 1972; Wretlind et al., 1974; Reynolds et al., 1974; Perkins et al., 1976; McAllister and Tait, 1976).

In early studies, some reports indicated that gentamicin-resistant Ps. aeruginosa strains (page 326) are usually susceptible to tobramycin (Black and Griffith, 1971; Del Bene and Farrar, 1972; Lockwood and Lawson, 1973), whilst in others these strains were found to be always tobramycin-resistant (Brusch et al., 1972). It is now known that cross-resistance with Ps. aeruginosa between these two drugs is not complete, so that gentamicin-resistant Ps. aeruginosa strains may or may not be tobramycin-resistant. In general strains with only low level gentamicin resistance (MIC 16–32 μg per ml) are still susceptible to tobramycin concentrations which are attainable in vivo (4–8 μg per ml). Ps. aeruginosa strains with a high degree of gentamicin resistance (MIC $\geqslant$ 128 μg per ml) are also usually, but not invariably, highly tobramycin-resistant (Kluge et al., 1974; Meyer et al., 1976; Houang and McKay-Ferguson, 1976; Moellering, 1977). Tobramycin-resistant strains of Ps. aeruginosa are usually highly gentamicin-resistant, but a proportion of these are sensitive to amikacin (page 378) (Kluge et al., 1974). As with the Enterobacteriaceae (page 359), resistance of Ps. aeruginosa to tobramycin is often due to R plasmid-mediated enzymes which inactivate the drug (Neu, 1976).

A tobramycin/carbenicillin (page 150) combination shows in vitro synergism against many isolates of Ps. aeruginosa, but the degree of susceptibility to tobramycin alone cannot be used to predict a synergistic effect (Klastersky et al., 1974b; Anderson et al., 1975; Marks et al., 1976). Similarly a tobramycin/ticarcillin (page 171) combination is synergistic in vitro against many strains of this organism (Comber et al., 1977).

Other Pseudomonas spp. such as Ps. stutzeri, Ps. maltophilia and Ps. cepacia may sometimes be tobramycin-sensitive, but the majority of strains are resistant (Uwaydah and Taqi-Eddin, 1976; Neu, 1976).

Among other Gram-negative bacteria, the Neisseria spp. (meningococci and gonococci), similar to gentamicin (page 327), are only moderately sensitive to tobramycin. H. influenzae is also only moderately sensitive (Neu, 1976). Acinetobacter calcoaceticus var. anitratus (Herellea vaginicola) is usually tobramycin-sensitive, but moderately or highly resistant strains occur. As with kanamycin (page 309) and gentamicin (page 328), tobramycin plus carbenicillin (page 151) often exhibits in vitro synergism against this organism, provided that the MIC of tobramycin for the strain is less than 31 μg per ml (Glew et al., 1977). Acinetobacter calcoaceticus var. lwoffi (Mima polymorpha) is also usually tobramycin-sensitive, but the Alcaligenes spp. are more commonly resistant (Uwaydah and Taqi-Eddin, 1976). The Flavobacterium spp. is always resistant to aminoglycosides including tobramycin (Drasar et al., 1976). The Legionnaires' disease bacterium is sensitive to tobramycin in vitro (Thornsberry et al., 1978).

Tobramycin, like gentamicin (page 328), is inactive against Bacteroides fragilis and most other anaerobic Gram-negative bacteria (McAllister, 1976; Moellering, 1977).

2. *Gram-positive bacteria.* Staph. pyogenes, including penicillin G-resistant

and methicillin-resistant strains, is highly tobramycin-sensitive (Neu, 1976; Jordan and Hoeprich, 1977). Gentamicin-resistant Staph. pyogenes strains (page 328) are usually also tobramycin-resistant ((Vogel et al., 1978). Staph. epidermidis is sensitive, but other Gram-positive cocci such as Strep. pyogenes, Group B streptococci, Strep. pneumoniae and the alpha-haemolytic streptococci (Strep. viridans) have only a low degree of sensitivity or are completely tobramycin-resistant (Britt et al., 1972; Meyers and Hirschman, 1972; Neu, 1976). The various enterococci, including Strep. faecalis and Strep. faecium, are also moderately resistant, being slightly more resistant to tobramycin than to gentamicin (Finland et al., 1976). Nevertheless, similar to gentamicin (page 329), tobramycin acts synergistically with penicillin G against nearly all Strep. faecalis strains (Basker et al., 1977; Gutschik et al., 1977; Calderwood et al., 1977). However Strep. faecium appears to be resistant to this combination, whereas penicillin G/gentamicin is effective against all Strep. faecium as well as all Strep. faecalis strains (Moellering et al., 1973).

Similar to gentamicin (page 329), tobramycin only has a low degree of activity against Gram-positive bacilli.

3. *Mycobacteria.* At clinically attainable concentrations, tobramycin has no activity against M. tuberculosis or other mycobacteria (Gangadharam and Candler, 1977).

In Vitro Sensitivities

The minimum inhibitory concentrations of tobramycin compared to those of gentamicin against some selected bacterial species are shown in Table 25.

TABLE 25

Condensed from Waterworth (1972)

ORGANISM	MIC (μg per ml)	
	Gentamicin	Tobramycin
Gram-positive bacteria		
Staph. pyogenes	0·03–0·12	0·12–0·25
Strep. faecalis (Enterococcus, Group D)	2·0–4·0	2·0–8·0
Gram-negative bacteria		
Esch. coli	0·25–1·0	0·25–1·0
Klebsiella spp.	0·06–0·25	0·12–1·0
Serratia marcescens	0·25–0·5	1·0–4·0
Proteus mirabilis	0·25–2·0	1·0–4·0
Pseudomonas aeruginosa	0·25–2·0	0·12–2·0

Mode of Administration and Dosage

Like gentamicin, tobramycin is not absorbed from the gastro-intestinal tract and it is administered either intramuscularly or intravenously.

1. *Intramuscular administration.* For the treatment of mild to moderate infections, tobramycin is usually administered in a dose of 3·0–4·5 mg per kg body weight per day, given in three or four divided doses. A common adult dosage is 80 mg every six or eight hours (Simon *et al.*, 1973; Neu, 1976). The dose can be increased to 5–8 mg per kg per day for serious infections (Lode *et al.*, 1975). These dosage schedules may also be suitable for the treatment of children (McCracken and Nelson, 1976), but young children with serious infections should receive at least 7·5 mg per kg per day (Neu, 1977). Recently Hoecker *et al.* (1978) evaluated the pharmacokinetics of tobramycin in 50 paediatric patients. They found that therapeutic non-toxic serum levels were only achieved if a high daily dose of 300 mg per M^2 (approximately 10 mg per kg every 24 h) was given, and this was administered in six divided doses every four hours. Accordingly these authors recommend that this tobramycin dose should be given to all children and adolescents under 18 years of age (*see also* amikacin, page 381).

The dose for newborn and premature infants is 2 mg per kg given every twelve hours (4 mg per kg per day), except that infants with birth weights higher than 2000 g and who are also aged more than seven days, should receive 2 mg per kg every eight hours (6 mg per kg per day) (Kaplan *et al.*, 1973; McCracken and Nelson, 1976; 1977).

2. *Intravenous administration.* The intravenous tobramycin dose is identical to the intramuscular dose (*vide supra*). Like gentamicin (page 331), it can be administered intermittently directly into the intravenous tubing over a period of two to three minutes (Stratford *et al.*, 1974), over one minute (Dobbs and Mawer, 1976), or even as rapidly as over 15 seconds (Gillett *et al.*, 1976a). After such rapid intravenous injections, peak serum concentrations usually exceed 10 μg per ml and sometimes even 20 μg per ml, but they are only transitory. Within 30 to 60 min serum levels are similar to the peak obtained after an intramuscular injection of the same dose; thereafter the half-life of the drug in serum is only slightly shorter than that which is obtained with intramuscular administration (*vide supra, see also* gentamicin, page 332). The transient high peak serum levels which follow rapid intravenous injections, are not associated with any immediate or delayed toxic effects on the eighth nerve or the kidney (Gillett *et al.*, 1976a; Dobbs and Mawer, 1976). It has been pointed out that if tobrainycin is administered by rapid intermittent intravenous injections, the serum level one hour after injection should still be 4–5 μg per ml, otherwise therapy may be inadequate (Gillett *et al.*, 1976a). These authors also found that serum levels were less than 2 μg per ml six hours after a 1·5 mg per kg intravenous dose. Accordingly they recommended that tobramycin should be given at intervals of six hours in a dose of 6 mg per kg per day, whenever the drug is administered by rapid intravenous injections.

Alternatively tobramycin, like gentamicin (page 332), may be administered intravenously as an intermittent infusion over 20–60 min, every six or eight hours (Lode *et al.*, 1975; Setia and Gross, 1976). This is the only method of intravenous administration recommended for neonates (McCracken and Nelson, 1977). If this method of administration is used for adults with normal renal function, a dose of at least 1·5 mg per kg every six hours is needed to produce mean peak serum concentrations of 4–9 μg per ml immediately after the infusion, and trough levels are usually less than 2 μg per ml (Setia and Gross,

1976). In some patients higher tobramycin doses such as 2 mg per kg body weight every six hours are required to obtain adequate mean peak concentrations and a satisfactory therapeutic result. Doses of tobramycin as high as 12 mg per kg per day may be necessary in patients with cystic fibrosis and severe burns, irrespective of the method of administration, as these patients appear to eliminate the drug from the body more rapidly (Setia and Gross, 1976; McCrae, 1976).

Continuous intravenous infusion of tobramycin is not recommended, because therapeutic serum levels may not be attained with the usual doses of the drug (Simon et al., 1973). Dosage can be increased to attain adequate serum levels, but this may be associated with increased toxicity. Animal studies indicate that continuous tobramycin (or gentamicin) infusion is associated with more nephrotoxicity than the injection once every 24 h of the same daily dose (Reiner et al., 1978). Furthermore an accurate constant infusion rate is difficult to obtain even with the use of infusion pumps (Bodey et al., 1975).

3. *Patients with renal failure.* The dose should be reduced in these patients as with gentamicin (page 332). This may be accomplished in two ways. Individual tobramycin doses may be left unchanged, but the usual interval between doses (6–8 h) is extended by multiplying it by the value of the patient's serum creatinine measured in mg per cent (for conversion of serum creatinine from mmol/l, *see* gentamicin, page 333). Alternatively the usual interval between doses (6–8 h) may be left unchanged and individual maintenance doses reduced by dividing them by the value of the patient's serum creatinine, measured in mg per cent (Naber et al., 1973; Jaffe et al., 1974; Neu, 1976; 1977). These dosage schedules are only rough approximations. The presumed linear relationship between serum creatinine and the tobramycin half-life in the body does not necessarily always hold true, especially at higher creatinine concentrations and particularly with those above 10 mg per cent (Jaffe et al., 1974; Neu, 1976). For this reason, the tobramycin dosage in patients with impaired renal function should always be governed by regular serum level estimations whenever possible. Ideally peak serum levels should be at least 4–5 μg per ml (or for serious infections 4–8 μg per ml), and trough levels should not exceed 2 μg per ml (Gillett et al., 1976a; Neu, 1976).

Nomograms developed to assist gentamicin prescribing in these patients (page 333) can also be used for tobramycin. The minimal input data for such nomograms are the patient's age, sex, weight and serum creatinine concentration. The gentamicin nomogram developed by Mawer et al. (1974) has been used to prescribe intravenous tobramycin to patients with acute leukaemia and suspected infection (Tobias et al., 1977). This was particularly helpful whenever large tobramycin doses were indicated for severe infections. However tobramycin serum level estimations are still advisable even if the dosage is prescribed according to a nomogram (*see* gentamicin, page 334).

Tobramycin, like gentamicin (page 334) is removed by haemodialysis; approximately 50 per cent of an administered dose is removed by a six-hour dialysis (Lockwood and Bower, 1973; Jaffe et al., 1974). In anephric patients maintained by regular haemodialysis, the usual single dose of 1·5–2·0 mg per kg, given after each dialysis will usually maintain therapeutic non-toxic serum levels. Removal of tobramycin by peritoneal dialysis is inefficient, and only about 50 per cent of an administered dose is recovered during 36 h of this procedure (Weinstein *et al.*, 1973; Jaffe *et al.*, 1974b). Nevertheless the tobramycin half-life in anephric patients of 53 h is reduced to 12–16 h when these patients undergo peritoneal dialysis. An approximate tobramycin dosage schedule for these patients is a loading dose of 2 mg per kg body weight followed by either the same dose once every 36 h or 1 mg per kg every 12 h (Malacoff *et al.*, 1975).

4. *Intrathecal and intraventricular administration*. In common with gentamicin (page 334), tobramycin can be administered intrathecally or intraventricularly to adults in a dose of 5–10 mg. Intrathecal administration produces adequate antibiotic concentrations in lumbar, but not in ventricular CSF. When it is given into the cerebral ventricles, adequate concentrations are attained in both lumbar and ventricular CSF (Kaiser and McGee, 1975).

Availability

For intramuscular or intravenous use.
  1. Ampoules: 40 mg in 1 ml and 80 mg in 2 ml.
  2. Disposable syringes: 80 mg in 2 ml.
  3. Paediatric ampoules: 20 mg in 2 ml.

Serum Levels in Relation to Dosage

After an 80 mg intramuscular injection of tobramycin is given to adults, an average peak serum level of $3 \cdot 7$ μg per ml is attained in thirty minutes. Six hours later the average serum level is $0 \cdot 56$ μg per ml, and after 8–12 h it is undetectable (Simon *et al.*, 1973). These serum levels are similar to those of gentamicin (page 335). The half-life of tobramycin after intramuscular injection is $1 \cdot 9$–$2 \cdot 2$ h (Neu, 1977).

If tobramycin is administered intravenously as a 30–60 min infusion, the peak serum level attained straight after the infusion and subsequent serum levels are similar to those obtained after an identical intramuscular dose (Lode *et al.*, 1975). When it is given intravenously by rapid intravenous injections, transient high peaks are reached soon after the injection, the height of the peak being proportional to the rate of injection (page 362). One hour after such an intravenous injection the serum level approximates to the peak level after an intramuscular injection of an identical dose (Gillett *et al.*, 1976a). However the serum half-life of the drug with this method (80 to 90 min) is shorter than that after intramuscular administration. Serum levels at 6 h are invariably below 1 μg per ml and often below $0 \cdot 1$ μg per ml (Neu, 1977).

When the drug is given by continuous intravenous infusion ($6 \cdot 6$ mg per h), the peak serum level is achieved $2 \cdot 5$–$3 \cdot 0$ h after commencement of the infusion. Thereafter a steady-state serum concentration which averages $0 \cdot 94$ μg per ml is maintained, and an almost identical result is achieved with gentamicin (Simon *et al.*, 1973) (page 331). If tobramycin is administered by constant infusion at 30 mg per hour, a steady-state concentration of $3 \cdot 6$–$4 \cdot 5$ μg per ml can be attained (Neu, 1977). To achieve steady-state serum levels of at least 3 μg per ml by continuous tobramycin infusion, a total daily dose of 7 mg per kg is needed (Bodey *et al.*, 1975).

With multiple dosing of tobramycin, gradually rising peak and trough serum levels sometimes occur even in patients with stable renal function. This can be probably explained on the basis of a slow tissue uptake and release of the antibiotic (*vide infra*). Later in the course of treatment, when the drug has already accumulated in tissues, a given dose is likely to produce a higher serum concentration (Schentag *et al.*, 1978).

Excretion

Tobramycin is excreted by the kidneys in an active unchanged form, producing high urinary concentrations. In patients with normal renal function, 60 per cent of an administered dose is excreted within six hours (Naber *et al.*, 1973), and 85 per cent within a 24 h period (Neu, 1977). Like gentamicin (page 336), some of the drug is not excreted and accumulates in the body, particularly in renal cortical tissue (page 337). Accumulated tobramycin is slowly excreted by the kidney for 10 to 20 days after the last dose (Schentag *et al.*, 1978). Excretion is only by glomerular filtration and therefore probenecid has no effect on its rate of elimination (Naber *et al.*, 1973).

In patients with impaired renal function, tobramycin excretion is reduced, but even in those with moderately severe renal failure, urine levels are adequate for the inhibition of tobramycin-sensitive Gram-negative bacilli (Weinstein *et al.*, 1973). The serum half-lives of tobramycin and gentamicin are virtually identical, being two hours in patients with normal kidneys and 53·4 h in anephric patients (Lockwood and Bower, 1973).

Distribution of the Drug in Body

The binding of tobramycin to serum proteins under normal conditions is very low, and it has been variously estimated to be virtually zero (Gordon *et al.*, 1972; Ullmann, 1976) to 25–30 per cent (Naber *et al.*, 1973).

Tobramycin appears to be distributed in human body fluids and tissues in a similar manner to gentamicin (page 337). It diffuses poorly into the CSF of patients with uninflamed meninges (Neu, 1976). Tobramycin levels are also low in the peritoneal fluid (Weinstein *et al.*, 1973; Gerding *et al.*, 1976), but they usually reach one half or more of the simultaneous serum level in patients with ascites and bacterial peritonitis (Gerding *et al.*, 1977). The drug penetrates well into the synovial fluid, even in the absence of bacterial infection, where concentrations consistently exceed 50 per cent of the serum level (Dee and Kozin, 1977). Tobramycin passes into the bronchial secretions to approximately the same extent as gentamicin (Pennington and Reynolds, 1973). In patients with cystic fibrosis, peak tobramycin sputum levels exceed the MIC's of many Ps. aeruginosa strains, provided that large doses of 5–10 mg per kg per day are used (McCrae *et al.*, 1976; Raeburn, 1976). Similar to gentamicin, tobramycin reaches satisfactory concentrations in non-inflamed human interstitial fluid (Tan and Salstrom, 1977). However in animal experiments its concentration in interstitial tissue fluid is low compared to that of gentamicin (Chisholm *et al.*, 1973; Carbon *et al.*, 1978). Tobramycin accumulates in kidney tissue, where it is selectively concentrated in renal cortical cells (Luft and Kleit, 1974; Bennett *et al.*, 1977). Some investigators have reported that tobramycin accumulates to a lesser extent than gentamicin in the renal cortex (Whelton *et al.*, 1978a and b), but others have found that they accumulate to about the same degree (Luft and Kleit, 1974; Gilbert *et al.*, 1978). These drugs are only slowly eliminated from renal tissue. Luft and Kleit (1974) found that the half-life of gentamicin in renal tissue was 109 h, whilst that of tobramycin was 74 h. This shorter renal half-life may partly explain the reports of slightly lower renal cortical concentrations of tobramycin compared to gentamicin.

The drug crosses the placenta but fetal serum levels are lower than those in the mother. This has been studied in detail by Bernard *et al.* (1977). After administering single 2 mg per kg body weight doses of tobramycin to pregnant women, the drug's half-life in fetal serum was $5 \cdot 2$ h, where levels did not exceed $0 \cdot 58 \mu$g per ml. For the subsequent 34 h the mean placental tissue concentration was $1 \cdot 4 \mu$g per g. Tobramycin was also detected in amniotic fluid, except in women during their first trimester. Fetal kidney tissue concentrations reached $7 \cdot 2 \mu$g per g 34 h after maternal drug administration; higher concentrations in this tissue were obtained when maturation of the fetal kidney was more advanced. Fetal urine concentrations estimated during second trimester ranged from $0 \cdot 1$ to $3 \cdot 4 \mu$g per ml. Very low tobramycin CSF concentrations $(0 \cdot 1 – 0 \cdot 7 \mu$g per ml) were found in fetuses at less than 17 weeks' gestation.

Mode of Action

This is probably similar to that of other aminoglycosides (*see* streptomycin, page 298).

Toxicity

1. *Ototoxicity.* Tobramycin, like gentamicin (page 338) can cause this complication, and it is prone to occur with prolonged serum levels of the drug. Wilson and Ramsdem (1977) performed electrocochleography on three patients who were receiving tobramycin by rapid intravenous injections. When peak serum tobramycin levels exceeded $8–10 \mu$g per ml, an immediate reduction in cochlear output was observed, which returned to normal as serum levels fell. These patients had no auditory or vestibular symptoms either during or after treatment.

Ototoxicity due to tobramycin has been relatively uncommon in clinical practice. Neu and Bendush (1976) found only 21 instances amongst 3506 patients treated by tobramycin. In 7 of these the effects were auditory only, in nine vestibular only and in five patients both auditory and vestibular. Subsequent progress of 18 patients was monitored; in 14 side-effects gradually subsided, in 3 a high frequency audiometric loss persisted and in the remaining patients there was a decrease in hearing. Analysis of the data suggested that pre-existing renal impairment, prior and/or concomitant therapy with other ototoxic drugs, and therapy for 10 days or more with a dose exceeding 3 mg per kg per day predisposed to ototoxicity.

Tobramycin may prove to be less ototoxic than gentamicin, but there is still insufficient information for this conclusion. Studies in animals suggest that tobramycin may cause less cochlear and vestibular damage (Brummett *et al.*, 1972; 1978; Federspil, 1978), but data from comparative human studies are very scanty. Fee *et al.* (1978) studied the results of administration of 23 courses of tobramycin and 45 courses of gentamicin, given separately to 60 patients. Serial audiograms and electronystagmograms were used to detect early cochlear or vestibular damage. Ototoxicity occurred in 4 patients (17 per cent) treated by tobramycin (3 cochlear, 1 vestibular), and in 11 gentamicin-treated patients (24 per cent), which was cochlear in 4, vestibular in 6 and combined in the other. There is a suggestion from these data that tobramycin may be slightly less ototoxic than gentamicin, but that its initial toxicity, unlike that of gentamicin, may be predominantly cochlear.

2. *Nephrotoxicity*. Tobramycin administration to animals produces changes in the proximal tubules similar to those produced by gentamicin (page 339). It causes renal impairment in man which is characterized by excretion of casts, oliguria, proteinuria and a progressive rise in blood urea and serum creatinine values (Appel and Neu, 1977). Serum levels of creatinine and, if possible, also of tobramycin itself, should be monitored during therapy (Neu, 1976).

To date nephrotoxicity has not been a frequent side-effect. In a review of 3506 patients treated by tobramycin, 53 (1·5 per cent) were considered to have developed nephrotoxicity as a result of its use, but this side-effect in another 105 (3 per cent) was of doubtful relation to tobramycin therapy (Bendush and Weber, 1976). Tobramycin related nephrotoxicity occurred primarily in patients receiving high doses for prolonged periods. Other predisposing factors appeared to be endotoxaemia, dehydration, consumptive coagulopathy and the use of other nephrotoxic drugs. Feld *et al.* (1977) used tobramycin to treat severe Gram-negative infections in cancer patients, and 22 per cent of patients developed nephrotoxicity.

As with gentamicin (page 340), a combination of tobramycin with cephalothin may be associated with a higher risk of nephrotoxicity than with the use of tobramycin alone (Klastersky *et al.*, 1975; Tobias *et al.*, 1976). However the role of cephalosporins in potentiating aminoglycoside nephrotoxicity is unresolved (Neu, 1977; Marsh, 1978). Similar to gentamicin (page 340), animal experiments show that cephalosporins do not potentiate, but actually protect against tobramycin nephrotoxicity (Barza *et al.*, 1978). Increased renal toxicity has not been observed when tobramycin has been used together with either carbenicillin (page 149) or ticarcillin (page 170) (Klastersky *et al.*, 1975, Neu, 1977; Appel and Neu, 1977).

Tobramycin may be less nephrotoxic than gentamicin (Bennett *et al.*, 1977). In animals gentamicin is more toxic to the renal tubules than tobramycin (Wick and Welles, 1968; Whelton *et al.*, 1978a and b; Gilbert *et al.*, 1978). Some preliminary clinical data also support this view. Walker and Gentry (1976) treated 80 patients with urinary tract infections randomly allocated to either a gentamicin or tobramycin regimen. Deterioration in renal function was observed in 7 gentamicin-treated, but only in 2 tobramycin-treated patients. Kamme *et al.* (1978) treated 38 consecutive patients randomly by either gentamicin or tobramycin. A progressive mean rise in serum creatinine and a reciprocal mean decrease in creatinine clearance occurred in the patients treated with gentamicin; these changes were much less pronounced in the tobramycin-treated patients. The abnormalities in all patients in this study rapidly returned to normal on cessation of therapy. Fee *et al.* (1978) who primarily studied comparative ototoxicity of these drugs (page 366), observed nephrotoxicity in 28 per cent of patients treated with gentamicin, but only in 9 per cent of those treated with tobramycin.

3. *Other side-effects*. These are uncommon and relatively unimportant. Local reactions may occur at the site of intramuscular injection and thrombophlebitis may occur after intravenous administration. Urticaria, eosinophilia or a maculopapular rash have been described but are rare. Elevated serum aspartate aminotransferase (SGOT) values have been noted in some patients, but other evidence of hepatotoxicity has not been reported (Neu, 1976; Bendush and Weber, 1976).

Clinical Uses of the Drug

1. *Pseudomonas aeruginosa infections*. Tobramycin is preferable to gentamicin for the treatment of confirmed Pseudomonas infections, and also for initial emergency treatment of patients with severe infections in whom Ps. aeruginosa is a likely pathogen, such as those with neutropenia, burns and cystic fibrosis (Neu, 1976; Moellering, 1977). Compared to gentamicin, tobramycin is more active *in vitro* against Ps. aeruginosa, and it is also active against a proportion of gentamicin-resistant strains of this organism (page (360). In one animal study tobramycin was more active than gentamicin for the treatment of infections with Ps. aeruginosa when results were analysed in terms of the therapeutic index (ratio of toxicity to efficacy) (Davis, 1975). In another study these two drugs appeared to be of about the same value for the treatment of induced Pseudomonas sepsis in monkeys (Saslaw *et al.*, 1972).

There have been few comparative clinical studies of gentamicin and tobramycin for severe Ps. aeruginosa infection. In one study the clinical effectiveness of the two drugs appeared about the same (Klastersky *et al.*, 1974a). In many uncontrolled studies, results of tobramycin treatment of severe Pseudomonas infections in general have been satisfactory. Tobramycin has been used with about the same success as gentamicin (page 341) to treat Pseudomonas septicaemia (Blair *et al.*, 1975; Feld *et al.*, 1977), pneumonia and purulent bronchial infections (Carmalt *et al.*, 1976; Altucci *et al.*, 1976) and respiratory infections in children with cystic fibrosis (Hoff *et al.*, 1974; McCrae *et al.*, 1976; McCrae, 1976). For the treatment of cystic fibrosis patients, large tobramycin doses are sometimes required to achieve satisfactory serum and sputum concentrations (page 363).

Likewise tobramycin has been used successfully to treat Pseudomonas urinary tract infections (Perkins *et al.*, 1976; Raine *et al.*, 1976; Bennett, 1976; Madsen *et al.*, 1976), soft tissue infections and osteomyelitis (Perkins *et al.*, 1976; Carmalt *et al.*, 1976). It has also been of value for surgical infections such as wound sepsis, infected burns and peritonitis, where Ps. aeruginosa is not infrequently involved in a mixed infection with other organisms (Ishiyama *et al.*, 1976). A small number of patients with Ps. aeruginosa endocarditis (Altucci *et al.*, 1976; Carmalt *et al.*, 1976) and meningitis (Bendush and Weber, 1976) have also been treated with a satisfactory result. Serious infections caused by gentamicin-resistant, but tobramycin-sensitive, strains of Ps. aeruginosa often respond satisfactorily to tobramycin (Moellering *et al.*, 1976).

For the initial treatment of severe infections in neutropenic patients with leukaemia or cancer, the combination of cephalothin and tobramycin has often been used with success (Klastersky *et al.*, 1975; Vincent *et al.*, 1976; Cohen and Miale, 1976; Papayannis *et al.*, 1977). Some authors prefer clindamycin (page 485) combined with tobramycin for this clinical situation (Gillet *et al.*, 1976b; Falk *et al.*, 1977). In confirmed severe Ps. aeruginosa infections, such as respiratory infections in patients with cystic fibrosis, tobramycin, like gentamicin (page 000), has often been successfully combined with either carbenicillin (Crozier and Khan, 1976) or ticarcillin (Parry and Neu, 1976). In experimental animal studies tobramycin, like gentamicin (page 342), when combined with carbenicillin is more effective against severe Pseudomonas sepsis (Andriole, 1974).

2. *Infections caused by other Gram-negative bacilli.* There is ample evidence that urinary tract infections, as well as more serious systemic infections such as pneumonia, soft tissue infections, osteomyelitis, meningitis and septicaemia, caused by the Enterobacteriaceae such as Esch. coli and the Enterobacter, Klebsiella and Proteus spp., also respond to tobramycin treatment (Jaffe *et al.*, 1974a; Queiroz *et al.*, 1976; Carmalt *et al.*, 1976; Perkins *et al.*, 1976; Walker and Gentry, 1976; Madsen *et al.*, 1976; Bennett, 1976; Bendush and Weber, 1976; Feld *et al.*, 1977).

At present most clinicians prefer to use the more familiar gentamicin (page 341) rather than tobramycin for the treatment of infections caused by these Enterobacteriaceae. Gentamicin is certainly indicated for Serratia marcescens infections, as it is about four times more active than tobramycin against this pathogen (page 359). In addition some strains of Esch. coli and of other Enterobacteriaceae may be about two-fold more sensitive to gentamicin than to tobramycin (page 359). For the treatment of infections caused by Enterobacteriaceae equally sensitive to both of these drugs, tobramycin can be used with success. Being a newer drug it may be used more extensively for these infections in the future, particularly if further studies confirm its lesser toxicity (pages 366, 367). There are no reasons why tobramycin should be considered as a 'reserve drug' for the treatment of infections due to Enterobacteriaceae resistant to gentamicin. There is almost complete cross-resistance between tobramycin and gentamicin with these bacteria and clinical use of gentamicin in a hospital environment selects organisms resistant to both these drugs (Moellering, 1977).

3. *Chemoprophylaxis in abdominal surgery.* Similar to gentamicin (page 345), tobramycin in adult doses of 80–160 mg, combined with lincomycin 600 mg, has been used to prevent post-operative sepsis in patients undergoing abdominal surgery. One dose of each drug is always given just before surgery, and in some trials no further antibiotics have been given (Griffiths *et al.*, 1976), but in others the same doses of both drugs were repeated eight hours later (Galland *et al.*, 1977). Some authors have administered a total of three doses, the second and third of which were given four and twelve hours after operation (Keighley and Crapp, 1976). All these regimens significantly reduced the post-operative sepsis rate, but lincomycin or clindamycin are no longer recommended for this purpose, because of their propensity to cause pseudomembranous colitis (page 481).

REFERENCES

Altucci, P., Abbate, G. F., Alagia, I. and Leonessa, V. (1976), 'Clinical evaluation of tobramycin in respiratory and systemic infections in immunodepressed and normal patients', *J. Infect. Dis.* (Suppl.), **134**, 182.

Anderson, E. L., Gramling, P. K., Vestal, P. R. and Farrar, W. E., Jr. (1975), 'Susceptibility of Pseudomonas aeruginosa to tobramycin or gentamicin alone and combined with carbenicillin', *Antimicrob. Ag. Chemother.*, **8**, 300.

Andriole, V. T. (1974), 'Antibiotic synergy in experimental infection with Pseudomonas. II. The effect of carbenicillin, cephalothin, or cephanone combined with tobramycin or gentamicin', *J. Infect. Dis.*, **129**, 124.

Appel, G. B. and Neu, H. C. (1977), 'The nephrotoxicity of antimicrobial agents (second of three parts), *New Engl. J. Med.*, **296, 722**.

Barza, M., Pinn, V., Tanguay, P. and Murray, T. (1978), 'Nephrotoxicity of newer cephalosporins and aminoglycosides alone and in combination in a rat model', *J. Antimicrob. Chemother.* (Suppl. A), **4**, 59.

Basker, M. J., Slocombe, B. and Sutherland, R. (1977), 'Aminoglycoside-resistant enterococci', *J. clin. Path.*, **30**, 375.

Bendush, C. L. and Weber, R. (1976), 'Tobramycin sulfate: A summary of worldwide experience from clinical trials', *J. Infect. Dis.* (Suppl.), **134**, 219.

Bennett, A. H. (1976), 'Evaluation of tobramycin in severe urinary tract infections', *J. Infect. Dis.* (Suppl.), **134, 156**.

Bennett, W. M., Plamp, C. and Porter, G. A. (1977), 'Drug-related syndromes in clinical nephrology', *Ann. Intern. Med.*, **87**, 582.

Bernard, B., Garcia-Cázares, S. J., Ballard, C. A., Thrupp, L. D., Mathies, A. W. and Wehrle, P. F. (1977), 'Tobramycin: Maternal-fetal pharmacology', *Antimicrob. Ag. Chemother.*, **11**, 688.

Black, H. R. and Griffith, R. S. (1971), 'Preliminary studies with nebramycin factor 6', *Antimicrob. Ag. Chemother.*—1970, p. 314.

Blair, D. C., Fekerty, F. R., Jr., Bruce, B., Silva, J. and Archer, G. (1975), 'Therapy of Pseudomonas aeruginosa infections with tobramycin', *Antimicrob. Ag. Chemother.*, **8**, 22.

Bodey, G. P. and Stewart, D. (1972), '*In vitro* studies of tobramycin', *Antimicrob. Ag. Chemother.*, **2**, 109.

Bodey, G. P., Chang, H.-Y., Rodriguez, V. and Stewart, D. (1975), 'Feasibility of administering aminoglycoside antibiotics by continuous intravenous infusion', *Antimicrob. Ag. Chemother.*, **8**, 328.

Britt, M. R., Garibaldi, R. A., Wilfert, J. N. and Smith, C. B. (1972), '*In vitro* activity of tobramycin and gentamicin', *Antimicrob. Ag. Chemother.*, **2**, 236.

Brummett, R. E., Himes, D., Saine, B. and Vernon, J. (1972), 'A comparative study of the ototoxicity of tobramycin and gentamicin', *Arch. Otolaryng.*, **96**, 505.

Brummett, R. D., Fox, K. E., Bendrick, T. W. and Himes, D. L. (1978), 'Ototoxicity of tobramycin, gentamicin, amikacin and sisomicin in the guinea pig', *J. Antimicrob. Chemother.* (Suppl. A), **4**, 73.

Brusch, J. L., Barza, M., Bergeron, M. G. and Weinstein, L. (1972), 'Cross-resistance of Pseudomonas to gentamicin and tobramycin', *Antimicrob. Ag. Chemother.*, **1**, 280.

Calderwood, S. A., Wennersten, C., Moellering, R. C., Jr., Kunz, L. J. and Krogstad, D. J. (1977), 'Resistance to six aminoglycosidic aminocyclitol antibiotics among entercococci: Prevalence, evolution and relationship to synergism with penicillin', *Antimicrob. Ag. Chemother.*, **12**, 401.

Carbon, C., Contrepois, A. and Lamotte-Barrillon, S. (1978), 'Comparative distribution of gentamicin, tobramycin, sisomicin, netilmicin and amikacin in interstitial fluid in rabbits', *Antimicrob. Ag. Chemother.*, **13**, 368.

Carmalt, E. D., Cortez, L. M. and Rosenblatt, J. E. (1976), 'Clinical experience with tobramycin in the treatment of infections due to Gram-negative bacilli', *Amer. J. Med. Sci.*, **271**, 285.

Chisholm, G. D., Waterworth, P. M., Calnan, J. S. and Garrod, L. P. (1973), 'Concentration of antibacterial agents in interstitial tissue fluid', *Brit. med. J.*, **1**, 569.

Cohen, J. D. and Miale, T. D. (1976), 'Tobramycin and cephalothin for treatment of suspected sepsis in neutropenic children with cancer', *J. Infect. Dis.* (Suppl.), **134**, 175.

Comber, K. R., Basker, M. J., Osborne, C. D. and Sutherland, R. (1977), 'Synergy between ticarcillin and tobramycin against Pseudomonas aeruginosa and Enterobacteriaceae *in vitro* and *in vivo*', *Antimicrob. Ag. Chemother.*, **11**, 956.

Crozier, D. N. and Khan, S. R. (1976), 'Tobramycin in treatment of infections due to Pseudomonas aeruginosa in patients with cystic fibrosis', *J. Infect. Dis.* (Suppl.), **134**, 187.

Davis, S. D. (1975), 'Activity of gentamicin, tobramycin, polymyxin B and colistimethate in mouse protection tests with Pseudomonas aeruginosa', *Antimicrob. Ag. Chemother.*, **8**, 50.

Dee, T. H. and Kozin, F. (1977), 'Gentamicin and tobramycin penetration into synovial fluid', *Antimicrob. Ag. Chemother.*, **12**, 548.

Del Bene, V. E. and Farrar, W. E., Jr. (1972), 'Tobramycin: *In vitro* activity and comparison with kanamycin and gentamicin', *Antimicrob. Ag. Chemother.*, **1**, 340.

Dienstag, J. and Neu, H. C. (1972), '*In vitro* studies of tobramycin, an aminoglycoside antibiotic', *Antimicrob. Ag. Chemother.*, **1**, 41.

Dobbs, S. M. and Mawer, G. E. (1976), 'Intravenous injection of gentamicin and tobramycin without impairment of hearing', *J. Infect. Dis.* (Suppl.), **134**, 114.

Drasar, F. A., Farrell, W., Maskell, J. and Williams, J. D. (1976), 'Tobramycin, amikacin, sisomicin and gentamicin resistant Gram-negative rods', *Brit. med. J.*, **2**, 1284.

Elwell, L. P., Inamine, J. M. and Minshew, B. H. (1978), 'Common plasmid specifying tobramycin resistance found in two enteric bacteria isolated from burn patients', *Antimicrob. Ag. Chemother.*, **13**, 312.

Falk, R. H., Gillett, A. P., Wise, R. and Melikian, V. (1977), 'Tobramycin and clindamycin in the treatment of febrile leukaemic patients', *J. Antimicrob. Chemother.*, **3**, 317.

Federspil, P. (1978), 'Comparative studies on the ototoxicity of tobramycin and the other aminoglycosides', *Assessment of Aminoglycoside Toxicity. A Symposium Sponsored by Eli Lilly and Company as a Service to Physicians*, Bürgenstock, Switzerland, September 24–25, 1977, p. 69.

Fee, W. E., Jr., Vierra, J. and Lathrop, G. R. (1978), 'Clinical evaluation of aminoglycoside toxicity: Tobramycin versus gentamicin, a preliminary report', *J. Antimicrob. Chemother.* (Suppl. A), **4**, 31.

Feld, R., Valdivieso, M., Bodey, G. P. and Rodriguez, V. (1977), 'Comparison of amikacin and tobramycin in the treatment of infection in patients with cancer', *J. Infect. Dis.*, **135**, 61.

Finland, M., Garner, C., Wilcox, C. and Sabath, L. D. (1976), 'Susceptibility of 'Enterobacteria' to aminoglycoside antibiotics: comparison with tetracyclines, polymyxins, chloramphenicol, and spectinomycin', *J. Infect. Dis.* (Suppl.), **134**, 57.

Galland, R. B., Mosley, J. G., Saunders, J. H. and Darrell, J. H. (1977), 'Prevention of wound infection in abdominal operations by peroperative antibiotics or povidone-iodine. A controlled trial', *Lancet*, **2**, 1043.

Gangadharam, P. R. J. and Candler, E. R. (1977), '*In vitro* anti-mycobacterial activity of some new aminoglycoside antibiotics', *Tubercle*, **58**, 35.

Gerding, D. N., Kromhout, J. P., Sullivan, J. J. and Hall, W. H. (1976), 'Antibiotic penetrance of ascitic fluid in dogs', *Antimicrob. Ag. Chemother.*, **10**, 850.

Gerding, D. N., Hall, W. H. and Schierl, E. A. (1977), 'Antibiotic concentrations in ascitic fluid of patients with ascites and bacterial peritonitis', *Ann. Intern. Med.*, **86**, 708.

Gilbert, D. N., Plamp, C., Starr, P., Bennett, W. M., Houghton, D. C. and Porter, G.

(1978), 'Comparative nephrotoxicity of gentamicin and tobramycin in rats', *Antimicrob. Ag. Chemother.*, **13**, 34.

Gillett, A. P., Falk, R. H., Andrews, J., Wise, R. and Melikian, V. (1976a), 'Rapid intravenous injection of tobramycin: suggested dosage schedule and concentrations in serum', *J. Infect. Dis.* (Suppl.), **134**, 110.

Gillett, P., Wise, R., Melikian, V. and Falk, R. (1976b), 'Tobramycin/cephalothin nephrotoxicity', *Lancet*, **1**, 547.

Glew, R. H., Moellering, R. C., Jr. and Buettner, K. R. (1977), '*In vitro* synergism between carbenicillin and aminoglycoside aminocyclitols against Acinetobacter calcoaceticus var. anitratus', *Antimicrob. Ag. Chemother.*, **11**, 1036.

Gordon, R. C., Regamey, C. and Kirby, W. M. M. (1972), 'Serum protein binding of the aminoglycoside antibiotics', *Antimicrob. Ag. Chemother.*, **2**, 214.

Griffiths, D. A., Shorey, B. A., Simpson, R. A., Speller, D. C. E. and Williams, N. B. (1976), 'Single-dose peroperative antibiotic prophylaxis in gastrointestinal surgery', *Lancet*, **2**, 325.

Gutschik, E., Jepsen, O. B. and Mortensen, I. (1977), 'Effect of combinations of penicillin and aminoglycosides on Streptococcus faecalis: A comparative study of seven aminoglycoside antibiotics', *J. Infect. Dis.*, **135**, 832.

Hammerberg, S., Sorger, S. and Marks, M. I. (1977), 'Antimicrobial susceptibilities of Yersinia enterocolitica Biotype 4, Serotype 0:3', *Antimicrob. Ag. Chemother.*, **11**, 566.

Hoecker, J. L., Pickering, L. K., Swaney, J., Kramer, W. G., van Eys, J., Feldman, S. and Kohl, S. (1978), 'Clinical pharmacology of tobramycin in children', *J. Infect. Dis.*, **137**, 592.

Hoff, G. E., Schiøtz, P. O. and Paulsen, J. (1974), 'Tobramycin treatment of Pseudomonas aeroginosa infections in cystic fibrosis', *Scand. J. Infect. Dis.*, **6**, 333.

Houang, E. T. and McKay-Ferguson, E. (1976), 'Activities of tobramycin and amikacin against gentamicin-resistant Gram-negative bacilli', *Lancet*, **1**, 423.

Ishiyama, S., Nakayama, I., Iwamoto, H., Iwai, S., Murata, I. and Ohashi, M. (1976), 'Clinical use of tobramycin in patients with surgical infections due to Gram-negative bacilli', *J. Infect. Dis.* (Suppl.), **134**, 178.

Jaffe, G., Ravreby, W., Meyers, B. R. and Hirschman, S. Z. (1974a), 'Clinical study of the use of the new aminoglycoside tobramycin for therapy of infections due to gram-negative bacteria', *Antimicrob. Ag. Chemother.*, **5**, 75.

Jaffe, G., Meyers, B. R. and Hirschman, S. Z. (1974b), 'Pharmacokinetics of tobramycin in patients with stable renal impairment, patients undergoing peritoneal dialysis, and patients on chronic hemodialysis', *Antimicrob. Ag. Chemother.*, **5**, 611.

Jordan, G. W. and Hoeprich, P. D. (1977), 'Susceptibility of three groups of Staphylococcus aureus to newer antimicrobial agents', *Antimicrob. Ag. Chemother.*, **11**, 7.

Kaiser, A. B. and McGee, Z. A. (1975), 'Aminoglycoside therapy of Gram-negative bacillary meningitis', *New Engl. J. Med.*, **293**, 1215.

Kamme, C., Kahlmeter, G. and Hallberg, T. (1978), 'Nephrotoxicity of gentamicin and tobramycin: A comparison in patients with serious infections'. In Siegenthaler, W. and Lüthy, R. (Ed.), *Current Chemotherapy: Proceedings of the 10th International Congress of Chemotherapy*, Zurich/Switzerland, 1977. American Society for Microbiology, Washington, D.C., p. 947.

Kaplan, J. M., McCracken, G. H., Jr., Thomas, M. L., Horton, L. J. and Davis, N. (1973), 'Clinical pharmacology of tobramycin in newborns', *Amer. J. Dis. Child.*, **125**, 656.

Karney, W., Holmes, K. K. and Turck, M. (1973), 'Comparison of five aminocyclitol antibiotics *in vitro* against Enterobacteriaceae and Pseudomonas', *Antimicrob. Ag. Chemother.*, **3**, 338.

Keighley, M. R. B. and Crapp, A. R. (1976), 'Short-term prophylaxis with tobramycin and lincomycin in bowel surgery', *Scot. med. J.*, **21**, 70.

Klastersky, J., Hensgens, C., Henri, A. and Daneau, D. (1974a), 'Comparative clinical study of tobramycin and gentamicin', *Antimicrob. Ag. Chemother.*, **5**, 133.

Klastersky, J., Nyamubeya, B. and Vandernborre, L. (1974b), 'Antimicrobial effectiveness of kanamycin, aminosidin, BB-K8, sisomicin, gentamicin and tobramycin combined with carbenicillin or cephalothin against Gram-negative rods', *J. Med. Microbiol.*, **7**, 465.

Klastersky, J., Hensgens, C. and Debusscher, L. (1975), 'Empiric therapy for cancer patients: Comparative study of ticarcillin-tobramycin, ticarcillin-cephalothin, and cephalothin-tobramycin', *Antimicrob. Ag. Chemother.*, **7**, 640.

Kluge, R. M., Standiford, H. C., Tatem, B., Young, V. M., Greene, W. H., Schimpff, S. C., Calia, F. M. and Hornick, R. B. (1974), 'Comparative activity of tobramycin, amikacin and gentamicin alone and with carbenicillin against Pseudomonas aeruginosa', *Antimicrob. Ag. Chemother.*, **6**, 442.

Levison, M. E., Knight, R. and Kaye, D. (1972), '*In vitro* evaluation of tobramycin, a new aminoglycoside antibiotic', *Antimicrob. Ag. Chemother.*, **1**, 381.

Lockwood, W. R. and Bower, J. D. (1973), 'Tobramycin and gentamicin concentrations in the serum of normal anephric patients', *Antimicrob. Ag. Chemother.*, **3**, 125.

Lockwood, W. R. and Lawson, L. A. (1973), 'Studies on the susceptibility of 150 consecutive clinical isolates of Pseudomonas aeruginosa to tobramycin, gentamicin, colistin, carbenicillin and five other antimicrobials', *Antimicrob. Ag. Chemother.*, **4**, 281.

Lode, H., Kemmerich, B. and Koeppe, P. (1975), 'Comparative clinical pharmacology of gentamicin, sisomicin and tobramycin', *Antimicrob. Ag. Chemother.*, **8**, 396.

Luft, F. C. and Kleit, S. A. (1974), 'Renal parenchymal accumulation of aminoglycoside antibiotics in rats', *J. Infect. Dis.*, **130**, 656.

McAllister, T. A. and Tait, S. C. (1976), 'Laboratory findings on tobramycin and their relation to clinical response', *J. Infect. Dis. (Suppl.)*, **134**, 20.

McAllister, T. A. (1976), 'Clinical bacteriology of tobramycin', *Scot. med. J.*, **21**, 64.

McCracken, G. H., Jr. and Nelson, J. D. (1976), 'Commentary: An appraisal of tobramycin usage in pediatrics', *J. Pediatrics*, **88**, 315.

McCracken, G. H., Jr. and Nelson, J. D. (1977), *Antimicrobial Therapy for Newborns: Practical Application of Pharmacology to Clinical Usage*, Grune & Stratton, New York, San Francisco, London, p. 38.

McCrae, W. M. (1976), 'Treatment of Pseudomonas infection in cystic fibrosis using tobramycin', *Scot. med. J.*, **21**, 68.

McCrae, W. M., Raeburn, J. A. and Hanson, E. J. (1976), 'Tobramycin therapy of infections due to Pseudomonas aeruginosa in patients with cystic fibrosis: Effect of dosage and concentration of antibiotic in sputum', *J. Infect. Dis. (Suppl.)*, **134**, 191.

Madsen, P. O., Kjaer, T. B. and Mosegaard, A. (1976), 'Comparison of tobramycin and gentamicin in the treatment of complicated urinary tract infections', *J. Infect. Dis. (Suppl.)*, **134**, 150.

Malacoff, R. F., Finkelstein, F. O. and Andriole, V. T. (1975), 'Effect of peritoneal dialysis on serum levels of tobramycin and clindamycin', *Antimicrob. Ag. Chemother.*, **8**, 574.

Marks, M. I., Hammerberg, S., Greenstone, G. and Silver, B. (1976), 'Activity of newer aminoglycosides and carbenicillin alone and in combination against gentamicin-resistant Pseudomonas aeruginosa', *Antimicrob. Ag. Chemother.*, **10**, 399.

Marsh, F. P. (1978), 'Do cephalosporins potentiate or antagonize aminoglycoside nephrotoxicity?', *J. Antimicrob. Chemother.*, **4**, 103.

Mawer, G. E., Ahmad, R., Dobbs, S. M., McGough, J. G., Lucas, C. B. and Tooth, J. A. (1974), 'Prescribing aids for gentamicin', *Brit. J. Clin. Pharmacol.*, **1**, 45.

Meyers, B. R. and Hirschman, S. Z. (1972), 'Tobramycin: *in vitro* antibacterial spectrum of a new aminoglycoside', *J. Clin. Pharmacol.*, **12**, 313.

Meyer, R. D., Lewis, R. P., Halter, J. and White, M. (1976), 'Gentamicin-resistant Pseudomonas aeruginosa and Serratia marcescens in a general hospital', *Lancet*, **1**, 580.

Minshew, B. H., Holmes, R. K., Sanford, J. P. and Baxter, C. R. (1974), 'Transferable resistance to tobramycin in Klebsiella pneumoniae and Enterobacter cloacae associated with enzymatic acetylation of tobramycin', *Antimicrob. Ag. Chemother.*, **6**, 492.

Moellering, R. C., Jr., Wennersten, C. and Weinsten, A. J. (1973), 'Penicillin-tobramycin synergism against enterococci: A comparison with penicillin and gentamicin', *Antimicrob. Ag. Chemother.*, **3**, 526.

Moellering, R. C., Jr., Wennersten, C. and Kunz, L. J. (1976), 'Emergence of gentamicin-resistant bacteria: Experience with tobramycin therapy of infections due to gentamicin-resistant organisms', *J. Infect. Dis.* (Suppl.), **134**, 40.

Moellering, R. C., Jr. (1977), 'Microbiological considerations in the use of tobramycin and related aminoglycosidic aminocyclitol antibiotics', *Med. J. Aust.* (Suppl.), **2**, 4.

Naber, K. G., Westenfelder, S. R. and Madsen, P. O. (1973), 'Pharmacokinetics of the aminoglycoside antibiotic tobramycin in humans', *Antimicrob. Ag. Chemother.*, **3**, 469.

Neu, H. C. and Bendush, C. L. (1976), 'Ototoxicity of tobramycin: A clinical overview', *J. Infect. Dis.* (Suppl.), **134**, 206.

Neu, H. C. (1976), 'Tobramycin: An overview', *J. Infect. Dis.* (Suppl.), **134**, 3.

Neu, H. C. (1977), 'The pharmacology of newer aminglycosides, with a consideration of the application to clinical situations', *Med. J. Aust.* (Suppl.), **2**, 13.

Papayannis, A. G., Thomopoulos, D., Voulgaris, E., Scliros, Ph. and Gardikas, C. (1977), 'Tobramycin-cephalothin treatment in leukaemic and neutropenic patients with severe infection', *J. Antimicrob. Chemother.*, **3**, 311.

Parry, M. F. and Neu, H. C. (1976), 'Tobramycin and ticarcillin therapy for exacerbations of pulmonary disease in patients with cystic fibrosis', *J. Infect. Dis.* (Suppl.), **134**, 194.

Pennington, J. E. and Reynolds, H. Y. (1973), 'Tobramycin in bronchial secretions', *Antimicrob. Ag. Chemother.*, **4**, 299.

Perkins, R. L., Saslaw, S., Fass, R. J., Prior, R. B., Scholand, J. F., Hodges, G. R., Tight, R. R. and Gardner, W. G. (1976), 'Tobramycin: *in vitro* and clinical evaluation in 30 patients', *Amer. J. Med. Sci.*, **271**, 297.

Preston, D. A. and Wick, W. E. (1971), 'Preclinical assessment of the antibacterial activity of nebramycin factor 6', *Antimicrob. Agents Chemother.*—1970, p. 322.

Queiroz, F. P., Oliveira, M. M. G. and Rocha, H. (1976), 'Tobramycin in chronic recurrent urinary tract infections', *Amer. J. Med. Sci.*, **271**, 29.

Raeburn, J. A. (1976), Leading article. 'Antibiotic management of cystic fibrosis', *J. Antimicrob. Chemother.*, **2**, 107.

Raine, P. A. M., Young, D. G., McAllister, T. A. and Tait, S. C. (1976), 'Tobramycin in pediatric use', *J. Infect. Dis.* (Suppl.), **134**, 165.

Reiner, N. E., Bloxham, D. D. and Thompson, W. L. (1978), 'Nephrotoxicity of gentamicin and tobramycin given once daily or continuously in dogs', *J. Antimicrob. Chemother.* (Suppl. A), **4**, 85.

Reynolds, A. V., Hamilton-Miller, J. M. T. and Brumfitt, W. (1974), 'Newer aminoglycosides-amikacin and tobramycin: An *in vitro* comparison with kanamycin and gentamicin', *Brit. med. J.*, **3**, 778.

Saslaw, S., Carlisle, H. N. and Moheimani, M. (1972), 'Comparison of tobramycin, gentamicin, colistin, and carbenicillin in Pseudomonas sepsis in monkeys', *Antimicrob. Ag. Chemother.*, **2**, 164.

Schentag, J. J., Lasezkay, G., Cumbo, T. J., Plaut, H. E. and Jusko, W. J. (1978), 'Accumulation pharmacokinetics of tobramycin', *Antimicrob. Ag. Chemother.*, **13**, 649.

Seligman, S. J. (1978), 'Frequency of resistance to kanamycin, tobramycin, netilmicin and amikacin in gentamicin-resistant Gram-negative bacteria', *Antimicrob. Ag. Chemother.*, **13**, 70.

Setia, U. and Gross, P. A. (1976), 'Administration of tobramycin and gentamicin by the intravenous route every 6 h in patients with normal renal function', *J. Infect. Dis.* (Suppl.), **134**, 125.

Simon, V. K., Mösinger, E. U. and Malerczy, V. (1973), 'Pharmacokinetic studies of tobramycin and gentamicin', *Antimicrob. Ag. Chemother.*, **3**, 445.

Stratford, B. C., Dixson, S. and Cobcroft, A. J. (1974), 'Serum levels of gentamicin and tobramycin after slow intravenous bolus injection', *Lancet*, **1**, 378.

Tan, J. S. and Salstrom, S. J. (1977), 'Levels of carbenicillin, ticarcillin, cephalothin, cefazolin, cefamandole, gentamicin, tobramycin and amikacin in human serum and interstitial fluid', *Antimicrob. Ag. Chemother.*, **11**, 698.

Thornsberry, C., Baker, C. N. and Kirven, L. A. (1978), '*In vitro* activity of antimicrobial agents on Legionnaires' disease bacterium', *Antimicrob. Ag. Chemother.*, **13**, 78.

Tobias, J. S., Whitehouse, J. M. and Wrigley, P. F. M. (1976), 'Severe renal dysfunction after tobramycin/cephalothin therapy', *Lancet*, **1**, 425.

Tobias, J. S., Wrigley, P. F. M., Korde, S. and Shaw, E. J. (1977), 'Nomogram-assisted dosage of tobramycin', *J. Antimicrob. Chemother.*, **3**, 305.

Ullmann, U. (1976), 'The protein binding of ticarcillin and tobramycin', *J. Antimicrob. Chemother.*, **2**, 213.

Uwaydah, M. and Taqi-Eddin, A. (1976), 'Susceptibility of non-fermentative Gram-negative bacilli to tobramycin', *J. Infect. Dis.* (Suppl.), **134**, 28.

Verbist, L., Vandepitte, J. and Vandeven, J. (1978), 'Activity of eight aminoglycosides against isolates of Serratia marcescens from four hospitals', *J. Antimicrob. Chemother.*, **4**, 47.

Vincent, P. C., Jennis, F., Hilmer, R. and Fabre, S. (1976), 'Tobramycin and cephalothin sodium in treatment of infected patients with acute leukemia', *J. Infect. Dis.* (Suppl.), **134**, 170.

Vogel, L., Nathan, C., Sweeney, H. M., Kabins, S. A. and Cohen, S. (1978), 'Infections due to gentamicin-resistant Staphylococcus aureus strain in a nursery for neonatal infants', *Antimicrob. Ag. Chemother.*, **13**, 466.

Walker, B. D. and Gentry, L. O. (1976), 'A randomized comparative study of tobramycin and gentamicin in treatment of acute urinary tract infections', *J. Infect. Dis.* (Suppl.), **134**, 146.

Waterworth, P. M. (1972), 'The *in vitro* activity of tobramycin compared with that of other aminoglycosides', *J. clin. Path.*, **25**, 979.

Weinstein, A. J., Karchmer, A. W. and Moellering, R. C., Jr. (1973), 'Tobramycin concentrations during peritoneal dialysis', *Antimicrob. Ag. Chemother.*, **4**, 432.

Wick, W. E. and Welles, J. S. (1968), 'Nebramycin, a new broad-spectrum antibiotic complex. IV. *In vitro* and *in vivo* laboratory evaluation', *Antimicrob. Ag. Chemother.—1967*, p. 341; quoted by Simon *et al.* (1973).

Wilson, P. and Ramsden, R. T. (1977), 'Immediate effects of tobramycin on human cochlea and correlation with serum tobramycin levels', *Brit. med. J.*, **1**, 259.

Whelton, A., Carter, G. G., Bryant, H. H., Cody, T. S., Craig, T. J. and Walker, W. G. (1978a), 'Tobramycin and gentamicin intrarenal kinetic comparisons: Therapeutic and toxicological answers'. In Siegenthaler, W. and Lüthy, R. (Ed.), *Current Chemotherapy: Proceedings of the 10th International Congress of Chemotherapy*, Zurich/Switzerland, 1977. American Society for Microbiology, Washington, D.C., p. 951.

Whelton, A., Carter, G. G., Craig, T. J., Bryant, H. H., Herbst, D. V. and Walker, W. G. (1978b), 'Comparison of the intrarenal disposition of tobramycin and gentamicin: Therapeutic and toxicologic answers', *J. Antimicrob. Chemother.* (Suppl.), **4,** 13.

Wretlind, B., Nord, C. E. and Wadström, T. (1974); '*In vitro* sensitivity of isolates of Pseudomonas aeruginosa to carbenicillin, gentamicin, tobramycin, and some other antibiotics', *Scand. J. Infect. Dis.*, **6,** 49.

Amikacin

Description

Amikacin (BB-K8) is a semisynthetic aminoglycoside aminocyclitol antibiotic (page 294). It was derived from kanamycin A by acetylation with an S-4-amino-2-hydroxybutyryl (AHB) side-chain at the 1-position of its deoxystreptamine moiety (Annotation, 1975; Kawaguchi, 1976). Amikacin is for practical purposes identical with kanamycin (page 308) in its physical, chemical, pharmacologic and toxicologic properties (Cabana and Taggart, 1973; Hewitt and Young, 1977). However it has an *in vitro* antibacterial spectrum which is broader than that of gentamicin (page 325) and tobramycin (page 359) (Ries *et al.*, 1973; Price *et al.*, 1974). The most important additional property of amikacin is that its AHB side-chain gives it stability against most of the bacterial R plasmid-mediated enzymes, which are responsible for resistance to aminoglycosides. For this reason amikacin is active against most gentamicin- and tobramycin-resistant Gram-negative bacilli (Price *et al.*, 1976; 1977; Davies and Courvalin, 1977).

Amikacin is marketed as amikacin sulphate with the trade name of 'Amikin' (Bristol).

Sensitive Organisms

1. *Gram-negative bacteria.* Amikacin is active against all the Enterobacteriaceae such as Esch. coli, the Enterobacter, Klebsiella, all Proteus, Salmonella, Shigella, Providencia, Serratia, Citrobacter, Hafnia, Edwardsiella, Arizona and Yersinia spp. (Yu and Washington, 1973; Bodey and Stewart, 1973; Young and Hewitt, 1973; Reynolds *et al.*, 1974; Kawaguchi, 1976; Drasar *et al.*, 1976; Schiffman, 1977; Hammerberg *et al.*, 1977).

Pseudomonas aeruginosa is also amikacin-sensitive (Yu and Washington, 1973; Kawaguchi, 1976; Davies and Courvalin, 1977). Pseudomonas stutzeri and Ps. fluorescens are also usually susceptible, but Ps. maltophilia and Ps. cepacia are more commonly resistant (Yu and Washington, 1973; Price *et al.*, 1976; Moellering *et al.*, 1977).

Amikacin, like kanamycin (page 309) is quite active against Neisseria spp. (meningococci and gonococci) and H. influenzae (Phillips *et al.*, 1977). Pasteurella multocida is also susceptible (Yu and Washington, 1973). Acinetobacter calcoaceticus var. anitratus (Herellea vaginicola), Acinetobacter calcoaceticus var. lwoffi (Mima polymorpha), and the Alcaligenes spp. are usually amikacin-sensitive, but resistant strains do occur (Yu and Washington, 1973; Drasar *et al.*, 1976; Phillips *et al.*, 1977). Flavobacterium spp. are always amikacin-resistant (Drasar *et al.*, 1976). The Legionnaires' disease bacterium is sensitive to amikacin *in vitro* (Thornsberry *et al.*, 1978). Campylobacter fetus is also sensitive to the aminoglycosides, including amikacin (median MIC 0·8 μg per ml) (*see also* gentamicin, page 328).

Similar to other aminoglycosides (pages 309, 328), amikacin is inactive against Bacteroides fragilis and most other anaerobic Gram-negative bacteria. The uptake of aminoglycosides by bacteria is an active process requiring oxygen, which can not occur in anaerobic bacteria (Moellering, 1977).

2. *Activity against gentamicin- and tobramycin-resistant Gram-negative bacteria*. The most important feature of amikacin is that it remains active against most strains of the Enterobacteriaceae and also a considerable proportion of Ps. aeruginosa strains, which have acquired resistance to gentamicin and/or other aminoglycosides. Many surveys have shown that most gentamicin-resistant Enterobacteriaceae (>80 per cent) and a smaller percentage of gentamicin-resistant Ps. aeruginosa strains (25–85 per cent in different series) are amikacin-sensitive (Reynolds *et al.*, 1974; 1976; Price *et al.*, 1974; 1976; 1977; Kluge *et al.*, 1974; Meyer *et al.*, 1976; Houang and McKay-Ferguson, 1976; Drasar *et al.*, 1976; Acar *et al.*, 1976; Moellering *et al.*, 1977; Kantor and Norden, 1977; Seligman, 1978; Verbist *et al.*, 1978).

The resistance of Enterobacteriaceae and Ps. aeruginosa to aminoglycosides may be chromosomally determined, but usually it is due to the action of R plasmid-mediated enzymes on the antibiotic in the outer layers of the bacterial cell wall (page 20). These enzymes do not inactivate the antibiotic but inhibit its transport into the cell (Davies and Courvalin, 1977). Enzyme modification of aminoglycosides occurs by either acetylation, adenylylation or phosphorylation. Gram-negative bacteria produce at least nine different enzymes, but only one, aminoglycoside 6'-N-acetyltransferase or AAC (6'), is known to modify and determine resistance to amikacin in clinical isolates (Jacoby, 1974; Kawabe *et al.*, 1975; Davies and Courvalin, 1977). Amikacin's AHB side-chain (page 377) prevents its modification by the majority of the plasmid-coded enzymes that determine resistance to other antibiotics. By contrast to amikacin, six enzymes affect gentamicin and sisomicin, five affect kanamycin and tobramycin and four affect netilmicin (Price *et al.*, 1977). This greater resistance to enzymes produced by Gram-negative bacilli explains why many of these organisms, which are resistant to gentamicin and other aminoglycosides, are still amikacin-sensitive.

3. *Amikacin-resistant Gram-negative bacteria*. These have been detected in relatively small numbers; some of them may be naturally occurring and others have acquired resistance. Jauregui *et al.* (1977) in a ten months' survey of 4640 strains of Gram-negative bacilli in one general hospital detected 37 strains (0·8 per cent) which were amikacin-resistant. These isolates comprised Ps. aeruginosa (6), Ps. cepacia (13) other Pseudomonas spp. (1) Serratia marcescens (6) and other Enterobacteriaceae (11). Moellering *et al.* (1977) surveyed 46 000 isolates of Gram-negative bacilli during a two-year period in another large general hospital, and also found a small percentage of amikacin-resistant bacteria. The majority of these were Acinetobacter and Flavobacterium spp. and Ps. maltophilia (*see* page 377), but there were also amikacin-resistant strains of Ps. aeruginosa and most Enterobacteriaceae.

There have been a number of reports of the emergence of amikacin-resistant organisms during treatment. Over a two-year period in a burns centre a number of isolates of Esch. coli, Kl. pneumoniae and Ps. aeruginosa with increased resistance to gentamicin, tobramycin and amikacin appeared (Minshew *et al.*, 1977). In one patient with Ps. aeruginosa bronchopneumonia, an amikacin-resistant strain emerged after only four days treatment with the drug (Amirak *et al.*, 1977). Amikacin was used to treat 19 patients with gentamicin-resistant Serratia marcescens infections by Craven *et al.* (1977). In four patients with pneumonia or other deep tissue infections, in whom the infection failed to clear promptly, Serratia strains became increasingly resistant to amikacin during therapy, and contributed to their death in two. It therefore seems likely that amikacin-resistant Gram-negative bacilli will become more prevalent with increased clinical use.

Although amikacin can be modified by one of the R plasmid-mediated enzymes (*vide supra*), over 90 per cent of amikacin-resistant bacteria owe their resistance to a different mechanism, presumably due to an increase in the permeability barrier to the drug (page 10). This type of resistance does not appear to be plasmid-mediated and it is not transferable to antibiotic-sensitive cells. Amikacin-resistant Gram-negative bacilli are usually, but not invariably, resistant to all other aminoglycosides (Price *et al.*, 1977; Moellering *et al.*, 1977).

4. *Synergy with other drugs*. Amikacin combined with carbenicillin or ticarcillin acts synergistically against most strains of Ps. aeruginosa *in vitro* (Marks *et al.*, 1976; Kelly and Matsen, 1976; Yoshikawa and Shibata, 1978). Carbenicillin in sub-inhibitory concentrations also enhances the action of amikacin on Serratia marcescens, provided the MBC of carbenicillin for the strain is not higher than 2000 μg per ml (Pogwizd and Lerner, 1976). Combinations of cephalothin or cephazolin with amikacin act synergistically against most strains of Klebsiella spp. (D'Alessandri *et al.*, 1976; Klastersky *et al.*, 1976a). Trimethoprim together with amikacin acts synergistically against many strains of Kl. pneumoniae, Serratia marcescens and Esch. coli, but not against those of Ps. aeruginosa (Parsley *et al.*, 1977).

5. *Gram-positive bacteria*. Staph. pyogenes, including penicillin G-resistant and methicillin-resistant strains, is amikacin-sensitive. Staph. pyogenes strains resistant to amikacin have been detected; these contain an R plasmid-mediated amikacin modifying enzyme, 4-adenylytransferase (Davies and Courvalin, 1977). In addition, an amikacin 3'phosphorylating enzyme is present in many clinical isolates of Staph. pyogenes, but surprisingly these strains are sensitive to the drug (Courvalin and Davies, 1977). Gentamicin-resistant Staph. pyogenes strains (page 328) are usually amikacin-sensitive, but their MIC's for amikacin may be four- to eight-fold higher than those for fully susceptible strains (Vogel *et al.*, 1978).

Staph. epidermidis is sensitive, but other Gram-positive cocci such as Strep. pyogenes, Strep. pneumoniae and Strep. faecalis are resistant (Schiffman, 1977; Hewitt and Young, 1977). Unlike penicillin G/gentamicin (page 329) and penicillin G/tobramycin (page 361), the combination of penicillin G and amikacin does not act synergistically against all Strep. faecalis strains. In general, Strep. faecalis strains unaffected by penicillin G/kanamycin (page 310) also do not exhibit synergism with penicillin G and amikacin (Gutschik *et al.*, 1977; Basker *et al.*, 1977; Calderwood *et al.*, 1977).

Gram-positive anaerobic bacilli such as the Clostridium and Actinomyces spp. are amikacin-resistant. Nocardia asteroides is sensitive, most strains being inhibited by 1·0 μg per ml or less (Dalovisio and Pankey, 1978b).

6. *Mycobacteria.* Mycobacterium tuberculosis is amikacin-sensitive (Sanders *et al.*, 1976; Gangadharam and Candler, 1977). Approximately 50 per cent of M. fortuitum strains and also some M. chelonei strains are susceptible to clinically attainable amikacin concentrations (Sanders *et al.*, 1977; Dalovisio and Pankey, 1978a). Most other Mycobacteria such as M. marinum, M. intracellulare and M. kansasii are moderately or completely amikacin-resistant, their MIC's being usually higher than 12·8 μg per ml (Gangadharam and Candler, 1977).

In Vitro Sensitivities

The minimum inhibitory concentrations of amikacin against some selected bacterial species are shown in Table 26. The intrinsic activity of amikacin against kanamycin-sensitive strains is generally equal to or greater than that of kanamycin (page 310) (Kawaguchi, 1976). Against gentamicin-sensitive strains, amikacin is two or four times less active than gentamicin (page 330) (Yu and Washington, 1973; Bodey and Stewart, 1973; Annotation, 1975). The majority of Gram-negative bacilli which are resistant to kanamycin, gentamicin and tobramycin are amikacin-sensitive. However, their amikacin MIC's may be greater than those of bacteria which are also sensitive to gentamicin and tobramycin (Hewitt and Young, 1977).

TABLE 26
(After Kawaguchi, 1976)

ORGANISM	MIC (μg per ml)
Gram-negative bacteria	
Escherichia coli	1·6–3·1
Klebsiella spp.	1·6–3·1
Enterobacter spp.	1·6–6·3
Serratia marcescens	0·8–3·1
Proteus mirabilis	3·1
Proteus morganii	3·1
Proteus rettgeri	1·6
Proteus vulgaris	1·6
Providencia stuartii	0·8–3·1
Pseudomonas aeruginosa	1·6–12·5
Gram-positive bacteria	
Staphylococcus pyogenes	0·4–3·1
Streptococcus pyogenes	12·5
Streptococcus pneumoniae	12·5
Mycobacteria	
Mycobacterium tuberculosis (H$_{37}$R strain)	0·6

Mode of Administration and Dosage

Amikacin is not absorbed from the gastro-intestinal tract and it is administered by either the intramuscular or intravenous route.

1. *Intramuscular administration to adults.* The common dosage schedule of amikacin, similar to that of kanamycin (page 311) is 15 mg per kg body weight per day, administered in either two or three divided doses (Gooding *et al.*, 1976). The drug is usually given in a dose of 7·5 mg per kg administered at 12-hourly intervals, which for most adults is approximately 0·5 g every twelve hours. For the treatment of serious infections higher doses of 7·5–8·0 mg per kg every eight hours have been used (Smith *et al.*, 1977; Lau *et al.*, 1977a). If this higher dose is used, serum level monitoring is advisable. The relationship between amikacin serum levels and toxicity has not yet been well defined, but present evidence indicates that peak serum levels should not exceed 30 μg per ml and the concentrations which prevail just prior to the next dose (trough levels), should not exceed 10 μg per ml (Black *et al.*, 1976; Hewitt and Young, 1977; Lau *et al.*, 1977a).

2. *Intravenous administration to adults.* Amikacin can be administered intravenously in the same total daily dosage and at the same intervals, as recommended for the intramuscular route. Manufacturers currently recommend that each individual amikacin dose should be dissolved in 100 ml of intravenous fluid, which is then infused over 30 min via a paediatric buretrol or a secondary intravenous bottle. Most clinical investigators to date have used this method and have found it satisfactory (Smith *et al.*, 1977; Yu *et al.*, 1977; Lau *et al.*, 1977a; Trenholme *et al.*, 1977). The serum level just after a 30 min infusion of a standard 7·5 mg per kg dose is usually higher than the peak after the same intramuscular dose, but the level 30 min after the completion of the infusion approximates to the peak obtained from intramuscular dosing (page 383). For the purposes of serum level monitoring, blood is usually taken 30 min after the completion of the infusion, and the result regarded as the 'peak' serum level (Lau *et al.*, 1977a; Trenholme *et al.*, 1977).

Similar to other aminoglycosides (pages 332, 362), amikacin can also probably be given by rapid intravenous injections. Vogelstein *et al.* (1977) administered individual doses over a period of five minutes; during the first hour after injection serum levels usually exceeded 30 μg per ml, and during the first fifteen minutes they averaged 59·6 μg per ml. One hour after administration, the serum concentration approximated the peak serum level attained after an intramuscular injection of the same dose. The transiently high serum levels obtained with this method do not appear to be associated with toxicity.

3. *Children and adolescents.* As with kanamycin (page 311) and gentamicin (page 331), younger subjects excrete more amikacin in proportion to their body weight, because of their higher glomerular filtration of this drug. Vogelstein *et al.* (1977) studied 20 patients aged 4–16 years, and found that many required an amikacin dosage as high as 10 mg per kg every eight hours, to produce satisfactory serum levels. Patients with small weight-to-surface area ratios, such as the young and debilitated, needed 15 mg or occasionally even 20 mg per kg every eight hours. Because of these variable requirements of dosage within the same age group, the authors considered that dosage based on body weight is unreliable for children. Dosage based on surface area, however, was

more satisfactory. From their studies, Vogelstein *et al.* (1977) concluded that an amikacin dose of 420 mg per M^2 administered intravenously every eight hours resulted in therapeutic non-toxic serum levels, and there was no accumulation of the drug after four doses.

These recommendations should be regarded as tentative at this stage. Nevertheless, it seems advisable to use the higher doses recommended either intravenously or intramuscularly, with serum level monitoring, whenever severe infections are treated in children. For milder infections the usual dose of 7·5 mg per kg 12-hourly may suffice. In clinical trials to date, many children with moderate or even severe infections have responded to this lower amikacin dose (Khan *et al.*, 1976; Yow, 1977).

4. *Newborn and premature infants.* For these a dose of 7·5 mg per kg, administered intramuscularly or intravenously (as a 20–30 min infusion), every twelve hours is recommended. Infants with birth weights of more than 2000 g and who are also older than seven days may require this dose every eight hours (Howard and McCracken, 1975; McCracken and Nelson, 1977). Many factors such as hypoxaemia affect the serum half-life of amikacin in neonates, so that routine monitoring of serum levels is advisable (Myers *et al.*, 1977).

5. *Patients with renal failure.* Dosage should be reduced in a similar manner to kanamycin (page 311) for such patients. The simplest approximate dosage schedule assumes a linear relationship between amikacin's serum half-life and the patient's serum creatinine in mg per cent (for conversion of creatinine values from SI units, *see* gentamicin, page 333). Normal individual amikacin doses can be used, but the interval between doses (in hours) is extended to a value which is obtained by multiplying the normal dosage interval (in hours) by the patient's serum creatinine in mg per cent. Alternatively the intervals between doses may be left unchanged, but after the loading dose, subsequent maintenance doses are calculated by dividing the usual dose by the patient's creatinine in mg per cent. These two approaches can also be combined (*see* kanamycin, page 312).

If amikacin dosage is calculated by these methods, frequent monitoring of serum levels is necessary, otherwise considerable errors can occur. This is because the relationship between the drug's half-life and serum creatinine is not always linear (McHenry *et al.*, 1976). Particularly in older patients, the creatinine clearance (and therefore amikacin clearance) is often considerably reduced without a corresponding increase in serum creatinine. These patients may thereby be overdosed with amikacin using the above dosage schedule (Pijck *et al.*, 1976). This simple formula is also likely to be quite inaccurate in patients with acute or unstable renal failure (Leroy *et al.*, 1976). There is a much better linear relationship between the amikacin serum half-life and the rate of creatinine clearance (McHenry *et al.*, 1976). This can be used to calculate a more accurate dosage schedule for patients with renal failure. A loading dose of 7·5 mg per kg body weight is used, and thereafter maintenance doses are given at the usual dosage intervals. The maintenance dose is obtained by dividing the observed creatinine clearance in ml per min by the normal creatinine clearance in ml per min, and then multiplying this result by the value of the calculated loading dose in milligrams (Schiffman, 1977). A disadvantage of this method is the difficulty in estimating the creatinine clearance in acutely ill patients. More accurate dosage schedules can be obtained from nomograms based on the rate of creatinine clearance, as in the case of kanamycin (page 312) (Pijck *et al.*, 1976). Even with nomogram prescribing of amikacin in patients with renal failure, several variables remain (*see* gentamicin, page 333), and serum level monitoring is still advisable.

Amikacin, like kanamycin (page 312), is removed by haemodialysis, and during this procedure its half-life decreases to less than 10 per cent of the pre-treatment value. A satisfactory dose for anephric patients undergoing twice-weekly haemodialysis, is 5·0–7·5 mg per kg body weight administered intravenously immediately after each dialysis (Regeur *et al.*, 1977). Peritoneal dialysis is less effective in removing amikacin; its serum half-life may be decreased to about 30 per cent of the pre-treatment value, but this may vary according to other factors such as peritoneal inflammation (Madhavan *et al.*, 1976; Regeur *et al.*, 1977). Individual dosage adjustment with serum level monitoring is required in patients undergoing peritoneal dialysis.

6. *Intrathecal administration.* Amikacin has been administered intrathecally as a supplement to systemic therapy to treat meningitis in two adults caused by gentamicin-resistant Klebsiella spp. In one patient the daily intrathecal dose was 4 mg (Hamory *et al.*, 1976), and in the other it was 20 mg (Block *et al.*, 1977). Intrathecal therapy was well tolerated and appeared to contribute to the recovery of both patients. Amikacin can probably also be administered intraventricularly (*see* gentamicin, page 334).

Availability
Vials containing 100 mg, 500 mg or 1·0 g in solution.

Serum Levels in Relation to Dosage

1. *Intramuscular administration.* Serum levels of amikacin are very similar to those of kanamycin (page 314). After a 0·5 g intramuscular dose, a peak serum concentration of about 20 μg per ml is attained approximately one hour (range 0·75–2·0 h) later. Thereafter the level falls and is approximately 10 μg per ml at four hours, 4 μg per ml at eight hours, and it is usually undetectable in serum twelve hours after administration. The half-life of amikacin after intramuscular injection is approximately 2·3 h (Cabana and Taggart, 1973; Kirby *et al.*, 1976; Dittert, 1977).

2. *Intravenous administration.* Following a 0·5 g intravenous infusion of amikacin given over 30 min to adults, serum levels as high as 34–48 μg per ml are attained immediately after the infusion (Schiffman, 1977; Dittert, 1977). After the infusion, a short (0·5 h) distribution phase occurs in most patients, during which serum levels fall to 20–30 μg per ml, a value similar to the peak level attained after intramuscular dosing (*vide supra*). Thereafter the serum level declines in a similar manner to that after intramuscular administration, and at 12 h very little if any amikacin can be detected in the serum (Dittert, 1977). For purposes of serum level monitoring during therapy, blood for the 'peak' level estimation is usually taken 0·5 h after the cessation of a 30 min infusion, and blood for the 'trough' level is collected shortly before the next infusion (*see* page 381).

When 0·5 g dose of amikacin is administered to adults by rapid intravenous injection (over 2–5 min), transient high peaks of up to 60 μg per ml are attained during first 15 min. These rapidly fall to 20–30 μg per ml at one hour, a value similar to the peak level attained after intramuscular administration (*vide supra*). Subsequent serum concentrations fall more slowly in a manner similar to the decline, which occurs after intramuscular administration (Vogelstein *et al.*, 1977).

Excretion

Like kanamycin (page 315), amikacin is eliminated from the body almost entirely by the kidney in an active unchanged form. High concentrations of the active drug are attained in urine. It is excreted entirely by glomerular filtration, but the rate of renal clearance of creatinine is higher than that of either amikacin or kanamycin, indicating that these antibiotics undergo appreciable tubular reabsorption (Kirby *et al.*, 1976). In patients with normal renal function approximately 94 per cent of an administered dose is excreted in the urine within 24 h (Cabana and Taggart, 1973; Kirby *et al.*, 1976). With impaired renal function the half-life of the drug is increased progressively as renal function deteriorates. The normal half-life of 2·3 h may be prolonged to 44 h in patients with minimal renal function and to 86 h in anephric patients (Regeur *et al.*, 1977).

Distribution of the Drug in Body

Serum protein binding of amikacin like that of kanamycin (page 315) is minimal (3·6 per cent) (Kirby *et al.*, 1976). Amikacin does not penetrate into the CSF of patients with normal meninges (Briedis and Robson, 1978), and even in those with bacterial meningitis CSF levels are low when usual parenteral doses are given. Hamory *et al.* (1976) treated an adult patient with *Klebsiella* meningitis, with amikacin 7·5 mg per kg intramuscularly every twelve hours, and concentrations in the spinal fluid were consistently less than 0·6 μg per ml. Badri *et al.* (1977) found CSF levels of <0·4–3·8 μg per ml in six neonates with bacterial meningitis, who were treated by parenteral amikacin.

The apparent volume of distribution of amikacin is approximately 23 per cent of body volume or 30 per cent of total body weight, suggesting that it is distributed primarily in extracellular fluids (Cabana and Taggart, 1973; Kirby *et al.*, 1976; Schiffman, 1977). Amikacin diffuses well into normal human interstitial fluid, but concentrations are lower than simultaneous serum levels (Tan and Salstrom, 1977). Muscle and fat concentrations of amikacin were determined in 41 children after intramuscular administration of a dose of 7·5 mg per kg body weight (Daschner *et al.*, 1977). After 1·5 h the concentrations peaked in serum (mean 14·9 μg per ml), as well as in muscle (2·2 μg per g) and fat tissue (1·89 μg per g). Thereafter all these concentrations declined, but they exceeded 1·0 μg per g in muscle and fat for at least three and four hours respectively. Amikacin crosses the placenta. When a single intravenous injection of 7·5 mg per kg was given to women in labour, amikacin levels of 0·5–6·0 μg per ml were detected in cord blood. Three hours later the babies' serum levels of amikacin were two to ten times lower than the mothers' (Mazzei *et al.*, 1976).

In animals, amikacin penetrates well into the exudate of experimental sterile peritonitis, where its concentrations approximately equate with serum levels at the time (MacGregor, 1977). In other animal experiments low concentrations of the drug (0·4–5·0 μg per g) have been detected in most body tissues such as liver, heart, lung and muscle, but not in brain, after seven daily injections of the drug (Kornguth and Kunin, 1977). As with other aminoglycosides (pages 337, 365), the major site of antibiotic deposition is the kidney, particularly the renal cortex, where concentrations may exceed 100 μg per g. Reabsorption in the proximal tubule (page 384), the major portion of which is located in the cortex, may explain the accumulation of the drug in renal tubular cells (Kornguth and Kunin, 1977). This accumulation, as with other aminoglycosides, appears to be related to nephrotoxicity (page 386).

High kidney concentrations were also found in five patients who died during therapy with amikacin (Edwards et al., 1976). Concentrations ranged from 365 to 1030 μg per g in the renal cortex and from 270 to 718 μg per g in the medulla. Tissue levels were high in patients with both normal and abnormal renal function.

Mode of Action

This is probably similar to that of other aminoglycosides (see streptomycin, page 298).

Toxicity

1. *Ototoxicity*. This can occur and like kanamycin (page 316) amikacin causes predominantly cochlear damage, although vestibular dysfunction can also happen in some patients (Black et al., 1976).

In an analysis of the case records of 1548 patients who had been treated with amikacin, high frequency hearing loss occurred in 71 (4·59 per cent), and conversational hearing loss in another 8 patients (0·52 per cent). A further 10 patients (0·65 per cent) had some vestibular damage, which was usually mild (Lane et al., 1977). In 328 of these patients pre- and post-treatment audiograms could be evaluated. In 11 patients a hearing loss of 15 decibels or greater occurred at least at one frequency; all of these had received approximately twice as much amikacin as those without audiometric changes. In addition, 8 of the 11 patients (72·8 per cent) had received previous aminoglycoside therapy compared to only 34·1 per cent of the 317 patients without cochlear damage. Differences between the mean ages of these groups were not significant.

The ototoxicity produced by amikacin has been compared with that due to gentamicin (page 338) in clinical studies. Lau et al. (1977a) treated 157 leucopenic patients with suspected severe Gram-negative organism sepsis, randomly by either an amikacin/carbenicillin or a gentamicin/carbenicillin regimen. During 105 courses of amikacin therapy, some hearing loss was documented by pre- and post-treatment audiograms in 21 patients (20 per cent), but only one had clinical hearing loss. Significant audiogram changes were observed following 13 of 96 (13·6 per cent) courses of gentamicin therapy; four of these patients also had tinnitus, but major vestibular symptoms did not occur. Smith et al. (1977) also used amikacin or gentamicin randomly to treat 174 patients, 64 of whom were evaluated for auditory toxicity. The frequency of this was similar in both groups, hearing loss developing in 10 per cent of 30 patients receiving gentamicin and in six per cent of the 34 receiving amikacin. Two additional patients receiving amikacin noted transient tinnitus. These two clinical studies suggest that ototoxicity of amikacin is similar to that of gentamicin. As only audiograms were used to assess ototoxicity, early vestibular damage, which is more likely to occur with gentamicin, may have been overlooked in some patients.

In comparative experiments in animals, amikacin has been used in a dose five times greater than gentamicin, the dose ratio with which these antibiotics are used clinically. In such experiments amikacin selectively produced an impairment of cochlear function, and gentamicin an impairment of vestibular function with also a significant degree of concurrent cochlear damage. The cochlear ototoxicity produced by amikacin was similar in degree and appeared after the same duration of drug administration as the vestibular ototoxicity produced by gentamicin. It could be concluded that amikacin was selectively toxic to the cochlea at five times the dose of gentamicin which produced both vestibular and cochlear damage (Hottendorf, 1977; Christensen et al., 1977).

As deafness is a potentially much more disabling defect than vestibular dysfunction, amikacin, like kanamycin (page 316), is a potentially more toxic drug than gentamicin. There are also no warning symptoms of early amikacin cochlear toxicity, and the performing of serial audiograms is often not feasible. Fortunately it appears that the hearing loss caused by amikacin, unlike that due to neomycin (page 409), is usually not progressive once the drug is stopped (Black et al., 1976).

2. *Nephrotoxicity.* Amikacin can cause this side-effect, the clinical features of which are similar to those of gentamicin nephrotoxicity (page 339). In a review, 8·7 per cent of 1548 patients treated with amikacin developed changes consistent with impairment of renal function (Lane et al., 1977). These changes were more frequent in patients whose initial serum creatinine values were high, in older patients, in those receiving a larger total dose of amikacin and in those who had also received other nephrotoxic agents, either previously or concurrently.

The nephrotoxic potential of amikacin appears to be similar to that of gentamicin (Schiffman, 1977). In two randomized clinical studies the frequency of nephrotoxicity in amikacin-treated and gentamicin-treated patients was about the same (Smith et al., 1977; Lau et al., 1977a). Also when amikacin and gentamicin are administered to animals in a dose ratio of five to one, the ratio with which these drugs are used clinically, there is no difference between their nephrotoxicity (Hottendorf, 1977).

3. *Other side-effects.* These are infrequent and relatively unimportant. They include hypersensitivity reactions, nausea and vomiting, headache, drug fever, tremor, paraesthesiae, arthralgia, eosinophilia, anaemia and mild abnormalities in liver function tests (Gooding et al., 1976; Schiffman, 1977).

Clinical Uses of the Drug

At present amikacin should be regarded as a 'reserve drug', only for the treatment of serious aerobic Gram-negative bacillary infections caused by organisms which are resistant to gentamicin and other aminoglycosides (Schiffman, 1977). Amikacin is the aminoglycoside of choice for the initial emergency treatment of serious, presumably Gram-negative, bacillary sepsis in hospitals, or units, where gentamicin-resistant Enterobacteriaceae or Ps. aeruginosa are known to occur (Hewitt and Young, 1977). In these circumstances it is usually used in combination with cephalothin or carbenicillin.

Several controlled studies have shown that amikacin is equally effective to gentamicin or tobramycin for the treatment of serious Gram-negative infections caused by organisms susceptible to all three drugs. Lau et al. (1977a) treated 157 leucopenic patients who had fever and evidence of Gram-negative infection, randomly by either an amikacin/carbenicillin or a gentamicin/carbenicillin regimen. The overall clinical response rate was 75 per cent for both groups. Similarly Smith et al. (1977) used amikacin or gentamicin randomly to treat 174 patients with suspected severe Gram-negative infections. Enteric Gram-negative bacilli were subsequently isolated from 71 of these patients, 39 of whom were treated with amikacin and 32 with gentamicin. A favourable response was obtained in 77 per cent of all the patients treated with amikacin and in 78 per cent of those treated by gentamicin. Feld et al. (1977) compared amikacin and tobramycin in a randomized study of the treatment of serious infections in 175 cancer patients. An aetiological agent was isolated from 74 patients which in 59 (80 per cent) was a Gram-negative bacillus, usually either Kl. pneumoniae, Esch. coli or Ps. aeruginosa: in these confirmed infections, the response rate was 60 per cent for tobramycin and 64 per cent for amikacin.

Amikacin has also been compared with gentamicin for the treatment of adults with urinary tract infections. In two randomized studies gentamicin was used in standard doses of 3–4 mg per kg per day, but amikacin was used in a reduced dose of 9 mg per kg per day (Cox, 1976; Gilbert et al., 1977). Results of treatment using both drugs in these doses were essentially the same.

Amikacin has been used in many uncontrolled studies to treat various infections caused by gentamicin-sensitive Gram-negative rods. In general it has been about as effective as would be expected from a gentamicin regimen. Mathias et al. (1976) treated 42 patients many of whom had pyelonephritis and/or a septicaemia. Most patients responded well, but in four with chronic urinary tract infection, Ps. aeruginosa isolates acquired amikacin resistance during therapy. Amikacin has been used successfully in Gram-negative bacillary pneumonias (van der Straeten et al., 1976; Trenholme et al., 1977), bone and joint Gram-negative infections (Schurman and Wheeler, 1977) and in exacerbations of Ps. aeruginosa infections in children and adults with cystic fibrosis (Lau et al., 1977b). It has also been valuable for the treatment of severe Gram-negative organism sepsis in neonates, but further clinical studies are needed to determine its efficacy in neonatal meningitis (Badri et al., 1977).

Many clinical studies have documented the efficacy of amikacin for the treatment of septicaemia and other serious infections caused by gentamicin-resistant aerobic Gram-negative bacilli. This is the prime indication for amikacin therapy. Amikacin appears to be just as effective for these infections as it is for the treatment of similar infections caused by gentamicin-sensitive bacilli. There have been a number of reports of the successful treatment of patients with septicaemia caused by gentamicin-resistant Gram-negative

388   THE USE OF ANTIBIOTICS

organisms (Tally *et al.*, 1975; 1976; Pollock *et al.*, 1977; Yu *et al.*, 1977; Guerrant *et al.*, 1977; Meyer *et al.*, 1975; 1977; Tally and Gorbach, 1977; Lewis *et al.*, 1977). It has also been useful for treatment of septicaemia and other serious infections due to Gram-negative gentamicin-resistant bacilli, in patients with cancer and neutropenia (Valdivieso *et al.*, 1977). Pulmonary infections caused by drug resistant Gram-negative bacilli also usually respond to amikacin (Bartlett, 1977). However in one trial in which 19 patients with Serratia infections were treated, only one of eight patients with pneumonia or other deep tissue infections was cured. In four of these treatment failures Serratia strains became increasingly amikacin-resistant during therapy (Craven *et al.*, 1977). Urinary tract infections caused by gentamicin-resistant organisms usually respond well to amikacin (Sharp *et al.*, 1974; Daikos *et al.*, 1976; Craven *et al.*, 1977). In one study of urinary tract infections caused by gentamicin-resistant Klebsiella aerogenes, amikacin treatment proved to be superior to treatment with colistin (page 541) (Speller *et al.*, 1977).

Amikacin is valuable for the treatment of serious infections, caused by multi-resistant aerobic Gram-negative bacilli, in children of all ages including neonates (Yow, 1977).

For neutropenic cancer patients with presumed infection, empiric emergency chemotherapy is often necessary. Combinations of either amikacin/carbenicillin (Lau *et al.*, 1977a) or amikacin/cephalothin (Hahn *et al.*, 1977) have been used with success in such patients. One of these two combinations may be worth continuing after isolation of the organism, provided that the two drugs show *in vitro* synergism against it (Klastersky *et al.*, 1976b).

If amikacin is used for the emergency treatment of sepsis following large bowel surgery, where infection by both aerobic and anaerobic Gram-negative organisms is possible, it should be combined with either chloramphenicol (page 442), clindamycin (page 484) or metronidazole (page 771).

REFERENCES

Acar, J. F., Witchitz, J. L., Goldstein, F., Talbot, J. N. and Le Goffic, F. (1976), 'Susceptibility of aminoglycoside-resistant Gram-negative bacilli to amikacin: Delineation of individual resistance patterns', *J. Infect. Dis.* (Suppl.), **134**, 280.
Amirak, I. D., Williams, R. J., Noone, P. and Wills, M. R. (1977), 'Amikacin resistance developing in a patient with Pseudomonas aeruginosa bronchopneumonia', *Lancet*, **1**, 537.
Annotation (1975), 'Amikacin', *Lancet*, **2**, 804.
Badri, M. D., Boysen, B. E., Chiu, T. W., Garrison, R. D. and Ayoub, E. M. (1977), 'Amikacin in neonatal infections, evaluation of efficacy and toxicity', *Amer. J. Med.*, **62** (Suppl.), US Amikacin Symposium, p. 172.
Bartlett, J. G. (1977), 'Amikacin treatment of pulmonary infections involving gentamicin-resistant Gram-negative bacilli', *Amer. J. Med.*, **62** (Suppl.), US Amikacin Symposium, p. 151.
Basker, M. J., Slocombe, B. and Sutherland, R. (1977), 'Aminoglycoside-resistant enterococci', *J. clin. Path.*, **30**, 375.
Black, R. E., Lau, W. K., Weinstein, R. J., Young, L. S. and Hewitt, W. L. (1976), 'Ototoxicity of Amikacin', *Antimicrob. Ag. Chemother.*, **9**, 956.
Block, C. S., Cassel, R., Koornhof, H. J. and Robinson, R. G. (1977), 'Klebsiella meningitis treated with intrathecal amikacin,' *Lancet*, **1**, 1371.

Bodey, G. P. and Stewart, D. (1973), '*In vitro* studies of BB-K8, a new aminoglycoside antibiotic', *Antimicrob. Ag. Chemother.*, **4**, 186.

Briedis, D. J. and Robson, H. G. (1978), 'Cerebrospinal fluid penetration of amikacin', *Antimicrob. Ag. Chemother.*, **13**, 1042.

Cabana, B. E. and Taggart, J. G. (1973), 'Comparative pharmacokinetics of BB-K8 and kanamycin in dogs and humans', *Antimicrob. Ag. Chemother.*, **3**, 478.

Calderwood, S. A., Wennersten, C., Moellering, R. C., Jr., Kunz, L. J. and Krogstad, D. J. (1977), 'Resistance of six aminoglycosidic aminocyclitol antibiotics among enterococci: Prevalence evolution and relationship to syngergism with penicillin', *Antimicrob. Ag. Chemother.*, **12**, 401.

Christensen, E. F., Reiffenstein, J. C. and Madissoo, H. (1977), 'Comparative ototoxicity of amikacin and gentamicin in cats', *Antimicrob. Ag. Chemother.*, **12**, 178.

Courvalin, P. and Davies, J. (1977), 'Plasmid mediated aminoglycoside phosphotransferase of broad substrate range that phosphorylates amikacin', *Antimicrob. Ag. Chemother.*, **11**, 619.

Cox, C. E. (1976), 'Amikacin therapy of urinary tract infections', *J. Infect. Dis.* (Suppl.), **134**, 362.

Craven, P. C., Jorgensen, J. H., Kaspar, R. L. and Drutz, D. J. (1977), 'Amikacin therapy of patients with multiply antibiotic-resistant Serratia marcescens infections. Development of increasing resistance during therapy', *Amer. J. Med.*, **62** (Suppl.), US Amikacin Symposium, p. 66.

Daikos, G. K., Kosmidis, J. C., Hamilton-Miller, J. M. T. and Brumfitt, W. (1976), 'Amikacin in treatment of infections caused by Gram-negative bacteria resistant to gentamicin and other aminoglycosides: Clinical and bacteriologic results', *J. Infect. Dis.* (Suppl.), **134**, 286.

D'Alessandri, R. M., McNeely, D. J. and Kluge, R. M. (1976), 'Antibiotic synergy and antagonism against clinical isolates of Klebsiella species', *Antimicrob. Ag. Chemother.*, **10**, 889.

Dalovisio, J. R. and Pankey, G. A. (1978a), '*In vitro* susceptibility of Mycobacterium fortuitum and Mycobacterium chelonei to amikacin', *J. Infect. Dis.*, **137**, 318.

Dalovisio, J. R. and Pankey, G. A. (1978b), '*In vitro* susceptibility of Nocardia asteroides to amikacin', *Antimicrob. Ag. Chemother.*, **13**, 128.

Daschner, F., Reiss, E. and Engert, J. (1977), 'Distribution of amikacin in serum, muscle, and fat in children after a single intramuscular injection', *Antimicrob. Ag. Chemother.*, **11**, 1081.

Davies, J. and Courvalin, P. (1977), 'Mechanisms of resistance to aminoglycosides', *Amer. J. Med.*, **62** (Suppl.), US Amikacin Symposium, p. 25.

Dittert, L. W. (1977), 'Pharmacokinetics of aminoglycosides: General considerations', *Amer. J. Med.*, **62** (Suppl.), US Amikacin Symposium, p. 77.

Drasar, F. A., Farrell, W., Maskell, J. and Williams, J. D. (1976), 'Tobramycin amikacin, sisomicin and gentamicin-resistant Gram-negative rods', *Brit. med. J.*, **2**, 1284.

Edwards, C. Q., Smith, C. R., Baughman, K. L., Rogers, J. F. and Lietman, P. S. (1976), 'Concentrations of gentamicin and amikacin in human kidneys', *Antimicrob. Ag. Chemother.*, **9**, 925.

Feld, R., Valdivieso, M., Bodey, G. P. and Rodriguez, V. (1977), 'Comparison of amikacin and tobramycin in the treatment of infection in patients with cancer', *J. Infect. Dis.*, **135**, 61.

Gangadharam, P. R. J. and Candler, E. R. (1977), '*In vitro* anti-mycobacterial activity of some new aminoglycoside antibiotics', *Tubercle*, **58**, 35.

Gilbert, D. N., Eubanks, N. and Jackson, J. (1977), 'Comparison of amikacin and gentamicin in the treatment of urinary tract infections', *Amer. J. Med.*, **62** (Suppl.), US Amikacin Symposium, p. 121.

Gooding, P. G., Berman, E., Lane, A. Z. and Agre, K. (1976), 'A review of results of clinical trials with amikacin', *J. Infect. Dis.* (Suppl.), **134**, 441.

Guerrant, R. L., Strausbaugh, L. J., Wenzel, R. P., Hamory, B. H. and Sande, M. A. (1977), 'Nosocomial bloodstream infections caused by gentamicin-resistant Gram-negative bacilli', *Amer. J. Med.*, **62** (Suppl.), US Amikacin Symposium, p. 58.

Gutschik, E., Jepsen, O. B. and Mortensen, I. (1977), 'Effect of combinations of penicillin and aminoglycosides on Streptococcus faecalis: A comparative study of seven aminoglycoside antibiotics', *J. Infect. Dis.*, **135**, 832.

Hahn, D. M., Schimpff, S. C., Young, V. M., Fortner, C. L., Standiford, H. C. and Wiernick, P. H. (1977), 'Amikacin and cephalothin: Empiric regimen for granulocytopenic cancer patients', *Antimicrob. Ag. Chemother.*, **12**, 618.

Hammerberg, S., Sorger, S. and Marks, M. I. (1977), 'Antimicrobial susceptibilities of Yersinia enterocolitica biotype 4, serotype 0:3', *Antimicrob. Ag. Chemother.*, **11**, 566.

Hamory, B., Ignatiadis, P. and Sande, M. A. (1976), 'Intrathecal amikacin administration. Use in the treatment of gentamicin-resistant Klebsiella pneumoniae meningitis', *JAMA*, **236**, 1973.

Hewitt, W. L. and Young, L. S. (1977), 'Symposium perspective', *Amer. J. Med.*, **62** (Suppl.), US Amikacin Symposium, p. 1.

Hottendorf, G. H. (1977), 'Comparative ototoxicity (cats) and nephrotoxicity (rats) of amikacin and gentamicin', *Amer. J. Med.*, **62** (Suppl.), US Amikacin Symposium, p. 97.

Houang, E. T. and McKay-Ferguson, E. (1976), 'Activities of tobramycin and amikacin against gentamicin-resistant Gram-negative bacilli', *Lancet*, **1**, 423.

Howard, J. B. and McCracken, G. H., Jr. (1975), 'Pharmacological evaluation of amikacin in neonates', *Antimicrob. Ag. Chemother.*, **8**, 86.

Huang, N. N., Laraya-Cuasay, L. R., Yasmin, N., Keith, H. H., Borden, M. and Cundy, K. R. (1977), 'Clinical experience with amikacin in patients with cystic fibrosis', *Amer. J. Med.*, **62** (Suppl.), US Amikacin Symposium, p. 186.

Jacoby, G. A. (1974), 'Properties of an R plasmid in Pseudomonas aeruginosa producing amikacin (BB-K8), butirosin, kanamycin, tobramycin and sisomicin resistance', *Antimicrob. Ag. Chemother.*, **6**, 807.

Jauregui, L., Cushing, R. D. and Lerner, A. M. (1977), 'Gentamicin/amikacin resistant Gram-negative bacilli at Detroit General Hospital, 1975–1976', *Amer. J. Med.*, **62** (Suppl.), US Amikacin Symposium, p. 39.

Kantor, R. J. and Norden, C. W. (1977), '*In vitro* activity of netilmicin, gentamicin, and amikacin', *Antimicrob. Ag. Chemother.*, **11**, 126.

Kawabe, H., Kondo, S., Umezawa, H. and Mitsuhashi, S. (1975), 'R factor-mediated aminoglycoside antibiotic resistance in Pseudomonas aeruginosa: A new aminoglycoside 6'-N-acetyltransferase', *Antimicrob. Ag. Chemother.*, **7**, 494.

Kawaguchi, H. (1976), 'Discovery, chemistry, and activity of amikacin', *J. Infect. Dis.* (Suppl.), **134**, 242.

Kelly, M. T. and Matsen, J. M. (1976), '*In vitro* activity, syngergism, and testing parameters of amikacin, with comparisons to other aminoglycoside antibiotics', *Antimicrob. Ag. Chemother.*, **9**, 440.

Khan, A. J., Evans, H. E., Jhaveri, R., Chang, C. T. and Hochstein, L. (1976), 'Amikacin pharmacokinetics in the therapy of childhood urinary tract infections', *Pediatrics*, **58**, 873.

Kirby, W. M. M., Clarke, J. T., Libke, R. D. and Regamey, C. (1976), 'Clinical pharmacology of amikacin and kanamycin', *J. Infect. Dis.* (Suppl.), **134**, 312.

Klastersky, J., Meunier-Carpenter, F., Prevost, J. M. and Staquet, M. (1976a), 'Syngerism between amikacin and cefazolin against Klebsiella: *In vitro* studies and effect on the bactericidal activity of serum', *J. Infect. Dis.*, **134**, 271.

Klastersky, J., Hensgens, C. and Meunier-Carpenter, F. (1976b), 'Comparative effectiveness of combinations of amikacin with penicillin G and amikacin with carbenicillin in Gram-negative septicaemia: Double-blind clinical trial', *J. Infect. Dis.* (Suppl.), **134**, 433.

Kluge, R. M., Standiford, H. C., Tatem, B., Young, V. M., Greene, W. H., Schimpff, S. C., Calia, F. M. and Hornick, R. B. (1974), 'Comparative activity of tobramycin, amikacin, and gentamicin alone and with carbenicillin against Pseudomonas aeruginosa', *Antimicrob. Ag. Chemother.*, **6**, 442.

Kornguth, M. L. and Kunin, C. M. (1977), 'Distribution of gentamicin and amikacin in rabbit tissues', *Antimicrob. Ag. Chemother.*, **11**, 974.

Lane, A. Z., Wright, G. E. and Blair, D. C. (1977), 'Ototoxicity and nephrotoxicity of amikacin. An overview of Phase 11 and Phase 111 experience in the United States', *Amer. J. Med.*, **62** (Suppl.), US Amikacin Symposium, p. 105.

Lau, W. K., Young, L. S., Black, R. E., Winston, D. J., Linne, S. R., Weinstein, R. J. and Hewitt, W. L. (1977a), 'Comparative efficacy and toxicity of amikacin/carbenicillin versus gentamicin/carbenicillin in leukopenic patients. A randomized prospective trial', *Amer. J. Med.*, **62** (Suppl.), US Amikacin Symposium, p. 212.

Lau, W. K., Young, L. S., Osher, A. B. and Dooley, R. R. (1977b), 'Amikacin therapy of exacerbations of Pseudomonas aeruginosa infections in patients with cystic fibrosis', *Pediatrics*, **60**, 372.

Leroy, A., Humbert, G., Oksenhendler, G. and Fillastre, J. P. (1976), 'Comparative pharmacokinetics of lividomycin, amikacin and sisomicin in normal subjects and in uraemic patients', *J. Antimicrob. Chemother.*, **2**, 373.

Lewis, R. P., Meyer, R. D. and Finegold, S. M. (1977), 'Amikacin therapy of patients with gentamicin-resistant Gram-negative bacillary infection', *Amer. J. Med.*, **62** (Suppl.), US Amikacin Symposium, p. 142.

McCracken, G. M., Jr. and Nelson, J. D. (1977), *Antimicrobial Therapy for Newborns. Practical Application of Pharmacology to Clinical Usage*, Grune and Stratton, New York, San Francisco, London, p. 41.

MacGregor, R. R. (1977), 'Comparative penetration of amikacin, gentamicin, and penicillin G into exudate fluid in experimental sterile peritonitis', *Antimicrob. Ag. Chemother.*, **11**, 110.

McHenry, M. C., Wagner, J. G., Hall, P. M., Vidt, D. G. and Gavan, T. L. (1976), 'Pharmacokinetics of amikacin in patients with impaired renal function', *J. Infect. Dis.* (Suppl.), **134**, 343.

Madhavan, T., Yaremchuk, K., Levin, N., Pohlod, D., Burch, K., Fisher, E., Cox, F. and Quinn, E. L. (1976), 'Effect of renal failure and dialysis on the serum concentration of the aminoglycoside amikacin', *Antimicrob. Ag. Chemother.*, **10**, 464.

Marks, M. I., Hammerberg, S., Greenstone, G. and Silver, B. (1976), 'Activity of newer aminoglycosides and carbenicillin, alone and in combination, against gentamicin-resistant Pseudomonas aeruginosa', *Antimicrob. Ag. Chemother.*, **10**, 399.

Mathias, R. G., Ronald, A. R., Gurwith, M. J., McCullough, D. W., Stiver, H. G., Berger, J., Cates, C. Y., Fox, L. M. and Lank, B. A. (1976), 'Clinical evaluation of amikacin in treatment of infections due to Gram-negative aerobic bacilli', *J. Infect. Dis.* (Suppl.), **134**, 394.

Mazzei, T., Paradiso, M., Nicoletti, I. and Periti, P. (1976), 'Amikacin in obstetric, gynaecologic, and neonatal infections: Laboratory and clinical studies', *J. Infect. Dis.* (Suppl.), **134**, 374.

Meyer, R. D., Lewis, R. P., Carmalt, E. D. and Finegold, S. M. (1975), 'Amikacin therapy for serious Gram-negative bacillary infections', *Ann. Intern. Med.*, **83**, 790.

Meyer, R. D., Lewis, R. P., Halter, J. and White, M. (1976), 'Gentamicin-resistant Pseudomonas aeruginosa and Serratia marcescens in a general hospital', *Lancet*, **1**, 580.

Meyer, R. D., Lewis, R. P. and Finegold, S. M. (1977), 'Amikacin therapy for Gram-negative septicaemia', *Amer. J. Med.*, **62** (Suppl.), US Amikacin Symposium, p. 127.

Minshew, B. H., Pollock, H. M., Schoenknecht, F. D. and Sherris, J. C. (1977), 'Emergence in a burn center of populations of bacteria resistant to gentamicin, tobramycin and amikacin: Evidence for the need for changes in zone diameter interpretive standards', *Antimicrob. Ag. Chemother.*, **12**, 688.

Moellering, R. C., Jr., Wennersten, C., Kunz, L. J. and Poitras, J. W. (1977), 'Resistance to gentamicin, tobramycin and amikacin among clinical isolates of bacteria', *Amer. J. Med.*, **62** (Suppl.), US Amikacin Symposium, p. 30.

Moellering, R. C., Jr. (1977), 'Microbiological considerations in the use of tobramycin and related aminoglycosidic aminocyclitol antibiotics', *Med. J. Aust.* (Suppl.), **2**, 4.

Myers, M. G., Roberts, R. J. and Mirhij, N. J. (1977), 'Effects of gestational age, birth weight and hypoxemia on pharmacokinetics of amikacin in serum of infants', *Antimicrob. Ag. Chemother.*, **11**, 1027.

Parsley, T. L., Provonchee, R. B., Glicksman, C. and Zinner, S. H. (1977), 'Synergistic activity of trimethoprim and amikacin against Gram-negative bacilli', *Antimicrob. Ag. Chemother.*, **12**, 349.

Phillips, I., Eykyn, S., King, B. A., Jenkins, C., Warren, C. A. and Shannon, K. P. (1977), 'The *in vitro* antibacterial activity of nine aminoglycosides and spectinomycin on clinical isolates of common Gram-negative bacteria', *J. Antimicrob. Chemother.*, **3**, 403.

Pijck, J., Hallynck, T., Soep, H., Baert, L., Daneels, R. and Boelaert, J. (1976), 'Pharmacokinetics of amikacin in patients with renal insufficiency: relation to half-life and creatinine clearance', *J. Infect. Dis.* (Suppl.), **134**, 331.

Pogwizd, S. M. and Lerner, S. A. (1976), '*In vitro* activity of gentamicin, amikacin and netilmicin alone and in combination with carbenicillin against Serratia marcescens', *Antimicrob. Ag. Chemother.*, **10**, 878.

Pollock, A. A., Berger, S. A., Richmond, A. S., Simberkoff, M. S. and Rahal, J. J., Jr. (1977), 'Amikacin therapy for serious Gram-negative infection', *JAMA*, **237**, 562.

Price, K. E., Pursiano, T. A., De Furia, M. D. and Wright, G. E. (1974), 'Activity of BB-KB (amikacin) against clinical isolates resistant to one or more aminoglycoside antibiotics', *Antimicrob. Ag. Chemother.*, **5**, 143.

Price, K. E., De Furia, M. D. and Pursiano, T. A. (1976), 'Amikacin, an aminoglycoside with marked activity against antibiotic-resistant clinical isolates', *J. Infect. Dis.* (Suppl.), **134**, 249.

Price, K. E., Casson, K., De Regis, R. G., Kresel, P. A., Pursianto, T. A. and Leitner, F. (1977), 'Amikacin: Antimicrobial properties and resistance mechanisms affecting its activity', *Amer. J. Med.*, **62** (Suppl.), US Amikacin Symposium, p. 14.

Reguer, L., Colding, H., Jensen, H. and Kampmann, J. P. (1977), 'Pharmacokinetics of amikacin during hemodialysis and peritoneal dialysis', *Antimicrob. Ag. Chemother.*, **11**, 214.

Reynolds, A. V., Hamilton-Miller, J. M. T. and Brumfitt, W. (1974), 'Newer aminoglycosides-amikacin and tobramycin: An *in vitro* comparison with kanamycin and gentamicin', *Brit. med. J.*, **3**, 778.

Reynolds, A. V., Hamilton-Miller, J. M. T. and Brumfitt, W. (1976), '*In vitro* activity of amikacin and ten other aminoglycoside antibiotics against gentamicin-resistant bacterial strains', *J. Infect. Dis.* (Suppl.), **134**, 291.

Ries, K., Levison, M. E. and Kaye, D. (1973), '*In vitro* evaluation of a new aminoglycoside derivative of kanamycin, a comparison with tobramycin and gentamicin', *Antimicrob. Ag. Chemother.*, **3**, 532.

Sanders, W. E., Jr., Cacciatore, R., Valdex, H., Schneider, N. and Hartwig, C. (1976), 'Activity of amikacin against mycobacteria *in vitro* and in experimental infections with M. tuberculosis', *Amer. Rev. Resp. Dis.* (Suppl.), **113**, 59.

Sanders, W. E., Jr., Hartwig, E. C., Schneider, N. J., Cacciatore, R. and Valdez, H. (1977), 'Susceptibility of organisms in the Mycobacterium fortuitum complex to antituberculous and other antimicrobial agents', *Antimicrob. Ag. Chemother.*, **12**, 295.

Schiffman, D. O. (1977), 'Evaluation of amikacin sulfate (amikin). A new aminoglycoside antibiotic', *JAMA*, **238**, 1547.

Schurman, D. J. and Wheeler, R. (1977), 'Bone and joint Gram-negative infection and amikacin treatment', *Amer. J. Med.*, **62** (Suppl.), US Amikacin Symposium, p. 160.

Seligman, S. J. (1978), 'Frequency of resistance to kanamycin, tobramycin, netilmicin and amikacin in gentamicin-resistant Gram-negative bacteria', *Antimicrob. Ag. Chemother.*, **13**, 70.

Sharp, P. M., Saenz, C. A. and Martin, R. R. (1974), 'Amikacin (BB-KB) treatment of multiple-drug-resistant Proteus infections', *Antimicrob. Ag. Chemother.*, **5**, 435.

Smith, C. R., Baughman, K. L., Edwards, C. Q., Rogers, J. F. and Lietman, P. S. (1977), 'Controlled comparison of amikacin and gentamicin', *New Engl. J. Med.*, **296**, 349.

Speller, D. C. E., Bint, A. J. and Stephens, M. (1977), 'Experience with amikacin and colistin in an outbreak of infection by resistant Klebsiella aerogenes', *J. Antimicrob. Chemother.*, **3**, 483.

Tally, F. P., Louie, T. J., Weinstein, W. M., Bartlett, J. G. and Gorbach, S. L. (1975), 'Amikacin therapy for severe Gram-negative sepsis. Emphasis on infections with gentamicin-resistant organisms', *Ann. Intern. Med.*, **83**, 484.

Tally, F. P., Louie, T. J., O'Keefe, J. P., Gorbach, S. L. and Bartlett, J. G. (1976), 'Amikacin therapy for severe Gram-negative sepsis: efficacy in infections involving gentamicin-resistant organisms', *J. Infect. Dis.* (Suppl.), **134**, 428.

Tally, F. P. and Gorbach, S. L. (1977), 'Review of 152 patients with bacteremias treated with amikacin', *Amer. J. Med.*, **62** (Suppl.), US Amikacin Symposium, p. 137.

Tan, J. S. and Salstrom, S. J. (1977), 'Levels of carbenicillin, ticarcillin, cephalothin, cefazolin, cefamandole, gentamicin, tobramycin and amikacin in human serum and interstitial fluid', *Antimicrob. Ag. Chemother.*, **11**, 698.

Thornsberry, C., Baker, C. N. and Kirven, L. A. (1978), '*In vitro* activity of antimicrobial agents on Legionnaires' disease bacterium', *Antimicrob. Ag. Chemother.*, **13**, 78.

Trenholme, G. M., McKellar, P. P., Rivera, N. and Levin, S. (1977), 'Amikacin in the treatment of Gram-negative pneumonia', *Amer. J. Med.*, **62** (Suppl.), US Amikacin Symposium, p. 155.

Valdivieso, M., Keating, M. J., Feld, R., Rodriguez, V. and Bodey, G. P. (1977), 'Review of experience with amikacin and other aminoglycoside antibiotics in the treatment of infectious complications in patients with cancer', *Amer. J. Med.*, **62** (Suppl.), US Amikacin Symposium, p. 204.

Van Der Straeten, M., Pauwels, R., Pijck, J., Van Nimmen, L., Kluyskens, P. and Soep, H. (1976), 'Amikacin in the treatment of Gram-negative bronchopulmonary infections', *J. Infect. Dis.* (Suppl.), **134**, 391.

Verbist, L., Vandepitte, J. and Vandeven, J. (1978), 'Activity of eight aminoglycosides against isolates of Serratia marcescens from four hospitals', *J. Antimicrob. Chemother.*, **4**, 47.

Vogel, L., Nathan, C., Sweeney, H. M., Kabins, S. A. and Cohen, S. (1978), 'Infections due to gentamicin-resistant Staphylococcus aureus strain in a nursery for neonatal infants', *Antimicrob. Ag. Chemother.*, **13**, 466.

Vogelstein, B., Kowarski, A. A. and Lietman, P. S. (1977), 'The pharmacokinetics of amikacin in children', *J. Pediatrics*, **91**, 333.

Yoshikawa, T. T. and Shibata, S. A. (1978), '*In vitro* antibacterial activity of amikacin and ticarcillin, alone and in combination, against Pseudomonas aeruginosa', *Antimicrob. Ag. Chemother.*, **13**, 997.

Young, L. S. and Hewitt, W. L. (1973), 'Activity of five aminoglycoside antibiotics *in vitro* against Gram-negative bacilli and Staphylococcus aureus', *Antimicrob. Ag.*

Chemother., **4**, 617.

Yow, M. D. (1977), 'An overview of pediatric experience with amikacin', *Amer. J. Med.*, **62** (Suppl.), US Amikacin Symposium, p. 167.

Yu, V. L., Rhame, F. S., Pesanti, E. L. and Axline, S. G. (1977), 'Amikacin therapy. Use against infections caused by gentamicin- and tobramycin-resistant organisms', *JAMA*, **238**, 943.

Yu, P. K. W. and Washington, J. A., 11 (1973), 'Comparative *in vitro* activity of three aminoglycosidic antibiotics: BB-K8, kanamycin and gentamicin', *Antimicrob. Ag. Chemother.*, **4**, 133.

Sisomicin and Netilmicin

Description

1. *Sisomicin*. This aminoglycoside is produced by Micromonospora inyoensis (Waitz *et al.*, 1972; Crowe and Sanders, 1973). In its antimicrobial spectrum and all other properties, it is very similar to gentamicin (page 325). Some investigators have reported that sisomicin is slightly more active than gentamicin against some Gram-negative bacilli, particularly Klebsiella and indole-positive Proteus spp. and Ps. aeruginosa (Crowe and Sanders, 1973; Hyams *et al.*, 1973; Meyers *et al.*, 1975). Others have found that gentamicin is slightly more active against all Gram-negative bacilli, except for Ps. aeruginosa (Drasar *et al.*, 1976; Phillips *et al.*, 1977a). Sisomicin is not as active as tobramycin (page 359) against Ps. aeruginosa (Levison and Kaye, 1974; Phillips *et al.*, 1977a).

There appears to be almost complete cross-resistance between gentamicin and sisomicin, most gentamicin-resistant Gram-negative bacilli being also sisomicin-resistant (Young and Hewitt, 1973; Meyer *et al.*, 1976; Drasar *et al.*, 1976; Flournoy, 1976; Verbist *et al.*, 1978). The probable reason for this is that sisomicin, like gentamicin, is affected by six of the nine R plasmid coded enzymes, which can be produced by Gram-negative bacteria (page 378) (O'Hara *et al.*, 1974).

Sisomicin does not offer any advantages over gentamicin, and it will probably not have a wide clinical usage. It has had limited clinical trials, and it is available commercially in Europe, but not in Australia, Britain and the United States. The dosage of sisomicin (3–6 mg per kg per day), its methods of administration and pharmacokinetics are similar to those of gentamicin (page 330) (Rodriguez *et al.*, 1975; Lode *et al.*, 1975; Pechere *et al.*, 1976; Leroy *et al.*, 1976). The toxicity of these two drugs is also probably about the same (Brummett *et al.*, 1978). Results of treatment of conditions such as urinary tract infections or Gram-negative organism septicaemias have in general been similar to what would be expected from an identical gentamicin regimen (Klastersky *et al.*, 1975; Makris *et al.*, 1978).

2. *Netilmicin* (*Sch 20569*). This newer aminoglycoside antibiotic is a semisynthetic derivative of sisomicin (*vide supra*), developed by the Schering Corporation. It is derived by ethylation of the 1-N position of the deoxystreptamine ring of sisomicin (Kabins *et al.*, 1976; Rahal *et al.*, 1976; Dhawan *et al.*, 1977). Netilmicin also has a similar *in vitro* antibacterial spectrum to that of gentamicin (page 325), but unlike sisomicin, it is active against a proportion of gentamicin-resistant Gram-negative bacilli (Miller *et al.*, 1976; Kabins *et al.*, 1976). While six of the nine R plasmid-mediated enzymes produced by Gram-negative bacilli affect gentamicin and sisomicin, netilmicin is only affected by

four (page 378). Netilmicin is mainly active against those gentamicin-resistant Gram-negative bacilli, which possess aminoglycoside adenylylating enzymes. It is ineffective against strains, some of which are sensitive to amikacin (page 378), which produce aminoglycoside acetylating enzymes (Kabins *et al.*, 1976; Miller *et al.*, 1976). Therefore netilmicin is not active against such a wide range of gentamicin-resistant Gram-negative bacilli as amikacin (page 378). Nevertheless, it may be indicated on occasions as an alternative to amikacin for the treatment of some infections caused by gentamicin-resistant but netilmicin-sensitive Gram-negative organisms.

The following details apply to netilmicin only.

Sensitive Organisms

1. *Gram-negative bacteria.* Netilmicin, like gentamicin (page 325), is active against all the Enterobacteriaceae such as Esch. coli, the Enterobacter, Klebsiella, all Proteus, Salmonella, Shigella, Providencia, Serratia, Citrobacter, Hafnia, Edwardsiella, Arizona and Yersinia spp. (Briedis and Robson, 1976; Eickhoff and Ehret, 1977; Chadwick *et al.*, 1977; Smith *et al.*, 1977; Hammerberg *et al.*, 1977). In general its effectiveness against gentamicin-susceptible strains of the Enterobacteriaceae appears to be roughly similar to that of gentamicin. However gentamicin is more active against Serratia spp. (Klastersky *et al.*, 1977; Eickhoff and Ehret, 1977; Kantor and Norden, 1977).

Pseudomonas aeruginosa is also netilmicin-sensitive, but most strains are approximately two-fold less sensitive than to gentamicin (Brown *et al.*, 1976; Smith *et al.*, 1977; Eickhoff and Ehret, 1977). Netilmicin, like gentamicin, is active against the Neisseria spp. (meningococci and gonococci) and H. influenzae (Eickhoff and Ehret, 1977). Acinetobacter spp. may be netilmicin-sensitive, but resistant strains occur (Meyers and Hirschman, 1977; Phillips *et al.*, 1977b).

In common with other aminoglycosides (pages 328, 360), netilmicin is inactive against Bacteroides fragilis and most other anaerobic Gram-negative bacteria.

2. *Gentamicin-resistant Gram-negative bacteria.* The most important feature of netilmicin is its activity against a percentage of strains of Enterobacteriaceae and also some strains of Ps. aeruginosa with acquired resistance to gentamicin and/or other aminoglycosides (Stewart *et al.*, 1977; Meyers and Hirschman, 1977; Kantor and Norden, 1977). Compared to amikacin, netilmicin is not active against as high a percentage of individual species strains, or as wide a range of gentamicin-resistant Gram-negative bacilli (Kantor and Norden, 1977; Seligman, 1978). This is due to its greater susceptibility to aminoglycoside-modifying enzymes (pages 378, 395).

Gentamicin-resistant strains of Esch. coli, Proteus mirabilis and the Enterobacter, Klebsiella, Citrobacter and Serratia spp. are usually netilmicin-sensitive, while gentamicin-resistant indole-positive Proteus and Providencia spp. are usually resistant to netilmicin (Kabins *et al.*, 1976; Miller *et al.*, 1976; Flournoy, 1976; Stewart *et al.*, 1977; Dhawan *et al.*, 1977; Kantor and Norden, 1977; Verbist *et al.*, 1978). Others have reported that a proportion of gentamicin-resistant strains of Esch. coli and Serratia marcescens are also resistant to netilmicin (Fu and Neu, 1976a; Meyers and Hirschman, 1977).

The majority of gentamicin-resistant Ps. aeruginosa strains are also netilmicin-resistant (Fu and Neu, 1976a; Kabins et al., 1976; Marks et al., 1976; Kantor and Norden, 1977; Mouton and de Kok-Broeren, 1977), but some investigators have reported a variable proportion of these strains to be netilmicin-sensitive (Stewart et al., 1977; Dhawan et al., 1977; Meyers and Hirschman, 1977). Strains of Acinetobacter spp. which are resistant to gentamicin are also usually netilmicin-resistant (Meyers and Hirschman, 1977).

3. *Synergy with other drugs against Gram-negative bacilli.* Fu and Neu (1976b) tested a number of drug combinations containing netilmicin *in vitro.* Synergy between netilmicin and carbenicillin occurred against approximately half of the Ps. aeruginosa isolates tested. The combination of a cephalosporin such as cephazolin with netilmicin was synergistic only against an occasional Klebsiella strain. A netilmicin/chloramphenicol combination usually demonstrated neither synergy nor antagonism against Esch. coli, and the same was true for a netilmicin/clindamycin combination against Esch. coli and Ps. aeruginosa.

4. *Gram-positive bacteria.* Staph. pyogenes, including penicillin G and methicillin-resistant strains, is netilmicin-sensitive. The drug acts synergistically with penicillinase-resistant penicillins such as nafcillin (page 93) or oxacillin (page 79) against most Staph. pyogenes strains (Watanakunakorn and Glotzbecker, 1977). Gentamicin-resistant staphylococci are generally more susceptible to netilmicin, but netilmicin MIC's for these strains are usually four- to eight-fold higher than those for fully susceptible strains. The suitability of netilmicin for treatment of infections caused by these staphylococci therefore depends on the susceptibility of the particular strain (Phillips et al., 1977b; Vogel et al., 1978).

Staph. epidermidis is netilmicin-sensitive, but other Gram-positive cocci such as Strep. pyogenes, Strep. pneumoniae and Strep. faecalis are relatively resistant (Eickhoff and Ehret, 1977). Activity of netilmicin against these organisms is comparable to that of gentamicin (page 329). Similar to penicillin G/gentamicin (page 329) and penicillin G/tobramycin (page 361) combinations, penicillin G and netilmicin act synergistically against most Strep. faecalis strains *in vitro* (Smith et al., 1977; Sanders, 1977). This combination is also effective for the treatment of experimental Strep. faecalis endocarditis in animals, caused by both 'streptomycin-susceptible' and 'streptomycin-resistant' (*see* page 294) Strep. faecalis strains (Korzeniowski et al., 1978; Carrizosa and Kaye, 1978).

In Vitro Sensitivities

The minimum inhibitory concentrations of netilmicin against some selected bacterial species are shown in Table 27.

Mode of Administration and Dosage

1. *Adults.* Netilmicin, like gentamicin (page 330), can be administered both intramuscularly or intravenously in the same dosage. In clinical trials the drug has been given in daily doses of either 3·0, 4·5, 6·0 or 7·5 mg per kg, administered in three divided doses at eight-hourly intervals (Welling et al., 1977;

TABLE 27

(After Fu and Neu, 1976a)

ORGANISM	MIC (μg per ml)
Gram-negative bacteria (*gentamicin-sensitive*)	
Escherichia coli	0·2 – 6·3
Enterobacter spp.	0·2 – 6·3
Klebsiella spp.	0·2 – 6·3
Salmonella spp.	0·2 – 1·6
Shigella spp.	0·2 – 1·6
Serratia marcescens	0·4 – 50·0
Citrobacter spp.	0·025– 0·8
Proteus mirabilis	0·2 – 25·0
Proteus, indole-positive	0·2 – 12·5
Providencia spp.	0·4 – 25·0
Pseudomonas aeruginosa	0·2 – 12·5
Acinetobacter spp.	0·2 – 25·0
Gram-negative bacteria (*gentamicin-resistant*)	
Escherichia coli	0·4 – 12·5
Enterobacter spp.	3·1 – 12·5
Klebsiella spp.	0·2 – 6·3
Serratia marcescens	3·1 –>100·0
Citrobacter spp.	0·4
Proteus mirabilis	50·0
Proteus, indole-positive	3·1 – 25·0
Pseudomonas aeruginosa	12·5 – 50·0
Gram-positive bacteria	
Staphylococcus pyogenes	0·05 – 0·8
Streptococcus faecalis	3·1 – 25·0

Klastersky *et al.*, 1977; Panwalker *et al.*, 1978; Edelstein and Meyer, 1978). The higher dosage schedules have been used for severely ill patients or for treatment of infections caused by organisms relatively resistant to netilmicin.

Netilmicin can be administered intravenously in the same manner as gentamicin (page 331), either by relatively rapid (3–5 min) intravenous injections (Riff and Moreschi, 1977), or by suitably diluting each dose in intravenous fluid for infusion over a 30 min period (Meyers *et al.*, 1977). It may also be feasible to give netilmicin by constant intravenous infusion using an infusion pump. To maintain constant serum concentrations of 4–6 μg per ml by this method, a higher total daily dose of the drug is needed, which may increase the risk of toxicity (Yap *et al.*, 1977).

2. *Patients with renal failure.* The netilmicin dose should be adjusted in a similar manner to that of gentamicin (Welling *et al.*, 1977) (*see* page 332).

3. *Newborn and premature infants.* Rubio *et al.* (1978) administered doses of 2·5 mg per kg intramuscularly to newborn infants. Peak serum concentrations attained at one hour, were 1·0–5·0 μg per ml, and these were usually at least six times the MIC's of netilmicin for susceptible organisms. The mean half-life of netilmicin in these patients was 4·18 h, compared to approximately

2 h in adults. Serum levels were low but detectable at 12 h ($0\cdot3$–$1\cdot4$ μg per ml). It is therefore possible that a dose of $2\cdot5$ mg per kg every 12 h may be suitable for newborn infants, but this is to be confirmed.

Serum Levels in Relation to Dosage

Serum netilmicin levels after both intramuscular and intravenous administration resemble those of gentamicin (page 335), with some minor differences.

1. *Intramuscular administration.* After an intramuscular dose of $1\cdot0$ mg per kg body weight to adults, a mean peak serum level of $3\cdot76$ μg per ml is reached in 30–40 min (Riff and Moreschi, 1977). These authors also studied serum levels after an identical dose of gentamicin, and although the mean peak serum level was the same, it was reached earlier. Netilmicin may be absorbed more slowly from intramuscular sites. After the peak, the serum level of netilmicin gradually falls with a half-life of $2\cdot0$–$2\cdot5$ h, reaching $1\cdot0$ μg per ml at 4 h and usually zero at 8 h. The mean gentamicin serum levels fall in a similar fashion, but individual subjects demonstrate more variability with gentamicin than with netilmicin (Riff and Moreschi, 1977).

2. *Intravenous administration.* Serum levels after the intravenous administration of $1\cdot0$ mg per kg doses of both gentamicin and netilmicin, administered over 3–5 min, have been compared (Riff and Moreschi, 1977). Mean peak serum levels 10 min after the injection were similar for both drugs ($5\cdot0$ μg per ml), but during the next 30 min (distribution phase) netilmicin serum levels fell more rapidly than those of gentamicin, so that at 40 min the netilmicin level was $2\cdot9$ μg per ml whilst that of gentamicin was still $3\cdot6$ μg per ml. It was postulated that netilmicin may be more quickly distributed to a larger extravascular area than gentamicin. From the second hour onwards after the injection (elimination phase), netilmicin and gentamicin had approximately the same half-life of two hours.

If a 2 mg per kg dose is infused intravenously over 30 min, the mean peak serum level 10 min after the infusion is $16\cdot56$ μg per ml. This falls to $12\cdot87$, $9\cdot75$, $7\cdot89$, $3\cdot25$, $1\cdot39$ and $0\cdot91$ μg per ml at 20 min, 40 min, 1 h, 2 h, 6 h and 8 h after the end of the infusion respectively (Meyers *et al.*, 1977).

Excretion

Like other aminoglycosides (pages 315, 336), netilmicin is excreted via the kidney by glomerular filtration and it is reabsorbed in the tubules to a limited extent (Chiu *et al.*, 1977). The drug appears in the urine in an unchanged active form, where high urinary concentrations are attained. Approximately 50 per cent of an administered dose is excreted in the urine during the first six hours (Yap *et al.*, 1977), and 70–80 per cent in the first twenty-four hours (Follath *et al.*, 1978). The urine excretion of netilmicin is almost the same regardless of the route of administration (Riff and Moreschi, 1977). Some netilmicin appears to be eliminated by non-renal mechanisms, but no metabolites have been identified (Welling *et al.*, 1977).

After intravenous administration of netilmicin, urinary excretion during the first two hours is slightly less than that after an identical dose of gentamicin. This suggests that the more rapid decline of netilmicin serum levels during the distribution phase (*vide supra*) is not due to its more rapid renal excretion, but due to a more rapid extravascular distribution (Riff and Moreschi, 1977).

Distribution of the Drug in Body

In common with other aminoglycosides (pages 315, 337), the serum protein binding of netilmicin is only very low (Welling *et al.*, 1977). The drug is probably distributed in various body fluids and tissues in a similar manner to gentamicin (page 337). Netilmicin does not penetrate into the CSF of patients with uninflamed meninges (Shah and Robson, 1978). In animal experiments it accumulates in the kidney in the same manner as gentamicin (page 337). The predominant site is the renal cortex (Chiu *et al.*, 1977), where the concentration of the antibiotic is similar to that of gentamicin (Luft *et al.*, 1976, Bowman *et al.*, 1977).

Mode of Action

This is presumably the same as that of other aminoglycosides (*see* streptomycin, page 298).

Toxicity

1. *Ototoxicity.* Characteristic of all aminoglycosides (pages 316, 338), netilmicin can cause this complication. Animal experiments indicate that cochlear toxicity of netilmicin on a weight for weight basis is less than one-fifth of that of gentamicin (Federspil, 1978). Reports of ototoxicity in humans have been uncommon, but netilmicin has only had a limited clinical use to date. Klastersky *et al.* (1977) treated 30 patients with doses of either 4·5, 6·0 or 7·5 mg per kg body weight per day, and ototoxicity was not encountered. Edelstein and Meyer (1978) used netilmicin to treat 25 patients; one patient developed reversible tinnitus during the drug infusion, but this was unaccompanied by audiogram changes. Dizziness was also noted in one of another 27 netilmicin treated patients, and this resolved when the drug was stopped (Buckwold *et al.*, 1978). Twenty-six patients, 20–77 years of age, were treated by Trestman *et al.* (1978) using netilmicin in a dose of 6 mg per kg body weight per day. Three of these developed ototoxicity which was only detected by audiograms. Panwalker *et al.* (1978) treated a further 27 patients with netilmicin and studied 21 by serial audiograms. One patient developed unilateral hearing loss, which was partially reversible. These authors also noted the absence of ototoxicity in two patients in whom very high netilmicin serum levels were maintained for more than a week; in one of these the range of peak serum levels was 15–36 μg per ml, and that of trough levels 10–24 μg per ml.

2. *Nephrotoxicity.* This is another characteristic side-effect of aminoglycosides (page 339), shared by netilmicin. Animal experiments indicate that netilmicin is less nephrotoxic than gentamicin, but this is not explicable by a difference in the concentrations of these antibiotics in the renal cortex (Luft *et al.*, 1976; Bowman *et al.*, 1977; Chiu *et al.*, 1977). In animals the concomitant administration of non-aminoglycoside antibiotics, such as ampicillin, carbenicillin, methicillin, cefamandole and clindamycin, does not

aggravate netilmicin nephrotoxicity (Hagstrom *et al.*, 1978).

Mild reversible nephrotoxicity has been encountered fairly frequently in clinical trials with netilmicin. Klastersky *et al.* (1977) noted granular casts in the urine and/or rises in blood urea and serum creatinine, in 7 of 10 patients treated by a netilmicin dose of 7·5 mg per kg body weight per day. These changes were not observed in patients receiving lower doses. Other authors also have reported rises in blood urea and serum creatinine, usually reversible, in a small number of patients (Edelstein and Meyer, 1978; Buckwold *et al.*, 1978; Trestman *et al.*, 1978). Nephrotoxicity appears to be more likely in older patients, after prolonged treatment and when a larger total amount of the drug is administered (Panwalker *et al.*, 1978).

3. *Other side-effects*. Elevated serum aspartate aminotransferase (SGOT) values have been noted in some patients (Edelstein and Meyer, 1978). An elevation of serum alkaline phosphatase occurred in 43 per cent of patients treated by Panwalker *et al.* (1978). There was no other evidence of hepatotoxicity in any of these patients.

Clinical Uses of the Drug

Netilmicin may have a place in therapeutics on occasions as an alternative to amikacin (page 386) for the treatment of those infections caused by gentamicin-resistant Gram-negative bacilli which remain netilmicin-sensitive.

In most clinical trials reported to date, netilmicin has been used to treat severe infections, such as pyelonephritis, biliary tract infections, peritonitis, pleuro-pulmonary infections and septicaemia, caused by gentamicin-sensitive Gram-negative bacilli. Results of treatment have usually been satisfactory and similar to those which would be expected from an identical gentamicin regimen (Klastersky *et al.*, 1977; Panwalker *et al.*, 1978; Buckwold *et al.*, 1978; Trestman *et al.*, 1978).

Edelstein and Meyer (1978) used netilmicin to treat 25 patients with serious Gram-negative bacillary infections, nine of which had gentamicin-resistant but netilmicin-susceptible pathogens. Previous therapy with gentamicin had been unsuccessful in six of these patients, but seven of the nine patients subsequently responded to netilmicin.

In a study of experimental Esch. coli meningitis in animals, Scheld *et al.* (1978) found that netilmicin and gentamicin penetrated into the CSF to the same extent, but that netilmicin achieved better *in vivo* bactericidal activity. Because of this finding and also its possible lesser toxicity (page 400), it was suggested that netilmicin may offer an advantage over gentamicin in the therapy of Gram-negative bacillary meningitis.

REFERENCES

Bowman, R. L., Silverblatt, F. J. and Kaloyanides, G. J. (1977), 'Comparison of the nephrotoxicity of netilmicin and gentamicin in rats', *Antimicrob. Ag. Chemother.*, **12**, 474.

Briedis, D. J. and Robson, H. G. (1976), 'Comparative activity of netilmicin, gentamicin, amikacin, and tobramycin against Pseudomonas aeruginosa and Enterobacteriaceae', *Antimicrob. Ag. Chemother.*, **10**, 592.

Brown, K. N., Benedictson, J. and Swanby, S. (1976), 'In vitro comparison of gentamicin, tobramycin, sisomicin and netilmicin', Antimicrob. Ag. Chemother., 10, 768.

Brummett, R. E., Fox, K. E., Bendrick, T. W. and Himes, D. L. (1978), 'Comparative ototoxicity of tobramycin, gentamicin, amikacin, and sisomicin'. In Siegenthaler, W. and Lüthy, R. (Ed.), Current Chemotherapy: Proceedings of the 10th International Congress of Chemotherapy, Zurich/Switzerland, 1977. American Society for Microbiology, Washington, D.C., p. 939.

Buckwold, F. J., Ronald, A. R., Lank, B. A., Fox, L., Harding, G. K. M. and Gurwith, M. J. (1978), 'Clinical trial of netilmicin'. In Siegenthaler, W. and Lüthy, R. (Ed.), Current Chemotherapy: Proceedings of the 10th International Congress of Chemotherapy, Zurich/Switzerland, 1977. American Society for Microbiology, Washington, D.C., p. 984.

Carrizosa, J. and Kaye, D. (1978), 'Penicillin and netilmicin in treatment of experimental enterococcal endocarditis', Antimicrob. Ag. Chemother., 13, 505.

Chadwick, P., Salmon, S. and Taylor, B. (1977), 'Activity of netilmicin compared with those of gentamicin and tobramycin against enterobacteria and Pseudomonas aeruginosa', Antimicrob. Ag. Chemother., 12, 301.

Chiu, P. J. S., Miller, G. H., Brown, A. D., Long, J. F. and Waitz, J. A. (1977), 'Renal pharmacology of netilmicin', Antimicrob. Ag. Chemother., 11, 821.

Crowe, C. C. and Sanders, E. (1973), 'Sisomicin: Evaluation in vitro and comparison with gentamicin and tobramycin', Antimicrob. Ag. Chemother., 3, 24.

Dhawan, V., Marso, E., Martin, W. J. and Young, L. S. (1977), 'In vitro studies with netilmicin compared with amikacin, gentamicin, and tobramycin', Antimicrob. Ag. Chemother., 11, 64.

Drasar, F. A., Farrell, W., Maskell, J. and Williams, J. D. (1976), 'Tobramycin, amikacin, sisomicin and gentamicin-resistant Gram-negative rods', Brit. med. J., 2, 1284.

Edelstein, P. H. and Meyer, R. D. (1978), 'Netilmicin therapy of serious Gram-negative bacillary infections'. In Siegenthaler, W. and Lüthy, R. (Ed.), Current Chemotherapy: Proceedings of the 10th International Congress of Chemotherapy, Zurich/Switzerland, 1977. American Society for Microbiology, Washington, D. C., p. 982.

Eickhoff, T. C. and Ehret, J. M. (1977), 'In vitro activity of netilmicin compared with gentamicin, tobramycin, amikacin, and kanamycin', Antimicrob. Ag. Chemother., 11, 791.

Federspil, P. J. (1978), 'Evaluation of ototoxicity of netilmicin'. In Siegenthaler, W. and Lüthy, R. (Ed.), Current Chemotherapy: Proceedings of the 10th International Congress of Chemotherapy, Zurich/Switzerland, 1977. American Society for Microbiology, Washington, D.C., p. 975.

Flournoy, D. J. (1976), 'Sisomicin versus netilmicin: In vitro susceptibility testing', Antimicrob. Ag. Chemother., 10, 864.

Follath, F., Spring, P., Wenk, M., Benet, L. Z. and Dettli, L. (1978), 'Comparative pharmacokinetics of sisomicin and netilmicin in healthy volunteers'. In Siegenthaler, W. and Lüthy, R. (Ed.), Current Chemotherapy: Proceedings of the 10th International Congress of Chemotherapy, Zurich/Switzerland, 1977. American Society for Microbiology, Washington, D.C., p. 979.

Fu, K. P. and Neu, H. C. (1976a), 'In vitro study of netilmicin compared with other aminoglycosides', Antimicrob. Ag. Chemother., 10, 526.

Fu, K. P. and Neu, H. C. (1976b), 'In vitro synergistic effect of netilmicin, a new aminoglycoside antibiotic', Antimicrob. Ag. Chemother., 10, 511.

Hagstrom, G. L., Luft, F. C., Yum, M. N., Sloan, R. S. and Maxwell, D. R. (1978), 'Nephorotoxicity of netilmicin in combination with non-aminoglycoside antibiotics', Antimicrob. Ag. Chemother., 13, 490.

Hammerberg, S., Sorger, S. and Marks, M. I. (1977), 'Antimicrobial susceptibilities of Yersinia enterocolitica biotype 4, serotype 0:3', *Antimicrob. Ag. Chemother.*, **11**, 566.

Hyams, P. J., Simberkoff, M. S. and Rahal, J. J., Jr. (1973), '*In vitro* bactericidal effectiveness of four aminoglycoside antibiotics', *Antimicrob. Ag. Chemother.*, **3**, 87.

Kabins, S. A., Nathan, C. and Cohen, S. (1976), '*In vitro* comparison of netilmicin, a semisynthetic derivative of sisomicin, and four other aminoglycoside antibiotics', *Antimicrob. Ag. Chemother.*, **10**, 139.

Kantor, R. J. and Norden, C. W. (1977), '*In vitro* activity of netilmicin, gentamicin, and amikacin', *Antimicrob. Ag. Chemother.*, **11**, 126.

Klastersky, J., Hensgens, C., Gerard, M. and Daneau, D. (1975), 'Comparison of sisomicin and gentamicin in bacteriuric patients with underlying diseases of the urinary tract', *Antimicrob. Ag. Chemother.*, **7**, 742.

Klastersky, J., Meunier-Carpentier, F., Coppens-Kahan, L., Daneau, D. and Prevost, J. M. (1977), 'Clinical and bacteriological evaluation of netilmicin in Gram-negative infections', *Antimicrob. Ag. Chemother.*, **12**, 503.

Korzeniowski, O. M., Wenndersten, C., Moellering, R. C., Jr. and Sande, M. A. (1978), 'Penicillin-netilmicin synergism against Streptococcus faecalis', *Antimicrob. Ag. Chemother.*, **13**, 430.

Leroy, A., Humbert, G., Oksenhendler, G. and Fillastre, J. P. (1976), 'Comparative pharmacokinetics of lividomycin, amikacin and sisomicin in normal subjects and in uraemic patients', *J. Antimicrob. Chemother.*, **2**, 373.

Levison, M. E. and Kaye, D. (1974), '*In vitro* comparison of four aminoglycoside antibiotics: sisomicin, gentamicin, tobramycin and BB-K8', *Antimicrob. Ag. Chemother.*, **5**, 667.

Lode, H., Kemmerich, B. and Koeppe, P. (1975), 'Comparative clinical pharmacology of gentamicin, sisomicin and tobramycin', *Antimicrob. Ag. Chemother.*, **8**, 396.

Luft, F. C., Yum, M. N. and Kleit, S. A. (1976), 'Comparative nephrotoxicities of netilmicin and gentamicin in rats', *Antimicrob. Ag. Chemother.*, **10**, 845.

Makris, A. T., Asper, R. F., Schanbacher, K. and Schwartz, A. R. (1978), 'Treatment of Gram-negative bacteremia with sisomicin'. In Siegenthaler, W. and Lüthy, R. (Ed.), *Current Chemotherapy: Proceedings of the 10th International Congress of Chemotherapy*, Zurich/Switzerland, 1977. American Society for Microbiology, Washington, D.C., p. 925.

Marks, M. I., Hammerberg, S., Greenstone, G. and Silver, B. (1976), 'Activity of newer aminoglycosides and carbenicillin, alone and in combination, against gentamicin-resistant Pseudomonas aeruginosa', *Antimicrob. Ag. Chemother.*, **10**, 399.

Meyer, R. D., Kraus, L. L. and Pasiecznik, K. A. (1976), '*In vitro* susceptibility of gentamicin-resistant Enterobacteriaceae and Pseudomonas aeruginosa to netilmicin and selected aminoglycoside antibiotics', *Antimicrob. Ag. Chemother.*, **10**, 677.

Meyers, B. R., Leng, B. and Hirschman, S. Z. (1975), 'Comparison of the antibacterial activities of sisomicin and gentamicin against Gram-negative bacteria', *Antimicrob. Ag. Chemother.*, **8**, 757.

Meyers, B. R. and Hirschman, S. Z. (1977), 'Antimicrobial activity *in vitro* of netilmicin and comparison with sisomicin, gentamicin and tobramycin', *Antimicrob. Ag. Chemother.*, **11**, 118.

Meyers, B. R., Hirschman, S. Z., Wormser, G. and Siegel, D. (1977), 'Pharmacokinetic study of netilmicin', *Antimicrob. Ag. Chemother.*, **12**, 122.

Miller, G. H., Arcieri, G., Weinstein, M. J. and Waitz, J. A. (1976), 'Biological activity of netilmicin, a broad-spectrum semisynthetic aminoglycoside antibiotic', *Antimicrob. Ag. Chemother.*, **10**, 827.

Mouton, R. P. and de Kok-Broeren, M. C. J. (1977), 'Activity of netilmicin against selected strains of Gram-negative bacteria and Staphylococcus aureus; Comparison with four other aminoglycosides', *J. Antimicrob. Chemother.*, **3**, 393.

O'Hara, K., Kono, M. and Mitsuhashi, S. (1974), 'Enzymatic inactivation of a new aminoglycoside antibiotic, sisomicin, by resistant strains of Pseudomonas aeruginosa', *Antimicrob. Ag. Chemother.*, **5**, 558.

Panwalker, A. P., Malow, J. B., Zimelis, V. M. and Jackson, G. G. (1978), 'Netilmicin: Clinical efficacy, tolerance, and toxicity', *Antimicrob. Ag. Chemother.*, **13**, 170.

Pechère, J.-C., Pechère, M.-M. and Dugal, R. (1976), 'Clinical pharmacokinetics of sisomicin: Dosage schedules in renal-impaired patients', *Antimicrob. Ag. Chemother.*, **9**, 761.

Phillips, I., Eykyn, S., King, B. A., Jenkins, C., Warren, C. A. and Shannon, K. P. (1977a), 'The *in vitro* antibacterial activity of nine aminoglycosides and spectinomycin on clinical isolates of common Gram-negative bacteria', *J. Antimicrob. Chemother.*, **3**, 403.

Phillips, I., Smith, A. and Shannon, K. (1977b), 'Antibacterial activity of netilmicin, a new aminoglycoside antibiotic, compared with that of gentamicin', *Antimicrob. Ag. Chemother.*, **11**, 402.

Rahal, J. J., Jr., Simberkoff, M. S., Kagan, K. and Moldover, N. H. (1976), 'Bactericidal efficacy of Sch 20569 and amikacin against gentamicin-sensitive and resistant organisms', *Antimicrob. Ag. Chemother.*, **9**, 595.

Riff, L. J. and Moreschi, G. (1977), 'Netilmicin and gentamicin: Comparative pharmacology in humans', *Antimicrob. Ag. Chemother.*, **11**, 609.

Rodriguez, V., Bodey, G. P., Valdiviesco, M. and Field, R. (1975), 'Clinical pharmacology of sisomicin', *Antimicrob. Ag. Chemother.*, **7**, 38.

Rubio, T., Wirth, F. and Wellman, L. (1978), 'Pharmacokinetics of netilmicin in newborn infants'. In Siegenthaler, W. and Lüthy, T. (Ed.), *Current Chemotherapy: Proceedings of the 10th International Congress of Chemotherapy*, Zurich/Switzerland, 1977. American Society for Microbiology, Washington, D.C., p. 977.

Sanders, C. C. (1977), 'Synergy of penicillin-netilmicin combinations against enterococci including strains highly resistant to streptomycin or kanamycin', *Antimicrob. Ag. Chemother.*, **12**, 195.

Scheld, W. M., Brown, R. S., Jr. and Sande, M. A. (1978), 'Comparison of netilmicin with gentamicin in the therapy of experimental Escherichia coli meningitis', *Antimicrob. Ag. Chemother.*, **13**, 899.

Seligman, S. J. (1978), 'Frequency of resistance to kanamycin, tobramycin, netilmicin and amikacin in gentamicin-resistant Gram-negative bacteria', *Antimicrob. Ag. Chemother.*, **13**, 70.

Shah, P. P. and Robson, H. G. (1978), 'Cerebrospinal fluid penetration of netilmicin'. In Siegenthaler, W. and Lüthy, R. (Ed.), *Current Chemotherapy: Proceedings of the 10th International Congress of Chemotherapy*, Zurich/Switzerland, 1977. American Society for Microbiology, Washington, D.C., p. 981.

Smith, J. A., Morgan, J. R. and Mogyoros, M. (1977), '*In vitro* activity of netilmicin', *Antimicrob. Ag. Chemother.*, **11**, 362.

Stewart, D., Bodey, G. P. and LeBlanc, B. (1977), '*In vitro* studies of netilmicin, a new aminoglycoside antibiotic', *Antimicrob. Ag. Chemother.*, **11**, 1017.

Trestman, I., Parsons, J., Santoro, J., Goodhart, G. and Kaye, D. (1978), 'Pharmacology and efficacy of netilmicin', *Antimicrob. Ag. Chemother.*, **13**, 832.

Verbist, L., Vandepitte, J. and Vandeven, J. (1978), 'Activity of eight aminoglycosides against isolates of Serratia marcescens from four hospitals', *J. Antimicrob. Chemother.*, **4**, 47.

Vogel, L., Nathan, C., Sweeney, H. M., Kabins, S. A. and Cohen, S. (1978), 'Infections due to gentamicin-resistant Staphylococcus aureus strain in a nursery for neonatal infants', *Antimicrob. Ag. Chemother.*, **13**, 466.

Waitz, J. A., Moss, E. L., Jr., Drube, C. G. and Weinstein, M. J. (1972), 'Comparative activity of sisomicin, gentamicin, kanamycin and tobramycin', *Antimicrob. Ag.*

Chemother., **2**, 431.

Watanakunakorn, C. and Glotzbecker, C. (1977), 'Enhancement of antistaphylococcal activity of nafcillin and oxacillin by sisomicin and netilmicin', *Antimicrob. Ag. Chemother.*, **12**, 346.

Welling, P. G., Baumueller, A., Lau, C. C. and Madsen, P. O. (1977), 'Netilmicin pharmacokinetics after single intravenous doses to elderly male patients', *Antimicrob. Ag. Chemother.*, **12**, 328.

Yap, B.-S., Stewart, D. and Bodey, G. P. *(1977), 'Clinical pharmacology of netilmicin', Antimicrob. Ag. Chemother.*, **12**, 717.

Young, L. S. and Hewitt, W. L. (1973), 'Activity of five aminoglycoside antibiotics *in vitro* against Gram-negative bacilli and Staphylococcus aureus', *Antimicrob. Ag. Chemother.*, **4**, 617.

Neomycin, Framycetin and Paromomycin

Description

These three aminoglycoside antibiotics are more toxic and, unlike strep-tomycin, kanamycin, gentamicin and the newer aminoglycosides, are not used systemically.

1. *Neomycin* was first described by Waksman and Lechevalier in 1949. In its marketed form it contains two chemically similar components (neomycin B and C).

2. *Framycetin* (*'Soframycin'*) was described in 1953 by Decaris in France, where subsequent purification was carried out by Roussel Laboratories. The drug is probably identical with neomycin B.

3. *Paromomycin* (*'Humatin', Parke Davis*) was isolated from a strain of Streptomyces rimosus in 1959.

These antibiotics are used clinically as sulphates, which produce stable solutions in water.

Sensitive Organisms

Neomycin, framycetin and paromomycin each have a spectrum of activity similar to that of kanamycin (page 308).

1. *Gram-negative bacteria.* Nearly all the medically important Gram-negative bacteria are sensitive to these drugs, with the exception of Pseudomonas aeruginosa and the anaerobic bacteria such as Bacteroides spp. Resistant strains of the usually sensitive organisms such as Esch. coli, Klebsiella and Proteus spp. may emerge, and these usually show complete cross-resistance with kanamycin (page 308). Long-term oral administration of neomycin particularly favours emergence of multi-resistant R plasmid carrying aerobic enteric bacteria. These enteric bacteria are usually also resistant to other drugs such as sulphonamides, tetracylines, streptomycin, ampicillin and carbenicillin. Such multi-resistant bacteria are capable of transferring their resistance to other aerobic enteric bacteria (Valtonen *et al.*, 1977). Neomycin-resistant strains of Shigella sonnei (Davies *et al.*, 1970) and the salmonellae (Bissett *et al.*, 1974) have also been encountered.

2. *Gram-positive bacteria.* Staphylococci are highly sensitive to these drugs, but all streptococci and the Gram-positive bacilli are relatively resistant. Neomycin-resistant strains of Staph. pyogenes have been reported, mainly in hospitals (Leading article, 1965; Rountree and Beard, 1965). These staphylococci are also always resistant to framycetin and kanamycin, and the majority are resistant to several other antibiotics including penicillin, strep-

tomycin, tetracycline and erythromycin. They may also become resistant to bacitracin (page 417), an antibiotic often used in combination with neomycin in topical applications (Rountree and Beard, 1965). When neomycin-containing topical preparations are used for short-term control of skin sepsis in conditions such as eczema, the risk of inducing neomycin-resistant strains of Staph. pyogenes is small. If these applications are used for weeks, months or intermittently, staphylococci resistant to neomycin may readily emerge. These may be implicated in further attacks of sepsis and be difficult to control (Smith *et al.*, 1975; Leading article, 1977).

3. *Mycobacterium tuberculosis.* That this organism is somewhat sensitive to these drugs is of no clinical importance.

4. *Entamoeba histolytica and Acanthamoebae.* Entamoeba histolytica has been reported to be sensitive to paromomycin (Courtney *et al.*, 1960), but not to neomycin and framycetin. Both neomycin and paromomycin are active *in vitro* against two species of Acanthamoebae, A. polyphaga and A. castellanii, which can cause eye infections (Nagington and Richards, 1976).

In Vitro Sensitivities

The minimum inhibitory concentrations of neomycin, framycetin and paromomycin against sensitive organisms are similar to those of kanamycin (*see* Table 21, page 310).

Mode of Administration and Dosage

1. *Intramuscular administration.* The use of neomycin by the intramuscular route is not recommended. Previously an intramuscular adult dose of 1 g or 15 mg per kg body weight given in two to four divided doses was used, but toxic effects were common (page 409).

2. *Oral administration.* These antibiotics are not significantly absorbed after oral administration, so they are only used orally to supress intestinal microbial flora or, nowadays rarely, for the treatment of intestinal infections (page 412). The usual adult dose of oral neomycin is 1 g every six hours (50–100 mg per kg body weight per day for children), but up to 2 g orally every six hours has been used. In newborn infants, doses of up to 100 mg per kg per day have been given for as long as three weeks (Yaffe, 1965). However oral neomycin may induce a malabsorption syndrome in babies (page 411) after five days' therapy (Nelson, 1971). The oral dosage of framycetin is 2–4 g per day for adults or 50 mg per kg body weight for children. Paromomycin has been used orally in a dose of 1–2 g daily in adults and 50 mg per kg body weight in children.

3. *Intraperitoneal administration.* Neomycin may be instilled into the peritoneal cavity after surgery for the treatment of peritonitis. A solution of 0·5 per cent neomycin in normal saline is suitable. The daily amount instilled in adults should not exceed 1 g (or 15 mg per kg body weight for children) and such treatment should not be continued longer than three days. Intraperitoneal framycetin has also been used in adult doses of up to 100 mg per day.

4. *Bladder irrigation or instillation.* For continuous bladder irrigation a solution containing 40 mg neomycin per litre has been recommended. Stronger

neomycin solutions (e.g. 40 to 100 ml of a 0·1 or 0·2 per cent solution) may be placed in the bladder for several hours following instrumentation (Fairley *et al.*, 1967; Clark, 1973). In patients with indwelling catheters, these instillations can be performed daily or more frequently, but the total dose of neomycin instilled should not exceed 0·5 g in a 24 h period. Framycetin in a daily dose of 200–500 mg dissolved in 100 ml (0·2 to 0·5 per cent solution) may also be used for instillation into the bladder. Solutions containing 1 per cent neomycin, 1 per cent bacitracin and 0·4 per cent polymyxin B, have been used in paraplegics for urethral irrigation prior to catheterization (McLeod *et al.*, 1963).

5. *Aerosols for respiratory infections.* Both neomycin and framycetin are used, and the daily dose is dissolved in 3–5 ml of normal saline. For prolonged aerosol therapy (longer than seven days) the daily dose of these drugs should not exceed 1·5 mg per kg or 100 mg for adults. A bronchodilator may be added to the solutions if required.

Availability

1. *Neomycin sulphate* ('*Mycifradin*', *Upjohn*). This is supplied as 500 mg tablets for oral administration and in vials containing 500 mg of sterile neomycin powder for preparation of solutions for bladder washout, etc., and rarely for parenteral administration. Neomycin is also available in creams, ointments, powders, eyedrops, sprays, etc., and is often combined with other antibacterial substances. 'Polybactrin Soluble', is a sterile powder, available in vials, each containing 2500 units bacitracin, 15 000 units polymyxin B and 4000 units of neomycin. The contents of each vial may be dissolved in 10 ml saline, to provide a solution for instillation or irrigation of infected wounds and sinuses. 'Polybactrin Soluble GU' is a similar freeze-dried sterile powder. Each vial of this preparation contains 75 000 units of polymyxin B, 1000 units of bacitracin and 20 000 units (about 30 mg) of neomycin sulphate. Solutions are prepared in the same manner as 'Polybactrin soluble' and are suitable for bladder instillations. One mg of neomycin is equivalent to 650 international units.

2. *Framycetin sulphate* ('*Soframycin*', *Roussel*) was previously available as 250 mg tablets and in vials containing 100 or 500 mg of framycetin sterile powder for the preparation of solutions. These preparations are no longer marketed commercially, and the drug is only available in various topical preparations such as creams and ointments, nasal sprays and eye and ear drops.

3. *Paromomycin sulphate* ('*Humatin*', *Parke Davis*.) Available previously for oral administration as 250 mg capsules and as a paediatric syrup, it is no longer marketed commercially.

Serum Levels in Relation to Dosage

Serum levels similar to those of kanamycin are attained after intramuscular injections of neomycin (*see* Fig. 20, page 314). After a 0·5 g intramuscular dose, a peak serum level of about 20 μg per ml is reached about one hour later. Although both neomycin and framycetin are generally classed as non-absorbable, some absorption from the gastro-intestinal tract does occur. A single oral dose of 4 g neomycin may produce a peak serum level of about 4·0 μg per ml (Kunin *et al.*, 1960). Enema administered neomycin is absorbed to about the same extent (Breen *et al.*, 1972). Prolonged oral administration of these drugs in high dosage may result in toxic blood levels, especially if renal impairment is present. Last and Sherlock (1960) reported neomycin blood level studies in 27 patients with acute and chronic hepatic insufficiency, treated with oral neomycin in a dose rarely exceeding 4 g daily. Detectable serum levels of neomycin were demonstrated in seven patients, which ranged from 0·5 to 40 μg per ml. The development of detectable blood levels correlated with the occurrence of oliguria. Intestinal ulceration does not appear to enhance neomycin absorption (Breen *et al.*, 1972).

These drugs are also absorbed from wounds, the peritoneum, bronchial tree, bladder and even from inflamed skin following cutaneous application (Trimble, 1969; Weinstein *et al.*, 1977). Significant serum levels may result if too large doses are administered at these sites (*see also* page 410).

Excretion

If these drugs are present in the serum, excretion is predominantly by the kidneys in a manner similar to kanamycin (page 315), and they may accumulate in the body if there is renal impairment.

Most of orally administered neomycin, framycetin or paromomycin appears in the faeces in an active unchanged form.

Distribution of Drugs in Body

Neomycin, administered parenterally, is distributed in the body in a similar fashion to kanamycin (page 315). Framycetin and paromomycin have not been used parenterally.

Mode of Action

Neomycin, framycetin and paromomycin act on bacteria like other aminoglycosides (*see* streptomycin, page 298).

Toxicity

1. *Ototoxicity*. These three antibiotics are capable of causing irreversible deafness rather than vestibular dysfunction. This is the principal reason why they are not used systemically. Neomycin, when first introduced, was used systemically, and with intramuscular doses of 0·5–1·0 g daily many patients became completely deaf after relatively short courses of seven to fifteen days (Welch, 1954). Neomycin is considerably more ototoxic than kanamycin (Leading article, 1963). Unfortunately the detection of early ototoxicity usually does not prevent further auditory loss, which often progresses to complete deafness, despite cessation of the drug. Sometimes hearing loss is first noted days or weeks after stopping the drug, and then progressively deteriorates (Kelly *et al.*, 1969; Leading article, 1969).

Sufficient absorption of these drugs may occur after prolonged oral administration (page 408) to cause ototoxicity, especially in the presence of renal impairment. This is most likely to occur in patients with liver failure, who often have associated renal functional impairment and are treated for prolonged periods with neomycin (A Co-operative Study, 1973). It is advisable to check neomycin serum levels regularly in such patients (Last and Sherlock, 1960). If serum levels higher than 5 or especially 10 μg per ml are detected, the drug should be stopped or the dose reduced.

Ototoxicity can also result from 'topical neomycin or framycetin therapy'. Kelly *et al.* (1969) reported deafness in a patient whose wound was irrigated four-hourly with 80 ml of a solution containing 0·5 per cent neomycin. Thus the total amount of neomycin used for the wound irrigation in this patient was 2·4 g daily. Following this report Trimble (1969) reviewed neomycin induced deafness, and showed that ototoxicity had occurred after use of this drug by all modes of administration—parenteral, aerosol, oral, wound and bowel irrigation, and cutaneous application. He also made the interesting observation that, whenever a new neomycin preparation became available, reports of ototoxicity following its use appeared.

Jawetz (1969) pointed out that the absorption of neomycin from a wound or granulating surface may be comparable to absorption after intramuscular injection. Neomycin is not absorbed after application to normal skin or instillation into a normal bladder, but it may be absorbed if the skin or bladder mucosa is inflamed. Weinstein *et al.* (1977) studied ten patients in whom neomycin wound irrigations were used during total hip replacement. A 1·0 per cent neomycin solution was used, and the volume of irrigation solution varied from 500 to 1400 ml in individual patients; it was calculated that these patients received a dose ranging from 67 to 203 mg per kg. Although ototoxicity was not observed, systemic absorption and significant neomycin serum levels occurred in all patients.

Neomycin toxicity after topical therapy may be avoided if the total daily amount of the drug administered is calculated, and this is restricted to a safe dose. The dose should not exceed 15 mg per kg per day or 1·0 g daily in adults, for longer than one to three days. A lower total daily dose should be used if 'topical therapy' is continued for longer periods. For instance in aerosol administration of neomycin to children with fibrocystic disease, the daily dose should probably not exceed 1·5 mg per kg per day.

Animal experiments have shown that many antibiotics such as neomycin, gentamicin, chloramphenicol, tetracycline, erythromycin and polymyxin B can cause deafness if instilled directly into the intact middle ear. Antibiotic ear drops may therefore be a potential cause of deafness in man, although sudden severe deafness from their use appears to be rare. Nevertheless, in view of their doubtful efficacy and the possibility of ototoxicity, antibiotic ear drops should seldom be prescribed, especially in the presence of large perforations and in patients undergoing ear surgery (Annotation, 1976).

2. *Nephrotoxicity.* These drugs may cause renal damage if administered systemically. In initial trials with intramuscular neomycin using daily doses of 0·5–1·0 g, a rising blood urea was observed after 7–15 days of treatment, and in many patients this renal damage was severe enough to warrant cessation of the drug (Welch, 1954). By contrast with neomycin ototoxicity, nephrotoxicity is usually reversible. Havard *et al.* (1959) described a patient with Strep. faecalis endocarditis, who developed renal damage after treatment by parenteral neomycin and penicillin, but this recovered after cessation of neomycin. Similarly de Beukelaer *et al.* (1971) described a 13-months-old infant who developed acute tubular necrosis and deafness following intramuscular neomycin. The nephrotoxicity was reversible, but hearing loss was not. A renal biopsy specimen from this infant showed vacuolization of proximal tubular epithelium similar to that observed in animal studies on

neomycin nephrotoxicity (*vide infra*). Krumlovsky *et al.* (1972) described a 39-year-old woman who developed severe but reversible nephrotoxicity following accidental intramuscular administration of neomycin. These authors found that neomycin could be removed from the body by haemodialysis, and this seems to be the treatment of choice for neomycin poisoning.

The danger of renal damage may not be very great when these drugs are used by the oral route. In 27 patients with liver disease treated by oral neomycin, there was no convincing evidence that sufficient quantities of neomycin had been absorbed to cause renal damage (Last and Sherlock, 1960). Nevertheless such patients should be monitored for declining renal function to avoid toxicity (Appel and Neu, 1977).

Animal studies show that neomycin is the most nephrotoxic of the commonly used aminoglycosides. Parenteral neomycin produces toxic lesions of the proximal renal tubules, which in the rat are manifested by glycosuria, aminoaciduria and proteinuria. These lesions are accompanied by a decrease of enzyme activity in the tubules, but are reversible. Renal toxicity in animals can also be demonstrated after very large oral doses of the drug (Emmerson and Pryse-Davies, 1964; Appel and Neu, 1977).

3. *Neuromuscular blockade.* Neomycin and framycetin can cause this complication similar to streptomycin (page 301) and kanamycin (page 317). Neomycin induced blockade is competitive in type, and may sometimes be reversed by neostigmine (Ross *et al.*, 1963). It has been observed most commonly after intraperitoneal administration of neomycin to children, probably because the danger of relative overdosage is greater in this age group. Intraperitoneal administration, especially if peritonitis is present, may result in rapid systemic absorption of the drug. This is of particular importance as these drugs are usually given intraperitoneally to patients undergoing anaesthesia, which potentiates neomycin neuromuscular blockade (Yow and Yow, 1961; Emery, 1963). Both ether anaesthesia and muscle relaxants such as tubocurarine have this effect. Neuromuscular blockade has also been observed when neomycin has been given by other routes. Thus Ross *et al.* (1963) reported post-operative apnoea in a man aged seventy with impaired renal function, who received 6 g oral neomycin prior to operation, but a small amount of the drug, probably less than 150 mg, was introduced into the peritoneal cavity during operation. Bush (1962) reported the same effect in a newborn baby, in whom a large area of subcutaneous tissue was sprayed with a neomycin and polymyxin B mixture. This neonate (wt 3·1 kg) probably received a total dose of 166 mg neomycin and 50 000 units of polymyxin B. The polymyxins may also cause neuromuscular blockade (page 540).

4. *Staphylococcal enterocolitis.* This is a rare, but dangerous complication of the oral use of these drugs. (Leading article, 1965). It has mainly occurred in surgical patients who have received pre-operative chemoprophylaxis (page 413), in whom the infection is caused by neomycin-resistant staphylococci.

5. *Gastro-intestinal side-effects.* Large oral doses of these drugs may cause vomiting or diarrhoea. Rubbo *et al.* (1966) found that doses of neomycin as high as 9 g per day used for pre-operative chemoprophylaxis, frequently caused these symptoms.

Prolonged oral administration of neomycin may also cause atrophic changes in the intestinal mucosa resulting in a malabsorption syndrome (Jacobson and

THE USE OF ANTIBIOTICS

Faloon, 1961). Malabsorption of fat, cholesterol, electrolytes, dissacharides, glucose, xylose, vitamin B_{12} and penicillin may result. Neomycin even in a single dose of $1 \cdot 0$ g depresses the rate and extent of the absorption of digoxin in man by an unknown mechanism (Lindenbaum et al., 1976).

In infants with Esch. coli gastro-enteritis, who were treated by oral neomycin, a mild form of malabsorption was commonly induced by relatively short courses of therapy. Nelson (1971) showed that diarrhoea was significantly prolonged and onset of weight gain was delayed in infants treated with neomycin for ten days, compared with infants treated for three days. The experimental studies of Emmerson and Pryse-Davies (1964) suggest that there are certain similarities in the responses of the alimentary and renal tubular epithelia to neomycin.

6. *Contact dermatitis.* Prolonged application of either neomycin or framycetin to skin lesions may cause sensitization. Kirton and Munro-Ashman (1965) described seventy cases of contact dermatitis due to these drugs. The patients had been treated for lesions such as leg ulcers, otitis externa, blepharitis and eczema. Sensitization was manifested by either an acute exacerbation of the disease or failure to respond to local treatment. In this latter group, the absence of an acute allergic reaction was ascribed to the concomitant use of topical corticosteroids. Patch testing showed that 65 patients were sensitive to neomycin and 50 to framycetin, and in 45 patients there was a 'cross-sensitivity' between these two antibiotics. Other studies also suggest that the risk of contact dermatitis is high, especially in eczema of the lower leg and when application is continued for long periods. By contrast short-term application of neomycin, particularly to children, carries little risk of sensitization (Leading article, 1977).

Clinical Uses of the Drugs

1. *Topical treatment of superficial infections.* Both neomycin and framycetin are valuable for local treatment of superficial infections due to staphylococci and many Gram-negative bacilli. These drugs are best used in combination with other antibiotics to avoid the development of resistant strains. Neomycin is often combined with polymyxin B and bacitracin in various creams, ointments, sprays and solutions, e.g. 'Neosporin ointment' and 'Polybactrin spray'. Neomycin in combination with chlorhexidine ('Naseptin Nasal-Carrier Cream') has been used to treat staphylococcal nasal carriers.

Neomycin is also often used in association with various corticosteroids in creams and ointment to treat allergic diseases with secondary bacterial infections. Many preparations are available, e.g. 'Synalar N' and 'Kenacomb'. These antibiotics have also been added to vasoconstrictor nose drops for treatment of sinusitis, e.g. 'Soframycin nose drops'. Eye and ear drops are also available containing neomycin or framycetin.

2. *Bacterial intestinal infections.* As these antibiotics are only slightly absorbed from the gastro-intestinal tract, they were used in the past to treat various bacterial intestinal infections. They are no longer recommended for this purpose.

Orally administered 'non-absorbable' drugs of this group (or any other antibiotics) are of no value in gastro-enteritis due to enteropathogenic Esch. coli (Ramsay, 1968; Edmond et al., 1969; Christie, 1973). Similarly antibiotics (absorbable or non-absorbable) are of little or no practical value for the treatment of Salmonella gastroenteritis. They do not shorten the clinical illness, and often prolong the Salmonella carrier state. This was confirmed to be the case in a controlled trial with neomycin (Joint Project, 1970). In patients with severe Salmonella gastro-enteritis in whom septicaemia is suspected or confirmed, treatment with either chloramphenicol (page 441), ampicillin (page 114) or co-trimoxazole (page 711) is indicated.

Neomycin and related drugs do not benefit mild to moderate cases of Shigella sonnei dysentery (Ramsey, 1968; Garrod et al., 1973), and these antibiotics are not used for this purpose at Fairfield Hospital. Severe Shigella dysentry with marked systemic symptoms, which occurs more frequently with Sh. flexneri and Sh. dysenteriae type 1 infections, may require chemotherapy, but absorbable antibiotics such as ampicillin (page 115), co-trimoxazole (page 713) or chloramphenicol (page 441) are preferred.

3. *Parasitic infections*. Oral paromomycin was found to be effective in amoebic dysentery, but it has no effect on hepatic amoebiasis (Courtney et al., 1960). As metronidazole (page 769) now appears to be the best drug for all forms of amoebiasis, paromomycin has little place in the treatment of this disease. Paromomycin is also effective for the treatment of Taenia saginata, T. solium, Hymenolepsis nana and Diphyllobothrium latum intestinal infestations. Tanowitz and Wittner (1973) used a single 4 g dose of the drug successfully to treat five patients with Diphyllobothrium latum infection. Nevertheless, at present niclosamide ('Yomesan') is regarded as the drug of choice for these infections.

4. *Pre-operative chemoprophylaxis in large bowel surgery*. Both oral neomycin and framycetin were often used in the past to suppress the normal flora of the large bowel prior to surgery. It was also doubtful whether such chemoprophylaxis reduced the post-operative sepsis rate (Rubbo et al., 1966; Annotation, 1970). Such use of non-absorbable antibiotics also encouraged the emergence of resistant organisms which occasionally resulted in bowel suprainfection. Severe enterocolitis due to neomycin-resistant staphylococci was described in patients given neomycin pre-operatively (Leading article, 1965; Annotation, 1970) (*see* page 411).

Nowadays it is generally accepted that non-absorbable antibiotics such as neomycin have little place in pre-operative chemoprophyiaxis. Post-operative infections can frequently be prevented in high risk patients by the use of other more appropriate antibiotics. However these must be in high concentrations in the tissues before bacterial contamination occurs, and this implies their intravenous or intramuscular use just before or at the beginning of an operation (Kune, 1978) (*see also* pages 345, 485).

5. *Hepatic failure*. Oral neomycin is commonly used for suppression of intestinal flora in this condition (Dawson et al., 1957), but framycetin or kanamycin (page 319) can also be used for this purpose.

6. *Suppression of intestinal flora in neutropenic patients*. Oral framycetin or a combination of oral framycetin, colistin and nystatin has been used to suppress intestinal bacteria in leukaemic patients during neutropenic episodes. This has met with some success in reducing the frequency of septicaemia, other infections and pyrexial episodes, because most of the causative organisms in such patients arise from the bowel (Keating and Pennington, 1973; Storring et

al., 1977).

7. *Respiratory infections.* Neomycin or framycetin solutions are sometimes used as aerosols for the treatment of chronic respiratory infections such as in mucoviscoidosis. Bronchodilators may be added to these solutions.

8. *Peritonitis.* Neomycin or framycetin may be introduced into the peritoneal cavity at operation for the prevention or treatment of peritonitis.

9. *Bladder infections.* Neomycin or framycetin solutions can be instilled into the bladder for prophylactic purposes after cystoscopy and other similar procedures. These solutions are also used for bladder washouts to treat or prevent infections in patients who have continuous catheter drainage (page 407).

10. *Hypercholesterolaemia.* Long-term administration of oral neomycin in a dose of 1·5 g daily has a serum cholesterol-lowering effect. This appears to be primarily due to inhibition of intestinal absorption of cholesterol, resulting in enhanced elimination of cholesterol as neutral sterols in the faeces (Miettinen and Toivonen, 1975). This long-term neomycin treatment, however, has a profound effect on the aerobic intestinal flora (page 406).

REFERENCES

A Cooperative Study (1973), 'Drug-induced deafness', *JAMA*, **224,** 515.

Annotation (1970), 'The colon and the surgeon', *Lancet*, **1,** 509.

Annotation (1976), 'Ear-drops', *Lancet*, **1,** 896.

Appel, G. B. and Neu, H. C. (1977), 'The nephorotoxicity of antimicrobial agents (second of three parts)', *New Engl. J. Med.*, **296,** 722.

Bissett, M. L., Abbott, S. L. and Wood, R. M. (1974), 'Antimicrobial resistance and R factors in Salmonella isolated in California (1971–1972)', *Antimicrob. Ag. Chemother.*, **5,** 161.

Breen, K. J., Bryant, R. E., Levinson, J. D. and Schenker, S. (1972), 'Neomycin absorption in man', *Ann. Intern. Med.*, **76,** 211.

Bush, G. H. (1962), 'Antibiotic paralysis', *Brit. med. J.*, **2,** 1062.

Christie, A. B. (1973), 'Treatment of gastro-intestinal infections; A clinician's viewpoint'. In Geddes, A. M. and Williams, J. D. (Ed.), *Current Antibiotic Therapy*, Churchill Livingstone, Edinburgh and London, p. 183.

Clark, L. W. (1973), 'Neomycin in the prevention of postcatheterization bacteriuria', *Med. J. Aust.*, **1,** 1034.

Courtney, K. O., Thompson, P. E., Hodgkinson, R. and Fitzsimmons, J. R. (1960), 'Paromomycin as a therapeutic substance for intestinal amebiasis and bacterial enteritis', *Antibiot. Annual*—1959–1960, p. 304.

Davies, J. R., Farrant, W. N. and Uttley, A. H. C. (1970), 'Antibiotic resistance of Shigella sonnei', *Lancet*, **2,** 1157.

Dawson, A. W., McLaren, J. and Sherlock, S. (1957), 'Neomycin in the treatment of hepatic coma', *Lancet*, **2,** 1263; quoted by Last and Sherlock (1960).

de Beukelaer, M. M., Travis, L. B., Dodge, W. F. and Guerra, F. A. (1971), 'Deafness and acute tubular necrosis following parenteral administration of neomycin', *Amer. J. Dis. Child.*, **121,** 250.

Emery, E. R. J. (1963), 'Neuromuscular blocking properties of antibiotics as a cause of post operative apnoea', *Anaesthesia*, **18,** 57.

Emmerson, B. T. and Pryse-Davies, J. (1964), 'Studies on the nephrotoxic effect of neomycin', *Aust. Ann. Med.*, **13,** 149.

Emond, R. T. D., Gray, J. A., Smith, H. and Young, S. E. J. (1969), 'Antibiotics in acute gastroenteritis', *Lancet*, **1,** 1312.

Fairley, K. F., Bond, A. G., Brown, R. B. and Habersberger, P. (1967), 'Simple test to determine the site of urinary-tract infection', *Lancet*, **2**, 427.

Garrod, L. P. and Waterworth, P. M. (1962), 'Methods of testing combined antibiotic bactericidal action and the significance of the results', *J. clin. Path.*, **15**, 328.

Garrod, L. P., Lambert, H. P. and O'Grady, F. (1973), *Antibiotic and Chemotherapy*, 4th edn., Churchill Livngstone, Edinburgh and London, p. 369.

Havard, C. W. H., Garrod, L. P. and Waterworth, P. M. (1959), 'Deaf or dead? A case of subacute bacterial endocarditis treated with penicillin and neomycin', *Brit. med. J.*, **1**, 688.

Jacobson, E. D. and Faloon, W. W. (1961), 'Malabsorptive effects of neomycin in commonly used doses', *JAMA*, **175**, 187.

Jawetz, E. (1969), 'Neomycin ototoxicity: Dossier and doses', *New Engl. J. Med.*, **281**, 219.

Joint Project by Members of the Association for the Study of Infectious Disease (1970), 'Effect of neomycin in non-invasive Salmonella infections of the gastrointestinal tract', *Lancet*, **2**, 1159.

Keating, M. J. and Penington, D. G. (1973), 'Prophylaxis against septicaemia in acute leukaemia: The use of oral framycetin', *Med. J. Aust.*, **2**, 213.

Kelly, D. R., Nilo, E. R. and Berggren, R. B. (1969), 'Deafness after topical neomycin wound irrigation', *New Engl. J. Med.*, **280**, 1338.

Kirton, V. and Munro-Ashman, D. (1965), 'Contact dermatitis from neomycin and framycetin', *Lancet*, **1**, 138.

Krumlovsky, F. A., Emmerman, J., Parker, R. H., Wisgerhof, M. and Del Greco, F. (1972), 'Dialysis in treatment of neomycin overdosage', *Ann. Intern. Med.*, **76**, 443.

Kune, G. A. (1978), 'Life-threatening surgical infection: Its development and prediction', *Ann. Royal College Surgeons England*, **60**, 92.

Kunin, C. M., Chalmers, T. C., Leevy, C. M., Sebastyen, S. C., Lieber, C. S. and Finland, M. (1960), 'Absorption of orally administered neomycin and kanamycin', *New Engl. J. Med.*, **262**, 380.

Last, P. M. and Sherlock, S. (1960), 'Systemic absorption of orally administered neomycin in liver disease', *New Engl. J. Med.*, **262**, 385.

Leading Article (1963), 'Antibiotic ototoxicity', *Brit. med. J.*, **2**, 68.

Leading Article (1965), 'Staphylococci resistant to neomycin and bacitracin', *Lancet*, **2**, 421.

Leading Article (1969), 'Deafness after topical neomycin', *Brit. med. J.*, **4**, 181.

Leading Article (1977), 'Steroid-antibiotic combinations', *Brit. med. J.*, **1**, 1303.

Lindenbaum, J., Maulitz, R. M. and Butler, V. P., Jr. (1976), 'Inhibition of digoxin absorption by neomycin', *Gastroenterology*, **71**, 399.

McLeod, J. W., Mason, J. M. and Pilley, A. (1963), 'Prophylactic control of infection of the urinary tract consequent on catheterisation', *Lancet*, **1**, 292.

Miettinen, T. A. and Toivonen, I. (1975), 'Treatment of severe and mild hypercholesterolaemia with probucol and neomycin', *Postgrad. Med. J.* (Suppl.), **51**, 71.

Nagington, J. and Richards, J. E. (1976), 'Chemotherapeutic compounds and Acanthamoebae from eye infections', *J. clin. Path.*, **29**, 648.

Nelson, J. D. (1971), 'Duration of neomycin therapy for enteropathogenic Escherichia coli diarrheal disease: A comparative study of 113 cases', *Pediatrics*, **48**, 248.

Powell, S. J. (1969), 'Metronidazole in the treatment of amoebic dysentery', *Medicine Today*, **3**, 48.

Ramsay, A. M. (1968), 'Acute infective diarrhoea', *Brit. med. J.*, **2**, 347.

Ross, E. D. T., Settle, J. A. D. and Telfer, A. B. M. (1963), 'Oral neomycin: A possible anaesthetic hazard', *Brit. med. J.*, **2**, 1109.

Rountree, P. M. and Beard, M. A. (1965), 'The spread of neomycin-resistant staphylococci in a hospital', *Med. J. Aust.*, **1**, 498.

Rubbo, S. D., Hughes, E. S. R., Blainey, B. and Russell, I. S. (1966), 'Role of preoperative chemoprophylaxis in bowel surgery', *Antimicrob. Ag.*

Chemother.—1965, p. 649.

Smith, R. J., Alder, V. G. and Warin, R. P. (1975), 'Pyogenic cocci in infantile eczema throughout one year', *Brit. med. J.*, **3,** 199.

Storring, R. A., McElwain, T. J., Jameson, B. and Wiltshaw, E. (1977), 'Oral non-absorbed antibiotics prevent infection in acute non-lymphoblastic leukaemia', *Lancet*, **2,** 837.

Tanowitz, H. B. and Wittner, M. (1973), 'Paromomycin in the treatment of Diphylobothrium latum infections', *J. Trop. Med.*, **76,** 151.

Trimble, G. X. (1969), 'Neomycin ototoxicity: Dossier and doses', *New Engl. J. Med.*, **281,** 219.

Valtonen, M. V., Suomalainen, R. J., Ylikahri, R. H. and Valtonen, V. V. (1977), 'Selection of multiresistant coliforms by long-term treatment of hyper-cholesterolaemia with neomycin', *Brit. med. J.*, **1,** 683.

Waksman, S. A. and Lechevalier, H. A. (1949), 'Neomycin, a new antibiotic active against streptomycin resistant bacteria, including tuberculosis organisms', *Science*, **109,** 305; quoted by Welch (1954).

Weinstein, A. J., McHenry, M. and Gavan, T. L. (1977), 'Systemic absorption of neomycin irrigating solution', *JAMA*, **238,** 152.

Welch, H. (1954), *Principles and Practice of Antibiotic Therapy*, Med. Encyc. Inc., New York, p. 158.

Yaffe, S. J. (1965), 'Antibiotic dosage in newborn and premature infants', *JAMA*, **193,** 818.

Yow, M. D. and Yow, E. M. (1961), 'Kanamycin, neomycin and paromomycin', *Pediat. Clin. North America*, **8,** 1043.

Bacitracin and Gramicidin

Description

Similar to the polymyxins (page 531), these are peptide antibiotics which are composed of peptide-linked amino acids.

1. *Bacitracin*. This was isolated from a strain of Bacillus spp. (Johnson *et al.*, 1945), which was originally classified as Bacillus subtilis, but now it is known as B. licheniformis (Katz and Demain, 1977). From the time of its discovery until about 1960, bacitracin was used systemically, mainly for the treatment of severe staphylococcal infections (Jawetz, 1968). Because of its toxicity and the availability of other antibiotics, it is now restricted to topical use. For this reason descriptions of its pharmacokinetics and detailed toxicology are not included.

2. *Gramicidin*. In 1939 an antibiotic named tyrothricin was isolated from Bacillus brevis by Dubos. Later it was shown that tyrothricin consisted of two antibiotics, gramicidin and tyrocidine. Gramicidin was the more active drug of the two, but it was too toxic to be used systemically. It is now used in a number of topical preparations.

Sensitive Organisms

Bacitracin is highly active against most Gram-positive bacteria, particularly Staph. pyogenes and Group A beta-haemolytic streptococci (Strep. pyogenes). Group C and G beta-haemolytic streptococci are usually less susceptible but Group B streptococci are usually resistant (Finland *et al.*, 1976; Baker *et al.*, 1976). Pathogenic Neisseria (meningococci and gonococci) are also sensitive, but Gram-negative bacilli are resistant.

Acquired bacterial resistance to bacitracin is unusual, but resistant Staph. pyogenes strains have been occasionally detected. In one hospital, where topical preparations containing both bacitracin and neomycin were commonly used, staphylococci resistant to both of these drugs were encountered (Rountree and Beard, 1965).

Gramicidin is also highly active against Gram-positive bacteria, but the Neisseria spp. are relatively resistant and Gram-negative bacilli are completely resistant.

Mode of Action

Bacitracin interferes with bacterial cell wall synthesis. It is a specific inhibitor of the dephosphorylation of a lipid pyrophosphate, a reaction which occurs during the second stage of bacterial cell wall synthesis (Strominger, 1973).

417

Bacitracin probably also damages the bacterial cytoplasmic membrane, and unlike the penicillins (page 23), it is active against protoplasts. Gramicidin acts on bacteria by altering the function of their cytoplasmic membrane (Carter and McCarthy, 1966). It may also be a potent and specific inhibitor of the transcription reaction and inhibit the binding of DNA-dependent RNA polymerase (transcriptase) to DNA (Dancer, 1977) (*see also* page 433).

Toxicity

Nephrotoxicity is the main toxic effect of bacitracin, if it is administered systemically, but it seldom causes side-effects when it is used topically. Applied locally to skin or mucous membranes the drug is non-irritating and allergic sensitization is rare.

By contrast to neomycin (page 410), there appear to be no reports of bacitracin toxicity caused by systemic absorption of the drug, when large amounts have been applied topically to inflamed areas. For example no side-effects were observed by Noon *et al.* (1967), who used 50 000 units bacitracin combined with kanamycin to irrigate the peritoneal cavity after surgery. In the past, when bacitracin was used systemically, 100 000 units was considered to be the maximum daily dose for adults.

Gramicidin also has virtually no side-effects when used topically.

Clinical Uses of the Drugs

1. *Bacitracin* is commonly used in various topical antibiotic applications such as creams, ointments, antibiotic sprays and powders and also in solutions for wound irrigation or bladder instillation, etc. Most commonly it is combined with both neomycin and polymyxin B, providing an effective 'cover' for all bacterial species (*see* pages 412, 543).

2. *Gramicidin* is also used in topical preparations such as eye and ear drops, creams and ointments, and like bacitracin, it is often combined with neomycin and polymyxin B.

REFERENCES

Baker, C. J., Webb, B. J. and Barrett, F. F. (1976), 'Antimicrobial susceptibility of Group B streptococci isolated from a variety of clinical sources', *Antimicrob. Ag. Chemother.*, **10**, 128.

Carter, W. and McCarthy, K. S. (1966), 'Molecular mechanisms of antibiotic action', *Ann. Intern. Med.*, **64**, 1087.

Dancer, B. N. (1977), 'Antibiotics and bacterial sporulation', *Nature*, **267**, 485.

Dubos, R. J. (1939), 'Studies on a bactericidal agent extracted from a soil bacillus', *J. Exper. Med.*, **70**, 11.

Finland, M., Garner, C., Wilcox, C. and Sabath, L. D. (1976), 'Susceptibility of beta-hemolytic streptococci to 65 antibacterial agents', *Antimicrob. Ag. Chemother.*, **9**, 11.

Jawetz, E. (1968), 'Polymyxins, colistin, bacitracin, ristocetin, and vancomycin', *Pediat. Clin. N. Amer.*, **15**, 85.

Johnson, B. A., Anker, H. and Meleney, F. L. (1945), 'Bacitracin: A new antibiotic produced by a member of the B. subtilis group', *Science*, **102,** 376; quoted by Welch (1954).

Katz, E. and Demain, A. L. (1977), 'The peptide antibiotics of bacillus: Chemistry, biogenesis, and possible functions', *Bacteriol. Rev.,* **41,** 449.

Noon, G. P., Beall, A. C., Jr., Jordan, G. L., Jr., Riggs, S. and De Bakey, M. E. (1967), 'Clinical evaluation of peritoneal irrigation with antibiotic solution', *Surgery,* **62,** 73.

Rountree, P. M. and Beard, M. A. (1965), 'The spread of neomycin-resistant staphylococci in a hospital', *Med. J. Aust.,* **1,** 498.

Strominger, J. L. (1973), 'The actions of penicillin and other antibiotics on bacterial cell wall synthesis', *Hopkins Med. J.,* **133,** 63.

Chloramphenicol and Thiamphenicol

Description

1. *Chloramphenicol*. Originally isolated from Streptomyces venezuelae (Ehrlich *et al*., 1947). this was the first 'broad-spectrum' antibiotic discovered. It has a benzene ring in its structure and has the chemical formula of D(-)-threo-p-nitrophenyl-2-dichloracetamido-1, 3-propanediol (Woodward and Wisseman, 1958). The chemical structure of chloramphenicol and a method for its synthetization were elucidated by Parke Davis Laboratories, who distribute the drug as 'Chloromycetin'.

2. *Thiamphenicol*. This is an analogue of chloramphenicol, in which the p-nitro group on the benzene ring is replaced by a methyl-sulphonyl group. It is more soluble and also more stable in solution than chloramphenicol. Unlike chloramphenicol (page 431), thiamphenicol is not conjugated with glucuronic acid in the liver to any extent, and in patients with normal renal function most of an administered dose is excreted in the urine in an active unchanged form. High urine levels of active thiamphenicol are attained (Ferrari and Della Bella, 1974; Tacquet *et al*., 1974; Furman *et al*., 1976). In patients with renal failure thiamphenicol dosage, unlike that of chloramphenicol (page 430), should be appropriately reduced (Dettli and Spring, 1974). The daily dose of thiamphenicol for patients with advanced renal failure is approximately 0·75 g, instead of the usual one of 3·0 g (Tacquet *et al*., 1974).

The antimicrobial spectrum of thiamphenicol is similar to that of chloramphenicol. In therapeutic doses thiamphenicol, like chloramphenicol, causes haemopoietic toxicity (page 437). Early bone marrow suppression mainly involving erythropoiesis is more severe with thiamphenicol than with chloramphenicol. However it has been claimed that thiamphenicol-induced bone marrow damage, even if severe, is always reversible, and that irreversible aplastic anaemia (page 436) has never been produced by this drug (Keiser, 1974a and b). There is insufficient evidence to accept this view-point at present (Yunis, 1974). Thiamphenicol is not currently used in the United States, Britain and Australia, but it is available commercially in Japan and certain European countries.

The following data only apply to chloramphenicol.

Sensitive Organisms

Chloramphenicol has a wide range of activity (Woodward and Wisseman, 1958).

1. *Gram-negative aerobic bacteria*. The Enterobacteriaceae are sensitive to chloramphenicol. Esch. coli and the Enterobacter, Klebsiella, Proteus, Serratia,

Citrobacter, Providencia, Hafnia, Edwardsiella and Arizona spp. are usually susceptible. Yersinia pestis (Butler *et al.*, 1974) and Y. enterocolitica (Kohl *et al.*, 1976; Hammerberg *et al.*, 1977; Raevuori *et al.*, 1978) are also usually chloramphenicol-sensitive.

The prevalence of chloramphenicol-resistant variants of these organisms has slowly increased over the years, but acute infections due to resistant strains are still uncommon unless hospital acquired. During a two-months' survey in a Boston hospital in 1967, Sabath (1969) found that 15 per cent of Esch. coli and 55 per cent of Klebsiella, 47 per cent of Enterobacter, 28 per cent of Proteus and 60 per cent of Serratia spp. strains isolated were chloramphenicol-resistant. The frequency of these resistant strains at that time was higher than that of kanamycin-resistant strains (page 308). More recent surveys indicate that approximately 80 per cent of clinical isolates of Serratia marcescens are still chloramphenicol-sensitive (Cooksey *et al.*, 1975; Mills and Drew, 1976). However in some nosocomial infections due to this organism, the epidemic strain has at times been resistant to chloramphenicol, and also to other antibiotics such as ampicillin, carbenicillin, tetracycline, streptomycin, kanamycin and gentamicin (Schaberg *et al.*, 1976; 1977). Such multiple drug resistance is often R plasmid-mediated (*see* page 422), and this resistance can be transferred in the urine or elsewhere from a multi-drug-resistant S. marcescens strain to other Enterobacteriaceae such as Esch. coli (Schaberg *et al.*, 1977).

The combination of chloramphenicol and gentamicin is now frequently used to cover the spectrum of infecting organisms in peritonitis (page 443). *In vitro* data suggest that these two drugs together may exhibit some antagonism against Enterobacteriaceae such as Esch. coli and Klebsiella spp. (D'Alessandri *et al.*, 1976). Such antagonism only occurs if the bacterial strain is sensitive to both chloramphenicol and gentamicin. Chloramphenicol appears to suppress the rapid bactericidal activity of gentamicin against these organisms (Klastersky and Husson, 1977). This antagonistic effect is not demonstrable *in vivo*, because in experimental animal infections the bacteristatic effect produced by the combination of drugs is not therapeutically inferior to the bactericidal effect of gentamicin alone (Hewitt *et al.*, 1978). *In vitro* synergism between chloramphenicol and a beta-lactam antibiotic such as cephaloridine has been reported against some strains of Enterobacteriaceae which are resistant to the beta-lactam antibiotic. This may occur because of chloramphenicol-induced inhibition of beta-lactamase production (Michel *et al.*, 1975; Sacks *et al.*, 1977). The clinical significance of this observation is not yet clear (*see also* page 103 re cloxacillin/ampicillin synergism).

Salmonella typhi, other salmonellae and the shigellae are usually chloramphenicol-sensitive, but over the years some drastic changes in the sensitivities of these organisms have occurred. Chloramphenicol-resistant shigellae were first observed in Japan (Suzuki *et al.*, 1956), and it was soon established that this resistance may be transferred from Esch. coli to shigellae. Such transfer has been demonstrated *in vitro* in laboratory animals and in human volunteers. Bacterial resistance to antibiotics acquired by this method is termed transferable drug resistance.

The transfer of resistance to an antibiotic (or to multiple antibiotics) from one bacterial species to another occurs during bacterial conjugation and is controlled by plasmids. Conjugation is the process which occurs when bacterial cells come in contact, and genetic material is passed from one organism to another. Plasmids are extrachromosomal genetic elements which are capable of independent replication and are stably inherited. Certain plasmids called 'resistance plasmids' (R plasmids) carry genetic information for resistance to antibiotics and/or other antibacterial drugs. In recently recommended nomenclature, 'R plasmid' supersedes 'R-factor' (Novick *et al.*, 1976). Other plasmids which bring about the transfer of DNA by conjugation are now called 'conjugative plasmids'; these were previously called infectious or transmissible plasmids. Many R plasmids are also conjugative plasmids, so that they have the additional ability to transfer their genetic information for antibiotic resistance by conjugation. Other R plasmids must be associated with conjugative plasmids before transfer of resistance from one organism to another can occur.

Transferable drug resistance mediated by R plasmids occurs amongst the Enterobacteriaceae, and many other organisms such as Pseudomonas aeruginosa (pages 149, 327), Vibrio cholerae (page 596), Haemophilus influenzae (page 102), and beta-lactamase producing Neisseria gonorrhoeae (page 8). DNA sequences carrying resistance genes can be transposed from one plasmid to another, or from plasmid to bacterial chromosome or to bacteriophage or *vice versa* (Datta, 1977). The specific lengths of DNA involved in such transpositions have been termed 'transposons' (Hedges and Jacob, 1974). The specific beta-lactamase (TEM enzyme) which confers resistance to the penicillins is plasmid-mediated. The genetic material confering this quality on the organism has been transferred by means of transposons from plasmids of enterobacteria to plasmids in N. gonorrhoeae and H. influenzae (Datta, 1977; Annotation, 1978). In this way ampicillin-resistant strains of H. influenzae (page 102) and penicillin-resistant strains of N. gonorrhoeae (page 8), have emerged.

R plasmid-mediated chloramphenicol-resistant shigellae have been common in Japan for many years, but until the last decade, rare in most other countries. During three large scale surveys of Shigella spp. isolated from patients in North America, chloramphenicol-resistant variants were either not detected or were very rare (Farrar and Eidson, 1971; Ross *et al.*, 1972; Neu *et al.*, 1975a). In Sweden, Urban (1972) found that 18 per cent of 94 Shigella flexneri and Sh. sonnei strains during 1970 were resistant to chloramphenicol. During 1969 and 1970 a major epidemic of bacillary dysentery due to Shigella dysenteriae type 1 (Shiga bacillus) occurred in Central America and this spread to Mexico in 1971. The Shigella strain involved possessed R plasmid-mediated resistance to chloramphenicol, tetracycline, streptomycin and sulphonamides (Thorne and Farrar, 1973; Balows, 1977). This pattern of resistance was similar to that found in the strain of Salm. typhi, which caused an extensive outbreak of typhoid fever in Mexico during 1972 (*vide infra*).

Surprisingly the R plasmids from the epidemic strains of Sh. dysenteriae type 1 and those from Salmonella typhi belonged to different compatibility groups, demonstrating that although these two epidemic organisms had similar antibiotic resistance patterns, their resistance was mediated by two unrelated R plasmids (Thorne and Farrar, 1974). During this dysentery epidemic, a small number of strains of Sh. dysenteriae type 1 were isolated from patients which were additionally resistant to ampicillin (*see* page 101). This ampicillin resistance was due to a separate plasmid. These strains with dual-plasmid resistance never became widespread in Central America. Only a very few 'imported' cases of Shiga dysentery were reported in the United States during the outbreak in Central America and Mexico (Balows, 1977).

Chloramphenicol resistance mediated by R plasmids can also be transmitted from Esch. coli to the salmonellae (Smith, 1973). Resistant strains of these organisms, including Salm. typhi, had been occasionally detected in the past (Oles and Stanio-Pyrkosz, 1964; Gill and Hook, 1966). It is of interest that chloramphenicol-resistant Salm. typhi was first detected in Britain (Colquhoun and Weetch, 1950). Large scale surveys indicated that such strains were very rare (Winshell et al., 1970; Morahan and Hawksworth, 1970). Later in a survey in California a higher prevalence of chloramphenicol-resistant salmonellae was detected. Sixteen per cent of Salm. typhi strains were resistant, but only 4 per cent or less of strains of other species were resistant, with most species being only 1 per cent or less resistant (Bissett et al., 1974). Some of the resistant Salm. typhi isolates detected in this survey were obtained from 'imported' typhoid cases during the 1972 epidemic in Mexico (vide infra).

From February 1972 until June 1973, an epidemic of typhoid fever involving over 10 000 cases, occurred in Mexico. The Salm. typhi strain concerned possessed transferable (R plasmid-mediated) resistance to chloramphenicol as well as resistance to tetracycline, streptomycin and sulphonamides (Vasquez et al., 1972; Leading article, 1972; Olarte and Galindo, 1973), which was mediated by a single R plasmid (Balows, 1977). The MIC of chloramphenicol for this strain was as high as 150 μg per ml, compared to 0·75–5·0 μg per ml for sensitive strains (WHO, 1974a; Anderson, 1975). During this epidemic a few Salm. typhi strains were isolated from patients, which were additionally resistant to ampicillin (page 101). This ampicillin resistance was mediated by a separate R plasmid (Balows, 1977). Fortunately strains with this dual resistance did not spread to any extent, and the vast majority of chloramphenicol-resistant organisms remained ampicillin-sensitive (Overturf et al., 1973; Datta and Olarte, 1974). After the epidemic in Mexico abated in 1973, typhoid remained endemic in the area, but surprisingly the previously resistant Salm. typhi strains were replaced by chloramphenicol-sensitive ones. In January 1973, 80 per cent of strains isolated in Mexico were chloramphenicol-resistant, but this fell to less than 10 per cent one year later (Annotation, 1975). It is not clear why the chloramphenicol-resistant Salm. typhi strain disappeared from the area. Perhaps it lost the R plasmid which coded for multiple antibiotic resistance. The possibility that chloramphenicol-resistant and even ampicillin-resistant typhoid might have remained endemic in Mexico, and be a source of importation for other countries, did not eventuate (Balows, 1977).

During the typhoid fever epidemic in Mexico, eighty cases of typhoid fever due to the Mexican epidemic strain were reported in the United States, and most of the patients concerned had recently travelled in Mexico (Lawrence et al., 1973; Overturf et al., 1973; Baine et al., 1977). Since mid-1973, when the epidemic subsided, no further cases of typhoid fever due to chloramphenicol-resistant organisms have been detected in the United States (Baines et al., 1977). Associated with the Mexican epidemic, a smaller number of 'imported' cases of typhoid were also detected in other countries such as Britain (Anderson and Smith, 1972), Switzerland and Canada (Balows, 1977). Imported cases of chloramphenicol-resistant typhoid fever can still be expected from time to time, but in developed countries such as the United States or Britain, the epidemic spread of these drug resistant organisms is unlikely (Leading article, 1972). It is of more concern that R plasmid-mediated chloramphenicol-resistant Salm. typhi strains have also been detected in countries such as South Vietnam (Butler *et al.*, 1973; Brown *et al.*, 1975), Thailand (Lampe and Man-suwan, 1973; WHO, 1974c), India (WHO, 1974b) and Indonesia (Sanborn *et al.*, 1975). Although precise data are not available, it appears likely that typhoid fever due to chloramphenicol-resistant Salm. typhi strains may be quite prevalent in South-East Asia, and that this prevalence may well be increasing (Anderson, 1975).

More recent surveys in the United States indicate that Salm. typhi strains resistant to chloramphenicol are now very rare. Chloramphenicol-resistant isolates of other salmonellae are also uncommon; the frequency of such strains being only approximately one per 1000 of Salmonella isolates (Neu *et al.*, 1975b; Cherubin *et al.*, 1977; Barros *et al.*, 1977). Surveillance of antibiotic resistance of salmonellae isolates from humans in the North Eastern United States has detected resistance to chloramphenicol in eight Salmonella strains. Five of these were isolated from individual patients, but the remaining three caused relatively large outbreaks in hospitals (Cherubin *et al.*, 1977). Seven strains were also ampicillin-resistant. Five of the resistant strains resulted from the administration of chloramphenicol to patients with sensitive strains, and these resistant strains emerged after treatment periods as short as one week. In one of the hospital outbreaks which involved a burns unit, a strain of Salm. typhimurium resistant to chloramphenicol, ampicillin, streptomycin, tetracycline, sulphonamides, mercuric chloride and silver nitrate appeared in three patients. The organism colonized the burned surfaces and also produced systemic infection and all three patients died (McHugh *et al.*, 1975; Cherubin *et al.*, 1977). Salmonella typhimurium strains with resistance to both chloramphenicol and ampicillin have also been noted in Canada. From January 1973 to July 1975, 12 per cent (6 of 51) of the infections due to this organism at the Hospital for Sick Children in Toronto were caused by such resistant strains (Grant *et al.*, 1976). Chloramphenicol-resistant strains of Salm. typhi and other salmonellae are still rare in North America, but they are more common in certain European countries such as Holland and France (Cherubin *et al.*, 1977). Chloramphenicol-resistant salmonellae are also still relatively uncommon in Japan (Tanaka *et al.*, 1976) and Korea (Chun *et al.*, 1977). During the 18 months' period ending June 1978, of 194 Salmonella strains (other than Salm. typhi or paratyphi) recovered from patients at Fairfield Hospital, Melbourne, with infective diarrhoea, only one (Salm. new-port) was resistant to chloramphenicol.

Most other Gram-negative bacteria are also sensitive to chloramphenicol. The Neisseria (meningococci and gonococci) are very sensitive. Strains of meningococci resistant to chloramphenicol have been reported, but are rare (less than 1·0 per cent) (Report, 1976). Gonococci, including penicillinase-producing strains (page 8), are always chloramphenicol-sensitive (Report, 1978). Haemophilus influenzae (Williams and Andrews, 1974) and H. parainfluenzae (Mayo and McCarthy, 1977) are also very sensitive. In tests of bactericidal action against H. influenzae type b strains, chloramphenicol is more rapidly effective than ampicillin (page 102) against both large and relatively small inocula (Turk, 1977). Furthermore chloramphenicol and ampicillin act synergistically against a proportion of both ampicillin-sensitive and ampicillin-resistant H. influenzae strains. Antagonism does not occur between these two drugs with any H. influenzae strains (Feldman, 1978). Haemophilus ducreyi, the causative organism of chancroid (page 445) is also consistently chloramphenicol-sensitive (Hammond et al., 1978).

In recent years occasional chloramphenicol-resistant isolates of Haemophilus spp. have been detected. Cavanagh et al. (1975) isolated a resistant strain of H. parainfluenzae from the pharynx of an adult patient. Chloramphenicol-resistant non-typable strains of H. influenzae have been isolated from the throat of a four-year-old girl (Manten et al., 1976) and from the blood of a woman with agammaglobulinaemia (Center for Disease Control, 1976). H. influenzae type b strains resistant to chloramphenicol were isolated from the CSF of two young children with meningitis, one of whom failed to respond to chloramphenicol therapy (Barrett et al., 1972; Kinmonth et al., 1978). Most of these chloramphenicol-resistant Haemophilus spp. isolates were also tetracycline-resistant. Resistance to both of these antibiotics is mediated by a single R plasmid, which can be transferred by conjugation. This plasmid codes for the production of an enzyme, an acetyltransferase, which inactivates chloramphenicol (Kattan, 1976; van Klingeren et al., 1977; Shaw et al., 1978). Fortunately chloramphenicol-resistant Haemophilus spp. remain very rare. In a recent survey of 952 H. influenzae strains in Britain, only two were resistant to chloramphenicol (Howard et al., 1978).

The Brucella spp., B. pertussis and Pasteurella multocida are always chloramphenicol-susceptible. The same is true for all Vibrio parahaemolyticus strains (Joseph et al., 1978). Vibrio cholerae is also sensitive, but rare resistant strains have been detected (page 596). The Moraxella spp. are chloramphenicol-sensitive (de Leys and Juni, 1977). Pseudomonas pseudomallei with a median MIC of $6 \cdot 4 \mu$g per ml is only sensitive to a degree (Eickhoff et al., 1970; Howe et al., 1971; Calabi, 1973), but Pseudomonas aeruginosa is always completely resistant. The Legionnaires' disease bacterium (MIC $0 \cdot 5 \mu$g per ml) is sensitive to chloramphenicol in vitro (Thornsberry et al., 1978), and the drug also prevents death of infected embryonated eggs (Lewis et al., 1978). However chloramphenicol is not as active as erythromycin (page 498) and especially rifampicin (page 553) against this bacterium; in one experiment chloramphenicol, unlike these other two drugs, did not prevent the death of guinea pigs infected intraperitoneally (Fraser et al., 1978). Campylobacter fetus is moderately sensitive to chloramphenicol (MIC $3 \cdot 1 \mu$g per ml) (Chow et al., 1978).

2. Gram-negative anaerobic bacteria. Chloramphenicol is one of the most active chemotherapeutic agents against these bacteria. Most Bacteroides fragilis strains are inhibited by $16 \cdot 0 \mu$g per ml or less, and over 80 per cent of strains are inhibited by $8 \cdot 0 \mu$g per ml or less (see table 28). Only occasional strains of B. fragilis are encountered which require up to $32 \cdot 0 \mu$g per ml of chloramphenicol for inhibition, and completely resistant strains are very rare. Bacteroides melaninogenicus, other Bacteroides spp. and the Fusobacterium and Veillonella spp. are also highly susceptible (Martin et al., 1972; Zabransky

et al., 1973; Blazevic, 1976; Sutter and Finegold, 1976; Nelson, 1976; Sutter, 1977). However an R plasmid coding for resistance to chloramphenicol, tetracycline and kanamycin has been recently identified in a strain of Bacteroides ochraceus, which normally resides in the oral cavity (Guiney and Davis, 1978). It is therefore possible that other Bacteroides spp. may acquire such plasmids and become resistant to chloramphenicol. When a gentamicin/chloramphenicol combination is used clinically to treat suspected mixed aerobic and anaerobic intra-abdominal infections (page 443), gentamicin does not interfere with activity of chloramphenicol against B. fragilis (Klastersky and Husson, 1977).

3. *Gram-positive cocci.* Staph. pyogenes (including penicillinase-producing strains), Staph. epidermidis, Strep. pyogenes, Strep. pneumoniae, alpha-haemolytic streptococci (Strep. viridans) and Strep. faecalis are usually sensitive. Group B streptococci are also nearly always chloramphenicol-sensitive; some authors have found 1·0–2·0 per cent of isolates to be resistant (Anthony and Concepcion, 1975; Baker *et al.*, 1976). Resistant strains of Staph. pyogenes (Sabath, 1969) and Staph. epidermidis (Bentley *et al.*, 1970) occur, but by contrast to the tetracyclines (page 593), chloramphenicol resistance is less common. In particular resistant strains of 'community staphylococci' have remained relatively uncommon (Bennett and Kucers, 1970; Hassam *et al.*, 1978). This is presumably mainly due to the lesser use of chloramphenicol, but there is also evidence that chloramphenicol resistance is acquired with more difficulty than tetracycline resistance (Fisher, 1960).

Chloramphenicol-resistant Strep. pyogenes strains have become common in Japan (Nakae *et al.*, 1977), but they appear to be rare elsewhere. Pneumococci resistant to chloramphenicol are still generally rare, but they have been detected in Poland, France, Britain, West Africa and Australia (Hansman, 1978; Howard *et al.*, 1978; Dang-Van *et al.*, 1978). Some of these resistant strains possess an R plasmid-mediated chloramphenicol acetyltransferase, which inactivates the drug (Dang-Van *et al.*, 1978). In South Africa pneumococci which were resistant to multiple antibiotics, including penicillin G and chloramphenicol, have been detected, and they were associated with serious infections (Center for Disease Control, 1977) (*see also* page 4). Chloramphenicol-resistant Strep. faecalis strains are not uncommon, and most of these variants show resistance to two or more antimicrobial agents. This resistance also appears to be R plasmid-mediated; one plasmid has been identified in Strep. faecalis, which codes for resistance to chloramphenicol and erythromycin and also for high level resistance to streptomycin and lincomycin (Marder and Kayser, 1977). The biochemical mechanism of chloramphenicol resistance in Strep. faecalis is enzymatic acetylation (Courvalin *et al.*, 1978).

Anaerobic Gram-positive cocci such as the Peptococcus and Peptostreptococcus spp. and the anaerobic streptococci are all susceptible to chloramphenicol (Sutter and Finegold, 1976).

4. *Gram-positive bacilli.* C. diphtheriae, Listeria monocytogenes and B. anthracis are nearly always sensitive. Similarly Cl. tetani, Cl. perfringens, other Clostridium spp. and the Actinomyces, Arachnia and Lactobacillus spp. are chloramphenicol-sensitive (Sutter and Finegold, 1976; Schwartzman *et al.*, 1977; Rood *et al.*, 1978). The Nocardia spp. are chloramphenicol-resistant.

5. T r e p o n e m a   p a l l i d u m ,   Leptospirae and Mycoplasmas are

chloramphenicol-sensitive. Mycobacteria, Fungi and Protozoa are resistant.

6. Chloramphenicol is active against the Rickettsiae which cause the various typhus fevers and Rocky Mountain spotted fever (Wisseman *et al.*, 1974). Coxiella burnetti, the agent causing Q fever, is also sensitive, as is the Chlamydia, a genus which includes the causative agents of psittacosis, lymphogranuloma venereum, trachoma and inclusion body conjunctivitis (*see also* page 626).

In Vitro Sensitivities

The minimum inhibitory concentrations of chloramphenicol against some selected bacterial species are shown in Table 28. Organisms inhibited by 5 μg per

TABLE 28

Compiled from data published by Welch (1954), Sutter and Finegold (1976) and Report (1978)

ORGANISM	MIC range (μg per ml)	MIC of most strains less than:
Gram-positive bacteria		
Staph. pyogenes (aureus)	1·0–5·0	12·5
Staph. epidermidis (albus)	1·0–6·25	2·5
Strep. pyogenes (Group A)	0·3–6·0	3·0
Strep. pneumoniae	0·06–12·5	2·5
Strep. viridans	0·6–2·5	1·0
Bacillus anthracis	0·75–5·0	3·0
Clostridium perfringens	2·0–4·0	4·0
Other Clostridium spp.	0·5–16·0	4·0
Actinomyces spp.	0·5–8·0	2·0
Peptococcus spp.	0·1–8·0	2·0
Gram-negative bacteria		
Escherichia coli	3·0–50·0	6·0
Enterobacter spp.	0·5–64·0	12·0
Klebsiella pneumoniae	0·5–25·0	3·1
Serratia marcescens	2·5–5·0	2·5
Proteus vulgaris	0·12–> 250	15·0
Salmonella typhi	0·75–5·0	1·56
Shigella sonnei	2·5–6·0	5·0
Neisseria gonorrhoeae	0·078–6·3	1·0
Neisseria gonorrhoeae (penicillinase-producing)	0·5–8·0	2·0
Neisseria meningitidis	0·78–6·25	1·5
Haemophilus influenzae	0·2–3·5	2·0
Bordetella pertussis	0·2–12·5	1·0
Brucella abortus	0·1–10·0	5·0
Pseudomonas aeruginosa	8·0–1000	Resistant
Bacteroides fragilis	0·5–16·0	8·0
Bacteroides melaninogenicus	0·1–4·0	1·0
Other Bacteroides spp.	0·1–16·0	2·0
Fusobacterium spp.	0·5–2·0	1·0

ml or less may be considered quite sensitive, those not susceptible to 25 μg per ml are resistant. Few organisms fall into an intermediate class, and chloramphenicol can often be used successfully for infections caused by these, provided large doses are given.

Mode of Administration and Dosage

1. Chloramphenicol can be administered orally, intramuscularly or intravenously. Oral administration is satisfactory for many conditions, but for severely ill patients, initial administration by one of the parenteral routes is preferable, because absorption of the oral drug may be poor in severely ill patients.

2. *Oral administration.* The usual adult oral dose is 3 g daily given in four divided doses. The corresponding dosage for children is 50 mg per kg per day given in four divided doses. For severe infections the dose can be increased to 80 mg per kg per day in children or to 4 g daily for adults.

3. *Chloramphenicol palmitate.* The oral administration of unaltered chloramphenicol is difficult in young children, because they cannot swallow capsules, and chloramphenicol elixir is exceedingly bitter. The tasteless compound, chloramphenicol palmitate, is used for children. This substance has no antibacterial activity, and must be hydrolysed by enzymes in the gut before absorption of liberated active chloramphenicol can occur. The initial preparations of this compound did not produce adequate serum levels after oral administration. These preparations contained large crystalline particles of palmitate ester, which were only slowly hydrolysed and absorbed. The particle size was controlled to produce satisfactory blood levels (Weiss *et al.*, 1960) and currently available chloramphenicol palmitate is satisfactory for clinical use (Hodgman, 1961; Ingall and Sherman, 1968; Snyder and Woodward, 1970; Garrod *et al.*, 1973). The recommended dose of chloramphenicol palmitate is usually the same as for other chloramphenicol preparations. However, Weiss *et al.* (1960) showed that the absorption of chloramphenicol palmitate was slower in newborn infants, probably because of reduced rate of hydrolysis in the intestinal tract. Also in older children sometimes up to 50 per cent of an administered dose of chloramphenicol palmitate may be lost in the faeces, and doses as high as 100 to 200 mg per kg per day may be required to produce adequate blood levels (Hodgman, 1961). It appears that, if chloramphenicol palmitate is used for the maintenance treatment of serious infections such as H. influenzae meningitis, it would be wise to check the serum levels obtained. From the evidence available the palmitate ester would probably be satisfactory for the majority, but it seems likely that there are individual variations in the rate of hydrolysis of this ester in the gastro-intestinal tract.

4. *Parenteral chloramphenicol.* Several forms of parenteral chloramphenicol have been available, but currently the ester, chloramphenicol sodium succinate is regarded as the most satisfactory. It is a highly soluble preparation which can be easily administered by either the intramuscular or intravenous route. This ester has no antibacterial activity, but after administration most of it is rapidly converted to active chloramphenicol (McCrumb *et al.*, 1958). For intramuscular administration the contents of a 2 g vial may be dissolved in as little as 2·5 ml of 'water for injection', resulting in a 40 per cent

solution. For intermittent intravenous injections, it is recommended that a more dilute 10 per cent solution be used, and the dose slowly injected into a vein or drip tubing over one minute. Rapid intravenous injection of a more concentrated solution is not dangerous, but the patient may experience an intensely bitter taste lasting a few minutes, and concentrated solutions may also cause thrombophlebitis. This chloramphenicol ester is stable in all commonly used intravenous fluids, so it can be added to intravenous bottles for continuous infusion, but incompatibility may occur in the presence of other intravenous additives. It has been generally recommended that the dose of intravenous or intramuscular chloramphenicol sodium succinate should be identical to oral chloramphenicol dosage, i.e. 3–4 g daily for adults and 50–80 mg per kg body weight per day in children, usually administered in four divided doses.

Initial studies with chloramphenicol sodium succinate showed that intravenous administration gave higher blood levels than identical intramuscular doses (McCrumb et al., 1958). This difference was not considered to be important, because patients treated intramuscularly had adequate serum levels and their clinical response was also satisfactory (McCrumb et al., 1958; Ross et al., 1958; Forbes, 1962). The efficacy of intramuscular chloramphenicol succinate for the treatment of induced typhoid fever and Rocky Mountain spotted fever was re-evaluated by Du Pont et al. (1970). They found that after intramuscular administration, serum levels of active chloramphenicol were about 50 per cent lower than those achieved after identical oral doses. Approximately one-third of the intramuscularly administered drug was present in serum in the form of antimicrobially inactive unhydrolysed ester, and the serum concentration of active chloramphenicol did not rise with continued intramuscular administration. Their typhoid fever patients responded more rapidly to oral chloramphenicol in a dose of 1 g eight-hourly, than to an identical intramuscular dosage of chloramphenicol sodium succinate. Accordingly Du Pont et al. (1970) recommended that when parenteral chloramphenicol sodium succinate is used for treatment of severe infections, the usually recommended dose should suffice if the intravenous route is used, but if the drug is given intramuscularly, the dose may need to be increased to 125–150 mg per kg per day. From this study it appears that it would be wise to monitor chloramphenicol serum levels if the succinate ester is used intramuscularly for serious infections. Some authors even consider that chloramphenicol must never be administered by the intramuscular route (Gleckman, 1975). However in our experience and that of others (Barrett et al., 1972), intramuscular chloramphenicol sodium succinate, administered in the usually recommended doses, gives good results in severe infections such as H. influenzae meningitis.

Several laboratory methods have been described for the estimation of chloramphenicol serum levels. These include a rapid microbiological assay (Louie et al., 1976), an enzymatic assay (Daigneault and Guitard, 1976), a simplified radioenzymatic assay (Robison et al., 1978) and a high-pressure liquid chromatographic method (Nilsson-Ehle et al., 1978).

5. *Newborn and premature infants.* In these a lower dosage should be used, and this usually should not exceed 25 mg per kg per day, given in one or two divided doses. However the rate of removal of chloramphenicol from the body varies in such infants, and in some this dosage may be toxic and in others it may be therapeutically ineffective. Hodgman and Burns (1961) reported two

infants aged less than four days, who developed serum levels over 50 μg per ml with toxic symptoms after daily doses of 25 mg per kg intramuscularly; they also observed another three prematures who when aged 12–22 days had inadequate levels with the same intramuscular dose. Black *et al.* (1978) treated one neonate with bacterial meningitis using intravenous chloramphenicol, which was commenced on the fifth day of life and continued for three weeks. Serum level monitoring showed that in order to maintain serum levels in the therapeutic range of 10–20 μg per ml, the daily chloramphenicol dose had to be progressively increased from 20 to 95 mg per kg with increasing age of the infant. It is apparent that serum level monitoring is highly advisable if chloramphenicol is used in this age group. If this is not possible, McCracken and Nelson (1977) recommend that intravenous chloramphenicol be given in a total daily dosage of 25 mg per kg to all infants weighing less than 2000 g and also to those who weigh more than 2000 g but are under 14 days of age. This dose can be administered as a single daily intravenous infusion, given over 15–30 min. Infants weighing more than 2000 g and who are 15–30 days old may be given 50 mg per kg body weight per day, which is usually administered intravenously in two divided doses. In children older than one month the dosage of 50 mg per kg is considered safe and therapeutically effective.

6. *Patients with renal failure.* Active chloramphenicol does not accumulate in these patients, and the drug may be administered in the usually recommended doses (Kunin, 1967). The drug may be more toxic to the bone marrow of uraemic patients, probably because of pre-existing bone marrow depression often associated with renal failure. Inactive chloramphenicol metabolites accumulate in the serum of patients with renal failure (page 432) but it is not known if these are toxic to the bone marrow. In using chloramphenicol to treat a severe infection in such patients, this increased risk of toxicity cannot be avoided, because dosage reduction results in inadequate serum levels of the active drug. Haemodialysis removes only small amounts of the active antibiotic, and peritoneal dialysis does not alter the serum half-life of active chloramphenicol (Greenberg and Sanford, 1967). Dosage modification of chloramphenicol is therefore not necessary in patients with renal failure undergoing these procedures.

7. *Patients with liver disease.* In severe liver disease the half-life of active chloramphenicol in the blood may be prolonged, and if the drug is used at all in such patients, appropriate dosage reduction with serum level monitoring is indicated (Kunin *et al.*, 1959).

Availability

For oral administration:
   (a) Chloramphenicol capsules: 125 and 250 mg.
   (b) Chloramphenicol palmitate suspension: 125 mg in 5 ml.
For intramuscular or intravenous administration:
   Chloramphenicol sodium succinate: 250 mg and 1·0 g vials.

Serum Levels in Relation to Dosage

Adequate serum levels of the active drug are attained after either intravenous or intramuscular administration of chloramphenicol sodium succinate (Fig.

22), but intravenous administration gives higher levels (*see* page 429). The blood level reaches its peak about two hours after an intramuscular dose, but the peak level of the active drug is attained immediately after intravenous injection. This latter finding indicates that a high proportion of the succinate ester is rapidly hydrolysed *in vivo* to form the active drug (McCrumb *et al.*, 1958).

Chloramphenicol, administered orally in capsules is rapidly and completely absorbed from the intestinal tract. The peak blood level after a 1 g oral dose in adults is about 10–13 μg per ml (Welch, 1954; DuPont *et al.*, 1970), which is about double the level attained after an identical dose given intramuscularly. The peak serum level after oral administration is approximately the same as that attained after a similar dose given intravenously, but the peak is not reached until about two hours after an oral dose. Doubling the usual oral dose, doubles the serum concentrations attained. The half-life of active chloramphenicol in serum is 1·6–3·3 h (Kunin *et al.*, 1959), but therapeutic levels may still be detected 6–8 h after the dose.

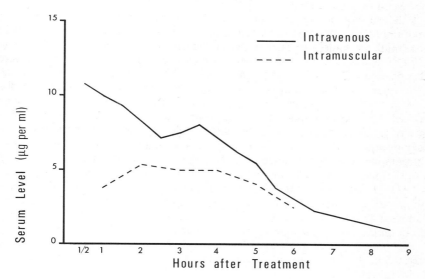

FIG. 22. Serum levels after single 1·0 g doses of chloramphenicol sodium succinate intravenously and intramuscularly. (Redrawn after McCrumb *et al.*, 1958.)

The serum levels achieved in children with an equivalent single oral dose (25 mg per kg) are of the same order. If the palmitate ester is used, some children, especially newborns, may attain lower peak blood levels, which may be only reached 6–12 h after the dose (Weiss *et al.*, 1960). There is considerable individual variation in the serum levels achieved when the palmitate ester is used (*see* page 427).

Excretion

1. About 90 per cent of administered chloramphenicol is excreted in urine, but only 5–10 per cent is in the unchanged active form. Chloramphenicol is

rapidly conjugated with glucuronic acid in the healthy human liver, and the conjugates are antibacterially inactive. Active chloramphenicol is excreted only by glomeruli, but the inactive derivatives are also eliminated by tubular secretion (Weiss *et al.*, 1960). Although most administered chloramphenicol is excreted in the form of inactive metabolites, urine concentrations of the active drug are still sufficiently high to be effective for treatment of urinary infections. Urine levels exceeding 200 μg per ml of the active drug have been found following a single oral dose of 1·5 g (Glazko *et al.*, 1949). However much less active chloramphenicol is excreted in the urine of patients with renal failure, and some of these patients may have no antibacterial effect in the urine (Lindberg *et al.*, 1966).

2. As most active chloramphenicol disappears from body primarily by conversion in liver, the active drug does not accumulate in the serum of anuric patients (Kunin *et al.*, 1959; Greenberg and Sanford, 1967). Inactive chloramphenicol metabolites, which are probably not toxic, do accumulate in the serum of such patients.

3. The immature liver of newborn and premature infants is deficient in chloramphenicol conjugating mechanisms, and the active drug accumulates in these patients, unless smaller doses are given (Weiss *et al.*, 1960) (*see* page 429). Similarly, active chloramphenicol may accumulate in adults with severe liver disease such as cirrhosis (Kunin *et al.*, 1959). In addition Weisberger *et al.* (1969) have suggested that some adults in the absence of any other liver disease, may have a genetic deficiency of glucuronyl transferase, an enzyme necessary for chloramphenicol conjugation. Such patients may develop high serum levels of the active drug, and would therefore be more prone to haemopoietic toxicity. The presence of an unusually high serum level of free chloramphenicol after a single intravenous test dose of the drug, may suggest that the patient has such an enzyme defect.

4. Only small amounts of chloramphenicol (2–3 per cent of the administered dose) are excreted in bile, mostly in the inactive form. The concentration of active chloramphenicol in bile is usually lower than that in the serum at the time (Woodward and Wisseman, 1958).

5. About 1 per cent of an orally administered dose of chloramphenicol is excreted in the faeces, mainly in the inactive form. It probably reaches the intestinal tract via the bile.

Distribution of the Drug in Body

Chloramphenicol diffuses into many body tissues and readily penetrates into pleural and ascitic fluids, and also crosses the placenta (Woodward and Wisseman, 1958). Concentrations of the drug in the ascitic fluid of patients with bacterial peritonitis usually exceed half of the serum level at the time (Gerding *et al.*, 1977). Also unlike many other antibiotics, it penetrates well into all parts of the eye, and into the CSF even in the absence of meningitis. The CSF concentration may be 50 per cent of that found in the serum of patients with normal meninges, a higher proportion than that attained with any other antibiotic. Dunkle (1978) used parenteral chloramphenicol to treat bacterial meningitis in four premature infants. Serum, CSF and ventricular fluid concentrations were measured frequently during therapy. Concentrations in the lumbar and ventricular fluid were in the therapeutic range (mean $23 \cdot 3 \pm 7 \cdot 7 \mu g$ per ml), and mean CSF levels were $66 \cdot 5$ per cent of peak serum levels in each patient. CSF chloramphenicol concentrations did not fall during treatment despite resolution of meningitis.

Chloramphenicol is protein bound to some extent, and as with other antibiotics this binding is probably readily reversible. Some authors have found that the drug is 50–60 per cent protein bound (Woodward and Wisseman, 1958), and others give a figure of 25 per cent (Kunin, 1967).

Mode of Action

Chloramphenicol is a potent inhibitor of bacterial protein synthesis (Goldberg, 1965). It is of some clinical importance to understand the mechanism of action of chloramphenicol and also that of the other antibiotics which interfere with bacterial protein synthesis. For this reason the following description of bacterial protein synthesis is included.

The basic mechanisms involved in the synthesis of bacterial and human proteins are similar. Fortunately there are sufficient differences between their metabolic processes to allow certain antibiotics to be selectively toxic to bacteria.

Deoxyribonucleic acid (DNA), contained in the nucleus, has the genetic control of the synthesis of all specific cellular proteins including enzymes. For this purpose DNA directs the formation of three types of ribonucleic acid (RNA).

(a) *Messenger RNA (m-RNA)*. The genetic code of DNA for the specific organism is copied onto m-RNA, the process being catalysed by a polymerase called DNA-dependent RNA polymerase (transcriptase). This 'transcription' of information onto m-RNA, determines the amino acid sequence of the proteins to be synthetized. Messenger RNA is an elongated strand consisting of many segments or codons, each of which is specific for a particular amino acid. This RNA migrates out into the cytoplasm, where in association with small organelles, the ribosomes, it acts as a template to direct synthesis of specific cellular proteins ('translation' of genetic message).

(b) *Transfer RNA (t-RNA)*. This RNA acts as a carrier to transport amino acids to the proper site on the template of m-RNA. For each amino acid to be incorporated into a protein molecule, there is a specific t-RNA molecule. The specific part of t-RNA for the amino acid carried is called the anticodon, and this is complementary to the codon on m-RNA for that particular amino acid.

(c) *Ribosome RNA (r-RNA)*. Ribosomes consist of this particular ribonucleic acid and various proteins. The ribosome can be considered as the 'work-bench' upon which various amino acids are joined in a predetermined arrangement to produce the polypeptide chains of the many proteins required for cell metabolism (Nomura, 1969). Ribosomes from bacteria can be distinguished from those of mammalian cells on the basis of their sedimentation coefficients ('S values'). Broadly speaking, bacteria contain 70 S ribosomes and mammalian cells 80 S ribosomes, and this distinction is useful in the context of antibiotic action, because many antibiotics selectively act against 70 S ribosomes. However some 70 S ribosomes are also found in mammalian mitochondria.

The first step in protein synthesis is activation of amino acids, which is carried out by activating enzymes specific for each amino acid, known as aminoacyl-RNA synthetases. These activated amino acid molecules are then attached to the specific t-RNA molecules which are coded for this purpose. This process is catalysed by specific enzymes known as aminoacyl-t-RNA synthetases. The resultant aminoacyl-t-RNA molecules then migrate to the ribosome-m-RNA complex for the synthesis of amino acid chains as specified by the m-RNA template.

The process by which polypeptide chains are manufactured from amino acids at the ribosomes is complicated. Bacterial 70 S ribosomes consist of two unequal portions, a larger '50 S' subunit and a smaller '30 S' subunit. Certain 'initiation factors' appear to be necessary for the commencement of polypeptide chain synthesis at the ribosomes. As a result it seems that m-RNA initially binds to the 30 S subunit and sequentially t-RNA and then the 50 S subunit to form the complete 70 S 'initiation complex' or active ribosome, necessary for protein synthesis.

The two parts of the aggregated or active ribosome particle have different functions. Messenger RNA is bound to the 30 S portion of the ribosome, whilst the 50 S subunit is a site for attachment of amino acids and a site for holding the growing peptide chains. These sites, known respectively as the acceptor ('A') site and the peptidyl donor ('P') site, are in close proximity to each other, and each site is also in juxtaposition to one m-RNA codon. The next step is the binding of individual aminoacyl-t-RNA molecules to each 'A' site on the ribosome as directed by the m-RNA codon in juxtaposition. This binding process is catalysed by a complex enzyme, called transfer factor, T.

Growth of peptide chains is achieved by the transfer and binding of a peptide chain from a nearby 'P' site, onto the amino acid at the 'A' site. This results in the release of the deacylated or old t-RNA which has lost its peptide chain at the 'P' site. The aminoacyl-t-RNA complex at the former 'A' site then becomes the carrier of the newly elongated peptide chain. This process called 'transpeptidation' is catalysed by an ezyme, peptidyl transferase, which is part of the 50 S subunit of the ribosome.

To enable further growth of the peptide chain, the newly elongated peptide chain is then moved into a donor or 'P' site, by a process called translocation. This involves the movement of the ribosome along the strand of RNA, resulting in the m-RNA codon for the next amino acid to be incorporated, to be brought into juxtaposition to the donor site, as the new acceptor site. Translocation is catalysed by a translocase enzyme called 'G' factor.

Protein synthesis occurs at the various ribosome-m-RNA complexes, and this enables multiple proteins to be synthetized at the same time. Other proteins are involved in the release of the completed polypeptide chains from the ribosome complexes.

Most of these steps in bacterial protein synthesis may be attacked by antibiotics with consequent disruption of cell metabolism.

The inhibitory action of chloramphenicol on bacterial protein synthesis is dependent on its ability to bind to the 50 S subunit of the ribosome (*vide supra*). It appears that chloramphenicol inhibits the transpeptidation reaction which occurs at the ribosomal acceptor site (Cundliffe and McQuillen, 1967; Hahn, 1968; Gale *et al.*, 1972; Vince *et al.*, 1975). In bacterial cells, which have been exposed to chloramphenicol for a short time, protein synthesis may resume when the drug is withdrawn. Peptide chains, whose synthesis was interrupted by chloramphenicol, can again be completed when the drug is removed. This explains the bacteristatic rather than bactericidal action which this drug has against certain bacteria (Green *et al.*, 1975). With more prolonged exposure, chloramphenicol has additional effects on bacteria resulting in excretion of cellular macromolecules, lysis of cells and degradation of ribosomes; these effects eventually lead to cell death. This bactericidal effect is dependent on the growth phase of the bacterial cells. Actively dividing cells rapidly lose viability, but resting or slowly dividing cells remain viable for long periods (Gupta, 1975; Bacchus and Javor, 1975). Ribosome located bacterial resistance to chloramphenicol is uncommon, and resistance of Gram-negative bacteria is usually acquired by means of R plasmids (page 422).

It was suggested that the haemopoietic toxicity of chloramphenicol (page 437) occurs because the drug inhibits human cell protein synthesis (Weisberger *et al.*, 1969). Immature or proliferating erythrocytes are much more susceptible to chloramphenicol than other mammalian cells. Furthermore the anamnestic antibody response to tetanus toxoid can be suppressed by chloramphenicol, suggesting that it may inhibit antibody synthesis (Daniel *et al.,* 1965). This inhibitory effect has been shown experimentally in tissue cultures of lymph node fragments (Ambrose and Coons, 1963). Chloramphenicol may be useful as an immunosuppressive drug for the treatment of diseases such as lupus glomerulonephritis or even for prevention of homograft rejection. This drug may be less toxic than other immunosuppressives because it inhibits antibody synthesis by a different mechanism and does not cause cellular necrosis (Weisberger *et al.*, 1969).

The mechanism by which chloramphenicol inhibits protein synthesis in mammalian cells is probably different from that operating in bacteria. It was suggested that the drug blocks the correct attachment of m-RNA to ribosomes in mammalian cells (Beard *et al.*, 1969), but it is now generally accepted that chloramphenicol does not inhibit ribosomal protein synthesis in mammals (Beard and Weisberger, 1972; Yunis, 1974). Mammalian cells contain 80 S ribosomes, and the protein synthesis in these, unlike that in bacterial 70 S ribosomes, appears to be unaffected by chloramphenicol. In human and other mammalian cells the mitochondria (which contain 70 S particles) are also capable of independent protein synthesis. Martelo *et al.* (1969) demonstrated that therapeutic concentrations of chloramphenicol inhibit protein synthesis by human and rabbit bone marrow mitochondria. Furthermore Yunis *et al.* (1970) observed mitochrondrial damage by electron microscopy in bone marrow cells obtained from patients treated with chloramphenicol. However, there is also some evidence suggesting that chloramphenicol only acts on human mitochrondria in experimental situations, as normally mitochondria are impermeable to this drug (Gale *et al.*, 1972). Nevertheless the effect of chloramphenicol on mitochondria appears to be the explanation of the dose related haemopoietic toxicity of the drug (page 437), but the pathogenesis of the rare aplastic anaemia (*vide infra*) remains unknown (Editorial, 1970; Yunis, 1974). It is possible that aplasia may be caused by cell-mediated immune mechanisms in man, but alternatively the stem cell may be directly damaged by the drug, and other mechanisms are also possible (Leading article, 1976).

Chloramphenicol is usually classed as a 'bacteristatic' agent, because *in vitro* this drug usually arrests the multiplication of bacteria, but does not reduce the number of living organisms. However chloramphenicol in high concentrations may be 'cidal' to some organisms, and it is even 'cidal' in relatively low concentrations to H. influenzae, which is a highly sensitive organism (Garrod and Waterworth, 1962). The distinction between so called 'bactericidal' and 'bacteristatic' agents is only relative, and many other factors influence the action of antibiotics on bacteria *in vivo* (*see also* pages 444, 612).

From a practical point of view it is wrong to assume that a 'bactericidal' drug will always be clinically superior to a 'bacteristatic' one. For example chloramphenicol is more effective than other drugs with a 'bactericidal action' in the treatment of typhoid fever. However one situation in which bactericidal drugs appear to be superior is in the treatment of bacterial endocarditis, an infection of a relatively avascular tissue.

Toxicity

1. *Bone marrow depression*. This is the most important toxic effect of chloramphenicol (Yunis and Bloomberg, 1964). Two forms of bone marrow depression occur:

   (a) *Aplastic anaemia*. This is a rare complication, but has a high mortality. Initially its frequency was variously estimated as 1 in 500 to 1 in 100 000 of treated patients (Willcox, 1967; Leading article, 1967). A survey in California showed that the calculated risk of dying from aplastic anaemia was 1 in 21 671 after an average adult course of 7·5 g of the drug. This chloramphenicol-associated fatal aplastic anaemia was 13 times more common than aplastic anaemia in the population not treated by chloramphenicol (Wallerstein *et al*., 1969; Wallerstein, 1969). Between 1965 and 1971 inclusive, 31 cases of aplastic anaemia following exposure to chloramphenicol were observed in Hamburg and surrounding districts. The frequency was estimated at 1 in 11 500 and the death rate as 1 in 18 500 (Hausmann and Skrandies, 1974). In Sweden during a six-year period 1966–1971, seven patients with chloramphenicol-induced aplastic anaemia were reported, and six of them died. In this study the risk of developing aplastic anaemia after a course of chloramphenicol was calculated to be 1 in 19 000 (Böttiger, 1974). It is apparent that the estimated risks of aplastic anaemia from chloramphenicol in these surveys from different countries are in accord. Some early publications gave the impression that this complication may be more common in Australia. In Melbourne, Shaw and McLean (1957) described seven cases in twelve months, and Hughes (1962) reported sixteen cases from a children's hospital in Sydney during an eight-year period. Subsequently there has been no evidence that there is an increased risk of chloramphenicol-induced aplastic anaemia in Australia. It has been claimed that chloramphenicol-induced aplastic anaemia is extremely rare in Israel (Sheba, 1967).

Bone marrow aplasia due to chloramphenicol usually results in aplastic anaemia with pancytopenia, and other forms, such as erythroid hypoplasia, selective leucopenia or thrombocytopenia are less common. The mortality in aplastic anaemia with pancytopenia has been in excess of 50 per cent (Davis and Rubin, 1972). Some recoveries have occurred after prolonged periods of bone marrow aplasia. This blood dyscrasia may develop during the first one or two weeks of chloramphenicol treatment, but in the majority of patients the disorder only becomes evident after a latent period of weeks or months. It has been difficult to correlate amounts of the drug administered and the frequency of aplastic anaemia (Best, 1967). Holt (1967) noted that there had been no recorded cases of marrow aplasia following the administration of the drug by parenteral routes alone. He hypothetized that a minority of people possess special intestinal Enterobacteriaceae which degrade chloramphenicol, and the absorption of by-products of this action, not chloramphenicol itself, is responsible for marrow toxicity. This hypothesis has not been confirmed, but it still appears to be true that aplastic anaemia has never resulted from the use of parenteral chloramphenicol alone (Gleckman, 1975). Some clinicians therefore now continue parenteral chloramphenicol even after a serious infection has responded and oral therapy is possible. A report of aplastic anaemia in identical twins given chloramphenicol is of considerable interest (Nagao and Mauer, 1969). In an attempt to explain this occurrence, Dameshek (1969) postulated that there may be a genetically determined defect in the bone marrow cells of some individuals, rendering them particularly susceptible to chloramphenicol bone marrow aplasia. Hodgkinson (1973) described five patients who developed aplastic anaemia after receiving chloramphenicol during the pre-icteric phase of hepatitis, presumed of viral aetiology. Viral hepatitis *per se* has been regarded as an important cause of aplastic anaemia, and it is possible that chloramphenicol and the hepatitis virus(es) may have an additive toxic effect on the bone marrow (Comments, 1973). Thus the risk of aplastic anaemia may be very much greater if the drug is used during viral hepatitis. This may also apply to some other virus infections. This could explain why parenteral chloramphenicol administration has not been associated with aplastic anaemia; the parenteral drug is used in hospitals for severe bacterial infections, and it would be unlikely for someone with a virus infection to receive this preparation.

(b) *Haemopoietic toxicity*. Side-effects grouped under this heading are much more common than aplastic anaemia and they appear to be dose related and reversible. There is some evidence from animal experiments that chloramphenicol suppresses the activity of ferrochelatase, an enzyme which normally catalyses haemoglobin synthesis within the mitochondria of bone marrow erythroid cells (Manyan *et al.*, 1972). Chloramphenicol in concentrations which are achieved in serum during therapy, also inhibits bone marrow colony formation *in vitro* (Howell *et al.*, 1975). A number of studies in humans (Scott *et al.*, 1965; Hughes, 1968; 1973) indicate that the administration of large doses of chloramphenicol for several weeks is sometimes associated with:

(1) Reduced iron utilization for haemoglobin synthesis as indicated by rising serum iron levels.

(2) Vacuolation of erythroblasts, or a progressive increase in the marrow myeloid-erythroid ratio, a low reticulocyte count and falling haemoglobin, suggesting interference with the production and maturation of erythroid cells. The use of phenylalanine reduces this vacuolation of the erythroblasts (Ingall *et al.*, 1965), but there is no evidence that this amino acid is useful for the treatment of patients with aplastic anaemia.

(3) Thrombocytopenia and leucopenia with vacuolation of marrow granulocyte precursors.

These changes occurred regularly when the serum levels of active chloramphenicol were 25 μg per ml or greater, suggesting that these toxic effects are a pharmacological property of the drug (Scott *et al.*, 1965) (*see also* mode of action, page 435). Similar changes occurred more rapidly in patients with hepatic diseases, especially in those with jaundice or ascites, who developed high active chloramphenicol serum levels more readily. Such side-effects are usually reversible after cessation of the drug; the serum iron falls abruptly, reticulocytosis appears, and the bone marrow and the peripheral blood returns to normal within a few days. In some cases erythropoietic recovery may occur even if chloramphenicol is continued (Hughes, 1973). This is more likely if the reticulocyte count exceeds 0·5 per cent and if the myeloid-erythroid ratio is less than 10:1. However, in other patients, especially if neutropenia and thrombocytopenia have already developed, more severe bone marrow depression may occur if the drug is continued (Hughes, 1973). Nevertheless the available evidence suggests that a different mechanism is responsible for the development of the rare and irreversible aplastic anaemia.

Some authors consider that this division of chloramphenicol induced blood dyscrasias into two separate categories is not always clear cut, and that a single pathogenic mechanism may be involved (Best, 1967). Chloramphenicol should be discontinued when the more benign haemopoietic toxicity is discovered, and regular blood examinations for all patients receiving chloramphenicol are advisable (Best, 1967; Weisberger *et al.*, 1969). Unfortunately these precautionary measures cannot reliably detect the rare patients liable to develop aplastic anaemia (Editorial, 1970).

2. *Other haemopoietic side-effects.* Chloramphenicol prevents the expected reticulocyte response in patients with pernicious anaemia treated by vitamin B_{12}. Similarly it prevents the expected response to iron in patients with iron deficiency anaemia. These phenomena are probably explicable in terms of the known mode of action of chloramphenicol on rapidly multiplying cells (Weisberger *et al.*, 1969) (*see also* page 435). Haemolytic anaemia developed in three patients with glucose-6-phosphate dehydrogenase deficiency who were treated by chloramphenicol for typhoid fever (McCaffrey *et al.*, 1971). The drug only caused a mild haemolytic reaction in two of these patients, when, free from the infection, they were studied one year later. *In vitro*,

chloramphenicol in therapeutic concentrations, markedly depresses leucocyte migration (Forsgren and Schmeling, 1977) and in high concentrations such as 200 μg per ml it also impairs phagocytosis (Melby and Midtvedt, 1977). The clinical significance of these observations is not yet clear.

3. *Grey syndrome.* This is a type of circulatory collapse, which can occur in premature and newborn infants receiving large doses of chloramphenicol (Burns *et al.*, 1959; Beveridge, 1961). In the trial reported by Burns *et al.* (1959) chloramphenicol was given to 61 premature infants in doses ranging from 100 to 165 mg per kg daily. Approximately 60 per cent of these infants died. Chloramphenicol serum levels (combined active and inactive drug) estimated in two of these children, rose to about 70 and 180 μg per ml, respectively, just before death. The syndrome was characterized by abdominal distension, vomiting, pallor, cyanosis and circulatory collapse, which usually resulted in death. The term 'grey syndrome' was coined from the appearance of these children. It is now known that babies aged less than four weeks have a defective capacity for both conjugating and excreting chloramphenicol. This syndrome has been clearly related to high toxic levels of the active drug, but if the recommended reduced dose for this age group is used (page 429), and serum active chloramphenicol levels do not rise higher than 20 μg per ml, this complication should not occur (Weiss *et al.*, 1960). As chloramphenicol readily crosses the placenta, it should be used with caution in late pregnancy or during labour, because of the risk of this toxic effect in the newborn. The use of chloramphenicol may also be best avoided during lactation, as the drug is excreted in human milk.

A similar syndrome has also been described in adults and older children who have received accidental chloramphenicol overdoses. Thompson *et al.* (1975) described three such patients. One patient, a 70-year-old woman who received one 20 g dose, died 11 h later. The second patient was a 26-year-old woman who received an initial 1·0 g dose followed in 7 and 12 h by two 10 g doses. Five hours after the last dose she developed severe shock, cyanosis and coma, but she responded slowly to fluids and dopamine and made a full recovery. The serum active chloramphenicol level 5·5 h after her last dose was 201 μg per ml. The third patient was a four-and-a-half-month-old infant, who following chloramphenicol overdosage became unresponsive with hypothermia and abdominal distension. The serum chloramphenicol level was 174 μg per ml. The infant recovered after an exchange transfusion and other measures.

4. *Optic neuritis.* This complication has been described in a small number of patients treated with chloramphenicol, and sometimes has resulted in optic atrophy and blindness (Leading article, 1965; Cocke *et al.*, 1966). Most of these patients were children with cystic fibrosis receiving prolonged chloramphenicol treatment for pulmonary infection. Blindness may occur without recognizable fundal changes. Vision may partly return after cessation of the drug, but this is not invariable. Large doses of B group vitamins have been used to treat this condition. This complication is an additional reason to avoid prolonged courses of chloramphenicol. Peripheral neuritis has also been described in association with optic neuritis (Joy *et al.*, 1960). Other neurotoxic symptoms, such as headache, depression, ophthalmoplegia, mental confusion and delirium have been occasionally attributed to chloramphenicol.

5. *Gastro-intestinal side-effects.* Nausea, vomiting and diarrhoea oc-

casionally occur, but these are much less common than with the tetracyclines. Pseudomembranous colitis (page 481) may occur, but this complication is rare with chloramphenicol. Glossitis and stomatitis, sometimes associated with thrush, may also be enccountered.

6. *Hypersensitivity reactions*. These are very rare, but contact dermatitis, rashes, drug fever, and even occasional instances of anaphylaxis and angioneurotic oedema have been reported. Jarisch-Herxheimer reactions have been described in patients treated for syphilis (Welch, 1954), and also during therapy for typhoid fever. Cahill (1962) reported a patient who developed a severe haemorrhagic reaction associated with chloramphenicol. There was no evidence of bone marrow depression, or coagulation defects, and bleeding appeared to be due to a capillary defect presumably due to hypersensitivity.

7. *Bleeding due to increase of prothrombin time*. This may occur as a result of prolonged oral administration of the drug. Decreased vitamin K synthesis results from a reduction of intestinal bacteria, and this defect can be rapidly corrected by the administration of parenteral vitamin K (Cahill, 1962).

8. *Ototoxicity*. Hearing loss has been noted in a few children with H. influenzae meningitis, who have been treated by chloramphenicol. This was almost certainly a sequel to their meningitis and not a drug toxicity (Svenungsson *et al.*, 1976). Animal experiments have shown that chloramphenicol ear drops can cause deafness, especially if the drops have a higher concentration than 5 per cent and if they are instilled in the middle ear cavity (Morizono and Johnstone, 1975). Chloramphenicol ear drops are seldom indicated, especially in the presence of large perforations (*see also* neomycin, page 410).

9. *Drug interactions*. Chloramphenicol inhibits the activity of certain liver enzymes, and it interferes with the biotransformation of tolbutamide, diphenylhydantoin, and dicoumarol. Toxicity due to these three drugs may occur if they are administered in usual doses to a patient who is also receiving chloramphenicol (Christensen and Skovsted, 1969; Rose *et al.*, 1977).

Clinical Uses of the Drug

1. *Salmonella infections*. Chloramphenicol remains the drug of choice for treatment of typhoid and paratyphoid fever, ampicillin (page 114) and co-trimoxazole (page 711) being less effective (Uwaydah, 1975; Snyder *et al.*, 1976). However for the treatment of typhoid fever caused by chloramphenicol-resistant Salm. typhi strains (page 423), other drugs are necessary; ampicillin is currently recommended but amoxycillin (page 142) or co-trimoxazole (page 711) appear to be equally effective (Herzog, 1976; Butler *et al.*, 1977). Ampicillin or possibly amoxycillin used alone or in combination with chloramphenicol is also indicated for the initial treatment of patients with suspected typhoid, acquired in South-East Asia or other areas where resistant typhoid bacilli are known to exist (Overturf *et al.*, 1973; Leading article, 1973). For infections due to Salm. typhi strains resistant to both chloramphenicol and ampicillin, co-trimoxazole is the only recommended alternative. Mecillinam (page 194), cefamandole (page 286) and possibly drug combinations (page 575) may also prove to be effective for the treatment of typhoid fever, but ampicillin-resistant strains of Salm. typhi are likely to be also mecillinam-

resistant. Typhoid fever is usually treated for a period of two weeks (Hoffman *et al.*, 1975; Snyder *et al.*, 1976). A second course of treatment for 10–14 days is given by some clinicians in order to prevent a relapse, which occurs in approximately 10 per cent of patients if only one two weeks' course of treatment is given.

Chloramphenicol is not indicated in salmonella gastro-enteritis, unless the infection is unduly severe or septicaemia is present. Septicaemias due to salmonellae such as Salm. cholerae-suis and Salm. typhimurium do not respond as well and predictably as typhoid fever (Christie, 1974), but chloramphenicol is still the best antibiotic available for their treatment. Chloramphenicol is of no value for the eradication of the salmonella carrier state, and this applies both to persistent typhoid carriers and the usually short lived carrier state due to other Salmonella species. In addition, treatment of patients with acute salmonella gastro-enteritis with chloramphenicol usually prolongs the period of excretion of salmonellae after clinical recovery (Aserkoff and Bennett, 1969).

2. *Arizona infections.* The disease spectrum in man caused by Arizona spp. is indistinguishable from that which occurs with the salmonellae. Patients with Arizona infections may present with gastro-enteritis, septicaemia or a localized infection. Chloramphenicol or ampicillin (page 99) are the antimicrobial agents of choice for severe systemic Arizona infections (Johnson *et al.*, 1976).

3. *Shigella infections.* For the vast majority of cases of shigella dysentery, chloramphenicol is not indicated, but it is a valuable drug for the rare severe case with extensive tissue involvement or associated septicaemia. If antibiotics are indicated in shigellosis, either ampicillin (page 115) or co-trimoxazole (page 713) are usually used. These two drugs are also effective alternatives for severe cases if chloramphenicol-resistant Shigella spp. strains (page 422) are involved.

4. *Rickettsial diseases.* Chloramphenicol is very effective for treatment of epidemic typhus fever, scrub typhus, murine typhus and Rocky Mountain spotted fever (Hazard *et al.*, 1969; Snyder and Woodward, 1970). The tetracyclines are equally effective (page 624), and are usually used in moderate cases, because they are potentially less toxic. Chloramphenicol is preferable for very ill patients, because parenteral forms of the tetracyclines are not as satisfactory and also most tetracyclines cannot be used in the presence of renal failure (page 602).

5. *Bacterial meningitis.* Penicillin G and chloramphenicol is a very useful combination for the initial treatment of this disease, before the causative organism is identified (Forbes, 1962; Lindberg *et al.*, 1977) (*see also* page 33). Chloramphenicol alone is very effective for the treatment of meningitis due to H. influenzae type b (Shackelford *et al.*, 1972; Lovell and Dugdale, 1973; Feigin *et al.*, 1976). Many clinicians, particularly in North America, consider that parenteral ampicillin is equally effective and preferable because of the potential toxicity of chloramphenicol (*see* page 116). However chloramphenicol (usually given for two weeks) is still used at Fairfield Hospital for this disease, and the emergence sometimes during treatment of H. influenzae strains resistant to ampicillin is an added reason for this preference (*see* page 102). Chloramphenicol is also very effective for rarer types of meningitis, such as those due to Staph. pyogenes and sensitive strains of Esch. coli. It is also an effective alternative drug for meningococcal and pneumococcal

meningitis in penicillin-allergic patients (Westenfelder and Paterson, 1969; Gleckman, 1975), although in many of these patients penicillin G can still be used if combined with corticosteroids (page 26). Chloramphenicol is now the best alternative drug to penicillin G for treatment of meningococcal meningitis (Whittle *et al.*, 1973), because cephalosporins are ineffective (page 216) and sulphonamide-resistant meningococci are now common (page 661). Some success in the treatment of pneumococcal meningitis has been obtained by cephaloridine (page 213), but chloramphenicol is a wiser choice if penicillin G cannot be used.

6. *Haemophilus influenzae infections.* Apart from meningitis (*vide supra*), H. influenzae type b may cause other severe infections, particularly in children, such as epiglottitis, osteomyelitis, cellulitis and pneumonia, all of which are usually associated with septicaemia. Chloramphenicol is very effective for these diseases, but some authors prefer parenteral ampicillin (page 117), provided the H. influenzae strain is sensitive. Chloramphenicol used alone may also succeed in Haemophilus endocarditis (Cooper and Lietman, 1977).

7. *Cerebral abscess.* Penicillin G combined with chloramphenicol appears to be the best initial chemotherapy for patients with this disease (Samson and Clark, 1973). Abscesses in the frontal lobe which are of sinusitic origin are usually caused by various types of streptococci; these may respond to penicillin G alone, but initially a penicillin G/chloramphenicol combination is advisable. Abscesses of otic origin which occur in the temporal lobe usually yield a mixed flora including anaerobes such as Bacteroides fragilis. Penicillin G/chloramphenicol is probably the best treatment of these, although it is possible that either clindamycin (page 484) or metronidazole (page 773) can be used instead of chloramphenicol. In post-traumatic abscesses and in spinal extradural abscesses, Staph. pyogenes is the predominant organism. These would also usually respond to chloramphenicol, but if the bacterial aetiology is known, a specific anti-staphylococcal agent such as cloxacillin (page 88) can be used (Ingham and Selkon, 1976; De Louvois *et al.*, 1977a and b; De Louvois, 1978; Ingham *et al.*, 1978).

8. *Staphylococcal infections.* Chloramphenicol is effective for many life-threatening Staph. pyogenes infections, but its use has been largely supplanted by the development of potent anti-staphylococcal agents, such as the penicillinase-resistant penicillins, cephalosporins, clindamycin and sodium fusidate. However it remains to be determined whether these drugs will be as effective as chloramphenicol in the treatment of staphylococcal meningitis.

9. *Pertussis.* Antibiotics including chloramphenicol, to which the organism is sensitive *in vitro*, do not influence the natural course of this disease except through control of secondary infection (page 116). Chloramphenicol is never indicated in uncomplicated pertussis. It may be required occasionally if there is associated severe secondary bacterial pneumonia, because the exact aetiology of these pneumonias is often difficult to determine.

10. *Gram-negative anaerobic bacterial infections.* The important role of Gram-negative anaerobes, particularly Bacteroides fragilis, as causative agents of a wide range of major infections in man is now established (Gleckman, 1975) (*see also* page 484). Bacteroides fragilis infections are particularly associated with intra-abdominal sepsis such as abscess or peritonitis, especially those following appendicitis or large bowel surgery. Similarly anaerobic

organisms are often involved in obstetric infections, septic abortions, other female genital tract infections or in infections which follow female genital tract surgery (Finegold *et al.*, 1975). The pulmonary infections in which there is usually mixed infection involving both aerobic and anaerobic Gram-negative and Gram-positive bacteria, include aspiration pneumonitis, lung abscess and necrotizing pneumonia (Bartlett *et al.*, 1974; Finegold *et al.*, 1975; Brook and Finegold, 1977). Bacteroides fragilis is an important pathogen in suppurative disease of the middle ear and mastoid, and in brain abscesses of otic origin (page 442), but other cerebral abscesses may also sometimes harbour Gram-negative anaerobes (Finegold *et al.*, 1975). Anaerobes such as B. fragilis may also cause bone and joint infections and occasionally endocarditis. These anaerobes may also sometimes be involved together with aerobic Gram-negative bacilli, in biliary tract infections, particularly in elderly patients with biliary obstruction (Shimada *et al.*, 1977). All of these infections can be associated with B. fragilis septicaemia, particularly those involving the lung and peritoneum (Finegold *et al.*, 1975; Olsen, 1976).

Many anaerobic infections need appropriate surgical treatment, but antibiotics are often also essential. Chloramphenicol is very effective for B. fragilis infections and it may well be the drug of choice (Masri and Grieco, 1972; Young *et al.*, 1977). Despite the development of other agents active against B. fragilis, such as clindamycin (page 484), metronidazole (page 771), carbenicillin (page 162) and cefoxitin (page 286), many clinicians still prefer chloramphenicol, particularly for treatment of serious anaerobic infections that are bacteriologically undefined, and for infections of the central nervous system (Finegold, 1977). Nevertheless there have been occasional cases which have failed to respond to chloramphenicol despite *in vitro* sensitivity of the organism concerned (Gorbach and Bartlett, 1974). In comparative studies, where severe infections such as Bacteroides septicaemia or infections of the female genital tract have been treated by either chloramphenicol or clindamycin, results of treatment have been approximately the same (Mathias *et al.*, 1977; Ledger *et al.*, 1977).

As many of the diseases associated with anaerobic bacteria are caused by a mixture of organisms, combination chemotherapy is often necessary. For conditions such as lung infections and brain abscess, chloramphenicol is usually combined with penicillin G, because both penicillin-sensitive aerobic and anaerobic Gram-positive cocci are often involved (*see also* page 34). Penicillin G and chloramphenicol are not antagonistic in the clinical setting (page 444). Chloramphenicol combined with gentamicin is often used for treatment of severe intra-abdominal sepsis to cover the possibility of mixed infection with anaerobic and aerobic Gram-negative bacilli. These two drugs are also not antagonistic *in vivo* (page 342), but animal experiments suggest that there may be some antagonism when the host's phagocytic function is reduced (Sande and Overton, 1973). In some instances a combination of chloramphenicol with both penicillin G and gentamicin may be needed to provide effective therapy for aerobic and anaerobic Gram-positive and Gram-negative bacteria. For instance, this may be necessary as emergency treatment for severe aspiration pneumonia or female genital tract infections, before identification of the organisms concerned.

11. *Gram-negative aerobic enteric bacterial infections.* Chloramphenicol is

effective in many severe infections due to these organisms, except those due to Ps. aeruginosa. It should never be used for uncomplicated urinary tract infections, which respond to safer drugs. For the treatment of severe infections caused by aerobic Gram-negative enteric bacteria, aminoglycosides such as kanamycin (page 317) or gentamicin (page 341) are usually preferred to chloramphenicol (Young et al., 1977). In some situations it may be reasonable to use chloramphenicol to treat infections such as an Esch. coli septicaemia, and accept the remote risk of aplastic anaemia, rather than the likelihood of ototoxicity with kanamycin or gentamicin (page 338). Thus chloramphenicol may be considered for an elderly patient, especially if facilities for monitoring serum levels of aminoglycosides are not available.

A combination of chloramphenicol with gentamicin is regarded as an effective treatment for difficult Serratia spp. infections, such as endocarditis (Mills and Drew, 1976) (see also pages 162, 344). Chloramphenicol is usually effective for Klebsiella pneumonia, provided the strain is sensitive. Other drugs such as one of the parenteral cephalosporins (page 215), kanamycin (page 318), gentamicin (page 342) or co-trimoxazole (page 710) may also be useful for the treatment of this infection. Chloramphenicol may be preferable to these drugs if anaerobic infection (page 442) coexists in such a pneumonia.

12. *Emergency treatment of severe infections*. Chloramphenicol in combination with penicillin G is valuable for the immediate treatment of life-threatening infections, such as septicaemia, fulminating pneumonia and possible severe Gram-negative anaerobic infections (page 442). Experience at Fairfield Hospital supports the opinion that antagonism between these drugs is of no clinical importance (Crofton, 1969; Derrington, 1971). Antagonism between penicillin G (bactericidal drug) and chloramphenicol (bacteristatic drug) can be demonstrated *in vitro* with marginal drug concentrations, but clinically these drugs are used in much higher doses. The effect of a high dose of a 'bactericidal' drug is not affected by the simultaneous administration of a 'bacteristatic' one (Jawetz, 1964) (see also page 612). The combination of penicillin G and chloramphenicol is particularly dependable for initial treatment of severe infections in previously healthy patients, who have acquired their infection in their home environment (Bennett and Kucers, 1970). The position is different for hospital-acquired infections, where chloramphenicol-resistant staphylococci and resistant aerobic Gram-negative bacilli may be encountered. In these patients different antibiotic regimens are necessary for emergency therapy, and may include kanamycin (page 317), gentamicin (page 341) or amikacin (page 387).

13. *Melioidosis*. This disease, caused by Pseudomonas pseudomallei, may be subacute or chronic, but sometimes presents as an acute septicamia, often with pulmonary involvement, and has a high mortality. Opinion on the ideal type of chemotherapy for this disease has not been uniform. For severe cases some authors favoured the use of large doses of chloramphenicol (sometimes as much as 3 g every six hours) combined with novobiocin and kanamycin (Sheehy et al., 1967; Weber et al., 1969). Others preferred tetracycline, either alone or in combination with novobiocin (Howe et al., 1971; Calabi, 1973). Gentamicin has also been used for the treatment of this disease page 345), and co-trimoxazole may prove of value (page 709). Nowadays tetracyclines (page 628), either alone or in combination with chloramphenicol, are most commonly

used for the treatment of this disease (Everett and Nelson, 1975).

14. *Bacterial eye infections*. Chloramphenicol penetrates into both the aqueous and vitreous humours after systemic administration, and is therefore useful for the treatment of intra-ocular infections. It also penetrates into the aqueous humour after topical application to eye (Hodgman, 1961).

15. *Chlamydial eye infections*. It has been claimed that topical chloramphenicol is effective against trachoma. Darougar *et al.* (1977) used one per cent chloramphenicol eye ointment for four to six weeks to treat patients with paratrachoma (*see* page 626). This appeared to reduce the severity of clinical signs and symptoms, but failed to eliminate the infection. Tetracyclines (page 626), sulphonamides (page 675) or erythromycin (page 499) are usually preferred for these infections.

16. *Venereal diseases*. Chloramphenicol is effective for chancroid, lymphogranuloma venereum and granuloma inguinale, but because of its potential toxicity it is regarded only as a 'back-up' drug for these diseases, and the tetracyclines (page 626) are the drugs of choice (Willcox, 1977).

17. *Leukaemia*. One study showed that chloramphenicol reduced the white cell and blast cell counts in a patient with chronic myeloid leukaemia in blastic transformation. It was therefore suggested that the drug may have a place in the management of acute leukaemia (Schwarz and Firkin, 1976).

18. *Parkinson's disease*. It has been noted that some patients with this disease markedly improved after a three to six weeks' course of chloramphenicol. It was postulated that the drug possibly inhibits some abnormal protein synthesis which may exist in parkinsonism. As chloramphenicol cannot be used for prolonged periods, its use for this purpose has not been pursued (Leading article, 1975).

REFERENCES

Ambrose, C. T. and Coons, A. H. (1963), 'Studies on antibody production: VIII. The inhibitory effect of chloramphenicol on the synthesis of antibody in tissue culture', *J. Exp. Med.,* **117**, 1075; quoted by Weisberger *et al.* (1969).

Anderson, E. S. and Smith, H. R. (1972), 'Chloramphenicol resistance in the typhoid bacillus', *Brit. med. J.,* **3**, 329.

Anderson, E. S. (1975), 'The problem and implications of chloramphenicol resistance in the typhoid bacillus', *J. Hyg., Camb.,* **74**, 289.

Annotation (1969), 'Chloramphenicol toxicity', *Lancet,* **2**, 476.

Annotation (1975). 'Typhoid fever in Mexico', *Lancet,* **1**, 1230.

Annotation (1978), 'Cephalosporins compared', *Lancet,* **1**, 863.

Anthony, B. F. and Concepcion, N. F. (1975), 'Group B streptococcus in a general hospital, *J. Infect. Dis.,* **132**, 561.

Aserkoff, B. and Bennett, J. V. (1969), 'Effect of antibiotic therapy in acute salmonellosis on the fecal excretion of salmonellae', *New Engl. J. Med.,* **281**, 636.

Bacchus, A. N. and Javor, G. T. (1975), 'Stability of Escherichia coli membrane proteins during chloramphenicol treatment', *Antimicrob. Ag. Chemother.,* **8**, 387.

Baine, W. B., Farmer, J. J. III, Gangarosa, E. J., Hermann, G. T., Thornsberry, C. and Rice, P. A. (1977), 'Typhoid fever in the United States associated with the 1972–1973 epidemic in Mexico', *J. Infect. Dis.,* **135**, 649.

Baker, C. J., Webb, B. J. and Barrett, F. F. (1976), 'Antimicrobial susceptibility of Group B streptococci isolated from a variety of clinical sources', *Antimicrob. Ag. Chemother.,* **10**, 128.

Balows, A. (1977), 'An overview of recent experiences with plasmid-mediated antibiotic resistance or induced virulence in bacterial diseases', *J. Antimicrob. Chemother.* (Suppl. C), **3**, 3.

Barrett, F. F., Taber, L. H., Morris, C. R., Stephenson, W. B., Clark, D. J. and Yow, M. D. (1972), 'A 12 year review of the antibiotic management of Hemophilus influenzae meningitis', *J. Pediatrics*, **81**, 370.

Barros, F., Korzeniowski, O. M., Sande, M. A., Martins, K., Santos, L. C. and Rocha, H. (1977), '*In vitro* antibiotic susceptibility of salmonellae', *Antimicrob. Ag. Chemother.*, **11**, 1071.

Bartlett, J. G., Gorbach, S. L. and Finegold, S. M. (1974), 'The bacteriology of aspiration pneumonia', *Amer. J. Med.*, **56**, 202.

Beard, N. S. Jr., Armentrout, S. A. and Weisberger, A. S. (1969), 'Inhibition of mammalian protein synthesis by antibiotics', *Pharmacol. Rev.*, **21**, 213.

Beard, N. S. Jr. and Weisberger, A. S. (1972), 'Protein synthesis by reticulocyte ribosomes. IV. Factors involved in formation of the mRNA-sRNA-ribosome complex and the absence of inhibition by chloramphenicol', *Amer. J. Med. Sci.*, **263**, 215.

Bennett, N. McK. and Kucers, A. (1970), 'Staphylococcal and Gram-negative septicaemia', *Aspects of Infection. Proc. Symp. Auckland, Sydney and Melbourne*, p. 123.

Bentley, D. W., Hahn, J. J. and Lepper, M. H. (1970), 'Transmission of chloramphenicol-resistant Staphylococcus epidermidis: Epidemiologic and laboratory studies', *J. Infect. Dis.*, **122**, 365.

Best, W. R. (1967), 'Chloramphenicol-associated blood dyscrasias', *JAMA*, **201**, 181.

Beveridge, J. (1961), 'Acute chloramphenicol poisoning in the new-born period', *Med. J. Aust.*, **1**, 93.

Bissett, M. L., Abbott, S. L. and Wood, R. M. (1974), 'Antimicrobial resistance and R factors in salmonella isolated in California (1971–1972)', *Antimicrob. Ag. Chemother.*, **5**, 161.

Black, S. B., Levine, P. and Shinefield, H. R. (1978), 'The necessity for monitoring chloramphenicol levels when treating neonatal meningitis', *J. Pediatrics*, **92**, 235.

Blazevic, D. J. (1976), 'Antibiotic susceptibility of the subspecies of Bacteroides fragilis', *Antimicrob. Ag. Chemother.*, **9**, 481.

Böttiger, L. E. (1974), 'Drug-induced aplastic anaemia in Sweden with special reference to chloramphenicol', *Postgrad. Med. J.* (Suppl. 5), **50**, 127.

Brook, I. and Finegold, S. M. (1977), 'Bacteriology of aspiration pneumonia in children', *Amer. Rev. Resp. Dis.* (Suppl.), **115**, 255.

Brown, J. D., Mo, D. H. and Rhoades, E. R. (1975), 'Chloramphenicol-resistant Salmonella typhi in Saigon', *JAMA*, **231**, 162.

Burns, L. E., Hodgman, J. E. and Cass, A. B. (1959), 'Fatal circulatory collapse in premature infants receiving chloramphenicol', *New Engl. J. Med.*, **261**, 1318.

Butler, T., Linh, N. N., Arnold, K. and Pollack, M. (1973), 'Chloramphenicol-resistant typhoid fever in Vietnam associated with R-factor', *Lancet*, **2**, 983.

Butler, T., Bell, W. R., Linh, N. N., Tiep, N. D. and Arnold, K. (1974), 'Yersinia pestis infection in Vietnam. I. Clinical and hemotologic aspects', *J. Infect. Dis.* (Suppl.), **129**, 78.

Butler, T., Linh, N. N., Arnold, K., Adickman, M. D., Chau, D. M. and Muoi, M. M. (1977), 'Therapy of antimicrobial-resistant typhoid fever', *Antimicrob. Ag. Chemother.*, **11**, 645.

Cahill, K. M. (1962), 'Chloramphenicol hypersensitivity. A severe haemorrhagic reaction', *Lancet*, **2**, 277.

Calabi, O. (1973), 'Bactericidal synergism of novobiocin and tetracycline against Pseudomonas pseudomallei', *J. Med. Microbiol.*, **6**, 293.

Cavanagh, P., Morris, C. A. and Mitchell, N. J. (1975), "Chloramphenicol resistance in Haemophilus species', *Lancet*, **1**, 696.

Center for Disease Control (1976), 'Chloramphenicol-resistant Haemophilus influenzae—Connecticut, Massachusetts', *Morbidity and Mortality Weekly Report*, **25**, 267.

Center for Disease Control (1977), 'Multiple-antibiotic resistance of pneumococci—South Africa', *Morbibidy and Mortality Weekly Report*, **26**, 285.

Cherubin, C. E., Neu, H. C., Rahal, J. J. and Sabath, L. D. (1977), 'Emergence of resistance to chloramphenicol in Salmonella', *J. Infect. Dis.*, **135**, 807.

Chow, A. W., Patten, J. and Bednorz, D. (1978), 'Susceptibility of Campylobacter fetus to twenty-two antimicrobial agents', Antimicrob. Ag. Chemother., **13**, 416.

Christensen, L. K. and Skovsted, L. (1969), 'Inhibition of drug metabolism by chloramphenicol', *Lancet*, **2**, 1397.

Christie, A. B. (1974), *Infectious Diseases: Epidemiology and Clinical Practice*, 2nd Edn., Churchill Livingstone, Edinburgh, London, and New York, p. 44.

Chun, D., Seol, S. Y., Cho, D. T. and Tak, R. (1977), 'Drug resistance and R plasmids in Salmonella typhi isolated in Korea', *Antimicrob. Ag. Chemother.*, **11**, 209.

Cocke, J. G. Jr., Brown, R. E. and Geppert, L. J. (1966), 'Optic neuritis with prolonged use of chloramphenicol', *J. Pediatrics*, **68**, 27.

Colquhoun, J. and Weetch, R. S. (1950), 'Resistance to chloramphenicol developing during treatment of typhoid fever', *Lancet*, **2**, 621.

Comments (1973), 'The hepatitis-aplastic anaemia syndrome', *Med. J. Aust.*, **1**, 918.

Cooksey, R. C., Bannister, E. R. and Farrar, W. E., Jr. (1975), 'Antibiotic resistance patterns of clinical isolates of Serratia marcescens', *Antimicrob. Ag. Chemother.*, **7**, 396.

Cooper, J. A. and Lietman, P. S. (1977), 'Chloramphenicol in Haemophilus endocarditis', *Lancet*, **2**, 871.

Courvalin, P. M., Shaw, W. V. and Jacob, A. E. (1978), 'Plasmid-mediated mechanisms of resistance to aminoglycoside-aminocyclitol antibiotics and to chloramphenicol in Group D streptococci', *Antimicrob. Ag. Chemother.*, **13**, 716.

Crofton, J. (1969), 'Some principles in the chemotherapy of bacterial infections', *Brit. med. J.*, **2**, 137 and 209.

Cundliffe, E. and McQuillen, K. (1967), 'Bacterial protein synthesis: The effects of antibiotics', *J. Mol. Biol.*, **30**, 137.

Daigneault, R. and Guitard, M. (1976), 'An enzymatic assay for chloramphenicol with partially purified chloramphenicol acetyltransferase', *J. Infect. Dis.*, **133**, 515.

D'Alessandri, R. M., McNeely, D. J. and Kluge, R. M. (1976), 'Antibiotic synergy and antagonism against clinical isolates of Klebisella species', *Antimicrob. Ag. Chemother.*, **10**, 889.

Dameshek, W. (1969), 'Chloramphenicol aplastic anaemia in identical twins—a clue to pathogenesis', *New Engl. J. Med.*, **281**, 42.

Dang-Van, A., Tiraby, G., Acar, J. F., Shaw, W. V. and Bouanchaud, D. H. (1978), 'Chloramphenicol resistance in Streptococcus pneumoniae: Enzymatic acetylation and possible plasmid linkage', *Antimicrob. Ag. Chemother.*, **13**, 577.

Daniel, T. M., Suhrland, L. G. and Weisberger, A. S. (1965), 'Suppression of the anamnestic response to tetanus toxoid in man by chloramphenicol', *New Engl. J. Med.*, **273**, 367.

Darougar, S., Viswalingam, M., Treharne, J. D., Kinnison, J. R. and Jones, B. R. (1977), 'Treatment of TRIC infection of the eye with rifampicin or chloramphenicol', *Brit. J. Ophthalmol.*, **61**, 255.

Datta, N. and Olarte, J. (1974), 'R factors in strains of Salmonella typhi and Shigella dysenteriae 1 isolated during epidemics in Mexico: Classification by compatibility', *Antimicrob. Ag. Chemother.*, **5**, 310.

Datta, N., (1977), 'Classification of plasmids as an aid to understanding their epidemiology and evolution', *J. Antimicrob. Chemother.* (Suppl. C), **3**, 19.

Davis, S. and Rubin, A. D. (1972), 'Treatment and prognosis in aplastic anaemia', *Lancet*, **1**, 871.

De Leys, R. J. and Juni, E. (1977), 'Unusual effects of penicillin G and chloramphenicol on the growth of Moraxella osloensis', *Antimicrob. Ag. Chemother.*, **12**, 573.

De Louvois, J., Gortvai, P. and Hurley, R. (1977a), 'Bacteriology of abscesses of the central nervous system: A multicentre prospective study', *Brit. med. J.*, **2**, 981.

De Louvois, J., Gortvai, P. and Hurley, R. (1977b), 'Antibiotic treatment of abscesses of the central nervous system', *Brit. med. J.*, **2**, 985.

De Louvois, J. (1978), 'The role of Bacteroides fragilis in abscesses of the central nervous system: Implications for therapy', *J. Antimicrob. Chemother.*, **4**, 97.

Derrington, A. W. (1971), 'Combinations of antibiotics', *Med. J. Aust.*, **2**, 238.

Dettli, L. and Spring, P. (1974), 'The dosage regimen of thiamphenicol in patients with kidney disease', *Postgrad. Med. J.* (Suppl. 5), **50**, 32.

Dunkle, L. M. (1978), 'Central nervous system chloramphenicol concentration in premature infants', *Antimicrob. Ag. Chemother.*, **13**, 427.

Du Pont, H. L., Hornick, R. B., Weiss, C. F., Snyder, M. J. and Woodward, T. E. (1970), 'Evaluation of chloramphenicol acid succinate therapy of induced typhoid fever and Rocky Mountain spotted fever', *New Engl. J. Med.*, **282**, 53.

Editorial (1970), 'Chloramphenicol-induced bone marrow suppression', *JAMA*, **213**, 1183.

Ehrlich, J., Bartz, Q. R., Smith, R. M., Joslyn, D. A. and Burkholder, P. R. (1947), 'Chloromycetin, a new antibiotic from a soil actinomycete', *Science*, **106**, 417; quoted by Welch (1954).

Eickhoff, T. C., Bennett, J. V., Hayes, P. S. and Feeley, J. (1970), 'Pseudomonas pseudomallei: Susceptibility to chemotherapeutic agents', *J. Infect. Dis.*, **121**, 95.

Everett, E. D. and Nelson, R. A. (1975), 'Pulmonary melioidosis. Observations in thirty-nine cases', *Amer. Rev. Resp. Dis.*, **112**, 331.

Farrar, W. E. Jr. and Eidson, M. (1971), 'Antibiotic resistence in Shigella mediated by R factors', *J. Infect. Dis.*, **123**, 477.

Feigin, R. D., Stechenberg, B. W., Chang, M. J., Dunkle, L. M., Wong, M. L., Palkes, H., Dodge, P. R. and Davis, H. (1976), 'Prospective evaluation of treatment of Hemophilus influenzae meningitis', *J. Pediatrics*, **88**, 542.

Feldman, W. E. (1978), 'Effect of ampicillin and chloramphenicol against Haemophilus influenzae', *Pediatrics*, **61**, 406.

Ferrari, V. and Della Bella, D. (1974), 'Comparison of chloramphenicol and thiamphenicol metabolism', *Postgrad. Med. J.* (Suppl. 5), **50**, 17.

Finegold, S. M., Bartlett, J. G., Chow, A. W., Flora, D. J., Gorbach, S. L., Harder, E. J. and Tally, F. P. (1975), 'Management of anaerobic infections', *Ann. Intern. Med.*, **83**, 375.

Finegold, S. M. (1977), 'Therapy for infections due to anaerobic bacteria: An overview', *J. Infect. Dis.* (Suppl.), **135**, 25.

Fisher, M. W. (1960), 'The susceptibility of staphylococci to chloramphenicol: A survey of experimental and clinical experiences', *Arch. Intern. Med.*, **105**, 413.

Forbes, J. A. (1962), 'Purulent meningitis: Principles and results of revised standardized treatment in 281 cases', *Aust. Ann. Med.*, **11**, 92.

Forsgren, A. and Schmeling, D. (1977), 'Effect of antibiotics on chemotaxis of human leukocytes', *Antimicrob. Ag. Chemother.*, **11**, 580.

Fraser, D. W., Wachsmuth, I. K., Bopp, C., Feeley, J. C. and Tsai, T. F. (1978), 'Antibiotic treatment of guinea-pigs infected with agent of Legionnaires' disease', *Lancet*, **1**, 175.

Furman, K. I., Koornhof, H. J., Kilroe-Smith, T. A., Landless, R. and Robinson, R. G. (1976), 'Peritoneal transfer of thiamphenicol during peritoneal dialysis', *Antimicrob. Ag. Chemother.*, **9**, 557.

Gale, E. F., Cundliffe, E., Reynolds, P. E., Richmond, M. H. and Waring, M. J. (1972), *The Molecular Basis of Antibiotic Action,* John Wiley & Sons Ltd., p. 332.

Garrod, L. P. and Waterworth, P. M. (1962), 'Methods of testing combined antibiotic bactericidal action and the significance of the results', *J. clin. Path.,* **15,** 328.

Garrod, L. P., Lambert, H. P. and O'Grady, F. (1973), *Antibiotic and Chemotherapy,* 4th edn., Churchill Livingstone, Edinburgh and London, p. 137.

Gerding, D. N., Hall, W. H. and Schierl, E. A. (1977), 'Antibiotic concentrations in ascitic fluid of patients with ascites and bacterial peritonitis', *Ann. Intern. Med.,* **86,** 708.

Gill, F. A. and Hook, E. W. (1966), 'Salmonella strains with transferable antimicrobial resistance', *JAMA,* **198,** 1267.

Glazko, A. J., Wolf, L. M., Dill, W. A. and Bratton, A. C., Jr. (1949), 'Biochemical studies on chloramphenicol (chloromycetin). II. Tissue distribution and excretion studies', *J. Pharmacol. Exper. Therap.,* **96,** 445; quoted by Woodward and Wisseman (1958).

Gleckman, R. A. (1975), 'Warning—chloramphenicol may be good for your health', *Arch. Intern. Med.,* **135,** 1125.

Goldberg, I. H. (1965), 'Mode of action of antibiotics II. Drugs affecting nucleic acid and protein synthesis', *Amer. J. Med.,* **39,** 722.

Gorbach, S. L. and Bartlett, J. G. (1974), 'Anaerobic infections (third of three parts)', *New Engl. J. Med.,* **290,** 1289.

Grant, R. B., Bannatyne, R. M. and Shapley, A. J. (1976), 'Resistance to chloramphenicol and ampicillin of Salmonella typhimurium in Ontario, Canada', *J. Infect. Dis.,* **134,** 354.

Green, C. E., Cameron, H. J. and Julian, G. R. (1975), 'Recovery of polysome function of T4-infected Escherichia coli after brief treatment with chloramphenicol and rifampin', *Antimicrob. Ag. Chemother.,* **7,** 549.

Greenberg, P. A. and Sanford, J. P. (1967), 'Removal and absorption of antibiotics in patients with renal failure undergoing peritoneal dialysis', *Ann. Intern. Med.,* **66,** 465.

Guiney, D. G., Jr. and Davis, C. E. (1978), 'Identification of a conjugative R plasmid in Bacteroides ochraceus capable of transfer to Escherichia coli', *Nature,* **274,** 181.

Gupta, R. S. (1975), 'Killing and lysis of Escherichia coli in the presence of chloramphenicol: Relation to cellular magnesium', *Antimicrob. Ag. Chemother.,* **7,** 748.

Hahn, F. E. (1968), 'Relationship between the structure of chloramphenicol and its action upon peptide synthetase', *Experimentia,* **24,** 856.

Hammerberg, S., Sorger, S. and Marks, M. I. (1977), 'Antimicrobial susceptibilities of Yersinia enterocolitica biotype 4, serotype 0:3', *Antimicrob. Ag. Chemother.,* **11,** 566.

Hammond, G. W., Lian, C. J., Wilt, J. C. and Ronald, A. R. (1978), 'Antimicrobial susceptibility of Haemophilus ducreyi', *Antimicrob. Ag. Chemother.,* **13,** 608.

Hansman, D. (1978), 'Chloramphenicol-resistant pneumococci in West Africa', *Lancet,* **1,** 1102.

Hassam, Z. A., Shaw, E. J., Shooter, R. A. and Caro, D. B. (1978), 'Changes in antibiotic sensitivity in strains of Staphylococcus aureus, 1952–78', *Brit. med. J.,* **2,** 536.

Hausmann, K. and Skrandies, G. (1974), 'Aplastic anaemia following chloramphenicol therapy in Hamburg and surrounding districts', *Postgrad. Med. J.* (Suppl. 5), **50,** 131.

Hazard, G. W., Ganz, R. N., Nevin, R. W., Nauss, A. H., Curtis, E., Bell, D. W. J. and Murray, E. S. (1969), 'Rocky Mountain spotted fever in the eastern United States', *New Engl. J. Med.,* **280,** 57.

Hedges, R. W. and Jacob, A. E. (1974), 'Transposition of ampicillin resistance from

RP4 to other replicons', *Molec. gen. Genet.,* **132,** 31.

Herzog, C. H. (1976), 'Drug treatment of typhoid fever', *Brit. med., J.,* **2,** 941.

Hewitt, W. L., O'Grady, F. W., Acar, J. F., McDonald, P. J. and Sande, M. A. (1978), 'The rational basis for chemotherapy'. In Siegenthaler, W. and Lüthy, R. (Ed.), *Current Chemotherapy: Proceedings of the 10th International Congress of Chemotherapy,* Zurich/Switzerland, 1977. American Society for Microbiology, Washington, D. C., p. 3.

Hodgkinson, R. (1973), 'The chloramphenicol-hepatitis-aplastic anaemia syndrome', *Med. J. Aust.,* **1,** 939.

Hodgman, J. E. and Burns, L. E. (1961), 'Safe and effective chloramphenicol dosages for premature infants', *Amer. J. Dis. Child.,* **101,** 140.

Hodgman, J. E. (1961), 'Chloramphenicol', *Pediat. Clin. North America,* **8,** 1027.

Hoffman, T. A., Ruiz, C. J., Counts, G. W., Sachs, J. M. and Nitzkin, J. L. (1975), 'Waterborne typhoid fever in Dade County, Florida—clinical and therapeutic evaluation of 105 bacteremic patients', *Amer. J. Med.,* **59,** 481.

Holt, R. (1967), 'The bacterial degradation of chloramphenicol', *Lancet,* **1,** 1259.

Howard, A. J., Hince, C. J. and Williams, J. D. (1978), 'Antibiotic resistance in Streptococcus pneumoniae and Haemophilus influenzae. Report of a study group on bacterial resistance', *Brit. med. J.,* **1,** 1657.

Howe, C., Sampath, A. and Spotnitz, M. (1971), 'The Pseudomallei group: A review', *J. Infect. Dis.,* **124,** 598.

Howell, A., Andrews, T. M. and Watts, R. W. E. (1975), 'Bone-marrow cells resistant to chloramphenicol in chloramphenicol-induced aplastic anaemia', *Lancet,* **1,** 65.

Hughes, D. W. O'G. (1962), 'Acquired aplastic anaemia in childhood: A review of 22 cases', *Med. J. Aust.,* **2,** 251.

Hughes, D. W. O'G. (1968), 'Studies on chloramphenicol: 1. Assessment of haemopoietic toxicity', *Med. J. Aust.,* **2,** 436.

Hughes, D. W. O'G. (1973), 'Studies on chloramphenicol. II. Possible determinants and progress of haemopoietic toxicity during chloramphenicol therapy', *Med. J. Aust.,* **2,** 1142.

Ingall, D., Sherman, J. D., Cockburn, F. and Klein, R. (1965), 'Amelioration by ingestion of phenylalanine of toxic effects of chloramphenicol on bone marrow', *New Engl. J. Med.,* **272,** 180.

Ingall, D. and Sherman, J. D. (1968), 'Chloramphenicol', *Pediat. Clin. North America,* **15,** 57.

Ingham, H. R. and Selkon, J. B. (1976), 'Cerebral abscess', *J. Antimicrob. Chemother.,* **2,** 224.

Ingham, H. R., Selkon, J. B. and Roxby, C. M. (1978), 'The role of Bacteroides fragilis in abscesses of the central nervous system: Implications for therapy', *J. Antimicrob. Chemother.,* **4,** 283.

Jawetz, E. (1964), *Modern Treatment,* **1,** 819; quoted by Crofton (1969).

Johnson, R. H., Lutwick, L. I., Huntley, G. A. and Vosti, K. L. (1976), 'Arizona hinshawii infections. New cases, antimicrobial sensitivities, and literature review', *Ann. Intern. Med.,* **85,** 587.

Joseph, S. W., DeBell, R. M. and Brown, W. P. (1978), '*In vitro* response to chloramphenicol, tetracycline, ampicillin, gentamicin, and beta-lactamase production by Halophilic Vibrios from human and environmental sources', *Antimicrob. Ag. Chemother.,* **13,** 244.

Joy, R. J. T., Scalettar, R. and Sodee, D. B. (1960), 'Optic and peripheral neuritis. Probable effect of prolonged chloramphenicol therapy', *JAMA,* **173,** 1731.

Kattan, S. (1976), 'Chloramphenicol-resistant Haemophilus', *Lancet,* **1,** 814.

Keiser, G. (1974a), 'Co-operative study of patients treated with thiamphenicol. Comparative study of patients treated with chloramphenicol and thiamphenicol', *Postgrad. Med. J.* (Suppl. 5), **50,** 143.

Keiser, G. (1974b), 'Concluding remarks. International symposium on chloramphenicol-thiamphenicol', *Postgrad. Med. J.* (Suppl. 5), **50**, 150.

Klastersky, J. and Husson, M. (1977), 'Bactericidal activity of the combinations of gentamicin with clindamycin or chloramphenicol against species of Escherichia coli and Bacteroides fragilis', *Antimicrob. Ag. Chemother.*, **12**, 135.

Kinmonth, A. L., Storrs, C. N. and Mitchell, R. G. (1978), 'Meningitis due to chloramphenicol-resistant Haemophilus influenzae type b', *Brit. med. J.*, **1**, 694.

Kohl, S., Jacobson, J. A. and Nahmias, A. (1976), 'Yersinia enterocolitica infections in children', *J. Pediatrics*, **89**, 77.

Kunin, C. M., Glazko, A. J. and Finland, M. (1959), 'Persistence of antibiotics in blood of patients with acute renal failure. II. Chloramphenicol and its metabolic products in the blood of patients with severe renal disease or hepatic cirrhosis', *J. Clin. Invest.*, **38**, 1498; quoted by Hodgman (1961).

Kunin, C. M. (1967), 'A guide to use of antibiotics in patients with renal disease', *Ann. Intern. Med.*, **67**, 151.

Lampe, R. M. and Mansuwan, P. (1973), 'Chloramphenicol-resistant Salmonella typhosa', *New Engl. J. Med.*, **289**, 1203.

Lawrence, R. M., Goldstein, E. and Hoeprich, P. D. (1973), 'Typhoid fever caused by chloramphenicol-resistant organisms', *JAMA*, **224**, 861.

Leading Article (1961), 'Mortality from chloramphenicol', *Brit. med. J.*, **1**, 1019.

Leading Article (1965), 'Chloramphenicol blindness', *Brit. med. J.*, **1**, 1511.

Leading Article (1967), 'Toxicity of chloramphenicol', *Brit. med. J.*, **1**, 649.

Leading Article (1975), 'Miracle cures in Parkinson's disease', *Brit. med. J.*, **3**, 1. **3**, 306.

Leading Article (1973), 'Chloramphenicol resistance in typhoid', *Lancet*, **2**, 1008.

Leading Article (1975), 'Miracle cures in Parkinson's disease', *Brit. med. J.*, **3**, 1.

Leading Article (1976), 'Mechanisms in aplastic anaemia', *Lancet*, **2**, 1179.

Ledger, W. J., Gee, C. L., Lewis, W. P. and Bobitt, J. R. (1977), 'Comparison of clindamycin and chloramphenicol in treatment of serious infections of the female genital tract', *J. Infect. Dis.* (Suppl.), **135**, 30.

Lewis, V. J., Thacker, W. L., Shepard, C. C. and McDade, J. E. (1978), '*In vivo* susceptibility of the Legionnaires' disease bacterium to ten antimicrobial agents', *Antimicrob. Ag. Chemother.*, **13**, 419.

Lindberg, A. A., Nilsson, L. H.: son, Bucht, H. and Kallings, L. O. (1966), 'Concentration of chloramphenicol in the urine and blood in relation to renal function', *Brit. med. J.*, **2**, 724.

Lindberg, J., Rosenhall, U., Nylén, O. and Ringnér, Å. (1977), 'Long-term outcome of Hemophilus influenzae meningitis related to antibiotic treatment', *Pediatrics*, **60**, 1.

Louie, T. J., Tally, F. P., Bartlett, J. G. and Gorbach, S. L. (1976), 'Rapid microbiological assay for chloramphenicol and tetracyclines', *Antimicrob. Ag. Chemother.*, **9**, 874.

Lovell, S. and Dugdale, A. E. (1973), 'The selection of antibiotics for the initial treatment of bacterial meningitis', *Med. J. Aust.*, **1**, 529.

Manten, A., van Klingeren, B. and Dessens-Kroon, M. (1976), 'Chloramphenicol resistance in Haemophilus influenzae', *Lancet*, **1**, 702.

Manyan, D. R., Arimura, G. K. and Yunis, A. A. (1972), 'Chloramphenicol-induced erythroid suppression and bone marrow ferrochelatase activity in dogs', *J. Lab. Clin. Med.*, **79**, 137.

Marder, H. P. and Kayser, F. H. (1977), 'Transferable plasmids mediating multiple-antibiotic resistance in Streptococcus faecalis subsp. liquefaciens', *Antimicrob. Ag. Chemother.*, **12**, 261.

Martelo, O. J., Manyan, D. R., Smith, U. S. and Yunis, A. A. (1969), 'Chloramphenicol and bone marrow mitochondria', *J. Lab. Clin. Med.*, **74**, 927.

Martin, W. J., Gardner, M. and Washington, J. A., II (1972), '*In vitro* antimicrobial susceptibility of anaerobic bacteria isolated from clinical specimens', *Antimicrob. Ag. Chemother.*, **1**, 148.

Masri, A. F. and Grieco, M. H. (1972), 'Bacteroides endocarditis. Report of a case', *Amer. J. Med. Sci.*, **263**, 357.

Mathias, R. G., Harding, G. K. M., Gurwith, M. J., Stiver, H. G., Sigurdson, E., Gratton, C. A. and Ronald, A. R. (1977), 'Bacteremia due to Bacteroidaceae: A review of 92 cases', *J. Infect. Dis.* (Suppl.), **135**, 69.

Mayo, J. B. and McCarthy, L. R. (1977), 'Antimicrobial susceptibility of Haemophilus parainfluenzae', *Antimicrob. Ag. Chemother.*, **11**, 844.

McCaffrey, R. P., Halsted, C. H., Wahab, M. F. A. and Robertson, R. P. (1971), 'Chloramphenicol-induced hemolysis in caucasian glucose-6-phosphate dehydrogenase deficiency', *Ann. Intern. Med.*, **74**, 722.

McCracken, G. H., Jr. and Nelson, J. D. (1977), *Antimicrobial Therapy for Newborns: Practical Application of Pharmacology to Clinical Usage*, Grune and Stratton, New York, San-Francisco, London, p. 45.

McCrumb, F. R., Jr., Snyder, M. J. and Hicken, W. J. (1958), 'The use of chloramphenicol acid succinate in the treatment of acute infections', *Antibiot. Ann.*—1957–1958, p. 837.

McHugh, G. L., Moellering, R. C., Hopkins, C. C. and Swartz, M. N. (1975), 'Salmonella typhimurium resistant to silver nitrate, chloramphenicol and ampicillin. A new threat in burns units?', *Lancet*, **1**, 235.

Melby, K. and Midtvedt, T. (1977), 'The effect of eight antibacterial agents on the phagocytosis of 32P-labelled Escherichia coli by rat polymorphonuclear cells', *Scand. J. Infect. Dis.*, **9**, 9.

Michel, J., Bornstein, H., Luboshitzky, R. and Sacks, T. (1975), 'Mechanism of chloramphenicol-cephaloridine synergism of Enterobacteriaceae', *Antimicrob. Ag. Chemother.*, **7**, 845.

Mills, J. and Drew, D. (1976), 'Serratia marcescens endocarditis: A regional illness associated with intravenous drug abuse', *Ann. Intern. Med.*, **84**, 29.

Morahan, R. J. and Hawksworth, D. N. (1970), 'Antibiotic and sulphadiazine sensitivities of New Guinea Salmonellas and Shigellas', *Med. J. Aust.*, **2**, 222.

Morizono, T. and Johnstone, B. M. (1975), 'Ototoxicity of chloramphenicol ear drops with propylene glycol as solvent', *Med. J. Aust.*, **2**, 634.

Nagao, T. and Mauer, A. M. (1969), 'Concordance for drug-induced aplastic anaemia in identical twins', *New Engl. J. Med.*, **281**, 7.

Nakae, M., Murai, T., Kaneko, Y. and Mitsuhashi, S. (1977), 'Drug-resistance in Streptococcus pyogenes isolated in Japan (1974–1975)', *Antimicrob. Ag. Chemother.*, **12**, 427.

Nelson, J. D. (1976), 'Odd creatures in the blood and cerebrospinal fluid', *Am. J. Dis. Child.*, **130**, 800.

Neu, H. C., Cherubin, C. E., Longo, E. D. and Winter, J. (1975a), 'Antimicrobial resistance of shigella isolated in New York City in 1973', *Antimicrob. Ag. Chemother.*, **7**, 833.

Neu, H. C., Cherubin, C. E., Longo, E. D., Flouton, B. and Winter, J. (1975b), 'Antimicrobial resistance and R-factor transfer among isolates of Salmonella in the Northeastern United States: A comparison of human and animal isolates', *J. Infect. Dis.*, **132**, 617.

Nilsson-Ehle, I., Kahlmeter, G. and Nilsson-Ehle, P. (1978), 'Determination of chloramphenicol in serum and cerebrospinal fluid with high-pressure liquid chromatography', *J. Antimicrob. Chemother.*, **4**, 169.

Nomura, M. (1969), 'Ribosomes', *Scientific American*, **221**, 28.

Novick, R. P., Clowes, R. C., Cohen, S. N., Curtiss, R. III, Datta, N. and Falkow, S. (1976), 'Uniform nomenclature for bacterial plasmids: A proposal', *Bacteriol. Rev.*, **40**, 168.

Olarte, J. and Galindo, E. (1973), 'Salmonella typhi resistant to chloramphenicol, ampicillin and other antimicrobial agents: Strains isolated during an extensive typhoid fever epidemic in Mexico', *Antimicrob. Ag. Chemother.*, **4**, 597.

Oles, A. and Stanio-Pyrkosz, B. (1964), 'Chloromycetin resistance of Salmonella typhi strains isolated from carriers and cases of typhoid fever', *J. Hyg. Epid Microb. and Immunol.*, **8**, 169.

Olsen, H. (1976), 'Bacteroides bacteraemia', *Scand. J. Infect. Dis.*, **8**, 107.

Overturf, G., Marton, K. I. and Mathies, A. W. Jr. (1973), 'Antibiotic resistance in typhoid fever', *New Engl. J. Med.*, **289**, 463.

Raevuori, M., Harvey, S. M., Pickett, M. J. and Martin, W. J. (1978), 'Yersinia enterocolitica: *In vitro* antimicrobial susceptibility', *Antimicrob. Ag. Chemother.*, **13**, 888.

Report of a WHO Study Group (1976), 'Cerebrospinal meningitis control', *Wld. Hlth. Org. Techn. Rep. Ser.*, No. **588**, p. 21.

Report of a WHO Scientific Group (1978), 'Neisseria gonorrhoeae and gonococcal infections', *Wld. Hlth. Org. Techn. Rep. Ser.*, N. **616**, p. 130.

Robison, L. R., Seligsohn, R. and Lerner, S. A. (1978), 'Simplified radioenzymatic assay for chloramphenicol', *Antimicrob. Ag. Chemother.*, **13**, 25.

Rood, J. I., Maher, E. A., Somers, E. B., Campos, E. and Duncan, C. L. (1978), 'Isolation and characterization of multiply antibiotic-resistant Clostridium perfringens strains from porcine feces', *Antimicrob. Ag. Chemother.*, **13**, 871.

Rose, J. Q., Choi, H. K., Schentag, J. J., Kinkel, W. R. and Jusko, W. J. (1977), 'Intoxication caused by interaction of chloramphenicol and phenytoin', *JAMA*, **237**, 2630.

Ross, S., Puig, J. R. and Zaremba, E. A. (1958), 'Chloramphenicol acid succinate (sodium salt). Some preliminary, clinical and laboratory observations in infants and children', *Antibiot. Ann.*—1957–1958, p. 803.

Ross, S., Controni, G. and Khan, W. (1972), 'Resistance of shigellae to ampicillin and other antibiotics', *JAMA*, **221**, 45.

Sabath, L. D. (1969), 'Current concepts: Drug resistance of bacteria', *New Engl. J. Med.*, **280**, 91.

Sacks, T., Michel, J., Durst, A. and Stessman, J. (1977), 'Inhibition of beta-lactamase: Synergistic bactericidal effect of combination of chloramphenicol-cephaloridine, *J. Antimicrob. Chemother.*, **3**, 525.

Samson, D. S. and Clark, K. (1973), 'A current review of brain abscess', *Amer. J. Med.*, **54**, 201.

Sanborn, W. R., Lesmana, M., Dennis, D. T., Trenggonowati, R. and Kadirman, L. I. (1975), 'Antibiotic-resistant typhoid in Indonesia', *Lancet*, **2**, 408.

Sande, M. A. and Overton, J. W. (1973), '*In vivo* antagonism between gentamicin and chloramphenicol in neutropenic mice', *J. Infect. Dis.*, **128**, 247.

Scott, J. L., Finegold, S. M., Belkin, G. A. and Lawrence, J. S. (1965), 'A controlled double-blind study of the hematologic toxicity of chloramphenicol', *New Engl. J. Med.*, **272**, 1137.

Schaberg, D. R., Alford, R. H., Anderson, R., Farmer, J. J. III, Melly, M. A. and Schaffner, W. (1976), 'An outbreak of nosocomial infection due to multiply resistant Serratia marcescens: Evidence of interhospital spread', *J. Infect. Dis.*, **134**, 181.

Schaberg, D. R., Highsmith, A. K. and Wachsmuth, I. K. (1977), 'Resistance plasmid transfer by Serratia marcescens in urine', *Antimicrob. Ag. Chemother.*, **11**, 449.

Schwarz, M. A. and Firkin, B. G. (1976), 'Chloramphenicol—a possible role in the treatment of leukaemia?', *Med. J. Aust.*, **1**, 687.

Schwartzman, J. D., Reller, L. B. and Wang, W.-L. (1977), 'Susceptibility of Clostridium perfringens isolated from human infections to twenty antibiotics', *Antimicrob. Ag. Chemother.*, **11**, 695.

Shackelford, P. G., Bobinski, J. E., Feigin, R. D. and Cherry, J. D. (1972), 'Therapy of

Haemophilus influenzae meningitis reconsidered', *New Engl. J. Med.*, **287**, 634.

Shaw, R. G. and McLean, J. A. (1957), 'Chloramphenicol and aplastic anaemia', *Med. J. Aust.*, **1**, 352.

Shaw, W. V., Bouanchaud, D. H. and Goldstein, F. W. (1978), 'Mechanism of transferable resistance to chloramphenicol in Haemophilus parainfluenzae', *Antimicrob. Ag. Chemother.*, **13**, 326.

Sheba, C. (1967), 'Risks of chloramphenicol?', *Lancet*, **1**, 1007.

Sheehy, T. W., Deller, J. J., Jr. and Weber, D. R. (1967), 'Melioidosis', *Ann. Intern. Med.*, **67**, 897.

Shimada, K., Inamatsu, T. and Yamashiro, M. (1977), 'Anaerobic bacteria in biliary disease in elderly patients', *J. Infect. Dis.*, **135**, 850.

Smith, H. W. (1973), 'Chloramphenicol resistance in Escherichia coli', *J. Med. Microbiol.*, **6**, 347.

Snyder, M. J. and Woodward, T. E. (1970), 'The clinical use of chloramphenicol', *Med Clin. North America*, **54**, 1187.

Snyder, M. J. *et al.* (1976), 'Comparative efficacy of chloramphenicol, ampicillin and co-trimoxazole in the treatment of typhoid fever', *Lancet*, **2**, 1155.

Sutter, V. L. and Finegold, S. M. (1976), 'Susceptibility of anaerobic bacteria to 23 antimicrobial agents', *Antimicrob. Ag. Chemother.*, **10**, 736.

Sutter, V. L. (1977), '*In vitro* susceptibility of anaerobes: Comparison of clindamycin and other antimicrobial agents', *J. Infect. Dis.* (Suppl.), **135**, 7.

Suzuki, S. A., Nakazawa, S. and Ushioda, T. (1956), 'Yearly changes of drug resistance of Shigella strains isolated in Kyoto for five years from 1951', *Chemotherapy*, **4**, 336; quoted by Farrar and Eidson (1971).

Svenungsson, B., Bengtsson, E., Fluur, E. and Siegborn, J. (1976), 'Hearing loss as a sequel to chloramphenicol and ampicillin treatment of Haemophilus influenzae meningitis', *Scand. J. Infect. Dis.*, **8**, 175.

Tacquet, A., Devulder, B., Cuvelier, D. and Legros, J. (1974), 'Pharmacokinetic aspects of thiamphenicol in subjects with normal renal function and in patients with chronic renal insufficiency, with or without haemodialysis', *Postgrad. Med. J.* (Suppl. 5), **50**, 36.

Tanaka, T., Ikemura, K., Tsunoda, M., Sasagawa, I. and Mitsuhashi, S. (1976), 'Drug resistance and distribution of R factors in Salmonella strains', *Antimicrob. Ag. Chemother.*, **9**, 61.

Thompson, W. L., Anderson, S. E., Jr., Lipsky, J. J. and Lietman, P. S. (1975), 'Overdoses of chloramphenicol', *JAMA*, **234**, 149.

Thorne, G. M. and Farrar, W. E., Jr. (1973), 'Genetic properties of R factors associated with epidemic strains of Shigella dysenteriae type I from central America and Salmonella typhi from Mexico', *J. Infect. Dis.*, **128**, 132.

Thorne, G. M. and Farrar, W. E., Jr. (1974), 'Superinfection compatibility of R factors in Shigella dysenteriae type I from Central America and Salmonella typhi from Mexico', *J. Infect. Dis.*, **130**, 284.

Thornsberry, C., Baker, C. N. and Kirven, L. A. (1978), '*In vitro* activity of antimicrobial agents on Legionnaires' diseases bacterium', *Antimicrob. Ag. Chemother.*, **13**, 78.

Turk, D. C. (1977), 'A comparison of chloramphenicol and ampicillin as bactericidal agents for Haemophilus influenzae type b', *J. Med. Microbiol.* **10**, 127.

Urban, T. (1972), 'Transferable multiple drug resistance of Shigella strains isolated in Sweden', *Scand. J. Infect., Dis.*, **4**, 221.

Uwaydah, M. (1975), 'Choice of antimicrobial agents in enteric fever', *J. Antimicrob. Chemother.*, **1**, 135.

Van Klingeren, B., Van Embden, J. D. A. and Dessens-Kroon, M. (1977), 'Plasmid-mediated chloramphenicol resistance in Haemophilus influenzae', *Antimicrob. Ag. Chemother.*, **11**, 383.

Vazquez, J., Calderon, E. and Rodriguez, R. S. (1972), 'Chloramphenicol-resistance strains of Salmonella typhosa', *New Engl. J. Med.*, **286**, 1220.

Vince, R., Almquist, R. G., Ritter, C. L. and Daluge, S. (1975), 'Chloramphenicol binding site with analogues of chloramphenicol and puromycin', *Antimicrob. Ag. Chemother.*, **8**, 439.

Wallerstein, R. O., Condit, P. K., Kasper, C. K., Brown, J. W. and Morrison, F. R. (1969), 'Statewide study of chloramphenicol therapy and fatal aplastic anemia', *JAMA*, **208**, 2045.

Wallerstein, R. O.(1969), 'Chloramphenicol toxicity', *Lancet*, **2**, 695.

Weber, D. R., Douglass, L. E., Brundage, W. G. and Stallkamp, T. C. (1969), 'Acute varieties of melioidosis occurring in U.S. soldiers in Vietnam', *Amer. J. Med.*, **46**, 234.

Weisberger, A. S., Wessler, S. and Avioli, L. V. (1969), 'Mechanisms of action of chloramphenicol', *JAMA*, **209**, 97.

Weiss, C. F., Glazko, A. J. and Weston, J. K. (1960), 'Chloramphenicol in the newborn infant: A physiologic explanation of its toxicity when given in excessive doses', *New Engl. J. Med.*, **262**, 787.

Welch, H. (1954), *Principles and Practice of Antibiotic Therapy*, Med. Encyc. Inc., New York, p. 205.

Westenfelder, G. O. and Paterson, P. Y. (1969), 'Life-threatening infection. Choice of alternate drugs when penicillin cannot be given', *JAMA*, **210**, 845.

Whittle, H. C., Davidson, N.McD., Greenwood, B. M., Warrell, D. A., Tomkins, A., Tugwell, P., Zalin, A., Bryceson, A. D. M., Parry, E. H. O., Brueton, M., Duggan, M. and Rajković, A. D. (1973), 'Trial or chloramphenicol for meningitis in Northern Savanna of Africa', *Brit. med. J.*, **3**, 379.

WHO (1974a), 'Transferable drug resistance in salmonella in South and Central America', *WHO Wkly epidem. Rec.*, **49**, 65.

WHO (1974b), 'Salmonella surveillance. Group H resistance factors in Southern Asia', *WHO Wkly epidem. Rec.*, **49**, 245.

WHO (1974c), 'Salmonella surveillance. Chloramphenicol-resistant Salmonella typhi in Viet-Nam (Rep. of) and Thailand', *WHO Wkly epidem. Rec.*, **49**, 295.

Willcox, P. H. A. (1967), 'Chloramphenicol', *Brit. med. J.*, **2**, 443.

Willcox, R. R. (1977), 'How suitable are available pharmaceuticals for the treatment of sexually transmitted diseases? (2) Conditions presenting as sores or tumours', *Brit. J. vener. Dis.*, **53**, 340.

Williams, J. D. and Andrews, J. (1974), 'Sensitivity of Haemophilus influenzae to antibiotics', *Brit. med. J.*, **1**, 134.

Winshell, E. B., Cherubin, C., Winter, J. and Neu, H. C. (1970), 'Antibiotic resistance of salmonella in the Eastern United States', *Antimicrob. Agents Chemother.*—1969, p. 86.

Wisseman, C. L., Jr., Waddell, A. D. and Walsh, W. T. (1974), '*In vitro* studies of the action of antibiotics on Rickettsia prowazeki by two basic methods of cell culture', *J. Infect. Dis.*, **130**, 564.

Woodward, T. E. and Wisseman, C. L., Jr., (1958), *Chloromycetin (Chloramphenicol)*, Med. Encyc. Inc., New York.

Young, L. S., Martin, W. J., Meyer, R. D., Weinstein, R. J. and Anderson, E. T. (1977), 'Gram-negative rod bacteremia: Microbiologic, immunologic, and therapeutic considerations', *Ann. Intern. Med.*, **86**, 456.

Yunis, A. A. and Bloomberg, G. R. (1964), 'Chloramphenicol toxicity: Clinical features and pathogenesis', *Progr. Hemat.*, **4**, 138.

Yunis, A. A., Smith, U. S. and Restrepo, A. (1970), 'Reversible bone marrow suppression from chloramphenicol: A consequence of mitochondrial injury', *Arch Intern. Med.*, **126**, 272.

Yunis, A. A. (1974), 'Concluding remarks. International symposium on chloramphenicol-thiamphenicol', *Postgrad. Med. J.* (Suppl. 5), **50,** 149.

Zabransky, R. J., Johnston, J. A. and Hauser, K. J. (1973), 'Bacteriostatic and bactericidal activities of various antibiotics against Bacteroides fragilis', *Antimicrob. Ag. Chemother.*, **3,** 152.

Cycloserine

Description

Cycloserine was isolated by independent investigators from cultures of Streptomyces orchidaceus (Harned *et al.*, 1955), and Streptomyces garyphalus (Harris *et al.*, 1955). The drug is a crystalline substance of low molecular weight with a chemical structure of D-4-amino-s-isoxazolidone. It is marketed in Australia with the trade name 'Closina' (Eli Lilly).

Sensitive Organisms

1. *Mycobacterium tuberculosis*. This is sensitive to cycloserine, and strains which have become resistant to streptomycin, isoniazid and PAS usually remain cycloserine-sensitive (Robson and Sullivan, 1963). However, strains of M. tuberculosis resistant to cycloserine emerge, if this drug is used singly for the treatment of tuberculosis (Storey and McLean, 1957).

2. *Other mycobacteria*. M. kansasii is usually sensitive (Elder *et al.*, 1977). M. intracellulare (Battey bacillus) is often resistant to all antituberculosis drugs except cycloserine (Bailey *et al.*, 1977).

3. *Other bacteria*. Bacteria such as Staph. pyogenes and Gram-negative enteric bacilli are cycloserine-sensitive to a variable degree (Hoeprich, 1964). Esch. coli is the most susceptible; Proteus and Klebsiella spp. are more resistant, and Pseudomonas aeruginosa is highly resistant (Murdoch *et al.*, 1966).

In Vitro Sensitivities

1. *Mycobacterium tuberculosis*. Most strains of M. tuberculosis are inhibited by cycloserine in a concentration of 10 to 20 μg per ml. The minimum inhibitory concentration of the standard H 37 RV strain is 10 μg per ml. Strains with MIC's higher than 40 μg per ml and resistance ratio >4 (*see* page 296) should be considered resistant.

2. *Esch. coli*. In terms of minimum inhibitory concentrations, cycloserine is not very active against this species, the MIC usually being greater than 50 μg per ml. However concentrations greater than this are readily obtained in the urine (but not in serum) with standard doses of the drug. Therefore for the purpose of treating Esch. coli urinary tract infections, organisms with MIC's of 100 μg per ml or lower have been regarded as 'sensitive' (Murdoch *et al.*, 1966). These authors tested 555 Esch. coli strains and on this basis found that 96 per cent were 'sensitive'. By contrast the majority of strains of Proteus and Klebsiella spp. and Pseudomonas aeruginosa were 'resistant'.

457

Mode of Administration and Dosage

Cycloserine can only be administered by the oral route.

1. *Treatment of tuberculosis.* For this purpose cycloserine is always administered with one or two other antituberculosis drugs. The dose is 20–30 mg per kg per day. The maximum daily dose of cycloserine for adults is 1·0 g administered in two divided doses. Many patients may not tolerate this dose for prolonged periods, and in these it may be necessary to reduce the daily dose to 0·75 g or even 0·5 g (*Today's Drugs*, 1963; 1968).

Appropriate doses for children are a quarter of the adult dose for those aged less than two years, and a half of the adult dose for those aged two to ten years.

Cycloserine should be avoided in patients with impaired renal function, but if it is used, the dosage should be reduced and serum levels monitored.

2. *Urinary tract infections.* A two weeks' course of cycloserine in a dose of 250 mg twice daily has been recommended for the treatment of acute Esch. coli urinary tract infections. For long-term suppressive treatment of patients with chronic Esch. coli bacteriuria, a cycloserine dose of 250 mg, administered on alternate evenings, has been advocated (Murdoch *et al.*, 1966). Children aged two to ten years should receive half, and younger children a quarter of these doses.

Cycloserine should not be used to treat urinary tract infections in patients with impaired renal function, because adequate urinary concentrations are not obtained with reduced doses of the drug.

Availability

Cycloserine is available in 250 mg capsules.

Serum Levels in Relation to Dosage

Cycloserine is well absorbed after oral administration. Following a 250 mg oral dose, the peak serum level of about 10 μg per ml is attained in 3–4 h (Storey and McLean, 1957; Truant, 1958). Doubling the dose doubles the peak serum level. Thereafter the plasma concentration falls rapidly, but some drug is still detectable in plasma after 12 h. With repeated doses of cycloserine, there is slight accumulation of the drug during the first three days of treatment (Storey and McLean, 1957).

Excretion

URINE: About 60–70 per cent of orally administered cycloserine is excreted by glomerular filtration in the urine in an unchanged active form. This excretion is not affected by probenecid. Most of the administered dose is excreted in urine during the first 24 h (Robson and Sullivan, 1963). High concentrations of active cycloserine are attained in urine. The drug given in usual doses will accumulate in patients with impaired renal function, because it is only slowly excreted in such patients.

INACTIVATION IN BODY: It appears that about 35 per cent of administered cycloserine is metabolized in the body. The metabolites have not been identified (Storey and McLean, 1957).

FAECES: Cycloserine is almost completely absorbed after oral administration, and only negligible amounts are excreted in the faeces.

Distribution of the Drug in Body

After absorption from the gastro-intestinal tract, cycloserine becomes widely distributed throughout the body. It penetrates well into the normal cerebrospinal fluid where concentrations may approximate those attained in serum (Storey and McLean, 1957). Animal studies have shown that the drug reaches significant concentrations in lymph, amniotic fluid and the fetal circulation (Anderson *et al.*, 1956).

Mode of Action

Cycloserine interferes with bacterial cell wall synthesis, but its mechanism of action differs from that of penicillin (page 19). During the early stages of cell wall synthesis D-alanine molecules are linked together. Cycloserine, being a structural analogue of D-alanine, acts as a competitive antagonist of the enzymes which link D-alanine molecules in the bacterial cell wall (Strominger *et al.*, 1959; Strominger and Tipper, 1965). In some cycloserine-resistant bacteria, similar to the tetracyclines (page 599), the resistance is due to a reduced uptake of the drug into the cell (Clark and Young, 1977).

Toxicity

1. *Neurotoxicity.* This is the most important toxic effect of cycloserine. Psychotic disturbances such as excitement, aggression, confusion and depression are not infrequent. In addition headache, drowsiness, tremor and epileptiform convulsions may occur. For these reasons the drug should be avoided in patients with mental instability or epilepsy. With a dose of 0·5 g twice daily, about eight per cent of patients have been reported to develop convulsions (Storey and McLean, 1957). These complications of cycloserine appear to be dose related, and their frequency is much higher if a peak serum level of 30 μg per ml is exceeded. Convulsions and other neurotoxic manifestations are less common if a smaller daily dose of 0·5 g is used (Storey and McLean, 1957). Cycloserine is also relatively safe if used in lower dosage schedules of 250 mg twice daily for the treatment of acute urinary tract infections, or 250 mg on alternate days for long-term suppression of bacteriuria (Murdoch *et al.*, 1966). These authors only observed neurotoxicity in 5 per cent of 404 patients treated in this manner. Two of their patients, who had impaired renal function, developed convulsions, seven complained of drowsiness, three of limb twitching and eight of depression. All these toxic effects disappeared when the drug was stopped.

Rarely, peripheral neuritis may result from cycloserine therapy.

Markedly reduced levels of cerebrospinal fluid calcium and magnesium have been found in patients taking large doses of cycloserine, and these changes may contribute to the toxicity of the drug (Murdoch, 1967). Neurotoxicity almost certainly results from a direct effect of the drug on the nervous system and the administration of various vitamins is unlikely to be beneficial. However, both pyridoxine and nicotinamide have been used to prevent these complications with apparent success (Swash *et al.*, 1972).

2. *Other side-effects*. Rarely drug fever, rashes (Kirshner, 1958) and cardiac arrhythmias have been reported. Murdoch *et al.* (1966) treated 27 pregnant women with cycloserine, and there was no evidence of teratogenicity.

Clinical Uses of the Drug

1. *Tuberculosis*. In this disease cycloserine is only used as a 'reserve drug'. It may occasionally replace a standard drug which is contraindicated either because of bacterial resistance or drug reactions. For example a combination of isoniazid and cycloserine has been used with moderate success (Kirshner, 1958; Truant, 1958). In general, however, cycloserine should be used together with two other drugs to which the strain of M. tuberculosis is still sensitive. A combination of isoniazid, PAS and cycloserine has been used continuously for three years for the treatment of renal tuberculosis (Comments, 1969). Nowadays with the advent of more effective and safer drugs such as ethambutol (page 832) and rifampicin (page 568), the role of cycloserine in the chemotherapy of tuberculosis is limited.

2. *Urinary tract infections*. Despite the good results reported by Murdoch *et al.* (1966), using cycloserine to treat Esch. coli urinary tract infections, most clinicians prefer other drugs. Long-term administration of cycloserine has also been reported to be effective as a suppressive in chronic Esch. coli bacteriuria (Murdoch, 1967). Cycloserine is ineffective in urinary tact infections caused by other bacterial species and also in systemic Esch. coli infections, because adequate serum levels are not attained (page 457).

REFERENCES

Anderson, R. C., Worth, H. M., Welles, J. S., Harris, P. N. and Chen, K. K. (1956), 'Pharmacology and toxicology of cycloserine', *Antibiot. Chemother.*, **6,** 360.

Bailey, W. C., Raleigh, J. W. and Turner, J. A. P. (1977), 'Treatment of mycobacterial disease', *Amer. Rev. Resp. Dis.*, **115,** 185.

Clark, V. L. and Young, F. E. (1977), 'Inducible resistance to D-cycloserine in Bacillus subtilis 168', *Antimicrob. Ag. Chemother.*, **11,** 871.

Comments (1969), 'Current treatment for renal tuberculosis', *Med. J. Aust.*, **2,** 1038.

Elder, J. L., Edwards, F. G. B. and Abrahams, E. W. (1977), 'Tuberculosis due to Mycobacterium kansasii', *Aust. N.Z. J. Med.*, **7,** 8.

Harned, R. L., Hidy, P. H. and Labaw, E. K. (1955), 'Cycloserine. I. A preliminary report', *Antib. & Chemo.*, **5,** 204; quoted by Storey and McLean (1957).

Harris, D. A., Ruger, M., Reagan, M. A., Wolf, F. J., Peck, R. L., Wallick, H. and Woodruff, H. B. (1955), 'Discovery, development, and antimicrobial properties of D-4-amino-3-isoxazolidone (oxamycin), a new antibiotic produced by Streptomyces garyphalus n. Sp.', *Antib. & Chemo.*, **5,** 183; quoted by Storey and McLean (1957).

Hoeprich, P. D. (1964), 'Alanine: cycloserine antagonism. I. Significance of phenomenon in testing susceptibility to cycloserine', *Amer. J. Clin. Path.*, **41,** 140.

Kirshner, J. J. (1958), 'Cycloserine with isoniazid in chronic pulmonary tuberculosis', *Antibiotic Annual, 1957–58*, p. 627.

Murdoch, J. McC., Geddes, A. M., Tulloch, W. S., Newsam, J. E., Thomson, W. N., Bidwell, D. and Wallace, E. T. (1966), 'The problem of pyelonephritis. A four-year study of a pyelonephritis unit', *The Practitioner*, **196,** 800.

Murdoch, J. McC. (1967), 'Panel discussion: clinical aspects of the therapy of systemic and urinary gram-negative infections', *Ann. N.Y. Acad. Sci.*, **145**, 354.

Robson, J. M. and Sullivan, F. M. (1963), 'Antituberculosis drugs', *Pharmacol. Rev.*, **15**, 169.

Storey, P. B. and McLean, R. L. (1957), 'A current appraisal of cycloserine', *Antibiot. Med. Clin. Ther.*, **4**, 223.

Strominger, J. L., Threnn, R. H. and Scott, S. S. (1959), 'Oxamycin, a competitive antagonist of the incorporation of D-alanine into a uridine nucleotide in Staphylococcus aureus', *J. Amer. Chem. Soc.*, **81**, 3803.

Strominger, J. L. and Tipper, D. J. (1965), 'Bacterial cell wall synthesis and structure in relation to the mechanism of action of penicillins and other antibacterial agents', *Amer. J. Med.*, **39**, 708.

Swash, M., Roberts, A. H. and Murnaghan, D. J. (1972), 'Reversible pellagra-like encephalopathy with ethionamide and cycloserine', *Tubercle*, **53**, 132.

Today's Drugs (1963), 'Drugs for tuberculosis', *Brit. med. J.*, **1**, 1593.

Today's Drugs (1968), 'Drugs for tuberculosis', *Brit. med. J.*, **3**, 664.

Truant, J. P. (1958), 'Studies on the *in vitro* and *in vivo* effect of cycloserine and isoniazid on tubercle bacilli', *Antibiotic Annual, 1957–58*, p. 630.

Fusidate Sodium ('Fucidin')

Description

Fusidic acid, obtained from the fungus Fusidium coccineum, has a steroid structure and is chemically related to cephalosporin P, which is one of the antibiotics formed by the mould Cephalosporium acremonium. The sodium salt of fusidic acid (sodium fusidate) is used clinically. This antibiotic was developed by Leo Laboratories in Copenhagen, and marketed with the trade name of 'Fucidin' (Smith Kline and French).

A number of derivatives of fusidic acid have been prepared, but their antibacterial activity is low compared to sodium fusidate (Godtfredsen et al., 1966).

Sensitive Organisms

1. *Gram-positive bacteria*. The most significant feature about sodium fusidate is its high degree of activity against Staph. pyogenes, including penicillinase-producing strains. Resistant strains of Staph. pyogenes can be readily produced by growing the organism in the presence of increasing concentrations of sodium fusidate (Godtfredsen et al., 1962; Hilson, 1962); however the development of resistance during treatment has been uncommon (Taylor and Bloor, 1962; Rao et al., 1972). Another important feature about this drug is that it is active against most methicillin-resistant staphylococci (Garrod, 1968; Hoeprich et al., 1970).

Compared to staphylococci, all other Gram-positive cocci are much less susceptible to sodium fusidate. The strains of Strep. pneumoniae resistant to multiple antibiotics, which were isolated in South Africa during 1977, were only partially resistant (MIC $2 \mu g$ per ml) to sodium fusidate (Center for Disease Control, 1977). Gram-positive bacteria such as C. diphtheriae, Cl. tetani and Cl. perfringens are quite sensitive.

2. *Gram-negative bacteria*. The Neisseria spp. (gonococci and meningococci) are susceptible. Bacteroides fragilis is commonly sensitive to fusidic acid (Stirling and Goodwin, 1977). All other Gram-negative bacilli are completely resistant.

3. Sodium fusidate has some action against Mycobacterium tuberculosis, but this is of no clinical importance. Fungi are completely resistant.

In Vitro Sensitivities

Table 29 shows the minimum inhibitory concentrations of sodium fusidate against some selected bacterial species. Staphylococci are almost a hundred times more sensitive than most streptococcal species.

462

TABLE 29

(Modified from Godtfredsen et al., 1962)

ORGANISM	Average concentration required for 50% inhibition (μg per ml)
Gram-positive bacteria	
Staph. pyogenes (non-penicillinase-producer	0·066
Staph. pyogenes (penicillinase-producer)	0·059
Strep. pyogenes (Group A)	6·8
Strep. pneumoniae (Dip. pneumoniae)	8·6
Strep. viridans spp.	1·6
Strep. faecalis (Enterococcus, Group D)	4·0
Clostridium tetani	0·016
Corynebacterium diphtheriae	0·0044
Gram-negative bacteria	
Esch. coli	>100·0
Klebsiella pneumoniae	35·0
Neisseria gonorrhoeae	0·66
Neisseria meningitidis	0·56
Miscellaneous	
Mycobacterium tuberculosis	1·0

Mode of Administration of Dosage

1. *Oral administration.* Sodium fusidate is usually administered by the oral route. The usual adult dose is 0·5 g eight-hourly, but for severe infections this dose can be doubled. For children the dose is 20–40 mg per kg body weight per day, given in three divided doses, but this may be increased to 50 mg per kg per day for treatment of severe infections. To reduce dyspepsia it may be taken with meals.

2. *Parenteral administration.* Another preparation of fusidic acid, diethanolamine fusidate is available solely for intravenous administration. It is marketed in 580 mg vials, each equivalent to 500 mg sodium fusidate. The drug is given by continuous infusion in isotonic saline in an adult dose of 580 mg eight-hourly. The dose for children is 20 mg per kg body weight daily. It has been suggested that it is preferable to infuse this drug into a wide bore vein with a good blood flow, because therapy may be complicated by venospasm and thrombosis (Webb *et al.*, 1968). However intravenous 'fucidin' has been administered to five neonates with severe staphylococcal infections without evidence of either local or systemic reactions (Liddy, 1973).

3. *Patients with renal failure.* Sodium fusidate may be administered in the usual doses to these patients.

Availability

1. Enteric coated tablets: 250 mg.
2. Suspension for oral use: 250 mg in 5 ml.

3. Intravenous preparation: vials containing 580 mg diethanolamine fusidate (equivalent to 500 mg sodium fusidate). The contents of the vial is dissolved in 50 ml of a phosphate-citrate buffer which is provided and then this is diluted in 250–500 ml saline for infusion.

Serum Levels in Relation to Dosage

1. Figure 23 shows the mean serum levels in ten subjects studied by Godt-fredsen *et al.* (1962). After a single oral dose of 0·5 g, the peak serum level is usually achieved in two hours, the level then gradually falls, and detectable amounts are still present after twenty-four hours. These authors also showed that there was considerable individual variation in the amount of the drug absorbed from the alimentary tract. At one hour the lowest level recorded was 0·7 μg per ml, and the highest 35 μg per ml, and although peak levels at two hours were more uniform, they still ranged from 14 to 38 μg per ml.

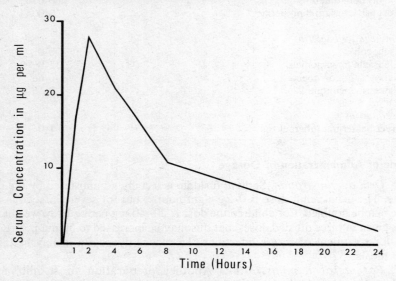

FIG. 23. Mean serum concentrations of sodium fusidate after a single oral dose of 0·5 g. (After Godtfredsen *et al.*, 1962.)

2. With a dosage of 0·5 g eight-hourly, the drug steadily accumulates in the body. After 96 h of such a regimen a mean serum level of 71 μg per ml was obtained, but some individuals showed serum levels just over 100 μg per ml (Godtfredsen *et al.*, 1962). With a lower dosage of 0·5 g twelve-hourly, there is usually no accumulation, and the serum concentration soon stabilizes at about 20 μg per ml. Stirling and Goodwin (1977) gave two volunteers two oral doses of 1 g at an interval of six hours, and serum concentrations of 54 and 59 μg per ml respectively were obtained.

Excretion

URINE: Very little active sodium fusidate is excreted by the kidneys, and only about 1 per cent of the administered dose can be recovered from urine. After four days treatment with standard doses, the urine only contains 0·8 μg per ml or less of the active drug (Godtfredsen *et al.*, 1962).

BILE: Some sodium fusidate is excreted and concentrated in bile. A fraction of the administered dose can be recovered in active form from the faeces, some of this may be non-absorbed drug, and some presumably due to biliary excretion.

INACTIVATION IN BODY: The total amounts of detectable drug excreted in the urine, faeces and bile does not account for all of the administered dose. It appears that some of the drug is converted to a microbiologically inactive form in the body.

Distribution of the Drug in Body

'Fucidin' is well distributed throughout the body. It has been demonstrated in samples of subcutaneous fat, kidney, muscle and prostate taken from patients undergoing surgery a few hours after administration. It also passes through the placenta and can be found in fetal tissue. Very little of the drug is detectable in the CSF of patients with normal meninges. Sodium fusidate is effective even in the presence of large collections of pus, possibly because of its ability to penetrate well into purulent collections (Crosbie, 1963). It also penetrates well into pus of a cerebral abscess (De Louvois *et al.*, 1977).

In vitro studies suggest that sodium fusidate is very highly protein bound; one study showed that the binding was as high as 97·2 per cent (Rolinson and Sutherland, 1965). The *in vitro* activity of the drug is reduced 64-fold in the presence of 50 per cent serum (Barber and Waterworth, 1962). Despite this very high degree of serum protein binding, the drug is quite effective clinically (Leading article, 1966). This can be partly explained by the wide margin between its MIC for staphylococci and the serum levels achieved after usual doses (compare MIC for Staph. pyogenes, Table 29 and serum levels, Fig. 23). However the exact clinical significance of protein binding of antibiotics remains somewhat uncertain (*see* page 86).

Mode of Action

Sodium fusidate is related chemically to cephalosporin P, but the cephalosporin antibiotics (pages 199, 225, 238) are derived from cephalosporin C. In contrast to the cephalosporins, which inhibit bacterial cell wall synthesis, sodium fusidate inhibits bacterial protein synthesis (Harvey *et al.*, 1966), by interfering with the 'G' factor (page 434) involved in translocation, and possibly by other mechanisms (Tanaka *et al.*, 1968). Mutants resistant to sodium fusidate have an altered 'G' factor (Tanaka *et al.*, 1971). This different mode of action probably explains the lack of cross-resistance between sodium fusidate and the penicillinase-resistant penicillins and cephalosporins. For this reason methicillin-resistant staphylococci are usually sensitive to fusidate sodium.

Gram-negative bacilli are 'fucidin'-resistant probably because the drug cannot penetrate their cell walls; sodium fusidate inhibits the protein synthesis of Esch. coli in cell free systems.

Results of *in vitro* tests with sodium fusidate illustrate that the distinction between the so called 'bactericidal' and 'bacteristatic' drugs is only relative.

Some investigators report that this drug is mainly bacteristatic (Hilson, 1962), whereas others have found it bactericidal (Newman *et al.*, 1962). These differing results appear to depend on such factors as the concentration of the drug used, the inoculum size and the sensitivity of the particular Staph. pyogenes strain (*see also* page 504).

Toxicity

1. In general 'fucidin' can be regarded as a non-toxic antibiotic. When administered orally, only mild upper gastro-intestinal discomfort and diarrhoea have been noted. Investigations have failed to show any evidence of hepatic, renal or haemopoietic toxicity. No severe allergic reactions have been observed, but occasional mild rashes have been reported. The drug appears to be safe in penicillin-allergic patients. In chronic infections 'fucidin' has been given continuously for several months without obvious toxic effects (Crosbie, 1963; Dodson, 1963).

2. Because of its steroid structure it was thought that this drug may possibly have some metabolic effects, unrelated to its antibacterial activity. Wynn (1965) showed that no significant metabolic changes were associated with 'fucidin' administration. It had a mild protein catabolic effect, lowered urinary calcium excretion, and also caused mild temporary impairment of bromsulphthalein excretion by the liver. However these mild biochemical effects appeared to be of no practical importance even after prolonged administration.

It is not known whether sodium fusidate accumulates in the presence of liver disease and therefore it should be used cautiously in patients with impaired liver function.

3. Human leucocytes incubated with sodium fusidate show markedly depressed migration (Forsgren and Schmeling, 1977). The clinical significance of this observation is unknown.

Clinical Uses of the Drug

1. *Staphylococcal infections.* The treatment of these infections is the main indication for sodium fusidate. It has been used for furunculosis, abscesses, infected wounds or burns, osteomyelitis, pneumonia, septicaemia and endocarditis. Most clinical studies show that the results of treatment of these diseases, including severe staphylococcal infection, have been good (Crosbie, 1963; Dodson, 1963; Jensen and Lassen, 1964; Matsaniotis *et al.*, 1967). The introduction of the parenteral form of fusidic acid in 1969 has overcome its previous disadvantage of using oral therapy for seriously ill patients. Sodium fusidate given intravenously has been used successfully to treat severe staphylococcal infections (Menday and Marsh, 1976).

Resistant Staph. pyogenes strains, which emerge very easily *in vitro* (page 462) have appeared *in vivo* during the treatment of burns (Lowbury *et al.*, 1962), but this has not been a common problem during treatment of other infections. Sodium fusidate has been used alone for the prolonged treatment of staphylococcal pulmonary infections complicating cystic fibrosis without the emergence of drug resistance (Norman, 1967).

However, many authors recommend that sodium fusidate should be combined with another anti-staphylococcal agent, particularly for treatment of infections due to methicillin-resistant staphylococci (Jensen, 1968; Jensen and Lassen, 1969). Some of the drugs which have been used for this purpose include methicillin, erythromycin, novobiocin and rifampicin. There is no convincing evidence that these combinations act synergistically, and the main clinical advantage is the prevention of emergence of 'fucidin'-resistant strains.

Several authors have shown that it is an advantage to combine sodium fusidate with penicillin G for treatment of severe staphylococcal infections (Scowen and Garrod, 1962; Taylor and Bloor, 1962). Penicillin G alone has no activity against penicillinase-producing Staph. pyogenes, but it appears that it may act synergistically with sodium fusidate. Sodium fusidate apparently reduces the number of staphylococci to a point, where there is insufficient penicillinase production to destroy penicillin G and interfere with its action (Taylor and Bloor, 1962). This combination also seems to prevent the emergence of 'fucidin'-resistant mutants, because these are killed by penicillin G (Waterworth, 1963). The synergism between these two agents varies *in vitro* according to the Staph. pyogenes strain tested, and is minimal when highly active penicillinase-producing organisms are examined (Barber and Waterworth, 1962; Waterworth, 1963). It is not known if penicillin G combined with 'fucidin' is useful clinically for the treatment of infections caused by these highly active penicillinase-producing staphylococci.

Conversely antagonism between sodium fusidate and penicillin G (or one of the semisynthetic penicillins such as methicillin) can be readily demonstrated *in vitro* with many staphylococcal strains, but this does not appear to have any clinical significance (O'Grady and Greenwood, 1973).

Sodium fusidate is an effective anti-staphylococcal agent but it is not usually recommended for the initial treatment of severe staphylococcal infections, other drugs such as penicillin G (page 34), methicillin (page 74) or cloxacillin (page 96) or a cephalosporin (page 213), being preferred. It is a useful drug for continuation oral therapy after the acute phase of the illness has responded and it is also a reserve drug for the treatment of infections due to methicillin-resistant strains.

Sodium fusidate has also been used topically as a cream to treat superficial staphylococcal soft tissue infections successfully (Pakrooh, 1968). Diethanolamine fusidate has been incorporated in bone cement; its use in this way has been suggested for prophylaxis against infection after total hip replacement (Gardner and Medcraft, 1974). Topical sodium fusidate has been used with some success to eradicate the staphylococcal nasal carrier state (Newman *et al.*, 1962).

2. *Other infections.* A combination of rifampicin and sodium fusidate was used to eradicate multiply resistant strains of Strep. pneumoniae in South Africa (page 5). Oral sodium fusidate in a high dose of 15 mg per kg (up to a maximum of $1 \cdot 0$ g) every eight hours was used to treat five patients successfully with Bacteroides fragilis infections (Stirling and Goodwin, 1977). As all meningococci are susceptible *in vitro* to $0 \cdot 5$ μg per ml of sodium fusidate, it has been suggested that this drug should be considered as a chemoprophylactic agent for those who may be at risk of meningococcal disease (Miles and Moyes, 1978).

REFERENCES

Barber, M. and Waterworth, P. (1962), 'Antibacterial activity *in vitro* of fucidin', *Lancet*, **1**, 931.

Center for Disease Control (1977), 'Multiple-antibiotic resistance of pneumo-cocci—South Africa', *Morbidity and Mortality Weekly Report*, **26**, 285.

Crosbie, R. B. (1963), 'Treatment of staphylococcal infections with "fucidin" ', *Brit. med. J.*, **1**, 788.

De Louvois, J., Gortvai, P. and Hurley, R. (1977), 'Antibiotic treatment of abscesses of central nervous system', *Brit. med. J.*, **2**, 985.

Dodson, B. (1963), 'Fusidic acid in the management of phage-type 80 staphylococcal infection', *Lancet*, **2**, 659.

Forsgren, A. and Schmeling, D. (1977), 'Effect of antibiotics on chemotaxis of human leukocytes', *Antimicrob. Ag. Chemother.*, **11**, 580.

Gardner, A. D. H. and Medcraft, J. W. (1974), 'Antibiotic/bone-cement mixtures in prevention of infection following total joint replacement', *Lancet*, **2**, 891.

Garrod, L. P. (1968), 'Methicillin-resistant staphylococci', *Lancet*, **2**, 871.

Godtfredsen, W., Roholt, K. and Tybring, L. (1962), 'Fucidin: A new orally active an-tibiotic', *Lancet*, **1**, 928.

Godtfredsen, W. O., Albrethsen, C., Daehne, W. V., Tybring, L. and Vengedal, S. (1966), 'Transformations of fusidic acid and the relationship between structure and antibacterial activity', *Antimicrob. Agents Chemother.*—1965, p. 132.

Harvey, C. L., Knight, S. G. and Sih, C. J. (1966), 'On the mode of action of fusidic acid', *Biochemistry*, **5**, 3320.

Hoeprich, P. D., Benner, E. J. and Kayser, F. H. (1970), 'Susceptibility of methicillin-resistant Staphylococcus aureus to 12 antimicrobial agents', *Antimicrob. Agents Chemother.*—1969, p. 104.

Hilson, G. R. F. (1962), '*In vitro* studies of a new antibiotic (Fucidin)', *Lancet*, **1**, 932.

Jensen, K. and Lassen, H. C. A. (1964), 'Fulminating staphylococcal infections treated with fucidin and penicillin or semisynthetic penicillin', *Ann. Intern. Med.*, **60**, 790.

Jensen, K. (1968), 'Methicillin-resistant staphylococci', *Lancet*, **2**, 1078.

Jensen, K. and Lassen, H. C. A. (1969), 'Combined treatment with antibacterial chemotherapeutical agents in staphylococcal infections', *Q.J. Med.*, New Series *XXXVIII*, **149**, 91.

Leading Article (1966), 'Serum binding of antibiotics', *Brit. med. J.*, **1**, 1059.

Liddy, N. (1973), 'Intravenous fusidic acid in the newborn', *Lancet*, **1**, 621.

Lowbury, E. J. L., Cason, J. S., Jackson, D. MacG. and Miller, R. W. S. (1962), 'Fucidin for staphylococcal infection of burns', *Lancet*, **2**, 478.

Matsaniotis, N., Messaritakis, J. and Anagnostakis, D. (1967), 'Fusidic acid for staphylococcal infections in children', *Brit. med. J.*, **1**, 564.

Menday, A. P. and Marsh, B. T. (1976), 'Intravenous fusidic acid ('Fucidin') in the management of severe staphylococcal infections: A review of 46 cases', *Curr. Med. Res. Opin.*, **4**, 132.

Miles, R. S. and Moyes, A. (1978), 'Comparison of susceptibility of Neisseria meningitis to sodium sulphadiazine and sodium fusidate *in vitro*', *J. clin. Path.*, **31**, 355.

Newman, R. L., Bhat, K. M., Hackney, R., Robinson, C. and Stewart, G. T. (1962), 'Fusidic acid; Laboratory and clinical assessment', *Brit. med. J.*, **2**, 1645.

Norman, A. P. (1967), 'Fusidic acid in cystic fibrosis', *Lancet*, **2**, 516.

O'Grady, F. and Greenwood, D. (1973), 'Interactions between fusidic acid and penicillins', *J. Med. Microbiol.*, **6**, 441.

Pakrooh. H. (1978), 'A comparison of sodium fusidate ointment ('Fucidin') alone ver-sus oral antibiotic therapy in soft tissue infections', *Curr. Med. Res. Opin.*, **5**, 289.

Rao, R., Webster, A. B. D., Sunderland, D. R., Smith, W. F., Ampalam, S. and

Lee, H. E. (1972), 'Cloxacillin and sodium fusidate in management of shunt infections', *Brit. med. J.*, **3**, 618.

Rolinson, G. N. and Sutherland, R. (1965), 'The binding of antibiotics to serum proteins', *Brit. J. Pharmacol.*, **25**, 638.

Scowen, E. F. and Garrod, L. P. (1962), 'A case of staphylococcal septicaemia treated with penicillin and fucidin', *Lancet*, **1**, 933.

Stirling, J. and Goodwin, S. (1977), 'Susceptibility of Bacteroides fragilis to fusidic acid', *J. Antimicrob. Chemother.*, **3**, 522.

Tanaka, N., Kinoshita, T. and Masukawa, H. (1968), 'Mechanism of protein synthesis inhibition by fusidic acid and related antibiotics', *Biochem. Biophys. Res. Commun.*, **30**, 278.

Tanaka, N., Kawano, G. and Kinoshita, T. (1971), 'Chromosomal location of a fusidic acid resistant marker in Escherichia coli', *Biochem. Biophys. Res. Commun.*, **42**, 564.

Taylor, G. and Bloor, K. (1962), 'Antistaphylococcal activity of fucidin', *Lancet*, **1**, 935.

Waterworth, P. M. (1963), 'Apparent synergy between penicillin and erythromycin or fusidic acid', *Clin. Med.*, **70**, 941.

Webb, J., Wilson, H. G. and Rao, A. (1968), 'Staphylococcal endocarditis treated by intravenous administration of fusidic acid and penicillin', *Med. J. Aust.*, **1**, 131.

Wynn, V. (1965), 'Metabolic effects of the steroid antibiotic fusidic acid', *Brit. med. J.*, **1**, 1400.

Lincomycin and Clindamycin

Description

Lincomycin, isolated from a strain of Streptomyces lincolnensis in the Upjohn Research Laboratories, is marketed with the trade name of 'Lincocin' (Lewis *et al.*, 1963). Lincomycin hydrochloride is used clinically because it is readily soluble in water. The drug is not chemically related to erythromycin, but there are certain similarities between lincomycin and the antibiotics of the macrolide group.

Several chemical modifications of the lincomycin molecule have been developed in an attempt to produce an improved antibiotic. Of these, clindamycin (7-chloro-7-deoxylincomycin), 'Dalcin-C' or 'Cleocin' (Upjohn) was the most promising (Magerlein *et al.*, 1967), and this drug is clinically superior to lincomycin. Initially in North America the generic name of clinimycin was adopted for this compound, but now the name clindamycin is used universally.

Sensitive Organisms

Both lincomycin and clindamycin have a similar antibacterial spectrum, but against sensitive microorganisms, clindamycin is the more active drug. Their antibacterial spectrum is also rather similar to that of erythromycin, with some important differences.

1. *Gram-positive bacteria*. Lincomycin and clindamycin are active against most of these bacteria. Staph. pyogenes (including penicillinase-producing strains), Staph. epidermidis, Strep. pyogenes, Strep. pneumoniae and Strep. viridans are usually susceptible. Unlike erythromycin, these drugs are inactive against Strep. faecalis. Of the other Group D streptococci (enterococci), Strep. faecium is resistant but Strep. durans is clindamycin-sensitive. Strep. bovis, a nonenterococcal Group D organism is also sensitive to clindamycin (Karchmer *et al.*, 1975). C. diphtheriae is highly sensitive to lincomycin and even more so to clindamycin (Zamiri and McEntegart, 1972). C. diphtheriae strains resistant to lincomycin (and erythromycin) have been reported (Jellard and Lipinski, 1973), but appear to be very rare. B. anthracis and the Nocardia spp. are sensitive (Keusch and Present, 1976). Gentamicin does not interfere with the activity of clindamycin against sensitive staphylococci, streptococci, pneumococci or clostridia, and in some instances these two drugs may show *in vitro* synergism (Sabath and Toftegaard, 1974; Fass *et al.*, 1974). *In vitro* synergism has been demonstrated with combinations of clindamycin with streptomycin (page 294) or gentamicin (page 325) against some of the viridans group streptococci such as Strep. sanguis and Strep. salivarius, but not against Strep. mutans (Duperval *et al.*, 1975).

Cl. tetani and Cl. perfringens (welchii) are sensitive. However some Cl. per-fringens strains and strains of less common human pathogens such as Cl. sporogenes, Cl. tertium, Cl. bifermentans, Cl. novyi, Cl. ramosum and Cl. sordellii may be lincomycin and clindamycin-resistant (Wilkins and Thiel, 1973; Staneck and Washington, 1974; Dornbusch et al., 1975; Sutter and Finegold, 1976). Amongst the other anaerobic Gram-positive organisms, the Peptococcus, Peptostreptococcus, Eubacterium, Propionibacterium, Bifidobacterium and Lactobacillus spp. are usually sensitive (Sutter and Finegold, 1976). Most strains of Actinomyces israelii and Arachnia propionica are sensitive to lincomycin and clindamycin (Mohr et al., 1970; Sutter and Finegold, 1976; Holmberg et al., 1977).

In clinical practice sensitivity testing is commonly not performed on the usually lincomycin-sensitive streptococci, but resistant strains have been detected amongst all these species. Strep. pyogenes resistant to lincomycin (Kohn et al., 1968; Sanders et al., 1968) and to clindamycin (Kohn and Evans 1970) have been reported. Dixon and Lipinski (1972; 1974) have made large scale surveys of the incidence of beta-haemolytic streptococci resistant to lincomycin (and erythromycin) in Canada. Of Group A strains isolated in a three-year period 1968–1970, 0·05 per cent were resistant but this percentage rose to 0·24 in 1971 and to 1·38 in 1972. During 1971 and 1972, 0·6 per cent of Group B, 1·2 per cent of Group C and 1·3 per cent of Group G beta-haemolytic streptococci were resistant to lincomycin (and erythromycin). Drapkin et al. (1976) described four patients from whom Group A streptococci were isolated from the blood, which were highly resistant to clindamycin but moderately susceptible to erythromycin; in two of these patients, the infection developed whilst they were receiving clindamycin. Similarly pneumococcal strains resistant to lincomycin have been reported (Dixon, 1967; Kislak, 1967), and in most instances these organisms are also erythromycin-resistant (Desmyter, 1968). A strain of Strep. pneumoniae which was resistant to clin-damycin (and erythromycin) has been detected (Champion et al., 1978). The penicillin-resistant pneumococci (page 4) isolated in South Africa during 1977, were also resistant to clindamycin (Center for Disease Control, 1977). Strains of the viridans group of streptococci resistant to lincomycin and clin-damycin (usually also to erythromycin) have been isolated from the pharynx (Sprunt et al., 1970) and from sutures taken from sockets of recently removed teeth (Phillips et al., 1976), of patients receiving these drugs.

Staphylococci resistant to lincomycin are more common, and sensitivity testing is always indicated in clinical practice. As with erythromycin, staphylococci resistant to lincomycin can be easily produced in vitro (Barber and Waterworth, 1964), and may occasionally emerge during treatment in vivo. There has been some disagreement about Staph. pyogenes cross-resistance between lincomycin and the macrolide antibiotics. Lewis et al. (1963) did not demonstrate such cross-resistance, but Barber and Waterworth (1964) observed it occasionally. If erythromycin-resistant and erythromycin-sensitive Staph. pyogenes strains are passaged in the presence of lincomycin, the erythromycin-resistant strains rapidly become lincomycin-resistant, whereas the erythromycin-sensitive ones slowly develop a lesser degree of lincomycin resistance (Duncan, 1968; McGehee et al., 1969). Lincomycin also exhibits the 'dissociated type of resistance' (page 497), characteristic of the macrolides, i.e.

strains of Staph. pyogenes, resistant to erythromycin but sensitive to lincomycin, are found to be lincomycin-resistant, if tested in the presence of erythromycin (Barber and Waterworth, 1964). These phenomena may be explicable by the mode of action of lincomycin and the macrolides (pages 480, 504). Lincomycin should not be selected for the treatment of infections due to Staph. pyogenes strains which are erythromycin-resistant but sensitive to lincomycin, because lincomycin resistance may develop *in vivo* (Duncan, 1968).

2. *Gram-negative aerobic bacteria.* Practically all the aerobic Gram-negative bacteria are resistant to both lincomycin and clindamycin. A difference between these drugs and erythromycin is that bacteria such as N. meningitidis, N. gonorrhoeae and H. influenzae, which are characteristically sensitive to erythromycin, are lincomycin and clindamycin-resistant (McGehee *et al.*, 1968; Hansman and Gibbs, 1972). Some authors have found that clindamycin is much more active against H. influenzae than lincomycin and suggest that it may be effective in human infections by this organism (Geddes *et al.*, 1970), but clinical results have usually been disappointing (*see* page 485) The microaerophilic organism Campylobacter fetus is sensitive to clindamycin (Chow *et al.*, 1978).

3. *Gram-negative anaerobic bacteria.* A clinically important property of lincomycin and clindamycin is that these bacteria are usually sensitive. Most Bacteroides spp. strains are inhibited by 6·2 μg per ml or less of lincomycin (Kitamoto, 1969; Martin *et al.*, 1972) and by 2 μg per ml or less of clindamycin (Kislak, 1972; Bodner *et al.*, 1972; Zabransky *et al.*, 1973; Sutter *et al.*, 1973). In particular B. fragilis is usually sensitive to clindamycin (Dornbusch *et al.*, 1974; Staneck and Washington, 1974; Blazevic, 1976; Sutter and Finegold, 1976; Sutter, 1977). The Fusobacterium spp., with the exception of Fusobacterium varium, are also usually sensitive to clindamycin (Staneck and Washington, 1974; Sutter and Finegold, 1976; Keusch and Present, 1976; Sutter, 1977). Strains of anaerobic Gram-negative bacilli resistant to lincomycin and clindamycin are still uncommon; in one study of 1067 strains of these bacteria isolated from patients only one was resistant to clindamycin (Mitchell, 1973). Clindamycin-resistant strains of B. fragilis have been isolated from the blood of two patients (Salaki *et al.*, 1976). Chloramphenicol (page 425) and metronidazole (page 761) are the only other chemotherapeutic agents which have as wide a spectrum of activity as clindamycin against anaerobes Sutter, 1977). The tetracyclines (page 595) and erythromycin (page 498) are now much less active.

Because there are clinical indications to combine clindamycin with an aminoglycoside, the interactions of these drugs against Gram-negative bacteria have been studied *in vitro*. Fass *et al.* (1974) did not detect antagonism between clindamycin and gentamicin, but found synergism with some strains of Enterobacteriaciae (a number being resistant to both drugs) and Pseudomonas aeruginosa. Leng *et al.* (1975) used combinations of either clindamycin or erythromycin with gentamicin or colistin against Enterobacteriaceae and Ps. aeruginosa and also demonstrated synergism and no antagonism. Klastersky and Husson (1977) demonstrated that gentamicin did not interfere with activity of clindamycin against B. fragilis, and that clindamycin did not influence the activity of gentamicin against Esch. coli. Moreover Okubadejo and Allen (1975) found *in vitro* synergism between clindamycin and gentamicin against

B. fragilis. Zinner *et al.* (1976), however, showed that clindamycin interferes with the bacterial killing of Esch. coli by amikacin or gentamicin during the first two to four hours of incubation. In one *in vivo* study in mice infected with Esch. coli, which were treated by clindamycin plus gentamicin or amikacin, there was no detectable antagonism (Ekwo and Peter, 1976).

4. *Mycoplasmas.* These are less susceptible to lincomycin and clindamycin than to erythromycin (page 499) and the tetracyclines (page 597). M. hominis is inhibited by 5 μg per ml of lincomycin, but M. pneumoniae (MIC 12·5 μg per ml) is resistant as are Mycoplasma T-strains (Ureaplasma urealyticum) (McGehee *et al.*, 1968; Csonka and Spitzer, 1969). Although clindamycin is more active against M. pneumoniae, this organism is still resistant to clinically attainable concentrations.

5. *Miscellaneous organisms.* The leptospirae appear to be susceptible to lincomycin when tested in experimental animals (Lewis *et al.*, 1963). The true fungi and mycobacteria are lincomycin-resistant. Clindamycin is much less active than erythromycin or penicillin for the treatment of established syphilitic lesions in rabbits (Brause *et al.*, 1976).

6. *Protozoa.* Clindamycin is effective in animals infected with chloroquine-resistant and -sensitive Plasmodium falciparum (Powers and Jacobs, 1972). It is also effective against P. vivax but not against the exo-erythrocytic parasites (Keusch and Present, 1976). Clindamycin is effective in experimental toxoplasmosis in mice (Araujo and Remington, 1974).

In Vitro Sensitivities

The minimum inhibitory concentrations of lincomycin and clindamycin for some selected bacterial species are shown in Table 30.

TABLE 30

(After McGehee *et al.*, 1968)

ORGANISM	MIC (μg per ml)			
	Lincomycin		Clindamycin	
	Range	Median	Range	Median
Gram-positive bacteria				
Staph. pyogenes	0·8 –3·1	1·6	0·04 –0·8	0·1
Strep. pyogenes (Group A)	0·04–0·2	0·04	0·02–0·1	0·04
Strep. pneumoniae	0·02–0·2	0·2	<0·002–0·04	0·01
Strep. viridans spp.	0·02–0·4	0·04	0·005–0·04	0·02
Strep. faecalis (Enterococcus, Group D)	25·0–>100·0	>100·0	12·5–>100·0	100·0
Gram-negative bacteria				
Esch. coli	>100·0	>100·0	>100·0	>100·0
Neisseria gonorrhoeae	<0·02–25·0	12·5	0·01–6·3	3·1
Neisseria meningitidis	100·0–>100·0	100·0	6·3–25·0	12·5
Haemophilus influenzae	6·3–50·0	25·0	6·3–50·0	12·5

Mode of Administration and Dosage

A. *Lincomycin*

1. *Oral administration.* Lincomycin is usually administered by the oral route, but it can also be given by intramuscular injection or intravenous infusion. It is acid stable and well absorbed after oral administration, provided it is given in the fasting state. Kaolin used for the treatment of diarrhoea, inhibits absorption of lincomycin (Nies, 1974). The usual adult dose is 0·5 g every six or eight hours. The dosage for children is 30 mg per kg body weight per day, given in three or four divided doses. Lincomycin is not recommended for newborn babies.

2. *Parenteral administration.* The recommended intramuscular dose for adults is 600 mg every 24 h, but for serious infections this dose can be given every 12 or 8 h. The dose for children is 10 mg per kg body weight every 24 h; this can also be administered more frequently for serious infections. The intravenous dose for adults is 600 mg every 8–12 h, and this should be dissolved in at least 250 ml of 5 per cent glucose in water for infusion. The equivalent dose for children is 10–20 mg per kg body weight per day which is given in divided doses by infusion every 8–12 h. The intravenous infusion of lincomycin solution should be relatively slow, because there are potential dangers with rapid infusion (*vide infra*).

3. *Dosage for serious infections.* The oral, intramuscular or intravenous dose of lincomycin may be doubled or even further increased. Adult doses as high as eight g daily intravenously have been used occasionally for treatment of severe infections such as bacterial endocarditis in penicillin-allergic patients (de Yeaza *et al.*, 1967; O'Connell and Plaut, 1969). No side-effects were noted with these high doses provided that a concentrated solution of the drug was not given by rapid intravenous injection. O'Connell and Plaut (1969) consider that a 2 g dose dissolved in 250 ml of intravenous fluid can be safely infused over 30 min. Novak *et al.* (1971) administered total daily doses of 8·4 g; a dose of 2·1 g was dissolved in 250 ml and infused over a two-hour period four times a day, without serious side-effects. Waisbren (1968) reported cardio-pulmonary arrest in four patients who received rapid intravenous injections of 4 g lincomycin. He recommended that if this drug is given intravenously in a dose of 4 g or more, it should be diluted in at least 500 ml of fluid, and the infusion rate should not exceed 100 ml per hour.

4. *Patients with renal failure.* The serum half-life of lincomycin in anuric patients is 10–13 h (normal 4–5 h) and dosage reduction is necessary for patients with severe renal failure (Kunin, 1967). Herrell (1969) recommends 25–30 per cent of the usual dose for these patients. Lincomycin is not removed from the body by either peritoneal or haemodialysis (Reinarz and McIntosh, 1966).

5. *Patients with liver disease.* In patients with a moderate degree of hepatic insufficiency the serum antibacterial activity of lincomycin is prolonged (Bellamy *et al.*, 1967). This drug is probably best avoided in these patients, but if it is used, appropriate dose reduction and serum level monitoring is indicated. Severe liver disease may be complicated by renal impairment ('hepato-renal syndrome') and the lincomycin half-life can be considerably prolonged in such patients.

B. *Clindamycin*

1. *Oral administration.* The hydrochloride salt of this drug is used for administration by the oral route. A dose of 150 mg every six hours is recommended for adults, but this may be increased to 300 or 450 mg six-hourly for the treatment of serious infections. Two dosage ranges are recommended for children depending on the severity of the infection, 8–16 mg or 16–20 mg per kg body weight per day, each given in three or four divided doses. Clindamycin is not recommended for infants aged less than one month. The ester clindamycin palmitate hydrochloride is available as a suspension for administration to children and elderly patients, who are unable to swallow capsules. This is a water soluble compound which is hydrolysed *in vivo* to the active base. The dosage of this preparation is similar to that of clindamycin hydrochloride.

2. *Parenteral administration.* Clindamycin is poorly soluble in solutions of neutral pH and it is too irritating for parenteral use, so that an ester, clindamycin-2-phosphate, is used for intramuscular and intravenous administration. The intramuscular dose for adults is 0·6–2·4 g per day, depending on the severity of the infection, given in two to four divided doses. The equivalent dose for children is 10–30 mg per kg body weight per day, given in two to four divided doses.

For intravenous infusion clindamycin phosphate must be diluted at least one part to 25 parts of infusion solution, and depending on the volume, this is infused over a period of 20–45 min. For example a 600 mg dose (available in 4 ml) should be diluted to 100 ml and infused over a minimum period of 20 min. The administration of more than 1·2 g intravenously in a single hour infusion is not recommended. The adult intravenous dose is 0·9–2·7 g per day, depending on the severity of the infection, given in two to four divided doses. For children a dose of 10–30 mg per kg body weight per day, depending on the severity of the infection, is given in two to four divided doses. An intravenous dose of 10 mg infused over two hours, two or three times a day produced high serum levels in newborn infants (Harrod and Stevens, 1974).

Clindamycin phosphate can also be administered to adults by constant intravenous infusion aiming to maintain constant serum levels. An initial rapid infusion is given and this is followed by a continuous infusion. The initial infusion should be given over 30 min and the dose for this purpose is 10–20 mg per min. The equivalent maintenance dose range is 0·75–1·25 mg per min. Depending on the dosage schedule selected, the resultant clindamycin serum levels in adults are maintained in a range of 4–6 μg per ml. Clindamycin phosphate can be diluted with most commonly used infusion solutions, but it is physically incompatible with a number of drugs including ampicillin.

3. *Patients with renal failure.* Although some clindamycin is excreted in urine, its main excretion pathway is probably by the liver (page 479). The clindamycin half-life (normally about 3 h) is not appreciably altered in patients with renal functional impairment (Eastwood and Gower, 1974; Malacoff *et al.*, 1975; Peddie *et al.*, 1975; Keusch and Present, 1976). For patients with mild to moderate renal failure, no dosage adjustments for clindamycin are necessary (Eastwood and Gower, 1974; Peddie *et al.*, 1975). In functionally anephric patients, Malacoff *et al.* (1975) found that peak serum levels were about two-

fold greater than those expected in normal patients after the same parenteral dosage. They therefore recommended that half the normal dose should be used in such patients. Clindamycin is not significantly removed by haemodialysis (Eastwood and Gower, 1974; Peddie *et al.*, 1975) or by peritoneal dialysis (Malacoff *et al.*, 1975).

4. *Patients with liver disease.* Some studies indicate that the clindamycin half-life may be prolonged up to five-fold in patients with severe liver disease (Brandl *et al.*, 1972; Keusch and Present, 1976), but Hinthorn *et al.* (1976) only found a 39 per cent increase in patients with cirrhosis. Williams *et al.* (1975) studying patients with moderate to severe hepatic dysfunction detected serum levels which were nearly three-fold higher than those found in patients with normal liver function. There was also an association between the serum levels after five hours and the degree of elevation of the serum aspartate aminotransferase (SGOT). These results indicate that clindamycin serum levels should be monitored in patients with liver disease, because sometimes appropriate dose reduction may be necessary.

Availability

Lincomycin hydrochloride is available as:

(a) Capsules: 250 and 500 mg.
(b) Paediatric syrup: 250 mg in 5 ml.
(c) Solution for intramuscular or intravenous use: 1 ml vials containing 300 mg, 2 ml vials or disposable syringes containing 600 mg.

Clindamycin is available as:

(a) Capsules: 75 and 150 mg clindamycin hydrochloride.
(b) Clindamycin palmitate hydrochloride granules for preparation of a suspension: 75 mg clindamycin base in 5 ml.
(c) Clindamycin-2-phosphate solution, suitable for intramuscular and intravenous administration: 150 mg per ml.

Serum Levels in Relation to Dosage

A. *Lincomycin*

1. *Oral administration.* After an oral dose of 0·5 g of lincomycin a peak serum level is reached in 2–4 h. Thereafter the level falls, and at 12 h very little lincomycin is present in the serum (Medina *et al.*, 1964). If the oral dose is increased to 1 g the peak level is higher, but not doubled. The presence of food in the stomach markedly impairs lincomycin absorption (Fig. 24).

2. *Parenteral administration.* If lincomycin is administered intramuscularly (Fig. 25), the peak serum level is achieved in 30 min, and serum levels are higher than those obtained after oral medication (Kaplan *et al.*, 1965; McCall *et al.*, 1967). With an intramuscular dosage of 600 mg every 8 h, lincomycin serum levels are maintained between 5·8 and 13·2 μg per ml.

After rapid intravenous administration of lincomycin, the peak serum level is achieved within minutes, and it is about double that attained after an identical intramuscular dose. This level falls rapidly during the first 2 h, declines slowly over the next 6 h, and usually there is no demonstrable lincomycin in the serum after 24 h (McCall *et al.*, 1967). If lincomycin is used intravenously, rapid in-

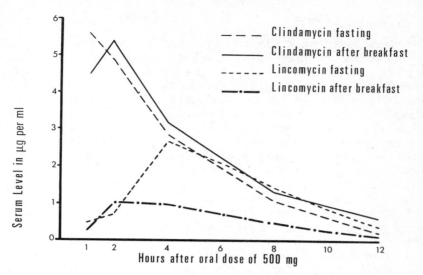

FIG. 24. Effect of food on serum concentrations of lincomycin and clindamycin after oral administration. (Redrawn after McGehee *et al.*, 1968.)

jections of large doses may be dangerous (*see* page 483). After an intravenous infusion of 2·1 g of lincomycin over 2 h, a peak serum level of about 37 μg per ml is attained after the infusion, which falls to about 12 μg per ml 4 h later (Novak *et al.*, 1971).

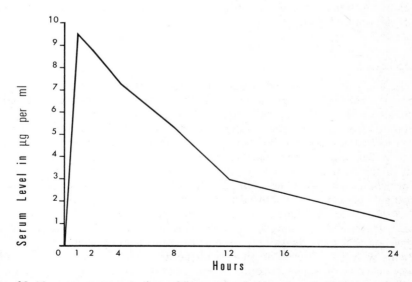

FIG. 25. Mean serum concentrations of lincomycin after intramuscular injection of 600 mg. (Redrawn after Kaplan *et al.*, 1965.)

B. *Clindamycin*

1. *Oral administration.* Clindamycin is more completely absorbed from the gastro-intestinal tract than lincomycin, and peak serum levels occur 1–2 h after administration. Following a single 150 mg oral dose to adults, peak serum levels are in the range 2·5–3·0 μg per ml (Peddie *et al.*, 1975). Peak levels after oral doses of 300 and 600 mg are about 4 and 8 μg per ml respectively (Keusch and Present, 1976). Serum levels achieved after an identical dose of clindamycin are approximately double those obtained with lincomycin (Fig. 24). Furthermore, the presence of food in the stomach does not significantly impair the absorption of clindamycin (McGehee *et al.*, 1968; Wagner *et al.*, 1968). Higher serum levels occur when clindamycin is given orally to patients with coeliac disease, jejunal diverticulosis and Crohn's disease (Keusch and Present, 1976). The ester, clindamycin palmitate hydrochloride, is also well absorbed from the gastro-intestinal tract, and serum levels attained with this compound are nearly the same as those with clindamycin capsules (Campbell *et al.*, 1973).

2. *Parenteral administration.* Satisfactory serum levels are attained with intramuscular or intravenous administration of clindamycin-2-phosphate. Following a 300 mg intramuscular dose a mean peak level of 4·9 μg per ml is attained at 2·5 h, and this falls to 2·8 μg per ml 8 h after administration. Diabetic patients tend to have lower serum clindamycin levels after intramuscular administration (Fass and Saslaw, 1972); a similar phenomenon occurs with penicillin G (page 16). The intravenous infusion of 300 mg over a 30 min period results in a mean peak serum level of 14·7 μg per ml, which falls to 4·9 μg per ml at 2–4 h, and to 3·9 μg per ml 8 h after the infusion (Fass and Saslaw, 1972). Maximum serum levels varying from 2·6 to 26·0 μg per ml after a 300 mg dose, and from 6·0 to 29·0 μg per ml after a 600 mg dose, both given by infusions over a period of 30–40 min, were detected in patients treated by Hugo *et al.* (1977).

Excretion

URINE: Both lincomycin and clindamycin are excreted in urine. In the canine model the kidneys are more important in this respect for lincomycin than clindamycin (Brown *et al.*, 1975). After a single oral dose of lincomycin, the amounts recovered from the urine in the first 24 h are 9·3 per cent of a dose given when fasting, but only 2·6 per cent of the dose given after food. After a single oral dose of clindamycin, administered either fasting or after food, 13 per cent of the administered dose can be recovered from the urine in the active form within 24 h (McGehee *et al.*, 1968). By contrast, in severe renal disease less than 1 per cent of the active drug may be detected in the urine in 24 h (Peddie *et al.*, 1975). Williams *et al.* (1975) found an increased urinary excretion after intravenous clindamycin in patients with severe hepatic dysfunction, suggesting that the kidneys may have some compensatory excretory ability in patients with liver disease. In those with normal renal function, high urinary concentrations of active lincomycin and clindamycin are obtained with the usual doses. The urinary activity is due to a mixture of the unchanged drug and the presence of active metabolites (*vide infra*).

After parenteral administration of lincomycin, approximately 30 per cent of the administered dose can be recovered from the urine in the first 24 h (McCall *et al.*, 1967); a large proportion of this is excreted in the first 4 h (75 per cent after intravenous injection and 45 per cent after intramuscular administration). With parenteral clindamycin administered every 8 h, eight per cent of an intramuscular dose and 28 per cent of an intravenous dose are recovered from the urine during the 8 h after each injection (Fass and Saslaw, 1972). The renal excretion of lincomycin and clindamycin are important clinically, because in the presence of severe renal impairment dosage reduction of these drugs is necessary (pages 474, 475).

BILE: Both lincomycin and clindamycin appear to be extensively eliminated by hepatic mechanisms. A bile level of 42 μg per ml was demonstrated 14 h after a single oral dose of 1·0 g lincomycin (Medina *et al.*, 1964). Biliary levels of 48 and 55 μg per ml of clindamycin have been detected in two patients receiving an intravenous dose of 600 mg every 6 h (Williams *et al.*, 1975).

INACTIVATION IN BODY: The excretion of lincomycin in urine and bile does not account for all of the administered dose, and a substantial proportion of the drug appears to be inactivated in the body, presumably mainly in the liver (Ma *et al.*, 1964). Studies by Bellamy *et al.* (1967) have shown that lincomycin metabolism is deranged in patients with liver disease (*see* page 474). Clindamycin is also metabolized in the body, presumably in the liver, and active metabolites (N-demethyl clindamycin and clindamycin sulphoxide) and inactive metabolites are excreted in urine. Clindamycin is metabolized at an increased rate in children (Leading article, 1975).

FAECES: After oral administration about 40 per cent of the dose of lincomycin can be recovered in its active form from the faeces, most probably being non-absorbed. Between 4 to 14 per cent of parenterally administered lincomycin can be recovered from faeces, and most of this probably results from biliary or intestinal excretion (McCall *et al.*, 1967). After a single oral dose of clindamycin, less than 5 per cent of the active drug is excreted in the faeces (Keusch and Present, 1976).

Distribution of the Drugs in Body

1. When lincomycin is administered in the recommended dosage, significant concentrations of the drug may be detected in most body tissues, pleural and peritoneal fluids, but not in the normal cerebrospinal fluid. In the presence of meningeal infection, the lincomycin concentration in CSF may reach 40 per cent of the simultaneous serum level (Kaplan *et al.*, 1965). Lincomycin appears to penetrate well into the pus of a cerebral abscess (De Louvois *et al.*, 1977). Clindamycin is probably distributed in the body in a similar manner to lincomycin. Concentrations in saliva are similar to those in serum (Keusch and Present, 1976) and satisfactory levels are reached in the sputum of patients with purulent chest infections (Raeburn and Devine, 1971). The penetration of clindamycin into the central nervous system and eye is poor (Keusch and Present, 1976). High biliary concentrations of clindamycin occur (*vide supra*) after intravenous clindamycin phosphate, and these may be two to three times higher than in the serum (Brown *et al.*, 1976). However, in the presence of obstruction of the common bile duct, no drug can be detected in bile, and there

is reduced clindamycin in the gall-bladder wall, but concentrations are a little higher in the liver than those detected in patients with no obstruction. Clindamycin penetrates well into ascitic fluid of patients with bacterial peritonitis (Gerding *et al.*, 1977).

2. Lincomycin crosses the placenta, and about one hour after intramuscular administration to the mother, the peak cord blood level is usually about a quarter of the maternal serum concentration (Duignan *et al.*, 1973). Lincomycin passage into the liquor is slower and more variable. Clindamycin also crosses the placenta (Philipson *et al.*, 1973). Lincomycin levels in human milk are about the same as those in maternal blood (Medina *et al.*, 1964).

3. High concentrations of lincomycin are found in specimens of bone (1·1–16·6 μg per g), suggesting that lincomycin may be valuable in the treatment of staphylococcal osteomyelitis (Holloway *et al.*, 1964; Norden and Kennedy, 1971; Parsons, 1976; Dornbusch *et al.*, 1977). Clindamycin also penetrates well into bone (Nicholas *et al.*, 1975; Smilack *et al.*, 1976; Dornbusch *et al.*, 1977).

4. Lincomycin, like many other antibiotics, is partly bound to serum proteins. Barber and Waterworth (1964) found that when Staph. pyogenes was tested in 90 per cent human serum instead of broth, the MIC's were doubled with a small inoculum and increased four-fold when a large inoculum was used. The percentage of lincomycin which is protein bound is not exactly known, and figures varying from 5–20 per cent (Kato *et al.*, 1966) to 80–90 per cent (Kunin, 1967) have been quoted. Clindamycin is about 60 per cent bound to proteins (Eastwood and Gower, 1974).

Mode of Action

Lincomycin and clindamycin inhibit bacterial protein synthesis and act specifically on the 50S subunit (page 434) of the bacterial ribosome, most likely by affecting the process of peptide chain initiation (page 434) (Cundliffe, 1969; Reusser, 1975).

The macrolide antibiotics (page 504) also bind to the 50S subunit of the ribosome to achieve their effect. Only one molecule either of erythromycin or lincomycin can be bound to a single ribosome (Weisblum, 1967), and it is therefore unwise to use these two drugs in combination. If the microorganism is resistant to erythromycin, and this drug becomes bound to the ribosomes, lincomycin may not gain attachment and be ineffective, even though the organism is susceptible to lincomycin in the absence of erythromycin (Anderson *et al.*, 1968). These observations may explain the 'dissociated type of resistance' (page 471) characteristic of these antibiotics.

Toxicity

1. *Gastro-intestinal side-effects*. Oral or parenteral administration of lincomycin or clindamycin may cause nausea, vomiting, abdominal cramps and diarrhoea (*vide infra*). A metallic taste in the mouth may follow intravenous administration of clindamycin.

Oesophageal ulceration due to temporary lodgement of a clindamycin capsule in the lower oesophagus has been reported (Sutton and Gosnold, 1977).

The mechanism of mucosal damage in this case was presumably similar to that which occurs with the tetracyclines (page 613).

2. *Pseudomembranous colitis.* Diarrhoea is a well recognized side-effect of lincomycin (Price *et al.*, 1968). Kaplan and Weinstein (1968) observed that lincomycin induced diarrhoea may occasionally be severe, simulate acute ulcerative colitis, and persist for one or two weeks after the drug is stopped. Subsequently there were numerous reports on the occurrence of pseudomembranous colitis following oral or parenteral lincomycin administration (Benner and Tellman, 1970; Scott *et al.*, 1973; Scott and Nicholson, 1974; Leading article, 1974; Le Frock *et al.*, 1975; Gibson *et al.*, 1975; Clark *et al.*, 1976; Munk *et al.*, 1976). Severe diarrhoea and pseudomembranous colitis have also occurred in association with either oral or parenteral clindamycin therapy (Cohen *et al.*, 1973; Wells *et al.*, 1974; Leading article, 1974; Tedesco *et al.*, 1974; Le Frock *et al.*, 1975; Dallos, 1975; Gibson *et al.*, 1975; Keusch and Present, 1976; Lemos *et al.*, 1976; Friedman *et al.*, 1976; Robertson *et al.*, 1977; Swartzberg *et al.*, 1977; Gurwith *et al.*, 1977; Lusk *et al.*, 1977; Neu *et al.*, 1977). In retrospective and prospective studies the frequency of clindamycin-associated diarrhoea has varied from 0·3 to 21 per cent and for pseudomembranous colitis from 1·9 to 10 per cent. In many reports there appeared to be geographical clustering of cases (Kabins and Spira, 1975), a greater frequency in older age groups and in patients who had undergone abdominal surgery (Clark *et al.*, 1976; Kappas *et al.*, 1978; Leading article, 1978). In most instances clindamycin diarrhoea and colitis were more common after oral than parenteral therapy but were not related to the duration of therapy. There was some evidence that atropine-diphenoxylate ('Lomotil') may increase the frequency of lincomycin-induced diarrhoea (Novak *et al.*, 1976).

Symptoms of colitis or pseudomembranous colitis associated with lincomycin or clindamycin usually appear 2–25 days after commencing treatment (Leading article, 1974). Diarrhoea may be mild, but is frequently profuse and watery but rectal bleeding is uncommon. It may be associated with cramp-like abdominal pain. A neutrophil leucocytosis is common. The disease may be complicated by dehydration, hypotension and hypoalbuminaemia; toxic megacolon, colonic perforation and fatalities have occurred. In patients who have undergone a laparotomy, a boggy, dilated colon associated with ascites has been found (Wells, 1974). Sigmoidoscopy, proctoscopy, or colonoscopy may only reveal a non-specific colitis with a red oedematous and friable mucosa (Gibson *et al.*, 1975), but the diagnostic feature of pseudomembranous colitis, white-yellow raised plaques of variable size, are usually visible. These plaques can sometimes be felt on digital examination. They consist of fibrin, mucus, epithelial debris and polymorphs. Underlying dilated mucous glands are often present in the mucosa. The plaques may slough and ulcerate into the muscle coat. Price and Davies (1977) consider that the earliest pathological lesion is focal epithelial necrosis or irregularity with polymorphs, and an eosinophilic exudate in the lamina propria. Barium studies may show widening and distortion of haustral folds, irregularities, ulceration, thumb-printing and a cobble-stone appearance (Scott and Nicholson, 1974; Le Frock *et al.*, 1975). Recovery usually occurs within three weeks of stopping the drug but prolonged diarrhoea and relapses have been reported (Lambert, 1975; Swartzberg *et al.*, 1977). In the past treatment was generally symptomatic; in severe cases resuscitation is necessary and at least two patients have had a subtotal colectomy (Boyd and Denbesten, 1976). There was no proof that corticosteroids were of value but the avoidance of lomotil (page 481) seemed prudent.

Pseudomembranous colitis is not a new disease and it had been described in the pre-antibiotic era (Keusch and Present, 1976; Gorbach and Bartlett, 1977). It was often associated with colonic obstruction (especially due to carcinoma) or as a sequel to abdominal surgery. It has long been recognized that antibiotics may be associated with the development of pseudomembranous colitis (Reiner et al., 1952; Goulston and McGovern, 1965). Pseudomembranous colitis has been described after the use of chloramphenicol (page 440), and the tetracyclines (page 612) (Reiner et al., 1952) and after ampicillin (page 112). The colitis associated with these antibiotics is indistinguishable from that caused by lincomycin and clindamycin. Pseudomembranous colitis should be distinguished from the now rare severe form of enterocolitis which is due to an overgrowth of staphylococci in the gut, and is also associated with antibiotic administration (pages 411, 614). That an identical clinical picture of pseudomembranous colitis could be caused by a variety of antibiotics and perhaps by physiological alterations in the bowel, indicated a common aetiological factor in this disease. Clustering of cases had suggested the possibility of an infective agent.

A variety of possibilities was considered for the aetiology of pseudomembranous colitis until Larson et al. (1977) detected a cytopathogenic toxin in the faeces of patients with the disease. At first this heat-labile toxin was thought to be elaborated from Clostridium sordellii (Rifkin et al., 1977; Larson and Price, 1977) but it was later shown to be produced by Clostridium difficile (Bartlett et al., 1978; Burdon and George, 1978; George et al., 1978a and b). A hypothesis has now evolved for the aetiology of antibiotic-induced pseudomembranous colitis in which the toxin of Cl. difficile plays an important role. This toxin may also be involved in the aetiology of non-antibiotic pseudomembranous colitis (Leading article, 1978; Annotation, 1978). Cl. difficile appears to be commonly present as a normal inhabitant of the gut but this may vary geographically, accounting for differences in reported incidence of pseudomembranous colitis. It is also possible that this organism may rapidly colonize the bowel of other patients in the ward environment, producing clustering of cases. There are several biotypes of Cl. difficile some of which are non-toxigenic. Normally the growth of Cl. difficile is limited by other intestinal bacteria and an insignificant amount of toxin is produced. Following the administration of certain antibiotics (or possibly after altered bowel physiology), the organism multiplies and produces larger amounts of toxin. The presence of Cl. difficile and its toxin is essential for the production of antibiotic-induced pseudomembranous colitis in hamsters. The exact mechanism of action of the toxin on the bowel wall is unknown, but human isolates of Cl. difficile can produce a powerful inflammatory agent, p-cresol, from tyrosine (Larson et al., 1978). Cl. difficile is often resistant to penicillins, cephalosporins, aminoglycosides, lincomycin, tetracycline and erythromycin (George et al., 1978a), although only a percentage of strains may be resistant to clindamycin (Larson et al., 1978). The survival of this organism in the gut at the expense of other intestinal organisms explains the occurrence of pseudomembranous colitis after the use of some antibiotics. Cl. difficile may be sensitive to metronidazole, sulphonamides and vancomycin (George *et al.*, 1978a). Vancomycin has been used with effect to treat patients with pseudomembranous colitis (Rifkin *et al.*, 1977) (*see also* page 651). This antibiotic also completely protects animals against colitis (Leading article, 1978). Metronidazole has also been used to treat pseudomembranous colitis (page 774). The final role of vancomycin and other chemotherapeutic agents to which Cl. difficile is susceptible, in the treatment or perhaps even for the prevention of pseudomembranous colitis, has yet to be established. Previous evidence suggesting that the anionic-exchange resin cholestyramine may be effective in this disease (Keusch and Present, 1976) may be related to the ability of this resin to bind the toxin of Cl. difficile (Chang *et al.*, 1978).

3. *Hypersensitivity reactions.* These are rare with lincomycin; some patients have developed a rash, and even anaphylaxis has been reported. Rashes may occur with clindamycin (Levison *et al.*, 1974) and in one study they occurred with a surprisingly high frequency of 10 per cent (Geddes *et al.*, 1970). Drug fever and eosinophilia may occur with clindamycin and one case of Stevens-Johnson syndrome has been attributed to it (Fulghum and Catalano, 1973). Lincomycin and clindamycin are not cross-allergenic with the penicillins, and may be safely used in penicillin-allergic patients.

4. *Hepatotoxicity.* Minor abnormalities of liver function tests, such as an elevated serum aspartate aminotransferase (SGOT) level, have been observed in patients receiving lincomycin (Bentley and Pollock, 1968) or clindamycin (Fass and Saslaw, 1972; Levison *et al.*, 1974; Williams *et al.*, 1975). Rarely jaundice has been associated with lincomycin or clindamycin therapy (Levison *et al.*, 1974; Elmore *et al.*, 1974). Clindamycin has been given parenterally to patients with liver disease without aggravation of their disease (Williams *et al.*, 1975; Hinthorn *et al.*, 1976). Elevations of aspartate aminotransferase (SGOT) occurring with intramuscular lincomycin or clindamycin may not be due to hepatotoxicity but to injection-produced muscle damage (Fass and Saslaw, 1972). In addition McGehee *et al.* (1968) showed that some of the apparently elevated SGOT levels observed in patients receiving either lincomycin or clindamycin were due to interference with the colorimetric method of estimating SGOT, by the drugs or their metabolites. If the SGOT was measured by a specific enzymatic method, no elevations could be detected. Similar observations have also been made in patients receiving erythromycin estolate (page 505).

5. *Side-effects from parenteral lincomycin and clindamycin.* Lincomycin may cause syncope or even cardio-pulmonary arrest if a large dose is injected rapidly by the intravenous route (Waisbren, 1968; O'Connell and Plaut, 1969). Intravenous lincomycin and clindamycin administration by the recommended method (page 474) is quite safe, but with high doses phlebitis can be a problem. Reversible glucose intolerance and hyperlipidaemia were noted in one patient receiving high doses of intravenous lincomycin (O'Connell and Plaut, 1969). Intramuscular lincomycin and clindamycin are usually well tolerated and injections are relatively painless.

6. *Miscellaneous side-effects.* Neutropenia has been occasionally noted in patients receiving lincomycin or clindamycin. The safety of these drugs in pregnancy has not been established but to date there is no evidence that they are harmful.

Clinical Uses of the Drugs

In view of their side-effects, particularly pseudomembranous colitis (page 481), the absolute indications for treatment with lincomycin or clindamycin are very few. For most diseases there are equal, if not more effective, drugs available which are safer than lincomycin and clindamycin.

Because it has a higher antibacterial activity, is better absorbed after oral administration and can also be given parenterally, clindamycin is now used in preference to lincomycin.

1. *Staphylococcal infections*. Both lincomycin (Geddes *et al.*, 1964; Kaplan *et al.*, 1965; Bentley and Pollock, 1968) and clindamycin (Geddes *et al.*, 1970; Fass and Saslaw, 1972) are effective even in severe staphylococcal infections, but they are not regarded as the drugs of first choice. Lincomycin (Geddes *et al.*, 1964; 1967; Holloway and Scott, 1965) and clindamycin (Kosmidis *et al.*, 1973; Feigin *et al.*, 1975; Wharton and Beddow, 1975; Finch *et al.*, 1975; Rodriguez *et al.*, 1977; Geddes *et al.*, 1977) are particularly effective for staphylococcal osteomyelitis and septic arthritis. Clindamycin has been used to treat staphylococcal endocarditis with some success but several failures have been described due to the development of *in vivo* resistance (Watanakunakorn, 1976; Cherubin and Nair, 1978). Methicillin-resistant staphylococci are usually lincomycin-sensitive, and therefore lincomycin or clindamycin may be useful for the treatment of infections due to these strains (Rountree and Beard, 1968).

2. *Streptococcal and pneumococcal infections*. Lincomycin or clindamycin may be occasionally indicated in these infections for patients allergic to penicillin G and the cephalosporins. They have been used successfully for the treatment of Strep. pyogenes throat and skin infections and pneumococcal pneumonia (Geddes *et al.*, 1970; Newell, 1970; Lines *et al.*, 1973; Breese *et al.*, 1974; Dillon and Derrick, 1975). Anderson *et al.* (1968) showed that intramuscular lincomycin was as effective as penicillin G in cases of mild and moderately severe pneumococcal pneumonia. Clindamycin also appears useful for the treatment of chronic suppurative ear infections (Cooke and Raghuvaran, 1974). A few cases of pneumococcal meningitis have also been treated by large doses of parenteral lincomycin with satisfactory results (Geddes *et al.*, 1967), and pneumococcal endocarditis has been successfully treated with intravenous clindamycin (Keane and Rose, 1973). Strep. viridans endocarditis also responds to parenteral lincomycin (de Yeaza *et al.*, 1967) and clindamycin (Freeman and Roberts, 1976).

3. *Gram-negative anaerobic bacterial infections*. Infections due to these bacteria occur in many parts of the body and Bacteroides fragilis is the most commonly encountered anaerobe (*see* page 442). The three drugs with the most consistent activity against anaerobes including B. fragilis are chloramphenicol (page 442), metronidazole (page 761) and clindamycin. Lincomycin and in particular clindamycin are effective for the treatment of severe Bacteroides infections including B. fragilis septicaemia (Tracy *et al.*, 1972; Bartlett *et al.*, 1972; Douglas and Kislak, 1973; Mitchell and Simpson, 1973). Many studies have shown that clindamycin is a very effective drug for the treatment of anaerobic infections of various types. Many of these infections also require appropriate surgical intervention. If a dual infection with added aerobic Gram-negative bacteria is suspected or confirmed, then another an-

tibiotic, usually an aminoglycoside, should be added to clindamycin therapy. A combination of clindamycin and gentamicin (page 342) is very effective for infections caused by a mixture of anaerobic and aerobic bacteria (Fass, 1977; Bartlett et al., 1977). Clindamycin is effective for pulmonary, intra-abdominal and pelvic anaerobic infections (Kapila et al., 1977; Levison et al., 1977; Leigh et al., 1977) and septicaemia and sepsis associated with decubitus ulcers (Chow et al., 1977b). Clindamycin has been found to be as effective as carbenicillin for the treatment of genital and intra-abdominal infections (Swenson and Lorber, 1977); it is equally effective to chloramphenicol for the treatment of pelvic infections (Ledger et al., 1977) and septicaemia due to Bacteroidaceae (Mathias et al., 1977). However a combination of penicillin G and chloramphenicol produced better results than clindamycin alone in the treatment of septic abortion, because the former drugs were active against aerobic Gram-negative bacteria (Chow et al., 1977a). A combination of clindamycin and tobramycin (page 368) produced good results in the treatment of leukaemic patients with bacterial infections (Falk et al., 1977). Clindamycin is as effective as tinidazole (page 786) for the treatment of anaerobic wound infections in patients with cancer (Klastersky et al., 1977). The choice between the use of chloramphenicol or clindamycin for severe anaerobic infections is one of individual preference, and depends on an assessment of the relative toxicity of these two antibiotics. Metronidazole (page 771) may prove to be an effective alternative to these drugs.

Lincomycin has been used alone to effectively reduce anaerobic infection after bowel surgery (Keighley et al., 1976; Leigh et al., 1976). It has also been combined with gentamicin for this purpose and was equally effective to a gentamicin/metronidazole combination (see also pages 345, 775). However a few patients receiving lincomycin/gentamicin developed pseudomembranous colitis (Feathers et al., 1977). The frequency of wound infections after gastrointestinal operations has also been reduced by the use of a combination of lincomycin and tobramycin (Griffiths et al., 1976; Galland et al., 1977). Nevertheless in view of the potential of lincomycin and clindamycin to produce pseudomembranous colitis (page 481), they should not be used prophylactically to prevent post-operative infection, particularly as abdominal surgery may predispose to this complication.

4. *Diphtheria*. A seven-day course of oral treatment with clindamycin (or erythromycin) was just as effective as a single injection of benzathine penicillin in eradicating C. diphtheriae from the nasopharynx of asymptomatic carriers (McCloskey et al., 1974).

5. *Actinomycosis*. This disease has been succesfully treated by prolonged (6–12 months) courses of lincomycin, and it has been suggested that this drug may be the most satisfactory alternative to penicillin G in penicillin-allergic patients (Mohr et al., 1970). Clindamycin is also effective in actinomycosis (Rose and Rytel, 1972; Fass and Saslaw, 1972).

6. *Chronic bronchitis due to H. influenzae*. Lincomycin has never been used for the treatment of this disease. Because clindamycin has a higher degree of *in vitro* activity against this pathogen (page 472), it was suggested that this drug may have a clinical use in chronic bronchitis (Geddes et al., 1970; Phillips et al., 1970). However in one study clindamycin usually failed to eradicate H. influenzae from the sputum of such patients (Ormonde et al., 1973).

7. *Mycoplasma pneumonia*. Lincomycin has not been used for the treatment of this disease, and variable results have been reported with clindamycin. Axelrod *et al.* (1972) observed good clinical response in nine patients, but three patients treated by Fass and Saslaw (1972) appeared to respond slowly if at all to clindamycin therapy. In a double blind study, clindamycin was compared with tetracycline and a placebo in 32 young men with mycoplasma pneumonia (Smilack *et al.*, 1974). Tetracycline was beneficial, but clindamycin was no more effective than the placebo. It appears that clindamycin should not be used for the treatment of this disease.

8. *Acne*. Some authors have found clindamycin, in a small dose of 150 mg daily, beneficial for this condition (Leading Article, 1973).

9. *Q fever endocarditis*. This infection has been treated by a combination of tetracycline (page 625) and lincomycin (Annotation, 1976; Turck, 1978).

10. *Malaria*. A three-day course of clindamycin given orally together with quinine sulphate in full dosage is very effective for chloroquine-resistant falciparum malaria (Hall *et al.*, 1975). However this regimen was associated with gastro-intestinal side-effects and a combination of quinine sulphate with sulfadoxine and pyrimethamine is the preferred treatment for this infection (page 676).

REFERENCES

Anderson, R., Bauman, M. and Austrian, R. (1968), 'Lincomycin and penicillin G in the treatment of mild and moderately severe pneumococcal pneumonia', *Amer. Rev. Resp. Dis.*, **97**, 914.

Annotation (1976), 'Chronic Q fever or Q fever endocarditis', *Lancet*, **1**, 1171.

Annotation (1977), 'Pseudomembranous enterocolitis', *Lancet*, **1**, 839.

Annotation (1978), 'Pseudomembranous colitis', *Lancet*, **1**, 1080.

Araujo, F. G. and Remington, J. S. (1974), 'Effect of clindamycin on acute and chronic toxoplasmosis in mice', *Antimicrob. Ag. Chemother.*, **5**, 647.

Axelrod, J., Meyers, B. R. and Hirschman, S. Z. (1972), '7-Chlorolincomycin therapy of pulmonary infections due to Mycoplasma pneumoniae', *Antimicrob. Ag. Chemother.*, **2**, 499.

Barber, M. and Waterworth, P. M. (1964), 'Antibacterial activity of lincomycin and pristinamycin: A comparison with erythromycin', *Brit. med. J.*, **2**, 603.

Bartlett, J. G., Sutter, V. L. and Finegold, S. M. (1972), 'Treatment of anaerobic infections with lincomycin and clindamycin', *New Engl. J. Med.*, **287**, 1006.

Bartlett, J. G., Miao, P. V. W. and Gorbach, S. L. (1977), 'Empiric treatment with clindamycin and gentamicin of suspected sepsis due to anaerobic and aerobic bacteria', *J. Infect. Dis.* (Suppl.), **135**, 80.

Bartlett, J. G., Chang, T. W. and Onderdonk, A. B. (1978), 'Will the real Clostridium species responsible for antibiotic-associated colitis please step forward', *Lancet*, **1**, 338.

Bellamy, H. M., Jr., Bates, B. B. and Reinarz, J. A. (1967), 'Lincomycin metabolism in patients with hepatic insufficiency: Effect of liver disease on lincomycin serum concentrations', *Antimicrob. Ag. Chemother.*—1966, p. 36.

Benner, E. J. and Tellman, W. H. (1970), 'Pseudomembranous colitis as a sequel to oral lincomycin therapy', *Amer. J. Gastroent.*, **54**, 55.

Bentley, J. F. R. and Pollock, D. (1968), 'Lincomycin in the treatment of penicillin-resistant staphylococcal infections in children', *Arch. Dis. Childh.*, **43**, 58.

Blazevic, D. J. (1976), 'Antibiotic susceptibility of the subspecies of Bacteroides fragilis', *Antimicrob. Ag. Chemother.*, **9**, 481.

Bodner, S. J., Koenig, M. G., Treanor, L. L. and Goodman, J. S. (1972), 'Antibiotic susceptibility testing of Bacteroides', *Antimicrob. Ag. Chemother.*, **2**, 57.

Boyd, W. C. and Denbesten, L. (1976), 'Subtotal colectomy for refractory Pseudomembranous enterocolitis', *JAMA*, **235**, 181.

Brandl, R. C., Arkenau, C., Simon, C., Malerczyk, V. and Eidelloth, G. (1972), 'Zur Pharmakokinetik von Clindamycin bei gestörter Leber-und Nierenfunktion', *Dtsch. Med. Wöckenschr.*, **97**, 1057.

Brause, B. D., Borges, J. S. and Roberts, R. B. (1976), 'Relative efficacy of clindamycin, erythromycin and penicillin in treatment of Treponema pallidum in skin syphilomas of rabbits', *J. Infect. Dis.*, **134**, 93.

Breese, B. B., Disney, F. A., Talpey, W., Green, J. L. and Tobin, J. (1974), 'Streptococcal infections in children. Comparison of the therapeutic effectiveness of erythromycin administered twice daily with erythromycin, penicillin phenoxymethyl, and clindamycin administered three times daily', *Am. J. Dis. Child.*, **128**, 457.

Brown, R. B., Barza, M., Brusch, J. L., Hashimoto, Y. and Weinstein, L. (1975), 'Pharmacokinetics of lincomycin and clindamycin phosphate in a canine model', *J. Infect. Dis.*, **131**, 252.

Brown, R. B., Martyak, S. N., Barza, M., Curtis, L. and Weinstein, L. (1976), 'Penetration of clindamycin phosphate into the abnormal human biliary tract', *Ann. Intern. Med.*, **84**, 168.

Burdon, D. W. and George, R. H. (1978), 'Pseudomembranous colitis', *Lancet*, **1**, 444.

Campbell, I. W., Hossack, D. J. N. and Munro, J. F. (1973), 'Absorption and urinary excretion of clindamycin palmitate in the elderly', *Curr. med. Res. Opin.*, **1**, 369.

Center for Disease Control (1977), 'Multiple-antibiotic resistance of pneumococci—South Africa', *Morbidity and Mortality Weekly Report*, **26**, 285.

Champion, L. A. A., Wald, E. R., Luddy, R. E. and Schwartz, A. D. (1978), 'Streptococcus pneumoniae resistant to erythromycin and clindamycin', *J. Pediatr.*, **92**, 505.

Chang, T. W., Onderdonk, A. B. and Bartlett, J. G. (1978), 'Anion-exchange resins in antibiotic-associated colitis', *Lancet*, **2**, 258.

Cherubin, C. E. and Nair, S. R. (1978), 'Clindamycin in infective endocarditis', *JAMA*, **239**, 626.

Chow, A. W., Marshall, J. R. and Guze, L. B. (1977a), 'A double-blind comparison of clindamycin with penicillin plus chloramphenicol in treatment of septic abortion', *J. Infect. Dis.* (Suppl.), **135**, 35.

Chow, A. W., Patten, V. and Bednorz, D. (1978), 'Susceptibility of Camiylobacter sepsis caused by decubitus ulcers', *J. Infect. Dis.* (Suppl.), **135**, 65.

Chow, A. W., Patten, V. and Bednorz, D. (1978), 'Susceptibility of campylobacter fetus to twenty-two antimicrobial agents', *Antimicrob. Ag. Chemother.*, **13**, 416.

Clark, C. E., Thompson, H., McLeisch, A. R., Powis, S. J. A., Dorricott, N. J. and Alexander-Williams, J. (1976), 'Pseudomembranous colitis following prophylactic antibiotics in bowel surgery', *J. Antimicrob. Chemother.*, **2**, 167.

Cohen, L. E., McNeill, C. J. and Wells, R. F. (1973), 'Clindamycin-associated colitis', *JAMA*, **223**, 1379.

Cooke, E. T. M. and Raghuvaran, G. (1974), 'Clindamycin in conjunction with surgery of the chronic suppurative ear', *Brit. J. Clin. Pract.*, **28**, 57.

Csonka, G. W. and Spitzer, R. J. (1969), 'Lincomycin, non-gonococcal urethritis and mycoplasmata', *Brit. J. vener. Dis.*, **45**, 52.

Cundliffe, E. (1969), 'Antibiotics and polyribosomes. II. Some effects of lincomycin, spiramycin, and streptogramin A *in vivo*', *Biochemistry*, **8**, 2063.

Dallos, V. (1975), 'Clindamycin—a retrospective study of its side-effects', *J. Antimicrob. Chemother.*, **1**, 411.

De Louvois, J., Gortvai, P. and Hurley, R. (1977), 'Antibiotic treatment of abscesses of central nervous system', *Brit. med. J.*, **2**, 985.

Desmyter, J. (1968), 'Lincomycin resistance of erythromycin-resistant cocci', *New Engl. J. Med.*, **278**, 967.

De Yeaza, J. J., Waisbren, B. A. and Goodman, J. S. (1967), 'Therapy of bacterial endocarditis in penicillin-hypersensitive patients', *Arch. Intern. Med.*, **120**, 361.

Dillon, H. C. and Derrick, C. W. (1975), 'Clinical experience with clindamycin hydrochloride 1. Treatment of streptococcal and mixed streptococcal-staphylococcal skin infections', *Pediatrics*, **55**, 205.

Dixon, J. M. S. (1967), 'Pneumococcus resistant to erythromycin and lincomycin', *Lancet*, **1**, 573.

Dixon, J. M. S. and Liponski, A. E. (1972), 'Resistance of Group A beta-hemolytic streptococci to lincomycin and erythromycin', *Antimicrob. Ag. Chemother.*, **1**, 333.

Dixon, J. M. S. and Lipinski, A. E. (1974), 'Infections with beta-hemolytic streptococcus resistant to lincomycin and erythromycin and observations on zonal-pattern resistance to lincomycin', *J. Infect. Dis.*, **130**, 351.

Dornbusch, K., Nord, C.-E. and Wadström, T. (1974), 'Biochemical characterization and *in vitro* determination of antibiotic susceptibility of clinical isolates of Bacteroides fragilis', *Scand. J. Infect. Dis.*, **6**, 253.

Dornbusch, K., Nord, C.-E. and Dahlbäck, A. (1975), 'Antibiotic susceptibility of Clostridium species isolated from human infections', *Scand. J. Infect. Dis.*, **7**, 127.

Dornbusch, K., Carlström, A., Hugo, H. and Lidström, A. (1977), 'Antibacterial activity of clindamycin and lincomycin in human bone', *J. Antimicrob. Chemother.*, **3**, 153.

Drapkin, M. S., Karchmer, A. W., Moellering, R. C., Jr. (1976), 'Bacteremic infections due to clindamycin-resistant streptococci', *JAMA*, **236**, 263.

Douglas, R. L. and Kislak, J. W. (1973), 'Treatment of Bacteroides fragilis bacteremia with clindamycin', *J. Infect. Dis.*, **128**, 569.

Duignan, N. M., Andrews, J. and Williams, J. D. (1973), 'Pharmacological studies with lincomycin in late pregnancy', *Brit. med. J.*, **3**, 75.

Duncan, I. B. R. (1968), 'Development of lincomycin resistance by staphylococci', *Antimicrob. Ag. Chemother.*—1967, p. 723.

Duperval, R., Bill, N. J., Geraci, J. E. and Washington, J. A. II (1975), 'Bactericidal activity of combinations of penicillin or clindamycin with gentamicin or streptomycin against species of viridans streptococci', *Antimicrob. Ag. Chemother.*, **8**, 673.

Eastwood, J. B. and Gower, P. E. (1974), 'A study of the pharmacokinetics of clindamycin in normal subjects and patients with chronic renal failure', *Postgrad. Med. J.*, **50**, 710.

Elmore, M., Rissing, J. P., Rink, L. and Brooks, G. F. (1974), 'Clindamycin-associated hepatotoxicity', *Amer. J. Med.*, **57**, 627.

Ekwo, E. and Peter, G. (1976), 'Effect of clindamycin on aminoglycoside activity in a murine model of invasive Escherichia coli infection', *Antimicrob. Ag. Chemother.*, **10**, 893.

Falk, R. H., Gillett, A. P., Wise, R. and Melikian, V. (1977), 'Tobramycin and clindamycin in the treatment of febrile leukaemic patients', *J. Antimicrob. Chemother.*, **3**, 317.

Fass, R. J. and Saslaw, S. (1972), 'Clindamycin: Clinical and laboratory evaluation of parenteral therapy', *Amer. J. Med. Sci.*, **263**, 369.

Fass, R. J., Rotilie, C. A. and Prior, R. B. (1974), 'Interaction of clindamycin and gentamicin *in vitro*', *Antimicrob. Ag. Chemother.*, **6**, 582.

Fass, R. J. (1977), 'Treatment of mixed bacterial infections with clindamycin and gentamicin', *J. Infect. Dis.* (Suppl.), **135**, 74.

Feathers, R. S., Lewis, A. A. M., Sagor, G. R., Amirak, I. D. and Noone, P. (1977), 'Prophylactic systemic antibiotics in colorectal surgery', *Lancet*, **2**, 4.

Feigin, R. D., Pickering, L. K., Anderson, D., Keeney, R. E. and Shackleford, P. G.

(1975), 'Clindamycin treatment of osteomyelitis and septic arthritis in children', *Pediatrics*, **55**, 213.

Finch, R. G., Phillips, I. and Geddes, A. M. (1975), 'A clinical, microbiological and toxicological assessment of clindamycin phosphate', *J. Antimicrob. Chemother.*, **1**, 297.

Freeman, R. and Roberts, D. W. (1976), 'A case of subacute bacterial endocarditis treated with parenteral clindamycin (clindamycin-2-phosphate)', *Postgrad. Med. J.*, **52**, 595.

Friedman, G. D., Gérard, M. J. and Ury, H. K. (1976), 'Clindamycin and diarrhea', *JAMA*, **236**, 2498.

Fulghum, D. D. and Catalano, P. M. (1973), 'Stevens–Johnson syndrome from clindamycin. A case report', *JAMA*, **223**, 318.

Galland, R. B., Saunders, J. H., Mosley, J. G. and Darrell, J. H. (1977), 'Prevention of wound infection in abdominal operations by peroperative antibiotics or povidone-iodine. A controlled trial', *Lancet*, **2**, 1043.

Geddes, A. M., Sleet, R. A. and Murdoch, J. McC. (1964), 'Lincomycin hydrochloride: Clinical and laboratory studies', *Brit. med. J.*, **2**, 670.

Geddes, A. M., Munro, J. F., Murdoch, J. McC., Begg, K. J. and Burns, B. A. (1967), 'Four years hospital experience with lincomycin hydrochloride', *Proceedings International Congress of Chemotherapy, Vienna, Austria*.

Geddes, A. M., Bridgwater, F. A. J., Williams, D. N., Oon, J. and Grimshaw, G. J. (1970), 'Clinical and bacteriological studies with clindamycin', *Brit. med. J.*, **2**, 703.

Geddes, A. M., Dwyer, N. St. J., Ball, A. P. and Amos, R. S. (1977), 'Clindamycin in bone and joint infections', *J. Antimicrob. Chemother.*, **3**, 501.

George, R. H., Symonds, J. M., Dimock, F., Brown, H. D., Arabi, Y., Shinagawa, N., Keighley, M. R. B., Alexander-Williams, J. and Burdon, D. W. (1978a), 'Identification of Clostridium difficile as a cause of pseudomembranous colitis', *Brit. med. J.*, **1**, 695.

George, W. L., Sutter, V. L., Goldstein, E. J. C., Ludwig, S. L. and Finegold, S. M. (1978b), 'Aetiology of antimicrobial-agent-associated colitis', *Lancet*, **1**, 802.

Gerding, D. N., Hall, W. H. and Schierl, E. A. (1977), 'Antibiotic concentrations in ascitic fluid of patients with ascites and bacterial peritonitis', *Ann. Intern. Med.*, **86**, 708.

Gibson, G. E., Rowland, R. and Hecker, R. (1975), 'Diarrhoea and colitis associated with antibiotic treatment', *Aust. N.Z. J. Med.*, **5**, 340.

Gorbach, S. L. and Bartlett, J. G. (1977), 'Pseudomembranous enterocolitis: A review of its diverse forms', *J. Infect. Dis.* (Suppl.), **135**, 89.

Griffiths, D. A., Shorey, B. A., Simpson, R. A., Speller, D. C. E. and Williams, N. B. (1976), 'Single-dose peroperative antibiotic prophylaxis in gastrointestinal surgery', *Lancet*, **2**, 325.

Goulston, S. J. M. and McGovern, V. J. (1965), 'Pseudomembranous colitis', *Gut*, **6**, 207.

Gurwith, M. J., Rabin, H. R., Love, K. and the Cooperative Antibiotic Diarrhea Study Group (1977), 'Diarrhea associated with clindamycin and ampicillin therapy: Preliminary results of a cooperative study', *J. Infect. Dis.* (Suppl.), **135**, 104.

Hall, A. P., Doberstyn, E. B., Nanakorn, A. and Sonkom, P. (1975), 'Falciparum malaria semi-resistant to clindamycin', *Brit. med. J.*, **2**, 12.

Hansman, D. and Gibbs, M. (1972), 'Lincomycin in meningococcal infection', *New Engl. J. Med.*, **287**, 201.

Harrod, J. R. and Stevens, D. A. (1974), 'Anaerobic infections in the newborn infant', *J. Pediatrics*, **85**, 399.

Herrell, W. E. (1969), *Lincomycin*, Modern Scientific Publications, Inc.

Hinthorn, D. R., Baker, L. H., Romig, D. A., Hassanein, K. and Liu, C. (1976), 'Use of clindamycin in patients with liver disease', *Antimicrob. Ag. Chemother.*, **9**, 498.

Holloway, W. J., Kahlbaugh, R. A. and Scott, E. G. (1964), 'Lincomycin: A clinical study', *Antimicrob. Ag. Chemother.*—1963, p. 200.

Holloway, W. J. and Scott, E. G. (1965), 'Clinical experience with lincomycin', *Amer. J. Med. Sci.*, **249**, 691.

Holmberg, K., Nord, C.-E. and Dornbusch, K. (1977), 'Antimicrobial *in vitro* susceptibility of Actinomyces israelii and Arachnia propionica', *Scand. J. Infect. Dis.*, **9**, 40.

Hugo, H., Dornbusch, K. and Sterner, G. (1977), 'Studies on the clinical efficacy, serum levels and side effects of clindamycin phosphate administered intravenously', *Scand. J. Infect. Dis.*, **9**, 221.

Jellard, C. H. and Lipinski, A. E. (1973), 'Corynebacterium diphtheriae resistant to erythromycin and lincomycin', *Lancet*, **1**, 156.

Kabins, S. A. and Spira, T. J. (1975), 'Outbreak of clindamycin-associated colitis', *Ann. Intern. Med.*, **83**, 830.

Kapila, R., Sen, P., Salaki, J. and Louria, D. B. (1977), 'Evaluation of clindamycin and other antibiotics in the treatment of anaerobic bacterial infections of the lung', *J. Infect. Dis.* (Suppl.), **135**, 58.

Kaplan, K., Chew, W. H. and Weinstein, L. (1965), 'Microbiological, pharmacological and clinical studies of lincomycin', *Amer. J. Med. Sci.*, **250**, 137.

Kaplan, E. and Weinstein, L. (1968), 'Lincomycin', *Pediat. Clin. North Amer.*, **15**, 131.

Kappas, A., Shinagawa, N., Arabi, Y., Thompson, H., Burdon, D. W., Dimock, F., George, R. H., Alexander-Williams, J. and Keighley, M. R. B. (1978), 'Diagnosis of pseudomembranous colitis', *Brit. med. J.*, **1**, 675.

Karchmer, A. W., Moellering, R. C., Jr. and Watson, B. K. (1975), 'Susceptibility of various serogroups of streptococci to clindamycin and lincomycin', *Antimicrob. Ag. Chemother.*, **7**, 164.

Kato, Y., Tomizawa, M., Chiba, A., Senshu, H., Kojima, A., Matsumoto, Y. and Sakuraba, T. (1966), 'Laboratory and clinical studies in lincomycin', *J. Antibiot.* (A), **5**, 234; quoted by Herrell (1969).

Keane, J. T. and Rose, H. D. (1973), 'Pneumococcal endocarditis treated with clindamycin', *JAMA*, **226**, 1120.

Keighley, M. R. B., Crapp, A. R., Burdon, D. W., Cooke, W. T. and Alexander-Williams, J. (1976), 'Prophylaxis against anaerobic sepsis in bowel surgery', *Br. J. Surg.*, **63**, 538.

Keusch, G. T. and Present, D. H. (1976), 'Summary of a workshop on clindamycin colitis', *J. Infect. Dis.*, **133**, 578.

Kislak, J. W. (1967), 'Brief recording: Type 6 Pneumococcus resistant to erythromycin and lincomycin', *New Engl. J. Med.*, **27**, 852.

Kislak, J. W. (1972), 'The susceptibility of Bacteroides fragilis to 24 antibiotics', *J. Infect. Dis.*, **125**, 295.

Kitamoto, O. (1969), 'Lincomycin: its dynamics and clinical effect', *Suppl. Bulletin of the Post-Graduate Committee in Medicine, University of Sydney*, **25**, XXXIV.

Klastersky, J. and Husson, M. (1977), 'Bactericidal activity of the combinations of gentamicin with clindamycin or chloramphenicol against species of Escherichia coli and Bacteroides fragilis', *Antimicrob. Ag. Chemother.*, **12**, 135.

Klastersky, J., Husson, M., Weerts-Ruhl, D. and Daneau, D. (1977), 'Anaerobic wound infections in cancer patients: Comparative trial of clindamycin, tinidazole, and doxycycline', *Antimicrob. Ag. Chemother.*, **12**, 563.

Kohn, J., Hewitt, J. H. and Fraser, C. A. M. (1968), 'Group A streptococci resistant to lincomycin', *Brit. med. J.*, **1**, 703.

Kohn, J. and Evans, A. J. (1970), 'Group A streptococci resistant to clindamycin, *Brit. med. J.*, **2**, 423.

Kosmidis, J. C., Corbett, V., Cole, A. J. L., Finch, R. G., Barker, J. E. and Geddes, A. M. (1973), 'The treatment of paediatric infections with the lincomycins', *Brit. J.*

Clin. Pract., **27**, 315.

Kunin, C. M. (1967), 'A guide to use of antibiotics in patients with renal disease', *Ann. Intern. Med.*, **67**, 151.

Lambert, H. P. (1975), 'Unwanted effects of antibiotics: Some recent additions', *J. Antimicrob. Chemother.*, **1**, 2.

Larson, H. E., Parry, J. V., Price, A. B., Davies D. R., Dolby, J. and Tyrrell, D. A. J. (1977), 'Undescribed toxin in pseudomembranous colitis', *Brit. med. J.*, **1**, 1246.

Larson, H. E. and Price, A. B. (1977), 'Pseudomembranous colitis: Presence of clostridial toxin', *Lancet*, **2**, 1312.

Larson, H. E., Price, A. B., Honour, P. and Borriello, S. P. (1978), 'Clostridium difficile and the aetiology of pseudomembranous colitis', *Lancet*, **1**, 1063.

Leading Article (1973), 'Antibiotics in acne vulgaris', *Brit. med. J.*, **1**, 65.

Leading Article (1974), 'Lincomycin and clindamycin colitis', *Brit. med. J.*, **4**, 65.

Leading Article (1975), 'Drug metabolism and increasing age', *Brit. med. J.*, **2**, 581.

Leading Article (1978), 'Antibiotic-associated colitis: A progress report', *Brit. med. J.*, **1**, 669.

Ledger, W. J., Gee, C. L., Lewis, W. P. and Bobitt, J. R. (1977), 'Comparison of clindamycin and chloramphenicol in treatment of serious infections of the female genital tract', *J. Infect. Dis.* (Suppl.), **135**, 30.

Le Frock, J. L., Klainer, A. S., Chen, S., Gainer, R. B., Omar, M. and Anderson, W. (1975), 'The spectrum of colitis associated with lincomycin and clindamycin therapy', *J. Infect. Dis.* (Suppl.), **131**, 108.

Leigh, D. A., Pease, R., Henderson, H., Simmons, K. and Russ, R. (1976), 'Prophylactic lincomycin in the prevention of wound infection following appendicectomy: A double blind trial', *Br. J. Surg.*, **63**, 973.

Leigh, D. A., Simmons, K. and Williams, S. (1977), 'The treatment of abdominal and gynaecological infections with parenteral clindamycin phosphate', *J. Antimicrob. Chemother.*, **3**, 493.

Lemos, L. B., Baba, N. and De Araujo, O. J. (1976), 'Clindamycin-induced pseudomembranous colitis', *Amer. J. Clin. Path.*, **65**, 455.

Leng, B., Meyers, B. R., Hirschman, S. Z. and Keusch, G. T. (1975), 'Susceptibilities of Gram-negative bacteria to combinations of antimicrobial agents *in vitro*', *Antimicrob. Ag. Chemother.*, **8**, 164.

Levison, M. E., Bran, J. L. and Ries, K. (1974), 'Treatment of anaerobic bacterial infections with clindamycin-2-phosphate', *Antimicrob. Ag. Chemother.*, **5**, 276.

Levison, M. E., Santoro, J., Bran, J. L., Ries, K. and Rubin, W. (1977), '*In vitro* activity and clinical efficacy of clindamycin in the treatment of infections due to anaerobic bacteria', *J. Infect. Dis.* (Suppl.), **135**, 49.

Lewis, C., Clapp, H. W. and Grady, J. E. (1963), '*In vitro* and *in vivo* evaluation of lincomycin, a new antibiotic', *Antimicrob. Ag. Chemother.*—1962, p. 570.

Lines, D. R. and Kernick, C. (1967), 'Lincomycin in childhood pneumonia', *Med. J. Aust.*, **1**, 551.

Lines, D. R., Vimpani, G. V. and Pearson, C. C. (1973), 'The use of 7-chlorolincomycin in the treatment of childhood respiratory disease', *Med. J. Aust.*, **1**, 439.

Lusk, R. H., Fekety, F. R., Jr., Silva, J., Jr., Bodendorfer, T., Devine, B. J., Kawanishi, H., Korff, L., Nakauchi, D., Rogers, S. and Siskin, S. B. (1977), 'Gastrointestinal side effects of clindamycin and ampicillin therapy', *J. Infect. Dis.* (Suppl.), **135**, 111.

Ma, P., Lim, M. and Nodine, J. H. (1964), 'Human pharmacological studies of lincomycin, a new antibiotic for gram-positive organisms', *Antimicrob. Ag. Chemother.*—1963, p. 183.

Magerlein, B. J., Birkenmeyer, R. D. and Kagam, F. (1967), 'Chemical modification of lincomycin', *Antimicrob. Ag. Chemother.*, 1966, p. 727.

Malacoff, R. F., Finkelstein, F. O. and Andriole, V. T. (1975), 'Effect of peritoneal dialysis on serum levels of tobramycin and lincomycin', *Antimicrob. Ag.*

Chemother., **8**, 574.

Martin, W. J., Gardner, M. and Washington, J. A., II (1972), '*In vitro* antimicrobial susceptibility of anaerobic bacteria isolated from clinical specimens', *Antimicrob. Ag. Chemother.*, **1**, 148.

Mathias, R. G., Harding, G. K. M., Gurwith, M. J., Stiver, H. G., Sigurdson, E., Gratton, C. A. and Ronald, A. R. (1977), 'Bacteremia due to bacteroidaceae: A review of 92 cases', *J. Infect. Dis.*, (Suppl.), **135**, 69.

McCall, C. E., Steigbigel, N. H. and Finland, M. (1967), 'Lincomycin: Activity *in vitro* and absorption and excretion in normal young men', *Amer. J. Med. Sci.*, **254**, 144.

McCloskey, R. V., Green, M. J., Eller, J. and Smilack, J. (1974), 'Treatment of diphtheria carriers: Benzathine penicillin, erythromycin, and clindamycin', *Ann. Intern. Med.*, **81**, 788.

McGehee, R. F., Jr., Smith, C. B., Wilcox, C. and Finland, M. (1968), 'Comparative studies of antibacterial activity *in vitro* and absorption and excretion of lincomycin and clinimycin', *Amer. J. Med. Sci.*, **256**, 279.

McGehee, R. F., Jr., Barrett, F. F. and Finland, M. (1969), 'Resistance of Staphylococcus aureus to lincomycin, clinimycin, and erythromycin', *Antimicrob. Ag. Chemother.*—1968, p. 392.

Medina, A., Fiske, N. Hjelt-Harvey, I., Brown, C. D. and Prigot, A. (1964), 'Absorption, diffusion and excretion of a new antibiotic, lincomycin', *Antimicrob. Ag. Chemother.*—1963, p. 189.

Mitchell, A. A. B. (1973), 'Incidence and isolation of Bacteroides species from clinical material and their sensitivity to antibiotics', *J. clin. Path.*, **26**, 738.

Mitchell, A. A. B. and Simpson, R. G. (1973), 'Bacteroides septicaemia', *Curr. med. Res. Opin.*, **1**, 385.

Mohr, J. A., Rhoades, E. R. and Muchmore, H. G. (1970), 'Actinomycosis treated with lincomycin', *JAMA*, **212**, 2260.

Munk, J. F., Collopy, B. T., Connell, J. L., McTeigue, J. J., Hughes, J. F., Hood, R. N. and Breen, K. J. (1976), 'Lincomycin-clindamycin-associated pseudomembranous colitis', *Med. J. Aust.*, **2**, 95.

Neu, H. C., Prince, A., Neu, C. O. and Garvey, G. J. (1977), 'Incidence of diarrhea and colitis associated with clindamycin therapy', *J. Infect. Dis.* (Suppl.), **35**, 120.

Newell, A. C. (1970), 'Clinical trial of a new antibiotic', *Med. J. Aust.*, **2**, 321.

Nicholas, P., Meyers, B. R., Levy, R. N. and Hirschman, S. Z. (1975), 'Concentration of clindamycin in human bone', *Antimicrob. Ag. Chemother.*, **8**, 220.

Nies, A. S. (1974), 'Drug interactions', *Med. Clin. North Amer.*, **58**, 965.

Norden, C. W. and Kennedy, E. (1971), 'Experimental osteomyelitis. II. Therapeutic trials and measurement of antibiotic levels in bone', *J. Infect. Dis.*, **124**, 565.

Novak, E., Vitti, T. G., Panzer, J. D., Schlagel, C. and Hearron, M. S. (1971), 'Antibiotic tolerance and serum levels after intravenous administration of multiple large doses of lincomycin', *Clin. Pharmacol. Ther.*, **12**, 793.

Novak, E., Lee, J. G., Seckman, C. E., Phillips, J. P. and Di Santo, A. R. (1976), 'Unfavourable effect of atropine-diphenoxylate (Lomotil) therapy in lincomycin-caused diarrhoea', *JAMA*, **235**, 1451.

O'Connell, C. J. and Plaut, M. E. (1969), 'Intravenous lincomycin in high doses', *Current Therap. Res.*, **11**, 478.

Okubadejo, O. A. and Allen, J. (1975), 'Combined activity of clindamycin and gentamicin on Bacteroides fragilis and other bacteria', *J. Antimicrob. Chemother.*, **1**, 403.

Ormonde, N. W. G., Gould, J. C., Degnen, F., Munro, A. H. G. and Munro, J. F. (1973), 'Treatment of acute exacerbations of chronic bronchitis with clindamycin', *Curr. med. Res. Opin.*, **1**, 390.

Parsons, R. L. (1976), 'Antibiotics in bone', *J. Antimicrob. Chemother.*, **2**, 228.

Peddie, B. A., Dann, E. and Bailey, R. R. (1975), 'The effect of impairment of renal function and dialysis on the serum and urine levels of clindamycin', *Aust. N.Z. J. Med.*, **5**, 198.

Phillips, I., Fernandes, R. and Warren, C. (1970), '*In vitro* comparison of erythromycin, lincomycin, and clindamycin', *Brit. med. J.*, **2**, 89.

Phillips, I., Warren, C., Harrison, J. M., Sharples, P., Ball, L. C. and Parker, M. T. (1976), 'Antibiotic susceptibilities of Streptococci from the mouth and blood of patients treated with penicillin or lincomycin and clindamycin', *J. Med. Microbiol.*, **9**, 393.

Philipson, A., Sabath, L. D. and Charles, D. (1973), 'Transplacental passage of erythromycin and clindamycin', *New Engl. J. Med.*, **288**, 1219.

Powers, K. G. and Jacobs, R. L. (1972), 'Activity of two chlorinated lincomycin analogues against chloroquine-resistant falciparum malaria in owl monkeys', *Antimicrob. Ag. Chemother.*, **1**, 49.

Price, D. J. E., O'Grady, F. W., Shooter, R. A. and Weaver, P. C. (1968), 'Trial of phenoxymethylpenicillin, phenethicillin, and lincomycin in treatment of staphylococcal sepsis in a casualty department', *Brit. med. J.*, **3**, 407.

Price, A. B. and Davies, D. R. (1977), 'Pseudomembranous colitis', *J. clin. Path.*, **30**, 1.

Raeburn, J. A. and Devine, J. D. (1971), 'Clindamycin levels in sputum in a patient with purulent chest disease due to cystic fibrosis', *Postgrad. Med. J.*, **47**, 366.

Reinarz, J. A. and McIntosh, D. A. (1966), 'Lincomycin excretion in patients with normal renal function, severe azotemia, and with hemodialysis and peritoneal dialysis', *Antimicrob. Ag. Chemother.*—1965, p. 232; quoted by Sanders (1970).

Reiner, L., Schlesinger, M. J. and Miller, G. M. (1952), 'Pseudomembranous colitis following aureomycin and chloramphenicol', *Arch. Path.*, **54**, 39.

Reusser, F. (1975), 'Effect of lincomycin and clindamycin on peptide chain initiation', *Antimicrob. Ag. Chemother.*, **7**, 32.

Rifkin, G. D., Fekety, F. R. and Silva, J., Jr. (1977), 'Antibiotic-induced colitis. Implication of a toxin neutralised by Clostridium sordellii antitoxin', *Lancet*, **2**, 1103.

Robertson, M. B., Breen, K. J., Desmond, P. V., Mashford, M. L. and McHugh, A. M. (1977), 'Incidence of antibiotic-related diarrhoea and pseudomembranous colitis. A prospective study of lincomycin, clindamycin and ampicillin', *Med. J. Aust.*, **1**, 243.

Rodriguez, W., Ross, S., Khan, W., McKay, D. and Moskowitz, P. (1977), 'Clindamycin in the treatment of osteomyelitis in children. A report of 29 cases', *Am. J. Dis. Child.*, **131**, 1088.

Rose, H. D. and Rytel, M. W. (1972), 'Actinomycosis treated with clindamycin', *JAMA*, **221**, 1052.

Rountree, P. M. and Beard, M. A. (1968), 'Hospital strains of Staphylococcus aureus, with particular reference to methicillin-resistant strains', *Med. J. Aust.*, **2**, 1163.

Sabath, L. D. and Toftegaard, I. (1974), 'Rapid microassays for clindamycin and gentamicin when present together and the effect of pH and of each on the antibacterial activity of the other', *Antimicrob. Ag. Chemother.*, **6**, 54.

Salaki, J. S., Black, R., Tally, F. P. and Kislak, J. W. (1976), 'Bacteroides fragilis resistant to the administration of clindamycin', *Amer. J. Med.*, **60**, 426.

Sanders, E., Foster, M. T. and Scott, D. (1968), 'Group A beta-hemolytic streptococci resistant to erythromycin and lincomycin', *New Engl. J. Med.*, **278**, 538.

Schwartzman, J. D., Reller, L. B. and Wang, W.-L. L. (1977), 'Susceptibility of Clostridium perfringens isolated from human infections to twenty antibiotics', *Antimicrob. Ag. Chemother.*, **11**, 695.

Scott, A. J., Nicholson, G. I. and Kerr, A. R. (1973), 'Lincomycin as a cause of pseudomembranous colitis', *Lancet*, **2**, 1232.

Scott, A. J. and Nicholson, G. I. (1974), 'The recognition of pseudomembranous colitis as a clinical entity', *Aust. N.Z. J. Med.*, **4**, 502.

Smilack, J. D., Burgin, W. W., Jr., Moore, W L., Jr. and Sanford, J. P. (1974), 'Mycoplasma pneumoniae pneumonia and clindamycin therapy. Failure to demonstrate efficacy', *JAMA*, **228**, 729.

Smilack, J. D., Flittie, W. H. and Williams, T. W., Jr. (1976), 'Bone concentrations of antimicrobial agents after parenteral administration', *Antimicrob. Ag. Chemother.*, **9**, 169.

Sprunt, K., Leidy, G. and Redman, W. (1970), 'Cross resistance between lincomycin and erythromycin in viridans streptococci', *Pediatrics*, **46**, 84.

Staneck, J. L. and Washington, J. A. II (1974), 'Antimicrobial susceptibilities of anaerobic bacteria: Recent clinical isolates', *Antimicrob. Ag. Chemother.*, **6**, 311.

Sutter, V. L., Kwok, Y-Y. and Finegold, S. M. (1973), 'Susceptibility of Bacteroides fragilis to six antibiotics determined by standardized antimicrobial disc susceptibility testing', *Antimicrob. Ag. Chemother.*, **3**, 188.

Sutter, V. L. and Finegold, S. M. (1976), 'Susceptibility of anaerobic bacteria to 23 antimicrobial agents', *Antimicrob. Ag. Chemother.*, **10**, 736.

Sutter, V. L. (1977), '*In vitro* susceptibility of anaerobes: Comparison of clindamycin and other antimicrobial agents', *J. Infect. Dis.* (Suppl.), **135**, 7.

Sutton, D. R. and Gosnold, J. K. (1977), 'Oesophageal ulceration due to clindamycin', *Brit. med. J.*, **1**, 1598.

Swartzberg, J. E., Maresca, R. M. and Remington, J. S. (1977), 'Clinical study of gastrointestinal complications associated with clindamycin therapy', *J. Infect. Dis.* (Suppl.), **135**, 99.

Swenson, R. M. and Lorber, B. (1977), 'Clindamycin and carbenicillin in treatment of patients with intraabdominal and female genital tract infection', *J. Infect. Dis.* (Suppl.), **135**, 40.

Tedesco, F. J., Barton, R. W. and Alpers, D. H. (1974), 'Clindamycin-associated colitis. A prospective study', *Ann. Intern. Med.*, **81**, 429.

Tracey, O., Gordon, A. M., Moran, F., Love, W. C. and McKenzie, P. (1972), 'Lincomycins in the treatment of Bacteroides infections', *Brit. med. J.*, **1**, 280.

Turck, W. P. G. (1978), 'Treatment of Q fever', *Brit. med. J.*, **1**, 1052.

Wagner, J. G., Novak, E., Patel, N. C., Chidester, C. G. and Lummis, W. L. (1968), 'Absorption, excretion and half-life of clinimycin in normal adult males', *Amer. J. Med. Sci.*, **256**, 25.

Waisbren, B. A. (1968), Lincomycin in larger doses', *JAMA*, **206**, 2118.

Watanakunakorn, C. (1976), 'Clindamycin therapy of Staphylococcus aureus endocarditis. Clinical relapse and development of resistance to clindamycin, lincomycin and erythromycin', *Amer. J. Med.*, **60**, 419.

Weisblum, B. (1967), 'Pneumococcus resistant to erythromycin and lincomycin', *Lancet*, **1**, 843.

Wells, R. F., Cohen, L. E. and McNeill, C. J. (1974), 'Clindamycin and pseudomembranous colitis', *Lancet*, **1**, 66.

Wells, R. F. (1974), 'Editorial. Clindamycin-associated colitis', *Ann. Intern. Med.*, **81**, 547.

Wharton, M. R. and Beddow, F. H. (1975), 'Clindamycin for acute osteomyelitis in children', *Postgrad. Med. J.*, **51**, 166.

Wilkins, T. D. and Thiel, T. (1973), 'Resistance of some species of clostridium to clindamycin', *Antimicrob. Ag. Chemother.*, **3**, 136.

Williams, D. N., Crossley, K., Hoffman, C. and Sabath, L. D. (1975), 'Parenteral clindamycin phosphate: Pharmacology with normal and abnormal liver function and effect on nasal staphylococci', *Antimicrob. Ag. Chemother.*, **7**, 153.

Zabransky, R. J., Johnston, J. A. and Hauser, K. J. (1973), 'Bacteriostatic and bactericidal activities of various antibiotics against Bacteroides fragilis', *Antimicrob. Ag. Chemother.*, **3**, 152.

Zamiri, I. and McEntegart, M. G. (1972), 'The sensitivity of diphtheria bacilli to eight antibiotics', *J. clin. Path.*, **25,** 716.

Zinner, S. H., Provonchee, R. B., Elias, K. S. and Peter, G. (1976), 'Effect of clindamycin on the *in vitro* activity of amikacin and gentamicin against Gram-negative
bacilli', *Antimicrob. Ag. Chemother.*, **9,** 661.

Erythromycin

Description

Erythromycin was isolated from a strain of Streptomyces erythreus (McGuire *et al.*, 1952), and it belongs to a group of antibiotics known as the 'macrolides', which have in common a macrocyclic lactone ring. They are all weak bases, only slightly soluble in water. There are many antibiotics in this group, but apart from erythromycin, only spiramycin, oleandomycin, kitasamycin (page 517) and josamycin (page 522) have been used clinically.

Erythromycin base is very bitter, insoluble in water and inactivated by acid. Originally erythromycin was marketed solely in this form. To prevent inactivation by gastric secretions erythromycin base has been manufactured in various 'acid-resistant' forms, such as 'enteric-coated' tablets and granules. Depending on the preparation, these acid-resistant forms are better absorbed and produce more consistent serum levels. Their absorption is still influenced by food and therefore they should be given at least one hour prior to meals.

Various erythromycin salts and esters subsequently became available for clinical use, which were more acid-resistant. Three of these are currently available commercially.

1. *Erythromycin stearate* (a salt).
2. *Erythromycin ethyl succinate* (an ester).

These two preparations are still susceptible to acid inactivation. Despite the fact that they are marketed with a buffering agent or as film-coated or enteric-coated tablets, they should be administered at least one hour before a meal.

3. *Propionyl erythromycin ester lauryl sulphate* (*erythromycin estolate*) (the salt of an ester).

This drug is much more resistant to inactivation by gastric acid and it can be administered in the fasting state or after food.

Sensitive Organisms

1. *Gram-positive bacteria*. Erythromycin is highly active against organisms such as Staph. pyogenes (including penicillinase producing strains), Staph. epidermidis, Strep. pyogenes, Strep. pneumoniae, and Strep. viridans. Penicillin combined with erythromycin is more effective that either drug alone for the treatment of staphylococcal infection in mice caused by a penicillin-sensitive strain (Steigbigel *et al.*, 1975).

Approximately 90 per cent of Strep. faecalis strains are also erythromycin-sensitive. In 1976 in Zurich up to 30 per cent of Strep. faecalis strains were resistant to erythromycin and chloramphenicol (Marder and Kayser, 1977).

These authors showed that resistance to erythromycin and chloramphenicol and also high-level resistance to streptomycin and lincomycin of Strep. faecalis, was transferable and mediated by an R plasmid (page 422).

Strains resistant to erythromycin are rare among the usually highly sensitive streptococci, and for this reason sensitivity tests, particularly against Strep. pyogenes and the pneumococci, are usually not performed in clinical practice. Strains of Strep. pyogenes (Group A) resistant to erythromycin (and lincomycin, page 471) were first reported in 1968 (Sanders et al., 1968; Dixon, 1968). The frequency of these resistant strains of Group A hemolytic streptococci has increased in northern Canada, where in 1972 1·38 per cent were resistant to erythromycin (and lincomycin) (Dixon and Lipinski, 1972; 1974). Also during 1971 and 1972 in northern Canada, 0·6 per cent of Group B, 1–2 per cent of Group C and 1·3 per cent of Group G streptococci were resistant to these antibiotics (Dixon and Lipinski, 1974). Of 707 clinical isolates of Group B streptococci from one hospital in California, 1–2 per cent were resistant to erythromycin or clindamycin, but cross-resistance between these two antibiotics was not absolute (Anthony and Concepcion, 1975). Strains of Strep. pneumoniae resistant to erythromycin remain rare (Kislak et al., 1965; Kislak, 1967; Dixon, 1967; Cooper et al., 1968; Champion et al., 1978). The multiply-antibiotic resistant strains of pneumococci isolated in South Africa during 1977 (page 4) were resistant to erythromycin (Center for Disease Control, 1977c). Resistant strains of Strep. viridans have been reported (Sprunt et al., 1970). Resistance to a strain of Strep. sanguis (one of the 'viridans group') to erythromycin (and lincomycin), which had been isolated from a patient who had received prolonged erythromycin therapy, was shown to be due to an R plasmid (Yagi et al., 1978).

Most staphylococci are still erythromycin-sensitive (Hassam et al., 1978), but resistant strains are encountered, particularly in hospitals. Staph. pyogenes strains resistant to erythromycin can be induced in vitro but these differ in certain respects from resistant strains isolated from patients, suggesting that in vivo resistance occurs by a different mechanism. On this basis Lacey (1977) considers that there is only a slight risk that sensitive staphylococci will mutate to resistant strains during prolonged therapy, so that erythromycin can be used freely in domiciliary patients without causing resistance. However in the hospital environment the extensive use of the drug is more likely to select naturally occurring resistant strains. In clinical practice sensitivity testing of staphylococci is always advisable. With staphylococci there is some cross-resistance between all the macrolides, and also to some extent between them and chemically unrelated lincomycin and clindamycin (page 471). Most staphylococcal strains resistant to lincomycin, oleandomycin and spiramycin are also resistant to erythromycin, but erythromycin-resistant strains are not always resistant to the other macrolides or lincomycin. A characteristic feature of the macrolide antibiotics is 'the dissociated type of resistance', which was first described by Garrod (1957). A staphylococcal strain resistant to erythromycin, but sensitive to the other antibiotics of this group, shows resistance to the other macrolides such as oleandomycin and spiramycin, if the sensitivity test is performed in the presence of erythromycin. This phenomenon also occurs with lincomycin (page 471).

B. anthracis and Listeria monocytogenes (Wiggins et al., 1978) are erythromycin-sensitive. C. diphtheriae is also very susceptible (Zamiri and McEntegart, 1972), but resistant strains have been detected on rare occasions (Jellard and Lipinski, 1973). The Nocardia are variable in their susceptibility. Bach *et al.* (1973) found that erythromycin in a concentration of 0·8 μg per ml inhibited 40 per cent of Nocardia asteroides strains tested, but the MIC's for most of the others were greater than 100 μg per ml (*see also* ampicillin, page 100).

Erythromycin also has a wide range of activity against Gram-positive anaerobic bacteria. It is active against Eubacterium, Propionibacterium, Bifidobacterium, Lactobacillus and Peptostreptococcus spp. and also against most strains of Peptococcus spp. (Sutter and Finegold, 1976). Clostridium tetani and Cl. perfringens (welchii) are sensitive. Occasional strains of Cl. perfringens are erythromycin-resistant (Wallace, 1977). Actinomyces israelii and Arachnia propionica (the causative agents of human actinomycosis) are sensitive to erythromycin (Sutter and Finegold, 1976; Holmberg *et al.*, 1977).

2. *Gram-negative bacteria.* Erythromycin is active against Neisseria meningitidis, H. influenzae (including ampicillin-resistant strains, page 102) and B. pertussis. N. gonorrhoeae is also sensitive, but strains with diminished sensitivity or which are completely resistant occur. Studies on clinical isolates of N. gonorrhoeae have demonstrated a positive correlation between the sensitivities of all possible pairs of the following antibiotics: penicillin, tetracycline, erythromycin and chloramphenicol (Report, 1978). Beta-lactamase producing strains of N. gonorrhoeae (page 8) isolated in East Asia, according to Report (1978), are inhibited by a concentration of 0·5 μg per ml of erythromycin. The Center for Disease Control (1978) however found that about 35 per cent of such strains isolated in the United States and East Asia were resistant to erythromycin in a concentration of 1·0 μg per ml. Some strains of the Brucella spp. are sensitive to erythromycin (Abbot Laboratories, 1966). Esch. coli, the Enterobacter, Klebsiella, Proteus, Salmonella and Shigella spp. and Ps. aeruginosa are erythromycin-resistant. However antibacterial activity of erythromycin against the Gram-negative bacilli is influenced by pH and it increases markedly as the pH rises to 8·5. Most Esch. coli and Klebsiella spp. strains can be inhibited by erythromycin concentrations attained in urine with ordinary therapeutic doses, provided the urine is made alkaline (Sabath *et al.*, 1968a and b). Combinations of either clindamycin or erythromycin with either gentamicin or colistin show *in vitro* synergism against Esch. coli (Leng *et.al.*, 1975).

Campylobacter fetus is an organism which is increasingly being implicated as a cause of gastro-enteritis but also of septicaemia, endocarditis, meningitis or arthritis. It is variable in its suceptibility to erythromycin and only 36 per cent of strains studied by Chow *et al.* (1978) were sensitive to a concentration of 1·6 μg per ml. Early *in vitro* and animal studies on the Legionnaires' disease bacterium indicated that erythromycin might be effective against this organism (Center for Disease Control, 1977a and b). Subsequent *in vitro* (Thornsberry *et al.*, 1978) and *in vivo* studies in guinea pigs (Fraser *et al.*, 1978) and embryonated eggs (Lewis *et al.*, 1978) have confirmed that erythromycin is one of the most active drugs against the Legionnaires' disease bacterium. Flavobacterium spp. may also be sensitive to erythromycin (Lee *et al.*, 1977).

Erythromycin has a variable activity against anaerobic Gram-negative bacteria. Most strains of Bacteroides spp. can be inhibited by moderately high erythromycin concentrations, but such high levels are only attained in the serum after parenteral administration (Zabransky *et al.*, 1973; Okubadejo *et al.*, 1973; Gorbach and Bartlett, 1974). Sutter and Finegold (1976) studied the susceptibility of a variety of anaerobic organisms to erythromycin. Although all strains of Bacteroides melaninogenicus and a high percentage of other Bacteroides spp. were susceptible to $1 \cdot 0 \mu$g per ml, B. fragilis and the Fusobacterium spp. were usually resistant. Erythromycin in concentrations easily attainable with oral therapy acts synergistically with cefamandole (page 270) against B. fragilis *in vitro*.

3. *Treponema pallidum*. Erythromycin is active against this organism. This has been confirmed experimentally in rabbits (Brause *et al.*, 1976).

4. *Rickettsiae*. The agents which cause epidemic and scrub typhus fevers are sensitive to erythromycin. The *in vitro* activity of erythromycin against Rickettsia prowazeki has been demonstrated in cell culture but the rate of killing of rickettsiae was slow (Wisseman *et al.*, 1974).

5. *Chlamydia trachomatis*. Various serotypes of this organism cause a variety of diseases (*see* page 626). Cell culture studies have indicated that tetracycline (page 597) and erythromycin are the most effective antibiotics against these organisms (Kuo *et al.*, 1977; Lee *et al.*, 1978).

6. *Mycoplasmas*. Mycoplasma pneumoniae is very susceptible to erythromycin (Jao and Finland, 1967). Erythromycin-resistant Mycoplasma pneumoniae variants can be obtained *in vitro* by serial subculture of the organism in the presence of the drug. Such erythromycin resistance is usually accompanied by resistance to other macrolides and lincomycin (Niitu *et al.*, 1974). There has been one report of a strain of Mycoplasma pneumoniae acquiring resistance to erythromycin during treatment; this strain was also resistant to oleandomycin, spiramycin, josamycin and lincomycin (Niitu *et al.*, 1970). Mycoplasma T-strains (Ureaplasma urealyticum) which can cause non-specific urethritis (page 627) are usually sensitive to erythromycin, but resistant strains occur (Spaepen *et al.*, 1976). Tetracycline-resistant strains of U. urealyticum may sometimes be sensitive to erythromycin (Ford and Smith, 1974). Erythromycin is not active against Mycoplasma hominis and in this respect it differs from lincomycin (Csonka and Spitzer, 1969).

7. Mycobacterium tuberculosis is resistant to erythromycin, but some atypical mycobacteria are erythromycin-sensitive (Molavi and Weinstein, 1971).

8. Erythromycin stearate probably has no antibacterial action, but in solution it rapidly dissociates into active erythromycin. Similarly, erythromycin estolate appears to have no antibacterial activity until it is hydrolysed to active erythromycin base (Braun, 1969; Tardrew *et al.*, 1969).

In Vitro Sensitivities

The minimum inhibitory concentrations of erythromycin against some selected bacterial species are shown in Table 31.

Mode of Administration and Dosage

1. *Oral administration*. Erythromycin is most commonly administered by

TABLE 31
(Modified after Abbott laboratories, 1966)

ORGANISM	MIC (μg per ml)
Gram-positive bacteria	
Staph. pyogenes	0·5
Staph. epidermidis	0·5
Strep. pyogenes (Group A)	0·04
Strep. pneumoniae	0·10
Strep. vidans spp.	0·5
Strep. faecalis (Enterococcus, Group D)	1·5
Bacillus anthracis	0·6
Clostridium tetani	0·09
Actinomyces israelii	0·3
Corynebacterium diphtheriae	1·6
Listeria monocytogenes	0·16
Gram-negative bacteria	
Neisseria gonorrhoeae	0·94
Neisseria meningitidis	0·78
Haemophilus influenzae	2·5
Bordetella pertussis	1·56
Brucella melitensis	1·6
Miscellaneous	
Mycoplasma pneumoniae	0·0125

the oral route. The usual dose is 30–50 mg per kg per day given in three or four divided doses. The usual adult dose is 0·5 g six-hourly. For severe infections higher doses can be used.

2. *Intramuscular administration.* Erythromycin can also be administered intramuscularly in the form of erythromycin ethyl succinate. The usual adult dose is 100 to 200 mg eight-hourly, but these injections are large and painful, so that this route of administration is rarely used.

3. *Intravenous administration.* The drug can be used intravenously for treatment of severe infections either as erythromycin lactobionate or gluceptate. The dose is 300 to 500 mg six-hourly for adults and 30 to 50 mg per kg for children. However a daily intravenous dose as high as 6 g has been given to adults without toxic effect. Erythromycin can be administered by either intermittent intravenous injections or continuous intravenous infusion. If erythromycin lactobionate is injected directly into the intravenous tubing, a 1 per cent solution should be used (the contents of a 500 mg vial dissolved in 50 ml of sterile water), and this should be injected slowly over five minutes to avoid pain along the vein. Being compatible with commonly used intravenous fluids, the drug can also be added to intravenous drip bottles and administered by continuous infusion, but possible incompatible additives should be avoided.

4. *Patients with renal failure.* The normal serum half-life of erythromycin of 1·4 h is only prolonged to 4·8–5·8 h in anuric patients, so that only minor, if any, dosage reduction of erythromycin is necessary in patients with severe renal failure (Kunin, 1967).

5. *Patients with liver disease.* Erythromycin may accumulate in patients with severe liver disease. If large doses are administered to such patients, serum level monitoring and perhaps dose reduction may be necessary.

6. *Newborn and premature infants.* The dose recommended for older children may be safely used in this age group. Burns and Hodgman (1963) administered 40 mg per kg per day of erythromycin estolate in four divided doses to 26 premature infants. Satisfactory serum levels, no evidence of accumulation and no toxic effects were observed.

7. *Pregnant patients.* Because of its propensity to cause hepatotoxicity (page 505), erythromycin estolate should not be used in such patients.

Availability (Australia)

For oral administration.
  1. *Erythromycin base:* ('EMU-V', Upjohn; 'Eryc' (Faulding). Enteric coated tablets and granules: 125 and 250 mg.
  2. *Erythromycin stearate:* ('Erythromycin oral', Abbot; 'Eratrex', Bristol; 'Ethryn', Faulding; 'Erostin', Knoll; 'E-MYCIN, Protea). Buffered in capsules, enteric- and film-coated tablets: 125 and 250 mg. An aqueous suspension containing 125 mg in 5 ml.
  3. *Erythromycin ethyl succinate:* ('Erythromycin oral' Abbot), Dulcets (chewable tablets): 200 mg.
  4. *Erythromycin estolate:* ('Eromycin', Dista; 'Ilosone', Eli Lilly). Suspension: each 5 ml containing 125 mg.
For intramuscular administration
  Erythromycin ethyl succinate: ('Erythrocin IM', Abbot). Ampoules: 100 mg in 2 ml.
For intravenous administration
  1. *Erythromycin lactobionate:* ('Erythrocin IV', Abbot). Vials of 300 mg and 1 g.
  2. *Erythromycin gluceptate:* ('Ilotycin Gluceptate IV', Eli Lilly). Ampoules containing 1 g.

Serum Levels in Relation to Dosage

1. *Erythromycin base* is destroyed by acid in the stomach, and tablets are manufactured with an acid-resistant coating, which subsequently dissolve in the duodenum.

2. *Erythromycin stearate* is less readily destroyed in the stomach, and it dissociates in the duodenum liberating active erythromycin, which is absorbed. The peak serum levels after oral administration of commercial preparations of erythromycin base and erythromycin stearate appear approximately the same, except that the absorption of the base may be slightly more delayed (Fig. 26). Triggs and Ashley (1978) showed in volunteers that although mean serum levels are low after a single dose of erythromycin stearate, these were considerably higher after repeated doses. Doubling the dose of these compounds approximately doubles the serum concentrations.

3. *Erythromycin estolate*, unlike the base and the stearate, is acid-stable and absorbed from the gastro-intestinal tract more completely. It is apparently absorbed mainly as the ester, and high serum concentrations are obtained rapidly and remain elevated for a prolonged period. The peak serum level obtained after erythromycin estolate is about three to four times higher than that obtained with a single dose of the base or stearate (Fig. 26). Furthermore food does not appreciably alter the absorption of estolate, whereas erythromycin stearate is poorly absorbed if given with food (Griffith and Black, 1962; 1964; Bell, 1970; 1971).

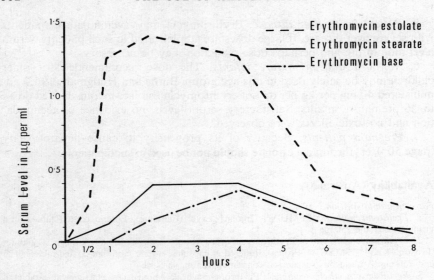

FIG. 26. Average serum concentrations in adults after oral administration of 250 mg erythromycin base, stearate and estolate. (Redrawn after Griffith and Black, 1962.)

The serum levels shown in Fig. 26 were obtained by using standard microbiological methods of assay. These assay methods unfortunately give spuriously high serum levels of active erythromycin when the estolate is used, because during incubation *in vitro* most of this ester hydrolyses to active erythromycin base. *In vivo* erythromycin estolate is only partially hydrolysed to active erythromycin base, and the estolate as such apparently has no antibacterial activity (Tardrew *et al.*, 1969). Using special chromatographic techniques at the Lilly Research Laboratories it has been estimated that 20–35 per cent of the total antibiotic in the blood appears as erythromycin base and the remainder as the estolate ester (Stephens *et al.*, 1969). On the basis of these figures higher serum levels of active erythromycin would still be obtained after ingestion of the estolate than after other oral erythromycin preparations. In addition these authors pointed out that erythromycin estolate in the blood may still be of value because later it may be hydrolysed to the active drug in the tissues. By contrast, Neaverson (1968), quoting unpublished data from Abbott Research Laboratories has claimed that as little as 10 per cent of absorbed erythromycin estolate may exist *in vivo* in the form of active erythromycin. Thus the controversy regarding the serum levels of active erythromycin attained after administration of the various oral erythromycins is not completely settled. Unfortunately this cannot at present be resolved by independent investigators, because the amount of erythromycin base in the serum after administration of estolate cannot be determined by current standard assay methods (Report, 1973).

Although it is generally accepted that the estolate form is better absorbed from the gastro-intestinal tract, it has the disadvantage of potential hepatotoxicity (page 505). Some authors have reported that clinical response with erythromycin estolate is about the same as that obtained with the stearate (Clapper *et al.*, 1960; Billow *et al.*, 1964), but this has not been confirmed by large scale controlled studies (Braun, 1969). In a more recent trial the estolate and stearate were compared for the treatment of 110 children with acute Strep. pyogenes throat infections (Ryan *et al.*, 1973). The disappearance of the pathogens from the pharynx was uniformly good with both preparations, but positive post-treatment cultures were more commonly obtained in the patients treated with the stearate. Overall there is little evidence of clinical superiority for the estolate, which has the clear disadvantage of hepatotoxicity (Report, 1973). Erythromycin estolate is not used at Fairfield Hospital.

4. Serum levels slightly at variance with those shown in Fig. 26 for erythromycin base and the stearate salt have been reported. The nature of the coating used for these tablets varies in commercial preparations, and this may influence the degree of absorption. Furthermore there is marked individual variation in the serum levels achieved after the administration of all forms of oral erythromycin (Clapper *et al.*, 1960; Griffith and Black, 1964; Lake and Bell, 1969).

5. *Parenteral erythromycin.* Satisfactory serum levels are achieved after parenteral erythromycin administration. After an intramuscular injection of 100 mg of erythromycin ethyl succinate in adults, the mean peak level after 1 h is 0·64 μg per ml; this level is maintained for nearly 6 h, and measurable serum concentrations persist for at least 12 h (Metzger *et al.*, 1959). Following a single intravenous injection of 200 mg of erythromycin lactobionate, the average serum level in adults is 3·0 μg per ml 1 h after the injection, and detectable levels persist for at least 6 h (Abott laboratories, 1966). If erythromycin lactobionate is given by continuous infusion at a rate of 1·0 g every 12 h, serum levels of about 4–6 μg per ml are maintained from 8 h onwards (Neaverson, 1976).

Excretion

URINE: Erythromycin is partly excreted in urine, and only about 2·5 per cent of an orally administered and 15 per cent of a parenterally administered dose is recoverable from the urine in the active form (Abbott laboratories, 1966). Urinary concentrations of the drug are usually low and variable. As renal excretion is not the main method of erythromycin elimination from the body, there is no significant accumulation of this drug in uraemic patients.

BILE: A considerable proportion of erythromycin is excreted in the bile, where high levels of the active drug are attained. Some erythromycin excreted in the bile is reabsorbed from the intestine.

INACTIVATION IN BODY: A large proportion of the erythromycin administered cannot be accounted for by combined renal and biliary excretion, and so a considerable amount appears to be inactivated in the body, probably in the liver (Garrod *et al.*, 1973).

Distribution of the Drug in Body

Erythromycin is widely distributed in the tissues, and is concentrated in the liver and spleen. It persists in the tissues for longer periods than in the serum.

The related macrolide antibiotic, spiramycin, is reported to produce even higher and better sustained tissue concentrations than erythromycin (page 519).

Adequate concentrations of erythromycin are found in pleural and ascitic fluids. The drug also enters middle ear exudates in sufficient concentration to inhibit the highly sensitive organisms Strep. pyogenes and Strep. pneumoniae, but not necessarily all strains of H. influenzae (Bass et al., 1971). Adequate levels of erythromycin are found in the tonsils after oral administration, the levels being higher after an estolate suspension than an ethyl succinate suspension (Ginsburg et al., 1976). Mean sputum levels of 2·6 μg per ml have been recorded when erythromycin lactobionate has been given by infusion in a dose of 1 g every 12 h (Neaverson, 1976). Erythromycin does not enter the cerebrospinal fluid in the absence of meningitis; however, as with many other antibiotics, the drug may be detectable in the CSF when the meninges are inflamed (Griffith and Black, 1970). Erythromycin crosses the placenta, but serum concentrations attained in the infant are considerably lower and less predictable than those in the mother (South et al., 1964; Philipson et al., 1973). The addition of 50 per cent serum has little effect on the minimum inhibitory concentrations of erythromycin indicating that its protein binding is low. It has been estimated that erythromycin is only 18 per cent protein bound (Kunin, 1967).

Mode of Action

Erythromycin interferes with bacterial protein synthesis at the ribosomes (Goldberg, 1965). This drug, similar to other macrolide antibiotics, becomes bound to the 50 S subunit of the ribosome. Chloramphenicol (page 434) and lincomycin (page 480) also become attached to this site (Weisblum, 1967). The exact stage of bacterial protein synthesis affected by erythromycin is not known with certainty, but it has been suggested that it may interfere with the 'translocation reaction' (page 434), which is catalysed by an enzyme, translocase (Cundliffe and McQuillen, 1967). During this reaction the growing peptide chain with its t-RNA moves from the 'acceptor site' to the 'donor site' on the ribosome. Erythromycin probably binds to the donor site, and, by competing for this site of attachment, prevents translocation of the peptide chain from the acceptor to the donor site (Oleinick and Corcoran, 1969).

It is probable that Gram-negative bacilli are resistant to erythromycin because it cannot penetrate their cell walls. Stable L-forms of Proteus mirabilis, which have no cell walls, are very susceptible to erythromycin (Guze and Kalmanson, 1964; Gutman et al., 1967). Resistant mutants of bacteria usually sensitive to erythromycin probably owe their resistance to some change in their ribosomal structure (Oleinick and Corcoran, 1969), but some genetic determinants of inducible resistance appear to be localized on plasmids (Weisblum et al., 1971) (see page 422).

Erythromycin is often classed as a 'bacteristatic' drug, but in vitro it is bacteristatic in low concentrations, and bactericidal in high concentrations (Garrod and Waterworth, 1962). This again illustrates that the differentiation between 'cidal' and 'static' antibiotics is only relative (Crofton, 1969) (see also page 466).

Toxicity

1. *Gastro-intestinal side-effects*. Symptoms such as nausea, vomiting and diarrhoea are fairly frequently encountered with oral erythromycin, but these are only occasionally severe.

2. *Hepatotoxicity*. This occurs after administration of erythromycin estolate, but not after other erythromycin preparations (Editorial, 1961; Masel, 1962; Sherlock, 1968; Braun, 1969). It appears that the propionyl ester linkage at the 2' position confers this property on the estolate, and cross-sensitivity with other erythromycin preparations does not occur (Tolman *et al.*, 1974). The administration of an oleandomycin ester, triacetyloleandomycin, also causes this complication (page 519). Jaundice usually occurs about ten to twelve days after starting treatment, but it may occur within one or two days in patients who have previously experienced the drug (Robinson, 1961; Gilbert, 1962; Braun, 1969). Another major symptom in these patients may be severe abdominal pain, which may lead to an erroneous diagnosis of cholelithiasis (Oliver *et al.*, 1973). Other symptoms include fever and pruritus and a rash may occasionally occur. Jaundice may be clinical or subclinical and hepatic enlargement is usually present. Eosinophilia is common, liver function tests usually indicate cholestasis, and together with other evidence this suggests that this jaundice is probably due to 'hypersensitivity cholestasis'. Circulating lymphocytes sensitized to erythromycin estolate have been detected in a patient who developed jaundice following its use (Cooksley and Powell, 1977). Many authors have also reported elevated serum asparate aminotransferase (SGOT) levels, and for this reason erythromycin estolate jaundice has often been considered to be of 'mixed origin', consisting of both a hypersensitivity cholestasis and a variable amount of liver cell necrosis (McKenzie and Doyle, 1966). However, liver histology usually reveals a picture of intrahepatic cholestasis without liver cell necrosis (Braun, 1969), and the reported SGOT elevations may not be due to liver cell necrosis. Spurious elevation of colorimetrically estimated SGOT can occur in patients taking erythromycin estolate. When the enzyme is measured by a specific enzymatic method, SGOT elevation is not detected, suggesting that some unidentified metabolite of this drug interferes with the colorimetric assay (Sabath *et al.*, 1968c).

The jaundice and other symptoms usually subside rapidly when the drug is stopped, but occasionally jaundice may persist for weeks, and in one case reported by Brown (1963) it persisted for about three months. In such cases the persistence of jaundice may lead to the consideration of laparotomy. There have been no deaths associated with erythromycin estolate jaundice, and the subsequent development of chronic liver disease has not been described. Many cases of erythromycin estolate jaundice have been reported, but the exact frequency of this complication is not known. The manufacturers claimed that only 33 cases had been reported to them during a period in which an estimated 15 million courses of erythromycin estolate had been distributed (Kohlstaedt, 1961). By contrast Ticktin and Robinson (1963) demonstrated some hepatic dysfunction in 15 of 93 patients treated for 14 days or longer with erythromycin estolate, and two of these patients developed jaundice. More recently McCormack *et al.* (1977) administered the estolate to pregnant patients and found a subclinical rise of serum asparate aminotransferase

(SGOT) as estimated by a fluorometic method, in 9·9 per cent. They estimated that 10–15 per cent of pregnant women given this drug for three weeks or longer would develop this subclinical reversible hepatotoxicity.

3. *Skin rashes* may occur as a single manifestation, but are rare.

4. *Ototoxicity*. Tinnitus and transient deafness have been described in a small number of patients, mainly in association with the intravenous administration of erythromycin lactobionate (Mintz *et al.*, 1973; Quinnan and McCabe, 1978), but also after oral administration (Eckman *et al.*, 1975; van Marion *et al.*, 1978). In a number of these patients renal failure and/or liver damage may have predisposed to high serum levels of erythromycin (Quinnan and McCabe, 1978; van Marion *et al.*, 1978).

5. Intramuscular erythromycin is painful and local irritation and sterile abscess formation may occur. Intravenous erythromycin is usually well tolerated. In general, apart from the special problem of hepatotoxicity associated with the estolate, erythromycin is a safe non-toxic drug.

Clinical Uses of the Drug

1. *Streptococcal and pneumococcal infections*. Erythromycin is an effective alternative to penicillin G for the treatment of many of these infections in penicillin-allergic patients. Streptococcal tonsillitis, scarlet fever and erysipelas can be successfully treated by erythromycin. Several studies have shown that erythromycin estolate given twice-daily is just as effective for streptococcal tonsillitis as when given six- or eight-hourly, provided that the same total daily dose is used (Breese *et al.*, 1974; Ginsburg and Eichenwald, 1976). A daily dose as low as 20 mg per kg of the estolate given in two divided doses for 10 days results in a high eradication rate of Strep. pyogenes from the throat (Derrick and Dillon, 1976).

The use of large doses of erythromycin intravenously is worth considering for the treatment of Strep. viridans or Strep. faecalis endocarditis, when it is impossible to use penicillin G or ampicillin. However in this disease one of the cephalosporins (page 213) may be a more suitable alternative for treatment of Strep. viridans infections, and vancomycin (page 650) for Strep. faecalis infections. The use of erythromycin alone, even in high doses, is unlikely to succeed in most cases of bacterial endocarditis and combination with another antibiotic is preferable. *In vitro* tests for combined antibiotic bactericidal action against the particular infecting strain may be helpful in the selection of the best antibiotic combination for the treatment of these severe infections (Garrod and Waterworth, 1962; Peard *et al.*, 1970). Erythromycin is recommended in certain situations for the prevention of bacterial endocarditis by the American Heart Association (Kaplan *et al.*, 1977). For prophylaxis against endocarditis by the viridans group of streptococci during dental procedures or surgical procedures and instrumentation of the upper respiratory tract, it is recommended for penicillin-allergic patients. It can be given alone in an oral dose of 1·0 g (children 20 mg per kg) 1·5 h to 2 h prior to the procedure, and then 0·5 g (children 10 mg per kg) every 6 h for eight doses. It can also be combined with vancomycin for this purpose; it is given after a vancomycin infusion (page 650), in a dose of 0·5 g every 6 h for eight doses.

Erythromycin is also an effective alternative to penicillin G for the treatment of pneumococcal pneumonia. Erythromycin can also be effective for severe infections such as pneumococcal meningitis, if it is used in large doses (2–6 g daily) intravenously, but chloramphenicol is preferable for this disease if penicillin G is contraindicated.

2. *Rheumatic fever chemoprophylaxis*. Erythromycin is the most suitable alternative to penicillin for this purpose (Ginsburg and Eichenwald, 1976). Suitable dosage is a single daily dose of 200 mg for children weighing more than 80 pounds (approximately 36·4 kg) and 100 mg for those weighing less than 80 pounds. This chemoprophylaxis has been used continuously for over four years without side-effects or the development of resistant strains of Strep. pyogenes.

Erythromycin-resistant strains of Strep. viridans often appear in the pharynx of patients receiving long-term erythromycin prophylaxis. In patients with rheumatic heart disease, who require temporary protection against endocarditis at the time of dental procedures, etc., treatment by an unrelated antibiotic such as cephaloridine is indicated. Lincomycin is not a suitable antibiotic for this purpose, as erythromycin-resistant Strep. viridans strains are also often lincomycin-resistant (Sprunt *et al.*, 1970).

3. *Bronchitis, otitis media and sinusitis*. Pneumococci and H. influenzae are the common pathogens in bacterial bronchitis and erythromycin is one of several effective drugs for the treatment of acute infections (*see also* pages 115, 621). Erythromycin is also an effective drug for the treatment of otitis media caused by pneumococci or Strep. pyogenes, but there is some doubt about its efficacy if this infection is caused by H. influenzae (Ginsburg and Eichenwald, 1976). This may be of particular significance if oral preparations other than the estolate are used, because they produce lower levels of the drug in the middle ear than the estolate. Triple sulphonamides (page 658) have been used together with erythromycin estolate in an attempt to provide a more adequate treatment for H. influenzae otitis media. The results of various studies comparing the efficacy of this regimen to erythromycin estolate alone have been contradictory (Ginsburg and Eichenwald, 1976). Overall erythromycin seems to be a suitable drug for the treatment of otitis media pending the result of bacteriological tests. Erythromycin penetrates well into the sinuses where its concentrations exceed the MIC's for Strep. pyogenes and pneumococci (Kalm *et al.*, 1975). These authors found that sinusitis responded well to erythromycin with the exception of those cases due to H. influenzae; this was possibly because the concentration of the drug in the sinuses only reached the MIC of 15–30 per cent of the H. influenzae strains examined.

4. *Staphylococcal infections*. Severe staphylococcal infections such as septiaemia can be successfully treated by large doses of intravenous erythromycin (Shoemaker and Yow, 1954), but nowadays other drugs are preferred for these infections. Prolonged chemotherapy is often necessary for patients with severe disseminated staphylococcal infections, particularly those with extensive osteomyelitis (Bennett and Kucers, 1970), and oral erythromycin is suitable for the extended treatment, though alternatives such as isoxazolyl penicillins (page 88) and sodium fusidate (page 466) are available. Erythromycin is also useful for treatment of staphylococcal diseases such as boils, carbuncles and wound infections. An oral dose of 1·0 g daily given for seven days is effective in eradicating staphylococci from healthy nasal carriers (Wilson *et al.*, 1977).

5. *Mycoplasma pneumonia.* Erythromycin and the tetracyclines (page 623) are both effective for the treatment of this disease (Foy *et al.*, 1970; Shames *et al.*, 1970; Wenzel *et al.*, 1976). Although treatment by either of these drugs reduces the length of illness, mycoplasmas may often persist in respiratory tract secretions both during and after therapy (Smith *et al.*, 1967; Shames *et al.*, 1970).

6. *Pertussis.* Erythromycin may prevent whooping cough in exposed susceptible individuals, and also may attenuate the illness if given early in the course of the disease (Linnemann *et al.*, 1975; Altemeier and Ayoub, 1977). However, once the paroxysmal stage is reached, erythromycin, like other antibiotics, does not influence the natural course of the illness. It may be useful in preventing secondary bacterial infection, and it also eliminates pertussis organisms from the nasopharynx, presumably rendering the patients non-infectious (Bass *et al.*, 1969; Nelson, 1969; Leading article 1970).

7. *Diphtheria.* Erythromycin is active against C. diphtheriae, but the administration of specific diphtheria antitoxin is essential for treatment of the disease itself. Many studies have indicated that erythromycin is effective in eliminating C. diphtheriae from carriers (Ginsburg and Eichenwald, 1976). Miller *et al.* (1974), however, found a 21 per cent relapse rate two weeks after a six-day course of treatment with erythromycin, but this may have been due to reinfection. Erythromycin given orally for seven days is somewhat more effective than treatment with benzathine penicillin (page 36) for the eradication of C. diphtheriae from nasopharyngeal carriers (Ginsburg and Eichenwald, 1976).

8. *Gas gangrene.* Erythromycin in large doses intravenously is an effective alternative to penicillin G for the treatment of this disease in penicillin-allergic patients. Occasionally strains of Cl. perfringens may be resistant to erythromycin. In such cases a cephalosporin (page 215), chloramphenicol (page 426) or metronidazole (page 773) would be indicated.

9. *Urinary tract infections.* Erythromycin is useful for these infections caused by Strep. faecalis and it is also quite effective for those due to Esch. coli and other Gram-negative bacilli, provided the urine is made alkaline (Sabath *et al.*, 1968a and b; Zinner *et al.*, 1970; 1971). These authors used erythromycin estolate, and the urine of their patients was rendered alkaline by the administration of either sodium bicarbonate or acetazolamine. However, other drugs are usually preferred for the treatment of urinary tract infections. Theoretically, erythromycin would not be effective for the treatment of prostatitis because of the acidity of prostatic tissue (*see* page 699).

Erythromycin may be a useful adjunct for treatment of relapsing urinary tract infections, in which bacterial L-forms play a role. The L-forms of Gram-negative bacilli such as Esch. coli or Pr. mirabilis are cell-wall deficient and spherical, and have a different antibiotic sensitivity pattern. The normal organism may be ampicillin-sensitive, but erythromycin-resistant, whilst the L-forms may be ampicillin-resistant and erythromycin-sensitive. In these cases a combination of ampicillin and erythromycin may eradicate an infection, which has repeatedly relapsed after ampicillin therapy alone (Guze and Kalmanson, 1964; Gutman *et al.*, 1967; Gnarpe, 1970). Alkalinization of urine and increased diuresis may also be helpful in such cases (Gnarpe, 1974).

10. *Gonorrhoea.* Erythromycin has been used as an alternative to penicillin G in this disease. However, the results of its use for treatment of penicillin-

allergic pregnant patients have been poorer than those obtained with other drugs (Willcox, 1977). In addition, when erythromycin (both estolate and base) was used in a trial to treat men with gonococcal urethritis (total of 9·0 g given over four days), there was a failure rate of 23–24 per cent (Brown *et al.*, 1977). Erythromycin can no longer be regarded as an effective drug for the treatment of gonorrhoea in penicillin-allergic patients; other drugs such as co-trimoxazole (page 710) or kanamycin (page 319) for non-pregnant patients, and perhaps cefuroxime (page 286) for pregnant patients are preferable (Willcox, 1977). Spectinomycin (page 589) should be restricted for the treatment of gonorrhoea due to beta-lactamase producing strains (page 8).

11. *Non-specific urethritis.* Tetracyclines are usually preferred for infection due to Chlamydia trachomatis (*see* page 626), but erythromycin in a dose of 0·5 g twelve-hourly for two weeks is also effective (Annotation, 1978). Erythromycin is also effective against Ureaplasma urealyticum (Mycoplasma T-strains) which may also cause non-specific urethritis (page 627).

12. *Syphilis.* Erythromycin, given in an adult dose of 3–4 g daily for at least 8–10 days is an effective 'second-choice' drug to penicillin G for the treatment of early syphilis in penicillin-allergic patients (Montgomery and Knox, 1959; Schroeter *et al.*, 1972). Currently in the United States a dose of 2·0 g daily for 15 days is recommended (Center for Disease Control, 1976). Little clinical data are available about the use of erythromycin in syphilis of more than one year duration. Erythromycin crosses the placenta, but fetal serum concentrations attained are lower than those in maternal blood at the time (page 504). The drug may be effective for treatment of syphilis during pregnancy (George, 1971), but cephaloridine (page 215) is another effective alternative for penicillin-allergic patients (Holder and Knox, 1972). Currently in the United States erythromycin is recommended for pregnant patients who are allergic to penicillin; if the disease is greater than one year duration, a dose of erythromycin (not estolate, *see* page 501 of 0·5 g four times a day for 30 days is advocated (Center for Disease Control, 1976). South *et al.* (1964) described a woman in the sixth month of pregnancy, who was treated for secondary syphilis with erythromycin estolate in a dose of 0·5 g three times a day for only ten days. Her syphilis was apparently cured, but she bore an infant with severe congenital disease.

13. *Actinomycosis.* Erythromycin or the tetracylines may be the best alternatives to penicillin G for the treatment of this disease in penicillin-allergic patients (Holmberg *et al.*, 1977).

14. *Pneumonia due to the Legionnaires' disease bacterium.* Clinical experience and the results of laboratory studies (page 498) indicate that erythromycin is one of the drugs of choice for this disease. A combination of rifampicin (page 575) and erythromycin may be justified for the treatment of seriously ill patients, who are not responding to erythromycin alone (Fraser *et al.*, 1978).

15. *Erythrasma.* This infection caused by Corynebacterium minutissimum causes a superficial dermatitis involving intertriginous areas, which may resemble a fungal infection. Erythrasma responds to systemic treatment with erythromycin (Sarkany *et al.*, 1961; Knox *et al.*, 1964; Kingery, 1965; Bowyer and McColl, 1966).

16. *Acne.* Erythromycin has been used for this disease on the same basis as

510   THE USE OF ANTIBIOTICS

the tetracyclines (page 629) (Ginsburg and Eichenwald, 1976).

17. *Campylobacter enteritis*. Erythromycin is apparently useful for the treatment of this disease, although milder cases respond equally well to symptomatic measures alone. For Campylobacter septicaemia, gentamicin (page 345) is regarded as the drug of choice (Leading article, 1978).

18. *Relapsing fever*. A single oral dose of 0·5 g erythromycin (or tetracycline) is considered optimal therapy for louse-borne relapsing fever due to Borrelia recurrentis (Butler *et al.*, 1978). Erythromycin is preferable to tetracycline for pregnant patients and children. Both of these drug regimens produce the Jarisch-Herxheimer reaction but the associated hypotension can be minimized by intravenous fluids.

REFERENCES

Abbot Laboratories (1966), *Erythromycin. A Review of Its Properties and Clinical Status*, Abbott Laboratories, Scientific Divisions North Chicago, Illinois.

Altemeier, W. A. III and Ayoub, E. M. (1977), 'Erythromycin prophylaxis for pertussis', *Pediatrics*, **59**, 623.

Annotation (1978), 'Treatment of Chlamydia trachomatis infections', *Lancet*, **1**, 192.

Anthony, B. F. and Concepcion, N. F. (1975), 'Group B streptococcus in a general hospital', *J. Infect. Dis.*, **132**, 561.

Bach, M. C., Sabath, L. D. and Finland, M. (1973), 'Susceptibility of Nocardia asteroides to 45 antimicrobial agents *in vitro*', *Antimicrob. Ag. Chemother.*, **3**, 1.

Bass, J. W., Klenk, E. L., Kotheimer, J. B., Linnemann, C. C. and Smith, M. H. D. (1969), 'Antimicrobial treatment of pertussis', *J. Pediatrics*, **75**, 768.

Bass, J. W., Steele, R. W., Wiebe, R. A. and Dierdorff, E. P. (1971), 'Erythromycin concentrations in middle ear exudates', *Pediatrics*, **48**, 417.

Bell, S. M. (1970), 'Supervision of antibiotic treatment—an important medical responsibility', *Aspects of Infection. Proc. Symp. Auckland, Sydney and Melbourne*, p. 107.

Bell, S. M. (1971), 'A comparison of absorption after oral administration of erythromycin estolate and erythromycin stearate', *Med. J. Aust.*, **2**, 1280.

Bennett, N. McK. and Kucers, A. (1970), 'Staphylococcal and Gram-negative septicaemia', *Aspects of Infection. Proc. Symp. Auckland, Sydney and Melbourne*, p. 123.

Billow, B. W., Thompson, E. A., Stern, A. and Florio, A. (1964), 'A clinical study of erythromycin: A comparative evaluation of several salts', *Curr. Ther. Res.*, **6**, 381.

Bowyer, A. and McColl, I. (1966), 'The role of erythromycin in pruritus ani', *Lancet*, **2**, 572.

Braun, P. (1969), 'Editorial: Hepatotoxicity of erythromycin', *J. Infect. Dis.*, **119**, 300.

Brause, B. D., Borges, J. S. and Roberts, R. B. (1976), 'Relative efficacy of clindamycin, erythromycin and penicillin in treatment of Treponema pallidum in skin syphilomas of rabbits', *J. Infect. Dis.*, **134**, 93.

Breese, B. B., Disney, F. A., Talpey, W., Green, J. L. and Tobin, J. (1974), 'Streptococcal infections in children. Comparison of the therapeutic effectiveness of erythromycin administered twice daily with erythromycin, penicillin phenoxymethyl, and clindamycin administered three times daily', *Am. J. Dis., Child.*, **128**, 457.

Brown, A. R. (1963), 'Two cases of untoward reaction after "Ilosone"', *Brit. med. J.*, **2**, 913.

Brown, S. T., Pedersen, A. H. B. and Holmes, K. K. (1977), 'Comparison of erythromycin base and estolate in gonococcal urethritis', *JAMA*, **238**, 1371.

Burns, L. and Hodgman, J. (1963), 'Studies of prematures, given erythromycin estolate', *Amer. J. Dis. Child.*, **106,** 280.

Butler, T., Jones, P. K. and Wallace, C. K. (1978), 'Borrelia recurrentis infection: Single-dose antibiotic regimens and management of the Jarisch-Herxheimer reaction', *J. Infect. Dis.*, **137,** 573.

Center for Disease Control (1976), 'Syphilis—CDC recommended treatment schedules, 1976, *Morbidity and Mortality Weekly Report*, **25,** 101.

Centre for Disease Control (1977a), 'Follow-up on Legionnaires' disease', *Morbidity and Mortality Weekly Report*, **26,** 111.

Center for Disease Control (1977b), 'Follow-up on Legionnaires' disease—Pennsylvania', *Morbidity and Mortality Weekly Report*, **26,** 152.

Center for Disease Control (1977c), 'Multiple-antibiotic resistance of pneumococci—South Africa', *Morbidity and Mortality Weekly Report*, **26,** 285.

Center for Disease Control (1978), 'Penicillinase-(beta-lactamase-) producing Neisseria gonorrhoeae-worldwide', *Morbidity and Mortality Weekly Report*, **27,** 10.

Champion, L. A. A., Wald, E. R., Luddy, R. E. and Schwartz, A. D. (1978), 'Streptococcus pneumoniae resistant to erythromycin and clindamycin', *J. Pediatrics*, **92,** 505.

Chow, A. W., Patten, V. and Bednorz, D. (1978), 'Susceptibility of Campylobacter fetus to twenty-two antimicrobial agents', *Antimicrob. Ag. Chemother.*, **13,** 416.

Clapper, W. E., Mostyn, M. and Meade, G. M. (1960), 'An evaluation of erythromycin stearate and propionyl erythromycin in normal and hospitalized subjects', *Antibiot. Med. Clin. Ther.*, **7,** 91.

Cooksley, W. G. E. and Powell, L. W. (1977), 'Erythromycin jaundice: Diagnosis by an *in vitro* challenge test', *Aust. N.Z. J. Med.*, **7,** 291.

Cooper, R. G., Rischbieth, H. G. and Vesey, B. (1968), 'Erythromycin-resistant pneumococcus', *Med. J. Aust.*, **1,** 1131.

Crofton, J. (1969), 'Some principles in the chemotherapy of bacterial infections', *Brit. med. J.*, **2,** 137 and 209.

Csonka, G. W. and Spitzer, R. J. (1969), 'Lincomycin, non-gonococcal urethritis, and mycoplasmata', *Brit. J. vener. Dis.*, **45,** 52.

Cundliffe, E. and McQuillen, K. (1967), 'Bacterial protein synthesis: The effect of antibiotics', *J. Mol. Biol.*, **30,** 137.

Derrick, C. W. and Dillon, H. C. (1976), 'Erythromycin therapy for Streptococcal pharyngitis', *Am. J. Dis., Child.*, **130,** 175.

Dixon, J. M. S. (1967), 'Pneumococcus resistant to erythromycin and lincomycin', *Lancet*, **1,** 573.

Dixon, J. M. S. (1968), 'Group A streptococcus resistant to erythromycin and lincomycin', *Can. Med. Assoc. J.*, **9,** 1093.

Dixon, J. M. S. and Lipinski, A. E. (1972), 'Resistance of Group A beta-hemolyic streptococci to lincomycin and erythromycin', *Antimicrob. Ag. Chemother.*, **1,** 333.

Dixon, J. M. S. and Lipinski, A. E. (1974), 'Infections with beta-hemolytic streptococcus resistant to lincomycin and erythromycin and observations on zonal-pattern resistance to lincomycin', *J. Infect. Dis.*, **130,** 351.

Eckman, M. R., Johnson, T. and Riess, R. (1975), 'Partial deafness after erythromycin', *New Engl. J. Med.*, **292,** 649.

Editorial (1961), 'Hepatosensitivity associated with erythromycin propionate lauryl sulphate', *JAMA*, **178,** 58.

Ford, D. K. and Smith, J. R. (1974), 'Non-specific urethritis associated with a tetracycline-resistant T-mycoplasma', *Brit. J. vener, Dis.*, **50,** 373.

Foy, H. M., Kenny, G. E., McMahan, R., Mansy, A. M. and Grayson, J. T. (1970), 'Mycoplasma pneumoniae pneumonia in an urban area', *JAMA*, **214,** 1666.

Fraser, D. W., Wachsmuth, I. K., Bopp, C., Feeley, J. C. and Tsai, T. F. (1978), 'Antibiotic treatment of guinea-pigs infected with agent of Legionnaires' disease', *Lancet*, **1,** 175.

Garrod, L. P. (1957), 'The erythromycin group of antibiotics', *Brit. med. J.*, **2**, 57.

Garrod, L. P. and Waterworth, P. M. (1962), 'Methods of testing combined antibiotic bactericidal action and the significance of the results', *J. clin. Path.*, **15**, 328.

Garrod, L. P., Lambert, H. P. and O'Grady, F. (1973), *Antibiotic and Chemotherapy*, 4th edn. Churchill Livingstone, Edinburgh and London, p. 173.

George, R. P., Jr. (1971), 'Therapy for syphilis during pregnancy', *New Engl. J. Med.*, **284**, 1271.

Gilbert, F. I. (1962), 'Cholestatic hepatitis caused by esters of erythromycin and oleandomycin', *JAMA*, **182**, 1048.

Ginsburg, C. M. and Eichenwald, H. F. (1976), 'Erythromycin: A review of its uses in pediatric practice', *J. Pediatrics*, **89**, 872.

Ginsburg, C. M., McCracken, G. H., Jr. and Culbertson, M. C., Jr. (1976), 'Concentrations of erythromycin in serum and tonsil: Comparison of the estolate and ethyl succinate suspensions', *J. Pediatrics*, **89**, 1011.

Gnarpe, H. (1974), 'Erythromycin, ampicillin, alkalization and increased diuresis in treatment of human L-phase urinary tract infections', *Scand. J. Infect. Dis.*, **6**, 75.

Gnarpe, H. (1970), 'Spheroplast infections of the urinary tract', *Scand J. Infect. Dis.*, **2**, 59.

Goldberg, I. H. (1965), 'Mode of action of antibiotics—II. Drugs affecting nucleic acid and protein synthesis', *Amer. J. Med.*, **39**, 722.

Gorbach, S. L. and Bartlett, J. G. (1974), 'Anaerobic infections (third of three parts)', *New Engl. J. Med.*, **290**, 1289.

Griffith, R. S. and Black, H. R. (1962), 'A comparison of blood levels after oral administration of erythromycin and erythromycin estolate', *Antibiot. Chemother.*, **12**, 398.

Griffith, R. S. and Black, H. R. (1964), 'Comparison of the blood levels obtained after single and mutliple doses of erythromycin estolate and erythromycin stearate', *Amer. J. Med. Sci.*, **247**, 69.

Griffith, R. S. and Black, H. R. (1970), 'Erythromycin', *Med. Clin. North America*, **54**, 1199.

Gutman, L., Schaller, J. and Wedgwood, R. J. (1967), 'Bacterial L-forms in relapsing urinary-tract infection', *Lancet*, **1**, 464.

Guze, L. B. and Kalmanson, G. M. (1964), 'Action of erythromycin on "protoplasts *in vivo*"', *Science*, **146**, 1299.

Hassam, Z. A., Shaw, E. J. and Shooter, R. A. (1978), 'Changes in antibiotic sensitivity in strains of Stapylococcus aureus, 1952–78', *Brit. med. J.*, **2**, 536.

Holder, W R. and Knox, J. M. (1972), 'Syphilis in pregnancy', *Med. Clin. North Amer.*, **56**, 1151.

Holmberg, K., Nord, C. -E. and Dornbusch, K. (1977), 'Antimicrobial *in vitro* susceptibility of Actinomyces israelii and Arachnia propionica', *Scand. J. Infect. Dis.*, **9**, 40.

Jao, R. L. and Finland, M. (1967), 'Susceptibility of Mycoplasma pneumoniae to 21 antibiotics *in vitro*', *Amer. J. Med. Sci.*, **253**, 639.

Jellard, C. H. and Lipinski, A. E. (1973), 'Corynebacterium diptheriae resistant to erythromycin and lincomycin', *Lancet*, **1**, 156.

Kalm, O., Kamme, C., Bergström, B., Löfkvist, T. and Norman, O. (1975), 'Erythromycin stearate in acute maxillary sinusitis', *Scand. J. Infect. Dis.*, **7**, 209.

Kaplan, E. L., Anthony, B. F., Bisno, A., Durack, D., Houser, H., Millard, H. D., Sanford, J., Schulman, S. T., Stillerman, M., Taranta, A. and Wenger, N. (1977), 'Prevention of bacterial endocarditis', *Circulation*, **56**, 139A.

Kingery, F. A. J. (1965), 'Imitators of athlete's foot', *JAMA*, **193**, 181.

Kislak, J. W., Razavi, L. M. B., Daly, A. K. and Finland, M. (1965), 'Susceptibility of pneumococci to nine antibiotics', *Amer. J. Med. Sci.*, **250**, 261.

Kislak, J. W. (1967), 'Type 6 pneumococcus resistant to erythromycin and lincomycin', *New Engl. J. Med.*, **276**, 852.

Knox, J. M., Richardson, J. B. and Montes, L. F. (1964), 'Superficial fungus diseases. Diagnosis and treatment', *Ind. Med. and Surgery*, **33**, 813.

Kohlstaedt, K. G. (1961), 'Propionyl erythromycin ester lauryl sulfate and jaundice', *JAMA*, **178**, 89.

Kunin, C. M. (1967), 'A guide to use of antibiotics in patients with renal disease', *Ann. Intern. Med.*, **67**, 151.

Kuo, C.-C., Wang, S.-P. and Grayston, J. T. (1977), 'Antimicrobial activity of several antibiotics and a sulfonamide against Chlamydia trachomatis organisms in cell culture', *Antimicrob. Ag. Chemother.*, **12**, 80.

Lacey, R. W. (1977), 'Lack of evidence for mutation to erythromycin resistance in clinical strains of Staphylococcus aureus', *J. clin. Path.*, **30**, 602.

Lake, B. and Bell, S. M. (1969), 'Variations in absorption of erythromycin', *Med. J. Aust.*, **1**, 449.

Leading Article (1970), 'Treatment of whooping-cough', *Brit. med. J.*, **2**, 619.

Leading Article (1978), 'Campylobacter enteritis', *Lancet*, **2**, 135.

Lee, E. L., Robinson, M. J., Thong, M. L., Puthucheary, S. D., Ong, T. H. and Ng, K. K. (1977), 'Intraventricular chemotherapy in neonatal meningitis', *J. Pediatrics*, **91**, 991.

Lee, C. K., Bowie, W. R. and Alexander, E. R. (1978), '*In vitro* assays of the efficacy of antimicrobial agents in controlling Chlamydia trachomatis propagation', *Antimicrob. Ag. Chemother.*, **13**, 441.

Leng, B., Meyers, B. R., Hirschman, S. Z. and Keusch, G. T. (1975), 'Susceptibilities of Gram-negative bacteria to combinations of antimicrobial agents *in vitro*', *Antimicrob. Ag. Chemother.*, **8**, 164.

Lewis, V. J., Thacker, W. L., Shepard, C. C. and McDade, J. E. (1978), '*In vivo* susceptibility of the Legionnaires' disease bacterium to ten antimicrobial agents', *Antimicrob. Ag. Chemother.*, **13**, 419.

Linnemann, C. C., Jr., Ramundo, N., Perlstein, P. H., Minton, S. D. and Englender, G. S. (1975), 'Use of pertussis vaccine in an epidemic involving hospital staff', *Lancet*, **2**, 540.

Marder, H. P. and Kayser, F. H. (1977), 'Transferable plasmids mediating multiple-antibiotic resistance in Streptococcus faecalis subsp. liquefaciens', *Antimicrob. Ag. Chemother.*, **12**, 261.

Masel, M. A. (1962), 'Erythromycin hepato-sensitivity: A preliminary report of two cases', *Med. J. Aust.*, **1**, 560.

McCormack, W. M., George, H., Donner, A., Kodgis, L. F., Alpert, S., Lowe, E. W. and Kass, E. H. (1977), 'Hepatotoxicity of erythromycin estolate during pregnancy', *Antimicrob. Ag. Chemother.*, **12**, 630.

McGuire, J. M., Bunch, R. L., Anderson, R. C., Boaz, H. E., Flynn, E. H., Powell, E. H. and Smith, J. W. (1952), '"Ilotycin", a new antibiotic', *Antibiot. Chemother.*, **2**, 281; quoted by Abbott Laboratories (1966).

McKenzie, I. and Doyle, A. (1966), 'Two cases of jaundice following "Ilosone"', *Med. J. Aust.*, **1**, 349.

Metzger, W. I., Jenkins, C. J., Jr., Harris, C. J., Broccolo, E. A. and Ade, R. D. (1959), 'Laboratory and clinical studies of intramuscular erythromycin', *Antibot. Annual*—1959–1959, p. 383.

Miller, L. W., Bickham, S., Jones, W. L., Heather, C. D. and Morris, R. H. (1974), 'Diphtheria carriers and the effect of erythromycin therapy', *Antimicrob. Ag. Chemother.*, **6**, 166.

Mintz, U., Amir, J., Pinkhas, J. and de Vries, A. (1973), 'Transient perceptive deafness due to erythromycin lactobionate', *JAMA*, **225**, 1122.

Molavi, A. and Weinstein, L. (1971), '*In vitro* activity of erythromycin against atypical mycobacteria', *J. Infect. Dis.*, **123**, 216.

Montgomery, C. H. and Knox, J. M. (1959), 'Antibiotics other than penicillin in the treatment of syphilis', *New Engl. J. Med.*, **261,** 277.

Neaverson, M. A. (1968), 'Erythromycin estolate', *Med. J. Aust.*, **1,** 741.

Neaverson, M. A. (1976), 'Intravenous administration of erythromycin: Serum, sputum and urine levels', *Curr. Med. Res. Opin.*, **4,** 359.

Nelson, J. D. (1969), 'Antibiotic treatment of pertussis', *Pediatrics*, **44,** 474.

Niitu, Y., Hasegawa, S., Suetake, T., Kubota, H., Komatsu, S. and Horikawa, M. (1970), 'Resistance of Mycoplasma pneumoniae to erythromycin and other antibiotics', *J. Pediatrics*, **76,** 438.

Niitu, Y., Hasegawa, S. and Kibota, H. (1974), '*In vitro* development of resistance to erythromycin, other macrolide antibiotics, and lincomycin in Mycoplasma pneumoniae', *Antimicrob. Ag. Chemother.*, **5,** 513.

Okubadejo, O. A., Green, P. J. and Payne, D. J. H. (1973), 'Bacteroides in the blood', *Lancet*, **1,** 147.

Oleinick, N. L. and Corcoran, J. W. (1969), 'Two types of binding of erythromycin to ribosomes from antibiotic-sensitive and -resistant Bacillus subtilis 168', *J. Biol. Chem.*, **244,** 727.

Oliver, L. E., Iser, J. H., Stening, G. F. and Smallwood, R. A. (1973), '"Biliary colic" and ilosone', *Med. J. Aust.*, **1,** 1148.

Peard, M. C., Fleck, D. G., Garrod, L. P. and Waterworth, P. M. (1970), 'Combined rifampicin and erythromycin for bacterial endocarditis', *Brit. med. J.*, **4,** 410.

Philipson, A., Sabath, L. D. and Charles, D. (1973), 'Transplacental passage of erythromycin and clindamycin', *New Engl. J. Med.*, **288,** 1219.

Quinnan, G. V., Jr. and McCabe, W. R. (1978), 'Ototoxicity of erythromycin', *Lancet*, **1,** 1160.

Report from the Australian Drug Evaluation Committee (1973), 'The erythromycins', *Med. J. Aust.*, **2,** 192.

Report of a WHO Scientific Group (1978), 'Neisseria gonorrhoeae and gonococcal infections', *Wld. Hlth. Org. techn. Rep. Ser.*, No. **616,** p. 99.

Robinson, M. M. (1961), 'Antibiotics increase incidence of hepatitis', *JAMA*, **178,** 89.

Ryan, D. C., Dreher, G. H. and Hurst, J. A. (1973), 'Estolate and stearate forms of erythromycin in the treatment of acute beta haemolytic streptococcal pharyngitis', *Med. J. Aust.*, **1,** 20.

Sabath, L. D., Lorian, V., Gerstein, D., Loder, P. B. and Finland, M. (1968a), 'Enhancing effect of alkalinization of the medium on the activity of erythromycin against Gram-negative bacteria', *Appl. Microbial.*, **16,** 1288.

Sabath, L. D., Gerstein, D. A., Loder, P. B. and Finland, M. (1968b), 'Excretion of erythromycin and its enhanced activity in urine against Gram-negative bacilli with alkalinization', *J. Lab. Clin. Med.*, **72,** 916.

Sabath, L. D., Gerstein, D. A. and Finland, M. (1968c), 'Serum glutamic oxalacetic transaminase. False elevations during administration of erythromycin', *New Engl. J. Med.*, **279,** 1137.

Sanders, E., Foster, M. T. and Scott, D. (1968), 'Group A beta-haemolytic streptococci resistant to erythromycin and lincomycin', *New Engl. J. Med.*, **278,** 538.

Sarkany, I., Taplin, D. and Blank, H. (1961), 'Erythrasma—common bacterial infection of the skin', *JAMA*, **177,** 130.

Schroeter, A. L., Lucas, J. B., Price, E. V. and Falcone, V. H. (1972), 'Treatment for early syphilis and reactivity of serologic tests', *JAMA*, **221,** 471.

Shames, J. M., George, R. B., Holliday, W. B., Rasch, J. R. and Mogabgab, W. J. (1970), 'Comparison of antibiotics in the treatment of Mycoplasma pneumonia', *Arch. Intern. Med.*, **125,** 680.

Sherlock, S. (1968), 'Drugs and the liver', *Brit. med. J.*, **1,** 227.

Shoemaker, E. H. and Yow, E. M. (1954), 'Clinical evaluation of erythromycin', *Arch. Intern. Med.*, **93,** 397.

Smith, C. B., Friedewald, W. T. and Chanock, R. M. (1967), 'Shedding of Mycoplasma pneumoniae after tetracycline and erythromycin therapy', *New Engl. J. Med.*, **276**, 1172.

South, M. A., Short, D. H. and Knox, J. M. (1964), 'Failure of erythromycin estolate therapy in *in utero* syphilis', *JAMA*, **190**, 70.

Spaepen, M. S., Kundsin, R. B. and Horne, H. W. (1976), 'Tetracycline-resistant T-mycoplasmas (ureaplasma urealyticum) from patients with a history of reproductive failure', *Antimicrob. Ag. Chemother.*, **9**, 1012.

Sprunt, K., Leidy, G. and Redman, W. (1970), 'Cross resistance between lincomycin and erythromycin in viridans streptococci', *Pediatrics*, **46**, 84.

Steigbigel, R. T., Greenman, R. L. and Remington, J. S. (1975), 'Antibiotic combinations in the treatment of experimental Staphylococcus aureus infection', *J. Infect. Dis.*, **131**, 245.

Stephens, V. C., Pugh, C. T., Davis, N. E., Hoehn, M. M., Ralston, S., Sparks, M. C. and Thompkins, L. (1969), 'A study of the behaviour of propionyl erythromycin in blood by a new chromatographic method', *J. Antibiotics*, **22**, 551.

Sutter, V. L. and Finegold, S. M. (1976), 'Susceptibility of anaerobic bacteria to 23 antimicrobial agents', *Antimicrob. Ag. Chemother.*, **10**, 736.

Tardrew, P. L., Mao, J. C. H. and Kenney, D. (1969), 'Antibacterial activity of 2'-esters of erythromycin', *Appl. Microbial.*, **18**, 159.

Thornsberry, C., Baker, C. N. and Kirven, L. A. (1978), '*In vitro* activity of antimicrobial agents on Legionnaires' disease bacterium', *Antimicrob. Ag. Chemother.*, **13**, 78.

Ticktin, H. E. and Robinson, M. M. (1963), 'Effects of some antimicrobial agents on the liver', *Ann. N.Y. Acad. Sci.*, **104**, 1080.

Today's Drugs (1963), 'Alternatives to penicillins. Erythromycin group—macrolides', *Brit. med. J.*, **1**, 1213.

Tolman, K. G., Sannella, J. J. and Freston, J. W. (1974), 'Chemical structure of erythromycin and hepatotoxicity', *Ann. Intern. Med.*, **81**, 58.

Triggs, E. J. and Ashley, J. J. (1978), 'Oral administration of erythromycin stearate: Effect of dosage form on plasma levels', *Med. J. Aust.*, **2**, 121.

van Marion, W. F., van der Meer, J. W. M., Kalff, M. W. and Schicht, S. M. (1978), 'Ototoxicity of erythromycin', *Lancet*, **2**, 214.

Wallace, J. G. (1977), 'Erythromycin-resistant Clostridium welchii', *Brit. med. J.*, **1**, 381.

Weisblum, B. (1967), 'Pneumococcus resistant to erythromycin and lincomycin', *Lancet*, **1**, 843.

Weisblum, B., Siddhikol, C., Lai, C. J. and Demohn, V. (1971), 'Erythromycin-inducible resistance in Staphylococcus aureus: Requirements for induction', *J. Bacteriol.*, **106**, 835.

Wenzel, R. P., Hendley, J. O., Dodd, W. K. and Gwaltney, J. M., Jr. (1976), 'Comparison of josamycin and erythromycin in the therapy of Mycoplasma pneumoniae pneumonia', *Antimicrob. Ag. Chemother.*, **10**, 899.

Wiggins, G. L., Albritton, W. L. and Feeley, J. C. (1978), 'Antibiotic susceptibility of clinical isolates of Listeria monocytogenes', *Antimicrob. Ag. Chemother.*, **13**, 854.

Willcox, R. R. (1977), 'How suitable are available pharmaceuticals for the treatment of sexually transmitted diseases? 1: Conditions presenting as genital discharges', *Brit. J. vener. Dis.*, **53**, 314.

Wilson, S. Z., Martin, R. R. and Putman, M. (1977), '*In vitro* effects of josamycin, erythromycin, and placebo therapy on nasal carriage of Staphylococcus aureus', *Antimicrob. Ag. Chemother.*, **11**, 407.

Wisseman, C. L., Jr., Waddell, A. D. and Walsh, W. T. (1974), '*In vitro* studies of the action of antibiotics on Rickettsia prowazeki by two methods of cell culture', *J. Infect. Dis.*, **130**, 564.

Yagi, Y., McLellan, T. S., Frez, W. A. and Clewell, D. B. (1978), 'Characterization of

a small plasmid determining resistance to erythromycin, lincomycin, and ver-
namycin B in a strain of Streptococcus sanguis isolated from dental plaque', *Antimicrob. Ag. Chemother.*, **13,** 884.

Zabransky, R. J., Johnston, J. A. and Hauser, K. J. (1973), 'Bacteriostatic and
bactericidal activities of various antibiotics against Bacteroides fragilis', *Antimicrob.
Ag. Chemother.*, **3,** 152.

Zamiri, I. and McEntegart, M. G. (1972), 'The sensitivity of diphtheria bacilli to eight
antibiotics', *J. clin. Path.*, **25,** 716.

Zinner, S. H., Sabath, L. D., Casey, J. I. and Finland, M. (1970), 'Erythromycin
plus alkalinization in treatment of urinary infections', *Antimicrob. Ag.
Chemother.*—1969, p. 413.

Zinner, S. H., Sabath, L. D., Casey, J. I. and Finland, M. (1971), 'Erythromycin and
alkalinization of the urine in the treatment of urinary-tract infections due to Gram-
negative bacilli', *Lancet,* **1** 1267.

Spiramycin, Oleandomycin and Kitasamycin

Description

Similar to erythromycin, these three antibiotics belong to the macrolide group (page 496).

1. *Spiramycin* was isolated from a strain of Streptomyces ambofaciens in 1954 at the Rhône Poulenc Laboratories in France. The antibiotic has been extensively used in France, but experience with it in Britain, North America and Australia has been limited.

2. *Oleandomycin* was isolated from a strain of Streptomyces antibioticus at Pfizer laboratories in 1954. The phosphate salt was found to be the most satisfactory preparation for clinical use, and an ester, triacetyloleandomycin has also been developed. The esters of oleandomycin and erythromycin are somewhat similar in respect to their absorption from the stomach and adverse effects. Oleandomycin and its ester are available in the United States but not in Australia.

3. *Kitasamycin* was isolated and described by Hata *et al.* in 1953, when it was better known by its generic name of leucomycin. This antibiotic has had limited use in Britain and Australia, but it appears to have been used fairly extensively in Japan. Kitasamycin is not commercially available in Australia or the United States.

Sensitive Organisms

1. The antibacterial spectrum of spiramycin, oleandomycin and kitasamycin is similar to that of erythromycin (page 496).

2. *Gram-positive cocci*. These drugs are active against bacteria such as Staph. pyogenes (including penicillinase-producing strains), Staph. epidermidis, Strep. pyogenes, Strep. pneumoniae, Strep. viridans and also most Strep. faecalis strains. Resistant strains of Staph. pyogenes occur, but they are less common than erythromycin-resistant strains. Kitasamycin is apparently active against most erythromycin-resistant staphylococci (Steinberg *et al.*, 1959; Welch *et al.*, 1959). These three antibiotics also show the 'dissociated type of resistance' against staphylococci, characteristic of all macrolide antibiotics (Waterworth, 1960) (*see also* page 497).

3. *Gram-positive bacilli* such as C. diphtheriae, Cl. tetani, Cl. perfringens and B. anthracis are also sensitive to these antibiotics.

4. *Gram-negative bacteria*. Spiramycin, oleandomycin and kitasamycin are active against Neisseria meningitidis, N. gonorrhoeae, H. influenzae and B. pertussis. Other Gram-negative bacilli such as Esch. coli are resistant.

517

In Vitro Sensitivities

The minimum inhibitory concentrations of these antibiotics and erythromycin, against a few selected bacterial species are shown in Table 32. Erythromycin has superior antibacterial activity to the other macrolides.

TABLE 32

Compiled from data published by *Today's drugs* (1968), Hata *et al.* (1953) and Waterworth (1960)

ORGANISM	MIC (μg per ml)			
	Erythromycin	Spiramycin	Oleandomycin	Kitasamycin
Staph. pyogenes	0·12	2·0	0·5	0·39
Strep. pyogenes (Group A)	0·03	0·25	0·25	0·39–0·78
Strep. pneumoniae	0·03	0·25	0·25	0·04–0·19
Strep. faecalis	0·5	2·0	2·0	2·0

Mode of Administration and Dosage

These antibiotics are usually administered by the oral route. Parenteral preparations of oleandomycin and kitasamycin have been marketed.

1. *Spiramycin.* The adult dose is 2 g per day, given in two or four divided doses. In severe infections the total daily dosage can be increased to 3–4 g. The dose for children is 50–100 mg per kg per day in two or four divided doses.

2. *Oleandomycin phosphate and triacetyloleandomycin.* The usual adult oral dose of either of these drugs is 1–2 g daily given in four divided doses. The dose for children is 30–50 mg per kg body weight per day.

3. *Kitasamycin.* The usual adult oral dose is 1–1·4 g daily given in four divided doses. This drug can also be given intravenously, and the recommended dose for adults is 200 mg every 6–8 h, administered by a slow infusion.

Serum Levels in Relation to Dosage

1. *Spiramycin.* Serum levels of this drug during continuous oral administration of 3 g per day in adults, range from 1·6 μg to 2·8 μg per ml (Chabbert, 1955). Hudson *et al.* (1956) administered oral spiramycin to 26 adults with a loading dose of 2 g followed by 1 g every six hours. Blood samples taken two, four and six hours after each dose showed serum levels ranging from 1·0 μg to 6·7 μg per ml. After the patients had received eleven doses, the lowest serum level detected was 2 μg per ml, indicating that some accumulation occurs after three days treatment.

2. *Oleandomycin and triacetyloleandomycin.* The average peak serum level two hours after a 0·5 g dose of oral oleandomycin is 0·8 μg per ml, whilst after an identical dose of triacetyloleandomycin the peak level is 2·0 μg per ml. Detectable serum levels may still be present twelve hours after this dose of triacetyloleandomycin (Busch and Lane, 1967).

3. *Kitasamycin.* The absorption of this drug from the gastro-intestinal tract is apparently satisfactory.

Excretion

1. *Oleandomycin*. This drug is excreted from the body in much the same way as erythromycin (page 503). Some of the drug is excreted in urine, and after a single oral dose of either oleandomycin or triacetyloleandomycin, about 10 per cent and 20 per cent of these drugs, respectively, can be recovered from the urine. Significant quantities are also excreted in the bile, but most of administered oleandomycin appears to be inactivated in the body.

2. *Spiramycin*. Similarly only 5–15 per cent of an orally administered dose of this drug can be recovered from the urine, and there is significant biliary excretion. Inactivation of the drug in the body accounts for most of the ingested dose, but this process is apparently slower than with erythromycin and oleandomycin.

3. *Kitasamycin*. Animal studies seem to indicate that this drug is excreted in much the same way as erythromycin and oleandomycin (Ayerst Research Laboratories, 1968).

Distribution of the Drugs in Body

The distribution of oleandomycin and kitasamycin in the body is similar to that of erythromycin (page 503). Spiramycin seems to have an exceptional property, in that high concentrations of this drug appear to persist in various organs and tissues for prolonged periods. Tissue concentrations of spiramycin may still be high at a time when serum spiramycin has fallen to a low level (Benazet and Dubost, 1959; Sutherland, 1962), whereas tissue concentrations of other macrolides decline more rapidly. This special pharmacological property may be the reason why spiramycin is clinically effective, despite antibacterial activity inferior to erythromycin.

Mode of Action

The mode of action of all macrolide antibiotics on bacteria is similar (*see* erythromycin, page 504).

Toxicity

1. *Spiramycin, oleandomycin phosphate and kitasamycin* are safe, non-toxic drugs. The only side-effects which have been noted after oral administration are:

   (a) *Gastro-intestinal side-effects*. Nausea, vomiting and diarrhoea are common if high oral doses are used.
   (b) *Skin rashes* are rarely encountered with these antibiotics.

2. *Triacetyloleandomycin*, in addition to the above minor toxic effects, causes jaundice similar to that of erythromycin estolate (page 505). Abnormalities of liver function tests have been reported in 34 per cent of patients receiving treatment for two weeks or longer (Ticktin and Zimmerman, 1962). Gilbert (1962) found abnormal liver function tests in 50 per cent of patients given triacetyloleandomycin for more than ten days, and 5 per cent of these

developed jaundice. Liver function tests and biopsy studies show that this hepatic abnormality has both hepatocellular and cholestatic features. It is possible, however, that, as in the case of erythromycin estolate jaundice (page 505), some of the serum aspartate aminotransferase (SGOT) elevations reported may be spurious. Liver function tests usually return to normal after the drug is discontinued. Readministration of triacetyloleandomycin reproduces hepatoxicity, often within 24–48 h (Gilbert, 1962; Ticktin and Zimmerman, 1962). This drug may also potentiate the action of car-bamazepine by interfering with its metabolism in the liver (Dravet *et al.*, 1977).

Clincal Uses of the Drugs

1. *Spiramycin* has been used for indications similar to those for oral erythromycin (page 506). It has been used as an alternative to penicillin G for streptococcal and pneumococcal infections, and also for treatment of staphylococcal infections. Despite the inferior antibacterial activity of spiramycin, compared to erythromycin, workers in France have obtained good results with spiramycin in all of these infections (*Today's Drugs,* 1968). This may be explained by the special pharmacological behaviour of this drug (page 519). Spiramycin has also been used for the treatment of gonorrhoea (David and Porter, 1959; Leading article, 1970), and has been claimed to be effective in the treatment of toxoplasmosis, but the evidence for this is conflicting (Beattie, 1967). In one prospective study of 378 pregnant women with high initial toxoplasma antibody titres or seroconversion during pregnancy, spiramycin treatment reduced the frequency of fetal toxoplasma infections (Desmonts and Couvreur, 1974). However, from this study it also appeared that spiramycin did not significantly influence the course of established fetal toxoplasmosis, possibly because the drug only crosses the placenta in low concentrations.

2. *Oleandomycin* has also been used for indications similar to those for erythromycin, but is less active than erythromycin and has no special advantages. The ester triacetyloleandomycin, which is better absorbed, but hepatotoxic (page 519) also is without advantages. For erythromycin-resistant staphylococcal infections other drugs such as the penicillinase-resistant penicillins are now preferred, and it appears that oleandomycin and triacetyloleandomycin no longer have any place in current therapeutics.

3. *Kitasamycin* also has been advocated for indications similar to those of erythromycin, but has no outstanding advantages.

REFERENCES

Ayerst Research Laboratories (1968), *Kitasamycin—a New Antibiotic*, Prospectus for clinical investigators.
Beattie, C. P. (1967), 'Toxoplasmosis'. In Waterson, A. P. (Ed.), *Recent Advances in Medical Microbiology*, J. & A. Churchill Ltd., p. 318.
Benazet, F. and Dubost, M. (1959), 'Apparent paradox of antimicrobial activity of spiramycin', *Antibiot. Annual—1958–1959*, p. 211.
Busch, H. and Lane, M. (1967), *Chemotherapy*, Year Book Medical Publishers, Inc., Chicago, p. 79.
Chabbert, Y. (1955), '*In vitro* studies with spiramycin', *Ann. Inst. Pasteur*, **89,** 434.

David, N. A. and Porter, G. A. (1959), 'Spiramycin in the treatment of hospitalized patients and in male patients with acute gonorrhoeal urethritis', *Antibiot. Annual*—1958–1959, p. 188.

Desmonts, G. and Couvreur, J. (1974), 'Congenital toxoplasmosis. A prospective study of 378 pregnancies', *New Engl. J. Med.*, **290**, 1110.

Dravet, C., Mesdjian, E., Cenraud, B. and Roger, J. (1977), 'Interaction between carbamazepine and triacetyloleandomycin', *Lancet*, **1**, 810.

Gilbert, F. I., Jr. (1962), 'Cholestatic hepatitis caused by esters of erythromycin and oleandomycin', *JAMA*, **182**, 1048.

Hata, T., Sano, Y., Ohki, N., Yokoyama, Y., Matsumae, A. and Ito, I. (1953), 'Leucomycin, a new antibiotic', *J. Antib.*, Ser. A., **6**, 87; quoted by Ayerst Research Laboratories (1968).

Hudson, D. G., Yoshihara, G. M. and Kirby, W. M. M. (1956), 'Spiramycin, clinical and laboratory studies', *Arch. Intern. Med.*, **97**, 57.

Leading Article (1970), 'Spiramycin in the treatment of gonorrhoea', *Brit. med. J.*, **2**, 129.

Steinberg, B. A., Muhlenpoh, J. A., Rushman, I. and Woodside, R. (1959), 'Antibiotic and resistance studies with leucomycin', *Antibiot. Annual*—1958–1959, p. 342.

Sutherland, R. (1962), 'Spiramycin: A reappraisal of its antibacterial activity', *Brit. J. Pharmacol.*, **19**, 99.

Ticktin, H. E. and Zimmerman, H. J. (1962), 'Hepatic dysfunction and jaundice in patients receiving triacetyloleandomycin', *New Engl. J. Med.*, **267**, 964.

Today's Drugs (1968), 'The macrolides and lincomycin', *Brit. med. J.*, **2**, 233.

Waterworth, P. M. (1960), 'The antibacterial properties of leucomycin', *Antibiot. Chemother.*, **10**, 101.

Welch, H., Wright, W. W., Oswald, E. J. and Wintermere, D. M. (1959), '*In vitro* studies with leucomycin', *Antibiot. Annual*—1958–1959, p. 337.

Josamycin and Rosamicin

Josamycin

This is a newer macrolide antibiotic which is structurally related to erythromycin and is produced from Streptomycin narbonensis var. josamyceticus (Osono *et al.*, 1967; Nitta *et al.*, 1967).

Josamycin has an *in vitro* activity similar to erythromycin against Strep. pyogenes, Strep. pneumoniae, Staph. pyogenes, Staph. epidermidis, viridans streptococci and enterococci (Strausbaugh *et al.*, 1976a; Westerman *et al.*, 1976). Other authors have found josamycin's activity against staphylococci and enterococci to be inferior to that of erythromycin and rosamicin (Shadomy *et al.*, 1976). Josamycin is also active against Haemophilus influenzae, Neisseria meningitidis, N. gonorrhoeae and B. pertussis.

Obligate anaerobes are sensitive to josamycin. Of the Gram-positive anaerobes, the Peptococcus, Peptostreptococcus, Propionibacterium and Eubacterium spp. are sensitive, but Clostridium spp. strains may be resistant (Long *et al.*, 1976). Josamycin is also active against Gram-negative anaerobes, particularly Bacteroides fragilis (Strausbaugh *et al.*, 1976a; Long *et al.*, 1976), but 60 per cent of Fusobacterium spp. strains tested by Long *et al.* (1976) were resistant to a concentration of 2 μg per ml. The activity of josamycin against anaerobes, particularly B. fragilis, has been compared to that of clindamycin (page 472). Westerman *et al.* (1976) considered that these two drugs had a comparable activity but others found that josamycin was not as active as clindamycin (Strausbaugh *et al.*, 1976a; Shadomy *et al.*, 1976). In another comparative *in vitro* study, josamycin and rosamicin had a similar inhibitory activity to metronidazole and clindamycin against B. fragilis. However, when the bactericidal activity of these drugs was tested, metronidazole was the most active, and the others had decreasing activity in the order of clindamycin, rosamicin, josamycin and erythromycin (Santoro *et al.*, 1976). Josamycin is active against Mycoplasma pneumoniae.

Pharmacological studies indicate that after oral administration, josamycin behaves similarly to erythromycin (Strausbaugh *et al.*, 1976b). By comparison to erythromycin there was a tendency for josamycin to accumulate over the first 48 h, resulting in higher peak and trough levels. Josamycin is metabolized in the liver and excreted in the bile in an inactive form (Mitsuhashi, 1971). Less than 20 per cent of the drug is excreted in the urine in the active form, but high urinary concentrations are obtained. The drug penetrates well into saliva, sweat and tears (Strausbaugh *et al.*, 1976b). Apart from mild gastro-intestinal side-effects, josamycin therapy has not been associated with any other toxic effects (Mitsuhashi, 1971; Strausbaugh *et al.*, 1976b).

Clinical trials with josamycin were started in Japan in 1967 (Mitsuhashi,

1971), but since then there are only a few reports concerning its clinical usage. In one controlled study josamycin and erythromycin both given in an oral dose of 2·0 g daily in four divided doses were equally effective for the treatment of adults with mycoplasma pneumonia (Wenzel *et al.*, 1976). Similarly josamycin (1·5 g per day) and erythromycin (1·0 g per day) were equally effective in reducing the nasal carrier rates of Staph. pyogenes (Wilson *et al.*, 1977). Josamycin has been used to treat a small number of anthraco-silicotic coalminers who had an exacerbation of chronic bronchitis, but the results were not as good as those obtained with either co-trimoxazole or ampicillin (Joly *et al.*, 1977).

Rosamicin

This new macrolide antibiotic, which is similar chemically and biologically to erythromycin, is produced by Micromonospora rosaria (Wagman *et al.*, 1972; Waitz *et al.*, 1972).

Its *in vitro* activity against Gram-positive bacteria such as Staph. pyogenes, Staph. epidermidis, enterococci, viridans streptococci and Strep. pyogenes is similar to erythromycin (Crowe and Sanders, 1974; Shadomy *et al.*, 1976). Erythromycin is more active against Strep. pyogenes (Saroglou and Bisno, 1978). Rosamicin is more active than erythromycin against the Enterobacteriaceae and Pseudomonas spp. particularly in an alkaline medium (Crowe and Sanders, 1974). It is very active against Haemophilus influenzae and the Neisseria spp. (Sanders and Sanders, 1977). The *in vitro* activity of rosamicin against H. influenzae (including ampicillin-resistant strains) is greater than that of chloramphenicol, erythromycin and ampicillin. Its activity against N. meningitidis is similar to penicillin G but greater than that of rifampicin, minocycline, erythromycin or chloramphenicol. Rosamicin is more active than penicillin G, erythromycin and tetracycline against N. gonorrhoeae; this activity also encompasses beta-lactamase producing strains.

Rosamicin is also active against anaerobes (Sutter and Finegold, 1976). Compared to erythromycin for Gram-positive anaerobes, it is more active against Peptococcus spp. but of about equal activity against others such as the Peptostreptococcus, Eubacterium, Arachnia, Propionibacterium, Actinomyces and Lactobacillus spp. Rosamicin is in general more active than erythromycin against Gram-negative anaerobes such as the Bacteroides and Fusobacterium spp. All strains of B. fragilis tested by Sutter and Finegold (1976) were inhibited at concentration of 4 μg per ml or less. Mycoplasmas are sensitive to rosamicin.

At present there is no information on the clinical use of this macrolide. The drug is concentrated in human prostatic tissue and therefore it has been suggested that it may be of use for the treatment of bacterial prostatitis (Baumueller *et al.*, 1977).

REFERENCES

Baumueller, A., Hoyme, U. and Madsen, P. O. (1977), 'Rosamicin—a new drug for the treatment of bacterial prostatitis', *Antimicrob. Ag. Chemother.*, **12**, 240.
Crowe, C. C. and Sanders, W. E., Jr. (1974), 'Rosamicin: Evaluation *in vitro* and com-

parison with erythromycin and lincomycin', *Antimicrob. Ag. Chemother.*, **5**, 272.

Joly, J., Ninane, G. and Kraytman, M. (1977), 'A double-blind comparative study of ampicillin, co-trimoxazole and josamycin in anthraco-silicotic miners, assessed by transtracheal puncture', *J. Antimicrob. Chemother.*, **3**, 429.

Long, S. S., Mueller, S. and Swenson, R. M. (1976), '*In vitro* susceptibilities of anaerobic bacteria to josamycin', *Antimicrob. Ag. Chemother.*, **9**, 859.

Mitsuhashi, S. (Ed.) (1971), *Drug Action and Drug Resistance in Bacteria*, University Park Press, Tokyo.

Nitta, K., Yano, K., Miyamoto, F., Hasegawa, Y., Sato, T., Kamotot, N. and Matsumoto, S. (1967), 'A new antibiotic, josamycin II. Biological studies', *J. Antibiot.* (*Tokyo*), **20**, 181.

Osono, T., Oka, Y., Watanabe, S., Numazaki, Y., Moriyama, K., Ishida, H., Suzaki, K., Okami, Y. and Umezawa, H. (1967), 'A new antibiotic, Josamycin I. Isolation and physico-chemical characteristics', *J. Antibio.* (*Tokyo*), **20**, 174.

Sanders, C. C. and Sanders, W. E., Jr. (1977), '*In vitro* activity of rosamicin against Neisseria and Haemophilus, including penicillinase-producing strains', *Antimicrob. Ag. Chemother.*, **12**, 293.

Santoro, J., Kaye, D. and Levison, M. E. (1976), '*In vitro* activity of josamycin and rosamicin against Bacteroides fragilis compared with clindamycin, erythromycin and metronidazole', *Antimicrob. Ag. Chemother.*, **10**, 188.

Saroglou, G. and Bisno, A. L. (1978), 'Susceptibility of skin and throat strains of Group A streptococci to rosamicin and erythromycin', *Antimicrob. Ag. Chemother.*, **13**, 701.

Shadomy, S., Tipple, M. and Paxton, L. (1976), 'Josamycin and rosamicin: *In vitro* comparisons with erythromycin and clindamycin', *Antimicrob. Ag. Chemother.*, **10**, 773.

Strausbaugh, L. J., Dilworth, J. A., Gwaltney, J. M., Jr. and Sande, M. A. (1976a), '*In vitro* susceptibility studies with josamycin and erythromycin', *Antimicrob. Ag. Chemother.*, **9**, 546.

Strausbaugh, L. J., Bolton, W. K., Dilworth, J. A., Guerrant, R. L. and Sande, M. A. (1976b), 'Comparative pharmacology of josamycin and erythromycin stearate', *Antimicrob. Ag. Chemother.*, **10**, 450.

Sutter, V. L. and Finegold, S. M. (1976), 'Rosamicin: *In vitro* activity against anaerobes and comparison with erythromycin', *Antimicrob. Ag. Chemother.*, **9**, 350.

Wagman, G. H., Waitz, J. A., Marquez, J., Murawski, A., Oden, E. M., Testa, R. T. and Weinstein, M. J. (1972), 'A new micromonospora-produced macrolide antibiotic, rosamicin', *J. Antibiot.* (*Tokyo*), **25**, 641.

Waitz, J. A., Drube, C. G., Moss, E. L., Jr. and Weinstein, M. J. (1972), 'Biological studies with rosamicin, a new micromonospora-produced macrolide antibiotic', *J. Antimicrob.* (*Tokyo*), **25**, 647.

Wenzel, R. P., Hendley, J. O., Dodd, W. K. and Gwaltney, J. M., Jr. (1976), 'Comparison of josamycin and erythromycin in the therapy of Mycoplasma pneumoniae pheumonia, *Antimicrob. Ag. Chemother.*, **10**, 899.

Wetserman, E. L., Williams, T. W., Jr. and Moreland, N. (1976), '*In vitro* activity of josamycin against aerobic Gram-positive cocci and anaerobes', *Antimicrob. Ag. Chemother.*, **9**, 988.

Wilson, S. Z., Martin, R. R. and Putman, M. (1977), '*In vivo* effects of josamycin, erythromycin, and placebo therapy on nasal carriage of Staphylococcus aureus', *Antimicrob. Ag. Chemother.*, **11**, 407.

Novobiocin

Description

Novobiocin was isolated from Streptomyces niveus in the Upjohn Research Laboratories and initially was given the generic name of 'Streptonivicin' (Smith *et al.*, 1956). It was also isolated almost simultaneously in other laboratories, and was given several other names. Novobiocin is no longer available commercially in Australia, but is available in the United States of America with the trade names of 'Albamycin' (Upjohn) and 'Cathomycin' (MSD).

Sensitive Organisms

1. *Gram-positive cocci*. Novobiocin is active against some of these bacteria, such as Staph. pyogenes (including penicillinase-producing strains) and the pneumococcus. However, Strep. pyogenes is much less sensitive, Strep. viridans strains vary in their sensitivity, and Strep. faecalis is usually resistant (Garrod *et al.*, 1973).

2. *Gram-positive bacilli* such as B. anthracis, Cl. tetani, Cl. perfringens and C. diphtheriae are also novobiocin-sensitive.

3. *Gram-negative bacteria*. Some of these, such as H. influenzae and the pathogenic Neisseria spp. are sensitive. Proteus vulgaris may be sensitive to moderate novobiocin concentrations, but other Proteus spp. are completely resistant. Other Gram-negative bacilli, such as Esch. coli, Enterobacter and Klebsiella spp., salmonellae, shigellae and Pseudomonas aeruginosa, are novobiocin-resistant. Novobiocin alone may inhibit Pseudomonas pseudomallei, but only in concentrations that can be attained with very high systemic doses. However *in vitro*, concentrations as low as $0 \cdot 2$ μg per ml, if combined with tetracycline, exert a bactericidal synergistic effect against this organism (Calabi, 1973). By contrast a chloramphenicol and novobiocin combination shows either only an additive or a moderate synergistic effect against Ps. pseudomallei. Novobiocin often potentiates the action of rifampicin against Salm. typhi *in vitro* (page 555).

4. *Acquired resistance*. Staph. pyogenes and many other bacteria usually sensitive to this drug readily acquire resistance following repeated subculturing *in vitro* in the presence of the antibiotic (Finland and Nichols, 1957).

In Vitro Sensitivities

The usual minimum inhibitory concentrations of novobiocin against some selected bacteria are shown in Table 33.

526

THE USE OF ANTIBIOTICS

TABLE 33

(Modified after *Today's Drugs*, 1963)

ORGANISM	MIC (μg per ml)
Staph. pyogenes	0·12– 1·0
Strep. pyogenes (Group A)	0·5 – 4·0
Strep. pneumoniae	0·5
Strep. faecalis	1·0 –16·0
Bacillus anthracis	2·0
Clostridium perfringens (welchii)	1·0
Neisseria gonorrhoeae	1·0 – 4·0
Haemophilus influenzae	1·0

Mode of Administration and Dosage

1. Novobiocin is most commonly administered by the oral route. The usual adult dose is 2 g per day, administered in four divided doses, and for children 30 mg per kg body weight per day, in four divided doses. The drug should not be administered to infants under one month of age, because it may cause hyperbilirubinaemia (*see* page 528).

2. Novobiocin may be given by intramuscular injection, and the usual adult dose is 0·5 g eight-hourly. These injections are painful, and solutions of novobiocin are incompatible with procaine.

3. The drug can also be given intravenously. If it is to be administered by continuous intravenous infusion, a 0·5 g dose should be dissolved in 5 ml of diluent, and then added to 500 ml isotonic saline for infusion in 6–8 h. Novobiocin is incompatible with 5 per cent dextrose. Novobiocin can also be administered by intermittent intravenous injections, and, for this purpose, a 0·5 g dose should be diluted in at least 30 ml, before injection slowly into the drip tubing over a period of 5–10 min.

4. The dose of novobiocin may be varied. Smaller doses have been used to treat mild infections, and larger doses (4 g per day in adults and up to 100 mg per kg per day in children) for serious infections (Finland and Nichols, 1957).

5. *Patients with renal failure.* Dosage modification is not necessary for these patients (Kunin, 1967).

6. *Patients with liver disease.* Novobiocin is best avoided in these patients, but if it is used, serum level monitoring and dose reduction may be necessary, because novobiocin is mainly excreted via the bile (page 527).

Serum Levels in Relation to Dosage

Novobiocin is well absorbed from the alimentary tract. After a single oral dose of 0·5 g to adults, a peak serum level of 10 to 20 μg per ml is attained in 1–4 h. Thereafter these levels fall slowly, but therapeutically effective levels may persist for 24 h or longer (Wright *et al.*, 1956). Doubling the dose doubles the serum concentrations. If a dose of 0·5 g is administered orally every 6 h, there is often some accumulation, and after four doses the peak serum level may reach 100 μg per ml (Martin *et al.*, 1955).

Excretion

URINE: Only about 3 per cent of administered novobiocin is excreted via the kidney, and urine concentrations of the active drug are usually lower than serum concentrations (Martin *et al.*, 1955).

BILE: Novobiocin is mainly excreted in the bile in which its concentration is usually high. Some of the drug excreted this way is reabsorbed from the bowel, which helps to maintain high serum levels. However, a large amount of the antibiotic is eventually excreted in the faeces (Larson *et al.*, 1956; Taylor *et al.*, 1956).

Distribution of the Drug in Body

Novobiocin slowly diffuses into most body tissues, but only small amounts penetrate into the cerebrospinal fluid when the meninges are uninflamed, and concentrations in pleural and ascitic fluids are usually lower than simultaneous serum levels. Of the tissues studied, the liver and large intestine have the highest novobiocin content (Taylor *et al.*, 1956).

Novobiocin is one of the antibiotics which is most highly bound to serum proteins. Over 90 per cent of the drug is reversibly bound to serum albumin, and some investigators have estimated its serum binding to be as high as 99·2 per cent (Rolinson and Sutherland, 1965). *In vitro* its antibacterial activity is markedly decreased in the presence of 10 per cent serum. Nevertheless the drug is therapeutically effective (Leading article, 1966). This may be partly because the serum levels of novobiocin are usually quite high in relation to the minimum inhibitory concentrations of highly susceptible organisms. The peak serum level of 'free novobiocin' after an oral dose of 0·5 g is 0·28 μg per ml (the total level being 35 μg per ml), which still exceeds the minimum inhibitory concentration (0·20 μg per ml) of a highly sensitive Staph. pyogenes strain (Rolinson, 1967). The significance of antibiotic serum binding is discussed on page 86).

Mode of Action

The mode of action of novobiocin on bacteria appears to be complex. It interferes with bacterial cell wall synthesis, but by contrast with the penicillins and cephalosporins, this does not appear to be its only site of action. The drug also inhibits bacterial protein and nucleic acid synthesis, and therefore it does not induce the formation of stable L-forms of susceptible bacteria (Molander *et al.*, 1964; Wishnow *et al.*, 1965; Smith and Davis, 1967). Novobiocin also seems to damage the bacterial cytoplasmic membrane (page 19) (Brock, 1962). Since cell wall precursors may be formed at, and transported across the membrane, and the bacterial chromosome is attached to the membrane before replication, all the effects of novobiocin may result from membrane damage (Morris and Russell, 1968).

Toxicity

1. *Gastro-intestinal side-effects.* Symptoms such as nausea, abdominal pain and diarrhoea are fairly common with oral novobiocin therapy, but are usually

not severe enough to necessitate cessation of treatment.

2. *Hypersensitivity reactions*. Erythematous or urticarial rashes are quite common, and may occur in 10–15 per cent of patients if treatment is continued for one week or longer. Drug fever may also occur. More serious allergic manifestations such as Stevens-Johnson syndrome have also been encountered (Martin and Wellman, 1967). Haemorrhagic cutaneous lesions have been described, possibly due to a coumarin-like effect of the drug. Rarely allergic pneumonitis or myocarditis may occur (Riley, 1970).

3. *Haematological changes*. Eosinophilia is common, and usually occurs in association with hypersensitivity reactions. Rarely anaemia, leucopenia, agranulocytosis, thrombocytopenia and pancytopenia have been reported (Martin and Wellman, 1967). Montgomery (1963) reported haemolytic anaemia with positive direct and indirect Coombs tests in a six-year-old girl in association with novobiocin administration.

4. *Interference with liver function*. Yellow discolouration of sclerae, commonly seen in patients treated by novobiocin, is usually due to transient deposition of a harmless pigment derivative of the drug. However, in young children novobiocin may interfere with bilirubin conjugation, resulting in hyperbilirubinaemia. This is particularly likely in newborns, in whom the enzyme systems for bilirubin conjugation are immature (Sutherland and Keller, 1961). For this reason novobiocin is contraindicated in infants under one month of age.

The serum bilirubin should be estimated if scleral discolouration appears in older children or adults. A normal bilirubin indicates that the yellow colour is due to novobiocin metabolites, and the drug need not be discontinued (Martin and Wellman, 1967).

Clinical Uses of the Drug

1. *Staphylococcal infections*. Novobiocin formerly had a role in the treatment of these infections. With the advent of the penicillinase-resistant penicillins and other anti-staphylococcal agents, novobiocin is no longer used for these infections, except perhaps as an adjunct to other drugs, for the treatment of methicillin-resistant staphylococcal infections. For instance novobiocin/sodium fusidate and novobiocin/rifampicin combinations have been used successfully to treat staphylococcal infections of this nature (Jensen, 1968). These combinations have only been used to prevent the emergence of further drug resistance among these strains, and there is no evidence that they act synergistically.

2. *Melioidosis*. This disease, caused by Pseudomonas pseudomallei, may present acutely as either pneumonia or septicaemia, and carries a high mortality. Novobiocin alone is ineffective in this disease, but some authors consider that it may potentiate the effect of other drugs (Sheehy et al., 1967; Calabi, 1973). For severe cases of melioidosis a combination of massive doses of chloramphenicol (10–12 g per day intravenously), novobiocin 2–4 g per day intravenously, and kanamycin 2–4 g per day intramuscularly is favoured by some (page 444), whilst others prefer tetracycline, either alone or in combination with novobiocin (page 628).

3. *Other infections*. Novobiocin does not appear to have any other role in

current therapeutics. It is effective for the treatment of pneumococcal pneumonia, but penicillin G is the drug of choice for this disease, and safer and more effective alternatives are now available for penicillin-allergic patients. Urinary tract infections due to either Strep. faecalis or Proteus spp. have been treated with novobiocin, but its use for these infections has now been superseded by other drugs.

REFERENCES

Brock, T. D. (1962), 'Effects of magnesium ion deficiency on Escherichia coli and possible relation to the mode of action of novobiocin', *J. Bacteriol.*, **84**, 679.

Calabi, O. (1973), 'Bacteridicdal synergism of novobiocin and tetracycline against Pseudomonas pseudomallei', *J. Med. Microbiol.*, **6**, 293.

Finland, M. and Nichols, R. L. (1957), 'Novobiocin', *The Practitioner,* **179**, 84.

Garrod, L. P., Lambert, H. P. and O'Grady, F. (1973), *Antibiotic and Chemotherapy,* 4th edn., Churchill Livingstone, Edinburgh and London, p. 214.

Jensen, K. (1968), 'Methicillin-resistant straphylococci', *Lancet*, **2**, 1078.

Kunin, C. M. (1967), 'A guide to use of antibiotics in patients with renal disease', *Ann. Intern. Med.*, **67**, 151.

Larson, E. J., Connor, N. D., Swoap, O. F., Runnells, R. A., Prestrud, M. C., Eble, T. E., Freyburger, W. A., Veldkamp, W. and Taylor, R. M. (1956), 'Novobiocin, a new antibiotic. VI. Toxicology', *Antibiot. Chemother.*, **6**, 226.

Leading Article (1966), 'Serum binding of antibiotics', *Brit. med. J.*, **1**, 1059.

Martin, W. J., Heilman, F. R., Nichols, D. R., Wellman, W. E. and Geraci, J. E. (1955), 'Streptonivicin (albamycin): A new antibiotic; preliminary report', *Proc. Mayo Clin.*, **30**, 540.

Martin, W. J. and Wellman, W. E. (1967), 'Clinically useful antimicrobial agents', *Postgraduate Medicine*, **42**, 350.

Molander, C. W., Kagan, B. M., Weinberger, H. J., Heimlich, E. M. and Busser, R. J. (1964), 'Induction by antibiotics and comparative sensitivity on L-phase variants of Staphylococcus aureus', *J. Bacteriol.*, **88**, 591.

Montgomery, J. R. (1963), 'Haemolytic reaction after novobiocin therapy', *New Engl. J. Med.*, **269**, 966.

Morris, A. and Russell, A. D. (1968), 'Studies on the mode of action of novobiocin', *Biochem. Pharmacol.*, **17**, 1923.

Riley, H. D. (1970), 'Vancomycin and novobiocin', *Med. Clin. North America*, **54**, 1277.

Rolinson, G. N. and Sutherland, R. (1965), 'The binding of antibiotics to serum proteins', *Brit. J. Pharmacol.*, **25**, 638.

Rolinson, G. N. (1967), 'The significance of protein binding of antibiotics *in vitro* and *in vivo*'. In Waterson, A. P. (Ed.), *Recent Advances in Medical Microbiology*, J. & A. Churchill, p. 254.

Sheehy, T. W., Deller, J. J., Jr. and Weber, D. R. (1967), 'Editorial. Melioidosis', *Ann. Intern. Med.*, **67**, 897.

Smith, C. G., Dietz, A., Sokolski, W. T. and Savage, G. M. (1956), 'Streptonivicin, a new antibiotic. I. Discovery and biologic studies', *Antibiot. Chemother.*, **6**, 135.

Smith, D. H. and Davis, B. D. (1967), 'Mode of action of novobiocin in Escherichia coli', *J. Bacteriol.*, **93**, 71.

Sutherland, J. M. and Keller, W. H. (1961), 'Novobiocin and neonatal hyper-bilirubinemia', *Amer. J. Dis. Child.*, **101**, 447.

Taylor, R. M., Miller, W. L. and Vander Brook, M. J. (1956), 'Streptonivicin, a new antibiotic. V. Absorption, distribution and excretion', *Antibiot. Chemother.*, **6**, 162.

Today's Drugs (1963), 'Alternatives to penicillins', *Brit. med. J.*, **1**, 1213.

Today's Drugs (1968), 'Novobiocin, fucidin and vancomycin', *Brit. med. J.*, **3**, 40.

Wishnow, R. M., Strominger, J. L., Birge, C. H. and Threnn, R. H. (1965), 'Biochemical effects of novobiocin on Staphylococcus aureus', *J. Bacterial.*, **89**, 1117.

Wright, W. W., Putnam, L. E. and Welch, H. (1956), 'Novobiocin: Serum concentrations and urinary excretion following oral administration in man', *Antibiot. Med.*, **2**, 311.

Polymyxins

Description

The polymyxins are a group of antibiotics, which were first isolated in 1947 from a spore-bearing soil bacillus (B. polymyxa). It was soon shown that a number of chemically different polymyxins, named A, B, C, D and E could be obtained from different strains of this bacillus. These compounds, like bacitracin (page 417) have a polypeptide structure.

Initially only polymyxin B in the form of its sulphate was commercially available. Polymyxin B is not available commercially in a pure form, and its activity and dosage are usually measured in units. One mg of pure polymyxin B is equivalent to 10 000 units, and commercial preparations contain not less than 6000 units per ml.

Colistin, which became available for clinical use in 1959, had been isolated in 1949 in Japan from Bacillus polymyxa var. colistinus. Initially it was thought to be a new antibiotic, but was soon shown to be identical with polymyxin E (Wilkinson, 1963). However, the drug was supplied in a new form as the sulphomethyl derivative (methane sulphonate) of polymyxin E, also known as colistimethate sodium. When polymyxin E (colistin) was marketed, a new unit was adopted, which was one-third the value of that used for polymyxin B. One mg of pure polymyxin E (colistin) is equivalent to 30 000 units. Hoeprich (1970) suggested that the generic name colistin should be replaced by polymyxin E which was the first name given to this compound. However the more widely known name of colistin is used in this book.

The other polymyxins (A, C and D) are too toxic for clinical use.

Colistin methane sulphonate, when introduced, was represented as a better drug than polymyxin B sulphate on the grounds of reduced toxicity. The methane sulphonates of both of these drugs are indeed less toxic, but they have an inferior antibacterial activity to the sulphates. Eickhoff and Finland (1965) showed that the sulphates had about eight times more activity than the methane sulphonates against Ps. aeruginosa. Nord and Hoeprich (1964) showed that polymyxin E (colistin) sulphate was less toxic to white mice than polymyxin B sulphate, and that the methane sulphonates of both drugs were even less toxic. The activity of these four derivatives against Ps. aeruginosa was found to be directly related to their toxicity, and so an equally toxic dose of each achieves about the same antibacterial effect. Therefore there appears to be no practical advantage in selecting a particular polymyxin derivative for parenteral use, and each clinician should choose the preparation with which he is most familiar.

Both polymyxin B and E have been available either as the sulphate or methane sulphonate for parenteral administration and other uses. In Australia and the United States of America there are now only two polymyxins available for parenteral use. Polymyxin B sulphate is marketed with the trade name of 'Aerosporin' (Burroughs Wellcome) and colistin (polymyxin E) methane sulphonate (colistimethate sodium) is marketed with the trade name of 'Coly-Mycin M Parenteral' (Warner).

Sensitive Organisms

1. All of the polymyxins have a similar antibacterial spectrum, but there are quantitative differences in their activity (*vide supra*).

2. *Gram-negative enteric bacilli*. The polymyxins are highly active against most of the important Gram-negative bacteria which are normal inhabitants of the human bowel. Esch. coli, Enterobacter and Klebsiella spp. and also Pseudomonas aeruginosa are highly susceptible, but all Proteus spp. are resistant (Schwartz *et al.*, 1960; Wright and Welch, 1960; Taylor and Allison, 1962). Serratia marcescens is also usually resistant (Greenfield and Feingold, 1970) and Bacteroides fragilis is invariably resistant (Kislak, 1972). Other Bacteroides and Fusobacterium spp. are much more sensitive (Hamilton-Miller, 1975).

3. *Other Gram-negative bacteria*. The polymyxins are also active against H. influenzae, B. pertussis, the salmonellae and shigellae. The pathogenic Neisseria spp. (meningococci and gonococci), and the Brucella spp. are resistant (Schwartz *et al.*, 1960). Classical Vibrio cholerae is sensitive to the polymyxins, but the El Tor biotype is resistant. Sensitivity to polymyxin is one of the laboratory tests, which can be used to distinguish these two strains (Mukerjee, 1964). Acinetobacter calcoaceticus is sensitive (Kuck, 1976), and so is the Legionnaires' disease bacterium (Thornsberry *et al.*, 1978).

4. *Gram-positive bacteria*. These are all resistant to the polymyxins.

5. *Acquired resistance*. An important property of the polymyxins is that the bacteria usually sensitive to these drugs do not readily acquire resistance. Occasionally resistant Ps. aeruginosa strains are encountered and these show complete cross-resistance between polymyxin B and colistin. Some Ps. aeruginosa strains, while developing resistance to polymyxins, have increased sensitivity to antibiotics such as chloramphenicol and in particular tetracycline, to which these organisms are normally insensitive (Brown *et al.*, 1972). The clinical significance of this observation is not clear.

6. *Synergy with other drugs*. The sulphonamides and trimethoprim, individually and in combination, enhance the activity of the polymyxins against certain bacteria. Simmons (1969) demonstrated that sulphamethoxazole and sulphamethizole potentiated the activity of colistin against 19 of 20 strains of Ps. aeruginosa; these 19 strains were all relatively sensitive to sulphonamides and the other one for which there was no potentiation was highly resistant. Furthermore, sulphonamides and polymyxins act synergistically against some Gram-negative bacilli, which are usually polymyxin-resistant, such as the Proteus spp. and Serratia marcescens. Holmgren and Möller (1970) demonstrated a marked synergistic action of colistin and sulphonamide against 78 of 100 strains of Proteus spp. by concentrations of the two drugs that could be easily obtained *in vivo*. Polymyxin/sulphonamide synergism can also be demonstrated against L-forms of Pr. mirabilis (Montgomerie *et al.*, 1973). In a

study of 23 strains of Serratia marcescens, Greenfield and Feingold (1970) found that 19 were inhibited by a sulphadiazine/polymyxin B conbination and the other four by a combination of trimethoprim and polymyxin B.

Adeniyi-Jones et al. (1973) reported that S. marcescens was sensitive to trimethoprim and that there was synergy between trimethoprim and sulphamethoxazole (co-trimoxazole, page 692). In a study of multiple drug-resistant S. marcescens strains, Thomas et al. (1976) showed that the addition of polymyxin to trimethoprim/sulphamethoxazole was synergistic and more rapidly bactericidal than co-trimoxazole alone. They also noted that polymyxin and rifampicin were synergistic against this organism (see also page 555). The triple drug combination of trimethoprim/sulphamethoxazole/polymyxin acts synergistically against a variety of Gram-negative bacilli. Simmons (1969) showed that the three drugs together were more active than a combination of any two of these drugs against 66 of 72 strains; organisms tested included Esch. coli, Ps. aeruginosa and the Klebsiella, Proteus, Shigella and Salmonella species. Rosenblatt and Stewart (1974) in a similar study tested Gram-negative bacilli resistant to multiple antimicrobials, including, not infrequently, gentamicin and carbenicillin. The organisms studied included strains of Enterobacter spp., Klebsiella pneumoniae, Serratia marcescens, Providencia and Proteus spp. and Pseudomonas aeruginosa. The majority of these were resistant to at least two of the three drugs, polymyxin B, sulphamethoxazole and trimethoprim. When these drugs were used in various combinations, enhanced activity (synergism or addition) was demonstrable most frequently with a polymyxin B/trimethoprim combination, but the majority of Enterobacter, Klebsiella and Serratia isolates were susceptible to enhanced activity of all combinations. Proteus and Providencia isolates were frequently susceptible but combined activity was indifferent or antagonistic against 60 per cent of Ps. aeruginosa strains. Optimal antibacterial activity was attained when all three drugs were used. Most strains of Pseudomonas cepacia and Ps. maltophilia are sensitive to co-trimoxazole (page 688). Nord et al. (1974) also showed that both of these organisms are susceptible to a combination of sulphamethoxazole, trimethoprim and colistin, even if the strains show resistance to these drugs when tested separately. They suggested that all the strains of Ps. cepacia and Ps. maltophilia, which they tested, would be susceptible to the combination in concentrations of these three drugs which are attainable clinically.

The polymyxins also potentiate the action of some drugs against fungi. In high concentrations polymyxin B affects the cell membrane of yeasts and inhibits their growth; at low concentrations it increases the permeability of the membrane to tetracycline which enters the cell to inhibit protein synthesis and cause cell death (Schwartz et al., 1972). By a similar mechanism polymyxin B also enhances the activity of amphotericin B against Coccidioides immitis (see page 866).

In Vitro Sensitivities

The minimum inhibitory concentrations of polymyxin B sulphate and colistin methane sulphonate against some bacterial species are shown in Table 34. Polymyxin B is more active, particularly against Ps. aeruginosa.

TABLE 34

(Condensed from Schwartz *et al.*, 1960)

ORGANISM	MIC (μg per ml)	
	Polymyxin B sulphate	Colistin methane sulphonate
Escherichia coli	0·02–11·1	0·04– 3·7
Enterobacter spp.	0·02–11·1	0·41–33·3
Klebsiella pneumoniae	0·02– 0·41	0·01– 3·7
Serratia marcescens	11·1	11·1
Proteus spp.	>100·0	>100·0
Salmonella typhi	0·02	0·14
Salmonella typhimurium	0·02	0·41
Shigella sonnei	0·02	0·14
Pseudomonas aeruginosa	0·02– 3·7	1·2 –33·3

Mode of Administration and Dosage

The polymyxins are not absorbed from the gastro-intestinal tract, and they are administered intramuscularly or intravenously for treatment of systemic infections.

1. *Polymyxin B sulphate.* The usual intramuscular adult dose of this drug is 150 mg (1 500 000 units) per day, given in three divided doses. A total daily dose of 200 mg (2 000 000 units) should not be exceeded. The dose for children is 2·5 mg (25 000 units) per kg of body weight per day, given in three divided doses. In newborn and premature infants a dose of 1·5 mg per kg per day is recommended (Yaffe, 1965). Intramuscular injections are quite painful, but this can be circumvented by adding procaine when preparing the drug for intramuscular injection.

Polymyxin B sulphate is given intravenously in the same dose as used by the intramuscular route. It can be given by continuous intravenous infusion provided incompatible additives are not present. For adults 50 mg of polymyxin B sulphate may be added to a 500 ml intravenous bottle for infusion over 8 h. The drug can also be given intermittently by this route, but rapid intravenous injections should be avoided, because of the risk of neuromuscular blockade (page 540). The recommended eight-hourly dose (50 mg for adults) should be added to at least 100 ml of fluid and infused over a period of not less than 20–30 min.

2. *Colistin (polymyxin E) methane sulphonate.* The usual intramuscular dose of this drug is 2·5–5·0 mg per kg per day, given in two or three divided doses. For severe infections the higher dose of 5·0 mg per kg per day should be used, which corresponds to an adult dose of 100–120 mg eight-hourly, or 150 mg twelve-hourly. The dosage of 2·5–5·0 mg per kg body weight per day is also safe for newborn infants (Lawson and Hewstone, 1964). Unlike most other antibiotics which are excreted from the body in the urine, colistin does not have a prolonged half-life in premature babies (Axline *et al.*, 1967; Weinstein and Dalton, 1968).

Colistin methane sulphonate is given intravenously in the same dose as used by the intramuscular route, 2·5–5·0 mg per kg body weight per day, given in two divided doses. Baines and Rifkind (1964) administered a dose of 2·0–2·5 mg per kg every 12 h by dissolving the dose in 100 ml of 5 per cent glucose which was then infused over 20–30 min. Cox and Harrison (1971) gave the drug intravenously in two stages. Half the daily dose (1·25 to 2·5 mg per kg) was given by rapid intravenous injection over 2–3 min, and the other half was administered as a slow infusion, lasting 20 h or longer, commencing 2 h after the loading dose. The rate of drug administration during this infusion was 5–6 mg per hour. Some patients experienced paraesthesiae, but no other adverse effects were noted. This latter method is currently recommended for the intravenous administration of colistin methane sulphonate.

3. *Patients with renal failure.* The polymyxins accumulate in these patients, so a modified dosage schedule with serum level monitoring is necessary (MacKay and Kaye, 1964).

One method of administration of these drugs to patients with renal failure is to use the usual recommended eight-hourly dose (50 mg polymyxin B or 100–120 mg colistin methane sulphonate for adults), but to adjust the intervals between doses according to the degree of renal functional impairment. In anuric patients in whom the serum half-life of polymyxin B or colistin methane sulphonate is two to three days, the interval between these doses, given either intramuscularly or intravenously, should be three to four days (Kunin, 1967). Curtis and Eastwood (1968) also suggest that colistin methane sulphonate in a dose of 2–3 mg per kg body weight, given intravenously once every three days is suitable for patients with severe renal failure. A corresponding dose of polymyxin B sulphate for this purpose is about 1·0 mg per kg body weight every three days. Curtis and Eastwood (1968) found that small, but significant amounts of colistin methane sulphonate were removed by haemodialysis, and recommended that a dose of 2–3 mg per kg body weight of the drug given at the end of each dialysis was suitable for patients undergoing bi-weekly haemodialysis. By contrast Goodwin and Friedman (1968) found that measurable quantities of the drug are not removed by Kiil or Kolff haemodialysis. The clearance of colistin methane sulphonate during peritoneal dialysis is insignificant, and there is no need to increase its dosage in patients undergoing this procedure (Greenberg and Sanford, 1967; Curtis and Eastwood, 1968; Goodwin and Friedman, 1968). A dosage schedule of colistin methane sulphonate for patients with renal impairment has been recommended by Goodwin and Friedman (1968), which differs somewhat from those of Kunin (1967) and Curtis and Eastwood (1968). Smaller doses at shorter intervals are used to avoid periods during which non-therapeutic serum levels may occur. They recommended the following dosage schedule for colistin methane sulphonate, assuming that the usual daily dose is 2·5 mg per kg per day (150 mg daily or 75 mg twelve-hourly for adults):

(a) *Patients with moderate renal impairment (creatinine clearance exceeding 20 ml per minute).*
   Dose: 75–100 per cent of the daily dose given in two divided doses every twelve hours. The duration of serum levels in these patients was almost the same as in subjects with normal renal function.

(b) *Patients with severe renal failure (creatinine clearance 5–20 ml per minute).*
    Dose: 50 per cent of the daily dose given in two divided doses every twelve hours.
(c) *Patients with negligible renal function (creatinine clearance less than 5 ml per minute).*
    Dose: 30 per cent of the daily dose given in two divided doses every twelve to eighteen hours.

The higher recommended daily dose of 5 mg per kg per day of colistin methane sulphonate should be used cautiously in the above schedule, because toxic blood levels may result in some patients with renal failure. Goodwin and Friedman (1968) did not study polymyxin B sulphate, but their dosage schedule can probably be applied to this drug (Kunin, 1968), assuming that the usual daily dose is 1·5–2·5 mg per kg. Nevertheless such dosage schedules are only an approximate guide and regular serum level monitoring is necessary in all patients with renal failure. In addition, the polymyxins are bound to various tissues, where they may persist when serum levels are already low. Current recommendations by the manufacturers for the use of colistin methane sulphonate in patients with renal failure are similar to those by Goodwin and Friedman (1968). For patients with pre-existing renal impairment, it is recommended that the maximum dose of polymyxin B should not exceed 15 000 units per kg per day.

4. *Intrathecal administration.* Polymyxin B sulphate can be administered intrathecally for the treatment of Ps. aeruginosa meningitis. A dose of 0·5 mg (5000 units) every one or two days has been used for infants (Clifford and Stewart, 1961), and for older children 2–4 mg (20 000 to 40 000 units) daily (Quintiliani and Lentneck, 1971), whilst for adults a dose as high as 10 mg (100 000 units) daily has been used. The current recommendations for intrathecal polymyxin B sulphate are: for children under two years, 20 000 units every day for three or four days followed by 25 000 units every alternate day; for children over two years and adults, 50 000 units given every day for three or four days, then this dose is continued on alternate days. This treatment should be continued for at least three days after the spinal fluid becomes sterile and sometimes it may be necessary for some weeks. For intrathecal or intraventricular injection, the contents of a 500 000 unit vial is dissolved in 10 ml sterile saline and the dose (0·4–1·0 ml) is injected as required.

5. *Aerosol administration.* Polymyxin B may be used as inhalation therapy for Pseudomonas aeruginosa bronchial infections, but this is usually not very effective (*see* page 542). The total daily aerosol dose of polymyxin B should not exceed the daily dose recommended for parenteral use. The drug is a bronchial irritant and concentrations higher than 10 mg per ml should not be used for inhalation (Marschke and Sarauw, 1971).

Availability

1. *Polymyxin B sulphate.* ('Aerosporin', Burroughs Wellcome.) This is marketed in vials containing 500 000 units, suitable for intramuscular or intravenous administration. Intramuscular injections are less painful if the solution is prepared by dissolving the contents of the vial in 1·0 ml of saline and 0·5 ml of 1 per cent precaine.

2. *Colistin* (*polymyxin E*) *methane sulphonate* (*Colistimethate sodium*). ('Coly-Mycin M Parenteral', Warner.) This preparation is suitable for both intramuscular and intravenous administration and is marketed in vials containing 20 or 150 mg of colistin base activity. In the United States this preparation is also available in vials containing 150 mg of colistin base activity mixed with a local anaesthetic for intramuscular use ('Coly-Mycin M Intramuscular', Warner).

3. *Polymyxin B sulphate* (and to a lesser extent polymyxin E sulphate) are also available in numerous topical preparations such as creams, ointments, solutions, sprays and eye-drops, and they are usually combined with other antibiotics such as neomycin and bacitracin (*see* pages 412, 418).

Serum Levels in Relation to Dosage

1. After a single intramuscular injection of 50 mg polymyxin B sulphate to adults, the peak serum level is reached after about 2 h. The peak serum level is subject to considerable individual variation, and it may be as high as 8 μg per ml or as low as 1–2 μg per ml. The serum level thereafter declines slowly, and detectable levels are usually present for about 8–12 h. The half-life of polymyxin B sulphate in serum is about 6 h (Kunin, 1967). Some accumulation of the drug usually occurs, and peak levels in patients given 2·5 mg per kg per day for over a week may reach 15 μg per ml.

2. After a single intramuscular injection of colistin methane sulphonate in a dose of 2·5 mg per kg body weight to children (about 150 mg for adults), a peak serum level of 5–7 μg per ml occurs in 1–2 h and detectable levels persist for 8–12 h (Fig. 27). The serum half-life of this drug is only 1·6–2·7 h (Kunin, 1967).

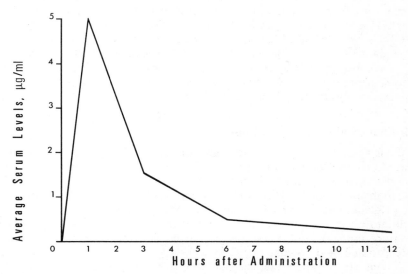

FIG. 27. Average serum levels of colistin methane sulphonate after a single intramuscular dose of 2·5 mg per kg body weight in children. (Redrawn after Ross *et al.*, 1960.)

As with polymyxin B sulphate, repeated administration yields higher serum levels. McMillan *et al.* (1962) measured serum levels in adult patients receiving 120 mg of colistin methane sulphonate intramuscularly at eight-hourly intervals. They found that a maximum level of 11–12 μg per ml, achieved 2–3 h after the injection, was maintained for 5–6 h and then fell progressively.

3. If colistin methane sulphonate is administered intravenously using an initial rapid injection, followed by a slow infusion (page 535), relatively constant serum levels of 5–6 μg per ml are maintained in most patients (Cox and Harrison, 1971).

Excretion

URINE: The polymyxins are mainly excreted by the kidney, but there is a time lag in the excretion of the sulphates after the initial dose. Only about 0·1 per cent of polymyxin B sulphate is recovered from urine during the first 12 h after injection, thereafter urinary excretion increases and with continuing administration in the usual dosage, the urinary concentration varies from 20 to 100 μg per ml. Overall about 60 per cent of the injected dose of polymyxin B sulphate can be recovered from the urine (Hoeprich, 1970).

The methane sulphonate derivatives are more rapidly excreted via the kidney. About 40 per cent of colistin methane sulphonate is excreted in the urine in the first 8 h following injection. The urine levels of colistin (and polymyxin B sulphate) vary according to fluid intake. Urinary colistin concentrations may reach more than 200 μg per ml after usual therapeutic doses, but when fluid intake is high, values of only 20 μg or less per ml may occur (McMillan *et al.*, 1962).

The polymyxins accumulate in patients with impaired renal function.

INACTIVATION IN BODY: The polymyxins are not excreted in bile. The fraction of the administered dose not recoverable from the urine is probably slowly inactivated in the body, possibly by normal tissues (Kunin and Edmondson, 1968). The serum half-life of the polymyxins in anuric patients is usually two to three days (Kunin, 1967), but Goodwin and Friedman (1968) showed that it may be considerably shorter in some patients with virtually no renal function. This suggests that there is considerable variation in the rate of inactivation of polymyxins by the 'non-renal mechanisms'.

Distribution of the Drugs in Body

Although reports conflict on the degree of dialysability of the polymyxins by haemodialysis (Curtis and Eastwood, 1968; Goodwin and Friedman, 1968), all authors agree that these drugs dialyse poorly by any method. This is probably due to the large molecular size of the polymyxins, rather than their protein binding (Kunin, 1967). For this reason the polymyxins do not appear to diffuse well into pleural or joint cavities or infective foci in general, but quantitative data are not available. These drugs also do not diffuse readily into normal cerebrospinal fluid (Wynne and Cooke, 1966).

Animal studies show that the polymyxins become bound to and persist in various body tissues such as the liver, kidney, brain, heart, muscle and lung (Kunin and Bugg, 1971). The drugs persist in these tissues for up to 72 h after single injections and for up to five days after a course of injections. Comparatively more colistin methane sulphonate than polymyxin B sulphate is localized in the kidney, lung and liver, but much higher levels of polymyxin B sulphate than colistin methane sulphonate are found in the brain. The clinical significance of these observations is uncertain.

According to Kunin (1967), the degree of the protein binding of the polymyxins is low.

Mode of Action

The polymyxins bind to and damage the bacterial cytoplasmic membrane (page 19) of susceptible Gram-negative bacteria (Kaye and Chapman, 1963). This membrane has specific transport systems, which determine the permeability characteristics of the cell. Damage to this osmotic barrier leads to leakage of intracellular components. The polymyxins affect the lipid containing cell membrane in a manner similar to a cationic detergent. Their attachment to the anionic binding sites and concentration at the interface of the phospholipid layer of the membrane allows essential cellular constituents to be lost. The toxic effects of the polymyxins may result from similar binding of these drugs to membranes of mammalian cells (Kunin and Edmondson, 1968; Kunin and Bugg, 1971).

In addition to this primary site of action, the polymyxins appear to have other effects on Gram-negative bacteria. For instance they markedly alter surface properties of Pr. mirabilis strains which are polymyxin B-resistant (Sud and Feingold, 1972). It is also possible that the polymyxins may penetrate into the cytoplasm of the cell and interact with nuclear material and ribosomes (Schindler and Teuber, 1975). Another interesting observation is that divalent cations such as calcium and magnesium antagonize the bactericidal effect of polymyxins against Ps. aeruginosa and Esch. coli. This effect seems to be exerted indirectly through interaction with the cell wall rather than at the bacterial plasma membrane, which is the primary site of polymyxin action (Chen and Feingold, 1972). This finding appears to have some clinical significance, as physiological concentrations of calcium inhibit the bactericidal activity of the polymyxins, and therefore these drugs may be less active *in vivo* than predicted by *in vitro* susceptibility studies (Davies *et al.*, 1971).

Toxicity

The polymyxins, even when administered in the recommended doses, frequently cause side-effects. For instance, in a study of 288 patients treated by colistin methane sulphonate (sodium colistimethate), untoward effects were observed in 25·1 per cent (Koch-Weser *et al.*, 1970).

1. *Nephrotoxicity*. This is the most serious toxic effect of the polymyxins. Polymyxin B compounds are more nephrotoxic than colistin (polymyxin E) compounds, and the sulphate derivatives of both these drugs are more toxic than their corresponding methane sulphonates. The antibacterial activity of these compounds is proportional to their toxicity, so that for a certain degree of antibacterial effect, the toxicity is the same whichever preparation is used (*see* page 531). Patients with pre-existing renal impairment can be treated by polymyxins if a modified dose is used, and renal function sometimes improves as the infection is controlled by polymyxin therapy.

Nephrotoxicity, occurring in 20·2 per cent of patients, was the most common side-effect observed by Koch-Weser *et al.* (1970) (*vide supra*). Proteinuria, haematuria and casts in the urine may occur, but rising blood urea and serum creatinine values are the most invariable features. These usually occur within the first four days of therapy. Acute tubular necrosis may result and this may not be preceded by progressive renal functional impairment. Renal impairment may sometimes continue to progress for one or two weeks after the drug has been stopped. Koch-Weser *et al.* (1970) also observed that, after excluding patients in whom dosage had not been appropriately reduced, the frequency of nephrotoxicity in patients with normal and in those with pre-existing renal impairment was the same. The simultaneous administration of cephalothin (page 211) was associated with a higher frequency of nephrotoxicity. The majority of the patients developing renal impairment had received sodium colistimethate in the recommended doses. However nephrotoxicity was more common in heavier patients, probably because a dose according to body weight tends to produce overdosage in such individuals, and surface area would correlate better with glomerular filtration rate and blood volume. In doses of 3 mg (30 000 units) per kg per day, polymyxin B may cause nephrotoxicity in patients with normal renal function, but lower doses may cause renal damage in patients with pre-existing renal impairment (Appel and Neu, 1977).

The use of polymyxins in doses higher than those recommended is dangerous and potentially fatal; this may result in oliguric renal failure due to acute tubular necrosis. Price and Graham (1970) reported 14 patients with refractory Klebsiella spp. infections treated by colistin in doses about six times higher than usually recommended, who all developed acute renal failure. This complication has also occurred in children who have received accidental colistin overdosages (Ryan *et al.*, 1969; Brown *et al.*, 1970). One child aged ten months, who had accidentally received 250 mg colistin intramuscularly (approximately 38·5 mg per kg), had a serum colistin level of 320 μg per ml a few hours later. This child subsequently developed oliguric renal failure, but eventually recovered. Peritoneal dialysis was ineffective in removing colistin from this patient, but exchange transfusion appeared to be effective (Brown *et al.*, 1970).

2. *Neurotoxicity*. The polymyxins can cause giddiness, disturbances of sensation, such as numbness and paraesthesiae mainly affecting the face, nausea and vomiting, muscle weakness and peripheral neuropathy (Koch-Weser *et al.*, 1970). These usually occur within the first four days of treatment and disappear when the drug is stopped. More severe neurotoxic disturbances such as mental confusion, coma, psychosis, convulsions or ataxia may also occur. These may be more frequent in patients receiving large doses or in those with renal functional impairment (Wolinsky and Hines, 1962).

Another serious neurotoxic effect is reversible neuromuscular blockade, which may result in respiratory paralysis (Perkins, 1964; Lindesmith *et al.*, 1968). This may appear quickly and be without premonitory minor side-effects of neurotoxicity (Koch-Weser *et al.*, 1970). The occurrence of paralysis due to polymyxins and other antibiotics has been reviewed by McQuillen *et al.* (1968). Neuromuscular blockade is related to the dose of the antibiotic given, but this is not the only factor. In most reported cases paralysis occurred post-operatively, and there were usually other potentiating factors such as ether anaesthesia, sedatives, neuromuscular blocking agents, hypocalcaemia, renal disease, hypoxia and chronic debilitating illnesses.

Polymyxin-induced neuromuscular blockade differs from that induced by the aminoglycosides (Lindesmith *et al.*, 1968). Neomycin, kanamycin and streptomycin apparently produce a competitive blockade (pages 411, 317, 301), which may be reversed by neostigmine, but the polymyxins cause a non-competitive blockade which is never reversed by neostigmine. Respiratory paralysis due to the polymyxins must be treated by artificial ventilation, and calcium administration may be helpful in some cases. Neuromuscular blockade usually improves within 24 h after the antibiotic is stopped.

It has been suggested that the polymyxins are particularly suitable for treatment of Ps. aeruginosa infections in anephric patients, because nephrotoxicity is not a consideration (Curtis and Eastwood, 1968). However neurotoxicity can be a serious hazard in chronically uraemic patients because their nervous system appears to be more susceptible to polymyxin toxicity compared to that of patients with either acute renal failure or normal renal function (Richet *et al.*, 1970).

Experiments in animals indicate that ear drops containing various antibiotics including polymyxins may be ototoxic and cause deafness. In view of this and the doubt about the efficacy of such treatment, the use of antibiotic ear drops has been discouraged, especially in the presence of large perforations, where ear surgery has been performed, or for pre-operative prophylaxis (Annotation, 1976).

3. *Hypersensitivity reactions.* Rashes, pruritus and drug fever have been observed with polymyxin therapy (Koch-Weser *et al.*, 1970; Hoeprich, 1970). Two patients have been reported who developed bronchospasm as a result of aerosol therapy with the usual doses of polymyxin B. This may have been due to an allergic reaction or bronchial irritation (Marschke and Sarauw, 1971). An interesting patient with aplastic anaemia and polymyxin allergy was reported by Lakin *et al.* (1975). After immunosuppression and receipt of a bone-marrow graft, and whilst lacking T cell activity, he developed a rash and fever attributed to intranasal polymyxin B which was associated with specific IgE antibody. These authors considered that there could be an increased frequency of type 1 hypersensitivity in immunosuppressed patients because the normal suppressor effect of T cells on B cell mediated IgE synthesis may be absent.

4. *Leucopenia* and *hepatotoxicity* have been observed during colistin therapy on rare occasions, but a definite causal relationship has not been established.

Clinical Uses of the Drug

1. *Pseudomonas aeruginosa infections.* In the past the polymyxins were the drugs of choice for the treatment of Ps. aeruginosa infections such as septicaemia, meningitis, pneumonia and wound, burn and urinary tract infections. Nowadays one of the aminoglycosides such as gentamicin (page 341), tobramycin (page 368) or amikacin (page 386) or a penicillin such as carbenicillin (page 160) or ticarcillin (page 180), either singly or in combination, are preferred for these infections. The efficacy of these latter drugs compared to polymyxins has been studied in Pseudomonas infections of animals. In one experiment with induced Pseudomonas sepsis in monkeys, a colistin/carbenicillin combination was found to be equally effective to either

drug given alone (Saslaw *et al.*, 1973). Other experimental Ps. aeruginosa infections have been studied in mice; gentamicin or tobramycin were more effective than colistin for most Ps. aeruginosa infections (Davis, 1974); tobramycin in terms of therapeutic index (ratio of toxicity to efficacy) was more active than gentamicin and the polymyxins (Davis, 1975). In the latter study colistin methane sulphonate had poor *in vivo* activity but polymyxin B was the most active and also the most toxic.

Pseudomonas septicaemia usually occurs in patients with severe associated diseases; nevertheless, some success has been obtained by the use of the polymyxins in this disease (Murdoch, 1964). Meningitis due to Pseudomonas has occasionally been cured by using polymyxin B methane sulphonate both intramuscularly and intrathecally (Clifford and Stewart, 1961). Pseudomonas has also been eliminated from infected burns by using one of the polymyxins both parenterally and locally. The treatment of chronic purulent Ps. aeruginosa bronchial infections by these drugs has usually been unsatisfactory (Pines *et al.*, 1967), though occasional successes have been reported (Lieberson *et al.*, 1969). In addition, in one study in which polymyxin B was administered by aerosol to critically ill patients in an attempt to prevent Ps. aeruginosa pneumonia, results were unfavourable. A number of these patients developed pneumonia due to organisms which were polymyxin-resistant and which were uncommon pathogens (Ps. maltophilia, Ps. cepacia, Flavobacterium spp., Serratia spp. and Strep. faecalis) (Feeley *et al.*, 1975).

Ps. aeruginosa urinary tract infections have also been treated, with reasonably satisfactory results (McMillan *et al.*, 1962; Edgar and Dickinson, 1962). It has been suggested that colistin methane sulphonate may be superior to polymyxin B sulphate for the treatment of these infections, because high urinary concentrations are more rapidly attained after administration (Goodwin, 1970). However the urine levels of polymyxin B sulphate also become adequate after a lag period of approximately 12 h and remain high with continuing treatment (page 537).

Because of the availability of effective and less toxic drugs, the polymyxins have now been relegated to the position of reserve drugs for the parenteral treatment of Ps. aeruginosa infections. If they are indicated, polymyxin B may be preferable to colistin methane sulphonate, because it is more effective *in vivo* in animal infections (*vide supra*).

2. *Infections due to other Gram-negative bacilli*. The polymyxins are not the drugs of choice for septicaemia, meningitis, pyelonephritis, etc., caused by organisms such as Esch. coli and Klebsiella spp., but they have been used when these bacteria are resistant to commonly used antibiotics. Colley and Frankel (1963) used colistin methane sulphonate with moderate success in 18 male paraplegic patients, who had chronic Klebsiella aerogenes infections of the urinary tract. The availability of gentamicin (page 325), the newer aminoglycosides (pages 359, 377) and co-trimoxazole (page 706) has virtually eliminated the use of polymyxins for these infections.

Advantage has been taken of the synergistic effects of the polymyxins with other chemotherapeutic agents to treat infections due to Gram-negative bacilli which are resistant to multiple antimicrobial agents. Polymyxin B has been used in combination with rifampicin to treat multi-resistant nosocomial Serratia marcescens infections (*see* page 574). Polymyxins have also been combined with co-trimoxazole to successfully treat Pseudomonas cepacia and Serratia marcescens infections (*see* page 708).

3. *Topical antibiotic therapy.* Polymyxin B sulphate is often combined with the two other commonly used topical antibiotics, neomycin and bacitracin, because the latter two are ineffective against Ps. aeruginosa. These three antibiotics are marketed in various creams, ointments, eye and ear drops, sprays, solutions for wound irrigation and bladder instillation, etc. (*see* pages 408, 412, 418). Polymyxin B sulphate is particularly suitable for topical therapy, because development of bacterial resistance to this drug is uncommon. Toxicity is not a problem with topical therapy, and therefore the polymyxin with the greatest therapeutic activity, polymyxin B sulphate, is always selected for this purpose.

4. *Prevention of infection in acute leukaemia.* In one trial the oral administration of colistin sulphate with framycetin (page 413) and nystatin (page 926) reduced the frequency of infections in patients with acute leukaemia who were neutropenic after receiving myelosuppressive therapy (Storring *et al.*, 1977) (*see also* pages 345, 651).

5. *Intestinal infections.* The polymyxins, administered orally, are of no clinical value for the treatment of any of these infections caused by bacteria (Marsden and Hyde, 1962; Gotoff and Lepper, 1965).

REFERENCES

Adeniyi-Jones, G., Neilly, S., Roberts, R. S. and Kaufmann, N. R. (1973), 'The susceptibility of Serratia marcescens to sulfamethoxazole, trimethoprim and trimethoprim-sulfamethoxazole', *J. Infect. Dis.* (Suppl.), **128**, 534.

Annotation (1976), 'Ear drops', *Lancet*, **1**, 896.

Appel, G. B. and Neu, H. C. (1977), 'The nephrotoxicity of antimicrobial agents (second of three parts)', *New Engl. J. Med.*, **296**, 722.

Axline, S. G., Yaffe, S. J. and Simon, H. J. (1967), 'Clinical pharmacology of antimicrobials in premature infants: II. Ampicillin, methicillin, oxacillin, neomycin, and colistin', *Pediatrics*, **39**, 97.

Baines, R. D. and Rifkind, D. (1964), 'Intravenous administration of sodium colistimethate', *JAMA*, **190**, 278.

Brown, J. M., Dorman, D. C. and Roy, L. P. (1970), 'Acute renal failure due to overdosage of colistin', *Med. J. Aust.*, **2**, 923.

Brown, M. R. W., Fenton, E. M. and Watkins, W. M. (1972), 'Tetracycline-sensitive/polymyxin-resistant Pseudomonas aeruginosa', *Lancet*, **2**, 86.

Chen, C.-C. H. and Feingold, D. S. (1972), 'Locus of divalent cation inhibition of the bactericidal action of polymyxin B', *Antimicrob. Ag. Chemother.*, **2**, 331.

Clifford, H. E. and Stewart, G. T. (1961), 'Intraventricular administration of a new derivative of polymyxin B in meningitis due to Ps. pyocyanea', *Lancet*, **2**, 177.

Colley, E. W. and Frankel, H. L. (1963), '"Colomycin" treatment of Klebsiella aerogenes infection of urinary tract in paraplegia', *Brit. med. J.*, **2**, 790.

Cox, C. E. and Harrison, L. H. (1971), 'Intravenous sodium colistimethate therapy of urinary-tract infections: Pharmacological and bacteriological studies', *Antimicrob. Ag. Chemother.*—1970, p. 296.

Curtis, J. R. and Eastwood, J. B. (1968), 'Colistin sulphomethate sodium administration in the presence of severe renal failure and during haemodialysis and peritoneal dialysis', *Brit. med. J.*, **1**, 484.

Davis, S. D., Iannetta, A. and Wedgwood, R. J. (1971), 'Activity of colistin against Pseudomonas aeruginosa: Inhibition by calcium', *J. Infect. Dis.*, **124**, 610.

Davis, S. D. (1974), 'Dissociation between results of *in vitro* and *in vivo* antibiotic susceptibility tests for some strains of Pseudomonas aeruginosa', *Antimicrob. Ag. Chemother.*, **5**, 281.

Davis, S. D. (1975), 'Activity of gentamicin, tobramycin, polymyxin B and colistimethate in mouse protection tests with Pseudomonas aeruginosa', *Antimicrob. Ag. Chemother.*, **8**, 50.

Edgar, W. M. and Dickinson, K. M. (1962), 'A trial of colistin methane sulphonate in urinary infection with Pseudomonas pyocyanea', *Lancet*, **2**, 739.

Eickhoff, T. C. and Finland, M. (1965), 'Polymyxin B and colistin: *In vitro* activity against Pseudomonas aeruginosa', *Amer. J. Med. Sci.*, **249**, 172.

Feeley, T. W., Du Moulin, G. C., Hedley-Whyte, J., Bushnell, L. S., Gilbert, J. P. and Feingold, D. S. (1975), 'Aerosol polymyxin and pneumonia in seriously ill patients', *New Engl. J. Med.*, **293**, 471.

Goodwin, N. J. and Friedman, E. A. (1968), 'The effects of renal impairment, peritoneal dialysis, and hemodialysis on serum sodium colistimethate levels', *Ann. Intern. Med.*, **68**, 984.

Goodwin, N. J. (1970), 'Colistin and sodium colistimethate', *Med. Clin. North America*, **54**, 1267.

Gotoff, S. P. and Lepper, M. H. (1965), 'Treatment of Salmonella carriers with colistin sulfate', *Amer. J. Med. Sci.*, **249**, 399.

Greenberg, P. A. and Sanford, J. P. (1967), 'Removal and absorption of antibiotics in patients with renal failure undergoing peritoneal dialysis', *Ann. Intern. Med.*, **66**, 465.

Greenfield, S. and Feingold, D. S. (1970), 'The synergistic action of the sulfonamides and the polymyxins against Serratia marcescens', *J. Infect. Dis.*, **121**, 555.

Hamilton-Miller, J. M. T. (1975), 'Antimicrobial agents acting against anaerobes', *J. Antimicrob. Chemother.*, **1**, 273.

Hoeprich, P. D. (1970), 'The polymyxins', *Med. Clin. North America*, **54**, 1257.

Holmgren, J. and Möller, O. (1970), 'Studies on the sensitivity of Proteus mirabilis and Proteus vulgaris to sulphonamide and colistin alone and in combination', *Scand. J. Infect. Dis.*, **2**, 121.

Kaye, J. J. and Chapman, G. B. (1963), 'Cytological aspects of antimicrobial antibiotics III. Cytologically distinguishable stages in antibiotic action of colistin sulfate on Escherichia coli', *J. Bacteriol.*, **86**, 536.

Kislak, J. W. (1972), 'The susceptibility of Bacteroides fragilis to 24 antibiotics', *J. Infect. Dis.*, **125**, 295.

Koch-Weser, J., Sidel, V. W., Federman, E. B., Kanarek, P., Finer, D. C. and Eaton, A. E. (1970), 'Adverse effects of sodium colistimethate. Mainfestations and specific reaction rates during 317 courses of therapy', *Ann. Intern. Med.*, **72**, 857.

Kuck, N. A. (1976), '*In vitro* and *in vivo* activities of minocycline and other antibiotics against Acinetobacter (Hercellea-Mina)', *Antimicrob. Ag. Chemother.*, **9**, 493.

Kunin, C. M. (1964), 'Clinical experience with the use of potentially nephrotoxic antibiotics in the treatment of infections in uremic patients', *Antimicrob. Ag. Chemother.*—1963, p. 793.

Kunin, C. M. (1967), 'A guide to use of antibiotics in patients with renal disease', *Ann. Intern. Med.*, **67**, 151.

Kunin, C. M. (1968), 'More on antimicrobials in renal failure', *Ann. Intern. Med.*, **69**, 397.

Kunin, C. M. and Edmondson, W. P. (1968), 'Inhibition of antibiotics in bacteriologic agar', *Proc. Soc. Exp. Biol. (N.Y.)*, **129**, 118.

Kunin, C. M. and Bugg, A. (1971), 'Binding of polymyxin antibiotics to tissues: The major determinant of distribution and persistence in the body', *J. Infect. Dis.*, **124**, 394.

Lakin, J. D., Strong, D. M. and Sell, K. W. (1975), 'Polymyxin B reactions, IgE antibody, and T-cell deficiency', *Ann. Intern. Med.*, **83**, 204.

Lawson, J. S. and Hewstone, A. S. (1964), 'Toxic effects of colistin methane sulphonate in the new-born', *Med. J. Aust.*, **1**, 917.

Lieberson, A. D., Winter, L. W., Behnke, R. H. and Martin, R. R. (1969), 'Extensive Pseudomonal pneumonia ultimately responding to polymyxin therapy', *Amer. Rev. Resp. Dis.*, **100**, 558.

Lindesmith, L. A., Baines, R. D., Jr., Bigelow, D. B. and Petty, T. L. (1968), 'Reversible respiratory paralysis associated with polymyxin therapy', *Ann. Intern. Med.*, **68**, 318.

MacKay, D. and Kaye, D. (1964), 'Serum concentrations of colistin in patients with normal and impaired renal function', *New Engl. J. Med.*, **270**, 394.

Marschke, G. and Sarauw, A. (1971), Polymyxin inhalation therapeutic hazard', *Ann. Intern. Med.*, **74**, 144.

Marsden, H. B. and Hyde, W. A. (1962), 'Colistin methane sulphonate in childhood infections', *Lancet*, **2**, 740.

McMillan, M., Price, T. M. L., MacLaren, D. M. and Scott, G. W. (1962), 'Pseudomonas pyocyanea infection treated with colistin methane sulphonate', *Lancet*, **2**, 737.

McQuillen, M. P., Cantor, H. E. and O'Rourke, J. R. (1968), 'Myasthenic syndrome associated with antibiotics', *Arch. Neurol.*, **18**, 402.

Montgomerie, J. Z., Kalmanson, G. M. and Guze, L. B. (1973), 'Syngergism of polymyxin and sulfonamides in L-forms of Staphylococcus aureus and Proteus mirabilis', *Antimicrob. Ag. Chemother.*, **3**, 523.

Mukerjee, S. (1964), 'Cholera El Tor in Calcutta', *Brit. med. J.*, **2**, 546.

Murdoch, J. McC. (1964), 'The treatment of severe Pseudomonas pyocyanea infections with colistin', *Proceedings Third International Congress of Chemotherapy, Stuttgart*, p. 319.

Nord, N. M. and Hoeprich, P. D. (1964), 'Polymyxin B and colistin, a critical comparison', *New Engl. J. Med.*, **270**, 1030.

Nord, C.-E., Wadström, T. and Wretlind, B. (1974), 'Synergistic effect of combinations of sulfamethoxazole, trimethoprim, and colistin against Pseudomonas maltophilia and Pseudomonas cepacia', *Antimicrob. Ag. Chemother.*, **6**, 521.

Perkins, R. L. (1964), 'Apnea with intramuscular colistin therapy', *JAMA*, **190**, 421.

Pines, A., Raafat, H. and Plucinski, K. (1967), 'Gentamicin and colistin in chronic purulent bronchial infections', *Brit. med. J.*, **2**, 543.

Price, D. J. E. and Graham, D. I. (1970), 'Effects of large doses of colistin sulphomethate sodium on renal function', *Brit. med. J.*, **4**, 525.

Quintiliani, R. and Lentneck, A. (1971), 'Polymyxin B in the treatment of Klebsiella pneumoniae meningoventriculitis', *Amer. J. Dis. Child.*, **121**, 239.

Richet, G., Lopez de Novales, E. and Verroust, P. (1970), 'Drug intoxication and neurological episodes in chronic renal failure', *Brit. med. J.*, **2**, 394.

Rosenblatt, J. E. and Stewart, P. R. (1974), 'Combined activity of sulfamethoxazole, trimethoprim and polymyxin B against Gram-negative bacilli', *Antimicrob. Ag. Chemother.*, **6**, 84.

Ross, S., Puig, J. R. and Zaremba, E. A. (1960), 'Colistin: Some preliminary laboratory and clinical observations in specific gastroenteritis in infants and children', *Antibiot. Annual*—1959–1960, p. 89.

Ryan, K. J., Schainuck, L. I., Hickman, R. O. and Striker, G. E. (1969), 'Colistimethate toxicity. Report of a fatal case in a previously healthy child', *JAMA*, **207**, 2099.

Saslaw, S., Carlisle, H. N. and Moheimani, M. (1973), 'Comparison of colistin-carbenicillin, colistin, and carbenicillin in Pseudomonas sepsis in monkeys', *Antimicrob. Ag. Chemother.*, **3**, 118.

Schindler, P. R. G. and Teuber, M. (1975), 'Action of polymyxin B on bacterial membranes: Morphological changes in the cytoplasm and in the outer membrane of Salmonella typhimurium and Escherichia coli B', *Antimicrob. Ag. Chemother.*, **8**, 95.

Schwartz, B. S., Warren, M. R., Barkley, F. A. and Landis, L. (1960), 'Micribiological and pharmacological studies of colistin sulfate and sodium colistin-methanesulfonate', *Antibiot. Annual*—1959–1960, p. 41.

Schwartz, S. N., Medoff, G., Kobayashi, G. S., Kwan, C. N. and Schlessinger, D. (1972), 'Antifungal properties of polymyxin B and its potentiation of tetracycline as an antifungal agent', *Antimicrob. Ag. Chemother.*, **2**, 36.

Simmons, N. A. (1969), 'Potentiation of inhibitory activity of colistin on Pseudomonas aeruginosa by sulphamethoxazole and sulphamethizole', *Brit. med. J.*, **3**, 693.

Storring, R. A., McElwain, T. J., Jameson, B. and Wiltshaw, E. (1977), 'Oral non-absorbed antibiotics prevent infection in acute non-lymphoblastic leukaemia', *Lancet*, **2**, 837.

Sud, I. J. and Feingold, D. S. (1972), 'Effect of polymyxin B on antibiotic-resistant Proteus mirabilis', *Antimicrob. Ag. Chemother.*, **1**, 417.

Sud, I. J. and Feingold, D. S. (1975), 'Detection of agents that alter the bacterial cell surface', *Antimicrob. Ag. Chemother.*, **8**, 34.

Taylor, G. and Allison, H. (1962), '"Colomycin"—laboratory and clinical investigations', *Brit. med. J.*, **2**, 161.

Thomas, F. E., Jr., Leonard, J. M. and Alford, R. H. (1976), 'Sulfamethoxazole-trimethoprim-polymyxin therapy of serious multiply drug-resistant Serratia infections', *Antimicrob. Ag. Chemother.*, **9**, 201.

Thornsberry, C., Baker, C. N. and Kirven, L. A. (1978), '*In vitro* activity of antimicrobial agents on Legionnaires' Disease bacterium', *Antimicrob. Ag. Chemother.*, **13**, 78.

Weinstein, L. and Dalton, A. C. (1968), 'Host determinants of response to antimicrobial agents', *New Engl. J. Med.*, **279**, 467.

Wilkinson, S. (1963), 'Identity of colistin and polymyxin E', *Lancet*, **1**, 922.

Wolinsky, E. and Hines, J. D. (1962), 'Neurotoxic and nephrotoxic effects of colistin in patients with renal disease', *New Engl. J. Med.*, **266**, 759.

Wright, W. and Welch, H. (1960), 'Chemical, biological and clinical observations on colistin', *Antibiot. Annual*—1959–1960, p. 61.

Wynne, J. M. and Cooke, E. M. (1966), 'Passage of chloramphenicol and sodium colistimethate into the cerebrospinal fluid; studies of hydrocephalic children', *Amer. J. Dis. Child.*, **112**, 422.

Yaffe, S. J. (1965), 'Antibiotic dosage in newborn and premature infants', *JAMA*, **193**, 818.

Rifamycin B Diethylamide (Rifamide)

Description

The rifamycins are a group of antibiotics which were isolated from Streptomyces mediterranei in the Lepetit laboratories in Italy. Rifamycin B, the most active of the naturally occurring compounds, was not itself active enough for clinical use without chemical modification. Of a number of new compounds rifamycin SV ('Rifocin'), produced in 1961, was the first one used clinically mainly in Italy (Bergamini and Fowst, 1965).

In 1962 rifamycin B diethylamide or rifamide, which has a superior antibacterial activity, was developed, and then superseded rifamycin SV (Sensi *et al.*, 1967). It is a mono-basic acid, which was marketed with the trade name of 'Rifocin-M' (Lepetit). Rifamide is not currently available in Australia, Great Britain or the United States of America. The following information only applies to rifamide.

Sensitive Organisms

1. *Gram-positive bacteria*. Rifamide is particularly active against Staph. pyogenes (including penicillin G- and methicillin-resistant strains), Strep. pyogenes, Strep. pneumoniae and Strep. viridans. It has a lower order of activity against Strep. faecalis (Pallanza *et al.*, 1965; Stratford and Dixson, 1966). B. anthracis is also sensitive to rifamide but the Nocardia spp. are resistant.

2. *Gram-negative bacteria*. The pathogenic Neisseria spp. are sensitive to rifamide in low concentrations. H. influenzae may be inhibited by $0 \cdot 25 - 0 \cdot 5$ μg per ml (Citron and May, 1969). Most strains of Bacteroides spp. are also inhibited by relatively low concentrations of this drug (Leading article, 1973). Other Gram-negative bacteria such as Esch. coli, the Enterobacter, Klebsiella, Proteus, Salmonella and Shigella spp. and Pseudomonas aeruginosa are inhibited only by high rifamide concentrations ($10-100$ μg per ml or more).

3. Mycobacterium tuberculosis is also highly susceptible to rifamide (Pallanza *et al.*, 1965). The drug is also active against Mycobacterium leprae.

4. Rifamide-resistant strains of usually sensitive bacteria such as Staph. pyogenes can be produced *in vitro*, but apparently this phenomenon is not common during treatment *in vivo* (Stratford and Dixson, 1966).

In Vitro Sensitivities

The minimum inhibitory concentrations of rifamide against some selected bacterial species are shown in Table 35. These values depend on the inoculum size used in the test; when a large inoculum is used, the MIC may be higher for some of these bacteria (Stratford and Dixson, 1966).

TABLE 35

**Compiled from data published by Pallanza *et al.* (1965)
and Stratford and Dixson (1966)**

ORGANISM	MIC (μg per ml)
Gram-positive bacteria	
Staph. pyogenes	0·01–0·15
Strep. pyogenes (Group A)	0·007–0·01
Strep. pneumoniae	0·02
Strep. faecalis (Enterococcus, Group D)	0·10–50·0
Bacillus anthracis	0·20
Gram-negative bacteria	
Esch. coli	10·0–100·0
Enterobacter spp.	20·0
Klebsiella pneumoniae	20·0–100·0
Klebsiella aerogenes	20·0–50·0
Proteus spp.	10·0–100·0
Salmonella spp.	20·0–50·0
Shigella spp.	10·0–50·0
Neisseria gonorrhoeae	0·05
Miscellaneous	
Mycobacterium tuberculosis	0·20

Mode of Administration and Dosage

1. Rifamide, not adequately absorbed from the alimentary tract, is administered by intramuscular injection. It is not suitable for intravenous administration.

2. The usual intramuscular dose for adults is 150 mg eight-hourly, but doses of 150 mg six-hourly or higher can be used for treatment of severe infections.

3. The dose for children is 10 mg per kg body weight per day, given in three divided doses. Rifamide has not been used in newborn and premature infants, and is not recommended for these age groups.

4. *Patients with renal failure.* Rifamide can be given in the usual doses to such patients, because it does not accumulate with impaired renal function.

5. *Patients with liver disease or biliary obstruction.* In these patients serum levels may rise substantially as a result of impaired biliary excretion (Fig. 28). A serum level of 9 μg per ml was observed following usual therapeutic doses in one patient with biliary obstruction due to a stone in the common bile duct (Stratford, 1966a). In such patients rifamide dosage should be reduced and serum levels monitored, and these levels should probably not exceed 2 μg per ml. However the use of rifamide in such reduced dosage is only satisfactory when infections other than those of the biliary tract are treated. Rifamide is not suitable for treatment of biliary infections in patients with impaired biliary excretion (page 551).

Serum Levels in Relation to Dosage

After intramuscular administration of 150–300 mg of rifamide, the peak serum level of about 1·0 μg per ml is usually attained about one hour after injection. Thereafter a therapeutic serum level against the majority of Gram-positive bacteria is maintained for 6–8 h. The serum level is higher and more prolonged in patients with poor liver function, and the biliary concentration of the drug is much lower than in patients with normal liver function (Fig. 28).

Excretion

URINE: Only about 4–7 per cent of the administered dose of rifamide is excreted in the active form by the kidneys. After a single 150 mg intramuscular dose in patients with normal renal function, urine levels of the active drug are in the range of 0·3–10 μg per ml for 24 h. These urinary concentrations exceed the MIC's of Gram-positive bacteria, but are not high enough to inhibit the common Gram-negative bacilli, which usually cause urinary tract infections.

BILE: Studies in patients with external biliary drainage after cholecystectomy show that 80 per cent or more of an administered dose of rifamide is eliminated in the bile (Acocella *et al.*, 1966). After a single intramuscular dose of 150 mg, the biliary concentration of rifamide may reach 1600 μg per ml, and a level of about 60 μg per ml may still be present 24 h later. Continued rifamide administration of 150 mg eight-hourly, produces maximum biliary concentrations in the range of 1100 to 2400 μg per ml. These concentrations easily exceed the minimum inhibitory concentrations of the Gram-negative organisms, which commonly cause biliary tract infections. However in patients with poor liver function or biliary tract obstruction, bile levels are much lower (Fig. 28).

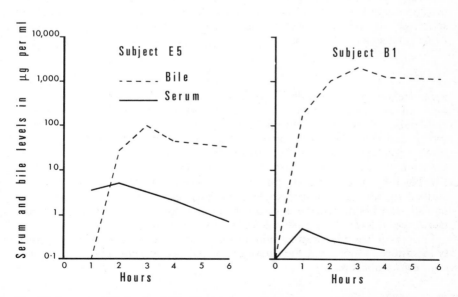

FIG. 28. Serum and bile levels of rifamide following the intramuscular injection of 300 mg of the drug in a patient (E5) with poor liver function and a patient (B1) with good liver function. (Redrawn after Khan and Scott, 1967)

INACTIVATION IN BODY: No appreciable metabolic inactivation of rifamide takes place in the body. Almost the entire administered dose of rifamide can be recovered from the urine and bile in animals.

Distribution of the Drug in Body

Rifamide is well distributed to all tissues, except the brain. Penetration of the drug into inflammatory exudates is also claimed to be good, but Citron and May (1969) failed to detect any antibiotic activity in the sputum of patients with chronic bronchitis treated with rifamide.

It has been emphasized that the drug is concentrated in the human gall bladder wall. An average tissue concentration of $39 \cdot 4$ μg per g was found in 16 patients who received 150 mg rifamide eight-hourly prior to cholecystectomy for gall stones, and in whom the cystic dust was not obstructed (Acocella et al., 1966). Such high rifamide concentrations in the gall bladder wall will probably not be attained in patients with acute cholecystitis, in whom the cystic duct is usually obstructed.

Rifamide apparently does not cross the placenta to any appreciable extent, and only negligible concentrations have been found in cord blood after administration of usual intramuscular doses to the mother.

Rifamide is about 70–80 per cent protein bound.

Mode of Action

The rifamycins (including rifamide) inhibit bacterial RNA synthesis by interfering with DNA directed RNA polymerase (page 433). The RNA polymerase of Esch. coli is very sensitive to the rifamycins, and these drugs are selectively damaging to bacteria because the corresponding mammalian enzyme is affected only by much higher concentrations (Hartmann et al., 1967).

Toxicity

Rifamide appears to be a drug with low toxicity. No toxic reactions have been reported from clinical studies, in particular there are no reports of hepatotoxicity in humans. Acute and chronic toxicity tests on many animal species have shown that rifamide is well tolerated (Lepetit Laboratories, 1968). Hypersensitivity reactions have not been reported, nor have they arisen in patients known to be allergic to the penicillins or other antibiotics.

It has been suggested that serum rifamide levels should not be allowed to rise above 2 μg per ml, but it is possible that higher serum levels are quite safe. One patient with a stone in the common bile duct reported by Stratford (1966a), had a serum level of 9 μg per ml, yet no toxic effects were noted.

Observations on laboratory animals have shown no evidence of teratogenicity (Stratford, 1966b), but the safety of rifamide during human pregnancy has not been established.

Clinical Uses of the Drug

Originally it was suggested that rifamide may be useful for staphylococcal, streptococcal and pneumococcal infections, but now a wide range of more effective drugs are available for these. Although high biliary levels of the drug sufficient to inhibit common Gram-negative organisms are attained in normal subjects (page 549), rifamide is not indicated for biliary tract infections. If there is significant biliary obstruction, therapeutic levels of the drug are not reached in the bile and also these infections are often associated with a septicaemia, so that a drug which produces therapeutic levels in the blood is indicated (Schoenfield, 1971). Rifamide is now largely of historical interest as a precursor of riampicin (page 552).

REFERENCES

Acocella, G., Lamarina, F., Tenconi, L. T. and Nicolis, F. B. (1966), 'Study of the excretion in bile and concentration in the gall bladder wall of rifamide', *Gut*, **7**, 380.

Bergamini, G. and Fowst, G. (1965), 'Rifamycin SV. A review', *Arzneimittel-Forsch.*, **15**, 951; quoted by Lepetit Laboratories (1968).

Citron, K. M. and May, J. R. (1969), 'Rifamycin antibiotics in chronic purulent bronchitis', *Lancet,* **2,** 982.

Hartmann, G., Honikel, K. O., Knüsel, F. and Nüesch, J. (1967), 'The specific inhibition of the DNA-directed RNA synthesis by rifamycin', *Biochim. Biophys. Acta,* **145,** 843.

Khan, G. A. and Scott, A. J. (1967), 'The place of rifamycin-B-diethylamide in the treatment of cholangitis complicating biliary obstruction', *Br. J. Pharmac. Chemother.,* **31,** 506.

Leading Article (1973), 'Bacteroides in the blood', *Lancet,* **1,** 27.

Lepetit Laboratories (1968), *Handbook on Rifamide (Rifocin-M),* Lepetit Pharmaceuticals Ltd.

Pallanza, R., Füresz, S., Timbal, M. T. and Carniti, G. (1965), '*In vitro* bacteriological studies on rifamycin B diethylamide (Rifamide)', *Arzneimittel-Forsch,* **15,** 800; quoted by Lepetit Laboratories (1968).

Schoenfield, L. J. (1971), 'Editorial. Biliary excretion of antibiotics', *New Engl. J. Med.,* **284,** 1213.

Sensi, P., Maggi, N., Füresz, S. and Maffii, G. (1967), 'Chemical modifications and biological properties of rifamycins', *Antimicrob. Ag. Chemother.*—1966, p. 699.

Stratford, B. C. and Dixson, S. (1966), 'Laboratory investigation of rifamycin diethylamide (rifamide), a new antibiotic', *Med. J. Aust.,* **1,** 1.

Stratford, B. C. (1966a), 'The treatment of acute cholecystitis and other diseases with rifamycin diethylamide (rifamide)', *Med. J. Aust.,* **1,** 7.

Stratford, B. F. (1966b), 'Observations on laboratory rodents treated with 'rifamide' during pregnancy', *Med. J. Aust.,* **1,** 10.

Rifampicin (Rifampin)

Description

After the discovery of rifamycin B (page 547), many modifications of the original compound were made in an attempt to obtain a drug suitable for oral administration and with greater activity against M. tuberculosis. One of these derivatives, rifampicin or rifampin (chemically 3-4(4-methylpiperazinyl-iminomethylidene)-rifamycin SV), appeared to conform to these requirements and was selected for clinical trials (Sensi et al., 1967). Rifampicin has now proved to be a most valuable 'first-line' drug for the treatment of tuberculosis, and it also has a place in the treatment of a number of other infections. Trade names include 'Rifadin' (Lepetit and British Schering) and 'Rimactane' (Ciba). There are also a number of commercial preparations available in which it is combined with isoniazid (page 802), such as 'Rifamate' (Dow), 'Rifinah' (Lepetit) and 'Rimactazid' (Ciba).

Sensitive Organisms

1. *Gram-positive bacteria*. Rifampicin, like rifamide (page 547) is highly active against Gram-positive cocci such as Staph. pyogenes (including penicillin G- and methicillin-resistant strains), Strep. pyogenes, Strep. pneumoniae and Strep. viridans. Strains of Strep. pneumoniae detected in South Africa in 1977, which were resistant to penicillin and many other antibiotics (page 4), were usually sensitive to rifampicin, but some developed resistance to this drug (Center for Disease Control, 1977; 1978). Most Strep. faecalis strains are only moderately sensitive. Gram-positive bacilli such as B. anthracis and the Clostridium spp. are sensitive (Sensi et al., 1967; Kunin et al., 1969; Dans et al., 1970). The Nocardia spp. are nearly always rifampicin-resistant (Tanzil et al., 1972).

2. *Gram-negative bacteria*. Meningococci are highly sensitive and H. influenzae including ampicillin-resistant strains (page 102) is also usually sensitive (Bannatyne and Cheung, 1978). N. gonorrhoeae is highly sensitive and this includes beta-lactamase-producing strains (page 4) which are inhibited by a concentration of 2 μg per ml or less (Report, 1978). Compared to rifamide, rifampicin has a higher degree of activity against the common Gram-negative bacilli, such as Esch. coli, the Enterobacter, Klebsiella, Proteus, Salmonella, Shigella and Bacteroides spp. and Ps. aeruginosa. The susceptibility of these Gram-negative bacteria to rifampicin is variable. Shanson and Leung (1976) found that 17 out of 18 strains of Salm. typhi were inhibited by 12 μg per ml of rifampicin. Although Pseudomonas pseudomallei is usually resistant *in vitro*, some animal studies suggest that rifampicin is effective

against it *in vivo* (Pattamasukon *et al.*, 1975). Most Bacteroides spp. strains are inhibited by 1·0 μg per ml (Leigh, 1974), and the Proteus spp. are also susceptible. By contrast some strains of Klebsiella spp. and Ps. aeruginosa are more resistant, and may have an MIC as high as 15 μg per ml (Atlas and Turck, 1968). Serratia marcescens and Providencia stuartii also may be sensitive. Kerry *et al.* (1975) found that the consistently most insensitive species was Ps. aeruginosa. Brucella spp. are sensitive and rifampicin is effective for the treatment of experimental brucellosis in animals (Philippon *et al.*, 1977). The susceptibility of the Legionnaires' disease bacterium to antimicrobial agents has been tested *in vitro* and *in vivo*; the most active agent was rifampicin (MIC ⩽ 0·01 μg per ml) (Thornsberry *et al.*, 1978; Lewis *et al.*, 1978). Nevertheless generally the activity of rifampicin against Gram-negative bacilli is of a much lower order than its activity against Gram-positive organisms and the Neisseria spp.

3. *Mycobacteria*. Rifampicin is highly active against M. tuberculosis (Sensi *et al.*, 1967; Clark and Wallace, 1967), and its activity is comparable to isoniazid under experimental conditions (Hobby, 1969). Subinhibitory amounts of rifampicin may increase the effectiveness of streptomycin or isoniazid and it may also prevent the emergence of mutants resistant to the other two drugs (Hobby and Lenert, 1972).

Some other mycobacteria (*see* page 832) may also be sensitive. M. kansasii is often rifampicin-sensitive, but others such as M. fortuitum, M. avium and M. intracellulare are almost always resistant (McClatchy *et al.*, 1969; Rynearson *et al.*, 1971; Woodley *et al.*, 1972). Sixty per cent of strains of M. kansasii obtained from patients with pulmonary infection in Texas between 1971 and 1974 were sensitive to rifampicin (Harris *et al.*, 1975). The majority of strains of M. kansasii isolated in Australia are also sensitive (Elder *et al.*, 1977).

M. marinum is commonly sensitive to rifampicin (Sage and Derrington, 1973; Van Dyke and Lake, 1975). Most strains of M. ulcerans are rifampicin-sensitive, and the drug is effective for the treatment of experimental M. ulcerans infection in mice footpads (Stanford and Phillips, 1972).

Mycobacterium leprae (including strains resistant to dapsone) is also susceptible to rifampicin, the MIC being 0·3 μg per ml when tested against human strains grown in mice. In this test system, it kills these bacilli more rapidly than other drugs used for treatment of leprosy, such as the sulphones (Rees *et al.*, 1970; Holmes and Hilson, 1972). Levy *et al.* (1976) studied the bactericidal effect of rifampicin in human volunteers with untreated multi-bacillary leprosy by taking repeated skin biopsies for mouse innoculation to determine the rate of killing of M. leprae. The organisms were killed equally rapidly by a daily dose of 600 mg or single doses of 1500 or 1200 mg; lower single doses or a daily dose of 300 mg were less effective but, even with these regimens, no viable organisms could be detected within one to two weeks, a result which can only be achieved by about three months' treatment with sulphones (dapsone). The effect of rifampicin or dapsone treatment on the bacteraemia associated with lepromatous leprosy has also been assessed by testing the ability of organisms taken from the blood to multiply in the mouse footpad. Leprosy bacilli could be detected in the blood by direct smears for at least 12–16 weeks with either form of therapy. However circulating viable M. leprae were only present for up to six weeks after initiation of dapsone treatment and for fewer than four weeks after rifampicin. It was concluded that either dead organisms had continued to circulate or their test system was not sufficiently sensitive to detect viable M. leprae (Drutz *et al.*, 1974).

Despite the rapid bactericidal action of rifampicin against M. leprae, it should not be concluded that all organisms are rapidly killed and that therefore there is no possibility of relapse after a short course of rifampicin. Pattyn *et al.* (1976) detected viable organisms in the nerve of a patient who had taken rifampicin at weekly intervals for three months. Viable organisms have also been recovered from nerve and muscle tissue after at least five years' daily treatment with rifampicin (Rees, 1975; Rees *et al.*, 1976; Waters *et al.*, 1978).

Collectively these studies indicate that the use of rifampicin results in rapid killing of M. leprae which reduces the period of the patient's infectivity. In addition, long-term chemotherapy of this disease is still necessary particularly for lepromatous and borderline-lepromatous leprosy. In these forms persisting M. leprae may be responsible for relapses after rifampicin therapy similar to that which may occur after dapsone therapy.

4. *Chlamydia*. Rifampicin is active *in vitro* against the agents causing trachoma, lymphogranuloma venereum and psittacosis (Binda *et al.*, 1971), and in this respect some authors have found that it is more active than tetracycline and erythromycin (Blackman *et al.*, 1977; Leading article, 1978). Mutant strains of Chlamydia trachomatis resistant to rifampicin can be induced *in vitro* (Keshishyan *et al.*, 1973).

5. *Rickettsiae*. Various *in vitro* studies show that rifampicin is very active against Rickettsia prowazeki (MIC 0·008–0·01 μg per ml) and although it is also cidal against this organism at a clinically attainable concentration, the rate of killing was slow (Wisseman *et al.*, 1974).

6. *Naegleria*. Rifampicin has been reported to have *in vitro* activity against the amoeboflagellate N. fowleri which can cause amoebic meningoencephalitis in humans (Thong *et al.*, 1977).

7. *Viruses*. It is of theoretical interest that rifampicin also has some activity against certain viruses (Heller *et al.*, 1969; Subak-Sharpe *et al.*, 1969). It has an inhibitory effect against Vaccinia virus, various other Poxviruses and the Adenoviruses. Rifampicin also interferes with the replication of Cytomegalovirus (Halstead *et al.*, 1972), but it has no effect against other Herpesviruses and a variety of RNA viruses. Unfortunately the concentration of rifampicin necessary for inhibition of the 'sensitive viruses' in tissue culture is 75–150 μg per ml, a level which cannot be attained in human body fluids. Rifampicin therefore has a 500–1000 fold lesser activity against viruses than against highly sensitive bacteria. In these studies antiviral activity was demonstrated by adding rifampicin to tissue cultures soon after virus inoculation, and this may be one of several reasons why it is ineffective in established virus infections (*Brit. med. J.* Leading article, 1969). In addition rifampicin-resistant strains of Vaccinia virus emerge readily (Subak-Sharpe *et al.*, 1969).

8. *Synergism with other drugs*. Rifampicin, when used in combination with several other chemotherapeutic agents, displays *in vitro* synergism against a wide variety of microorganisms.

Rifampicin and erythromycin was shown in one study to be the most bactericidal combination against a particular strain of Staph. pyogenes by extensive *in vitro* antibiotic testing (Peard *et al.*, 1970); this combination was used to treat a patient with endocarditis successfully (see page 572). In a study of Staph. pyogenes strains isolated from patients with endocarditis, Tuazon *et al.* (1978) found that a combination of rifampicin and nafcillin (page 93) was synergistic against 12 of 20 strains. A combination of rifampicin and vancomycin was also synergistic against five of the isolates. Arioli *et al.* (1970) showed that rifampicin plus tetracycline increased the survival rate of mice injected intra-peritoneally with Gram-negative organisms, compared to the survival rate when either drug was used alone. This effect was demonstrable with strains of Salm. typhimurium, Esch. coli, Pr. vulgaris and Sh. dysenteriae. *In vitro* synergism between rifampicin and novobiocin has been demonstrated with Salm. typhi; the optimal ratio for novobiocin:rifampicin was 13:1. Synergy was maximal at concentrations of both drugs which are easily attainable in serum and in bile (pages 559, 560) with therapeutic doses. It may be possible to use this combination for the treatment of typhoid due to strains resistant to chloramphenicol, co-trimoxazole and ampicillin (Shanson and Leung, 1976). The *in vitro* action of polymyxin B and rifampicin against multi-drug-resistant Serratia marcescens strains has been demonstrated to be additive in one study (Traub and Kleber, 1975) and synergistic in others (Ostenson *et al.*, 1977; *see* page 533). There have been a number of other *in vitro* studies showing that rifampicin in combination with other chemotherapeutic agents produces synergism and sometimes antagonism against Gram-positive and Gram-negative bacteria (Binda *et al.*, 1971). The modes of action of erythromycin, tetracycline, novobiocin and polymyxin B, differing as they do from that of rifampicin, may account for synergistic effects.

Because trimethoprim and rifampicin act at different points in the biosynthesis of nucleic acids, they were tested for possible synergism against a broad spectrum of common hospital pathogens (Kerry *et al.*, 1975). Synergism or additive effect was almost always observed. Synergism was most marked against Strep. pyogenes, Strep. faecalis, Proteus rettgeri and Pr. morganii. An additive or synergistic effect occurred against all strains of Kl. aerogenes, Esch. coli, Enterobacter spp., Ps. aeruginosa, Bacteroides fragilis and Salm. typhimurium. Antagonism was only observed against Staph. pyogenes and this occurred at very low concentrations of rifampicin. Arioli *et al.* (1977) confirmed an *in vitro* synergism of rifampicin and trimethoprim in various concentrations against Gram-negative bacteria such as Sh. dysenteriae, Pr. vulgaris, Salm. typhimurium and Esch. coli. They also showed that this combination was more effective than either drug alone in increasing the percentage of surviving mice infected with these bacteria. A further advantage of this combination is that the frequency of rifampicin-resistant mutants is decreased in the presence of subinhibitory levels of trimethoprim. Synergism may also sometimes be demonstrable when the organism is resistant to trimethoprim and/or rifampicin. In a study of this drug combination on 100 urinary pathogens, synergism occurred with 16 strains. Of these, two strains of Strep. faecalis were sensitive to both drugs, nine other (5 Strep. faecalis, 3 Staph. epidermidis and 1 Pr. mirabilis) were resistant to trimethoprim only, whilst five (2 Strep. faecalis, 2 Staph. epidermidis and 1 Esch. coli) were resistant to both drugs (Grüneberg and Emmerson, 1977). Rifampicin and trimethoprim have also been tested together *in vitro* against 61 Gram-negative rods resistant to gentamicin. Strains of various Enterobacteriaceae, Ps. aeruginosa and

Acinetobacter, Alcaligenes and Flavobacterium spp. were studied (Farrell *et al.*, 1977). Although synergy was demonstrable with only two strains at concentrations of the drugs readily obtainable in serum, it was demonstrable with 24 strains at concentrations of the drugs attainable in the urine. The combination of rifampicin and trimethoprim was also shown to be uniformly synergistic *in vitro* against 15 strains of Serratia marcescens (Hamilton-Miller *et al.*, 1977). Various pharmacokinetic studies of the use of these drugs together have been made in man. Hamilton-Miller and Brumfitt (1976) used daily doses of rifampicin 300 mg and trimethoprim 160 mg; Acocella and Scotti (1976) used daily doses of rifampicin 600 mg and trimethoprim 160 mg. Both studies showed that after single doses of the combination, serum levels and excretion of each drug was unaffected by the other, and the ratio of their serum concentrations were similar to those which produce *in vitro* synergism. After seven days' treatment with the two drugs, there was some reduction in the serum half-life of trimethoprim. Nevertheless these kinetic studies were considered to be favourable enough to warrant a clinical trial of a rifampicin/trimethoprim combination.

Rifampicin used together with amphotericin B is more effective than either drug alone when tested *in vitro* and *in vivo* against a number of fungi (*see* page 866). Amphotericin B by its action on the fungal cytoplasmic membrane (page 871), apparently allows penetration of rifampicin into the cell.

9. *Acquired resistance.* Mutants resistant to rifampicin can be detected both *in vitro* and *in vivo* amongst most of the bacteria usually sensitive to this drug, such as Staph. pyogenes, Strep. pyogenes, Strep. pneumoniae, Esch. coli, Proteus spp. and Ps. aeruginosa (Atlas and Turck, 1968; McCabe and Lorian, 1968; Kunin *et al.*, 1969; Binda *et al.*, 1971). Such resistant mutants appear rapidly when rifampicin is used alone, usually as a result of one-step mutation i.e. a change from sensitivity to resistance occurs in one generation. Resistance of a number of bacteria is due to the development of a DNA-dependent RNA polymerase which will not bind rifampicin (Binda *et al.*, 1971). Investigations on a strain of M. intracellulare which exhibited natural resistance to rifampicin showed that it contained RNA polymerase susceptible to the drug. This suggested that rifampicin resistance in naturally occurring strains of mycobacteria may be due to permeability barriers which may vary between species and strains of bacteria (Hui *et al.*, 1977). The rate at which resistant mutants appear is reduced if rifampicin is used with another chemotherapeutic agent. Jensen (1968) used fusidic acid or novobiocin with rifampicin for this purpose when treating infections by methicillin-resistant staphylococci. Kerry *et al.* (1975) showed that the frequency of rifampicin-resistant mutants was reduced by subinhibitory levels of trimethoprim (*vide supra*).

The rate of spontaneous development of rifampicin-resistant mutants of M. tuberculosis *in vitro* is low (McClatchy *et al.*, 1969). Such mutants show a high degree of resistance to the drug, and there are no intermediate levels between sensitive and highly resistant strains (Tsukamura, 1972). In one trial rifampicin was used alone for 45 days to treat 11 patients with pulmonary tuberculosis; resistant strains were detected in two patients and strains with diminished sensitivity to rifampicin in another four (Baronti and Lukinovich, 1968). Emergence of rifampicin-resistant M. tuberculosis during treatment of patients has not been a major problem, but in nearly all trials rifampicin has been used together with one or two other antituberculosis drugs (Lancet, Leading article, 1969). Primary rifampicin resistance in tuberculosis is still uncommon. In Australia, during the five-year period 1972–1976, its incidence has remained less than 0·4 per cent (Commonwealth Dept. Health, 1973–1977). In the United States of America primary rifampicin resistance in tuberculosis has also been uncommon (Woodley *et al.*, 1972); in a continuing study amongst veterans from 1969 to 1973, the incidence has remained less than two per cent and has not increased (Hobby *et al.*, 1971; 1974). An increasing incidence of rifampicin resistant strains (reaching a percentage of 1·96) was found in Massachusetts in the years 1971 to 1974, mainly amongst patients who had had previous treatment for tuberculosis (acquired or secondary resistance); with the exception of two strains which were isolated from patients who had not received prior chemotherapy, the remainder were also resistant to other antituberculosis drugs (Stottmeier, 1976). Strains of M. tuberculosis isolated from countries where rifampicin is used for both tuberculosis and non-tuberculous conditions (Italy, Argentina, Brazil and Spain) do not show a higher incidence of primary resistance than strains from other countries (France, Britain and the United States), where rifampicin use is confined to tuberculosis (Acocella *et al.*, 1977). These findings have been proffered as an argument for the use of rifampicin in combination with other chemotherapeutic agents for the treatment of certain non-tuberculous infections.

Acquired resistance of rifampicin by M. kansasii has been described in two patients with pulmonary disease. Both had failed to respond to chemotherapy to which the organisms were resistant, one had received isoniazid and the other isoniazid and ethambutol; rifampicin was added to these regimens, this being in effect rifampicin monotherapy (Davidson and Waggoner, 1976). Strains of M. leprae resistant to rifampicin have been confirmed by mouse foot-pad studies; these occurred in patients who were receiving rifampicin alone for the treatment of their disease (Jacobson and Hastings, 1976).

In Vitro Sensitivities

The minimum inhibitory concentrations of rifampicin against some selected bacterial species are shown in Table 36. Naturally occurring strains of M. tuberculosis, both sensitive and resistant to other antituberculosis drugs, are usually inhibited by 0·5 μg per ml or less of rifampicin. However the MIC of M. tuberculosis varies with the *in vitro* technique used, being between 0·005 and 0·5 μg per ml in liquid media, and 2·5 to 5·0 μg per ml in Lowenstein-Jensen medium (*Lancet*, Leading article, 1969).

Mode of Administration and Dosage

Rifampicin is administered orally in a dosage of 10–20 mg per kg per day given in one, two or three divided doses. For elderly or underweight patients smaller doses of 8 mg per kg per day are given. The daily adult dose which has been used in clinical trials has ranged from 450 to 900 mg. A common dosage schedule for the treatment of tuberculosis is 600 mg per day for adults administered as a single dose, preferably before breakfast (Proust and Evans, 1972). The dose for children is 10 mg per kg per day but this may be increased

TABLE 36

Compiled from data published by Sensi et al. (1967) and Kerry et al. (1975)

ORGANISM	MIC (μg per ml)
Gram-positive bacteria	
Staph. pyogenes	0·02
Strep. pyogenes	0·099
Strep. pneumoniae (Dip. pneumoniae)	0·01
Strep. faecalis	4·12
Gram-negative bacteria	
Esch. coli	5·3
Klebsiella pneumoniae	10·0
Klebsiella aerogenes	11·9
Enterobacter spp.	11·3
Proteus mirabilis	3·85
Proteus vulgaris	4·28
Proteus rettgeri	5·8
Proteus morganii	11·4
Salmonella typhimurium	7·16
Pseudomonas aeruginosa	19·95
Bacteroides fragilis	0·26
Miscellaneous	
Mycobacterium tuberculosis (H37 RV)	0·5

to 20 mg per kg for serious infections. Although serum levels are slightly lower if the drug is given with food (page 559), the duration of therapeutically active serum levels is unchanged (Siegler *et al.*, 1974). Nevertheless, the failure of a number of patients to respond to short-term chemotherapy of tuberculosis with a rifampicin-based regimen has been attributed to giving rifampicin after breakfast. Therefore this drug should be given on waking and as long as possible before breakfast (Gill, 1976). Rifampicin is not recommended as routine chemotherapy for children under two years of age but it may be used for serious infections (*see* page 570).

This drug is used in regimens for the intermittent chemotherapy of tuberculosis (page 569). A rifampicin dose of 1200 mg twice-weekly is no longer recommended because of severe side-effects (page 563). The frequency of side-effects is much lower with a dosage of 900 mg (15 mg per kg) twice-weekly (Citron, 1972; Anastasatu *et al.*, 1973). This and a lower dose of 600 mg twice-weekly have been satisfactory for intermittent regimens (*see* page 569). Rifampicin in a dose of 600 mg or even 450 mg given on alternate days has also been used.

Rifampicin does not accumulate in patients with impaired renal function and for these the usually recommended doses are suitable. The drug may accumulate in the presence of liver disease or biliary tract obstruction, and so it should be used with caution in patients with chronic alcoholism or known liver disease. The elimination of rifampicin is not affected by haemodialysis or peritoneal dialysis (Binda *et al.*, 1971).

It appears that rifampicin can be used during pregnancy if the appropriate indications are present, and that termination of the pregnancy because of rifampicin therapy is unjustified (Jentgens, 1975; Stern and Stainton-Ellis, 1977; Commonwealth Dept. Health Australia, 1977). Nevertheless the American Thoracic Society currently prefers a combination of isoniazid and ethambutol when treatment during pregnancy is necessary (Bailey *et al.*, 1977).

Serum Levels in Relation to Dosage

Rifampicin is well absorbed from the gastro-intestinal tract, and a peak serum concentration of about 8 μg per ml is reached $1 \cdot 5$–$3 \cdot 0$ h after an oral dose of 600 mg. Serum levels are lower if the drug is taken immediately after food (Fig. 29). A wide range of serum levels following this dose have been obtained in different studies, some of which are considerably higher than those depicted in Fig. 29 (Binda *et al.*, 1971). There is also a disproportion between peak serum

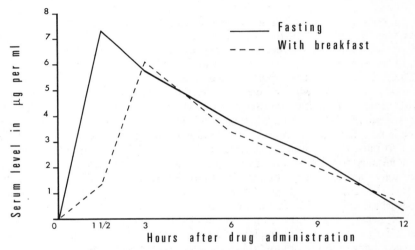

FIG. 29. Rifampicin serum concentrations in adult humans after a single oral dose of 600 mg on an empty stomach and 600 mg in addition to breakfast. (Redrawn after Verbist and Gyselen, 1968.)

levels and the size of the dose, because larger doses result in greater than proportional peak levels. In addition after a high dose the elimination of rifampicin 4–8 h later is slower than expected, possibly due to saturation of the mechanism for biliary excretion of the drug (Dickinson *et al.*, 1974).

Changes in the serum levels also occur with continuation treatment (Acocella *et al.*, 1971; Acocella and Scotti, 1976). During the first six days of treatment, although peak serum levels are unaffected, the levels at 12 h show a definite decrease. The serum half-life also becomes shorter during the first six days and this is most evident with daily doses of 900 mg; the half-lives following 600 mg and 900 mg daily doses are then nearly the same (about $2 \cdot 5$–$3 \cdot 0$ h). An increased rate of biliary excretion during the first six days of treatment occurs, because during this period rifampicin induces enzymes in the liver which increase its own metabolism and hence its excretion (page 567).

The concomitant administration of para-amino salicylic acid interferes with the absorption of rifampicin from the gastro-intestinal tract, and if these two drugs are used together, their administration should be separated by an interval of about 8–12 h (Boman *et al.*, 1971). Adequate serum levels also may not be attained if barbiturates are administered concomitantly, presumably as a result of induction of liver enzymes, which metabolize rifampicin (*vide supra*) (Council on Drugs, 1972).

Excretion

URINE: Some active rifampicin is excreted in the urine. Murdoch *et al.* (1969) found that with daily oral doses of 900 mg, 200–400 mg of the active drug could be recovered from urine in the next 24 h. Kunin *et al.* (1969) showed in five male volunteers given a single dose of 300 mg rifampicin, that 6 per cent of the total dose was excreted in the urine in the active form, and peak urine concentrations of 10–70 μg per ml were obtained within 4–8 h. With small oral doses of 150 mg or less the drug is nearly all excreted in bile; at doses of 300 mg or more the excretory capacity of the liver is exceeded, rifampicin serum levels rise and the drug appears in the urine (Girling, 1977).

BILE: A considerable proportion of a dose of rifampicin is eliminated in the bile and it competes with bilirubin for excretion. Its rate of biliary excretion is slower than that of rifamide (Sensi *et al.*, 1967). Rifampicin levels attained in bile are about 100 times higher than those in the serum at the time, provided there is no biliary obstruction or impaired liver function (Keberle *et al.*, 1968). Prior to biliary excretion, the drug is partly deacetylated in the liver by an enzyme induced in the first few days of treatment. The deacetylated compound is also active antibacterially but less so than the parent drug (Dickinson *et al.*, 1974). The unchanged rifampicin excreted in bile is readily reabsorbed from the gut but its deacetylated form is poorly absorbed. Eventually about 60 per cent of a single dose of the drug is excreted in the faeces (Keberle *et al.*, 1968). The biliary excretion of rifampicin is impaired in patients with either liver disease or biliary obstruction, and this may lead to increased serum levels (Lancet, Leading article, 1969).

The concomitant administration of probenecid increases serum levels in man probably by depressing the hepatic uptake of rifampicin, thereby slowing its deacetylation in the liver and excretion via the bile. Studies by Kenwright and Levi (1973) indicated that the peak serum level could be almost doubled when a 300 mg dose of rifampicin is preceded by 2 g probenecid given 30 min earlier. Subsequent investigations by Fallon *et al.* (1975), whilst confirming that probenecid does increase rifampicin serum levels, showed that this effect is so uncommon and inconsistent that probenecid has no place as an adjunct to routine rifampicin therapy.

INACTIVATION IN BODY: In addition to deacetylation in the liver, rifampicin, unlike rifamide, appears to be inactivated in the body to some extent, as a proportion of the dose has remained undetected in excretion studies (Hobby, 1969).

Distribution of the Drug in Body

Rifampicin, like rifamide, apparently penetrates well into most tissues. Studies in man show that concentrations in the lungs, liver, stomach wall, pleural exudate, ascitic fluid and bone usually exceed simultaneous serum levels (Sensi et al., 1967). Therapeutically active concentrations are also attained in tears and saliva (Hoeprich, 1971). A concentration of about 0.5 μg per ml may be attained in normal cerebrospinal fluid following the administration of the usual oral doses. There may be a four- to eight-fold increase in this concentration if the meninges are inflamed, and in patients with tuberculous meningitis therapeutic CSF concentrations can be easily maintained during the first one to two months of treatment (Curci et al., 1969; D'Oliveira, 1972). In a more recent study rifampicin was not detected in the cerebrospinal fluid of normal subjects 3 h after a dose of 25 mg per kg, but in patients with tuberculous meningitis significant CSF concentrations were reached in 3 h and maintained for 24 h (Sippel et al., 1974).

Sputum levels of $1-3$ μg per ml have been reported when fairly large doses of rifampicin were given to patients with chronic bronchitis (Citron and May, 1969).

Rifampicin crosses the placenta producing clinically significant levels of the drug in the fetus and amniotic fluid (Binda et al., 1971).

Rifampicin, unlike many other antibiotics, is lipid soluble and therefore it can penetrate the cell membrane and kill intracellular organisms. Rifampicin therefore may be of special value in the treatment of patients whose leucocytes are unable to kill ingested bacteria, e.g. in chronic granulomatous disease (Mandell and Vest, 1972; Lobo and Mandell, 1972).

Rifampicin is about 80 per cent bound to serum proteins (Boman, 1973).

Mode of Action

In studies using Esch. coli, rifampicin inhibits bacterial RNA synthesis by binding to DNA-dependent RNA polymerase (page 433). Its mechanism of action on mycobacteria is similar, and rifampicin-resistant strains may possess an altered DNA-dependent RNA polymerase (Konno et al., 1973) (see also page 556). Mammalian cells also contain RNA polymerase, but rifampicin is selectively toxic to bacteria, because the mammalian cell enzyme is much less sensitive to the drug than its bacterial counterpart (Hartmann et al., 1967; Staehelin et al., 1968). The polymerase in mammalian mitochondria is sensitive to rifampicin, but is probably unaffected by the drug in vivo because it appears that intact mitochondria are impermeable to rifampicin (Gadaleta et al., 1970). Rifampicin also inhibits fungal RNA synthesis, provided the drug is used with amphotericin B, which acts on the fungal plasma membrane (page 871) thereby increasing cell permeability to rifampicin (Battaner and Kumar, 1974).

On theoretical grounds it was considered that rifampicin might also inhibit certain DNA viruses such as Poxviruses and Adenoviruses, which also induce the formation of DNA-dependent RNA polymerases (transcriptases) in infected cells. The rifamycin group of antibiotics do inhibit DNA-dependent RNA polymerase activity associated with viral particles and also inhibit the viral enzyme, RNA-dependent DNA polymerase (reverse transcriptase), which is capable of synthetizing DNA from a RNA template (Gurgo et al., 1971;

Gale *et al.*, 1972). High concentrations of rifampicin (but not other rifamycins) indeed do inhibit Poxviruses and Adenoviruses (Heller *et al.*, 1969; Subak-Sharpe *et al.*, 1969). However its mode of action on viruses may not be the same as that on bacteria (Annotation, 1969). It has been suggested that the antiviral activity of rifampicin may be due to its side chain, because other rifamycins, whilst having a similar action on bacteria, have no antiviral activity (Annotation, 1970).

Toxicity

1. *Hypersensitivity reactions.* Severe generalised hypersensitivity reactions can occur but are rare (Girling, 1977). One of the most common side-effects of rifampicin is the 'cutaneous syndrome'; this may occur in patients receiving daily or intermittent rifampicin therapy and it usually becomes apparent early in the course of treatment. It consists of flushing and/or itching of the skin with or without a rash, involving particularly the face and scalp and redness and watering of the eyes may also occur. Symptoms usually occur 2–3 h after a rifampicin dose, are generally self-limiting and only require symptomatic treatment (Girling and Fox, 1971; Aquinas *et al.*, 1972). On rare occasions an acute shock-like state, probably due to anaphylaxis, has followed rifampicin administration (Nessi *et al.*, 1973). The drug is not cross-allergenic with the penicillins or any other antibiotics.

2. *Gastro-intestinal side-effects.* Anorexia, nausea, abdominal pain, vomiting and diarrhoea ('abdominal syndrome') are uncommon side-effects. These symptoms may occur with both daily and intermittent rifampicin therapy and, if unaccompanied by other side-effects, seldom necessitate change in therapy (Girling, 1977).

3. *Hepatotoxicity.* Liver damage has been reported in up to 20 per cent of patients treated with rifampicin, but it has been difficult to determine whether this has been solely due to rifampicin, because the drug has been commonly used with other antituberculosis drugs (Lancet, Leading article, 1969; Scheuer *et al.*, 1974; Leading article, 1975). Many patients receiving rifampicin alone or in combination with other drugs, develop elevations of serum transaminase levels, particularly during the first few weeks of chemotherapy, but most of these are asymptomatic and the transaminase levels return to normal whether rifampicin is stopped or not (Newman *et al.*, 1974). In a small percentage of patients, the use of rifampicin together with other antituberculosis drugs has been associated with clinical 'toxic hepatitis' characterized by jaundice and raised serum transaminase levels (Proust, 1971). Elderly patients may be more prone to such liver damage (Lees *et al.*, 1970), but severe hepatotoxicity has also been described in children (Casteels-Van Daele *et al.*, 1975). Pre-existing liver disease or alcoholism appears to predispose to symptomatic hepatitis. Thompson (1976) studied 36 patients with alcoholism who were receiving rifampicin plus isoniazid for tuberculosis. Fifteen of these with pre-existing liver disease, studied by serial liver biopsies, developed further morphological abnormalities not attributable to alcoholism, and one patient appeared to develop chronic active hepatitis after irregular rifampicin treatment. Patients with normal pre-treatment liver function and biopsies did not develop histological abnormalities. Thompson (1976) suggested that rifampicin is contraindicated in

alcoholics with initial abnormal liver function tests. Girling (1977) considers that pre-existing liver disease or alcoholism are not absolute contraindications to rifampicin treatment, provided that the patient's liver function is monitored and the dosage is reduced if liver function deteriorates. The frequency of hepatotoxicity in patients receiving high dosage intermittent rifampicin therapy does not appear to be higher than in those receiving daily rifampicin (Aquinas et al., 1972).

Ideally rifampicin should not be used in combination with other antituberculosis drugs which have a propensity to cause liver damage, namely ethionamide, pyrazinamide, PAS and isoniazid (Proust, 1971). Some studies indicated that there was an increased frequency of hepatotoxicity when isoniazid was used in combination with rifampicin (Lees et al., 1971; Lal et al., 1972) (see page 807). Subsequent studies in Chinese patients in which daily rifampicin was added for the first four months of a six-month course of isoniazid and pyrazinamide did not reveal an increased frequency of hepatotoxicity (Hong Kong/BMRC, 1976). Baron and Bell (1974) showed that biochemical liver disturbances were common with a daily regimen of streptomycin plus isoniazid and rifampicin but these were not more common than with a similar regimen in which PAS was substituted for rifampicin. Experience with the combined use of rifampicin and isoniazid in daily or intermittent regimens (pages 568, 569) now indicates that this combination may be safely used in patients with normal liver function, because hepatotoxicity appears to be mild and uncommon.

It may be concluded that mild transient abnormalities of liver function not uncommonly occur in the early weeks of rifampicin treatment, but the risk of overt hepatitis during chemotherapy is small (Girling, 1977).

4. *Thrombocytopenia and other haematological changes*. Thrombocytopenic purpura sometimes associated with bleeding usually occurs with intermittent rifampicin therapy, but it may also occur during supervised daily treatment (Hong Kong/BMRC, 1975).

Blajchman et al. (1970) reported a patient in whom severe thrombocytopenia with bleeding occurred during administration and re-administration of rifampicin. The thrombocytopenia had an immunological basis, because the patient's serum contained both IgG and IgM antibodies, which could only fix complement to platelets in the presence of rifampicin. These authors also referred to seven similar cases communicated to them. They noted that in all patients thrombocytopenia was associated with high dosage intermittent rifampicin therapy (1200 mg twice-weekly). Poole et al. (1971) also observed the same complication in three patients under similar circumstances. In view of these reports high intermittent doses of rifampicin should be avoided, and where possible monthly platelet counts should be performed on all patients receiving rifampicin. Thrombocytopenia and other side-effects of intermittent therapy (*vide infra*) are much less common when lower rifampicin doses of 900 mg or 600 mg twice-weekly are used (page 569). All side-effects from intermittent rifampicin therapy are more frequent and severe when either the individual dose or the interval between doses is increased. These complications may also occur in patients who have been prescribed daily rifampicin, if they do not take the drug regularly and interrupt their medication for several days at a time (Flynn et al., 1974).

Thrombocytopenia usually becomes apparent within three hours of a dose and in the absence of further rifampicin the platelet count returns to normal within 36 h. Fatalities have been recorded due to cerebral haemorrhage when the drug has been continued (Girling, 1977). The occurrence of thrombocytopenia or purpura is a contraindication to the further use of rifampicin.

Blajchman *et al.* (1970) demonstrated weak serum antibodies against red cells in 10 of 41 other patients receiving rifampicin, but these did not appear to be associated with any haematological complications. These rifampicin-dependent antibodies, which bind complement to the surface of red cells, appear to be more common in patients receiving intermittent rifampicin therapy, either in high doses (Poole *et al.*, 1971), or in the lower dose of 600 mg twice-weekly (Poole *et al.*, 1973). However rifampicin, unlike penicillin G (page 29), does not combine firmly with red cells, and haemolytic anaemia due to this drug, although reported, appears to be rare (Worlledge 1973a; Girling, 1977). Haemolysis usually becomes evident within two to three hours after a rifampicin dose and recovery occurs when the drug is stopped. Severe haemolysis with renal failure has been described. Massive haemolysis has been reported in one patient who received rifampicin therapy for nearly a year (Lakshminarayan *et al.*, 1973).

Human leucocytes incubated with rifampicin (or with chloramphenicol, sodium fusidate or tetracyclines) show markedly depressed migration (Forsgren and Schmeling, 1977). The clinical significance of this observation is not known.

5. *Immunosuppression.* Rifampicin has been reported to affect both humoral and cell-mediated immunity in animals and man, but results have been inconsistent. For instance, Graber *et al.* (1973) found that rifampicin interfered with the anamnestic response to Salm. typhi vaccine in patients with tuberculosis, but Bassi *et al.* (1975) and Miller (1978), studying similar patients, found no interference with antibody response after administration of killed influenza vaccine. Other studies in humans have suggested that rifampicin may suppress cell-mediated immunity, as tested for by delayed cutaneous hypersensity to purified protein derivative (PPD) of M. tuberculosis or by *in vitro* lymphocyte responses. The drug has been observed to cause a decreased cutaneous reaction to PPD in some patients treated with rifampicin (Mukerjee *et al.*, 1973). In high concentrations rifampicin suppresses *in vitro* lymphocyte responses to PPD and inhibits the blastic transformation of lymphocytes cultured in the presence of phytohaemagglutinin (PHA) (Nilsson, 1971; Grassi and Pozzi, 1972).

Other investigators have found differing results in studies of patients with tuberculosis receiving rifampicin. Ruben *et al.* (1974) noted that suppression of *in vitro* lymphocyte responses to PHA and PPD only occurred in such patients after 12 to 16 weeks' treatment. Gupta *et al.* (1975) demonstrated suppression of T-lymphocyte rosettes in 8 out of 18 patients, which usually occurred after a period of eight weeks; they were also able to demonstrate similar changes in some healthy subjects who had received rifampicin for two to three weeks and these changes were reversible after cessation of the drug. Goldstein *et al.* (1976) only found depression of lymphocyte responses to PHA in patients with tuberculosis who had received the drug for 4–24 months and in whom *in vitro* and *in vivo* responses to PPD remained normal. These authors pointed out that

the divergent conclusions which have been reached about the immunosuppressive effect of rifampicin can be explained by the diversity of the patients
with tuberculosis who have been tested, some of whom may have been anergic
due to their disease, and to the variety of test systems used. It was concluded
that most studies have not shown any consistent alterations in humoral immune responses and the influence of rifampicin therapy on cell-mediated immune responses in patients with tuberculosis is minimal. Certainly there is no
evidence so far that immunosuppressive effects of the drug hinder its effectiveness in the treatment of tuberculosis in man (Gupta et al. 1975).

6. *Renal failure*. Sudden onset of fever and lumbar pain followed by oliguria
and then anuria has been described in patients treated with rifampicin
(Kleinknecht et al., 1972; Cordonnier and Muller, 1972; Flynn et al., 1974).
All of these patients had temporarily discontinued daily rifampicin therapy and
their symptoms occurred one to two hours after readministration of the drug.
The anuria usually persisted for several days necessitating haemodialysis, but
ultimately recovery was complete. Rothwell and Richmond (1974) reported a
patient who took rifampicin intermittently of her own accord and who
developed acute reversible renal failure in association with moderately severe
hepatocellular damage. Renal failure has also occurred when rifampicin administration had been resumed after an interval. In two patients reported by
Seufert (1973), acute renal failure was associated with haemolysis, but this did
not appear to be the direct cause of the renal damage. Renal failure may also
result from shock associated with rifampicin therapy (*vide supra*). The
pathological changes commonly described with renal failure due to rifampicin
have usually been acute tubular necrosis possibly caused by a period of tubular
ischaemia (Chan et al., 1975). Studies in other patients have revealed changes
of interstitial nephritis (Flynn et al., 1974; Stone et al., 1976; Gabow et al.,
1976). An acute interstitial nephritis, similar to that which may be caused by
the penicillins (page 29), has been described as a rare complication of rifampicin; this hypersensitivity reaction is characterized by fever and often by
nausea, diarrhoea, myalgia, rash, eosinophilia, abnormal liver function tests
and renal failure (Nessi et al., 1976). The patient described by Gabow et al.
(1976) is of interest, because he developed renal failure which was detected by
a rising serum creatinine level in the absence of symptoms when rifampicin was
readministered after a gap of 36 days; renal biopsy showed interstitial and
glomerular changes and antibody deposited about the renal tubules. Perma-
ment renal damage occurred in a 42-year-old woman who resumed rifampicin
therapy after a period of nine months; two renal biopsies showed severe cortical necrosis (Cochran et al., 1975). Some of the pathological changes which
have been described, together with the detection of circulating rifampicin-
dependent antibodies in high titre in some patients (Chan et al., 1975), suggests
that the renal complications of rifampicin have an immunological basis.

Acute renal failure due to rifampicin therapy is uncommon but is more
prone to occur in patients receiving intermittent therapy or those taking the
drug irregularly. If the drug is recommenced after an interval, special care
should be taken and it may be advisable to reintroduce it in small gradually increasing daily doses (Girling, 1977). If renal failure develops, further use of the
drug is contraindicated.

7. '*Influenza syndrome*'. This is a collection of symptoms which is common

with certain regimens of intermittent rifampicin therapy (Aquinas *et al.*, 1972; Zierski, 1973). The features of this syndrome have been delineated during various clinical trials on patients with tuberculosis (Hong Kong/Brompton Hospital/BMRC, 1974; 1975; Hong Kong/BMRC, 1974; 1975; Singapore/BMRC, 1975); these have been summarised by Girling (1977).

The 'flu' syndrome is peculiar to intermittent therapy; it consists of fever, headache, malaise and bone pain beginning 1–2 h after a dose of rifampicin and these usually subside spontaneously within 12 h. Features of the syndrome usually do not appear until after three to six months of intermittent rifampicin therapy, and they may be accompanied by other side-effects of rifampicin. The frequency of the 'flu' syndrome is much higher both in patients receiving higher doses of the drug (especially 1200 mg or more), and also in patients receiving the drug at weekly intervals compared to others given the same dosage twice a week. Some authors have noted that this syndrome is more frequent in females (Eule *et al.*, 1974), and it is commoner in men, but not women with increasing age (Hong Kong/BMRC, 1975). Therapy with rifampicin may be continued in most patients, either by using a lower dosage for intermittent therapy or by substituting a daily rifampicin regimen (Girling and Fox, 1971; Aquinas *et al.*, 1972). Attempts to reduce the frequency of this side-effect by adding a small daily supplement of rifampicin to the larger intermittent doses have not been successful enough for practical application (Hong Kong/BMRC, 1974; Singapore/BMRC, 1975). The syndrome appears to be mild and infrequent if rifampicin is given in doses of 600 mg or 450 mg three times a week or 900 mg, 600 mg or 450 mg twice a week or 600 mg once a week.

An immunological reaction appears to be involved because many patients with the syndrome develop serum rifampicin-dependent antibodies (Worlledge, 1973b; Hong Kong/Brompton Hospital/BMRC, 1974; Singapore/BMRC, 1975). These antibodies are affected by the rhythm of rifampicin administration. They are rarely detectable with daily administration, possibly because this causes immune tolerance, whereas intermittent therapy favours sensitization. Bassi *et al.* (1976) studied rifampicin antibodies in patients with tuberculosis, one day, one week, three weeks and eight weeks after discontinuation of daily therapy; the greatest number of patients with antibodies was found in the third week. These findings were considered to be more consistent with a hypothesis that continuous rifampicin treatment results in continuous neutralization of antibodies, rather than induction of tolerance. The dose size is also important in determining the presence of antibodies; doses of 450 mg or 600 mg three times a week are much less liable to produce antibodies than doses of 900 mg or 600 mg twice or once a week (Girling, 1977). There is no evidence from studies in Hong Kong and Singapore that the presence of antibodies to rifampicin affects the therapeutic response to the drug (Hong Kong/Singapore/BMRC, 1976).

8. '*Respiratory syndrome*'. This syndrome is a less common complication of intermittent rifampicin administration (Aquinas *et al.*, 1972; Hong Kong/Brompton Hospital/BMRC, 1974). It consists of dyspnoea with or without a wheeze and sometimes a fall in blood pressure and shock. This side-effect is usually managed in a similar manner to the 'flu' syndrome, with which it may be associated and share a common mechanism.

9. *Fetal abnormalities*. These have been observed in rats and mice when

large doses of rifampicin are used (Stern and Stainton-Ellis, 1977). Although the manufacturers warn that the drug is contraindicated in pregnancy, particularly during the first trimester because of possible teratogenicity, experience to date indicates that it may be used under appropriate indications (*see* page 559).

10. *Interference with metabolism of other drugs.* Rifampicin competes with and thereby decreases the biliary excretion of some substances such as bilirubin, bromsulphalein (BSP) and certain contrast media used in cholecystography (Binda *et al.*, 1971).

There is also evidence that rifampicin induces a gradual proliferation of hepatic cell smooth endoplasmic reticulum in man, which is thought to be a locus for microsomial enzymes responsible for drug metabolism (Jezeguel *et al.*, 1971). In this way rifampicin causes enhancement of its own metabolism during the first six days of treatment, resulting in lowering of serum levels and half-life values for the drug (*see* page 559). This also seems to be the main mechanism by which it accelerates the metabolism of a number of other drugs in man. The half-life of tolbutamide is shortened in patients with tuberculosis treated by rifampicin (Syvälahti *et al.*, 1974). The efficacy of oral contraceptive medication may be impaired, resulting in disturbances of the menstrual cycle and unplanned pregnancy (Skolnick *et al.*, 1976). Induction of liver enzymes by rifampicin causes an increased breakdown of oestrogenic hormones (Bolt *et al.*, 1974). An increase in cortisol catabolism is probably caused by a similar mechanism (Yamada and Iwai, 1976). In rifampicin-treated patients with pulmonary tuberculosis, the rate of cortisol production is increased. In addition, one patient with Addison's disease in whom the half-life of cortisol was reduced required increased corticosteroid dosage during concomitant rifampicin administration (Edwards *et al.*, 1974). Buffington *et al.* (1976) described three patients with renal transplants, who developed progressive loss of renal allograft function during treatment of tuberculosis by rifampicin; investigations suggested that this was due to a decreased glucocorticosteroid effect because of its increased degradation. If it is necessary to use rifampicin in a renal transplant patient, to counteract the effect of rifampicin on cortisol catabolism, it may be necessary to double the usual daily dose of corticosteroids.

Rifampicin also diminishes the activity of anticoagulants. Studies by O'Reilly (1974; 1975) indicate that rifampicin markedly decreases the effect of warfarin during long-term therapy by enhancing its elimination from plasma, presumably mainly by liver enzyme induction. In patients receiving therapy with both warfarin and rifampicin, an unusually high maintenance dose of warfarin may be required to achieve a therapeutic effect. Romankiewicz and Ehrman (1975) described a patient in whom this effect on warfarin appeared to be maximal five to seven days after commencing rifampicin therapy, and it persisted for a similar period of time after rifampicin was stopped. Symptoms of methadone withdrawal have been described in patients receiving rifampicin, which have been attributed to enhanced methadone metabolism in the liver (Kreek *et al.*, 1976; Bending and Skacel, 1977). In the report by Kreek *et al.* (1976), of 30 patients receiving rifampicin (600–900 mg per day) and also methadone maintenance, symptoms of narcotic withdrawal developed in 21 patients 1–33 days after commencing rifampicin. In pharmacological studies of six of these patients, concomitant administration of rifampicin lowered methadone plasma concentrations and increased the urinary excretion of its major metabolite, consistent with an enhancement of methadone metabolism in the liver.

11. *Other side-effects*. There have been single case reports of severe exudative conjunctivitis (Cayley and Majumdar, 1976), and Stevens-Johnson syndrome (Nyirenda and Gill, 1977), which have been attributed to rifampicin usage. A nine-year-old patient developed polyarthritis, rash and hepatitis in association with anti-native DNA antibodies and a positive antinuclear factor after nine months continuous treatment with rifampicin and ethambutol. It was considered that rifampicin was the most likely cause of this illness (Grennan and Sturrock, 1976).

The presence of rifampicin in serum interferes with serum vitamin B_{12} and folate assays. This problem may be overcome either by using a rifampicin-resistant organism in such assays or by collecting specimens for assay from patients just before redosing, when the serum rifampicin level should be low (Cole *et al.*, 1973).

Rifampicin causes a red discoloration of the urine and other body fluids, but this is harmless. The pleural fluid in rifampicin-treated patients may also be stained red, and this can be mistaken for blood.

Clinical Uses of the Drug

1. *Standard chemotherapy for active pulmonary tuberculosis*. Rifampicin is the most effective companion drug for isoniazid in the treatment of tuberculosis. In developed countries where cost is not such a significant factor, it is now nearly always included in initial therapy (*see* page 810).

In one early study rifampicin was used alone to treat eleven patients in whom previous chemotherapy had been ineffective. After 45 days' treatment the number of bacilli in sputum smears had decreased considerably in most patients, and in three patients both smears and cultures became negative. However at the end of this course, strains of M. tuberculosis less sensitive to rifampicin than pre-treatment strains were isolated from five of the eight patients with persistent positive cultures (Baronti and Lukinovich, 1968). This experience indicates that rifampicin should not be used as a single agent for the treatment of pulmonary tuberculosis.

Results of numerous controlled trials are available comparing the efficacy of drug combinations containing rifampicin with previous 'first-line' drug combinations (Newman *et al.*, 1971; 1974; Nitti *et al.*, 1971; Raleigh, 1972; BMRC, 1973; O'Connell *et al.*, 1973). Isoniazid and rifampicin were combined with either streptomycin or ethambutol for a period of two to four months, followed by maintenance therapy with isoniazid and rifampicin. These regimens were compared with classical therapy consisting of isoniazid, streptomycin and PAS for two to four months, followed by isoniazid and PAS. Regimens containing rifampicin were either found to be equally effective or marginally superior to classical therapy. However in all these trials maintenance therapy with isoniazid and rifampicin produced fewer side-effects and less interruptions to treatment than such therapy with isoniazid and PAS. Other authors have treated new tuberculosis patients satisfactorily with an isoniazid/rifampicin combination alone (Lees *et al.*, 1972b; Clarke *et al.*, 1972).

Nowadays standard chemotherapy in Australia consists of isoniazid and rifampicin for 18 months plus streptomycin or ethambutol for the first two to four months. If streptomycin is selected as a third drug it is suggested that it be replaced by ethambutol after eight weeks to avoid injections (Commonwealth Dept. Health Australia, 1977). In the United States the most frequently used regimen has been isoniazid and ethambutol for 18 months, to which streptomycin may be added for the first three months if there is extensive disease or if the patient is from an area where drug-resistant tuberculosis is prevalent. The American Thoracic Society considers that rifampicin and isoniazid is as effective as any three-drug regimen for treatment of extensive cavitary disease (Bailey *et al.*, 1977).

2. *Intermittent chemotherapy for pulmonary tuberculosis*. Regimens in which antituberculosis drugs are given intermittently have certain advantages (page 811). Rifampicin is quite suitable for such regimens provided that large individual doses are not used (page 558). Intermittent therapy consisting of rifampicin and a companion drug is usually preceded by two to three months of daily therapy with three drugs. A regimen of rifampicin 900 or 600 mg plus isoniazid in a dose of 15 mg per kg body weight, given twice-weekly, has been used successfully; these drugs were also used in once-weekly regimens but the therapeutic response was not as good as in the twice-weekly regimens (Singapore/BMRC, 1975). Another commonly used combination for intermittent chemotherapy is 900 mg rifampicin plus ethambutol 45–50 mg per kg body weight, twice-weekly (Anastasatu *et al.*, 1973; Hong Kong/Brompton Hospital/BMRC, 1974). Rifampicin may also be used effectively with one of these companion drugs in a lower dose of 450 mg or 600 mg, if it is given on alternate days or thrice-weekly. Intermittent regimens containing rifampicin have also been used in short-course chemotherapy of tuberculosis and for the retreatment of tuberculosis (*vide infra*).

3. *Short-course chemotherapy for pulmonary tuberculosis*. The background leading to the development of short-course chemotherapy and the results of recent clinical trials are summarised on page 812. At this time the inclusion of rifampicin in short-course regimens appears to be the most important factor in their success. Rifampicin is of special value because of its role in the sterilizing phase of treatment of tuberculosis (page 847). Trials of short-course chemotherapy have been carried out in a number of countries including the United States, France and the United Kingdom. Treatment has consisted of isoniazid and rifampicin either given daily or twice-weekly, sometimes accompanied by a third drug for the whole period of treatment or just for the first two months. These drug regimens used for a total period of 9–10 months have been effective for the treatment of pulmonary tuberculosis. It is anticipated that such short courses of chemotherapy will be used in most countries of the world in the near future.

4. *Retreatment of pulmonary tuberculosis*. Rifampicin is a very useful drug for the treatment of patients with pulmonary tuberculosis, who are excreting bacilli resistant to one or several of the older 'first-line' drugs, such as isoniazid, streptomycin or PAS. For this purpose rifampicin is always combined with one or more other antituberculosis drugs. The best results have been obtained when it has been used with ethambutol, a combination which is both effective and well tolerated (Gyselen *et al.*, 1968; Pines, 1969; Proust and Evans, 1972; Lees

et al., 1972a). Capreomycin has sometimes been used in conjunction with these two drugs for the initial period of treatment (*see* page 851). Rifampicin and ethambutol have also been used intermittently with success for the retreatment of tuberculosis (*see* page 837).

5. *Other forms of tuberculosis.* These in general should be treated with triple drug therapy for an initial period and then maintenance therapy with two drugs for 18–24 months (*see* page 810). Under optimal circumstances rifampicin should always be included in such regimens.

In life-threatening forms of tuberculosis such as miliary disease or meningitis the use of four drugs initially, including rifampicin, has been advocated (*see* page 814). The addition of rifampicin to existing regimens for the treatment of tuberculous meningitis is valuable (Curci *et al.*, 1969; D'Oliveira, 1972). Although there have been no controlled studies to compare regimens containing rifampicin with other regimens for the treatment of tuberculous meningitis, the results obtained by Visudhiphan and Chiemchanya (1975) are very encouraging. They compared children in Bangkok with meningitis who were treated with streptomycin, isoniazid and PAS with others treated with isoniazid and rifampicin; the mortality and sequelae in the patients treated with the rifampicin regimen were less. There are theoretical reasons why rifampicin should be used in tuberculous meningitis. Fox and Mitchison (1975) describe isoniazid and rifampicin as 'complete bactericidal drugs' against the entire population of M. tuberculosis. Streptomycin is active in tissues with an alkaline pH, and pyrazinamide is active in an acid pH, and each of these is said to be equivalent to half a bactericidal drug. It has therefore been suggested that the most bactericidal regimen which can be used in tuberculous meningitis would be pyrazinamide, isoniazid and rifampicin, with or without streptomycin or ethambutol (Leading article, 1976a). The efficacy and drug toxicity of such a regimen has yet to be determined by controlled trials. Despite the fact that little is known about the pharmacology of rifampicin in infants and children, on the information available, the drug should not be withheld from such patients with tuberculous meningitis (Sifontes, 1975).

6. *Leprosy.* Rifampicin is more rapidly bactericidal than the sulphone drugs against M. leprae and it is also effective against strains of M. leprae resistant to sulphones (page 553). Nevertheless M. leprae bacilli have been detected in the body after at least five years therapy with rifampicin, indicating that despite the use of this drug, treatment of leprosy particularly the multi-bacillary form, should still be prolonged.

Wilkinson *et al.* (1972) used rifampicin to treat 20 patients with lepromatous leprosy; they obtained a good clinical response in 15 patients and considered that a small daily dose of 150 mg of rifampicin was as effective as a 450 mg daily dose. Rees (1975) showed that even lower doses of rifampicin (20 mg daily) are still bactericidal, but as measured by the viability of M. leprae in the mouse footpad test, such doses are not as rapidly killing as one of 600 mg daily. Waters *et al.* (1978) have described the use of rifampicin daily in over a hundred patients with lepromatous leprosy; they confirmed the rapid bactericidal effect of the drug and noted that sometimes clinical improvement becomes apparent as early as 14 days after the start of treatment. A few patients were also given rifampicin weekly, one developed fever and abdominal symptoms without rifampicin-dependent antibodies, and another patient developed antibodies without toxicity. Other trials are presently being conducted to determine the efficacy of intermittent rifampicin therapy for leprosy; no rifampicin-dependent antibodies or adverse effects were detected in some 30 patients who have received 600 mg rifampicin on two consecutive days once a month, over a period of approximately 12 months (Rees, 1975).

Secondary dapsone resistance to M. leprae has become increasingly common throughout the world, occurring in lepromatous and borderline types of leprosy (WHO, 1977). It is for this reason that dapsone combined with another drug has been recommended for these forms of the disease. Taking into account effectiveness, toxicity, cost and availability, WHO (1977) recommends that the other drug should be clofazimine ('Lamprene') given for the first four to six months of treatment. Alternatively dapsone can be combined with rifampicin in a dosage of 300–600 mg daily for a minimum of two weeks. In developed countries, particularly for patients with light-coloured skins, rifampicin is preferred to avoid skin discolouration which occurs with clofazimine; rifampicin therapy is usually continued for some months. For the treatment of patients with dapsone-resistant M. leprae, WHO (1977) recommends combined therapy with rifampicin 600 mg and clofazimine 100 mg daily.

7. *Other mycobacterial infections.* Harris et al. (1975) reviewed the outcome of 59 patients with pulmonary infection due to M. kansasii in Texas, during the period 1971–1974. Overall, in 92 per cent of patients sputum cultures became negative during chemotherapy and only one patient required a surgical resection. One group of these patients received isoniazid and streptomycin and usually also ethambutol, and another group rifampicin combined with either isoniazid and streptomycin or isoniazid and ethambutol. A high proportion of patients from both groups had bacteriologically negative sputa after four months' chemotherapy; the difference between the groups was not significant. Similar regimens were used to retreat patients who had persistently positive sputum despite previous chemotherapy (without ethambutol or rifampicin) or after failure of current chemotherapy; in this comparison rifampicin containing regimens were superior. *In vitro* resistance to isoniazid and ethambutol did not adversely affect the results of treatment with these drugs. These authors also compared their results to previous reported series in which 20–54 per cent of patients had required surgical intervention for control of the disease. They concluded that initial treatment of patients with pulmonary disease due to M. kansasii should be with isoniazid, ethambutol and streptomycin. Rifampicin should be reserved for retreatment programmes and it should be substituted if cultures remain positive after four to six months' treatment. They also recommended that treatment should be continued for at least 18 months, or for 6 months beyond any evidence of activity demonstrated either by positive sputum culture or changing chest X-rays.

Elder et al. (1977) in a study of patients with pulmonary infections due to M. kansasii in Queensland, Australia, also noted radiological clearing and sputum conversion within six months with a variety of chemotherapeutic regimens, a number of which included rifampicin. Other experience suggests that various combinations of rifampicin, isoniazid, ethambutol and streptomycin may obviate the need for surgery and be successful for the treatment of tendinitis and fasciitis (Parker and Irwin, 1975) and arthritis (Saphyakhajon et al., 1977) caused by infection with M. kansasii.

Rifampicin has been used successfully as a single chemotherapeutic agent to treat four children with atypical mycobacterial cervical adenitis (Mandell and Wright, 1975). Culture was positive in two (one each for M. avium and M. intracellulare) and rapid regression of the lymph nodes occurred; in three patients who had been followed at the time, total resolution had occurred after six to eleven months' therapy. Other experience in which strains of M. kansasii developed resistance following rifampicin monotherapy (page 557) indicates that rifampicin should always be combined with one or two other antituberculosis drugs for the treatment of these infections.

Rifampicin has been used with some success to treat infections due to M. marinum, although lesions due to this organism often resolve spontaneously (page 838). Van Dyke and Lake (1975) treated two patients with an aquarium granuloma with rifampicin and ethambutol (one also with isoniazid) with apparent improvement. This drug combination was of more apparent value for the treatment of a patient reported by Sage and Derrington (1973). This 70-year-old man with lymphosarcoma developed multiple cutaneous lesions due to M. marinum; complete resolution of all lesions followed a prolonged course of therapy with rifampicin and ethambutol.

8. *Staphylococcal infections*. Rifampicin, like rifamide, although effective, is not advocated for the routine treatment of these infections. However there are some special circumstances in which its use can be justified. For example Jensen (1968) used rifampicin successfully in combination with at least one other anti-staphylococcal drug for treatment of infections due to methicillin-resistant staphylococci. Peard *et al.* (1970) reported the case of a three-year-old child with staphylococcal endocarditis who failed to respond to cloxacillin, cephaloridine and kanamycin, but subsequently responded to rifampicin and erythromycin in combination. Special *in vitro* studies for combined bactericidal action predicted that the latter combination would be effective against the particular Staph. pyogenes strain involved.

Studies in a tuberculosis hospital showed that rifampicin is effective in eliminating the nasal carriage of Staph. pyogenes; a carriage rate of 1·7 per cent was found in 227 patients receiving rifampicin, compared to a rate of 7·8 per cent in 190 patients receiving other antituberculosis drugs and 14·2 per cent in 98 hospital employees. All four strain isolated from the rifampicin treated patients were resistant to this drug, as was one other strain isolated from a hospital employee (Sande and Mandell, 1975). Rifampicin should never be used as a single drug for the treatment of staphylococcal infections because resistant staphylococci emerge readily both *in vitro* and *in vivo* (Jensen, 1968; McCabe and Lorian, 1968) (*see also* page 556).

9. *Respiratory tract infections*. There are a number of reasons why rifampicin should not be used for non-tuberculous respiratory tract infections. Although this drug may be effective for the treatment of diseases such as streptococcal tonsillitis and pneumococcal pneumonia, there are a number of other effective antibiotics, which can be used as alternatives to penicillin G to treat these infections in penicillin-allergic patients (pages 213, 484, 506). In addition, there is some evidence from *in vitro* studies that Strep. pyogenes may develop resistance to rifampicin (Kunin *et al.*, 1969). Furthermore the large scale use of this drug for the initial treatment of diseases such as bronchitis and pneumonia seems most undesirable because it may mask underlying tuberculosis. Also

rifampicin is not effective for the treatment of chronic bronchitis due to H. influenzae (Citron and May, 1969).

10. *Gonorrhoea.* Cobbold *et al.* (1968) used single oral doses of 900 mg rifampicin to treat 103 patients with acute uncomplicated gonorrhoea. Follow-up studies in 89 patients showed that this treatment had been ineffective in only ten (11·2 per cent). It was concluded that rifampicin gives results which compare favourably with those from similar regimens of orally administered antibiotics, and that it is a suitable alternative for 'single session' therapy for patients in whom penicillin G is contraindicated. Rajan *et al.* (1977) obtained similar results. However other authors have recorded less satisfactory results and conclude that rifampicin should not be used for this disease (Hatos and Tuza, 1972). There are other suitable alternatives to penicillin G for the treatment of gonorrhoea (pages 286, 319, 588, 625, 710), and the use of this effective antituberculosis drug should be restricted (Report, 1978).

11. *Chemoprophylaxis of meningococcal infection.* Rifampicin is of no value for the treatment of meningococcal meningitis and septicaemia, but it has been used successfully in an adult dose of 300–600 mg daily (according to weight) for four days, to eradicate meningococci from chronic pharyngeal carriers (Deal and Sanders, 1969; Devine *et al.*, 1970; Eickhoff, 1971; Kaiser *et al.*, 1974; Sivonen *et al.*, 1978). This is probably related to the drug's ability to produce therapeutically active concentrations in saliva (page 561). Although penicillin G is excellent for the treatment of meningococcal diseases, it is not satisfactory in eradicating the carrier state. Sulphonamides are no longer generally suitable for this purpose, as many meningococcal strains are now sulphonamide-resistant (page 661). Minocycline, though effective as a chemoprophylactic agent for meningococcal disease, is unfortunately associated with a high frequency of vestibular reactions (page 621). Although rifampicin has been highly effective (85–100 per cent) in eradicating meningococci in field trials, rifampicin-resistant strains have been detected in trials in which their presence was sought (Eickhoff, 1975). Meningococcal mutants highly resistant to rifampicin can be easily selected *in vitro* (Ivler *et al.*, 1970), and frequently emerge during treatment *in vivo* (Guttler *et al.*, 1971; Weidmer *et al.*, 1971; Devine *et al.*, 1972; Sivonen *et al.*, 1978). Failure to eradicate meningococci has been attributed to one-step development of rifampicin resistance. Rifampicin-resistant meningococci have been found in untreated individuals but such strains have not persisted in a population without continuing rifampicin administration and clinical disease caused by them has not been recorded (Eickhoff, 1975; McCormick and Bennett, 1975). It is most improbable that the use of rifampicin for meningococcal chemoprophylaxis will result in resistant strains of M. tuberculosis; the chance of a recipient being infected with M. tuberculosis is low and it is unlikely that a four-day course of rifampicin would cause resistance (McCormick and Bennett, 1975). Also should widespread resistance of meningococci to rifampicin occur, the efficacy of penicillin G for the established disease would be unaffected. For these reasons rifampicin is now recommended as the chemoprophylactic agent of choice for meningococcal infections in the United States (McCormick and Bennett, 1975; Center for Disease Control, 1976). A recommended dosage schedule is 600 mg rifampicin every 12 h for four doses in adults, 10 mg per kg body weight every 12 h for four doses in children aged 1–12 years, and 5 mg

per kg body weight per dose every 12 h for four doses in children aged less than 12 months.

12. *Urinary tract infections*. High urinary concentrations are achieved with usual rifampicin doses (page 560), but clinical data indicate that rifampicin is of no value for treatment of these infections. Atlas and Turck (1968) treated 27 patients with urinary tract infections with rifampicin in a dose of 300 mg three times a day for 14 days. Results of treatment were unsatisfactory and in many patients the organisms became more highly rifampicin-resistant. Murdoch *et al.* (1969) gave rifampicin in a dose of 900 mg daily to 19 female patients with urinary tract infections. Treatment failed in 11; with continuing treatment, the MIC's of rifampicin against the causative organisms rapidly rose to 600 μg per ml. The remaining 8 patients appeared to be cured after this course of rifampicin, but their infection soon relapsed. It was concluded that rifampicin is of no value in the treatment of urinary tract infections.

13. *Other infections*. Rifampicin in combination with fusidic acid was used to eradicate multiple-antibiotic resistant pneumococci in South Africa (Center for Disease Control, 1977; 1978) (*see also* page 5). The drug has been used in conjunction with amphotericin B to treat disseminated histoplasmosis (Seriki *et al.*, 1975) (*see* page 876). Rifampicin plus streptomycin have been successfully combined to treat mycetoma (*see* page 303). A number of cures were obtained when polymyxin B was used in combination with rifampicin to treat nosocomial infections due to multi-drug-resistant strains of Serratia marcescens; the infections which responded included septic thrombophlebitis, urinary tract infections, pneumonia and osteomyelitis (Ostenson *et al.*, 1977). Rifampicin was used successfully to eradicate Haemophilus influenzae type b from the pharynx of three children in a day-care centre, where there had been outbreaks of serious disease due to this organism (Ward *et al.*, 1978).

Rifampicin eye ointment (one per cent) used three times a day for five or six weeks is highly effective for the treatment of hyperendemic trachoma and sexually transmitted C. trachomatis (TRIC agent) infections of the eye (Annotation, 1977; Darougar *et al.*, 1977). A trial on patients with endemic trachoma in which treatment with a one per cent ophthalmic ointment of either tetracycline or rifampicin were compared, showed that both antibiotics were effective and that rifampicin offered no advantage over tetracycline (Dawson *et al.*, 1975).

14. *Potential use for other infections*. Because rifampicin is such a valuable drug for the treatment of tuberculosis, its use for other infections has not been encouraged (Lancet Leading article, 1969; Morrison-Smith, 1975). However rifampicin in concentrations attainable in the body is effective against many pathogenic bacteria, it is freely diffusible and excreted in urine and bile. Because of these attributes it has been considered for other infections (Leading article, 1976b). In addition, in countries where rifampicin has been used for both tuberculous and non-tuberculous infections, the incidence of M. tuberculosis resistant to rifampicin has not increased (page 557). In this respect it is similar to streptomycin which was used extensively for non-tuberculous conditions without an increase in resistant strains of M. tuberculosis. One of the disadvantages of rifampicin is that if it is used alone, one-step mutation to high level resistance rapidly occurs. For this reason a number of *in vitro* studies have been carried out using rifampicin in combination with some other

chemotherapeutic agent (page 554). Apart from the rifampicin combinations which have already been used for clinical purposes, a combination of rifampicin with novobiocin or particularly with trimethoprim may prove of value. The former may be useful to treat typhoid fever due to strains resistant to chloramphenicol, co-trimoxazole and ampicillin. A combination of rifampicin and trimethoprim is synergistic against a wide range of organisms and the two drugs are compatible pharmacologically. The value of such combinations remains to be tested by appropriate clinical trials.

Results of studies in animals (page 553) suggests that rifampicin may have a role in the treatment of human brucellosis. Both rifampicin and erythromycin prevent the death of guinea pigs injected intra-peritoneally with the agent causing Legionnaires' disease (Fraser *et al.*, 1978). Legionnaires' disease bacterium is also very sensitive to rifampicin *in vitro* (page 553). Therefore a rifampicin/erythromycin combination has been suggested for patients with this disease not responding to erythromycin alone (page 509).

15. *Virus diseases.* There is experimental evidence that rifampicin in high concentrations can inhibit certain viruses (page 554), but this has little or no practical application for the treatment of human diseases (Hirschman, 1971). It has been shown that locally applied rifampicin ointment prevents the smallpox vaccination reaction in about 50 per cent of volunteers, but orally administered rifampicin has no effect (Moshkowitz *et al.*, 1971).

REFERENCES

Acocella, G., Pagani, V., Marchetti, M., Baroni, G. C. and Nicolis, F. B. (1971), 'Kinetic studies on rifampicin', *Chemotherapy*, **16**, 356.

Acocella, G. and Scotti, R. (1976), 'Kinetic studies on the combination rifampicin-trimethoprim in man. I. Absorption and urinary excretion after administration to healthy volunteers of single doses of the two compounds alone and in combination, and the combination over a period of 1 week', *J. Antimicrob. Chemother.*, **2**, 271.

Acocella, G., Hamilton-Miller, J. M. T. and Brumfitt, W. (1977), 'Can rifampicin use be safely extended? Evidence for non-emergence of resistant strains of Mycobacterium tuberculosis', *Lancet*, **1**, 740.

Anastasatu, C., Bungeteanu, Gh. and Sibila, S. (1973), 'The intermittent chemotherapy of tuberculosis with rifampicin regimens on ambulatory basis', *Scand. J. resp. Dis. Suppl.*, **84**, 136.

Annotation (1969), 'Rifampicin', *Lancet*, **1**, 976.

Annotation (1970), 'Antiviral action of rifampicin', *Lancet*, **1**, 399.

Annotation (1977), 'Chlamydial infections of the eye', *Lancet*, **2**, 857.

Arioli, V., Pallanza, R., Nicolis, F. B. and Furesz, S. (1970), 'Experimental data on the interaction between rifampicin and tetracycline. Progress in antimicrobial and anticancer chemotherapy'. *Proceedings of the 6th International Congress of Chemotherapy*. University of Tokyo Press, Tokyo, p. 339.

Arioli, V., Berti, M., Carniti, G., Rossi, E. and Silvestri, L. G. (1977), 'Interaction between rifampicin and trimethoprim *in vitro* and in experimental infections', *J. Antimicrob. Chemother.*, **3**, 87.

Atlas, E. and Turck, M. (1968), 'Laboratory and clinical evaluation of rifampicin', *Amer. J. Med. Sci.*, **256**, 247.

Aquinas, M., Allan, W. G. L., Horsfall, P. A. L., Jenkins, P. K., Wong Hung-Yan, Girling, D., Tall, R. and Fox, W. (1972), 'Adverse reactions to daily and intermittent rifampicin regimens for pulmonary tuberculosis in Hong Kong', *Brit. med. J.*, **1**, 765.

Bailey, W. C., Raleigh, J. W. and Turner, J. A. P. (1977), 'Treatment of mycobacterial disease', *Amer. Rev. Resp. Dis.*, **115**, 185.

Bannatyne, R. M. and Cheung, R. (1978), 'Susceptibility of Haemophilus influenzae type b to rifampicin and sulfisoxazole', *Antimicrob. Ag. Chemother.*, **13**, 969.

Baron, D. N. and Bell, J. L. (1974), 'Serum enzyme changes in patients receiving antituberculosis therapy with rifampicin or *p*-aminosalicylic acid, plus isoniazid and streptomycin', *Tubercle*, **55**, 115.

Baronti, A. and Lukinovich, N. (1968), 'A pilot trial of rifampicin in tuberculosis', *Tubercle (Lond.)*, **49**, 180.

Bassi, L., Di Berardino, L., Perna, G. and Silvestri, L. G. (1975), 'Lack of effect of rifampicin on the antibody response to a viral antigen in patients with tuberculosis', *Amer., Rev. Resp. Dis.*, **112**, 739.

Bassi, L., Di Berardino, L., Perna, G. and Silvestri, L. G. (1976), 'Antibodies against rifampin in patients with tuberculosis after discontinuation of daily treatment', *Amer. Rev. Resp. Dis.*, **114**, 1189.

Battaner, E. and Kumar, B. V. (1974), 'Rifampin: Inhibition of ribonucleic acid synthesis after potentiation by amphotericin B in Saccharomyces cerevisiae', *Antimicrob. Ag. Chemother.*, **5**, 371.

Bending, M. R. and Skacel, P. O. (1977), 'Rifampicin and methadone withdrawal', *Lancet*, **1**, 1211.

Binda, G., Domenichini, E., Gottardi, A., Orlandi, B., Ortelli, E. Pacini, B. and Fowst, G. (1971), 'Rifampicin, a general review', *Arzneim. Forsch.*, **21**, 1907.

Blackman, H. J., Yoneda, C., Dawson, C. R. and Schachter, J. (1977), 'Antibiotic susceptibility of Chlamydia trachomatis', *Antimicrob. Chemother.*, **12**, 673.

Blajchman, M. A., Lowry, R. C., Pettit, J. E. and Stradling, P. (1970), 'Rifampicin-induced immune thrombocytopenia', *Brit. med. J.*, **3**, 24.

Bolt, H. M., Kappus, H. and Bolt, M. (1974), 'Rifampicin and oral contraception', *Lancet*, **1**, 1280.

Boman, G., Hanngren, A., Malmborg, A., Borga, O. and Sjöqvist, F. (1971), 'Drug interaction: Decreased serum concentrations of rifampicin when given with PAS', *Lancet.*, **1**, 800.

Boman, G. (1973), 'Protein binding of rifampicin. A review', *Scand. J. resp. Dis. Suppl.*, **84**, 40.

British Medical Research Council Co-operative Study (1973), 'Co-operative controlled trial of a standard regimen of streptomycin, PAS and isoniazid and three alternative regimens of chemotherapy in Britain', *Tubercle*, **54**, 99.

Buffington, G. A., Dominguez, J. H., Piering, W. F., Hebert, L. A., Kauffman, M., Jr. and Lemann, J., Jr. (1976), 'Interaction of rifampicin and glucocorticoids. Adverse effect on renal allograft function', *JAMA*, **236**, 1958.

Casteels-van Daele, M., Igodt-Ameye, L., Corbeel, L. and Eeckels, R. (1975), 'Hepatotoxicity of rifampicin and isoniazid in children', *J. Pediatrics*, **86**, 739.

Cayley, F. E. and Majumdar, S. K. (1976), 'Ocular toxicity due to rifampicin', *Brit. med. J.*, **1**, 199.

Center for Disease Control (1976), 'Analysis of endemic meningococcal disease by serogroup and evaluation of chemoprophylaxis', *J. Infect. Dis.*, **134**, 201.

Center for Disease Control (1977), 'Multiple-antibiotic resistance of pneumococci—South Africa', *Morbidity and Mortality Weekly Report*, **26**, 285.

Center for Disease Control (1977), 'Multiple-antibiotic resistance of pneumococci—pneumococci—South Africa', *Morbidity and Mortality Weekly Report*, **27**, 1.

Chan, W. C., O'Mahoney, M. G., Yu, D. Y. C. and Yu, R. Y. H. (1975), 'Renal failure during intermittent rifampicin therapy', *Tubercle*, **56**, 191.

Citron, K. M. and May, J. R. (1969), 'Rifamycin antibiotics in chronic purulent bronchitis', *Lancet*, **2**, 982.

Citron, K. M. (1972), 'Tuberculosis-chemotherapy', *Brit. med. J.*, **1**, 426.

Clark, J. and Wallace, A. (1967), 'The susceptibility of mycobacteria to rifamide and rifampicin', *Tubercle (Lond.)*, **48**, 144.

Clarke, G. B. M., Cuthbert, J., Cuthbert, R. J. and Lees, A. W. (1972), 'Isoniazid plus rifampicin in the initial treatment of pulmonary tuberculosis', *Brit. J. Dis. Chest*, **66**, 268.

Cobbold, R. J. C., Morrison, G. D. and Willcox, R. R. (1968), 'Treatment of gonorrhoea with single oral doses of rifampicin', *Brit. med. J.*, **4**, 681.

Cochran, M., Moorhead, P. J. and Platts, M. (1975), 'Permanent renal damage with rifampicin', *Lancet*, **1**, 1428.

Cole, A. J. L., Bate, J. and Gyde, O. H. B. (1973), 'Rifampicin and folate and vitamin B_{12} assays', *Brit. med. J.*, **2**, 53.

Commonwealth Department of Health Australia (1977), *Treatment of Tuberculosis with particular reference to Chemotherapy*, 4th edn., Australian Government Publishing Service, Canberra.

Commonwealth Department of Health Australia (1973–1977), *Tuberculosis Statistics*, Canberra.

Cordonnier, D. and Muller, J. M. (1972), 'Acute renal failure after rifampicin', *Lancet*, **2**, 1364.

Council on Drugs (1972), 'Evaluation of a new antituberculosis agent rifampin (rifadin, rimactane)', *JAMA*, **220**, 414.

Curci, G., Cava, F. D. and Vitalo, L. (1969), 'Distribution of rifamycin AMP in blood and cerebro-spinal fluid', *Minerva Medica*, **60**, 2399.

Dans, P. E., McGehee, R. F., Jr., Wilcox, C. and Finland, M. (1970), 'Rifampin: Antibacterial activity *in vitro* and absorption and excretion in normal young men', *Amer. J. Med. Sci.*, **259**, 120.

Darougar, M. S., Viswalingam, M., Treharne, J. D., Kinnison, J. R. and Jones, B. R. (1977), 'Treatment of TRIC infection of the eye with rifampicin or chloramphenicol', *Br. J. Ophthalmol.*, **61**, 255.

Davidson, P. T. and Waggoner, R. (1976), 'Acquired resistance to rifampicin by Mycobacterium kansasii', *Tubercle*, **57**, 271.

Dawson, C. R., Hoshiwara, I., Daghfous, T., Messadi, M., Vastine, D. W. and Schachter, J. (1975), 'Topical tetracycline and rifampicin therapy of endemic trachoma in Tunisia', *Am. J. Ophthalmol.*, **79**, 803.

Deal, W. B. and Sanders, E. (1969), 'Efficacy of rifampin in treatment of meningococcal carriers', *New Engl. J. Med.*, **281**, 641.

Devine, L. F., Johnson, D. P., Hagerman, C. R., Pierce, W. E., Rhode, S. L. and Peckinpaugh, R. O. (1970), 'Rifampin. Levels in serum and saliva and effect on the meningococcal carrier state', *JAMA*, **214**, 1055.

Devine, L. F., Springer, G. L., Frazier, W. E., Rhode, S. L., III, Pierce, W. E., Johnson, D. P. and Peckinpaugh, R. O. (1972), 'Selective minocycline and rifampin treatment of Group C meningococcal carriers in a new naval recruit camp', *Amer. J. Med. Sci.*, **263**, 79.

Dickinson, J. M., Aber, V. R., Allen, B. W., Ellard, G. A. and Mitchison, D. A. (1974), 'Assay of rifampicin in serum', *J. clin. Path.*, **27**, 457.

D'Oliveira, J. J. G. (1972), 'Cerebrospinal fluid concentrations of rifampin in meningeal tuberculosis', *Amer. Rev. Resp. Dis.*, **106**, 432.

Drutz, D. J., O'Neill, S. M. and Levy, L. (1974), 'Viability of blood-borne Mycobacterium leprae', *J. Infect. Dis.*, **130**, 288.

Edwards, O. M., Courtenay-Evans, R. J., Galley, J. M., Hunter, J. and Tait, A. D. (1974), 'Changes in cortisol metabolism following rifampicin therapy', *Lancet*, **2**, 549.

Eickhoff, T. C. (1971), '*In vitro* and *in vivo* studies of resistance to rifampin in meningococci', *J. Infect. Dis.*, **123,** 414.

Eickhoff, T. C. (1975), 'Meningococcal prophylaxis', *JAMA,* **234,** 150.

Elder, J. L., Edwards, F. G. B. and Abrahams, E. W. (1977), 'Tuberculosis due to Mycobacterium kansasii', *Aust. N.Z. J. Med.,* **7,** 8.

Eule, H., Werner, E., Winsel, K. and Iwainsky, H. (1974), 'Intermittent chemotherapy of pulmonary tuberculosis using rifampicin and isoniazid for primary treatment: the influence of various factors on the frequency of side-effects', *Tubercle,* **55,** 81.

Fallon, R. J., Lees, A. W., Allan, G. W., Smith, J. and Tyrrell, W. F. (1975), 'Probenecid and rifampicin serum levels', *Lancet,* **2,** 792.

Farrell, W., Wilks, M. and Drasar, F. A. (1977), 'The action of trimethoprim and rifampicin in combination against Gram-negative rods resistant to gentamicin', *J. Antimicrob. Chemother.,* **3,** 459.

Flynn, C. T., Rainford, D. J. and Hope, E. (1974), 'Acute renal failure and rifampicin: Danger of unsuspected intermittent dosage', *Brit. med. J.,* **2,** 482.

Forsgren, A. and Schmeling, D. (1977), 'Effect of antibiotics on chemotaxis of human leukocytes', *Antimicrob. Ag. Chemother.,* **11,** 580.

Fox, W. and Mitchison, D. A. (1975), 'Short-course chemotherapy for pulmonary tuberculosis', *Amer. Rev. Resp. Dis.,* **111,** 325.

Fraser, D. W., Wachsmuth, I. K., Bopp, C., Feeley, J. C. and Tsai, T. F. (1978), 'Antibiotic treatment of guinea-pigs infected with agent of Legionnaires' disease', *Lancet,* **1,** 175.

Gabow, P. A., Lacher, J. W. and Neff, T. A. (1976), 'Tubulointerstitial and glomerular nephritis associated with rifampicin', *JAMA,* **235,** 2517.

Gadaleta, M. N., Greco, M. and Saccone, C. (1970), 'The effect of rifampicin on mitochondrial RNA polymerase from rat liver', *FEBS Letters,* **10,** 54.

Gale, E. F., Cundliffe, E., Reynolds, P. E., Richmond, M. H. and Waring, M. J. (1972), *The Molecular Basis of Antibiotic Action,* John Wiley and Sons Ltd.

Gill, G. V. (1976), 'Rifampicin and breakfast', *Lancet,* **2,** 1135.

Girling, D. J. and Fox, W. (1971), 'Side effects of intermittent rifampicin', *Brit. med. J.,* **4,** 231.

Girling, D. J. (1977), 'Adverse reactions to rifampicin in antituberculosis regimens', *J. Antimicrob. Chemother.,* **3,** 115.

Goldstein, R. A., Ang, U. H., Foellmer, J. W. and Janicki, B. W. (1976), 'Rifampin and cell-mediated immune responses in tuberculosis', *Amer. Rev. Resp. Dis.,* **113,** 197.

Graber, C. D., Jebaily, J., Galphin, R. L. and Doering, E. (1973), 'Light chain proteinuria and humoral immunoincompetence in tuberculosis patients treated with rifampin', *Amer. Rev. Resp. Dis.,* **107,** 713.

Grassi, G. G. and Pozzi, E. (1972), 'Effect of rifampicin on delayed-hypersensitivity reactions', *J. Infect. Dis.,* **126,** 542.

Grennan, D. M. and Sturrock, R. D. (1976), 'Polyarthritis, hepatitis and anti-native DNA antibodies after treatment with ethambutol and rifampicin', *Tubercle,* **57,** 259.

Grüneberg, R. N. and Emmerson, A. M. (1977), 'The interactions between rifampicin and trimethoprim: An *in vitro* study', *J. Antimicrob. Chemother.,* **3,** 453.

Gupta, S., Grieco, M. H. and Siegel, I. (1975), 'Suppression of T-lymphocyte rosettes by rifampin. Studies in normals and patients with tuberculosis', *Ann. Intern. Med.,* **82,** 484.

Gurgo, C., Ray, R. K., Thiry, L. and Green, M. (1971), 'Inhibitors of the RNA and DNA dependent polymerase activities of RNA tumour viruses', *Nature New Biol.,* **229,** 111.

Guttler, R. B., Counts, G. W., Avent, C. K. and Beaty, H. N. (1971), 'Effects of rifampin and minocycline on meningococcal carrier rates', *J. Infect. Dis.,* **124,** 199.

Gyselen, A., Verbist, L., Cosemans, J., Lacquet, L. M. and Vandenbergh, E. (1968), 'Rifampin and ethambutol in the retreatment of advanced pulmonary tuberculosis', *Amer. Rev. Resp. Dis.,* **98,** 933.

Halsted, C. C., Minnefor, A. B. and Lietman, P. S. (1972), 'Inhibition of cytomegalovirus by rifampin', *J. Infect. Dis.*, **125**, 552.

Hamilton-Miller, J. M. T. and Brumfitt, W. (1976), 'Trimethoprim and rifampicin: Pharmacokinetic studies in man', *J. Antimicrob. Chemother.*, **2**, 181.

Hamilton-Miller, J. M. T., Kerry, D. W. and Brumfitt, W. (1977), 'The use of antibiotic combinations in the treatment of Serratia marcescens infections', *J. Antimicrob. Chemother.*, **3**, 193.

Harris, G. D., Johanson, W. G., Jr. and Nicholson, D. P. (1975), 'Response to chemotherapy of pulmonary infection due to Mycobacterium kansasii', *Amer. Rev. Resp. Dis.*, **112**, 31.

Hartmann, G., Honikel, K. O., Knüsel, F. and Nüesch, J. (1967), 'The specific inhibition of the DNA—directed RNA synthesis by rifamycin', *Biochim. Biophys. Acta*, **145**, 843.

Hatos, G. and Tuza, F. L. C. (1972), 'Treatment of gonorrhoea with trimethoprim-sulphamethoxazole and with rifampicin', *Med. J. Aust.*, **1**, 1197.

Hirschman, S. Z. (1971), 'Editorial. Approaches to antiviral chemotherapy', *Amer. J. Med.*, **51**, 699.

Heller, E., Argaman, M., Levy, H. and Goldblum, N. (1969), 'Selective inhibition of vaccinia virus by the antibiotic rifampicin', *Nature*, **222**, 273.

Hoeprich, P. D. (1971), 'Prediction of antimeningococcic chemoprophylactic efficacy', *J. Infect. Dis.*, **123**, 125.

Hobby, G. L. (1969), Editorial. 'Rifampin, a powerful new antimicrobial agent', *J. Infect. Dis.*, **119**, 195.

Hobby, G. L., Johnson, P. M. and Boytar-Papirnyik, V. (1971), 'Primary drug resistance: A continuing study of drug resistance in tuberculosis in a veteran population within the United States. IX. September 1969–September 1970', *Amer. Rev. Resp. Dis.*, **103**, 842.

Hobby, G. L. and Lenert, T. F. (1972), 'Observations on the action of rifampin and ethambutol alone and in combination with other antituberculous drugs', *Amer. Rev. Resp. Dis.*, **105**, 292.

Hobby, G. L., Johnson, P. M. and Boytar-Papirnyik, V. (1974), 'Primary drug resistance: A continuing study of drug resistance in tuberculosis in a veteran population within the United States. X. September 1970–September 1973', *Amer. Rev. Resp. Dis.*, **110**, 95.

Holmes, I. B. and Hilson, G. R. F. (1972), 'The effect of rifampicin and dapsone on experimental Mycobacterium leprae infections: minimum inhibitory concentrations and bactericidal action', *J. Med. Microbiol.*, **5**, 251.

Hong Kong Tuberculosis Treatment Services/British Medical Research Council (1974), 'A controlled clinical trial of small daily doses of rifampicin in the prevention of adverse reactions to the drug in a once-weekly regimen of chemotherapy in Hong Kong: Second report. The results at 12 months', *Tubercle*, **55**, 193.

Hong Kong Tuberculosis Treatment Services/Brompton Hospital/British Medical Research Council Investigation (1974), 'A controlled clinical trial of daily and intermittent regimens of rifampicin plus ethambutol in the retreatment of patients with pulmonary tuberculosis in Hong Kong', *Tubercle*, **55**, 1.

Hong Kong Tuberculosis Treatment Services/British Medical Research Council (1975), 'The influence of age and sex on the incidence of the 'flu' syndrome and rifampicin-dependent antibodies in patients on intermittent rifampicin for tuberculosis', *Tubercle*, **56**, 173.

Hong Kong Tuberculosis Treatment Services/Brompton Hospital/British Medical Research Council (1975), 'A controlled trial of daily and intermittent rifampicin plus ethambutol in the retreatment of patients with pulmonary tuberculosis: Results up to 30 months', *Tubercle*, **56**, 179.

Hong Kong Tuberculosis Treatment Services/British Medical Research Council

(1976), 'Adverse reactions to short-course regimens containing streptomycin, isoniazid, pyrazinamide and rifampicin in Hong Kong', *Tubercle*, **57**, 81.

Hong Kong Tuberculosis Treatment Services, Singapore Tuberculosis Service, Royal Postgraduate Medical School, Brompton Hospital, British Medical Research Council (1976), 'Lack of association between rifampicin-dependent antibodies and bacteriological response during intermittent rifampicin treatment', *J. Antimicrob. Chemother.*, **2**, 265.

Hui, J., Gordon, N. and Kajioka, R. (1977), 'Permeability barrier to rifampicin in mycobacteria', *Antimicrob. Ag. Chemother.*, **11**, 773.

Ivler, D., Leedom, J. M. and Mathies, A. W., Jr. (1970), '*In vitro* susceptibility of Neisseria meningitidis to rifampicin', *Antimicrob. Ag. Chemother.*—1969, p. 473.

Jacobson, R. R. and Hastings, R. C. (1976), 'Rifampin-resistant leprosy', *Lancet*, **2**, 1304.

Jensen, K. (1968), 'Methicillin-resistant staphylococci', *Lancet*, **2**, 1078.

Jentgens, H. (1975), 'Antituberkulotische Therapie mit Ethambutol und Rifampicin in der Schwangerschaft', *Prox. Pneumol.*, **30**, 42.

Jezeguel, A. M., Orlandi, F. and Tenconi, L. T. (1971), 'Changes of the smooth endoplasmic reticulum induced by rifampicin in human and guinea-pig hepatocytes', *Gut*, **12**, 984.

Kaiser, A. B., Hennekens, C. H., Saslaw, M. S., Hayes, P. S. and Bennett, J. V. (1974), 'Seroepidemiology and chemoprophylaxis of disease due to sulfonamide-resistant Neisseria meningitidis in a civilian population', *J. Infect. Dis.*, **130**, 217.

Keberle, H., Schid, K. and Meyer-Brunot, H. G. (1968), 'The metabolic fate of rimactane in the animal and in man', in *A Symposium on Rimactane, Ciba, Basle,* 20; quoted by Proust (1971).

Kenwright, S. and Levi, A. J. (1973), 'Impairment of hepatic uptake of rifamycin antibiotics by probenecid, and its therapeutic implications', *Lancet*, **2**, 1401.

Kerry, D. W., Hamilton-Miller, J. M. T. and Brumfitt, W. (1975), 'Trimethoprim and rifampicin: *In vitro* activities separately and in combination', *J. Antimicrob. Chemother.*, **1**, 417.

Keshishyan, H., Hanna, L. and Jawetz, E. (1973), 'Emergence of rifampin-resistance in Chlamydia trachomatis', *Nature*, **244**, 173.

Kleinknecht, D., Homberg, J. C. and Decroix, G. (1972), 'Acute renal failure after rifampicin', *Lancet*, **1**, 1238.

Konno, K., Oizumi, K. and Oka, S. (1973), 'Mode of action of rifampin on mycobacteria', *Amer. Rev. Resp. Dis.*, **107**, 1006.

Kreek, M. J., Garfield, J. W., Gutjahr, C. L. and Giusti, L. M. (1976), 'Rifampin-induced methadone withdrawal', *New Engl. J. Med.*, **234**, 1104.

Kunin, C. M., Brandt, D. and Wood, H. (1969), 'Bacteriologic studies of rifampin, a new semisynthetic antibiotic', *J. Infect. Dis.*, **119**, 132.

Lakshminarayan, S., Sahn, S. A. and Hudson, L. D. (1973), 'Massive haemolysis caused by rifampicin', *Brit. med. J.*, **2**, 282.

Lal, S., Singhal, S. N., Burley, D. M. and Crossley, G. (1972), 'Effect of rifampicin and isoniazid on liver function', *Brit. med. J.*, **1**, 148.

Leading Article (1969), 'Rifampicin and viruses', *Brit. med. J.*, **2**, 588.

Leading Article (1969), 'New drugs against tuberculosis', *Lancet*, **1**, 1081.

Leading Article (1973), 'Rifampicin or ethambutol in the routine treatment of tuberculosis', *Brit. med. J.*, **4**, 568.

Leading Article (1975), 'Antituberculous drugs and the liver', *Brit. med. J.*, **2**, 522.

Leading Article (1976a), 'Treatment of tuberculous meningitis', *Lancet*, **1**, 787.

Leading Article (1976b), 'Rifampicin: for tuberculosis only?', *Lancet*, **1**, 290.

Leading Article (1978), 'Treatment of Chlamydia trachomatis infections', *Lancet*, **1**, 192.

Lees, A. W., Asgher, B., Hashem, M. A. and Sinha, B. N. (1970), 'Jaundice after rifampicin', *Brit. J. Dis. Chest.*, **64**, 90.

Lees, A. W., Allan, G. W., Smith, J., Tyrrell, W. F. and Fallon, R. J. (1971), 'Toxicity from rifampicin plus isoniazid and rifampicin plus ethambutol therapy', *Tubercle*, **52**, 182.

Lees, A. W., Allan, G. W., Smith, J., Tyrrell, W. F. and Fallon, R. J. (1972a), 'Retreatment of pulmonary tuberculosis with rifampin and ethambutol', *Amer. Rev. Resp. Dis.*, **105**, 129.

Lees, A. W., Allan, G. W., Smith, J., Tyrrell, W. F. and Fallon, R. J. (1972b), 'Rifampin and isoniazid in previously un-treated patients with pulmonary tuberculosis', *Amer. Rev. Resp. Dis.*, **105**, 132.

Leigh, D. A. (1974), 'Clinical importance of infections due to Bacteroides fragilis and role of antibiotic therapy', *Brit. med. J.*, **3**, 225.

Levy, L., Shepard, C. C. and Fasal, P. (1976), 'The bactericidal effect of rifampicin on M. leprae in man: (a) single doses of 600, 900 and 1200 mg; and (b) daily doses of 300 mg', *Int. J. Leprosy*, **44**, 183.

Lewis, V. J., Thacker, W. L., Shepard, C. C. and McDade, J. E. (1978), '*In vivo* susceptibility of the Legionnaires' disease bacterium to ten antimicrobial agents', *Antimicrob. Ag. Chemother.*, **13**, 419.

Lobo, M. C. and Mandell, G. L. (1972), 'Treatment of experimental staphylococcal infection with rifampin', *Antimicrob. Ag. Chemother.*, **2**, 195.

Mandell, G. L. and Vest, T. K. (1972), 'Killing of intraleukocytic Staphylococcus aureus by rifampin: *In vitro* and *in vivo* studies', *J. Infect. Dis.*, **125**, 486.

Mandell, F. and Wright, P. F. (1975), 'Treatment of atypical mycobacterial cervical adenitis with rifampin', *Pediatrics*, **55**, 39.

McCabe, W. R. and Lorian, V. (1968), 'Comparison of the antibacterial activity of rifampicin and other antibiotics', *Amer. J. Med. Sci.*, **256**, 255.

McClatchy, J. K., Waggoner, R. F. and Lester, W. (1969), '*In vitro* susceptibility of mycobacteria to rifampin', *Amer. Rev. Resp. Dis.*, **100**, 234.

McCormick, J. B. and Bennett, J. V. (1975), 'Public health considerations in the management of meningococcal disease', *Ann. Intern. Med.*, **83**, 883.

Miller, W. T. (1978), 'Long-term therapy with rifampin and the secondary antibody response to killed influenza vaccine', *Amer. Rev. Resp. Dis.*, **117**, 605.

Morrison-Smith, J. (1975), 'Rifampicin in clinical use', *J. Antimicrob. Chemother.*, **1**, 353.

Moshkowitz, A., Goldblum, N. and Heller, E. (1971), 'Studies on the antiviral effect of rifampicin in volunteers', *Nature*, **229**, 422.

Mukerjee, P., Schuldt, S. and Kasik, J. E. (1973), 'Effect of rifampin on cutaneous hypersensitivity to purified protein derivative in humans', *Antimicrob. Ag. Chemother.*, **4**, 607.

Murdoch, J. McC., Speirs, C. F., Wright, N. and Wallace, E. T. (1969), 'Rifampicin', *Lancet*, **1**, 1094.

Nessi, R., Domenichini, E. and Fowst, G. (1973), '"Allergic" reactions during rifampicin treatment: A review of published cases', *Scand. J. resp. Dis. Suppl.*, **84**, 15.

Nessi, R., Bonoldi, G. L., Redaelli, B. and Di Filippo, G. (1976), 'Acute renal failure after rifampicin: A case report and survey of the literature', *Nephron*, **16**, 148.

Newman, R., Doster, B., Murray, F. J. and Ferebee, S. (1971), 'Rifampin in initial treatment of pulmonary tuberculosis', *Amer. Rev. Resp. Dis.*, **103**, 461.

Newman, R., Doster, B. E., Murray, F. J. and Woolpert, S. F. (1974), 'Rifampin in initial treatment of pulmonary tuberculosis. A U.S. Public Health Service tuberculosis trial', *Amer. Rev. Resp. Dis.*, **109**, 216.

Nilsson, B. S. (1971), 'Rifampicin: an immunosuppressant?', *Lancet*, **2**, 374.

Nitti, V., Catena, E., Veneri, F. D., de Michele, G. and Marra, A. (1971), 'Rifampin in association with isoniazid, streptomycin and ethambutol, respectively, in the initial treatment of pulmonary tuberculosis', *Amer. Rev. Resp. Dis.*, **103**, 329.

Nyirenda, R. and Gill, G. V. (1977), 'Stevens-Johnson syndrome due to rifampicin', *Brit. med. J.*, **2,** 1189.

O'Connell, J., Campbell, A. H., Cowen, K. and Verins, A. (1973), 'Initial treatment of tuberculosis with rifampicin', *Med. J. Aust.*, **2,** 881.

O'Reilly, R. A. (1974), 'Interaction of sodium warfarin and rifampin. Studies in man', *Ann. Intern. Med.*, **81,** 337.

O'Reilly, R. A. (1975), 'Interaction of chronic daily warfarin therapy and rifampin', *Ann. Intern. Med.*, **83,** 506.

Ostenson, R. C., Fields, B. T. and Nolan, C. M. (1977), 'Polymyxin B and rifampin: New regimen for multiresistant Serratia marcescens infections', *Antimicrob. Ag. Chemother.*, **12,** 655.

Parker, M. D. and Irwin, R. S. (1975), 'Mycobacterium kansasii tendinitis and fasciitis', *J. Bone Joint Surg.*, **57-A,** 557.

Pattamasukon, P., Pichyangkura, C. and Fischer, G. W. (1975), 'Melioidosis in childhood', *J. Pediatrics*, **87,** 133.

Pattyn, S. R., Dockx, P., Rollier, M. T., Rollier, R. and Saerens, E. J. (1976), 'Mycobacterium leprae persisters after treatment with dapsone and rifampicin', *Int. J. Leprosy*, **44,** 154.

Peard, M. C., Fleck, D. G., Garrod, L. P. and Waterworth, P. M. (1970), 'Combined rifampicin and erythromycin for bacterial endocarditis', *Brit. med. J.*, **4,** 410.

Philippon, A. M., Plommet, M. G., Kazmierczak, A., Marly, J. L. and Nevot, P. A. (1977), 'Rifampin in the treatment of experimental brucellosis in mice and guinea pigs', *J. Infect. Dis.*, **136,** 482.

Pines, A. (1969), 'Preliminary results with rifampicin in the treatment of drug-resistant tuberculosis', *Tubercle* (Suppl.), **50,** 50.

Poole, G., Stradling, P. and Worlledge, S. (1971), 'Potentially serious side-effects of high-dose twice-weekly rifampicin', *Brit. med. J.*, **3,** 343.

Poole, G., Stradling, P. and Worlledge, S. (1973), 'Side-effects observed during intermittent rifampicin therapy', *Scand. J. resp. Dis. Suppl.*, **84,** 129.

Proust, A. J. (1971), 'The Australian rifampicin trial', *Med. J. Aust.*, **2,** 85.

Proust, A. and Evans, C. (1972), 'The Australian rifampicin trial', *Med. J. Aust.*, **2,** 861.

Raleigh, J. W. (1972), 'Rifampin in treatment of advanced pulmonary tuberculosis. Report of a VA cooperative pilot study', *Amer. Rev. Resp. Dis.*, **105,** 397.

Rajan, V. S., Tan, N. J., Tan, T., Khoo, R., Sng, E. H. and Pang, G. P. (1977), 'Treatment of gonorrhoeae: The Singapore experience', *Asian J. Infect. Dis.*, **1,** 71.

Rees, R. J. W., Pearson, J. M. H. and Waters, M. F. R. (1970), 'Experimental and clinical studies on rifampicin in treatment of leprosy', *Brit. med. J.*, **1,** 89.

Rees, R. J. W. (1975), 'Rifampicin: Investigation of a bactericidal antileprosy drug', *Lepr. Rev.* (Suppl.), **46,** 121.

Rees, R. J. W., Waters, M. F. R., Pearson, J. M. H., Helmy, H. S. and Laing, A. B. G. (1976), 'Long-term treatment of dapsone-resistant leprosy with rifampicin: Clinical and bacteriological studies', *Int. J. Leprosy*, **44,** 159.

Report of a WHO Scientific Group (1978), 'Neisseria gonorrhoeae and gonococcal infections', *Wld. Hlth. Org. techn. Rep. Ser.*, No. 616.

Romankiewicz, J. A. and Ehrman, M. (1975), 'Rifampicin and warfarin: A drug interaction', *Ann. Intern. Med.*, **82,** 224.

Rothwell, D. L. and Richmond, D. E. (1974), 'Hepatorenal failure with self-initiated intermittent rifampicin therapy', *Brit. med, J.*, **2,** 481.

Ruben, F. L., Winkelstein, A. and Fotiadis, I. G. (1974), 'Immunological responsiveness of tuberculosis patients receiving rifampin', *Antimicrob. Ag. Chemother.*, **5,** 383.

Rynearson, T. K., Shronts, J. S. and Wolinsky, E. (1971), 'Rifampin: *In vitro* effect on atypical mycobacteria', *Amer. Rev. Resp. Dis.*, **104,** 272.

Sage, R. E. and Derrington, A. W. (1973), 'Opportunistic cutaneous Mycobacterium marinum infection mimicking Mycobacterium ulcerans in lymphosarcoma', *Med. J. Aust.*, **2**, 434.

Sande, M. A. and Mandell, G. L. (1975), 'Effect of rifampin on nasal carriage of Staphylococcus aureus', *Antimicrob. Ag. Chemother.*, **7**, 294.

Saphyakhajon, P., Mukhopadhyay, D., Spiegel, P. and Grossman, B. J. (1977), 'Mycobacterium kansasii arthritis of the knee joint', *Amer. J. Dis. Child.*, **131**, 573.

Scheuer, P. J., Summerfield, J. A., Lal, S. and Sherlock, S. (1974), 'Rifampicin hepatitis. A clinical and histological study', *Lancet*, **1**, 421.

Sensi, P., Maggi, N., Füresz, S. and Maffii, G. (1967), 'Chemical modifications and biological properties of rifamycins', *Antimicrob. Ag. Chemother.*—1966, p. 699.

Seriki, O., Aderele, W. I., Johnson, A. and Smith, J. A. (1975), 'Disseminated histoplasmosis due to Histoplasma capsulatum in two Nigerian children', *J. Trop. Med. Hyg.*, **78**, 248.

Seufert, C. D. (1973), 'Acute renal failure after rifampicin therapy', *Scand. J. resp. Dis. Suppl.*, **84**, 174.

Shanson, D. C. and Leung, T. (1976), 'Susceptibility of Salmonella typhi to rifamycins and novobiocin', *J. Antimicrob. Chemother.*, **2**. 81.

Siegler, D. I., Bryant, M., Burley, D. M., Citron, K. M. and Standen, S. M. (1974), 'Effect of meals on rifampicin absorption', *Lancet*, **2**, 197.

Sifontes, J. E. (1975), 'Rifampin in tuberculous meningitis', *J. Pediatrics*, **87**, 1015.

Singapore Tuberculosis Service/British Medical Research Council (1975), 'Controlled trial of intermittent regimens of rifampicin plus isoniazid for pulmonary tuberculosis in Singapore', *Lancet*, **2**, 1105.

Sippel, J. E., Mikhail, I. A., Girgis, N. I. and Youssef, H. H. (1974), 'Rifampin concentrations in cerebrospinal fluid of patients with tuberculous meningitis', *Amer. Rev. Resp. Dis.*, **109**, 579.

Sivonen, A., Renkonen, O.-V., Weckström, P., Koskenvuo, K., Raunio, V. and Mäkelä, P. H. (1978), 'The effect of chemoprophylactic use of rifampin and minocycline on rates of carriage of Neisseria meningitidis in army recruits in Finland', *J. Infect. Dis.*, **137**, 238.

Skolnick, J. L., Stoler, B. S., Katz, D. B. and Anderson, W. H. (1976), 'Rifampin, oral contraceptives, and pregnancy', *JAMA*, **236**, 1382.

Staehelin, M., Knusel, F. and Wehrli, W. (1968), 'The mechanism of action of rimactane', *A Symposium on Rimactane, Ciba, Basle*, 18; quoted by Proust (1971).

Stanford, J. L. and Phillips, I. (1972), 'Rifampicin in experimental Mycobacterium ulcerans infection', *J. Med. Microbiol.*, **5**, 39.

Stern, J. S. M. and Stainton-Ellis, D. M. (1977), 'Rifampicin in pregnancy', *Lancet*, **2**, 604.

Stone, W. J., Waldron, J. A., Dixon, J. H., Jr., Primm, R. K. and Horn, R. G. (1976), 'Acute diffuse interstitial nephritis related to chemotherapy of tuberculosis', *Antimicrob. Ag. Chemother.*, **10**, 164.

Stottmeier, K. D. (1976), 'Emergence of rifampin-resistant Mycobacterium tuberculosis in Massachusetts', *J. Infect. Dis.*, **133**, 88.

Subak-Sharpe, J. H., Timbury, M. C. and Williams, J. F. (1969), 'Rifampin inhibits the growth of some mammalian viruses', *Nature*, **222**, 341.

Syvälahti, E. K. G., Pihlajamäki, K. K. and Iisalo, E. J. (1974), 'Rifampicin and drug metabolism', *Lancet*, **2**, 232.

Tanzil, H. O. K., Chatim, A., Utomo, R. R. and Harun, H. (1972), 'Sensitivity of various species of nocardia to rifampin *in vitro*', *Amer. Rev. Resp. Dis.*, **105**, 455.

Thompson, J. E. (1976), 'The effect of rifampicin on liver morphology in tuberculous alcoholics', *Aust. N.Z. J. Med.*, **6**, 111.

Thong, Y. H., Rowan-Kelly, B., Shepherd, C. and Ferrante, A. (1977), 'Growth inhibition of Naegleria fowleri by tetracycline, rifampicin, and miconazole', *Lancet*, **2**, 876.

Thornsberry, C., Baker, C. N. and Kirven, L. A. (1978), '*In vitro* activity of antimicrobial agents on Legionnaires' disease bacterium', *Antimicrob. Ag. Chemother.*, **13**, 78.

Traub, W. H. and Kleber, I. (1975), '*In vitro* additive effect of polymyxin B and rifampin against Serratia marcescens', *Antimicrob. Agents Chemother.*, **7**, 874.

Tsukamura, M. (1972), 'The pattern of resistance development to rifampicin in Mycobacterium tuberculosis', *Tubercle*, **53**, 111.

Tuazon, C. U., Lin, M. Y. C. and Sheagren, J. N. (1978), '*In vitro* activity of rifampicin alone and in combination with nafcillin and vancomycin against pathogenic strains of Staphylococcus aureus', *Antimicrob. Ag. Chemother.*, **13**, 759.

Van Dyke, J. J. and Lake, K. B. (1975), 'Chemotherapy for aquarium granuloma', *JAMA*, **233**, 1380.

Verbist, L. and Gyselen, A. (1968), 'Antituberculous activity of rifampin *in vitro* and *in vivo* and the concentrations attained in human blood', *Amer. Rev. Resp. Dis.*, **98**, 923.

Visudhiphan, P. and Chiemchanya, S. (1975), 'Evaluation of rifampicin in the treatment of tuberculous meningitis in children', *J. Pediatrics*, **87**, 983.

Ward, J. I., Gorman, G. Phillips, C. and Fraser, D. W. (1978), 'Hemophilus influenzae type b disease in a day-care center', *J. Pediatr.*, **92**, 713.

Waters, M. F. R., Rees, R. J. W., Pearson, J. M. H., Laing, A. B. G., Helmy, H. S. and Gelber, R. H. (1978), 'Rifampicin for lepromatous leprosy: Nine years' experience', *Brit. med. J.*, **1**, 133.

Weidmer, C. E., Dunkel, T. B., Pettyjohn, F. S., Smith, C. D. and Leibovitz, A. (1971), 'Effectiveness of rifampicin in eradicating the meningococcal carrier state in a relatively closed population: Emergence of resistant strains', *J. Infect. Dis.*, **124**, 172.

WHO (1977), 'WHO expert committee on leprosy', *Wld, Hlth. Org. techn. Rep. Ser.*, No. 607.

Wilkinson, F. F., Gago, J. and Santabaya, E. (1972), 'Therapy of leprosy with rifampicin', *International Journal of Leprosy*, **40**, 53.

Wisseman, C. L., Jr., Waddell, A. D. and Walsh, W. T. (1974), '*In vitro* studies of the action of antibiotics on Rickettsia prowazeki by two basic methods of cell culture', *J. Infect. Dis.*, **130**, 564.

Woodley, C. L., Kilburn, J. O., David, H. L. and Silcox, V. A. (1972), 'Susceptibility of mycobacteria to rifampin', *Antimicrob. Ag. Chemother.*, **2**, 245.

Worlledge, S. (1973a), 'The detection of rifampicin-dependent antibodies', *Scand. J. resp. Dis. Suppl.*, **84**, 60.

Worlledge, S. (1973b), 'Correlation between the presence of rifampicin-dependent antibodies and the clinical data', *Scand. J. resp. Dis. Suppl.*, **84**, 125.

Yamada, S. and Iwai, K. (1976), 'Induction of hepatic cortisol-6-hydroxylase by rifampicin', *Lancet*, **2**, 366.

Zierski, M. (1973), 'Clinical aspects of side-effects on intermittent rifampicin regimen', *Scand. J. resp. Dis. Suppl.*, **84**, 166.

Spectinomycin

Description

Spectinomycin is an aminocyclitol compound which has some structural similarities to the aminocyclitol streptomycin, but it differs by not being an aminoglycoside (*see* page 294). Spectinomycin was isolated in 1960 from Streptomyces spectabilis in the Upjohn Research Laboratories (Mason *et al.*, 1961). It was orginally known as actinospectacin and was manufactured as the sulphate salt. Now it is manufactured as the more soluble dihydrochloride salt and as spectinomycin dihydrochloride pentahydrate it has the trade name of 'Trobicin' (Upjohn). The clinical use of this drug is at present restricted to the treatment of gonorrhoea.

Sensitive Organisms

1. *Gram-positive bacteria*. Many of these bacteria such as Strep. pyogenes, Strep. pneumoniae and Staph. epidermidis are usually sensitive (McCormack and Finland, 1976; Fass and Prior, 1977). Only a small percentage of Staph. pyogenes and Strep. viridans strains are sensitive to concentrations easily obtainable in serum. The *in vitro* sensitivity of the Clostridia (perfringens and ramosum) depends on the pH of the medium used (Rosenblatt and Gerdts, 1977).

2. *Gram-negative bacteria*. Spectinomycin has a wide range of activity against these bacteria (Mason *et al.*, 1961; Lewis and Clapp, 1961; Washington and Yu, 1972; McCormack and Finland, 1976; Fass and Prior, 1977). Esch. coli, Klebsiella pneumoniae and the Enterobacter, Salmonella and Shigella spp. are usually sensitive. Proteus mirabilis and to a lesser extent indole-positive Proteus spp. are often sensitive. Serratia and Citrobacter spp. are sometimes sensitive whilst Providencia spp. and Pseudomonas aeruginosa are always resistant. A high percentage of the Enterobacteriaceae are inhibited by a concentration of $\leqslant 128\,\mu$g per ml, a concentration which is easily attainable in the urine with normal spectinomycin doses (Fass and Prior, 1977). Spectinomycin is active against a higher percentage of Enterobacteriaceae than ampicillin (page 100) or tetracycline (page 594), but is less active than gentamicin (page 325). Some of these bacteria have developed resistance to spectinomycin *in vivo* when it was used to treat urinary tract infections (Vineyard *et al.*, 1963).

Spectinomycin is highly active against Haemophilus influenzae. Its greatest activity is against Neisseria gonorrhoeae (Lewis and Clapp, 1961; Levy *et al.*, 1973; McCormack and Finland, 1976). Nearly all strains of N. gonorrhoeae in the United States are inhibited by a concentration of $6\cdot3\,\mu$g or less (McCormack and Finland, 1976). Some studies indicate that gonococcal strains relatively resistant to penicillin G (page 7) show no increased resistance to spectinomycin (Maness and Sparling, 1973), but others have found that there is a weak correlation between their sensitivities (Report, 1978). Beta-lactamase producing strains of N. gonorrhoeae (page 8) remain sensitive to spectinomycin; all such strains isolated in East Asia were sensitive to 12 μg per ml or less of spectinomycin (Report, 1978). Gonococci with increased resistance to spectinomycin can be produced *in vitro* by serial passage of the organisms in media containing increasing amounts of the drug (Pedersen *et al.*, 1972). The development of resistance to spectinomycin is of the one-step type, similar to streptomycin (page 295) and rifampicin (page 556) (Report, 1978). Gonococcal strains which are highly resistant to spectinomycin have only been isolated from a few patients in Denmark (Reyn *et al.*, 1973) and the United States (Thornsberry *et al.*, 1977; Center for Disease Control, 1978). This resistance to spectinomycin occurred in non-beta-lactamase producing gonococcal strains. Total resistance to spectinomycin results from a chromosomal mutation which affects the ribosomal structure of N. gonorrhoeae (Report, 1978), thereby preventing spectinomycin from inhibiting protein synthesis by its action on the ribosome (page 587). Spectinomycin resistant strains remain sensitive to the aminoglycosides, streptomycin, kanamycin, amikacin, gentamicin, tobramycin and sisomicin (Thornsberry *et al.*, 1977). There is concern that the widespread use of spectinomycin may lead to an increase in resistant strains by the additional mechanism of transfer of R plasmids (page 422) from resistant enteric bacteria (Report, 1978). An R plasmid has been found in strains of Esch. coli, which codes for the production of an adenylylating enzyme which inactivates spectinomycin (Benveniste *et al.*, 1970).

Varying results have been obtained in tests for susceptibility of Gram-negative anaerobic bacteria to spectinomycin. Phillips and Warren (1975) reported that most strains of Bacteroides fragilis are inhibited by a concentration of 16 μg per ml or less of spectinomycin. However, other authors, using different techniques, have not confirmed this degree of susceptibility of B. fragilis (Ferguson and Smith, 1975; Okubadejo, 1975; Churcher and Human, 1977). Rosenblatt and Gerdts (1977) also showed that B. fragilis, B. melaninogenicus and Fusobacterium spp. vary in their susceptibility to spectinomycin *in vitro,* the results being particularly dependent on the initial pH of the medium used.

3. *Agents causing non-specific urethritis.* Aetiological agents of this disease include Chlamydia trachomatis and Ureaplasma urealyticum (Mycoplasma T-strains) (*see* page 627). Spectinomycin is inactive against C. trachomatis but Ureaplasma urealyticum is sensitive (Bowie *et al.*, 1976; McCormack and Finland, 1976; Oriel *et al.*, 1977; Report, 1978).

4. *Treponema pallidum.* Spectinomycin has no curative effect on syphilis (Report, 1978) and used in a single dose it will not abort incubating syphilis but it may prolong the incubation period (McCormack and Finland, 1976).

In Vitro Sensitivities

The minimum inhibitory concentrations of spectinomycin for a few selected bacterial species are shown in Table 37. Organisms inhibited by 31·2 μg per ml or less may be considered as sensitive and organisms for which concentrations in excess of 125 μg per ml are required as resistant. Organisms with MIC's between these limits belong to an intermediate category (Washington and Yu, 1972).

TABLE 37

(After Lewis and Clapp, 1961)

ORGANISM	MIC (μg per ml)
Staph. pyogenes	6·2–25
Strep. pneumoniae	12·5–25
Neisseria gonorrhoeae	7·8
Esch. coli	12·5–50

Mode of Administration and Dosage

1. Spectinomycin is only administered by intramuscular injection. Adult doses of 2–4 g given by deep intramuscular injection have been used for 'single-session' therapy of gonorrhoea. Originally the higher dose was used for females but now a 2 g dose is recommended for both females and males (McCormack and Finland, 1976; Report, 1978).

2. No dosage recommendations are available for children.

3. The drug would presumably accumulate in patients with renal disease if repeated doses were given, but as it is administered only as a single injection, dosage modification is not necessary in such patients.

4. The safety of spectinomycin has not been established in pregnancy, but no ill-effects have been observed so far (McCormack and Finland, 1976; Report, 1978).

Availability

Spectinomycin dihydrochloride pentahydrate is supplied in 2 and 4 g vials which when reconstituted with diluent, provide volumes of 3·2 and 6·5 ml respectively for intramuscular injection.

Serum Levels and Excretion

Spectinomycin is poorly absorbed after oral administration but it is well absorbed from intramuscular injection sites. A peak blood level of about 100 μg per ml is attained about one hour after a 2 g dose (Wagner et al., 1968). Doubling the dose nearly doubles the serum concentration. A detectable serum level persists for about 8 h after a dose. Most of the injected drug (70–80 per cent) is excreted in the urine within 48 h in a microbiologically active form. Urinary concentrations of the active drug may reach 1000 μg per ml. Probenecid does not delay the excretion of spectinomycin. The drug is little bound to serum proteins (Wagner et al., 1968).

Mode of Action

Similar to streptomycin (page 298), spectinomycin acts at the 30S ribosomal subunit (page 434), thereby inhibiting protein synthesis. Unlike streptomycin, it causes no detectable misreading of polyribonucleotide code and at high concentration it is not bactericidal to Esch. coli (Davies *et al.*, 1965). However in studies using N. gonorrhoeae, Ward (1977), showed that spectinomycin is more bactericidal than penicillin, tetracycline and kanamycin. Spectinomycin also produces alterations in the surface morphology of gonococci, leading to their lysis. This possibly results from the action of spectinomycin on the ribosomes resulting in inhibition of the cytoplasmic membrane proteins and interference with the osmotic integrity of the cell (Ward, 1977).

Toxicity

Spectinomycin given as a single dose daily only appears to be of low toxicity. Willcox (1962) treated 101 patients and observed no side-effects. Its low toxicity has been confirmed by others (Tiedeman *et al.*, 1965; Platts, 1970; Duncan *et al.*, 1972). Occasionally patients have noted transient dizziness after the injection (Labowitz *et al.*, 1970). A few patients have also developed either transient fever, nausea, headache or moderate discomfort at the injection site. No cases of ototoxicity or nephrotoxicity have been reported (Savage, 1973). Rarely an erythematous rash has been noted (Pedersen *et al.*, 1972.)

When spectinomycin was given in a dose of 2 g four times a day for 21 days to volunteers, no evidence of ototoxicity or nephrotoxicity was detected (Novak *et al.*, 1974).

Spectinomycin is not cross-allergenic with the penicillins.

Clinical Uses of the Drug

1. *Gonorrhoea.* At present uncomplicated gonorrhoea is the only clinical indication for the use of spectinomycin. It is given as 'single-injection' therapy in a dose of 2 g. Such 'single-injection' treatment is not ideal, but it is practical for the treatment of large numbers of unreliable patients who attend venereal disease clinics (Tiedeman *et al.*, 1965). Results of spectinomycin treatment of uncomplicated gonorrhoea caused by non-beta-lactamase producing strains in both sexes are good and comparable with those obtained by 'single-injection' treatment with penicillin G (Willcox, 1962; Sparling *et al.*, 1966; Cornelius and Domescik, 1970; Duncan *et al.*, 1972; Pedersen *et al.*, 1972; Duančić *et al.*, 1974; Judson *et al.*, 1974; Annotation, 1974; Finger, 1975; Porter and Rutherford, 1977). Spectinomycin treatment failures are not usually attributable to the presence of gonococcal strains resistant to spectinomycin (Report, 1978). Anorectal gonorrhoea also responds to 'single-injection' treatment with spectinomycin to successfully treat gonococcal proctitis in male homosexual patients. Gonococcal infections of the pharynx do not respond to single-dose spectinomycin (McCormack and Finland, 1976; Report, 1978). Multiple doses of penicillin G (page 37), ampicillin (page 119), co-trimoxazole (page 710) or tetracycline (page 625) over several days, are required for the treatment of gonococcal pharyngitis (Report, 1978). It is possible that spectinomycin in a dose of 4–8 g per day for 7–10 days may be effective in disseminated gonococcal infections (McCormack and Finland, 1976).

With the advent of beta-lactamase producing strains of N. gonorrhoeae (page 8), it is now recommended that the use of spectinomycin in gonorrhoea should be restricted (Willcox, 1977; Report, 1978). The widespread use of this drug could otherwise lead to a greater prevalence of spectinomycin-resistant gonococci (*see* page 586). Spectinomycin is now advocated for patients infected with beta-lactamase producing gonococcal strains and for those patients who are allergic to penicillin. It is also the drug of choice for those in whom treatment with other drugs has failed, irrespective of whether the strain is beta-lactamase producing or not. Possible alternative drugs to spectinomycin in non-pregnant patients are kanamycin (page 319) and co-trimoxazole (page 710), whilst for pregnant patients cefuroxime (page 286) may prove of value, erythromycin (page 508) being less reliable.

2. *Non-specific urethritis.* The majority of cases of non-specific (non-gonococcal or post-gonococcal) urethritis are caused by Chlamydia trachomatis and a smaller number are due to Ureaplasma urealyticum (Mycoplasma T-strains) (page 627). A disadvantage of spectinomycin is that it is ineffective against infections due to C. trachomatis (page 586) though infections due to U. urealyticum respond (Bowie *et al.*, 1976; McCormack and Finland, 1976).

3. *Other infections.* Although spectinomycin is active against a variety of Gram-positive and Gram-negative bacteria, other chemotherapeutic agents are preferred for infections due to these organisms. Gram-negative bacteria tend to become resistant to spectinomycin (page 585) and the drug can only be administered parenterally. Of more importance is the need to restrict the use of spectinomycin to delay the further emergence of strains of N. gonorrhoeae resistant to this drug (page 586).

REFERENCES

Annotation (1974), 'Spectinomycin for gonorrhoea', *Lancet,* **2,** 1239.

Benveniste, R., Yamada, T. and Davies, J. (1970), 'Enzymatic adenylyation of strep-tomycin and spectinomycin by R-factor-resistant Escherichia coli', *Infect. Immun.,* **1,** 109.

Bowie, W. R., Alexander, E. R., Floyd, J. F., Holmes, J., Miller, Y. and Holmes, K. K. (1976), 'Differential response of chlamydial and ureaplasma—associated urethritis to sulphafurazole (sulfisoxazole) and aminocyclitols', *Lancet,* **2,** 1276.

Center for Disease Control (1978), 'Penicillinase-(beta-lactamase-) producing Neisseria gonorrhoeae-worldwide', *Morbidity and Mortality Weekly Report,* **27,** 10.

Churcher, G. H. and Human, R. P. (1977), 'Assessment of the *in vitro* activity against Bacteroides spp. of spectinomycin, metronidazole and clindamycin', *J. Antimicrob. Chemother.,* **3,** 363.

Cornelius, C. E., III and Domescik, G. (1970), 'Spectinomycin hydrochloride in the treatment of uncomplicated gonorrhoea', *Brit. J. vener. Dis.,* **46,** 212.

Davies, J., Anderson, P. and Davis, B. D. (1965), 'Inhibition of protein synthesis by spectinomycin', *Science,* **149,** 1096.

Dunančić, A., Fiumara, N. J., Alpert, S., Lee, Y., Tarr, P. I., Rosner, B. and McCor-mack, W. M. (1974), 'Comparison of spectinomycin hydrochloride and aqueous procaine penicillin G in the treatment of uncomplicated gonorrhoea', *Antimicrob. Ag. Chemother.,* **6,** 512.

Duncan, W. C., Holder, W. R., Roberts, D. P. and Knox, J. M. (1972), 'Treatment of gonorrhoea with spectinomycin hydrochloride: Comparison with standard penicillin schedules', *Antimicrob. Ag. Chemother.,* **1,** 210.

Fass, R. J. and Prior, R. B. (1977), '*In vitro* activity of spectinomycin against recent urinary tract isolates', *Antimicrob. Ag. Chemother.*, **12**, 551.

Ferguson, I. R. and Smith, L. L. (1975), 'Bacteroides fragilis and spectinomycin', *J. Antimicrob. Chemother.*, **1**, 245.

Finger, A. H. (1975), 'Spectinomycin in the treatment of gonorrhoea in females and males', *Brit. J. vener. Dis.*, **51**, 38.

Fiumara, N. J. (1978), 'The treatment of gonococcal proctitis. An evaluation of 173 patients treated with 4 g of spectinomycin', *JAMA, 239*, 735.

Judson, F. N., Allaman, J. and Dans, P. E. (1974), 'Treatment of gonorrhea. Comparison of penicillin G procaine doxycycline, spectinomycin and ampicillin', *JAMA, 230*, 705.

Karney, W. W., Pedersen, A. H. B., Nelson, M., Adams, H., Pfeifer, R. T. and Holmes, K. K. (1977), 'Spectinomycin versus tetracycline for the treatment of gonorrhoea', *New Engl. J. Med.,* **296**, 889.

Labowitz, R., Porter, W. L. and Holloway, W. J. (1970), 'The treatment of gonorrhoea with spectinomycin and rifampicin', *Delaware Medical Journal*, **42**, 353.

Levy, J., Wicher, K. and Rose, N. R. (1973), '*In vitro* susceptibility of Neisseria gonorrhoeae to spectinomycin examined by a broth dilution method', *Antimicrob. Ag. Chemother.*, **3**, 335.

Lewis, C. and Clapp, H. W. (1961), 'Actinospectacin, a new antibiotic. III. *In vitro* and *in vivo* evaluation', *Antibiot. Chemother.*, **11**, 127.

Maness, M. J. and Sparling, P. F. (1973), 'Multiple antibiotic resistance due to a single mutation in Neisseria gonorrhoeae', *J. Infect. Dis.*, **128**, 321.

Mason, D. J., Dietz, A. and Smith, R. M. (1961), 'Actinospectacin, a new antibiotic. I. Discovery and biological properties', *Antibiot. Chemother.*, **11**, 118.

McCormack, W. M. and Finland, M. (1976), 'Drugs five years later. Spectinomycin', *Ann. Intern. Med.,* **84**, 712.

Novak, E., Gray, J. E. and Pfeifer, R. T. (1974), 'Animal and human tolerance of high-dose intramuscular therapy with spectinomycin', *J. Infect. Dis.,* **130**, 50.

Okubadejo, O. A. (1975), 'Susceptibility of Bacteroides fragilis to spectinomycin', *J. Antimicrob. Chemother.*, **1**, 347.

Oriel, J. D., Ridgway, G. L., Tchamouroff, S. and Owen, J. (1977), 'Spectinomycin hydrochloride in the treatment of gonorrhoea: Its effect on associated Chlamydia trachomatis infections', *Brit. J. vener, Dis.*, **53**, 226.

Phillips, I. and Warren, C. (1975), 'Susceptibility of Bacteroides fragilis to spectinomycin', *J. Antimicrob. Chemother.*, **1**, 91.

Pedersen, A. H. B., Wiesner, P. J., Holmes, K. H., Johnson, C. J. and Turck, M. (1972), 'Spectinomycin and penicillin G in the treatment of gonorrhea. A comparative evaluation', *JAMA, 220*, 205.

Platts, W. M. (1970), ' "Trobicin" in the treatment of gonorrhoea', *Med. J. Aust.*, **2**, 500.

Porter, I. A. and Rutherford, H. W. (1977), 'Treatment of uncomplicated gonorrhoea with spectinomycin hydrochloride (Trobicin)', *Brit. J. vener. Dis.*, **53**, 115.

Report of a WHO Scientific Group (1978), 'Neisseria gonorrhoeae and gonococcal infections', *Wld. Hlth. Org. techn. Rep. Ser.*, No. 616.

Reyn, A., Schmidt, H., Trier, M. and Bentzon, M. W. (1973), 'Spectinomycin hydrochloride (Trobicin) in the treatment of gonorrhoea. Observations of resistant strains of Neisseria gonorrhoeae', *Brit. J. vener. Dis.*, **49**, 54.

Rosenblatt, J. E. and Gerdts, A. M. (1977), 'Activity of spectinomycin against anaerobes', *Antimicrob. Ag. Chemother.*, **12**, 37.

Savage, G. M. (1973), 'Spectinomycin related to the chemotherapy of gonorrhea', *Infection, 1*, 227.

Sparling, P. F., Yobs, A. R., Billings, T. E. and Hackney, J. F. (1966), 'Spectinomycin sulfate and aqueous procaine penicillin G in treatment of female gonorrhea', *An-*

timicrob. Ag. Chemother.—1965, p. 689.

Thornsberry, C., Jaffee, H., Brown, S. T., Edwards, T., Biddle, J. W. and Thompson, S. E. (1977), 'Spectinomycin-resistant Neisseria gonorrhoeae', *JAMA,* **237,** 2405.

Tiedemann, J. H., Hackney, J. F. and Price, E. V. (1965), 'Acute gonorrheal urethritis in men. Treatment with spectinomycin sulfate', *JAMA,* **191,** 101.

Vineyard, J. P., Mays, B. M. and Sanford, J. P. (1963), 'Evaluation of actinospectacin in urinary tract infections', *Clin. Pharmacol. Ther.,* **4,** 622.

Wagner, J. G., Novak, E., Leslie, L. G. and Metzler, C. M. (1968), 'Absorption, distribution and elimination of spectinomycin dihydrochloride in man', *Int. J. clin. Pharmacol.,* **1,** 261.

Ward, M. E. (1977), 'The bactericidal action of spectinomycin on Neisseria gonorrhoeae', *J. Antimicrob. Chemother.,* **3,** 323.

Washington, J. A., II and Yu, P. K. W. (1972), '*In vitro* antibacterial activity of spectinomycin', *Antimicrob. Ag. Chemother.,* **2,** 427.

Willcox, R. R. (1962), 'Trobicin (actinospectacin) a new injectable antibiotic in the treatment of gonorrhoea', *Brit. J. vener. Dis.,* **38,** 150.

Willcox, R. R. (1977), 'How suitable are available pharmaceuticals for the treatment of sexually transmitted diseases? 1: Conditions presenting as genital discharges', *Brit. J. vener. Dis.,* **53,** 314.

Tetracyclines

Description

Numerous tetracycline compounds with a similar molecular structure (four benzene rings) and about the same spectrum of activity are currently available.

1. *Chlortetracycline* ('*Aureomycin*'), the first tetracycline to be discovered, was isolated from Streptomyces aureofaciens in 1944 (Duggar *et al.*, 1948).
2. *Oxytetracycline* ('*Terramycin*'), derived from Streptomyces rimosus, was reported in 1950.
3. *Tetracycline* ('*Achromycin*', '*Tetracyn*'), first described in 1953, was prepared from chlortetracycline at Lederle laboratories and was also independently derived from oxytetracycline at Pfizer laboratories.
4. *Demethylchlortetracycline or demeclocycline* ('*Ledermycin*') was obtained from a mutant of Duggar's original strain of Streptomyces aureofaciens and reported in 1957.

Five more recent additions to the tetracycline group of drugs are:

1. *Methacycline* (*6-methylene-5-hydroxytetracycline or* '*Rondomycin*') was prepared in the Pfizer laboratories.
2. *Lymecycline* (*Tetracycline-L-methylene-lysine or* '*Tetralysal*') is a compound of tetracycline and an amino acid (Whitby and Black, 1964). It was developed in Italy and has not been available in Australia.
3. *Clomocycline* (*N-methylolchlortetracycline*, '*Megaclor*' or '*Pharmax*') is also an Italian product, not available in Australia.
4. *Doxycycline* (*alpha-6-deoxytetracycline or* '*Vibramycin*'), developed by Pfizer laboratories, is available as both doxycycline monohydrate and doxycycline hyclate. Its main advantage is increased oral absorption and a prolonged serum half-life.
5. *Minocycline* (*7-dimethylamino-6-demethyl-6-deoxytetracycline*) is the most recent tetracycline developed (Redin, 1967).

All of these tetracycline compounds are mainly marketed for oral administration, but intravenous and intramuscular preparations of tetracycline and oxytetracycline and intravenous preparations of doxycycline and minocycline are also available. In addition two more soluble compounds have been introduced specially for parenteral use.

1. *Rolitetracycline* (*Pyrrolidino-methyl-tetracycline or* '*Reverin*') (Dimmling, 1960).
2. *Rolitetracycline nitrate* (*Pyrrolidino-methyl-tetracycline nitrate or* '*Bristacin A*') (Kaplan *et al.*, 1960).

Sensitive Organisms

These antibiotics have a wide range of activity.

1. *Gram-positive bacteria*. The tetracyclines are active against most of these organisms such as Staph. pyogenes (including penicillinase-producing strains), Staph. epidermidis, Strep. pyogenes (Group A), Strep. pneumoniae, Strep. viridans, Strep. faecalis and also the anaerobic streptococci. Group B streptococci are commonly resistant (*vide infra*). Gram-positive bacilli such as B. anthracis, Cl. tetani, Cl. perfringens and Listeria monocytogenes (Wiggins *et al.*, 1978) are tetracycline-sensitive. Actinomyces israelii and Arachnia propionica, the causative organisms of human actinomycosis, are also sensitive to tetracycline (Holmberg *et al.*, 1977). Minocycline is quite active against the Nocardia, most N. asteroides strains being inhibited by $1 \cdot 6 - 3 \cdot 1$ μg per ml (Bach *et al.*, 1973), but all other tetracyclines are much less active against this species.

2. *Acquired resistance of Gram-positive bacteria*. Most of these bacteria may acquire resistance to the tetracyclines. Staphylococci readily become tetracycline-resistant, so that sensitivity testing is important if these drugs are used for the treatment of staphylococcal infections. The prevalence of staphylococci resistant to tetracyclines may be quite high in hospitals. In a survey in one Boston hospital, of 482 Staph. pyogenes strains isolated, $38 \cdot 2$ per cent were resistant (Sabath, 1969). Nevertheless community staphylococci often remain sensitive; in a study of out-patients attending a London hospital the percentage of tetracycline-resistant Staph. pyogenes in 1968 was $6 \cdot 5$ and this had only increased to 8 per cent in 1978 (Hassam *et al.*, 1978).

Strains of Strep. pyogenes (Group A) resistant to tetracycline occur. This was first observed in isolates from burned patients in Birmingham, England (Lowbury and Cason, 1954; Lowbury and Hurst, 1956). Kuharic *et al.* (1960) found 20 per cent of 218 strains and Mitchell and Baber (1965) 32 per cent of 640 strains examined to be tetracycline-resistant. Subsequent surveys showed a lower prevalence of resistant strains, possibly resulting from a more selective use of the tetracyclines. Kahlmeter and Kamme (1972) found only 6 per cent of 130 strains of Strep. pyogenes to be resistant, and Robertson (1973) observed a decrease in the prevalence of resistant strains in South-west Essex from a peak of 35 per cent in 1965 to $9 \cdot 2$ per cent in 1972. The majority of Group A beta-haemolytic streptococci collected in 1972 in Massachusetts were sensitive to tetracyclines (Finland *et al.*, 1976a). A more recent nation-wide survey in Britain during 1975, showed that overall 36 per cent of Group A streptococci were resistant, but the percentage of resistant strains in different localities ranged from 15 to 62; additionally resistance to tetracyclines was commoner amongst in-patients and patients aged 50 years or more and in isolates from sites other than the respiratory tract (Report, 1977). Group B haemolytic streptococci are frequently resistant to tetracyclines. In California during 1971–1973, of 607 isolates, mainly from urine, cervico-vaginal swabs or from neonates, 72 per cent were resistant to tetracycline (Anthony and Concepcion, 1975). Similarly, $87 \cdot 5$ per cent of 244 isolates of Group B streptococci during 1970–1975 in Houston, were resistant (Baker *et al.*, 1976).

Tetracycline-resistant pneumococci were first recognized in Australia in 1962 (Evans and Hansman, 1963). Since that time they have been frequently isolated from patients (Richards and Rycroft, 1963; Turner, 1963; Schaedler *et al.*, 1964; Hansman and Andrews, 1967). Subsequent surveys showed that the prevalence of tetracycline-resistant pneumococci was about 3 per cent (Holt *et al.*, 1969; Kahlmeter and Kamme, 1972), but a frequency of 23 per cent was reported from one Liverpool hospital (Percival *et al.*, 1969). A survey conducted in the United Kingdom during 1975 showed that overall 13 per cent of pneumococci were resistant to tetracyclines, but there was great geographic variation, the percentage resistant varying from 2 to 32 according to locality (Report, 1977). In a similar survey during 1977 in the United Kingdom, 6·8 per cent of Strep. pneumoniae strains studied were resistant to tetracycline (Howard *et al.*, 1978). Pneumococcal strains resistant to tetracyclines appear to be uncommon in the United States (Finland *et al.*, 1976b; Neu, 1978). Strep. viridans and Strep. faecalis strains can also acquire tetracycline resistance.

Resistance has also been described with Gram-positive anaerobic organisms. Johnstone and Cockcroft (1968) tested 102 strains of Cl. perfringens (welchii) and found that 11 had some degree of resistance to tetracycline. In a similar study of 43 strains of Cl. perfringens, Sapico *et al.* (1972) found that only 53 per cent were highly sensitive, the others being intermediate in sensitivity. However all the strains tested at that time were quite sensitive to doxycycline and minocycline. More recently Chow *et al.* (1975) found 54 per cent of strains of Cl. perfringens resistant to tetracycline and comparable percentages were resistant to minocycline and doxycycline. In another study Sutter and Finegold (1976) showed that about 40 per cent of Cl. perfringens strains were inhibited by clinically achievable concentrations and a slightly higher percentage of strains were inhibited by minocycline and particularly by doxycycline. Schwartzman *et al.* (1977) tested 57 strains of Cl. perfringens and found a higher susceptibility to tetracyclines; 81 per cent were inhibited by 4 μg per ml or less of tetracycline and 96 per cent by 2 μg per ml or less of doxycycline. Of the other Gram-positive anaerobes, such as the Peptococcus, Peptostreptococcus, Eubacterium, Acidaminococcus, Propionibacterium, Lactobacillus, Bifidobacterium and Actinomyces spp., a variable but significant proportion are resistant to the tetracycline drugs. Overall doxycycline and minocycline are somewhat more active than tetracycline against these anaerobes, with minocycline being the most active against some Peptococcus and Peptostreptococcus spp. (Chow *et al.*, 1975; Sutter and Finegold, 1976).

3. *Gram-negative bacteria.* Tetracyclines are active against Enterobacteriaceae such as Esch. coli and the Enterobacter, Klebsiella, Yersinia, Salmonella and Shigella spp. However Serratia marcescens and the Proteus spp. are usually resistant. Although the salmonellae are usually sensitive *in vitro*, tetracycline drugs are not usually effective for the treatment of infections due to these bacteria. Sometimes minocycline acts synergistically with gentamicin against certain Enterobacteriaceae, in particular against Esch. coli (Fass *et al.*, 1976). Vibrio cholerae (both classical and El tor biotypes) is susceptible. The halophilic vibrios, Vibrio parahaemolyticus and V. alginolyticus, which cause food-borne gastroenteritis, are nearly always sensitive to tetracycline (Joseph *et al.*, 1978). Campylobacter fetus is tetracycline-sensitive (Chow *et al.*, 1978).

Many other Gram-negative bacteria are also susceptible, including N. meningitidis, H. influenzae, B. pertussis, Pasteurella multocida and Francisella tularensis. The Brucella spp. are always highly and uniformly tetracycline-sensitive (Robertson *et al.*, 1973). N. gonorrhoeae may be sensitive but its sensivity varies in different parts of the world (page 596). Beta-lactamase-producing strains of N. gonorrhoeae are often moderately resistant to tetracyclines (*see* page 8). Pseudomonas aeruginosa is invariably tetracycline-resistant, but Pseudomonas pseudomallei is usually susceptible to tetracycline and to a slightly lesser extent to minocycline (Eickhoff *et al.*, 1970; Howe *et al.*, 1971). In addition, tetracycline and novobiocin display *in vitro* synergism against Ps. pseudomallei (Calabi, 1973), whereas a tetracycline/kanamycin combination is antagonistic (Eickhoff *et al.*, 1970). Most strains of Acinetobacter calcoaceticus var. antitratus (Herellea vaginicola) are susceptible to tetracycline, but all strains are susceptible to minocycline (Maderazo *et al.*, 1975; Kuck, 1976; Montgomerie *et al.*, 1976). The Legionnaires' disease bacterium is of intermediate sensitivity to tetracycline but it is quite sensitive *in vitro* to doxycline and minocycline (Thornsberry *et al.*, 1978). Minocycline also seems to be effective *in vivo* in studies using guinea pigs infected with this organism (Nash *et al.*, 1978).

The Bacteroides spp. may be sensitive, but many strains are moderately and others highly resistant to tetracyclines (Martin *et al.*, 1972; Overman *et al.*, 1974; Gorbach and Bartlett, 1974). Only 40–60 per cent of B. fragilis strains are now sensitive to tetracycline in clinically achievable concentrations; doxycycline is somewhat more active and minocycline inhibits 70–80 per cent of strains at clinically achievable concentrations (Leigh and Simmons, 1975; Chow *et al.*, 1975; Sutter and Finegold, 1976). Gentamicin acts synergistically with minocycline against 20 per cent of those B. fragilis strains which are sensitive to minocycline in clinically attainable concentrations (Fass *et al.*, 1976). Other Bacteroides spp. and the Fusobacterium spp. are more sensitive to tetracycline and even more so to doxycycline and particularly to minocycline (Chow *et al.*, 1975; Sutter and Finegold, 1976). In one *in vivo* study, minocycline was more effective than tetracycline in experimental infections in mice due to certain Fusobacterium spp. (Hill, 1977).

4. *Acquired resistance of Gram-negative bacteria.* Many Gram-negative bacteria, particularly those Enterobacteriaceae which are normal inhabitants of the human bowel, may acquire tetracycline resistance. In many cases this resistance is transferable by R plasmids (page 422), and it may be multiple against a number of chemotherapeutic agents. For instance, of 300 Esch. coli strains isolated from patients in the general community in Britain, 24 per cent were resistant to one or more antibiotics, 16 per cent of all strains were tetracycline resistant and in 60 per cent of the latter, resistance was transferable (Lewis, 1968). In another study in the United Kingdom enteropathogenic strains of Esch. coli were studied; all strains isolated between 1948 and 1951 were susceptible to tetracycline (MIC $\leqslant 5\ \mu$g per ml) but 17·5 per cent of strains isolated between 1957 and 1960 and 22 per cent of those isolated between 1967 and 1968 were resistant (MIC $> 12\cdot5\ \mu$g per ml). During the latter two periods, in 60 and 68 per cent respectively of the tetracycline-resistant strains, resistance was transferable (Slocombe and Sutherland, 1973). Very similar results were obtained in a study of Esch. coli isolates from hospital patients in Buffalo in the United States. Of 759 strains, 48 per cent were resistant to one or more of ampicillin, chloramphenicol, kanamycin, streptomycin and sulphonamide and multiple resistance occurred

in 53 per cent of the resistant strains. Tetracycline-resistant strains accounted for 25 per cent of all strains and 53 per cent of the resistant strains; 79 per cent of tetracycline-resistant strains were resistant to multiple drugs. In 50 per cent of tetracycline-resistant strains, resistance was transferable, and in 61 per cent it was associated with streptomycin resistance (Camiolo et al., 1975).

Resistant strains of Enterobacteriaceae are particularly common in hospitals. In a survey in a Boston hospital, 61 per cent of Esch. coli and 62 per cent Klebsiella, 58 per cent Enterobacter, 91 per cent Proteus and 97 per cent Serratia spp. strains were tetracycline-resistant (Sabath, 1969). In another survey of Esch. coli strains isolated from patients at a children's hospital in Oklahoma, 25 per cent were highly resistant to tetracycline (MIC > 50 µg per ml) (Yoshioka et al., 1977). Sensitivity testing is obviously important if tetracyclines are used for the treatment of infections caused by these bacteria. Following administration of the tetracyclines, faecal organisms of the recipients often become resistant to these drugs. Some studies have indicated that doxycycline causes a lower percentage of resistant Esch. coli strains in the faeces than tetracycline (Bartlett et al., 1975; Alestig and Lidin-Janson, 1975), but others have been unable to show any difference between these drugs with regard either to the emergence of resistant strains or the occurrence of R plasmids (Jonsson and Tunevall, 1976). In 1973, 67 per cent of Shigella spp. strains tested at Washington were resistant to tetracycline but this percentage fell to 27 in 1976 (Controni et al., 1978).

In a study of antibiotic sensitivities of 1156 Vibrio cholerae strains from various parts of the world, O'Grady et al. (1976) only detected six, all from Indonesia or the Philippines, which had increased resistance to tetracycline (MIC > 2 µg per ml). These six strains also showed increased resistance to chloramphenicol, and four of them had increased resistance to sulphonamides and the other two increased resistance to ampicillin. Some strains of V. alginolyticus may also be resistant to tetracycline and these are also resistant to ampicillin and chloramphenicol (Joseph et al., 1978).

Strains of N. gonorrhoeae which are resistant or have a reduced sensitivity to tetracyclines are not uncommon. The pattern of resistance varies in different parts of the world (Report, 1978). Resistant strains have decreased in frequency in the United States of America between 1972 and 1976. In South-East Asia and the Western Pacific the incidence of N. gonorrhoeae strains with reduced sensitivity to tetracyclines has ranged from 30 to 60 per cent. The sensitivity of strains from northern Europe has been fairly stable in recent years; for instance 9·0–12·6 per cent of strains isolated in Denmark in 1976 were less sensitive to tetracycline. Treatment failures with the usual recommended tetracycline regimen for gonorrhoea (page 625) are commonly associated with gonococcal strains with a tetracycline MIC of 1 µg per ml or greater (Karney et al., 1977; Report, 1978). Over 50 per cent of beta-lactamase-producing gonococcal strains isolated in the United States and East Asia have a tetracycline MIC of 1 µg per ml or greater (Center for Disease Control, 1978; Report, 1978). Beta-lactamase-producing gonococcal strains isolated in West Africa are usually more sensitive to tetracyclines (page 9). Increased resistance to tetracycline is often associated with increased resistance to other antibiotics such as penicillin, erythromycin, streptomycin and chloramphenicol, suggesting a common genetic basis (Maness and Sparling, 1973; Maier et al., 1974; Report, 1978) (*see also* page 8). Common chromosomal loci for resistance ave been detected for some of these antibiotics (Report, 1978). For instance, genes for high-level resistance to streptomycin and spectinomycin and for low-level resistance to tetracycline and chloramphenicol are linked.

Non-encapsulated strains of H. influenzae may occasionally become resistant to the tetracyclines when these drugs are used for prolonged periods in patients with chronic bronchitis (Gould and Murdock, 1960), and the prevalence of such strains has been increasing (Williams and Andrews, 1974). In Australia four strains of Haemophilus influenzae type b have been isolated from patients which were highly resistant to tetracycline (Hansman and Pidgeon, 1971; Hansman, 1975). The first of these was isolated from a 25-year-old woman with a post-operative respiratory infection and the other three from children, two with meningitis and one with epiglottitis. The latter three strains were all resistant to doxycycline but two of them were sensitive to minocycline. In a survey conducted in the United Kingdom during 1977, 2·7 per cent of H. influenzae strains (two type b and 26 untypable strains) were resistant to tetracycline (Howard *et al.*, 1978). Strains of Haemophilus ducreyi resistant to tetracyclines have been encountered in South-East Asia and Canada (Hammond *et al.*, 1978).

5. *Mycobacterium tuberculosis.* That the tetracyclines have a low degree of activity against this organism is of no clinical importance. Apparently minocycline is more active than the other tetracyclines against the standard H 37 RV strain of the tubercle bacillus.

6. *Mycoplasma pneumoniae* is sensitive to tetracycline (Jao and Finland, 1967).

7. *Ureaplasma urealyticum (Mycoplasma T-strains).* These are usually sensitive (Csonka and Spitzer, 1969), but resistant strains occur naturally (Ford and Smith, 1974; Spaepen *et al.,* 1977). Evans and Taylor-Robinson (1978) studied 141 ureaplasma strains isolated from men with non-specific urethritis attending London venereal disease clinics between 1973 and 1976, and who had been treated with tetracyclines; 9·9 per cent of these strains were resistant to tetracyclines. They also showed that resistance could be induced *in vitro.* Evans and Taylor-Robinson (1978) found that all naturally occurring tetracycline-resistant ureaplasmas were sensitive to erythromycin, a different finding to that of Spaepen *et al.* (1976). Comparative studies on the *in vitro* susceptibilities of Ureaplasma urealyticum to various tetracyclines show that their activity decreases in the order of minocycline, demethylchlortetracycline, doxycycline and tetracycline (Spaepen *et al.*, 1976; Spaepen and Kundsin, 1977). Nevertheless, when their MIC's are related to clinically achievable serum concentrations, all these tetracyclines are comparable in activity and cross-resistance occurs between them.

8. *Rickettsiae and Chlamydia.* The tetracyclines are active against the Rickettsiae such as those causing the various typhus fevers and Rocky Mountain spotted fever. *In vitro* studies with Rickettsia prowazeki in cell culture show that doxycycline, minocycline and tetracycline have comparable activity, so that the apparent greater efficacy of the two former drugs in typhus fever (page 624) is probably due to their greater persistence in tissues (Wisseman *et al.*, 1974). Coxiella burnetti (the agent causing Q fever) is also sensitive. Chlamydia trachomatis which causes trachoma and various genital infections

(page 626) is sensitive to tetracycline (Kuo *et al.*, 1977; Blackman *et al.*, 1977). Chlamydia psittaci which causes psittacosis is also sensitive.

9. *Miscellaneous*. The malarial parasites are sensitive to tetracyclines. Minocycline unlike other tetracyclines also inhibits Candida albicans and C. tropicalis *in vitro* (Waterworth, 1974), but *in vivo* there is no significant difference between the actions of tetracycline and minocycline on vaginal yeast flora (Oriel and Waterworth, 1975). All other fungi are tetracycline-resistant. Doxycycline has a synergistic effect with amphotericin B against Candida albicans *in vitro*, probably because amphotericin B increases cell permeability for doxycycline (Ånséhn *et al.*, 1976). Tetracycline also potentiates the action of the polymyxins against fungi (page 533). *In vitro* tetracyclines suppresses the growth of Naegleria fowleri, the causative agent of primary amoebic meningoencephalitis (Thong *et al.*, 1977). The addition of tetracycline to amphotericin B therapy also increases survival of mice with experimental amoebic meningoencephalitis (*see* page 866).

10. *Differences between tetracyclines*. There is usually cross-resistance between the various tetracyclines and therefore it is only necessary to use one member of the group, such as tetracycline, for sensitivity testing. However the newer tetracycline analogues, doxycycline and minocycline, differ from the older tetracyclines in a number of respects. Some of these differences have already been described in the preceding sections.

Minocycline is more active than other tetracyclines against Staph. pyogenes, being active against a significant percentage of strains which are resistant to tetracycline (Steigbigel *et al.*, 1968b; Bach *et al.*, 1972; Mitchell, 1974; Minuth *et al.*, 1974; Leigh and Simmons, 1974; Chattopadhyay and Harding, 1975). Doxycycline is also active against a proportion of tetracycline-resistant Staph. pyogenes strains (Minuth *et al.*, 1974). Minocycline is also more active than tetracycline against penicillin-resistant Staph. pyogenes; of 200 strains, 13·5 per cent were resistant to tetracycline, but susceptible to minocycline (Candanoza and Ellner, 1975). Thirteen methicillin-resistant strains of Staph. pyogenes and Staph. epidermidis were found to be resistant to tetracycline and doxycycline but six had a minocycline MIC of $\leqslant 2$ μg per ml (Minuth *et al.*, 1974). Similarly, Rich and Davidson (1975) found that of 34 cloxacillin-resistant Staph. pyogenes strains isolated from a hospital, one was resistant, one was fully sensitive and the other 32 had MIC's in the range 1·25–2·5 μg per ml for minocycline; all of these strains were resistant to tetracycline. These concentrations of minocycline are just obtainable in the serum after standard doses (page 607), so that minocycline is of doubtful efficacy for infections due to such strains.

Against beta-haemolytic streptococci, minocycline is the most active of the tetracyclines. In one study 16 of 33 Group A strains were inhibited by tetracycline (MIC $\leqslant 2·5$ μg per ml) whereas 22 of these were inhibited by minocycline (MIC $\leqslant 1·25$ μg per ml); the susceptibility of strains from Groups B, C and G were identical (McGill, 1974). Finland *et al.* (1976a) studied 29 Group A, 4 Group C and 2 Group C strains of beta-haemolytic streptococci. Their results showed that the majority were sensitive to all of seven tetracycline drugs tested but a few strains were sensitive to minocycline (MIC 0·2–1·6 μg per ml), but resistant to other tetracyclines. In another study minocycline was not found to be as active against Strep. pyogenes (Group A); with tetracycline-sensitive strains the MIC's of minocycline and tetracycline were similar, but with tetracycline-resistant strains although minocycline was more active its MIC's were never below 4 μg per ml (Wood et al., 1975). Minocycline is active against tetracycline-sensitive pneumococci (Steigbigel et al., 1968b) and it is usually active against tetracycline-resistant strains in concentrations which are clinically achievable (Wood et al., 1975).

Some Gram-negative organisms resistant to tetracycline are sensitive to minocycline. In a study of 311 clinical isolates of tetracycline-resistant Enterobacteriaceae 48 (24 per cent) were sensitive to minocycline; these included Esch. coli, Proteus mirabilis, Klebsiella, Enterobacter and Serratia spp. (Candanoza and Ellner, 1975). The reason for this difference in the case of Esch. coli appears to be a difference in bacterial cell penetration; resistance to tetracycline in R plasmid bearing cells is due to decreased transport of tetracycline into the cell, but in such cells the transport of minocycline is by a different mechanism (Del Bene and Rogers, 1975). In clinically achievable concentrations minocycline is more active than tetracycline against both tetracycline-sensitive and tetracycline-resistant Haemophilus species (Wood et al., 1975). Although the majority of Brucella spp. strains are sensitive to the tetracyclines, there are differences in their activity. Farrell et al. (1976) tested 100 Brucella strains (B. abortus, melitensis and suis). Demethylchlortetracycline was the most active, although mean MIC values for lymecycline, doxycycline and tetracycline were always < 1 μg per ml. Minocycline was also very active with methacycline followed by chlortetracycline and oxytetracycline being the least active against Brucella spp.

In Vitro Sensitivities

1. The minimum inhibitory concentrations of four tetracycline antibiotics against some selected bacterial species are shown in Table 38. This table is condensed from a study in which the majority of organisms tested were isolated from patients, and therefore also includes strains with acquired tetracycline resistance. For practical purposes organisms inhibited by 1 μg per ml or less can be regarded as highly sensitive, those inhibited by 1–5 μg per ml as intermediate, and those not inhibited by 5 μg per ml as resistant. With doxycycline and minocycline serum levels are lower than with other tetracyclines (pages 606, 607); organisms with an MIC greater than 2–3 μg per ml should be regarded as probably resistant.

2. The differences in antibacterial activity between individual tetracyclines are relatively minor, and usually their activity does not differ by more than two-fold from that of tetracycline.

3. *Chlortetracycline.* Compared to tetracycline, this drug is slightly less active against most bacteria with the exception of the Gram-positive cocci.

4. *Oxytetracycline* is also slightly less active than tetracycline against most bacteria.

5. *Demethylchlortetracycline* was reported to be twice as active as tetracycline against most bacteria (Finland and Garrod, 1960), but Steigbigel et al. (1968b) showed that this only applied to some bacterial species such as

Strep. viridans, N. gonorrhoeae and H. influenzae (Table 38).

6. *Methacycline* has an activity closely similar to that of demethylchlortetracycline.

7. *Lymecycline*. The activity of this drug is very similar to that of tetracycline (Whitby and Black, 1964).

8. *Doxycycline* is about twice as active against most bacteria as tetracycline. Steigbigel *et al.* (1968b) showed that Strep. faecalis strains relatively resistant to all the tetracyclines, were less resistant to doxycycline (Table 38).

9. *Minocycline* has a higher activity against most Gram-positive and Gram-negative bacteria (Table 38), and it is active against some bacteria with acquired tetracycline resistance (page 599).

10. The two parenteral tetracyclines (rolitetracycline and rolitetracycline nitrate) have the same antibacterial activity *in vitro* as tetracycline (Dimmling, 1960).

Mode of Administration and Dosage

The tetracyclines are usually administered by mouth.

1. *Tetracycline*. The dose for children is 25–50 mg per kg body weight per day, given in four divided doses. The adult dose is 250 mg six-hourly, or 0·5 g six-hourly for more serious infections. Doses larger than 0·5 g six-hourly are usually of no additional benefit because higher serum levels are not obtained and the excess tetracycline is excreted in the faeces.

2. *Oxytetracycline and chlortetracycline*. The dosages of these compounds are the same as for tetracycline.

3. *Demethylchlortetracycline*. The dosage of this drug is 12 mg per kg per day for children given in two to four divided doses, and 150 mg six-hourly or 300 mg twelve-hourly for adults.

4. *Methacycline*. The dose for children is 10 mg per kg body weight per day, given in two to four divided doses and for adults either 150 mg six-hourly or 300 mg twelve-hourly.

5. *Lymecycline*. This drug is marketed in 200 mg capsules (each containing 150 mg of tetracycline base). It is claimed that it is better absorbed from the intestinal tract than tetracycline, and the recommended dose for adults is 200 or 400 mg six-hourly.

6. *Doxycycline*. The usual adult dosage of doxycycline is a single dose of 200 mg (or 100 mg every twelve hours) on the first day of treatment, followed by a maintenance dose of 100 mg per day. For severe infections the maintenance dose can be increased to 100 mg twelve-hourly. The dose for children is 4·0 mg per kg of body weight given in two equal doses on the first day, followed by 2·0 mg per kg given as a single daily maintenance dose.

7. *Minocycline*. The recommended dosage for adults consists of an initial loading dose of 200 mg followed by a maintenance dose of 100 mg every twelve hours.

8. *Rolitetracycline*. The usual daily intravenous dose for adults is 275 mg, and for children 10 mg per kg body weight. The manufacturers recommend that this daily dose should be given as one direct intravenous injection, but the dose can probably be added to an intravenous flask for a slow infusion, provided that there are no incompatible additives. For the treatment of severe

TABLE 38

(Condensed from Steigbigel *et al.*, 1968b)

ORGANISM	Minimum Inhibitory Concentrations in μg per ml							
	Tetracycline		Demethylchlor-tetracycline		Doxycycline		Minocycline	
	Range	Median	Range	Median	Range	Median	Range	Median
Gram-positive bacteria								
Staph. pyogenes	1·6->100	3·1	0·78->100	3·1	0·39->100	1·6	0·39-12·5	0·78
Strep. pyogenes (Group A)	0·19-50	0·78	0·19-25	0·78	0·09-25	0·39	0·09-25	0·39
Strep. pneumoniae	0·19-3·1	0·39	0·09-1·6	0·39	0·04-0·39	0·19	0·04-0·78	0·09
Strep. viridans spp.	3·9-100	3·1	0·39-50	1·6	0·09-50	0·39	0·09-50	0·39
Strep. faecalis (Enterococcus, Group D)	6·3->100	>100	1·6->100	100	1·6->100	50	1·6->100	100
Gram-negative bacteria								
Escherichia coli	3·1-500	12·5	3·1->500	12·5	1·6-500	12·5	3·1-500	6·3
Enterobacter aerogenes	6·3-50	25	6·3-25	25	12·5-25	25	6·3-12·5	12·5
Klebsiella spp.	6·3-500	50	6·3-500	100	6·3-300	50	3·1-500	25
Serratia spp.	200	200	100-200	100	50	50	25	25
Proteus mirabilis	50->100	>100	25->100	50	50->100	>100	50->100	>100
Neisseria gonorrhoeae	0·39-6·3	0·78	0·39-3·1	0·78	0·09-3·1	0·39	0·19-3·1	0·39
Haemophilus influenzae	3·1-12·5	6·3	1·6-6·3	3·1	1·6-6·3	1·6	1·6-6·3	3·1
Pseudomonas aeruginosa	50-300	200	25-100	100	25-300	100	100-200	100

infections the recommended doses can be doubled for short periods. The usual adult intramuscular dose of rolitetracycline is a single daily injection of 350 mg, but similarly this dose can be doubled for short periods for treatment of severe infections. The intramuscular dose for children is 10 mg per kg per day, but the intramuscular use of this preparation is not recommended for children during the first year of life.

9. *Rolitetracycline nitrate*. This drug is said to be preferable to rolitetracycline for intramuscular administration, because it apparently causes less pain. The usual adult intramuscular dose is 350 mg given once a day, but 350 mg twelve-hourly can be used for short periods for the treatment of severe infections. The recommended dose for children is 10–15 mg per kg daily given singly or in two divided doses. Rolitetracycline nitrate can also be given intravenously in an adult dose of 350 mg daily, and similar to rolitetracycline, the manufacturers recommend that it be given as a single intravenous injection.

10. *Parenteral tetracycline and oxytetracycline*. Intravenous and intramuscular preparations of these drugs have also been available. The adult daily intravenous dose of either of these is 0·5 g or a maximum of 1·0 g (*see* page 618). The solubility of these compounds is poor compared to the rolitetracyclines, so the contents of each 250 mg ampoule must be dissolved in at least 100 ml of saline for administration by infusion. These infusions frequently cause thrombophlebitis.

The adult intramuscular dose of tetracycline or oxytetracycline is 100 mg eight- or twelve-hourly. These intramuscular preparations appear to cause more local irritation than the more soluble rolitetracyclines. A parenteral preparation of oxytetracycline with incorporated polyvinylpyrrolidone ('Vendarcin') is available. This is said to cause less tissue irritation than the older parenteral oxytetracycline preparations, and it is suitable for both intramuscular and intravenous administration. The adult dose of this drug is 250 mg daily or 250 mg 12-hourly for severe infections.

11. *Parenteral doxycycline*. An intravenous preparation of this drug is also available. The adult dose is either 100 mg daily or 100 mg twice-daily for more severe infections. It is recommended that the 100 mg dose should be diluted in at least 200 ml of intravenous fluid, and its infusion should take a minimum of 15 min. However 100 mg of doxycycline in 5 ml of solvent has been administered as a slow direct intravenous injection without adverse effects (Klastersky *et al.*, 1972).

12. *Parenteral minocycline*. This preparation is suitable for intravenous administration; the adult dose is 200 mg initially, followed by 100 mg every 12 h. It is recommended that each dose be dissolved in 500 or 1000 ml of glucose/saline fluid for slow intravenous infusion.

13. *Patients with renal failure*. Tetracycline therapy should be avoided in such patients, as these drugs may cause further deterioration of renal function (page 618). In addition most of the tetracycline compounds accumulate in patients with renal failure if the usual doses are given. Accumulation of oxytetracycline, tetracycline, demethylchlortetracycline, methacycline and the rolitetracyclines can be avoided in anuric patients by administering individual doses every 3–4 days (Kunin, 1967), but this is not recommended because renal disease may still be aggravated (Leading article, 1972b; Ribush and Morgan, 1972).

Chlortetracycline is rapidly inactivated in the body by non-renal mechanisms, and it does not accumulate if usual therapeutic doses are given. Nevertheless it should not be used in patients with renal disease, because it can cause further deterioration of renal function (Kunin, 1967). By contrast, doxycycline which also does not accumulate in these patients, appears to be safe in the presence of renal failure (Mérier et al., 1969; Mahon et al., 1970; Whelton et al., 1974). Unlike other tetracyclines, its use, either oral or intravenous, is not associated with significant further rises of the blood urea and serum creatinine in azotaemic patients (Little and Bailey, 1970; George and Evans, 1971; Alestig, 1973; Stenbaek et al., 1973; Mahony and Lloyd-Jones, 1975). Doxycycline does not accumulate in the serum of such patients because it is eliminated by an alternate non-renal gastro-intestinal pathway (page 609). Doxycycline has the same effect on mammalian protein synthesis as other tetracyclines (page 611), but its antianabolic effect is rarely manifested in uraemic patients, apparently because it does not accumulate to toxic levels (Morgan and Ribush, 1972). Nevertheless other studies by Mahon et al. (1976) suggest that doxycycline should be used cautiously in patients with renal failure. They observed that although the serum half-life of doxycycline is only slightly increased and the drug does not accumulate in the plasma compartment of these patients, up to 30 per cent of an administered dose accumulates in some other unknown part of the body, which could conceivably produce side-effects (see also page 618).

The evidence concerning the safety of minocycline in patients with impaired renal function is conflicting. Because the drug is excreted in faeces and is mainly metabolized in the body and only a small amount is excreted in urine (page 608), it could be expected that only minor dose adjustments are required in such patients. Some investigators have found that minocycline excretion is not significantly reduced in patients with renal failure (McHenry et al., 1972; Carney et al., 1974). By contrast Bernard et al. (1971) showed that there was a prolongation of the drug's serum half-life from 18 to 68 h, which was in direct relationship to the severity of the patient's renal failure. In addition, George et al. (1973) demonstrated that minocycline administration caused exacerbation of pre-existing renal insufficiency. More recently Welling et al. (1975) have further studied the pharmacokinetics of minocycline in patients with renal failure. After a single intravenous infusion of 100 mg minocycline given over 30 min, resultant serum levels in patients with normal renal function and those with various grades of renal function impairment, including two who were essentially anephric, were similar. Five patients with normal renal function and four with mild impairment (creatinine clearance 18–45 ml per min) were each given an initial oral dose of 200 mg minocycline followed by 100 mg every 12 h for five days; after the initial dose serum levels in patients with impaired renal function tended to be higher, but there were no differences in serum levels in the two groups after single or repeated doses of the drug. Although these results suggest that minocycline may be used safely in the presence of mild renal failure, further studies are required to confirm this and to establish whether the drug can be safely used in patients with severe renal failure. At this time minocycline should be used cautiously in patients with severe renal impairment; in particular the normal recommended dose of 200 mg per day should not be exceeded because the protein catabolic effect (page 611) of the drug is dose dependent, and in such patients a resultant small increase in urea production may be sufficient to aggravate uraemia (Carney *et al.*, 1974).

The tetracyclines are slowly removed from the body by haemodialysis, but the rate of removal by peritoneal dialysis is poor (Greenberg and Sanford, 1967). This also applies to doxycycline (Whelton *et al.*, 1974) and minocycline (Carney *et al.*, 1974). The addition of tetracyclines to peritoneal dialysis fluids is not recommended because they are well absorbed from the peritoneal cavity (Kunin, 1967).

14. *Patients with liver diseases.* The tetracyclines should be administered cautiously in such patients, because liver damage may occur as a complication of high-dosage tetracycline therapy (page 617). Although tetracyclines are excreted in the bile, this mode of excretion is not a major pathway for their excretion (page 609) and patients with pre-existing liver damage do not appear to be more prone to the toxic effects of tetracyclines (Alestig, 1974).

Availability (Australia)

1. *Chlortetracycline ('Aureomycin', Lederle, 'Chlortet', Langley)* 250 mg capsules.
2. *Oxytetracycline ('Terramycin', Pfizer and 'Oxycycline', Protea).*
   (a) Capsules: 250 mg.
   (b) Suspension: each 5 ml containing 125 mg.
   (c) Capsules containing 250 mg oxytetracycline and 250 000 units nystatin ('Terrastatin', Pfizer).
   (d) Oxytetracycline with incorporated polyvinylpyrrolidone, for either intramuscular or intravenous administration ('Vendarcin', Gist-Brocades), syringes of 250 mg.
3. *Tetracycline ('Achromycin' and 'Achromycin V', Lederle; 'Austramycin' and 'Austramycin V', CSL; 'Tetracyn' and 'Tetracyn V', G.P.; 'Panmycin', Upjohn; 'Tetracaps', Protea; 'Steclin V', Squibb; 'Hostacycline', Hoechst; 'Hydracycline', Fawns and McAllan).*
   (a) Capsules: 125 and 250 mg.
   (b) Suspension: 125 mg in 5 ml.
   (c) For intramuscular administration, vials of 250 mg.

   Tetracycline capsules designated with the suffix 'V', contain the buffering substances glucosamine or sodium hexametaphosphate. These additions are said to enhance the absorption of tetracyclines, but they are of doubtful value.
4. *Tetracycline phosphate complex ('Tetrex', Bristol; 'Panmycin M', Upjohn; 'Hostacycline P', Hoechst).* Capsules of 250 mg and other preparations.
5. *Tetracycline and Nystatin combinations ('Mysteclin' and 'Mysteclin V', Squibb; 'Tetrex F', Bristol; 'Achrostatin', Lederle; 'Comycin', Upjohn).*
   Capsules containing 250 mg tetracycline and 250 000 units nystatin, and other preparations.
6. *Demethylchlortetracycline ('Ledermycin', Lederle).*
   (a) Capsules: 150 mg.
   (b) Capsules containing 150 mg demethylchlortetracycline and 250 000 units nystatin ('Lederstatin', Lederle).
7. *Methacycline ('Rondomycin', G.P.).*
   (a) Capsules: 150 and 300 mg.
   (b) Suspension: 75 mg in 5 ml.
8. *Lymecycline ('Tetralysal', Carlo Erba).*
   Capsules containing the equivalent of 150 mg tetracycline base. This drug is not available in Australia.
9. *Doxycycline ('Vibramycin', Pfizer; 'Doxin', G.P.).*
   (a) Capsules: 100 mg.
   (b) Suspension: 10 mg in 1 ml.
   (c) Intravenous preparation, vials of 100 mg ('Vibramycin IV', Pfizer).

10. *Minocycline ('Minomycin', Lederle).*
    (a) Capsules: 100 mg.
    (b) Intravenous preparation ('Vectrin IV', Parke-Davis in United States).
11. *Rolitetracycline ('Reverin', Hoechst).*
    (a) For intramuscular administration, vials of 150 and 350 mg (lignocaine hydrochloride added).
    (b) For intravenous administration, vials of 110 and 275 mg.
12. *Rolitetracycline nitrate ('Bristacin A', Bristol).*
    (a) For intramuscular administration, vials 350 mg (lignocaine hydrochloride added).
    (b) For intravenous administration, vials of 350 mg.
  The Australian Department of Health withdrew marketing approval for paediatric formulations of all tetracyclines in 1977.

It is difficult to recommend any one of the many tetracyclines as the best for clinical use, because there are only marginal differences between these preparations. However it may be more convenient to use one of the newer compounds which can be administered at less frequent intervals for the treatment of out-patients.

The latest tetracycline minocycline, being more active *in vitro* against some pathogens (page 599), appears to have advantages over other tetracyclines for the treatment of some infections (page 623), but it causes vestibular side-effects (page 621). Doxycycline on the other hand has definite advantages for patients with impaired renal function (page 618).

For parenteral administration the more soluble tetracyclines, rolitetracycline and rolitetracycline nitrate appear to be preferable to the older parenteral preparations of tetracycline and oxytetracycline. The intravenous preparation of doxycycline also appears quite satisfactory for clinical use (Beneventi, 1972; Klastersky *et al.*, 1972).

Phosphate is now commonly included in tetracycline capsules to enhance absorption, either as an addition or in chemical combination as a tetracycline phosphate complex. The superiority of these compounds has not yet been clearly established. The use of tetracycline in combination with nystatin or amphotericin B is discussed on page 613.

Serum Levels in Relation to Dosage

1. *Tetracycline*, administered orally, produces higher blood levels than oxy- or chlortetracycline (Fig. 31). Following repeated doses of 250 or 500 mg tetracycline at six-hourly intervals, the drug accumulates and the serum level gradually increases. With a continuous dosage of 0·5 g tetracycline every six hours, the serum level stabilizes at about 4–5 μg per ml after about twenty-four hours, which is approximately double the serum level achieved with a dosage of 250 mg orally six-hourly (Fig. 30).

Further increase of the dosage to 1 g or more orally every six hours does not produce significantly higher serum levels. The tetracyclines are better absorbed if the patient is fasting. By comparison to the fasting state, serum levels obtained when tetracycline hydrochloride is administered with a meal are reduced by approximately 50 per cent (Welling *et al.*, 1977). The presence of divalent and trivalent cations such as calcium and aluminium, antacids, mild or milk products in the gastro-intestinal tract also reduces the absorption of these drugs. In addition, the simultaneous administration of ferrous sulphate greatly impairs the absorption of all tetracyclines from the intestinal tract (Neuvonen

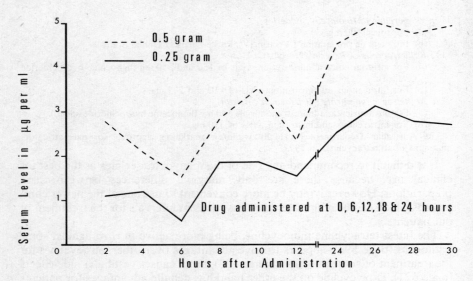

FIG. 30. Average serum concentrations following oral administration of 0·25 g and 0·5 g of tetracycline to adults six-hourly. (Redrawn after Welch, 1954.)

et al., 1970). The serum half-life of tetracycline after oral administration is about seven hours (Wood *et al.*, 1975).

2. *Demethylchlortetracycline.* The serum level of this drug rises and falls at a slower rate than that of tetracycline (Fig. 31), and is still detectable after 48 or even 72 h (Finland and Garrod, 1960).

3. *Methacycline* serum levels are similar to those attained after an identical oral dose of demethylchlortetracycline, except that methacycline levels are slightly higher during the first eight hours (Steigbigel *et al.*, 1968a).

4. *Doxycycline* is almost completely absorbed in the duodenum after oral administration, and it has a more prolonged serum half-life (18–22 h). After oral administration the peak serum level is usually obtained two to three hours later. Neuvonen *et al.* (1970) obtained a peak serum level of 3·0 µg per ml after an oral dose of 200 mg doxycycline. After an identical dose, Welling *et al.* (1977) detected peak serum levels of 5·0–5·4 µg per ml at 3–4 h in fasted subjects and these levels fell to 2·9–4·0 and 1·3–2·2 µg per ml after 8 and 24 h respectively. These authors also noted that serum levels of doxycycline were only reduced by 20 per cent if the dose was given with a meal, whereas serum levels of tetracycline were reduced by about 50 per cent. Welling *et al.* (1977) estimated that the mean serum doxycycline level obtained on a regimen of 200 mg daily taken on an empty stomach would be 4·4 µg per ml, and this would only drop to 4·0 µg per ml if the drug was taken with meals. All tetracyclines form complexes with metal ions in food but doxycycline complexes are unstable in the acid contents of the stomach, so that this drug enters the duodenum in a free state where it is absorbed. However metal complexes formed in the alkaline contents of the small bowel, into which doxycycline diffuses as part of its mode of excretion (page 609), are stable and are not absorbed. This explains why simultaneous ingestion of food does not inhibit the

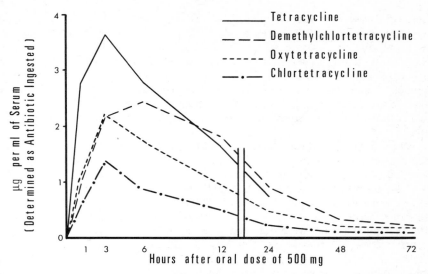

Fig. 31. Mean concentrations of four tetracycline antibiotics in serum of normal subjects after single oral doses of 0·5 g equivalents of their hydrochlorides. (Redrawn after Finland and Garrod, 1960.)

absorption of doxycycline from the upper gastro-intestinal tract (Whelton *et al.*, 1974). However the absorption of doxycycline is impaired by the presence of ferrous sulphate (Neuvonen *et al.*, 1970).

When a single oral dose of 0·5 g was administered after breakfast, a mean peak serum level of 15·29 μg per ml was obtained at 4 h and this fell to levels of 6·60, 3·42, 1·24 and 1·00 μg per ml after 24, 48, 72 and 96 h respectively (Adadevoh *et al.*, 1976). The fluorometric method used in this study may have resulted in higher serum levels than those obtained by microbiological assay. After a 200 mg intravenous infusion of doxycycline, a peak serum level of 5–10 μg per ml is usually attained (Alestig, 1973), which falls slowly and levels ranging between 1–2 μg per ml persist for 24 h (Klastersky *et al.*, 1972). Gnarpe *et al.* (1976) studied serial serum levels after a 200 mg dose given by infusion over 30–45 min; following this infusion mean serum levels of 8·32, 2·98 and 1·32 μg per ml were obtained at 2, 24 and 48 h respectively.

5. *Minocycline,* similar to doxycycline, is essentially completely absorbed after oral administration. Its absorption also does not seem to be significantly impaired by administration with food or milk. After a 150 mg oral dose in adults, an average peak serum level of 2·19 μg per ml is reached in 2 h, which progressively falls to 1·85 μg per ml at 4 h, 1·40 μg per ml at 8 h, and 0·53 μg per ml at 24 h. The drug may be detected in serum for up to 48 h after this single oral dose (Steigbigel *et al.*, 1968a). After an oral loading dose of 200 mg minocycline, peak serum levels occur after two to four hours and are usually in the range of 2–4 μg per ml (Cartwright *et al.*, 1975; Wood *et al.*, 1975). Following this dose a serum level of about 1 μg per ml is still detectable after 24 h (Cartwright *et al.*, 1975). If after an initial oral dose of 200 mg a dose of 100 mg every 12 h is continued, serum levels are maintained in the range of

2·3–3·5 μg per ml (Macdonald *et al.*, 1973). Very similar results were obtained by Carney *et al.* (1974). When an oral dose of 100 mg minocycline is given twice a day, peak serum levels are reached after five days and these are significantly higher in women (mean 3·4 μg per ml) than in men (mean 2·45 μg per ml) (Fanning *et al.*, 1977). This is probably related to the smaller size of women. A significant inverse correlation has been demonstrated between body surface area and serum concentrations (Bernard *et al.*, 1971; Fanning *et al.*, 1977), but in another study this was not always demonstrable (Gump *et al.*, 1977).

When a 100 mg dose of minocycline dissolved in 200 ml of 5 per cent dextrose in water is infused over 30 min, a mean peak serum of 8·75 μg per ml is attained immediately after infusion and levels of 3·37, 1·96, 1·32 and 0·81 μg per ml are detected 4, 12, 24 and 36 h later respectively (Welling *et al.*, 1975). If a dose of 200 mg dissolved in 500 ml is infused daily over a period of an hour, serum levels of 1–4 μg per ml are maintained (Macdonald *et al.*, 1973). Similar results were obtained when the same dose was infused over six hours but mean serum levels of 6·2 μg per ml were reached immediately on cessation of the infusion (Carney *et al.*, 1974). The serum half-life of minocycline is approximately 13 h which is about the same or even longer than that of demethylchlortetracycline (Bernard *et al.*, 1971; Carney *et al.*, 1974; Cartwright *et al.*, 1975).

6. *Rolitetracycline and rolitetracycline nitrate.* After a single intravenous injection of 275 mg of rolitetracycline, the initial serum level is almost ten times higher than the peak level attained after oral administration of 250 mg of tetracycline. This serum level falls rapidly to about 2–4 μg per ml two hours after injection. However therapeutically useful levels are still present in the serum as late as 24 h after the injection (Dimmling, 1960).

After a single intramuscular dose of 350 mg of rolitetracycline nitrate, the average serum concentration at one hour is 3·94 μg per ml, which progressively falls to 2·76 μg per ml at three hours and 2·45 μg per ml at six hours. Adequate therapeutic concentrations persist in serum for at least 24 h (Kaplan *et al.*, 1960).

Excretion

URINE: All the tetracyclines are excreted by the kidneys and this occurs solely by glomerular filtration. Urinary excretion accounts for about 20 per cent of an orally administered dose of most of the tetracyclines. More than 50 per cent of a parenterally administered tetracycline is excreted in the urine within 24 h (Dimmling, 1960). Between 60 and 70 per cent of a parenterally administered dose of tetracycline or oxytetracycline is excreted in the urine (Kunin *et al.*, 1959). By comparison only 4–9 per cent of an orally or parenterally administered dose of minocycline (Macdonald *et al.*, 1973; Welling *et al.*, 1975; Wood *et al.*, 1975) and 35–40 per cent of a similarly administered dose of doxycycline (Alestig, 1973; 1974; Mahon *et al.*, 1976) are excreted in the urine. High concentrations of the tetracyclines (about 300 μg per ml) appear in the urine during the first two hours after an oral dose, and persist for 6–12 h. The rate of renal excretion of demethylchlortetracycline is about half that of tetracycline, and therapeutic concentrations of this drug are maintained in the blood for longer. The rate of renal excretion of methacycline is about the same as that of demethylchlortetracycline, but the rates of excretion of doxycycline and minocycline are slower still. The urinary concentrations attained after parenteral administration of the rolitetracyclines are much higher than those attained with any of the oral drugs.

Tetracycline, oxytetracycline, demethylchlortetracycline, methacycline and rolitetracycline accumulate in the body in the presence of renal failure. By contrast chlortetracycline, doxycycline and probably minocycline do not accumulate in the serum of such patients (*see* page 603).

BILE: The tetracyclines are also excreted in bile, where in the absence of biliary obstruction, concentrations reached may be 10–25 times those found in the blood (Barza *et al.*, 1975). High concentrations of doxycycline, up to 14 μg per ml, are also attained in bile, but this route of elimination only accounts for a small percentage of an administered dose (Mahon *et al.*, 1970; Alestig, 1974). High concentrations (76 μg per ml) of minocycline have also been detected in bile (Macdonald *et al.*, 1973).

A large proportion of the tetracyclines excreted in the bile is reabsorbed from the intestine.

FAECES: With the exceptions of doxycycline and minocycline, the tetracyclines are incompletely absorbed from the gastro-intestinal tract and the unabsorbed percentage rises with increased dosage. The faecal concentrations of these tetracyclines may reach 1000 μg per g after oral administration. After parenteral administration, much smaller amounts conveyed by the bile are excreted in the faeces.

With doxycycline, that part of an administered dose which is not excreted in the urine is excreted in the faeces. Blood-borne doxycycline diffuses across the small bowel wall into the lumen, where cationic chelation occurs preventing reabsorption (Whelton *et al.*, 1974). The contents of the small bowel, being constantly added to from the stomach and other secretions, easily copes with the binding of successive amounts of doxycycline. Biliary excretion only contributes a small amount to the faecal excretion of doxycycline (*vide supra*). In the presence of renal functional impairment increased amounts of doxycycline are excreted in the faeces thereby preventing accumulation of the drug in the serum (Whelton *et al.*, 1974; Alestig, 1974; Mahon *et al.*, 1976). For instance Whelton *et al.* (1974) found that 77 per cent of an orally administered dose given to anephric patients was excreted in the faeces.

Despite the fact that minocycline is almost completely absorbed (page 607), a considerable amount of an orally administered dose is also excreted in the faeces (Macdonald *et al.*, 1973). In patients with renal failure the urinary excretion of minocycline is reduced in proportion to renal function (Welling *et al.*, 1975), but it is not clear whether increased faecal excretion or metabolism (*vide infra*) prevents accumulation of the drug in the serum of such patients.

INACTIVATION IN BODY: Only relatively small amounts of most tetracyclines are metabolized to bacteriologically inactive derivatives in the liver. Therefore most of the tetracyclines depend largely on the kidney and to a lesser extent on the biliary system for their elimination. Chlortetracycline is an exception, because it is rapidly inactivated in the body, so that it does not accumulate in patients with renal functional impairment (page 603). Although the main non-renal route for excretion of doxycycline is via the gastro-intestinal tract (*vide supra*), it is possible that a small proportion of the drug is metabolized in the body (Whelton *et al*., 1974; Mahon *et al*., 1976). The concomitant administration of barbiturates (Neuvonen and Penttilä, 1974), diphenylhydantoin or carbamazepine (Penttilä *et al*., 1974) shortens the serum half-life of doxycycline, suggesting that these drugs, which are inducers of liver enzymes, increase the metabolism of doxycycline. It is also possible that these drugs interfere with the protein binding of doxycycline thereby encouraging its excretion. A small study by Alestig (1974) did not demonstrate an increased metabolism of doxycycline with the concomitant administration of barbiturates. By comparison, a proportion of an administered dose of minocycline appears to be metabolized in the body (Macdonald *et al*., 1973).

Distribution of the Drugs in Body

1. All the tetracyclines are protein bound to some extent, but quoted figures vary. According to Kunin (1967) tetracycline is about 24 per cent, chlortetracycline 47 per cent, oxytetracycline 20 per cent, demethylchlortetracycline 41 per cent and methacycline 78·5 per cent protein bound, when estimated by a method of equilibrium dialysis. Higher values for tetracycline 65 per cent, oxytetracycline 35 per cent, demethylchlortetracycline and methacycline 90 per cent have been reported when ultrafiltration has been used. The values for doxycycline and minocycline are 82 and 76 per cent respectively (Macdonald *et al*., 1973).

2. The older tetracyclines penetrate fairly well into various body fluids and tissues. Tetracyclines can be readily demonstrated in pleural, ascitic, and synovial fluids and cord serum. They also appear to pass into maxillary sinus secretions, where concentrations almost equal to serum levels may be reached if repeated doses are used (Lundberg and Malmborg, 1973; 1974). Most of the tetracyclines can be detected only in low concentrations in tears and saliva. Following an oral dose of 250 mg tetracycline three times a day, sputum levels in the range 0·4–2·6 μg per ml have been detected (Ruhen and Tandon, 1976). The tetracyclines penetrate into normal cerebrospinal fluid, but to a lesser extent than chloramphenicol (page 432). The concentration of tetracycline in CSF is about one tenth of the simultaneous serum concentration. Demethylchlortetracycline CSF levels are lower, and in the absence of meningitis are only one twentieth to one fiftieth of those in the serum at the time (Finland and Garrod, 1960). After administration of intravenous rolitetracycline, higher CSF concentrations are obtained (Dimmling, 1960) in association with high serum levels (page 608).

3. The newer tetracycline analogues, doxycycline and in particular minocycline, are more highly lipid soluble. This lipophilic property is an important factor determining their better tissue penetration. In dogs, the lipophilicity of the tetracyclines has been correlated with many of their transport characteristics; it facilitates their transport across lipid-rich cell membranes and therefore the newer tetracyclines penetrate more readily into the brain, eyes and intestinal epithelium.

There have been many studies on the tissue penetration of doxycycline. In humans, concentrations of the drug in thoracic duct lymph and peritoneal fluid are maintained at about 75 per cent of simultaneous serum levels (Andersson *et al*., 1976), and those in colonic tissue and particularly ileal tissue approximate to or exceed the serum levels (Höjer and Wetterfors, 1976). The concentration of doxycycline reached in prostatic tissue may also reach 60 per cent of that in the serum (Eliasson and Malmborg, 1976; Oosterlinck *et al*., 1976). Lower concentrations of the drug are achieved in bone (Dornbusch, 1976), skin, subcutaneous fat and tendon tissue but levels in muscle are higher (Gnarpe *et al*., 1976). Therapeutic concentrations of doxycycline may occur in the aqueous humour but CSF concentrations do not exceed 1 μg per ml in subjects with non-inflamed meninges (Andersson and Alestig, 1976). The penetration of doxycycline (and the older tetracyclines) into sputum is poor (MacCulloch *et al*., 1974; Ruhen and Tandon, 1975; 1976; Hartnett and Marlin, 1976).

Studies by Macdonald *et al*. (1973) have shown that minocycline has a better penetration into most tissues than all other tetracyclines, and in most instances its tissue levels exceed simultaneous serum levels. The highest concentrations are found in the tissues of thyroid, lung, intestinal tract, liver, gallbladder and also in bile. Concentrations exceeding those in the serum are also obtained in the prostate, uterus, ovaries, fallopian tubes, breast, skin and sinuses, but lower concentrations are found in sweat and sebum. Although minocycline penetrates into the CSF of subjects with non-inflamed meninges better than doxycycline (Macdonald *et al*., 1973) and other tetracyclines, the levels achieved are low (Macdonald *et al*., 1973; Carney *et al*., 1974). Minocycline (and to a lesser extent, doxycycline) achieve higher concentrations in tears and saliva than other tetracyclines (Hoeprich and Warshauer, 1974). This probably explains why minocycline is effective for the treatment of meningococcal carriers (page 628), whilst other tetracyclines are not. Minocycline sputum levels are also quite high and may reach 60 per cent of simultaneous serum levels (MacCulloch *et al*., 1974; Ruhen and Tandon, 1975; 1976; Brogan *et al*., 1977).

4. The tetracycline antibiotics become markedly bound to bones, teeth and neoplasms, causing yellow fluorescence (*see* toxicity, page 615).

Mode of Action

The tetracyclines inhibit bacterial protein synthesis. They bind principally to the 30 S subunits of bacterial ribosomes (*see* page 434) and specifically inhibit the enzyme binding of aminoacyl-t-RNA to the adjacent ribosomal acceptor site (Cundliffe and McQuillen, 1967; Lucas-Lenard and Haenni, 1968). There is also some evidence that tetracyclines may cause alterations in the cytoplasmic membrane (page 19) thereby allowing leakage of nucleotides and other compounds from the cell. This action would explain the rapid inhibition of DNA replication (which occurs at a site on the membrane) that ensues when cells are exposed to concentrations of tetracycline in excess of that needed for protein inhibition (Pato, 1977).

In higher concentrations the tetracyclines also inhibit mammalian protein synthesis (Beard *et al*., 1969). This antianabolic effect is of clinical significance because it may aggravate pre-existing renal functional impairment (page 618). In addition these drugs may interfere with parenteral nutrition in post-operative patients by inhibiting the utilization of amino acids for protein synthesis (Korkeila, 1971).

The tetracyclines are usually described as 'bacteristatic', but they are 'bactericidal' in low concentrations against some bacterial species such as Strep. pyogenes and Strep. pneumoniae (Steigbigel *et al.*, 1968b). Tetracycline and minocycline also have a slow bactericidal effect upon Staph. pyogenes including their cell wall-defective variants (Carleton and Phair, 1972). Jawetz and Gunnison (1952) divided chemotherapeutic drugs into those whose effect is mainly bactericidal (e.g. penicillin) and those with mainly a bacteristatic effect (e.g. tetracyclines). *In vitro* they showed that whereas two bactericidal drugs were often synergistic, a combination of bactericidal and bacteristatic antibiotics often resulted in antagonism. As a result, it was generally believed for many years that so-called bactericidal and bacteristatic drugs should not be combined *in vivo*. This appeared to be substantiated by a number of reports of apparent antagonism especially between the penicillins and chloramphenicol or tetracycline, occurring during the treatment of patients (Lepper and Dowling, 1951; Ström, 1955; McCabe and Jackson, 1965; Mathies *et al.*, 1968). The demonstration of *in vitro* antagonism between different chemotherapeutic agents is however subject to many technical variables. For instance, Daschner (1976) using a checkerboard dilution technique to test drug sensitivities of Esch. coli and Staph. pyogenes could not demonstrate antagonism between penicillin or cephalothin and rolitetracycline; instead he showed an additive or synergistic activity of each drug combination against 40–50 per cent of the strains tested. Other clinical studies have failed to demonstrate decreased clinical efficacy by combining penicillin with chlortetracycline (Ahern and Kirby, 1953) or with chloramphenicol (Walker, 1953) (*see also* page 444). Moreover extensive clinical experience over many years has failed to reveal any clinical antagonism when these so-called bactericidal and bacteristatic drugs are used in combination. Throughout this book there are numerous examples of the successful use of drug combinations which under certain laboratory conditions could be demonstrated to be antagonistic. Nevertheless *in vitro* testing is sometimes valuable for selecting the best drug combination to treat infections due to certain resistant organisms (pages 532, 555). New drug combinations which show *in vitro* antagonism will not necessarily be antagonistic *in vivo,* but their clinical use should be cautiously assessed.

Toxicity

1. *Gastro-intestinal side-effects.* Symptoms such as nausea, heartburn, epigastric pain, vomiting and diarrhoea are more common with tetracyclines than with most other orally administered antibiotics. Diarrhoea is probably mainly due to direct chemical irritation of the bowel by unabsorbed tetracycline (page 609), but induced changes in the bowel flora may also be contributory. These gastro-intestinal symptoms usually subside quickly when the tetracycline is stopped. A severe pseudomembranous enterocolitis, similar to that caused by lincomycin (page 481) and other antibiotics, may rarely occur (Gorbach and Barlett, 1974). This clinical entity appears to be due to the overgrowth of Clostridium difficile in the bowel (page 482), and is quite different from tetracycline-induced staphylococcal enterocolitis (page 614).

It was anticipated that demethylchlortetracycline, which is used in lower dosage, would cause fewer intestinal side-effects, but this has not been confirmed. Methacycline and in particular doxycycline are also claimed to be less prone to cause these side-effects because of their lower dosages. A few limited studies suggest that gastro-intestinal side-effects are indeed less common with doxycycline therapy (Grossan, 1968; Aitchison et al., 1968; Clendinnen, 1974). Minocycline produces more side-effects of all types (including gastro-intestinal) in women than in men (Fanning et al., 1977), and this does not appear to be related to the higher serum levels attained in women (page 608) (Gump et al., 1977). Nausea is the most common gastro-intestinal symptom which occurs with minocycline, and this has occurred in 40–50 per cent of female volunteers, but vomiting and diarrhoea are much less common (Fanning et al., 1977; Gump et al., 1977). Whitby and Black (1964) found that the frequency of gastro-intestinal side-effects with lymecycline was the same as with tetracycline.

Four young women have been reported who developed oesophageal ulceration in association with oral doxycycline or tetracycline therapy (Bokey and Hugh, 1975; Crowson et al., 1976). Each of these patients had taken their capsule just before retiring to bed, one felt at the time that the capsule 'did not go right down' and three had an associated hiatus hernia. It was postulated that either the capsules had lodged in the oesophagus or had been refluxed from the stomach, and the high acidity of tetracycline in solution caused oesophageal ulceration. It was recommended therefore that oral tetracyclines should not be given to patients with oesophageal obstruction or compression (including patients with cardiac enlargement), capsules should not be taken within one hour of going to bed, particularly if symptoms of oesophageal reflux are present, and capsules should be swallowed with adequate quantities of water. One case report has suggested that sensitization to a metabolite of tetracycline present in certain foods, as a result of using the drug for growth promotion in stock feeds, led to excessive flatus with alternating diarrhoea and constipation (Anthony, 1977).

2. *Candida albicans (Monilia) suprainfections.* The term 'antibiotic-induced suprainfection' rather than 'superinfection' has been suggested to describe secondary infections that arise during treatment with antimicrobial drugs (Weinstein and Musher, 1969). Monilia often increases in the stools of patients treated by tetracyclines, but their causal relationship to diarrhoea is not well defined. Commercial combinations containing tetracycline and nystatin (page 604) or amphotericin B (page 878) have been manufactured and advertised on the assumption that monilial bowel suprainfection is the main cause of tetracycline gastro-intestinal side-effects. These antifungal agents effectively prevent monilial overgrowth, but there is little evidence that this has any bearing on the gastro-intestinal side-effects of tetracycline therapy (Leading article, 1968). The British Tuberculosis Association (Report, 1968) carried out a controlled trial on 111 patients with respiratory infections, using either tetracycline or tetracycline plus nystatin ('Mysteclin'). The frequency of gastro-intestinal symptoms was high in both groups before treatment was started. After ten days' treatment 50 per cent of patients in the 'Mysteclin' group and 34 per cent in the tetracycline group had gastro-intestinal symptoms, a difference which was not considered significant. The frequency of Candida albicans in the stools after ten days in the 'Mysteclin' group was 9·1 per cent, which was significantly lower than that in the tetracycline group (37·1 per

cent), but this was not associated with a reduction in gastro-intestinal symptoms. The authors concluded 'that the addition of nystatin to tetracycline cannot be justified at present on the grounds that it suppresses the upgrowth of Candida in the bowel and hence symptoms caused by Candida'.

Nystatin therapy however is indicated when oral or vaginal moniliasis occurs as a complication of the use of the tetracyclines.

In debilitated patients treated with tetracyclines or other antibiotics, there is the additional danger that the fungus may spread to involve the bronchi, oesophagus and other sites, or even result in a fungaemia with widespread dissemination of monilial infection. If the gut is heavily colonized by C. albicans, these organisms may pass through the intestinal wall and cause a temporary fungaemia (Krause *et al.*, 1969). For this reason it has been suggested that in severely ill patients, oral nystatin therapy is indicated, whenever it seems that excessive C. albicans proliferation in the gut may lead to disseminated fungaemia (Leading article, 1968).

3. *Staphylococcal enterocolitis.* Tetracycline-resistant staphylococci often appear in the stools of patients treated with a tetracycline, but staphyloccal enterocolitis with severe fulminating diarrhoea, dehydration and circulatory collapse is a rare complication (Thaysen and Eriksen, 1956). In this disease superficial necrosis of large areas of intestinal mucosa occurs, and the faeces usually contain large numbers of staphylococci. This enterocolitis occurs more commonly as a post-operative complication, and may be associated with either oral or parenteral tetracycline therapy. Lundsgaard-Hansen *et al.* (1960) reported six cases of staphylococcal enterocolitis with two fatalities, all in surgical patients, who were given intravenous rolitetracycline post-operatively. These authors pointed out that after parenteral tetracycline administration, sufficient tetracycline reaches the intestinal lumen via the bile to inhibit the normal flora, thus predisposing to staphylococcal supra-infection.

Treatment of staphylococcal enterocolitis consists of stopping tetracycline therapy, administering a reliable anti-staphylococcal agent such as cloxacillin and fluid replacement. The mortality from this complication is high.

4. *Other suprainfections.* The use of the tetracyclines may also result in colonization of the respiratory tract and bowel with Gram-negative organisms such as Proteus spp. and Ps. aeruginosa. Usually the presence of these organisms is of no clinical significance, but occasionally they may cause suprainfections of the respiratory tract (page 710). Rarely bowel colonization may cause diarrhoea, but severe disease, similar to staphylococcal enterocolitis, has not been reported.

5. *Hypersensitivity reactions.* These are uncommon, and usually take the form of urticaria, asthma or facial oedema, and contact dermatitis has also been described (Shelley and Heaton, 1973). Rare cases of acute anaphylaxis have been reported (Fellner and Baer, 1965; Furey and Tan, 1969). Copperman (1967) reported two patients who developed hypothermia, apparently due to tetracycline hypersensitivity. The development of lupus erythematosus has been observed after the administration of oxytetracycline and also tetracycline (Mull, 1966), but no clear cause and effect relationship has been established.

The Jarisch-Herxheimer reaction (page 27) may occur when tetracyclines are used to treat spirochaetal infections such as louse-borne relapsing fever and leptospirosis, and other infections such as brucellosis and tularaemia. The mechanism of this reaction is probably related to the release of pyrogen and/or endotoxin from phagocytosed dead organisms (Bryceson, 1976).

6. *Photosensitivity*. This side-effect is more common in hot climates. It consists of erythema which if severe may be associated with oedema, papules, vesiculation and onycholysis (Bethell, 1977). This is a 'phototoxic reaction' (page 736), because the rash does not spread to areas of skin not exposed to sun. Demethylchlortetracycline has the greatest propensity to cause this reaction. Photosensitivity has also been reported in patients taking doxycycline (Council on Drugs, 1969), and according to Ory (1970) any tetracycline may occasionally provoke this reaction. Minocycline and methacycline may be less likely to cause this side-effect (Allen, 1976).

7. *Teeth pigmentation and effect on bones*. All the tetracyclines are deposited in calcifying areas of bones and teeth and this may cause a yellow discolouration. Teeth discolouration was first noted during an assessment of long-term tetracycline therapy in children with fibrocystic disease (Shwachman et al., 1959). The observation was subsequently confirmed by many workers (Wallman and Hilton, 1962; Porter et al., 1966; Leading article, 1966a). The main disadvantage of tetracycline deposition in teeth is purely a cosmetic one.

Tetracycline may be deposited in the deciduous teeth in children if they receive these drugs early in life, or if their mother is treated by tetracyclines during pregnancy, because these drugs cross the placenta (Kline et al., 1964). The period of mineralization of the anterior deciduous teeth extends from 14 weeks *in utero* until two to three months after birth. However it appears that deciduous teeth staining is more likely if the mother is treated after the twenty-fifth week of gestation (Toaff and Ravid, 1966). The tetracyclines may also produce a life-long discolouration of the permanent teeth if they are administered to children aged less than six to seven years. The mineralization of these teeth commences about four to six months after birth, and it is completed at about the age of five to six years. The frequency of tetracycline staining may be particularly high during the first year of life because immature kidneys are unable to excrete these drugs efficiently (Medical News, 1977).

The type of discolouration varies somewhat according to the particular tetracycline used (Weyman, 1965, Leading article, 1966a). Chlortetracycline tends to produce grey brown teeth, but tetracycline, oxytetracycline and demethylchlortetracycline cause yellow discolouration. There is some evidence that oxytetracycline causes less discolouration than the other older tetracyclines (Weyman, 1965). For this reason it has been suggested that if the use of a tetracycline is unavoidable during pregnancy or in children aged less than six to seven years, oxytetracycline should be selected (Weyman, 1965; Gästrin and Josephson, 1966; Annotation, 1968). The propensity of the newer tetracyclines (methacycline, doxycycline and minocycline) to cause teeth discolouration is unknown (Medical News, 1977).

The degree of teeth discolouration depends on the amount of tetracyclines administered, and discolouration is usually only obvious in children who have received several courses of these drugs (Annotation, 1968). In one study it was found that only a very mild, cosmetically trivial, darkening of permanent incisor teeth occurred in children who had been given up to five six-day courses of either tetracycline or demethylchlortetracycline in the first five years of life (Grossman et al., 1971). Nevertheless the degree of discolouration increases with increasing numbers of teeth crown deposits of tetracycline. According to Baker (1975) if there are more than seven tetracycline lines per crown, severe discolouration is unavoidable.

Various studies have shown that the frequency of teeth discolouration in children in the community has been high. Brearley *et al.* (1968) examined 1168 Melbourne children aged from eighteen months to seven years, and found teeth discolouration in 20·1 per cent and in 4·0 per cent both discolouration and hypoplasia. Brearley and Storey (1968) examined 1000 deciduous molar teeth extracted from patients attending the pre-school clinic of the Royal Dental Hospital of Melbourne. Fluorescent yellow bands, characteristic of the tetracyclines, were found in 8 per cent of these teeth. These investigators also found that 61 per cent of permanent teeth extracted from patients aged 6–18 years were affected by tetracycline (Baker and Storey, 1970). A similar study from this clinic showed that during 1972, 75 per cent of permanent teeth from patients of the same age group had characteristic tetracycline fluorescence (Baker, 1975). However when these teeth were analysed in yearly growth zones and the frequency of fluorescence was related to serial ages, a continuing decreasing incidence of tetracycline affected teeth was found. This decrease was almost certainly due to an increasing awareness of doctors to the dental side-effects of tetracyclines. In a British study, Stewart (1973) found that 70 per cent of primary molars, extracted from 505 children aged three to five years, were also affected by tetracyclines given during their first three years of life. Other authors reported a much lower prevalence of tetracycline discolouration in both deciduous and permanent teeth (Martin and Barnard, 1969). Nevertheless tetracycline discolouration of teeth is still prevalent, and has been considered a significant public health problem (Comments, 1972).

The role of the tetracyclines in the production of defective teeth and enamel hypoplasia has been disputed (Leading article, 1966a). Their effect in causing enamel hypoplasia is difficult to assess, because several factors predispose to this condition (Storey, 1963; McIntosh and Storey, 1970). Enamel hypoplasia associated with tetracycline administration has been most commonly described in premature infants (Wallman and Hilton, 1962), but such hypoplasia is known to occur in association with prematurity, neonatal jaundice and febrile illnesses. Similar hypoplasia has also been described in older children in association with tetracycline therapy, but these children also had suffered from diseases which are known to cause this defect (Witkop and Wolf, 1963). Animal experiments have shown that the tetracyclines *per se* can cause enamel hypoplasia (McIntosh and Storey, 1970). Tetracycline, demethylchlortetracycline and lymecycline produced severe effects on the enamel, but chlortetracycline, oxytetracycline and methacycline were less damaging, and doxycycline had no apparent effect on enamel structure. It is not known whether these results from animal studies are wholly applicable to humans. According to Baker (1975), if there are seven fluorescent tetracycline lines per crown, severe discolouration, enamel hypomineralization and hypoplasia are unavoidable.

The deposition of tetracycline in the bones of infants causes temporary inhibition of bone growth. The administration of tetracycline to premature infants produces a 40 per cent depression of normal skeletal growth, as measured by the inhibition of fibula growth (Cohlan *et al.*, 1963). This effect was rapidly reversible after cessation of tetracycline therapy, and permanent effects on the human skeleton have not been observed.

In view of these side-effects and others (*vide infra*) which may affect children, it has been concluded that there are few, if any, reasons for using tetracycline drugs in children aged less than eight years (Committee on Drugs, 1975; Yeager, 1977). One of the few remaining indications for their use in children is for treatment of Rocky Mountain spotted fever (Lapp, 1977; Wight, 1977; Duma, 1977). Because of the effect of tetracyclines on teeth and bone, the Australian Department of Health withdrew marketing approval for all paediatric preparations of these drugs in 1977.

8. *Teratogenicity*. Animal experiments have suggested that the tetracyclines may be teratogenic (Leading article, 1965), but there is no evidence that this occurs in humans. The frequency of congenital abnormalities in children whose mothers received tetracycline therapy during pregnancy is no higher than in children whose mothers received penicillin G (Carter and Wilson, 1963).

9. *Hepatotoxicity*. This complication was first described by Lepper *et al.* (1951). These authors showed that this effect was dose related occurring particularly when these drugs were given intravenously in a total daily dose exceeding 1–2 g.

Subsequently a series of reports indicated that overdosage with intravenous tetracyclines is particularly dangerous during pregnancy (Schultz *et al.*, 1963; Whalley *et al.*, 1964; Dowling and Lepper, 1964; Kunelis *et al.*, 1965). Most of these pregnant patients were treated with intravenous tetracycline for acute pyelonephritis, and in some the daily dose was as high as 3·5–6·0 g. Initial symptoms consisted of nausea, vomiting and fever, which were followed by jaundice. The disease was often severe and was associated with haematemesis and malaena, renal failure with acidosis, and in the fatal cases coma and terminal hypotension. Six fatal cases reported by Schultz *et al.* (1963) had all received 3·5–6·0 g intravenous tetracycline daily, whereas in the five cases reported by Whalley *et al.* (1964), which included only one fatality, the daily intravenous tetracycline dosage was only 1–2 g. In fatal cases the liver showed extensive fine vacuolar fatty infiltration, and in addition pathological changes were found in the pancreas, kidneys and brain (Whalley *et al.*, 1964; Kunelis *et al.*, 1965).

The findings of Kunelis *et al.* (1965) are of considerable interest. They described twelve cases of 'fatty liver of pregnancy' associated with the intravenous administration of large doses of tetracycline, but in addition reported four similar cases of 'fatty liver in late pregnancy' in women who had not received tetracyclines. 'Tetracycline-induced fatty liver of pregnancy' appears to be a very similar illness to the rare 'acute fatty liver of pregnancy', which may occur during the last trimester, and was first described by Sheehan (1940) as 'idiopathic obstetric acute yellow atrophy'. It is probable that this disease may be associated with several aetiological factors, one of which may be the administration of tetracyclines in high doses.

A similar syndrome can also occur in non-pregnant patients if excessive doses of tetracyclines are used (Dowling and Lepper, 1964). There are also isolated reports of fatalities due to 'fatty liver' in non-pregnant adult patients, in whom the tetracycline dose was not excessive (Damjanov *et al.*, 1968; Hanson, 1968). This complication was also described in three children with obstructive uropathy, all of whom received intravenous tetracycline post-operatively and two died (Lloyd-Still *et al.*, 1974). It appears that all the patients who developed this complication following normal tetracycline doses had renal functional impairment, which probably resulted in high tetracycline serum levels.

In view of these findings it is advisable that the total daily intravenous dose of tetracycline should not exceed 1·0 g in adults, and that these drugs should not be used in patients with renal disease or in pregnant patients especially during the third trimester.

10. *Nephrotoxicity*. Four types of renal damage due to tetracycline therapy have been described.

(a) *Aggravation of pre-existing renal failure*. This is an important toxic effect because it is fairly common and often unrecognised (Edwards *et al.*, 1970; Eastwood *et al.*, 1970; Leading article, 1972b). In patients with impaired renal function the tetracyclines may cause further rises in the blood urea and creatinine (Lew and French, 1966). The associated clinical deterioration may be so severe that peritoneal or haemodialysis may be required, which occasionally has to be continued until renal transplantation is available (Phillips *et al.*, 1974). The known antianabolic effect of the tetracyclines (Shils, 1963) is probably the main cause of this complication (*see also* page 611). These drugs interfere with human protein synthesis, so that the kidneys need to excrete an additional load from amino acid metabolism. Some authors consider that this is the only mechanism by which tetracyclines aggravate azotaemia (Van Ypersele de Strihou, 1970), whilst others maintain that they also have a direct toxic effect on the kidneys (Roth *et al.*, 1967; Eastwood *et al.*, 1970). The exact mechanism is difficult to determine in individual patients, and in some, indirect effects of nausea, vomiting, diarrhoea and polyuria, caused at times by tetracyclines, may be contributory (Eastwood *et al.*, 1970). Water and salt loss, caused by concomitant diuretic administration, aggravates tetracycline nephrotoxicity (Report, 1972). It also appears that the combination of methoxyflurane anaesthesia with tetracycline therapy may predispose to the development of renal failure (Proctor and Barton, 1971). Doxycycline and possibly minocycline, unlike other tetracyclines, can usually be used safely in patients with renal failure. Nevertheless even doxycline should be used cautiously in these patients. Orr *et al.* (1978) described a patient whose stable renal failure deteriorated during doxycyline treatment, possibly due to impairment of the non-renal excretory pathway for this drug (*see* page 603).

(b) *Tetracycline nephrotoxicity associated with 'acute fatty liver'*. Features of liver failure usually predominate in this syndrome (page 617), but renal and electrolyte abnormalities are also often severe (Lew and French, 1966). These authors described a pregnant woman, treated by intravenous tetracycline in a dose of 2–4 g daily, who developed acute hepatic and renal failure without oliguria. They pointed out that this unusual type of renal failure with normal or even increased volumes of urine had been noted in other reported cases (Schultz *et al.*, 1963). By contrast, the acute renal failure which occurs in 'idiopathic fatty liver of pregnancy' without the administration of tetracyclines is usually associated with oliguria. Apparently the deterioration of renal function caused by tetracyclines in patients with pre-existing renal damage is not usually associated with oliguria (*vide supra*).

(c) *Renal tubular damage*. The oral administration of degraded tetracyclines may cause a 'Fanconi-like syndrome', consisting of nausea, acidosis, proteinuria, glycosuria and aminoaciduria (Frimpter *et al.*, 1963). This complication occurred with earlier preparations of tetracycline, because the capsules contained an acid excipient, which led to degradation of the antibiotic during storage. Since this formulation has been discontinued, this complication is no longer likely to occur.

(d) *Demethylchlortetracycline-induced nephrogenic diabetes insipidus and renal failure*. First reported by Castell and Sparks (1965), nephrogenic diabetes insipidus is now a well recognised side-effect of treatment with demethylchlortetracycline (demeclocycline) (Roth *et al.*, 1967; Singer and Rotenberg, 1973; Hayek and Ramirez, 1974). In doses of 600 to 1200 mg per day to adults, demethylchlortetracycline produces a reversible partial nephrogenic diabetes insipidus syndrome in normal subjects. This effect is dose-dependent and a daily dose of 1200 mg consistently induces this syndrome. The polyuria which occurs is vasopressin-resistant. Studies with toad urinary bladders show that demethylchlortetracycline reversibly impairs both antidiuretic hormone (ADH)-induced and cyclic adenosine-3^1, 5^1-monophosphate-induced water flow (Singer and Rotenberg, 1973). In human renal medulla demethylchlortetracycline impairs ADH-stimulated adenylate cyclase (Dousa and Wilson, 1973). Because the polyuria induced by demethylchlortetracycline was unresponsive to ADH, Singer and Rotenberg (1973) suggested that this tetracycline may be of value in the treatment of clinical states associated with excessive ADH activity.

There have been numerous reports of effectiveness of demethylchlortetracycline for the treatment of patients with inappropriate secretion of ADH. The drug inhibits the action of ADH in patients with inappropriate hypersecretion of ADH associated with lung carcinoma (Cherrill *et al.*, 1975; De Troyer and Demanet, 1975; Perks *et al.*, 1976; De Troyer, 1977a). The response to the drug, similar to that in normal subjects, takes several days so that it is of limited value in acute water intoxication due to excess ADH secretion. Demethylchlortetracycline has also been used with success to treat patients with water retention in congestive cardiac failure who were unresponsive to usual therapy (Cox *et al.*, 1977; Zegers de Beyl *et al.*, 1978). Similarly it has also been used with effect in a number of patients with alcoholic cirrhosis with sodium and water retention (De Troyer *et al.*, 1976; De Troyer, 1977b; Oster and Epstein, 1977; Carrilho *et al.*, 1977; Kirkpatrick, 1978). In a comparative trial, Forrest *et al.* (1978) showed that treatment with demethylchlortetracycline was superior to treatment with lithium carbonate for patients with the chronic syndrome of inappropriate secretion of ADH. In a number of publications evidence has been presented which indicates that demethylchlortetracycline also increases the excretion of sodium (De Troyer *et al.*, 1976; Cox *et al.*, 1977; Zegers de Beyl *et al.*, 1978).

Notwithstanding these successful reports of the efficacy of demethylchlortetracycline in syndromes of excess ADH secretion or for patients with water retention presumed to have inappropriate secretion of ADH, its use for this purpose has been associated with various degrees of renal impairment with elevations of the blood urea and serum creatinine (Roth *et al.*, 1967; Cherrill *et al.*, 1975; De Troyer *et al.*, 1976; Cox *et al.*, 1977; De Troyer, 1977a; Zegers de Beyl *et al.*, 1978). Renal impairment has been particularly noticeable when demethylchlortetracycline has been used to treat patients with cirrhosis and water retention, perhaps because of the tendency for renal failure to occur in such patients (De Troyer *et al.*, 1976; Oster and Epstein, 1977; Carrilho *et al.*, 1977; Kirkpatrick, 1978). In many of these patients azotaemia necessitated stopping treatment with demethylchlortetracycline, but the renal failure was always reversible. The mechanism of demethylchlortetracycline-induced renal failure is unknown. It is unlikely that it is due to resultant hypovolaemia or due to its antianabolic effect and it may be due to direct drug-induced nephrotoxicity (Carrilho *et al.*, 1977). The frequency of nephrotoxicity due to demethylchlortetracycline in patients with the syndrome of inappropriate secretion ADH has yet to be determined. Meanwhile the drug should be used cautiously for this purpose and regular monitoring of renal function and serum demethylchlortetracycline levels should be performed. The dose of the drug should be reduced in the presence of renal functional impairment, because it is in this clinical situation that overdosage with the tetracyclines and subsequent toxicity is likely to occur.

11. *Vitamin depletion and effects on leucocyte function.* There is an increased urinary excretion of vitamin C during tetracycline therapy, leucocytes are thereby depleted of ascorbic acid, and this may interfere with their phagocytic activity (Windsor *et al.*, 1972). *In vitro* tetracyclines in concentrations which are usually attained during treatment of humans *in vivo* markedly depress leucocyte migration (Martin *et al.*, 1974; Forsgren and Schmeling, 1977). The ability of human leucocytes to phagocytose yeasts and bacteria is also decreased by the tetracyclines (Forsgren *et al.*, 1974). The clinical significance of these effects is unknown, but they could possibly be important when patients with impaired defense mechanisms are treated. Tetracyclines also cause a reduction in serum B_{12}, B_6 and pantothenic acid levels, and therefore it is possible that long-term therapy with these drugs may cause vitamin deficiencies, particularly in the elderly (Windsor *et al.*, 1972).

12. *Malignant change.* Sadoff and Eckberg (1973) described a 16-year-old girl, who developed a malignant lymphoepithelioma, while receiving long-term tetracycline therapy for acne. The significance of this report is uncertain.

13. *Haematological side-effects.* Mild leucopenia can occur with tetracycline therapy, but is rare (Fanning *et al.*, 1977). Tetracycline also very rarely appears to cause vascular purpura, sometimes associated with thrombocytopenia (Kounis, 1975). In these cases a lowered leucocyte ascorbic acid level (*vide supra*) may be a contributory factor. The tetracyclines may modify some coagulation factors and cause impaired blood clotting if administered in high doses intravenously (Searcy *et al.*, 1965).

14. *Bulging fontanelle syndrome*. This uncommon complication has been observed in infants receiving usual doses of tetracycline, and is characterized by irritability, vomiting and a tense bulging fontanelle. The cerebrospinal fluid pressure is raised, but the fluid is otherwise normal, similar to 'benign intracranial hypertension' (Mull, 1966). All these signs resolve rapidly when the drug is discontinued. This 'benign intracranial hypertension' has also been described in one adult patient (Koch-Weser and Gilmore, 1967), a 16-year-old girl (Ohlrich and Ohlrich, 1977), and in one seven-year-old boy (Maroon and Mealy, 1971). All of these patients developed severe headache, blurring of vision and papilloedema while receiving tetracycline therapy. The symptoms subsided after withdrawal of the drug.

15. *Vestibular disturbance*. Minocycline, but not other tetracyclines, can cause reversible dizziness, ataxia, vertigo, tinnitus associated with weakness, nausea and vomiting. Prior to 1974 symptoms of vestibular dysfunction attributed to minocycline were reported at an average rate of 4·5–7·2 per cent (Allen, 1976). Williams *et al.* (1974) reported that 17 (89 per cent) of 19 patients receiving minocycline developed vestibular side-effects. Subsequently a number of small studies in the United States of America confirmed a high frequency (86–96 per cent) of vestibular symptoms, which in 12–52 per cent were so severe that treatment with the drug had to be stopped (Center for Disease Control, 1975; Jacobson and Daniel, 1975). The frequency of vestibular side-effects appeared to be less in the United Kingdom (Masterton and Schofield, 1974; Center for Disease Control, 1976a). More recently side-effects due to minocycline have been studied in controlled trials using volunteers (Fanning *et al.*, 1977; Gump *et al.*, 1977). All toxic effects (including vestibular symptoms) were more common in women, with vestibular side-effects occurring in 70·4 per cent (Fanning *et al.*, 1977). This did not seem to be related to the higher minocycline serum levels which occur in women (page 608). Most side-effects occur on the third day of therapy at a time which coincides with peak minocycline serum levels. A second trial showed that there was no significant difference in vestibular symptoms with a daily dose of 150 compared to one of 200 mg minocycline, these occurring at rates of 53·3 and 66·7 per cent, respectively (Gump *et al.*, 1977). Two additional symptoms were observed in this trial, lightheadedness in 53·3 per cent and a feeling of dissociation in about 50 per cent of volunteers. Because of these vestibular side-effects, the widespread use of minocycline is unlikely.

16. *Miscellaneous side-effects*. There have been a few case reports suggesting that tetracyclines may precipitate lactic acidosis in diabetic patients receiving phenformin (Aro *et al.*, 1978). Coma in a 67–year-old woman with diabetes treated by diet alone has been ascribed to oxytetracycline (Jung and Rowntree, 1977). A macroscopically black thyroid was observed at the autopsy of a patient who had been taking minocycline for nearly a year up to four months before death (Attwood and Dennett, 1976).

Clinical Uses of the Drugs

1. *Respiratory tract infections*. Tetracyclines are frequently used for pneumonia, bronchitis and especially for acute exacerbations of chronic

bronchitis, a disease in which non-encapsulated strains of H. influenzae are frequently pathogens. They have also been used continuously during the winter for patients with chronic bronchitis.

The role of antibiotics in the management of chronic bronchitis has been reviewed by Tager and Speizer (1975) and Hughes (1976). Some early large-scale controlled trials showed that tetracyclines used prophylactically decrease the number of days lost from work due to exacerbations of chronic bronchitis, and in other trials, the number of exacerbations of this disease in patients prone to these were reduced. Many other uncontrolled studies have shown conflicting results from both the prophylactic use of antibiotics in chronic bronchitis and from their short-term use for acute exacerbations of the disease. Nevertheless Hughes (1976) considers that chemoprophylaxis with a tetracycline or co-trimoxazole (page 709) should be considered in patients with chronic bronchitis subject to frequent exacerbations. Patients can also be advised to begin antibiotics themselves when they develop signs of infection; various drugs such as erythromycin (page 507), tetracyclines, co-trimoxazole (page 709), ampicillin (page 115) or amoxycillin (page 142) can be used in rotation. The newer tetracyclines, doxycycline and minocycline, have the advantage of only requiring single daily dosing. Although sputum concentrations of doxycycline are low (page 611), the drug was beneficial in one uncontrolled study of patients with various forms of bronchitis (Swarz, 1977). Higher sputum levels are attained with minocycline (page 611), but long-term chemoprophylaxis with this drug is contraindicated because of its vestibular side-effects (page 621).

In a controlled trial in which doxycycline was used to treat otherwise healthy patients with only a cough and purulent sputum, there was no advantage over treatment with a placebo (Stott and West, 1976). Tetracycline is usually in-effective for the prevention of bacterial pneumonia in patients with viral respiratory diseases (Ellenbogen et al., 1974). Patients with pneumonia or bronchitis do not always respond to tetracycline therapy, because tetracycline-resistant strains of streptococci, staphylococci, pneumococci and H. influenzae occur. Minocycline, and to a lesser extent doxycycline, are sometimes active in vitro against some strains of these organisms, which are resistant to the older tetracyclines.

Doxycycline has been used with favourable results to treat anaerobic lung infections. However in a number of adult patients higher intravenous doses of 100 mg every eight hours or 200 mg every twelve hours were necessary to obtain a therapeutic response (Thadepalli et al., 1978).

These drugs are not advised for the treatment of acute tonsillitis, because some strains of Strep. pyogenes are resistant. Penicillin G remains the drug of choice for this infection, and in penicillin-allergic patients there are other suitable alternatives such as erythromycin (page 506) or a suitable cephalosporin (pages 213, 232).

2. *Pertussis*. For many years the tetracyclines were extensively used for the treatment of this disease, but since the observation of the teeth staining effects in children, other drugs such as erythromycin, ampicillin or amoxycillin are indicated. Like other antibiotics, the tetracyclines do not modify the natural course of this disease. They have been alleged to eliminate pertussis organisms, presumably rendering patients non-infectious (Bass et al., 1969). They may

also prevent secondary pulmonary infections.

3. *Mycoplasma pneumonia.* The tetracyclines are effective for the treatment of this disease (Smith *et al.*, 1967; Foy *et al.*, 1970). In one study, tetracycline, demethylchlortetracycline and methacycline were equally effective to erythromycin (page 508) in reducing the length of illness in pneumonia caused by Mycoplasma pneumoniae (Shames *et al.*, 1970). The organism was cultured from the pharynx of a number of patients following antibiotic treatment, despite a reduction in the duration of their symptoms.

4. *Brucellosis.* The combination of one of the tetracyclines with streptomycin is still regarded as the best treatment for this disease. These drugs are usually administered for a 2–3 week period, and this course is often repeated after an interval of one week. The tetracyclines alone are effective, but the combined therapy is recommended for severe or prolonged cases (Joint FAO/WHO Expert Committee, 1971).

5. *Staphylococcal infections.* Relatively minor staphylococcal infections may be treated by the tetracyclines, if sensitivity testing indicates organism susceptibility. The newer tetracycline minocycline is effective in staphylococcal soft tissue skin infections (Phair *et al.*, 1974), including those which are caused by tetracycline-resistant but minocycline-sensitive staphylococci (Allen, 1976). Other drugs are preferable for the treatment of serious staphylococcal infections such as septicaemia.

6. *Surgical infections.* Tetracyclines were often used as adjuncts to surgery in the treatment of peritonitis due to a perforated viscus. They were also used to treat wound infections and other types of post-operative sepsis. However, many Staph. pyogenes strains and Gram-negative bacilli are now tetracycline-resistant, particularly in hospital-acquired infections (pages 593, 595). Doxycycline has been used for some abdominal infections because of its somewhat better activity against Gram-negative anaerobic bacteria. Favourable results have been reported when doxycycline was used to treat peritonitis and other intra-abdominal infections in uncontrolled studies (Hengeveld, 1977), and also when it was used prophylactically in colorectal surgery (Wetterfors and Höjer, 1976; Leandoer *et al.*, 1976). Doxycycline was used alone or in conjunction with gentamicin (page 341) to treat a small number of patients undergoing surgery for intra-abdominal infection with less favourable results (Klein *et al.*, 1977). Anaerobic infections occurred in both groups of patients and one developed a septicaemia due to a doxycycline-resistant strain of Bacteroides fragilis. It was concluded that doxycycline is not indicated for cases of serious intra-abdominal infection unless the infecting bacteria are known to be susceptible. In another study doxycycline was not effective in a number of anaerobic infections occurring in patients with cancer, because of the occurrence of resistant strains, especially B. fragilis (Klastersky *et al.*, 1977). It is now apparent that tetracyclines alone should not be used for the treatment of severe post-operative infections, such as septicaemia, before the results of sensitivity tests are available. In addition it is doubtful whether the prophylactic use of tetracyclines for surgical patients serves any useful purpose.

7. *Biliary infections.* Acute cholangitis and acute cholecystitis can be treated successfully by one of the tetracyclines, provided the causative organism is sensitive to these drugs. The tetracyclines have been especially

advocated for the treatment of biliary infections because they are excreted and concentrated in bile. However they have no special advantage in the presence of biliary tract obstruction, because in this situation they may not be significantly concentrated in the bile (Schoenfield, 1971). In addition, in acute cholangitis the most important pre-operative measure is the control of the associated septicaemia.

8. *Urinary tract infections.* Nowadays the tetracyclines are only occasionally used to treat these infections. If they are used, sensitivity testing is important, as Esch. coli and the other Gram-negative bacilli readily acquire tetracycline resistance. Tetracyclines, unlike many other drugs, are more active in acid urine. They may be useful for the treatment of those urinary tract infections in which L-phase organisms play a role (Gnarpe, 1973) (*see also* erythromycin, page 508). Tetracycline, and to a lesser extent doxycycline and minocycline, are excreted in high concentrations in the urine (page 608). Musher *et al.* (1975) examined the sensitivity of 171 urinary pathogens, which were tetracycline-resistant, by standard disc testing to concentrations of tetracycline attained in the urine with normal oral doses. Eighty-four per cent of these organisms were sensitive to 200 μg per ml of tetracycline and these included Ps. aeruginosa, Strep. faecalis, Proteus spp. and Esch. coli. Musher *et al.* (1975) also treated successfully two patients with a chronic urinary infection due to Pseudomonas and twelve other patients. These authors considered that tetracycline may be useful to treat hospitalized patients with urinary infection without clinical evidence of sepsis. Once clinical evidence of sepsis appears, drugs which produce inhibitory serum levels against the causative organisms are necessary. Tetracyclines should not be used to treat urinary tract infections in patients with impaired renal function, because they may cause a further rise in blood urea and serum creatinine (*see* page 618).

9. *Cholera.* In this disease correction of dehydration is the most important measure. Controlled studies have demonstrated that oral tetracycline therapy is effective in eradicating vibrios from stools and also in diminishing the volume and duration of diarrhoea (Carpenter *et al.*, 1965; Leading article, 1966b). The tetracyclines may also be useful for prophylactic purposes during a cholera epidemic and for cholera contacts (McCormack *et al.*, 1968). A three-day course of tetracycline has also been reported to effectively eliminate the organism from cholera carriers (Joint Study, 1971). However in another study of cholera carriers among children, the carrier rate was considerably reduced but not eliminated (Benčić *et al.*, 1976). A single oral dose of doxycycline (300 mg for adults) is nearly as effective as 0·5 g tetracycline given every six hours for two days for the treatment of cholera (De *et al.*, 1976). If a daily oral dose of doxycycline is given for four days then the results of treatment are as effective as those obtained by tetracycline given six-hourly for four days, the only difference being that faeces are cleared of vibrios within three days with doxycycline compared to two days with tetracycline (Rahaman *et al.*, 1976). Minocycline is also as effective as tetracycline for the treatment of cholera but similarly it does not clear the faeces of vibrios as rapidly as tetracycline (Mazumder *et al.*, 1974).

10. *Rickettsial infections.* The tetracyclines are the drugs of choice for the treatment of epidemic typhus, murine typhus, scrub typhus, rickettsialpox and Rocky Mountain spotted fever (Mull, 1966; Berman and Kundin, 1973). For

the treatment of typhus fever single doses of doxycycline or minocycline may be as effective as a dose of 1–2 g of tetracycline per day given for several days (Wisseman *et al.*, 1974). Chloramphenicol is also very effective for these diseases, and is sometimes preferred for very severe infections (page 441).

11. *Q fever.* Acute Q fever is usually a self-limited febrile illness, in which the value of any antibiotic therapy is hard to assess. Tetracyclines are the best form of treatment for chronic Q fever. The most difficult chronic Q fever infection to treat successfully is Q fever endocarditis. Prolonged tetracycline therapy has proved to be of some benefit for most patients with this complication, but complete eradication of infection has been unusual. Kristinsson and Bentall (1967) reported the complete cure of six patients with Q fever endocarditis using prolonged tetracycline therapy, but in four of these the infected heart valve was replaced by a valve prosthesis. Some authors prefer a combination of tetracycline and lincomycin for Q fever endocarditis (Annotation, 1976). Treatment of this disease should be prolonged and valve replacement may also become necessary for mechanical reasons.

12. *Relapsing fever, tularaemia and bubonic plague.* A single dose of 0·5 g tetracycline (or erythromycin) is considered to be the optimal treatment of relapsing fever (*see* page 510). Streptomycin is effective for the treatment of tularaemia, but a two weeks' course of tetracycline is now regarded as the treatment of choice (Leading article, 1971). The tetracyclines are effective in bubonic plague (Mull, 1966), but streptomycin (page 303) is usually preferred (Butler *et al.*, 1974).

13. *Gonorrhoea.* Tetracyclines have been used extensively for the treatment of this disease, and some authors have considered them preferable to penicillin G (Jones, 1972). Usually a four to six day course of tetracycline is recommended. Good results have been obtained with doxycycline, 200 mg initially, followed by 100 mg twice a day for three days (Neumann and Baecker, 1972). Attempts to use doxycycline 300 mg as 'single-session therapy' have resulted in a high rate of therapeutic failure, and a single dose of any oral tetracycline cannot be recommended (Wiesner *et al.*, 1973). Minocycline in a single-dose of 300 mg is also only about 50 per cent effective (Baytch, 1974).

Tetracycline in a dose of 0·5 g four times a day for four-and-a-half days has been recommended for the treatment of gonorrhoea in penicillin-allergic patients, who are not pregnant (Willcox, 1977a; Report, 1978). This regimen is also effective for the treatment of acute pelvic inflammatory disease due to N. gonorrhoeae (Cunningham *et al.*, 1977). For pregnant patients who are allergic to penicillin, erythromycin (page 509) has been preferred. Karney *et al.* (1977) in a comparative study found that a four-day course of tetracycline was as effective as single dose treatment with spectinomycin (page 588), both producing a minimum cure rate of 94 per cent in anogenital gonorrhoea. Tetracycline failure correlated with resistance to the drug; one-fifth of the isolates resistant to 1 μg per ml of tetracycline were not eradicated.

The level of resistance to tetracycline in parts of South-East Asia may be so high that tetracyclines are ineffective (Karney *et al.*, 1977). These drugs are also not recommended for the treatment of disease due to beta-lactamase-producing gonococci (page 8) (Willcox, 1977a; Center for Disease Control, 1978). Failure rates of 30–40 per cent have occurred when patients infected with these strains have been treated with tetracycline (Center for Disease Control, 1978). Over 50 per cent of beta-lactamase producing gonococci isolated in the United States and East Asia have a tetracycline MIC of 1 μg per ml or greater, indicating that tetracyclines would be ineffective in therapy (page 596). Thirty-five per cent of these strains are also resistant to erythromycin (page 498). At present it is recommended that spectinomycin (page 589) should be restricted for the treatment of infections due to beta-lactamase producing strains. Alternatives to spectinomycin for the treatment of infection by such strains have not been defined; kanamycin (page 319) and co-trimoxazole (page 710) may be satisfactory for non-pregnant patients and cefuroxime (page 286) may prove satisfactory for pregnant patients (Willcox, 1977a).

14. *Chlamydial infections*

(a) *Psittacosis.* The tetracyclines are the most effective drugs against this disease, which is caused by C. psittaci (Jawetz, 1969). A daily dose of 1 g tetracycline for 21 days has been advocated for treatment and prevention of relapse (WHO, 1977).

(b) *Lymphogranuloma venereum.* This is caused by particular serotypes of C. trachomatis (Annotation, 1977) and responds to treatment with the tetracyclines (Jawetz, 1969). Treatment is usually required for an average of two weeks (Willcox, 1977b). Minocycline has been used to treat this disease and it is effective in courses lasting 15–21 days (Velasco *et al.*, 1972).

(c) *Trachoma.* Both hyperendemic trachoma and paratrachoma are caused by various serotypes of C. trachomatis (Annotation, 1977). Hyperendemic trachoma is transmitted from eye to eye and responds to topical treatment with tetracycline or rifampicin (page 574) eye ointment given for five to six weeks. Oral tetracycline in a dose of 0·75 g twice-daily for 21 days (Dawson *et al.*, 1971), and a daily dose of doxycycline (2·5–4·0 mg per kg body weight) given for five days each week for a total of 28 doses in 40 days (Hoshiwara *et al.*, 1973) also result in significant suppression of trachomatous activity. Chloramphenicol eye ointment is not effective. Paratrachoma is transmitted sexually and includes TRIC ophthalmia neonatorum in the newborn, inclusion conjunctivitis, TRIC punctate keratoconjunctivitis and endemic trachoma. These latter eye infections are transmitted to the eyes from infections in the genital tract (cervicitis or urethritis, *vide infra*). Because of this associated genital infection in adults, systemic treatment with tetracycline 1 g or doxycycline 100 mg daily (or a sulphonamide, page 675) is recommended for three weeks (Annotation, 1977). TRIC ophthalmia neonatorum responds well to topical tetracycline therapy alone (Goscienski and Sexton, 1972). Sequelae of this infection are prevented if treatment is commenced before the thirteenth day of life and it may require treatment for five to six weeks (Dunlop, 1977).

(d) *Non-specific urethritis and other infections.* The chlamydia are important causes of non-specific (non-gonoccal) urethritis (Dunlop, 1977; Schachter, 1978a) and may cause infection of the rectum and throat of sexual partners. They have also been implicated as causes of salpingitis and pneumonitis of infants (Leading article, 1978). The most effective drugs for the treatment of non-specific urethritis are the tetracyclines (Csonka and Spitzer, 1969; Willcox, 1977a; Schachter, 1978b), whilst spiramycin (page 520) and streptomycin plus a sulphonamide are not quite as effective (Willcox, 1977a). Tetracyclines including minocycline administered for six to seven days are effective in eradicating chlamydia from the female and male genital tract (Prentice *et al.*, 1976; Waugh and Nayyar, 1977). Erythromycin is preferable for the treatment of these infections in pregnant or lactating women (Dunlop, 1977). A two-week course of 250 mg oxytetracycline every six hours or 0·5 g erythromycin stearate twelve-hourly results in an 86 per cent cure rate (Leading article, 1978). A seven-day course of tetracycline 2 g daily also eradicates the infection and is clinically effective (Schachter, 1978b). Female sexual partners of men with non-specific urethritis should also be treated (Dunlop, 1977). There may be grounds for using a drug regimen for the treatment of gonorrhoea which is also effective against C. trachomatis because these infections often co-exist. Penicillin (page 11), ampicillin (page 99), gentamicin (page 325) and spectinomycin (page 586) are all ineffective against C. trachomatis infections (Leading article, 1978).

15. *Non-specific urethritis due to Ureaplasma urealyticum (Mycoplasma T-strains)*. Although chlamydia (*vide supra*) are the major cause of non-specific urethritis, there is accumulating evidence that the ureaplasma are also important causes of this disease (Bowie *et al.*, 1976; Taylor-Robinson *et al.*, 1977). Infection due to these organisms usually responds to the tetracyclines. Sometimes the tetracyclines, including minocycline and doxycycline, fail to eradicate Ureaplasma urealyticum from patients because of the presence of resistant strains (Prentice *et al.*, 1976; Spaepen *et al.*, 1976). Infections due to these organisms also respond to the aminocyclitols, streptomycin and spectinomycin (Bowie *et al.*, 1976). Ureaplasma are also usually sensitive to erythromycin *in vitro* (page 499).

16. *Chancroid and granuloma inguinale*. Tetracyclines given for two weeks are effective in these diseases (Willcox, 1977b). Minocycline is also effective (Velasco *et al.*, 1972). Some strains of H. ducreyi (the cause of chancroid) acquired in the Far East may be resistant to tetracyclines and treatment with sulphonamides (page 675) or even chloramphenicol (page 445) may be necessary (Willcox, 1977b).

17. *Syphilis*. Penicillin G is the best drug for treatment of this disease (page 38). Tetracycline given for a period of two weeks is an effective alternative for the treatment of early syphilis in penicillin-allergic patients (Montgomery and Knox, 1959). Minocycline in a dose of 100 mg twice-daily for 15 days also appears to be satisfactory for primary and secondary syphilis (Velasco *et al.*, 1972). Cephaloridine (page 215) and erythromycin (page 509) are probably as effective as the tetracyclines for this purpose. The United States Public Health Service recommends tetracycline for the treatment of syphilis in penicillin-allergic patients (Center for Disease Control, 1976b). For early syphilis (less than one year's duration) a dose of 0·5 g four times a day for 15 days is recommended, whilst for disease of greater than one year's duration this treatment should be continued for 30 days. For pregnant patients identical dosage regimens of erythromycin are advocated (*see* page 509).

18. *Actinomycosis, gas gangrene, anthrax and leptospirosis*. The tetracyclines can be used as alternatives to penicillin G for the treatment of these diseases in penicillin-allergic patients, but nowadays they are not

necessarily the drugs of second choice. For instance, clindamycin has been suggested as an alternative drug for the treatment of actinomycosis (page 485), tetracycline-resistant Cl. welchii strains have been detected (page 594). There is some controversy as to whether any antibiotic is beneficial in leptospirosis (page 39).

19. *H. influenzae meningitis*. Chloramphenicol (page 441) is now the preferred treatment for this disease, as ampicillin-resistant H. influenzae strains are prevalent (page 102). Nelson *et al.* (1972) demonstrated that satisfactory results can be obtained in this meningitis by using intravenous tetracycline in a dose of 50 mg per kg per day. A combination of streptomycin and sulfisoxazole has also been used (page 303).

20. *Chemoprophylaxis of meningococcal infections*. Minocycline administered to adults in a dose of 200 mg initially, then 100 mg 12-hourly for five days, is moderately effective for the elimination of sulphonamide-resistant meningococci from nasopharyngeal carriers (Devine *et al.*, 1971; Guttler and Beaty, 1972; Devine *et al.*, 1972). A study in Finland indicated that minocycline was nearly as good as rifampicin (page 573) in eradicating both sulphonamide-sensitive and -resistant meningococcal strains (Sivonen *et al.*, 1978). Minocycline-resistant meningococcal strains usually do not emerge after treatment, but the drug only eliminates meningococci from about 60 per cent of carriers. Sequential treatment of carriers with minocycline followed by rifampicin may be a more effective regimen (Devine *et al.*, 1973), whilst the simultaneous use of these two drugs may reduce the emergence of rifampicin-resistant meningococci (Munford *et al.*, 1974).

Despite its clinical efficacy, minocycline is no longer advocated for chemoprophylaxis of meningococcal infections because of its propensity to cause vestibular symptoms (Drew *et al.*, 1976) (page 621). In the United States rifampicin is preferred (page 573), but in areas where meningococcal strains are sulphonamide-sensitive, sulphonamides have still been recommended (page 674).

21. *Melioidosis*. This disease, caused by Pseudomonas pseudomallei, can either present as subacute pneumonitis or as a fulminating septicaemia with a high mortality. Large doses of tetracycline (3 g daily for at least 30 days) have been effective for the treatment of subacute pneumonitis (Sponitz *et al.*, 1967). Everett and Nelson (1975) treated 39 patients with subacute disease including pulmonary melioidosis and found that tetracycline alone or in combination with chloramphenicol (page 444) were equally effective. No drug is universally active against all strains of Ps. pseudomallei. Tetracycline alone or in combination with chloramphenicol (page 444), novobiocin (page 528) or co-trimoxazole (page 709) may be indicated for the septicaemic form of this disease.

22. *Shigella dysentery*. One study in adults showed that a single oral dose of 2·5 g tetracycline is effective in shigellosis (Pickering *et al.*, 1978). This treatment resulted in a high clinical cure rate and elimination of the organisms (Sh. flexneri, Sh. boydii and Sh. sonnei) from the stools of symptomatic and asymptomatic patients 48 h after therapy. This occurred irrespective of the sensitivity of the organisms, 59 per cent being resistant to tetracycline.

23. *Traveller's diarrhoea*. In one controlled trial a 100 mg daily dose of doxycycline, given for three weeks, was very effective in reducing the incidence

of traveller's diarrhoea amongst Peace Corps volunteers in Kenya (Sack *et al.*, 1978). Tetracyclines were used because the enterotoxigenic strains of Esch. coli in the area were nearly all uniformly sensitive to the drug. Doxycycline was selected because of its once-daily dosage and unique excretion into the bowel (page 609).

24. *Yersinia enterocolitica infections.* Eriksson and Olcén (1975) described one patient with a septicaemia, who failed to respond to co-trimoxazole but who recovered when tetracycline was used; the strain of Y. enterocolitica was sensitive to these two drugs and also to streptomycin, gentamicin and chloramphenicol.

25. *Acne and rosacea.* Tetracyclines are beneficial for many patients with acne (Pochi, 1976; Leading article, 1976). An initial daily dose at 0·5–1·0 g is often used and, after improvement occurs, a daily dose of 0·25—0·5 g may be continued for months or even years. Tetracyclines probably inhibit Corynebacterium acne which is a lipase-producing bacterium in the skin, thereby reducing free acid in sebum which causes inflammation. Long-term therapy with tetracyclines is well tolerated in this disease probably because of the low-dosage used and the age of the patients. Such treatment increases the numbers of intestinal bacteria with resistance to tetracycline mediated by R plasmids (page 422), and there is a progressive tendency for this resistance to develop against a number of drugs (Møller *et al.*, 1977). A higher daily dose of 2·0 g tetracycline is associated with more side-effects (Baer *et al.*, 1976). Treatment of acne with erythromycin (page 509) or co-trimoxazole (page 687) is also effective and these drugs are sometimes used when tetracycline therapy fails. Clindamycin is also effective but it is not recommended because its long-term use in acne has been associated with the development of pseudomembranous colitis (page 481) (Leading article, 1976). Tetracyclines may also benefit some patients with rosacea (Marks and Ellis, 1971), and the keratitis often associated with this disease may also respond (Leading article, 1975).

26. *Amoebic dysentery.* The tetracyclines have been used in conjunction with other drugs to treat amoebic dysentery. They have no effect on Entamoeba histolytica *in vitro,* but appear to be beneficial in amoebic dysentery by interfering with the bacterial flora of the bowel necessary for the nutrition of these parasites. Tetracyclines are of no value in hepatic or other forms of systemic amoebiasis. Metronidazole (page 769) is now the best drug for all forms of amoebiasis, and the tetracyclines only have a very minor place in the treatment of amoebic dysentery.

27. *Malaria.* Because of their activity against malarial parasites, the tetracyclines have been used for the treatment of chloroquine-resistant falciparum malaria. This malaria responds rather slowly to tetracycline therapy alone (Clyde *et al.*, 1971), and a regimen of quinine sulphate combined with tetracycline has been much more successful (Colwell *et al.,* 1972; Leading article, 1972a). Usually a regimen of quinine sulphate 600 mg three times daily for three days, followed by tetracycline 250 mg four times daily for ten days, has been used (Colwell *et al.*, 1972; Benson *et al.*, 1972). Doxycycline in a dose of 200 mg daily has also been used in these regimens. The recommended treatment for chloroquine-resistant falciparum malaria now consists of triple therapy with quinine sulphate, a long-acting sulphonamide and pyrimethamine (page 676).

28. *Toxoplasmosis*. Based on the treatment of a few patients only, it has been suggested that tetracycline may be useful in this disease (Fertig *et al.*, 1977). Although some animal experiments indicate a possible effect of various tetracyclines in toxoplasmosis, there is no evidence at present of their value in human disease (Grossman and Remington, 1977). The recommended treatment for toxoplasmosis is a combination of sulphadiazine and pyrimethamine (page 675).

29. *Balantidiasis*. A 10–14 day course of tetracyclines has been reported to be effective for the diarrhoeal disease caused by Balantidium coli (Hoekenga, 1953; Areán and Koppisch, 1956).

30. *Tropical sprue*. Long-term tetracycline administration is beneficial in patients suffering from this disease (Rickles *et al.*, 1972). Most patients show definite improvement after a four weeks' course of tetracycline (Tomkins *et al.*, 1974).

31. *Whipple's disease* (*Intestinal lipodystrophy*). Patients with this disease may respond to treatment with tetracyclines. Clancy *et al.* (1975) isolated a cell wall deficient alpha-haemolytic streptococcus from a patient with the disease, which has been postulated as a possible aetiological agent (Lie, 1976).

32. *Detection of mycocardial infarction by radioisotopic scanning*. In addition to bone (page 611) tetracycline accumulates in malignant tumours, necrotic tissue, liver and infarcted myocardium (Meyers and Goldstein, 1974). Studies by Holman *et al.* (1974) indicate that radioisotopic scanning after the intravenous administration of a compound in which technetium is coupled with tetracycline may be useful for detection and sizing of myocardial infarcts.

REFERENCES

Adadevoh, B. K., Ogunnaike, I. A. and Bolodeoku, J. O. (1976), 'Serum levels of doxycycline in normal subjects after a single oral dose', *Brit. med. J.*, 1, 880.

Ahern, J. J. and Kirby, W. M. M. (1953), 'Lack of interference of aureomycin with penicillin in treatment of pneumococcal pneumonia', *Arch. Intern. Med.*, 91, 197.

Aitchison, W. R. C., Grant, I. W. B. and Gould, J. C. (1968), 'Treatment of acute exacerbations in chronic bronchitis', *Brit. J. Clin. Practice*, 22, 343.

Alestig, K. (1973), 'Studies on doxycycline during intravenous and oral treatment with reference to renal function', *Scand. J. Infect. Dis.*, 5, 193.

Alestig, K. (1974), 'Studies on the intestinal excretion of doxycycline', *Scand. J. Infect. Dis.*, 6, 265.

Alestig, K. and Lidin-Janson, G. (1975), 'The effect of doxycycline and tetracycline hydrochloride on the aerobic fecal flora', *Scand. J. Infect. Dis.*, 7, 265.

Allen, J. C. (1976), 'Drugs five years later: Minocycline', *Ann. Intern. Med.*, 85, 482.

Andersson, K.-E., Mårdh, P.-A. and Åkerlund, M. (1976), 'Passage of doxycycline into extracellular fluid', *Scand. J. Infect. Dis.* (Suppl.), 9, 7.

Andersson, H. and Alestig, K. (1976), 'The penetration of doxycycline into CSF', *Scand. J. Infect. Dis.* (Suppl.), 9, 17.

Annotation (1968), 'Tetracyclines and teeth', *Lancet,* 1, 1360.

Annotation (1976), 'Chronic Q fever or Q fever endocarditis', *Lancet,* 1, 1171.

Annotation (1977), 'Chlamydial infections of the eye', *Lancet,* 2, 857.

Ånséhn, S., Granström, S., Höjer, H., Nillson, L., Åkesson, E., Lundin, A. and Thore,

A. (1976), 'In-vitro effects on Candida albicans of amphotericin B combined with other antibiotics. Preliminary observations', Scand. J. Infect. Dis. (Suppl.), 9, 62.

Anthony, B. F. and Concepcion, N. F. (1975), 'Group B streptococcus in a general hospital', J. Infect. Dis., 132, 561.

Anthony, H. M. (1977), 'Tetracycline sensitivity as a cause of excessive flatus', Brit. med. J., 2, 1632.

Areán, V. M. and Koppisch, E. (1956), 'Balantidiasis. A review and report of cases', Amer. J. Path., 32, 1089.

Aro, A., Korhonen, T. and Halinen, M. (1978), 'Phenformin-induced lacticacidosis precipitated by tetracycline', Lancet, 1, 673.

Attwood, H. D. and Dennett, X. (1976), 'A black thyroid and minocycline treatment', Brit. med. J., 2, 1109.

Bach, M. C., Zinner, S. H., Wilcox, C. and Finland, M. (1972), 'Efficacy of standard disc-diffusion test as applied to susceptibility of Staphylococcus aureus to tetracycline and minocycline', J. Lab. Clin. Med., 79, 316.

Bach, M. C., Sabath, L. D. and Finland, M. (1973), 'Susceptibility of Nocardia asteroides to 45 antimicrobial agents in vitro', Antimicrob. Ag. Chemother., 3, 1.

Baer, R. L., Leshaw, S. M. and Shalita, A. R. (1976), 'High-dose tetracycline therapy in severe acne', Arch. Dermatol., 112, 479.

Baker, K. L. and Storey, E. (1970), 'Tetracycline-induced tooth changes, part 3: Incidence in extracted first permanent molar teeth', Med. J. Aust., 1, 109.

Baker, K. L. (1975), 'Tetracycline-induced tooth changes: Part 5. Incidence in extracted first permanent molar teeth: A resurvey after four years', Med. J. Aust., 2, 301.

Baker, C. J., Webb, B. J. and Barrett, F. F. (1976), 'Antimicrobial susceptibility of Group B streptococci isolated from a variety of clinical sources', Antimicrob. Ag. Chemother., 10, 128.

Bartlett, J. G., Bustetter, L. A., Gorbach, S. L. and Onderdonk, A. B. (1975), 'Comparative effect of tetracycline and doxycycline on the occurrence of resistant Escherichia coli in fecal flora', Antimicrob. Ag. Chemother., 7, 55.

Barza, M., Brown, R. B., Shanks, C., Gamble, C. and Weinstein, L. (1975), 'Relation between lipophilicity and pharmacological behaviour of minocycline, doxycycline, tetracycline and oxytetracycline in dogs', Antimicrob. Ag. Chemother., 8, 713.

Bass, J. W., Klenk, E. L., Kotheimer, J. B., Linnemann, C. C. and Smith, M. H. D. (1969), 'Antimicrobial treatment of pertussis', J. Pediatrics, 75, 768.

Baytch, H. (1974), 'Minocycline in single dose therapy in the treatment of gonococcal urethritis in male patients', Med. J. Aust., 1, 831.

Beard, N. S. Jr., Armentrout, S. A. and Weisberger, A. S. (1969), 'Inhibition of mammalian protein synthesis by antibiotics', Pharmacol. Rev., 21, 213.

Benčic, Z., Witjaksona, H., Hondro, S. and De Witt, W. E. (1976), 'Use of tetracycline for the elimination of Vibrio cholerae from an infected community', Tropical Doctor, 6, 2.

Beneventi, F. A. (1972), 'Intravenously administered doxycycline in urological and surgical infections', Curr. Ther. Res., 14, 367.

Benson, L. E., Siegel, A. J., Lynch, R. E., Colwell, E. J. and Canby, J. P. (1972), 'Drug resistance in malaria', Lancet, 1, 743.

Berman, S. J. and Kundin, W. D. (1973), 'Scrub typhus in South Vietnam. A study of 87 cases', Ann. Intern. Med., 79, 26.

Bernard, B., Yin, E. J. and Simon, H. J. (1971), 'Clinical pharmacologic studies with minocycline', J. Clin. Pharmacol., 11, 332.

Bethell, H. J. N. (1977), 'Photo-onycholysis caused by demethylchlortetracycline', Brit. med. J., 2, 96.

Blackman, H. J., Yoneda, C., Dawson, C. R. and Schachter, J. (1977), 'Antibiotic susceptibility of Chlamydia trachomatis', Antimicrob. Ag. Chemother., 12, 673.

Bokey, L. and Hugh, T. B. (1975), 'Oesophageal ulceration associated with doxycycline therapy', *Med. J. Aust.,* **1**, 236.

Bowie, W. R., Alexander, E. R., Floyd, J. F., Holmes, J., Miller, Y. and Holmes, K. K. (1976), 'Differential response of chlamydial and ureaplasma-associated urethritis to sulphafurazole (sulfisoxazole) and aminocyclitols', *Lancet,* **2**, 1276.

Brearley, L. J., Stragis, A. A. and Storey, E. (1968), 'Tetracycline-induced tooth changes: Part I. Prevalence in pre-school children', *Med. J. Aust.,* **2**, 653.

Brearley, L. J. and Storey, E. (1968), 'Tetracycline-induced tooth changes: Part 2. Prevalence, localization and nature of staining in extracted deciduous teeth', *Med. J. Aust.,* **2**, 714.

Brogan, T. D., Neale, L., Ryley, H. C., Davies, B. H. and Charles, J. (1977), 'The secretion of minocycline in sputum during therapy of bronchopulmonary infection in chronic chest diseases', *J. Antimicrob. Chemother.,* **3**, 247.

Bryceson, A. D. M. (1976), 'Clinical pathology of the Jarisch-Herxheimer reaction', *J. Infect. Dis.,* **133**, 696.

Butler, T., Bell, W. R., Linh, N. N., Tiep, N. D. and Arnold, K. (1974), 'Yersinia pestis infection in Vietnam. I. Clinical and hematological aspects', *J. Infect. Dis. (Suppl.),* **129**, 78.

Calabi, O. (1973), 'Bactericidal synergism of novobiocin and tetracycline against Pseudomonas pseudomallei', *J. Med. Microbiol.,* **6**, 293.

Camiolo, S. M., Beck, M. E. and Reynard, A. M. (1975), 'Tetracycline resistance in Escherichia coli isolates from hospital patients', *Antimicrob. Ag. Chemother.,* **8**, 488.

Candanoza, C. and Ellner, P. D. (1975), 'Differences in susceptibility of Enterobacteriaceae and penicillin-resistant Staphylococcus aureus to tetracycline and minocycline', *Antimicrob. Ag. Chemother.,* **7**, 227.

Carleton, J. and Phair, J. P. (1972), 'The slow bactericidal effect of tetracycline and monocycline on wall-defective Staphylococcus', *J. Infect. Dis.,* **126**, 457.

Carney, S., Butcher, R. A., Dawborn, J. K. and Pattison, G. (1974), 'Minocycline excretion and distribution in relation to renal function in man', *Clin. Exp. Pharmacol. Physiol.,* **1**, 299.

Carpenter, C. C. J., Wallace, C. K., Mitra, P. P., Sack, R. B., Mondal, A., Wells, S. A., Dans, P. E., Lewis, G. W. and Chaudhuki, R. N. (1965), 'Antibiotic therapy in cholera', *Proc. Chol. Res. Symp., U.S. Dept. Health, Ed. Welfare,* p. 190.

Carrilho, F., Bosch, J., Arroyo, V., Mas, A., Viver, J. and Rodes, J. (1977), 'Renal failure associated with demeclocycline in cirrhosis', *Ann. Intern. Med.,* **87**, 195.

Carter, M. P. and Wilson, F. (1963), 'Antibiotics and congenital malformations', *Lancet,* **1**, 1267.

Cartwright, A. C., Hatfield, H. L., Yeadon, A. and London, E. (1975), 'A comparison of the bioavailability of minocycline capsules and film-coated tablets', *J. Antimicrob. Chemother.,* **1**, 317.

Castell, D. O. and Sparks, H. A. (1965), 'Nephrogenic diabetes insipidus due to demethylchlortetracycline hydrochloride', *JAMA,* **193**, 237.

Center for Disease Control (1975), 'Vestibular reactions to minocycline-follow up', *Morbidity and Mortality Weekly Report,* **24**, 55.

Center for Disease Control (1976a), 'Vestibular reactions to minocycline—Scotland', *Morbidity and Mortality Weekly Report,* **25**, 31.

Center for Disease Control (1976b), 'Syphilis—CDC recommended treatment schedules, 1976', *Morbidity and Mortality Weekly Report,* **25**, 101.

Center for Disease Control (1978), 'Penicillinase-(beta-lactamase-) producing Neisseria gonorrhoeae-worldwide', *Morbidity and Mortality Weekly Report,* **27**, 10.

Chattopadhyay, B. and Harding, E. (1975), '*In-vitro* minocycline activity against tetracycline-resistant Staphylococcus aureus', *Lancet,* **1**, 405.

Cherrill, D. A., Stote, R. M., Birge, J. R. and Singer, I. (1975), 'Demeclocycline treatment in the syndrome of inappropriate antidiuretic hormone secretion', *Ann. Intern.*

Med., 83, 654.

Chow, A. W., Pattern, V. and Guze, L. B. (1975), 'Comparative susceptibility of anaerobic bacteria to minocycline, doxycycline, and tetracycline', *Antimicrob. Ag. Chemother.*, **7**, 46.

Chow, A. W., Patten, V. and Bednorz, D. (1978), 'Susceptibility of Campylobacter fetus to twenty-two antimicrobial agents', *Antimicrob. Ag. Chemother.*, **13**, 416.

Clancy, R. L., Tomkins, W. A. F., Muckle, T. J., Richardson, H. and Rawls, W. E. (1975), 'Isolation and characterization of an aetiological agent in Whipple's disease', *Brit. med. J.*, **3**, 568.

Clendinnen, I. J. (1974), 'Doxycycline in the treatment of chronic lung infections', *Med. J. Aust.*, **1**, 9.

Clyde, D. F., Miller, R. M., DuPont, H. L. and Hornick, R. B. (1971), 'Antimalarial effects of tetracyclines in man', *J. Trop. Med.*, **74**, 238.

Cohlan, S. Q., Bevelander, G. and Tiamsic, T. (1963), 'Growth inhibition of prematures receiving tetracycline', *Amer. J. Dis. Child.*, **105**, 453.

Colwell, E. J., Hickman, R. L. and Kosakal, S. (1972), 'Tetracycline treatment of chloroquine-resistant falciparum malaria in Thailand', *JAMA*, **220**, 684.

Comments (1972), 'Tooth discoloration and tetracyclines', *Med. J. Aust.*, **1**, 954.

Committee on Drugs (1975), 'Requiem for tetracyclines', *Amer. Acad. Pediatrics*, **55**, 142.

Controni, G., Friedman, G. and Ficke, M. (1978), 'Update of Shigella gastroenteritis: Changing patterns of antibiotic resistance, 1964–1976' In Siegenthaler, W. and Lüthy, R. (Ed.), *Current Chemotherapy: Proceedings of the 10th International Congress of Chemotherapy*, Zurich/Switzerland, 1977. American Society for Microbiology, Washington, D.C., p. 169.

Copperman, I. J. (1967), 'Hypersensitivity to tetracycline', *Lancet*, **2**, 610.

Council on Drugs (1969), 'Evaluation of a new antibacterial agent: Doxycycline monohydrate and doxycycline hyclate (vibramycin)', *JAMA*, **209**, 549.

Cox, M., Guzzo, J., Morrison, G. and Singer, I. (1977), 'Demeclocycline and therapy of hyponatraemia', *Ann. Intern. Med.*, **86**, 113.

Crowson, T. D., Head, L. H. and Ferrante, W. A. (1976), 'Esophageal ulcers associated with tetracycline therapy', *JAMA*, **235**, 2747.

Csonka, G. W. and Spitzer, R. J. (1969), 'Lincomycin, non-gonococcal urethritis, and mycoplasmata', *Brit. J. Vener. Dis.*, **45**, 52.

Cundliffe, E. and McQuillen, K. (1967), 'Bacterial protein synthesis: The effects of antibiotics', *J. Mol. Biol.*, **30**, 137.

Cunningham, F. G., Hauth, J. C., Strong, J. D., Herbert, W. N. P., Gilstrap, L. C., Wilson, R. H. and Kappus, S. S. (1977), 'Evaluation of tetracycline or penicillin and ampicillin for treatment of acute pelvic inflammatory disease', *New Engl. J. Med.*, **296**, 1380.

Damjanov, I., Arnold, R. and Faour, M. (1968), 'Tetracycline toxicity in a nonpregnant woman', *JAMA*, **204**, 934.

Daschner, F. D. (1976), 'Combination of bacteriostatic and bactericidal drugs: Lack of significant *in vitro* antagonism between penicillin, cephalothin and rolitetracycline', *Antimicrob. Ag. Chemother.*, **10**, 802.

Dawson, C. R., Ostler, H. B., Hanna, L., Hoshiwara, I. and Jawetz, E. (1971), 'Tetracyclines in the treatment of chronic trachoma in American Indians', *J. Infect. Dis.*, **124**, 255.

De, S., Chaudhuri, A., Dutta, P., Dutta, D., De, S. P. and Pal, S. C. (1976), 'Doxycycline in the treatment of cholera', *Bull. Wld. Hlth. Org.*, **54**, 177.

Del Bene, V. E. and Rogers, M. (1975), 'Comparison of tetracycline and minocycline transport in Escherichia coli', *Antimicrob. Ag. Chemother.*, **7**, 801.

De Troyer, A. and Demanet, J.-C. (1975), 'Correction of antidiuresis by demeclocycline', *New Engl. J. Med.*, **293**, 915.

De Troyer, A., Pilloy, W., Broeckaert, I. and Demanet, J.-C. (1976), 'Demeclocycline treatment of water retention in cirrhosis', *Ann. Intern. Med.,* **85,** 336.

De Troyer, A. (1977a), 'Demeclocycline. Treatment for syndrome of inappropriate antidiuretic hormone secretion', *JAMA,* **237,** 2723.

De Troyer, A. (1977b), 'Demeclocycline and therapy of hyponatraemia, in comment', *Ann. Intern. Med.,* **86,** 114.

Devine, L. F., Johnson, D. P., Hagerman, C. R., Pierce, W. E., Rhode, S. L. and Peckinpaugh, R. O. (1971), 'The effect of minocycline on meningococcal nasopharyngeal carrier state in naval personnel', *Amer. J. Epidemiol.,* **93,** 337.

Devine, L. F., Springer, G. L., Frazier, W. E., Rhode, S. L. III, Pierce, W. E., Johnson, D. P. and Peckinpaugh, R. O. (1972), 'Selective monocycline and rifampin treatment of group C meningococcal carriers in a new naval recruit camp', *Amer. J. Med. Sci.,* **263,** 79.

Devine, L. F., Pollard, R. B., Krumpe, P. E., Hoy, E. S., Mammen, R. E., Miller, C. H. and Peckinpaugh, R. O. (1973), 'Field trial of the efficacy of a previously proposed regimen using minocycline and rifampin sequentially for the elimination of meningococci from healthy carriers', *Amer. J. Epidemiol.,* **97,** 394.

Dimmling, T. (1960), 'Experimental and clinical investigations with pyrrolidinomethyl tetracycline', *Antibiot. Annual*—1959–1960, p. 350.

Dornbusch, K. (1976), 'The detection of doxycycline activity in human bone', *Scand. J. Infect. Dis.* (Suppl.), **9,** 47.

Dousa, T. P. and Wilson, D. M. (1973), 'Tetracyclines: Interference with ADH-responsive cyclic AMP system in human renal medulla', *Clin. Res.,* **21,** 75.

Dowling, H. F. and Lepper, M. H. (1964), 'Hepatic reactions to tetracycline', *JAMA,* **188,** 307.

Drew, T. M., Altman, R., Black, K. and Goldfield, M. (1976), 'Minocycline for prophylaxis of infection with Neisseria meningitidis: High rate of side-effects in recipients', *J. Infect. Dis.,* **133,** 194.

Duggar, B. M. *et al.* (1948), 'Aureomycin: Product of continuing search for new antibiotic', *Ann. N.Y. Acad. Sci.,* **51,** 177; quoted by Ory (1970).

Duma, R. J. (1977), 'Prescribing of tetracycline to children', *JAMA,* **238,** 579.

Dunlop, E. M. C. (1977), 'Treatment of patients suffering from chlamydial infections', *J. Antimicrob. Chemother.,* **3,** 377.

Eastwood, J. B., Bailey, R. R., Curtis, J. R., Gower, P. E. and De Wardener, H. E. (1970), 'Tetracycline in renal failure', *Lancet,* **2,** 39 and 262.

Edwards, O. M., Huskisson, E. C. and Taylor, R. T. (1970), 'Azotaemia aggravated by tetracycline', *Brit. med. J.,* **1,** 26.

Eickhoff, T. C., Bennett, J. V., Hayes, P. S. and Feeley, J. (1970), 'Pseudomonas pseudomallei: Susceptibility to chemotherapeutic agents', *J. Infect. Dis.,* **121,** 95.

Ellenbogen, C., Graybill, J. R., Silva, J., Jr. and Homme, P. J. (1974), 'Bacterial pneumonia complicating adenoviral pneumonia', *Amer. J. Med.,* **56,** 169.

Eliasson, R. and Malmborg, A.-S. (1976), 'Concentrations of doxycycline in human seminal plasma', *Scand. J. Infect. Dis.* (Suppl.), **9,** 32.

Eriksson, M. and Olcén, P. (1975), 'Septicaemia due to Yersinia enterocolitica in a non-compromised host', *Scand. J. Infect. Dis.,* **7,** 78.

Evans, W. and Hansman, D. (1963), 'Tetracycline-resistant pneumococcus', *Lancet,* **1,** 451.

Evans, R. T. and Taylor-Robinson, D. (1978), 'The incidence of tetracycline-resistant strains of Ureaplasma urealyticum', *J. Antimicrob. Chemother.,* **4,** 57.

Everett, E. D. and Nelson, R. A. (1975), 'Pulmonary melioidosis. Observations in thirty-nine cases', *Amer. Rev. Resp. Dis.,* **112,** 331.

Fanning, W. L., Gump, D. W. and Sofferman, R. A. (1977), 'Side-effects of minocycline: A double blind study. *Antimicrob. Ag. Chemother.,* **11,** 712.

Farrell, I. D., Hinchliffe, P. M. and Robertson, L. (1976), 'Sensitivity of Brucella spp.

to tetracycline and its analogues', *J. clin. Path.*, **29**, 1097.

Fass, R. J., Ruiz, D. E., Prior, R. B. and Perkins, R. L. (1976), '*In vitro* activity of gentamicin and minocycline alone and in combination against bacteria associated with intra-abdominal sepsis', *Antimicrob. Ag. Chemother.*, **10**, 34.

Fellner, M. J. and Baer, R. L. (1965), 'Anaphylactic reaction to tetracycline in a penicillin-allergic patient. Immunologic studies', *JAMA*, **192**, 997.

Fertig, A., Selwyn, S. and Tibble, M. J. K. (1977), 'Tetracycline treatment in a foodborne outbreak of toxoplasmosis', *Brit. med. J.*, **1**, 1064.

Finland, M. and Garrod, L. P. (1960), 'Demethylchlortetracycline', *Brit. med. J.*, **2**, 959.

Finland, M., Garner, C., Wilcox, C. and Sabath, L. D. (1976a), 'Susceptibility of beta-hemolytic streptococci to 65 antibacterial agents', *Antimicrob. Ag. Chemother.*, **9**, 11.

Finland, M., Garner, C., Wilcox, C. and Sabath, L. D. (1976b), 'Susceptibility of pneumococci and Haemophilus influenzae to antibacterial agents', *Antimicrob. Ag. Chemother.*, **9**, 274.

Ford, D. K. and Smith, J. R. (1974), 'Non-specific urethritis associated with a tetracycline-resistant T-mycoplasma', *Brit. J. vener. Dis.*, **50**, 373.

Forrest, J. N., Cox, M., Hong, C., Morrison, G., Bia, M. and Singer, I. (1978), 'Superiority of demeclocycline over lithium in the treatment of chronic syndrome of inappropriate secretion of antidiuretic hormone', *New Engl. J. Med.*, **298**, 173.

Forsgren, A., Schmeling, D. and Quie, P. G. (1974), 'Effect of tetracycline on the phagocytic function of human leukocytes', *J. Infect. Dis.*, **130**, 412.

Forsgren, A. and Schmeling, D. (1977), 'Effect of antibiotics on chemotaxis of human leukocytes', *Antimicrob. Ag. Chemother.*, **11**, 580.

Foy, H. M., Kenny, G. E., McMahan, R., Mansy, A. M. and Grayson, J. T. (1970), 'Mycoplasma pneumoniae pneumonia in an urban area', *JAMA*, **214**, 1666.

Frimpter, G. W., Timpanelli, A. E., Eisenmenger, W. J., Stein, H. S. and Ehrlich, L. I. (1963), 'Reversible Fanconi syndrome caused by degraded tetracycline', *JAMA*, **184**, 111.

Furey, W. W. and Tan, C. (1969), 'Anaphylactic shock due to oral demethylchlortetracycline', *Ann. Intern. Med.*, **70**, 357.

Gästrin, U. and Josephson, S. (1966), 'Tetracyclines and the teeth', *Lancet*, **2**, 492.

George, C. R. P. and Evans, R. A. (1971), 'Tetracycline toxicity in renal failure', *Med. J. Aust.*, **1**, 1271.

George, C. R. P., Guinness, M. D. G., Lark, D. J. and Evans, R. A. (1973), 'Minocycline toxicity in renal failure', *Med. J. Aust.*, **1**, 640.

Gnarpe, H. (1973), 'Treatment of experimental L-phase infections of the urinary tract', *J. Med. Microbiol.*, **6**, 53.

Gnarpe, H., Dornbusch, K. and Hägg, O., (1976), 'Doxycycline concentration levels in bone, soft tissue and serum after intravenous infusion of doxycycline', *Scand. J. Infect. Dis.* (Suppl.), **9**, 54.

Gorbach, S. L. and Bartlett, J. G. (1974), 'Anaerobic infections (third of three parts)', *New Engl. J. Med.*, **290**, 1289.

Goscienski, P. J. and Sexton, R. R. (1972), 'Follow-up studies in neonatal inclusion conjunctivitis', *Amer. J. Dis. Child.*, **124**, 180.

Gould, J. C. and Murdoch, J. McC. (1960), 'The long-term management of chronic bronchitis with antibiotics', *Antibiot. Annual*—1959–1960, p. 190.

Greenberg, P. A. and Sanford, J. P. (1967), 'Removal and absorption of antibiotics in patients with renal failure undergoing peritoneal dialysis: Tetracycline, chloramphenicol, kanamycin, and colistimethate', *Ann. Intern. Med.*, **66**, 465.

Grossan, M. (1968), 'Management of infections of the ear, nose, and throat with a new tetracycline antibiotic, doxycycline', *The Eye, Ear, Nose and Throat Monthly*, **47**, 56.

Grossman, E. R., Walchek, A. and Freedman, H. (1971), 'Tetracyclines and permanent teeth: The relation between dose and tooth colour', *Pediatrics*, **47**, 567.

Grossman, P. L. and Remington, J. S. (1977), 'Tetracycline and toxoplasmosis', *Brit. med. J.*, **1**, 1664.

Gump, D. W., Ashikaga, T., Fink, T. J. and Radin, A. M. (1977), 'Side effects of minocycline: Different dosage regimens', *Antimicrob. Ag. Chemother.*, **12**, 642.

Guttler, R. B. and Beaty, H. N. (1972), 'Minocycline in the chemoprophylaxis of meningococcal disease', *Antimicrob. Ag. Chemother.*, **1**, 397.

Hammond, G. W., Lian, C. J., Wilt, J. C. and Ronald, A. R. (1978), 'Antimicrobial susceptibility of Haemophilus ducreyi', *Antimicrob. Ag. Chemother.*, **13**, 608.

Hansman, D. and Andrews, G. (1967), 'Hospital infection with pneumococci resistant to tetracycline', *Med. J. Aust.*, **1**, 498.

Hansman, D. and Pidgeon, M. (1971), 'Chemotherapy of bronchitis', *Brit. med. J.*, **2**, 467.

Hansman, D. (1975), 'Haemophilus influenzae Type b resistant to tetracycline', *Lancet*, **2**, 893.

Hanson, G. C. (1968), 'A death from tetracycline', *Postgrad. Med. J.*, **44**, 870.

Hartnett, B. J. S. and Marlin, G. E. (1976), 'Doxycycline in bronchial secretions', *Med. J. Aust.*, **1**, 280.

Hassam, Z. A., Shaw, E. J. and Shooter, R. A. (1978), 'Changes in antibiotic sensitivity in strains of Staphylococcus aureus, 1952–78', *Brit. med. J.*, **2**, 536.

Hayek, A. and Ramirez, J. (1974), 'Demeclocycline-induced diabetes insipidus', *JAMA*, **229**, 676.

Hengeveld, W. L. (1977), 'A multi-centre surgical trial of intravenous doxycycline ('Vibravenous') in the Netherlands', *Curr. Med. Res. Opin.*, **4**, 505.

Hill, G. B. (1977), 'Therapeutic evaluation of minocycline and tetracycline for mixed anaerobic infection in mice', *Antimicrob. Ag. Chemother.*, **11**, 625.

Hoekenga, M. T. (1953), 'Terramycin treatment of balantidiasis in Honduras', *Amer. J. Trop. Med.*, **2**, 271.

Hoeprich, P. D. and Warshauer, D. M. (1974), 'Entry of four tetracyclines into saliva and tears', *Antimicrob. Ag. Chemother.*, **5**, 330.

Höjer, H. and Wetterfors, J. (1976), 'Concentration of doxycycline in bowel tissue and postoperative infections' *Scand. J. Infect. Dis.* (Suppl.), **9**, 100.

Holman, B. L., Lesch, M., Zweiman, F. G., Temte, J., Lown, B. and Gorlin, R. (1974), 'Detection and sizing of acute myocardial infants with 99 mm Tc (SN) tetracycline', *New Engl. J. Med.*, **291**, 159.

Holmberg, K., Nord, C.-E. and Dornbusch, K. (1977), 'Antimicrobial *in vitro* susceptibility of Actinomyces israelii and Arachnia propionica', *Scand. J. Infect. Dis.*, **9**, 40.

Holt, R., Evans, T. N. and Newman, R. L. (1969), 'Tetracycline-resistant pneumococci', *Lancet*, **2**, 545.

Hoshiwara, I., Ostler, H. B., Hanna, L., Cignetti, F., Coleman, V. R. and Jawetz, E. (1973), 'Doxycycline treatment of chronic trachoma', *JAMA*, **224**, 220.

Howard, A. J., Hince, C. J. and Williams, J. D. (1978), 'Antibiotic resistance in Streptococcus pneumoniae and Haemophilus influenzae. Report of a study group on bacterial resistance', *Brit. med. J.*, **1**, 1657.

Howe, C., Sampath, A. and Spotnitz, M. (1971), 'The Pseudomallei group: A review', *J. Infect. Dis.*, **124**, 598.

Hughes, D. (1976), 'Chemoprophylaxis in chronic bronchitis', *J. Antimicrob. Chemother.*, **2**, 320.

Jacobson, J. A. and Daniel, B. (1975), 'Vestibular reactions associated with minocycline', *Antimicrob. Ag. Chemother.*, **8**, 453.

Jao, R. L. and Finland, M. (1967), 'Susceptibility of Mycoplasma pneumoniae to 21 antibiotics *in vitro*', *Amer. J. Med. Sci.*, **253**, 639.

Jawetz, E. and Gunnison, J. B. (1952), 'Studies on antibiotic synergism and antagonism: A scheme of combined antibiotic action', *Antibiot. Chemother.*, **2**, 243.

Jawetz, E. (1969), 'Chemotherapy of chlamydial infections', *Advances in Pharmacol. Chemother.*, **7**, 253.

Johnstone, F. R. C. and Cockcroft, W. H. (1968), 'Clostridium welchii resistance to tetracycline', *Lancet*, **1**, 660.

Joint FAO/WHO Expert Committee on Brucellosis (1971), *Wld. Hlth. Org. techn. Rep. Ser.*, No. 464, 35.

Joint ICMR-GWB-WHO Cholera Study Group, Calcutta, India (1971), 'Effect of tetracycline on cholera carriers in households of cholera patients', *Bull. Wld. Hlth. Org.*, **45**, 451.

Jones, P. H. (1972), 'Treatment of choice for uncomplicated gonorrhea', *JAMA*, **219**, 619.

Jonsson, M. and Tunevall, G. (1976), 'Selective pressure of tetracyclines on the faecal flora. A comparison between tetracycline and doxycycline', *Scand. J. Infect. Dis.* (Suppl.), **9**, 89.

Joseph, S. W., DeBell, R. M. and Brown, W. P. (1978), '*In vitro* response to chloramphenicol, tetracycline, ampicillin, gentamicin, and beta-lactamase production by Halophilic vibrios from human and environmental sources', *Antimicrob. Ag. Chemother.*, **13**, 244.

Jung, R. T. and Rowntree, C. A. (1977), 'Case report: Coma due to oxytetracycline', *Curr. Med. Res. Opin.*, **5**, 210.

Kahlmeter, G. and Kamme, C. (1972), 'Tetracycline-resistant Group A streptococci and pneumococci', *Scand. J. Infect. Dis.*, **4**, 193.

Kaplan, M. A., Albright, H. and Buckwalter, F. H. (1960), 'A new tetracycline antibiotic for parenteral use', *Antibiot. Annual*—1959–1960, p. 365.

Karney, W. W., Pedersen, A. H. B., Nelson, M., Adams, H., Pfeifer, R. T. and Holmes, K. K. (1977), 'Spectinomycin versus tetracycline for the treatment of gonorrhea', *New Engl. J. Med.*, **296**, 889.

Kirkpatrick, R. (1978), 'Demeclocycline and renal insufficiency', *JAMA*, **239**, 616.

Klastersky, J., Cappel, R., Rens, B. and Daneau, D. (1972), 'Clinical and bacteriological evaluation of intravenous doxycycline in severe hospital infections', *Curr. Ther. Res.*, **14**, 49.

Klastersky, J., Husson, M., Weerts-Ruhl, D. and Daneau, D. (1977), 'Anaerobic wound infections in cancer patients: Comparative trial of clindamycin, tinidazole, and doxycycline', *Antimicrob. Ag. Chemother.*, **12**, 563.

Klein, R. A., Busch, D. F., Wilson, S. E., Flora, D. J. and Finegold, S. M. (1977), 'Doxycycline in abdominal surgery', *JAMA*, **238**, 1933.

Kline, A. H., Blattner, R. J. and Lunin, M. (1964), 'Transplacental effect of tetracyclines on teeth', *JAMA*, **188**, 178.

Koch-Weser, J. and Gilmore, E. B. (1967), 'Benign intracranial hypertension in an adult after tetracycline therapy', *JAMA*, **200**, 345.

Korkeila, J. (1971), 'Antianabolic effect of tetracyclines', *Lancet*, **1**, 974.

Kounis, N. G. (1975), 'Oxytetracycline-induced thrombocytopenic purpura', *JAMA*, **231**, 734.

Krause, W., Matheis, H. and Wulf, K. (1969), 'Fungaemia and funguria after oral administration of Candida albicans', *Lancet*, **1**, 598.

Kristinsson, A. and Bentall, H. H. (1967), 'Medical and surgical treatment of Q-fever endocarditis', *Lancet*, **2**, 693.

Kuck, N. A. (1976), '*In vitro* and *in vivo* activities of minocycline and other antibiotics against Acinetobacter (Herellea-Mima)', *Antimicrob. Ag. Chemother.*, **9**, 493.

Kuharic, H. A., Roberts, C. E. and Kirby, W. M. M. (1960), 'Tetracycline resistance of Group A beta haemolytic streptococci', *JAMA*, **174**, 1779.

Kunelis, C. T., Peters, J. L. and Edmondson, H. A. (1965), 'Fatty liver of pregnancy and its relationship to tetracycline therapy', *Amer. J. Med.*, **38**, 359.

Kunin, C. M., Dornbush, A. C. and Finland, M. (1959), 'Distribution and excretion of four tetracycline analogues in normal young men', *J. Clin. Invest.*, **38**, 1950.

Kunin, C. M. (1967), 'A guide to use of antibiotics in patients with renal disease', *Ann. Intern. Med.*, **67**, 151.

Kuo, C.-C., Wang, S.-P. and Grayston, J. T. (1977), 'Antimicrobial activity of several antibiotics and a sulfonamide against Chlamydia trachomatis organisms in cell culture', *Antimicrob. Ag. Chemother.*, **12**, 80.

Lapp. C. W. (1977), 'Prescribing of tetracycline to children', *JAMA*, **238**, 579.

Leading Article (1965), 'Tetracyclines in pregnancy', *Brit. med. J.*, **1**, 743.

Leading Article (1966a), 'Tetracyclines and the teeth', *Lancet*, **1**, 917.

Leading Article (1966b), 'Antibiotics in cholera', *Lancet*, **1**, 801.

Leading Article (1968), 'Tetracycline diarrhoea', *Brit. med. J.*, **4**, 402.

Leading Article (1971), 'Tularaemia', *Brit. med. J.*, **4**, 4.

Leading Article (1972a), 'Tetracyclines for malaria', *Brit. med. J.* **3**, 487.

Leading Article (1972b), 'Tetracycline and blood urea', *Brit. med. J.*, **3**, 370.

Leading Article (1975), 'The problem of rosacea', *Brit. med. J.*, **4**, 366.

Leading Article (1976), 'Pills for pimples', *Brit. med. J.*, **1**, 1423.

Leading Article (1978), 'Treatment of Chlamydia trachomatis infections', *Lancet*, **1**, 192.

Leandoer, L., Ekelund, G., Genell, S. and Olson, S. (1976), 'Antibiotic prophylaxis in colorectal surgery. Doxycycline compared to a combination of benzylpenicillin and streptomycin. A preliminary report'. *Scand. J. Infect. Dis.* (Suppl.), **9**, 106.

Leigh, D. A. and Simmons, K. (1974), 'Effect of minocycline on tetracycline-resistant Staphylococcus aureus', *Lancet*, **1**, 1006.

Leigh, D. A. and Simmons, K. (1975), 'Activity of minocycline against Bacteroides fragilis', *Lancet*, **1**, 51.

Lepper, M. H. and Dowling, H. F. (1951), 'Treatment of pneumococcal meningitis with penicillin compared with penicillin plus aureomycin', *Arch. Intern. Med.*, **88**, 489.

Lepper, M. H., Wolfe, C. K., Zimmerman, H. J., Caldwell, E. R., Jr., Spies, H. W. and Dowling, H. F. (1951), 'Effect of large doses of aureomycin on human liver', *Arch. Intern. Med.*, **88**, 271.

Lew. H. T. and French, S. W. (1966), 'Tetracycline nephrotoxicity and nonoliguric acute renal failure', *Arch. Intern. Med.*, **118**, 123.

Lewis, M. J. (1968), 'Transferable drug resistance and other transferable agents in strains of Escherichia coli from two human populations', *Lancet*, **1**, 1389.

Lie, J. T. (1976), 'The Whipple riddle', *JAMA*, *235*, 1148.

Little, P. J. and Bailey, R. R. (1970), 'Tetracyclines and renal failure', *N.Z. med. J.*, **72**, 183.

Lloyd-Still, J. D., Grand, R. J. and Vawter, G. F. (1974), 'Tetracycline hepatotoxicity in the differential diagnosis of postoperative jaundice', *J. Pediatrics*, **84**, 366.

Lowbury, E. J. L. and Cason, J. S. (1954), 'Aureomycin and erythromycin therapy for Str. pyogenes in burns', *Brit. med. J.*, **2**, 914.

Lowbury, E. J. L. and Hurst, L. (1956), 'Atypical anaerobic forms of Streptococcus pyogenes associated with tetracycline resistance', *J. clin. Path.*, **9**, 59.

Lucas-Lenard, J. and Haenni, A.-L. (1968), 'Requirement of guanosine 5-triphosphate for ribosomal binding of aminoacyl-SRNA', *Proc. nat. Acad. Sci.* (*Wash.*), **59**, 554.

Lundberg, C. and Malmborg, A-S. (1973), 'Concentration of penicillin V and tetracycline in maxillary sinus secretion after repeated doses', *Scand. J. Infect. Dis.*, **5**, 123.

Lundberg, C. and Malmborg, A.-S. (1974), 'Concentration of penicillin and tetracycline in maxillary sinus secretion after a single dose', *Scand. J. Infect. Dis.*, **6**, 79.

Lundsgaard-Hansen, P., Senn, A., Roos, B. and Waller, U. (1960), 'Staphylococcic enterocolitis. Report of six cases with two fatalities after intravenous administration of N-(pyrrolidinomethyl) tetracycline', *JAMA*, **173**, 1008.

MacCulloch, D., Richardson, R. A. and Allwood, G. K. (1974), 'The penetration of doxycycline, oxytetracycline and minocycline into sputum', *N.Z. Med. J.*, **80**, 300.

MacDonald, H., Kelly, R. G., Allen, E. S., Noble, J. F. and Kanegis, L. A. (1973), 'Pharmacokinetic studies on minocycline in man', *Clin. Pharmacol. Ther.*, **14**, 852.

Maderazo, E. G., Quintiliani, R., Tilton, R. C., Bartlett, R., Joyce, N. C. and Andriole, V. T. (1975), 'Activity of minocycline against Acinetobacter calcoaceticus var. anitratus (Syn. Herellea vaginicola) and Serratia marcescens', *Antimicrob. Ag. Chemother.*, **8**, 54.

Mahon, W. A., Wittenberg, J. V. P. and Tuffnel, P. G. (1970), 'Studies on the absorption and distribution of doxycycline in normal patients and in patients with severely impaired renal function', *C.M.A. Journal*, **103**, 1031.

Mahon, W. A., Johnson, G. E., Endrenyi, L., Kelly, M. F. and Fenton, S. S. A. (1976), 'The elimination of tritiated doxycycline in normal subjects and in patients with severely impaired renal function', *Scand. J. Infect. Dis.* (Suppl.), **9**, 24.

Mahony, J. F. and Lloyd-Jones, D. (1975), 'Serum doxycycline levels after intravenous administration in haemodialysis patients', *Med. J. Aust.*, **2**, 673.

Maier, T. W., Beilstein, H. R. and Zubrzycki, L. (1974), 'Multiple antibiotic resistance in Neisseria gonorrhoeae', *Antimicrob. Ag. Chemother.*, **6**, 22.

Maness, M. J. and Sparling, P. F. (1973), 'Multiple antibiotic resistance due to a single mutation in Neisseria gonorrhoeae', *J. Infect. Dis.*, **128**, 321.

Marks, R. and Ellis, J. (1971), 'Comparative effectiveness of tetracycline and ampicillin in rosacea. A controlled trial', *Lancet*, **2**, 1049.

Maroon, J. C. and Mealy, J., Jr. (1971), 'Benign intracranial hypertension. Sequel to tetracycline therapy in a child', *JAMA*, **216**, 1479.

Martin, N. D. and Barnard, P. D. (1969), 'Prevalence of tetracycline staining in erupted teeth', *Med. J. Aust.*, **1**, 1286.

Martin, R. R., Warr, G. A., Couch, R. B., Yeager, H. and Knight, V. (1974), 'Effects of tetracycline on leukotaxis', *J. Infect. Dis.*, **129**, 110.

Martin, W. J., Gardner, M. and Washington, J. A. II (1972), '*In vitro* antimicrobial susceptibility of anaerobic bacteria isolated from clinical specimens', *Antimicrob. Ag. Chemother.*, **1**, 148.

Masterton, G. and Schofield, C. B. S. (1974), 'Side-effects of minocycline hydrochloride', *Lancet*, **2**, 1139.

Mathies, A. W., Jr., Leedom, J. M., Ivler, D., Wehrle, P. F. and Portnoy, B. (1968), 'Antibiotic antagonism in bacterial meningitis', *Antimicrob. Ag. Chemother.*—1967, p. 218.

Mazumder, D. N. G., Sirkar, B. K. and De, S. P. (1974), 'Minocycline in the treatment of cholera. A comparison with tetracycline', *Indian J. Med. Res.*, **62**, 712.

McCabe, W. R. and Jackson, G. G. (1965), 'The treatment of pyelonephritis. Bacterial, drug and host factors in success or failure among 252 patients', *New Eng. J. Med.*, **272**, 1037.

McCormack, W. M., Chowdhury, A. M., Jahangir, N., Fariduddin Ahmed, A. B. and Mosley, W. H. (1968), 'Tetracycline prophylaxis in families of cholera patients', *Bull. Wld. Hlth. Org.*, **38**, 787.

McGill, R. E. T. (1974), 'Minocycline and beta-haemolytic streptococci', *Brit. med. J.*, **3**, 625.

McHenry, M. C., Gavan, T. L., Vidt, D. G., Jameson, S. and Wagner, J. G. (1972), 'Minocycline in renal failure', *Clin. Pharmacol. Ther.*, **13**, 146.

McIntosh, H. A. and Storey, E. (1970), 'Tetracycline-induced tooth changes, Part 4: Discoloration and hypoplasia induced by tetracycline analogues', *Med. J. Aust.*, **1**, 114.

Medical News (1977), 'Tetracycline stained teeth in children', *JAMA*, **237**, 636.

Mérier, G., Laurencet, F. L., Rudhardt, M., Chuit, A. and Fabre, J. (1969), 'Behaviour of doxycycline in renal insufficiency', *Helvetica Medica Acta*, **35**, 124.

Meyers, R. W. and Goldstein, R. E. (1974), 'Radioisotopic assessment of myocardial infarction', *New Engl. J. Med.*, **291**, 203.

Minuth, J. N., Holmes, T. M. and Musher, D. M. (1974), 'Activity of tetracycline, doxycycline, and minocycline against methicillin-susceptible and -resistant staphylococci', *Antimicrob. Ag. Chemother.*, **6**, 411.

Mitchell, R. G. and Baber, K. G. (1965), 'Infections by tetracycline-resistant haemolytic streptococci', *Lancet*, **1**, 25.

Mitchell, A. A. B. (1974), 'Comparative activity of minocycline and tetracycline', *Brit. med. J.*, **1**, 576.

Møller, J. K., Leth Bak, A., Stenderup, A., Zachariae, H. and Afzelius, H. (1977), 'Changing patterns of plasmid-mediated drug resistance during tetracycline therapy', *Antimicrob. Ag. Chemother.*, **11**, 388.

Montgomerie, J. Z., Pickett, M. J., Yoshimori, R. N., Chow, A. W. and Guze, L. B. (1976), 'Susceptibility of Acinetobacter calcoaceticus var. anitratus (Herellea vaginicola) to minocycline', *Antimicrob. Ag. Chemother.*, **10**, 102.

Montgomery, C. H. and Knox, J. M. (1959), 'Antibiotics other than penicillin in the treatment of syphilis', *New Engl. J. Med.*, **261**, 277.

Morgan, T. and Ribush, N. (1972), 'The effect of oxytetracycline and doxycycline on protein metabolism', *Med. J. Aust.*, **1**, 55.

Mull, M. M. (1966), 'The tetracyclines, a critical reappraisal', *Amer. J. Dis. Child.*, **112**, 483.

Munford, R. S., de Vasconcelos, Z. J. S., Phillips, C. J., Gelli, D. S., Gorman, G. W., Risi, J. B. and Feldman, R. A. (1974), 'Eradication of carriage of Neisseria meningitidis in families: A study in Brazil', *J. Infect. Dis.*, **129**, 644.

Musher, D. M., Minuth, J. N., Thorsteinsson, S. B. and Holmes, T. (1975), 'Effectiveness of achievable urinary concentrations of tetracyclines against 'tetracycline-resistant', pathogenic bacteria', *J. Infect. Dis.* (Suppl.), **131**, 40.

Nash, P., Sideman, L., Pidcoe, V. and Kleger, B. (1978), 'Minocycline in Legionnaires' disease', *Lancet*, **1**, 45.

Neu, H. C. (1978), 'A symposium on the tetracyclines: A major appraisal. Introduction', *Bull. N.Y. Acad. Med.*, **54**, 141.

Nelson, K. E., Levin, S., Spies, H. W. and Lepper, M. H. (1972), 'Treatment of Hemophilus influenzae meningitis: A comparison of chloramphenicol and tetracycline', *J. Infect. Dis.*, **125**, 459.

Neumann, H. H. and Baecker, J. M. (1972), 'Treatment of gonorrhea. Penicillin or tetracyclines?', *JAMA*, **219**, 471.

Neuvonen, P. J., Gothoni, G., Hackman, R. and af Björksten, K. (1970), 'Interference of iron with the absorption of tetracyclines in man', *Brit. med. J.*, **4**, 532.

Neuvonen, P. J. and Penttilä, O. (1974), 'Interaction between doxycycline and barbiturates', *Brit. med. J.*, **1**, 535.

O'Grady, F., Lewis, M. J. and Pearson, N. J. (1976), 'Global surveillance of antibiotic sensitivity of Vibrio cholerae', *Bull. Wld. Hlth. Org.*, **54**, 181.

Ohlrich, G. D. and Ohlrich, J. G. (1977), 'Papilloedema in an adolescent due to tetracycline', *Med. J. Aust.*, **1**, 334.

Oosterlinck, W., Wallijn, E. and Wijndaele, J. J. (1976), 'The concentration of doxycycline in human prostate gland and its role in the treatment of prostatitis', *Scand. J. Infect. Dis.*, (Suppl.), **9**, 85.

Oriel, J. D. and Waterworth, P. M. (1975), 'Effects on minocycline and tetracycline on the vaginal yeast flora', *J. clin. Path.*, **28**, 403.

Orr, L. H., Jr., Rudisill, E., Jr., Brodkin, R. and Hamilton, R. W. (1978), 'Exacerbation of renal failure associated with doxycycline', *Arch. Intern. Med.*, **138**, 793.

Ory, E. M. (1970), 'The tetracyclines', *Med. Clin. North America,* **54,** 1173.

Oster, J. R. and Epstein, M. (1977), 'Democlocycline-induced renal failure', *Lancet,* **1,** 52.

Overman, S. B., Lambe, D. W., Jr. and Bennett, J. V. (1974), 'Proposed standardized method for testing and interpreting susceptibility of Bacteroides fragilis to tetracycline', *Antimicrob. Ag. Chemother.,* **5,** 357.

Pato, M. L. (1977), 'Tetracycline inhibits propagation of deoxyribonucleic acid replication and alters membrane properties', *Antimicrob. Ag. Chemother.,* **11,** 318.

Penttilä, O., Neuvonen, P. J., Aho, K. and Lehtovaara, R. (1974), 'Interaction between doxycycline and some antiepileptic drugs', *Brit. med. J.,* **2,** 470.

Percival, A., Armstrong, E. C. and Turner, G. C. (1969), 'Increased incidence of tetracycline-resistant pneumococci in Liverpool in 1968', *Lancet,* **1,** 998.

Perks, W. H., Mohr, P. and Liversedge, I. A. (1976), 'Demeclocycline in inappropriate A.D.H. syndrome', *Lancet,* **2,** 1414.

Phair, J. P., Hartman, R. E. and Carleton, J. (1974), 'Evaluation of the efficacy of minocycline therapy for staphylococcal soft-tissue infection', *Antimicrob. Ag. Chemother.,* **6,** 551.

Phillips, M. E., Eastwood, J. B., Curtis, J. R., Gower, P. E. and de Wardener, H. E. (1974), 'Tetracycline poisoning in renal failure', *Brit. med. J.,* **2,** 149.

Pickering, L. K., DuPont, H. L. and Olarte, J. (1978), 'Single-dose tetracycline therapy for shigellosis in adults', *JAMA,* **239,** 853.

Pochi, P. E. (1976), 'Editorial. Antibiotics in acne', *New Engl. J. Med.,* **294,** 43.

Porter, P. J., Sweeney, E. A., Golan, H. and Kass, E. H. (1966), 'Controlled study of the effect of prenatal tetracycline on primary dentition', *Antimicrob. Ag. Chemother.—*1965, p. 668.

Prentice, M. J., Taylor-Robinson, D. and Csonka, G. W. (1976), 'Non-specific urethritis. A placebo-controlled trial of minocycline in conjunction with laboratory investigations', *Brit. J. vener. Dis.,* **52,** 269.

Proctor, E. A. and Barton, F. L. (1971), 'Polyuric acute renal failure after methoxyflurane and tetracycline', *Brit. med. J.,* **4,** 661.

Redin, G. S. (1967), 'Antibacterial activity in mice of minocycline, a new tetracycline', *Antimicrob. Ag. Chemother.—*1966, p. 371; quoted by Steigbigel *et al.* (1968).

Rahaman, M. M., Majid, M. A., Alam, A. K. M. J. and Islam, M. R. (1976), 'Effects of doxycycline in actively purging cholera patients: A double-blind clinical trial', *Antimicrob. Ag. Chemother.,* **10,** 610.

Report to the Research Committee of the British Tuberculosis Association by the Clinical Trials Subcommittee (1968), 'Comparison of side-effects of tetracycline and tetracycline plus nystatin', *Brit. med. J.,* **4,** 411.

Report from the Boston Collaborative Drug Surveillance Program (1972), 'Tetracycline and drug-attributed rises in blood urea nitrogen', *JAMA,* **220,** 377.

Report of an Ad-Hoc Study Group on Antibiotic Resistance (1977), 'Tetracycline resistance in pneumococci and Group A streptococci', *Brit. med. J.,* **1,** 131.

Report of a WHO Scientific Group (1978), 'Neisseria gonorrhoeae and gonococcal infections', *Wld. Hlth. Org. techn. Rep. Ser.,* No. 616.

Ribush, N. and Morgan, T. (1972), 'Tetracyclines and renal failure', *Med. J. Aust.,* **1,** 53.

Rich, G. and Davidson, J. (1975), 'Minocycline sensitivity related to the phage type of multiply resistant staphylococci', *J. clin. Path.,* **28,** 450.

Richards, J. D. M. and Rycroft, J. A. (1963), 'Tetracycline-resistant pneumococci', *Lancet,* **1,** 553.

Rickles, F. R., Klipstein, F. A., Tomasini, J., Corcino, J. J. and Maldonado, N. (1972), 'Long-term follow-up of antibiotic-treated tropical sprue', *Ann. Intern. Med.,* **76,** 203.

Robertson, L., Farrell, I. D. and Hinchcliffe, P. M. (1973), 'The sensitivity of Brucella abortus to chemotherapeutic agents', *J. Med. Microbiol.,* **6,** 549.

Robertson, M. H. (1973), 'Tetracycline-resistant beta-haemolytic streptococci in South-west Essex: Decline and fall', *Brit. med. J.,* **4,** 84.

Roth, H., Beckler, K. L., Shalhoub, R. J. and Katz, S. (1967), 'Nephrotoxicity of demethylchlortetracycline hydrochloride', *Arch. Intern. Med.,* **120,** 433.

Ruhen, R. W. and Tandon, M. K. (1975), 'Minocycline, doxycycline and tetracycline levels in serum and bronchial secretions of patients with chronic bronchitis', *Pathology,* **7,** 193.

Ruhen, R. W. and Tandon, M. K. (1976), 'Comparative effectiveness of tetracycline, minocycline and doxycycline in treatment of acute-on-chronic bronchitis. A study based on sputum levels', *Med. J. Aust.,* **2,** 151.

Sabath, L. D. (1969), 'Current concepts: Drug resistance of bacteria', *New Engl. J. Med.,* **280,** 91.

Sack, D. A., Kaminsky, D. C., Sack, R. B., Itotia, J. N., Arthur, R. R., Kapikian, A. Z., Ørskov, F. and Ørskov, I. (1978), 'Prophylactic doxycycline for Travelers' diarrhea. Results of a prospective double-blind study of Peace Corps Volunteers in Kenya', *N. Engl. J. Med.,* **298,** 758.

Sadoff, L. and Eckberg, T. (1973), 'Lymphoepithelioma after long-term tetracycline for acne', *Lancet,* **1,** 675.

Sapico, F. L., Kwok, Y.-Y., Sutter, V. L. and Finegold, S. M. (1972), 'Standardized antimicrobial disc susceptibility testing of anaerobic bacteria: *In vitro* susceptibility of clostridium perfringens to nine antibiotics', *Antimicrob. Ag. Chemother.,* **2,** 320.

Schachter, J. (1978a), 'Chlamydial infections (first of three parts)', *New Engl. J. Med.,* **298,** 428.

Schachter, J. (1978b), 'Chlamydial infections (second of three parts)', *New Engl. J. Med.,* **298,** 490.

Schaedler, R. W., Choppin, P. W. and Zabriskie, J. B. (1964), 'Pneumonia caused by tetracycline-resistant pneumococci', *New Engl. J. Med.,* **270,** 127.

Schoenfield, L. J. (1971), 'Editorial. Biliary excretion of antibiotics', *New Engl. J. Med.,* **284,** 1213.

Schultz, J. C., Adamson, J. S., Jr., Workman, W. W. and Norman, T. D. (1963), 'Fatal liver disease after intravenous administration of tetracycline in high dosage', *New Engl. J. Med.,* **269,** 999.

Schwartzman, J. D., Reller, L. B. and Wang, W.-L. L. (1977), 'Susceptibility of Clostridium perfringens isolated from human infections to twenty antibiotics', *Antimicrob. Ag. Chemother.,* **11,** 695.

Searcy, R. L., Simms, N. M., Foreman, J. A. and Bergquist, L. M. (1965), 'Evaluation of the blood-clotting mechanism in tetracycline-treated patients', *Antimicrob. Ag. Chemother.—*1964, p. 179.

Shames, J. M., George, R. B., Holliday, W. B., Rasch, J. R. and Mogabgab, W. J. (1970), 'Comparison of antibiotics in the treatment of mycoplasmal pneumonia', *Arch. Intern. Med.,* **125,** 680.

Sheehan, H. L. (1940), 'The pathology of acute yellow atrophy and delayed chloroform poisoning', *J. Obst. Gynaec. Brit. Emp.,* **47,** 49; quoted by Kunelis *et al.* (1965).

Shelley, W. B. and Heaton, C. L. (1973), 'Minocycline sensitivity', *JAMA,* **224,** 125.

Shils, M. E. (1963), 'Renal disease and the metabolic effects of tetracycline', *Ann. Intern. Med.,* **58,** 389.

Shwachman, H., Fekete, E., Kulczycki, L. L. and Foley, G. E. (1969), 'The effect of long-term antibiotic therapy in patients with cystic fibrosis of the pancreas', *Antibiot. Annual—*1958–1959, p. 692.

Singer, I. and Rotenberg, D. (1973), 'Demeclocycline-induced nephrogenic diabetes insipidus. *In-vivo* and *in-vitro* studies', *Ann. Intern. Med.,* **79,** 679.

Sivonen, A., Renkonen, O.-V., Weckström, P., Koskenvuo, K., Raunio, V. and

Mäkelä, P. H. (1978), 'The effect of chemoprophylactic use of rifampin and minocycline on rates of carriage of Neisseria meningitidis in army recruits in Finland', *J. Infect. Dis.*, **137**, 238.

Slocombe, B. and Sutherland, R. (1973), 'Transferable antibiotic resistance in enteropathogenic Escherichia coli between 1948 and 1968', *Antimicrob. Ag. Chemother.*, **4**, 459.

Smith, C. B., Friedewald, W. T. and Chanock, R. M. (1967), 'Shedding of Mycoplasma pneumoniae after tetracycline and erythromycin therapy', *New Engl. J. Med.*, **276**, 1172.

Spaepen, M. S., Kundsin, R. B. and Horne, H. W. (1976), 'Tetracycline-resistant T-Mycoplasmas (Ureaplasma urealyticum) from patients with a history of reproductive failure', *Antimicrob. Ag. Chemother.*, **9**, 1012.

Spaepen, M. S. and Kundsin, R. B. (1977), 'Simple, direct broth-disk method for antibiotic susceptibility testing of Ureaplasma urealyticum', *Antimicrob. Ag. Chemother.*, **11**, 267.

Sponitz, M., Rudnitzky, J. and Rambaud, J. J. (1967), 'Melioidosis pneumonitis', *JAMA*, **202**, 950.

Steigbigel, N. H., Reed, C. W. and Finland, M. (1968a), 'Absorption and excretion of five tetracycline analogues in normal young men', *Amer. J. Med. Sci.*, **255**, 296.

Steigbigel, N. H., Reed, C. W. and Finland, M. (1968b), 'Susceptibility of common pathogenic bacteria to seven tetracycline antibiotics *in vitro*', *Amer. J. Med. Sci.*, **255**, 179.

Stenbaek, Ø, Myhre, E. and Berdal, B. P. (1973), 'The effect of doxycycline on renal function in patients with advanced renal insufficiency', *Scand. J. Infect. Dis.*, **5**, 199.

Stewart, D. J. (1973), 'Prevalence of tetracyclines in children's teeth—study II: A resurvey after five years', *Brit. med. J.*, **3**, 320.

Storey, E. (1963), 'Tetracycline antibiotics and their effects on calcified and non-calcified tissues', *Aust., Ann. Med.*, **12**, 325.

Stott, N. C. H. and West, R. R. (1976), 'Randomised controlled trial of antibiotics in patients with cough and purulent sputum', *Brit. med. J.*, **2**, 556.

Ström, J. (1955), 'The question of antagonism between penicillin and chlortetracycline illustrated by therapeutical experiments in scarlatina', *Antibiot. Med.*, **1**, 6.

Sutter, V. L. and Finegold, S. M. (1976), 'Susceptibility of anaerobic bacteria to 23 antimicrobial agents', *Antimicrob. Ag. Chemother.*, **10**, 736.

Swarz, H. (1977), 'Doxycycline in bronchitis: Results of a multicentre study', *Curr. Med. Res. Opin.*, **5**, 234.

Tager, I. and Speizer, F. E. (1975), 'Role of infection in chronic bronchitis', *New Engl. J. Med.*, **292**, 563.

Taylor-Robinson, D., Csonka, G. W. and Prentice, M. J. (1977), 'Chlamydial and ureaplasma—associated urethritis', *Lancet*, **1**, 903.

Thadepalli, H., Webb, D. and Huang, J. T. (1978), Anaerobic lung infections treated with doxycycline, *Bull N.Y. Acad. Med.*, **54**, 165.

Thaysen, E. H. and Eriksen, K. R. (1956), 'Staphylococcal enteritis following administration of the tetracyclines', *Antibiot. Ann.*—1955–1956, p. 867.

Thong, Y. H., Rowan-Kelly, B., Shepherd, C. and Ferrante, A. (1977), 'Growth inhibition of Naegleria fowleri by tetracycline, rifamycin, and miconazole', *Lancet*, **2**, 876.

Thornsberry, C., Baker, C. N. and Kirven, L. A. (1978), '*In vitro* activity of antimicrobial agents on Legionnaires' disease bacterium', *Antimicrob. Ag. Chemother.*, **13**, 78.

Toaff, R. and Ravid, R. (1966), 'Tetracyclines and the teeth', *Lancet*, **2**, 281.

Tomkins, A. M., James, W. P. T., Walters, J. H. and Cole, A. C. E. (1974), 'Malabsorption in overland travellers to India', *Brit. med. J.*, **3**, 380.

Turner, G. C. (1963). 'Tetracycline-resistant pneumococci in a general hospital',

Lancet, **2,** 1292.

Van Ypersele de Strihou, C. (1970), 'Tetracycline in renal failure', *Lancet,* **2,** 208.

Velasco, J. E., Miller, A. E. and Zaias, N. (1972), 'Minocycline in the treatment of venereal disease', *JAMA,* **220,** 1323.

Walker, S. H. (1953), 'A study of the possible interference of chloramphenicol with penicillin in acute streptococcal pharyngitis', *Antibiot. Chemother.,* **3,** 677.

Wallman, I. S. and Hilton, H. B. (1962), 'Teeth pigmented by tetracycline', *Lancet,* **1,** 827.

Waterworth, P. M. (1974), 'The effect of minocycline on Candida albicans', *J. clin. Path.,* **27,** 269.

Waugh, M. A. and Nayyar, K. C. (1977), 'Triple tetracycline (Deteclo) in the treatment of chlamydial infection of the female genital tract', *Brit. J. vener. Dis.,* **53,** 96.

Weinstein, L. and Musher, D. M. (1969), 'Antibiotic-induced suprainfection', *J. Infect. Dis.,* **119,** 662.

Welch, H. (1954), *Principles and Practice of Antibiotic Therapy,* Med. Encyc. Inc., New York, p. 255.

Welling, P. G., Shaw, W. R., Uman, S. J., Tse, F. L. S. and Craig, W. A. (1975), 'Pharmacokinetics of minocycline in renal failure', *Antimicrob. Ag. Chemother.,* **8,** 532.

Welling, P. G., Koch, P. A., Lau, C. C. and Craig, W. A. (1977), 'Bioavailability of tetracycline and doxycycline in fasted and nonfasted subjects', *Antimicrob. Ag. Chemother.,* **11,** 462.

Wetterfors, J. and Höjer, H. (1976), 'Systemic prophylaxis with doxycycline in surgery of the colon and rectum', *Scand. J. Infect. Dis.* (Suppl.), **9,** 94.

Weyman, J. (1965), 'The clinical appearances of tetracycline staining of the teeth', *Brit. Dent. J.,* **118,** 289.

Whalley, P. J., Adams, R. H. and Combes, B. (1964), 'Tetracycline toxicity in pregnancy', *JAMA,* **189,** 357.

Whelton, A., Schach von Wittenau, M., Twomey, T. M., Walker, W. G. and Bianchine, J. R. (1974), 'Doxycycline pharmacokinetics in the absence of renal function', *Kidney Int.,* **5,** 365.

Whitby, J. L. and Black, H. J. (1964), 'Comparison of lymecycline with tetracycline hydrochloride', *Brit. med. J.,* **2,** 1491.

WHO (1977), 'Chlamydia surveillance', *Wkly. Epidem. Rec.,* **52,** 230.

Wiesner, P. J., Holmes, K. K., Sparling, P. F., Maness, M. J., Bear, D. M., Gutman, L. T. and Karney, W. W. (1973), 'Single doses of methacycline and doxycycline for gonorrhea: A cooperative study of the frequency and cause of treatment failure', *J. Infect. Dis.,* **127,** 461.

Wiggins, G. L., Albritton, W. L. and Feeley, J. C. (1978), 'Antibiotic susceptibility of clinical isolates of Listeria monocytogenes', *Antimicrob. Ag. Chemother.,* **13,** 854.

Wight, J. (1977), 'Prescribing of tetracycline to children', *JAMA,* **238,** 579.

Willcox, R. R. (1977a), 'How suitable are available pharmaceuticals for the treatment of sexually transmitted diseases? 1. Conditions presenting as genital discharges', *Brit. J. vener. Dis.,* **53,** 314.

Willcox, R. R. (1977b), 'How suitable are available pharmaceuticals for the treatment of sexually transmitted diseases? 2. Conditions presenting as sores or tumours', *Brit. J. vener. Dis.,* **53,** 340.

Williams, D. N., Laughlin, L. W. and Yhu-Hsiung Lee (1974), 'Minocycline: Possible vestibular side-effects', *Lancet,* **2,** 744.

Williams, J. D. and Andrews, J. (1974), 'Sensitivity of Haemophilus influenzae to antibiotics', *Brit. med. J.,* **1,** 134.

Windsor, A. C. M., Hobbs, C. B., Treby, D. A. and Cowper, R. A. (1972), 'Effect of tetracycline on leucocyte ascorbic acid levels', *Brit. med. J.,* **1,** 214.

Wisseman, C. L., Jr., Waddell, A. D. and Walsh, W. T. (1974), '*In vitro* studies of the action of antibiotics on Rickettsia prowazeki by two basic methods of cell culture',

J. Infect. Dis., **130,** 564.

Witkop, C. J. and Wolf, R. O. (1963), 'Hypoplasia and intrinsic staining of enamel following tetracycline therapy', *JAMA,* **185,** 1008.

Wood, M. J., Farrell, W., Kattan, S. and Williams, J. D. (1975), 'Activity of minocycline and tetracycline against respiratory pathogens related to blood levels', *J. Antimicrob. Chemother.,* **1,** 323.

Yeager, A. S. (1977), 'Editorial. Why now? Use of tetracycline in young children', *JAMA,* **237,** 2101.

Yoshioka, H., Rudoy, P., Riley, H. D., Jr. and Yoshida, K. (1977), 'Antimicrobial susceptibility of Escherichia coli isolated at a children's hospital', *Scand. J. Infect. Dis.,* **9,** 207.

Zegers, De Beyl, D., Naeije, R. and De Troyer, A. (1978), 'Demeclocycline treatment of water retention in congestive heart failure', *Brit. med. J.,* **1,** 760.

Vancomycin

Description

Vancomycin was isolated from Streptomyces orientalis in the Lilly Research Laboratories (McCormick *et al.*, 1956). Vancomycin hydrochloride which is soluble in water, is used for clinical purposes, and is marketed as 'Vancocin'.

Sensitive Organisms

1. *Gram-positive bacteria.* Vancomycin is highly effective against Gram-positive cocci such as Staph. pyogenes (including penicillin G- and methicillin-resistant strains), Staph. epidermidis, Strep. pyogenes, Strep. pneumoniae, Strep. viridans and Strep. faecalis (McCormick *et al.*, 1956; Griffith and Peck, 1956). The multiply-antibiotic resistant strains of Strep. pneumoniae which were isolated in South Africa during 1977 (page 4) were sensitive to vancomycin (Center for Disease Control, 1977). The drug has a marked inhibitory activity against Strep. faecalis but it is usually not bactericidal in concentrations which can be easily attained *in vivo* (Harwick *et al.*, 1973). A bactericidal effect can be obtained with a synergistic vancomycin/streptomycin combination against most Strep. faecalis strains (Westenfelder *et al.*, 1973), or with a vancomycin/gentamicin combination against virtually all of these strains (Watanakunakorn and Bakie, 1973; Harwick *et al.*, 1974). Such a bactericidal effect may be important in the treatment of Strep. faecalis endocarditis (page 650). A combination of vancomycin with rifampicin is sometimes synergistic against Staph. pyogenes (page 555).

Gram-positive bacilli such as B. anthracis, C. diphtheriae, Cl. tetani and Cl. perfringens (welchii) are also sensitive to this drug.

Vancomycin-sensitive bacteria do not readily develop resistance *in vitro* or *in vivo*, but resistant strains of Staph. pyogenes have been produced by passaging sensitive strains in graded vancomycin concentrations *in vitro* (Geraci *et al.*, 1957). However the emergence of resistant staphylococci has not been observed during the treatment of patients, and also there is no cross-resistance between vancomycin and other antibiotics (Riley, 1961).

2. *Gram-negative bacteria.* Occasional strains of Neisseria spp. may be susceptible to vancomycin (Griffith and Peck, 1956), but all other Gram-negative bacteria are resistant.

3. The *Mycobacteria* and *fungi* are vancomycin-resistant.

In Vitro Sensitivities

The minimum inhibitory concentrations of vancomycin against some bacterial

646

species are shown in Table 39. Usually an organism is considered to be vancomycin-resistant if the MIC is 10 μg per ml or higher.

TABLE 39
(After Griffith and Peck, 1956)

ORGANISM	MIC (μg per ml)
Staph. pyogenes (aureus)	0·156–1·87
Staph. epidermidis (albus)	0·39 –1·56
Strep. pyogenes (Group A)	0·156–2·5
Strep. pneumoniae (Dip. pneumoniae)	0·29
Strep. viridans spp.	0·312–1·25
Strep. faecalis (Enterococcus, Group D)	0·312–2·5
Esch. coli	>10·0

Mode of Administration and Dosage

1. Vancomycin must be administered intravenously for the treatment of systemic infections, being poorly absorbed after oral administration and there being no satisfactory intramuscular preparation available.

2. The usual adult intravenous dose is 2 g per day given in two to four divided doses. A higher daily dose of 3–4 g may only be used for short periods in severely ill patients. The usual daily intravenous dose for children is 40 mg per kg (Jawetz, 1968). Vancomycin is stable in all commonly used intravenous fluids for at least 24 h, and therefore it can be administered by continuous intravenous infusion, provided that incompatible additives are avoided. However, most authors prefer intermittent infusions of concentrated vancomycin solutions. Kirby et al. (1960) administered this drug to adults in 1 g doses every 12 h. This dose was diluted in 100–200 ml of 5 per cent dextrose in water, and the resultant solution was infused over a period of 20–30 min. Direct intravenous injection of undiluted vancomycin solution into the drip tubing causes flushing, itching of skin, and other discomforts (Spears and Koch, 1960).

3. *Patients with renal failure.* Vancomycin accumulates in these patients, and a modified dosage schedule with serum level monitoring is necessary. The serum half-life of vancomycin which in patients with normal renal function is six hours, is prolonged to nine days in anuric patients (Kunin, 1967). Lindholm and Murray (1966) suggested that a dose of 1 g of intravenous vancomycin every ten to fourteen days may be sufficient for anuric patients, but Eykyn et al. (1970), who treated six anuric patients with staphylococcal infections of the shunt site, found that this dose was necessary every seven days to maintain effective serum levels. Vancomycin may be administered more frequently to patients with less severe renal failure. Serum level monitoring of the drug is necessary to adjust the dose in individual patients, and these levels should be maintained in a range of 2·5–25 μg per ml. Serum levels greater than 50 μg per ml at 1 h or 25 μg per ml at 2 h after an intravenous infusion of 1·0 g should probably be avoided.

Vancomycin is not removed from the body by haemodialysis (Lindholm and

Murray, 1966; Eykyn *et al.*, 1970) or by peritoneal dialysis (Appel and Neu, 1977).

4. *Newborn and premature infants.* In these patients a daily dose of 12–15 mg per kg has been recommended (Riley, 1961).

Availability

Vancomycin hydrochloride is available in 10 ml ampoules, each containing 0·5 g.

Serum Levels in Relation to Dosage

After a single intravenous injection or infusion of 0·5 g of vancomycin in adults, adequate serum levels are maintained for at least 6 h (Table 40). After an infusion of a 1·0 g dose, serum levels are approximately doubled, and therapeutic concentrations persist for at least 12 h. A therapeutic regimen of 1·0 g administered twelve-hourly is satisfactory (Kirby *et al.*, 1960). There may be slight accumulation of vancomycin in the serum when this regimen is used, even in patients with normal renal function (Geraci *et al.*, 1957). The serum half-life is 6 h.

TABLE 40

Average serum levels of vancomycin in normal healthy adults after a single intravenous injection of 0·5 g, administered during a four-minute period. (After Geraci *et al.*, 1957)

Time after injection	1 minute	1 hour	3 hours	6 hours	12 hours	24 hours
Serum level in μg per ml	33·0	7·3	4·3	2·8	1·5	0·7

Excretion

URINE: Vancomycin is excreted by the kidneys in its active unchanged form. About 80–90 per cent of an intravenously administered dose can be recovered from the urine during the first 24 h. Urine concentrations of 90–300 μg per ml are maintained for 24 h after a single 0·5 g intravenous dose in healthy adults (Geraci *et al.*, 1957).

BILE: Only a very small quantity of vancomycin is excreted in the bile (Geraci *et al.*, 1957).

INACTIVATION IN BODY: This process is very slow, and vancomycin has a very prolonged half-life in anuric patients (page 647).

Distribution of the Drug in Body

Vancomycin diffuses readily into pleural, pericardial, ascitic and synovial fluids (Geraci *et al.*, 1957). It does not diffuse into the cerebrospinal fluid with normal meninges, but therapeutic concentrations may be reached in this fluid in patients with acute meningitis (Riley, 1970).

Vancomycin is only about 10 per cent bound to serum proteins (Kunin, 1967).

Mode of Action

Vancomycin is bound rapidly and irreversibly to the cell walls of sensitive bacteria (Sinha and Neuhaus, 1968) thereby inhibiting cell wall synthesis. It appears to have this effect by forming complexes with peptide side-chains ending in acyl-D-ala-D-ala of the mucopeptide (page 19), which is contained in the cell wall (Nieto and Perkins, 1971a, b and c). This is a different mechanism to that of the penicillins and cephalosporins on bacterial cell walls (page 21). Vancomycin further differs from these drugs in that it inhibits the growth of spheroplasts, possibly by an additional action on the bacterial cytoplasmic membrane (Riley, 1970).

These differing mechanisms of action seem to explain the activity of vancomycin against 'methicillin-resistant staphylococci' (page 64), the cell wall synthesis of which are unaffected by the penicillins and cephalosporins.

Toxicity

1. *Ototoxicity*. Deafness is the most serious toxic effect of vancomycin. This may be preceded by tinnitus and it is more common in elderly patients. Ototoxicity is related to excessively high serum levels, and deafness has occurred in patients in whom serum concentrations of over 80 μg per ml were exceeded for several days (Lindholm and Murray, 1966). In some, hearing improves after cessation of therapy, in others the loss may progress despite withdrawal of the drug (Riley, 1970).

2. *Nephrotoxicity*. Proteinuria, haematuria, and occasionally a rise in blood urea have been described (Jawetz, 1968; Riley, 1970). Whether or not vancomycin is nephrotoxic appears to be debatable, some authors ascribing kidney damage to the drug and others finding no deterioration in renal function with its use (Appel and Neu, 1977). Regular determinations of vancomycin serum levels are advisable for patients receiving the drug parenterally.

3. *Allergy and other reactions*. Eosinophilia and urticarial rashes are fairly frequent with vancomycin. A severe anaphylactic reaction has been described in one patient about 10 min after the infusion of 1·0 g of vancomycin (Rothenberg, 1959).

Other unpleasant reactions, such as nausea, transient flushing and itching of skin may occur after intravenous infusion of the drug (Spears and Koch, 1960).

Drug fever and thrombophlebitis were apparently very common with early vancomycin preparations, but with the elimination of impurities these side-effects became less common (Kirby et al., 1959).

Clinical Uses of the Drug

1. *Staphylococcal infections*. Prior to the development of the penicillinase-resistant penicillins and other potent anti-staphylococcal agents, vancomycin was used fairly extensively for the treatment of severe staphylococcal infections

such as septicaemia and endocarditis. Many clinical studies confirmed that this drug was effective for these diseases (Geraci *et al.*, 1957; Geraci *et al.*, 1958; Dutton and Elmes, 1959; Kirby *et al.*, 1960).

Vancomycin is rather toxic, can only be administered intravenously, and is now regarded as a 'reserve drug' for the treatment of severe staphylococcal infections. It has been advocated for the treatment of severe infections caused by methicillin-resistant staphylococci (Benner and Morthland, 1967), although other safer drugs or drug combinations are available for this purpose (page 66). It has also been suggested that vancomycin may be useful for severe staphylococcal infections such as endocarditis, if the infection fails to respond to treatment with other antibiotics, which are active against the organism *in vitro* (Jawetz, 1968; Riley, 1970; Garrod *et al.*, 1973). In experimental Staph. pyogenes endocarditis in rabbits, vancomycin killed bacteria at a rate equal to that obtained using a combination of gentamicin plus penicillin (Sande and Johnson, 1975). In one patient described by Gopal *et al.* (1976), vancomycin alone failed to eradicate Staph. pyogenes from the blood although the strain was sensitive. This was ascribed to a lack of bactericidal effect by the drug because there was a great disparity between the MIC and the MBC of vancomycin for the organism. The patient eventually recovered with treatment by vancomycin, gentamicin and methicillin, a combination which was synergistic against the organism *in vitro*. Intravenous vancomycin has been successfully used to treat a child with staphylococcal meningitis, who failed to respond to other antibiotics (Hawley and Gump, 1973).

Vancomycin may also be of value to treat serious infections due to methicillin- and cephalosporin-resistant strains of Staph. epidermidis (Cook and Farrar, 1978).

2. *Streptococcal endocarditis.* Vancomycin is a useful 'reserve drug' for treatment of Strep. faecalis endocarditis (Friedberg *et al.*, 1968). It may be indicated when the usual treatment (a combination of penicillin G or ampicillin with streptomycin or gentamicin) is ineffective clinically or when the penicillins cannot be used because of allergy. In experimental enterococcal (Strep. faecalis) endocarditis in rabbits and *in vitro*, a vancomycin/streptomycin combination is more rapidly bactericidal than vancomycin alone when the strain used is 'sensitive' to streptomycin (Hook *et al.*, 1975). Although a combination of vancomycin with either streptomycin or gentamicin appears to be the most effective alternative therapy for Strep. faecalis endocarditis in penicillin-allergic patients (Mandell *et al.*, 1970; Harwick *et al.*, 1973), it is preferable to avoid the combination of two ototoxic drugs, if possible.

Similarly vancomycin is effective for the treatment of Strep. viridans endocarditis (Friedberg *et al.*, 1968). It may be selected for this disease if the strain concerned is highly resistant to the penicillins and cephalosporins, or if these drugs cannot be used because of allergy.

3. *Chemoprophylaxis of bacterial endocarditis.* Intravenous vancomycin has been suggested for the prevention of Strep. viridans endocarditis in susceptible patients, prior to dental extractions (Leading article, 1975). The American Heart Association recommends vancomycin as an alternative in penicillin-allergic patients to prevent endocarditis (Kaplan *et al.*, 1977). For dental procedures and surgery of the upper respiratory tract, chemoprophylaxis with various penicillin regimens, some combined with strep-

tomycin, are recommended (page 34); for penicillin-allergic patients alternative prophylaxis with either erythromycin (page 506) or vancomycin is recommended. The dose of vancomycin is 1·0 g for adults and 20 mg per kg body weight for children, which is given intravenously over a period of 30–60 min, 30–60 min before the procedure. For chemoprophylaxis against enterococcal endocarditis (e.g. Strep. faecalis) in patients with prosthetic heart valves, who are undergoing gastro-intestinal or genito-urinary tract surgery and instrumentation, penicillin or ampicillin plus gentamicin or streptomycin is recommended (page 35). For penicillin-allergic patients vancomycin (the same regimen as for Strep. viridans endocarditis prophylaxis) is recommended, plus a 1·0 g (20 mg per kg for children) intramuscular dose of streptomycin, 30 min before the procedure. During prolonged procedures these doses of vancomycin and streptomycin may be repeated in 12 h.

4. *Suppression of intestinal flora.* Oral vancomycin in a dose of 0·5 g six-hourly, combined with oral gentamicin and nystatin, has been administered to patients with acute leukaemia throughout the period of their induction chemotherapy. Intestinal bacteria were suppressed in most cases, and the overall frequency of bacterial infections appeared to be reduced (Levi *et al.*, 1973) (*see also* gentamicin, page 345).

5. *Pseudomembranous colitis.* This disease when associated with antibiotic therapy, appears to be due to overgrowth of Clostridium difficile and production of a heat-labile toxin in the bowel (page 481). An oral dose of vancomycin 2 g daily appeared to result in rapid recovery of one patient with pseudomembranous colitis (Modigliani and Delchier, 1978) (*see also* page 483). Larson *et al.* (1978) treated another patient with vancomycin in an oral dose of 0·5 g every six hours, and correlated clinical recovery with the disappearance of both Cl. difficile and its toxin from her faeces. Tedesco *et al.* (1978) used the same dose of vancomycin to treat nine patients with prolonged diarrhoea (10 days to 8 weeks) associated with pseudomembranous colitis; all patients showed a good clinical recovery after 7–10 days' treatment and this was associated with a rapid decrease in concentrations of toxin in their stools. Minimal absorption of vancomycin from the bowel occurred but faecal concentrations of the drug of about 3 mg per g were nearly 1000 times the highest MIC of Cl. difficile strains isolated.

REFERENCES

Appel, G. B. and Neu, H. C. (1977), 'The nephrotoxicity of antimicrobial agents (second of three parts)', *New Engl. J. Med.*, **296**, 722.

Benner, E. J. and Morthland, V. (1967), 'Methicillin-resistant Staphylococcus aureus. Antimicrobial susceptibility', *New Engl. J. Med.*, **277**, 678.

Center for Disease Control (1977), 'Multiple-antibiotic resistance of pneumococci—South Africa', *Morbidity and Mortality Weekly Report*, **26**, 285.

Cook, F. V. and Farrar, W. E., Jr. (1978), 'Vancomycin revisited', *Ann. Intern. Med.*, **88**, 813.

Dutton, A. A. C. and Elmes, P. C. (1959), 'Vancomycin: Report on treatment of patients with severe staphylococcal infections', *Brit. med. J.*, **1**, 1144.

Eykyn, S., Phillips, I. and Evans, J. (1970), 'Vancomycin for staphylococcal shunt site infections in patients on regular haemodialysis', *Brit. med. J.*, **3**, 80.

Friedberg, C. K., Rosen, K. M. and Bienstock, P. A. (1968), 'Vancomycin therapy for Enterococcal and Streptococcus viridans endocarditis', *Arch. Intern. Med.*, **122**, 134.

Garrod, L. P., Lambert, H. P. and O'Grady, F. (1973), *Antibiotic and Chemotherapy*, 4th edn., Churchill Livingstone, Edinburgh and London, p. 226.

Geraci, J. E., Heilman, F. R., Nichols, D. R., Wellman, W. E. and Ross, G. T. (1957), 'Some laboratory and clinical experiences with a new antibiotic, vancomycin', *Antibiot. Annual—1956–1957*, p. 90.

Geraci, J. E., Heilman, F. R., Nichols, D. R. and Wellman, W. E. (1958), 'Antibiotic therapy of bacterial endocarditis. VII. Vancomycin for acute Micrococcal endocarditis', *Proc. Mayo Clin.*, **33**, 172.

Gopal, V., Bisno, A. L. and Silverblatt, F. J. (1976), 'Failure of vancomycin treatment in Staphylococcus aureus endocarditis', *JAMA*, **236**, 1604.

Griffith, R. S. and Peck, F. B., Jr. (1956), 'Vancomycin, a new antibiotic. III. Preliminary clinical and laboratory studies', *Antibiot. Annual—1955–1956*, p. 619.

Harwick, H. J., Kalmanson, G. M. and Guze, L. B. (1973), '*In vitro* activity of ampicillin or vancomycin combined with gentamicin or streptomycin against Enterococci', *Antimicrob. Ag. Chemother.*, **4**, 383.

Harwick, H. J., Kalmanson, G. M. and Guze, L. B. (1974), 'Pyelonephritis. XVII. Comparison of combinations of vancomycin, ampicillin, streptomycin, and gentamicin in the treatment of Enterococcal infection in rats', *J. Infect. Dis.*, **129**, 358.

Hawley, H. B. and Gump, D. W. (1973), 'Vancomycin therapy of bacterial meningitis', *Amer. J. Dis. Child.*, **126**, 261.

Hook, E. W. III, Roberts, R. B. and Sande, M. A. (1975), 'Antimicrobial therapy of experimental Enterococcal endocarditis', *Antimicrob. Ag. Chemother.*, **8**, 564.

Jawetz, E. (1968), 'Polymyxins, colistin, bacitracin, ristocetin, and vancomycin', *Pediat. Clin. N. Amer.*, **15**, 85.

Kaplan, E. L., Anthony, B. F., Bisno, A., Durack, D., Houser, H., Millard, H. D., Sanford, J., Shulman, S. T., Stillerman, M., Taranta, A. and Wenger, N. (1977), 'Prevention of bacterial endocarditis', *Circulation*, **56**, 139A.

Kirby, W. M. M., Perry, D. M. and Lane, J. L. (1959), 'Present status of vancomycin therapy of staphylococcal and streptococcal infections', *Antibiot. Annual—1958–1959*, p. 580.

Kirby, W. M. M., Perry, D. M. and Bauer, A. W. (1960), 'Treatment of staphylococcal septicemia with vancomycin. Report of thirty-three cases', *New Engl. J. Med.*, **262**, 49.

Kunin, C. M. (1967), 'A guide to use of antibiotics in patients with renal disease', *Ann. Intern. Med.*, **67**, 151.

Larson, H. E., Levi, A. J. and Borriello, S. P. (1978), 'Vancomycin for pseudomembranous colitis', *Lancet*, **2**, 48.

Leading Article (1975), 'Antibiotic cover for dental extraction', *Brit. med. J.*, **3**, 191.

Levi, J. A., Vincent, P. C., Jennis, F., Lind, D. E. and Gunz, F. W. (1973), 'Prophylactic oral antibiotics in the management of acute leukaemia', *Med. J. Aust.*, **1**, 1025.

Lindholm, D. D. and Murray, J. S. (1966), 'Persistence of vancomycin in the blood during renal failure and its treatment by haemodialysis', *New Engl. J. Med.*, **274**, 1047.

Mandell, G. L., Kaye, D., Levison, M. E. and Hook, E. W. (1970), 'Enterococcal endocarditis', *Arch. Intern. Med.*, **125**, 258.

McCormick, M. H., Stark, W. M., Pittenger, G. E., Pittenger, R. C. and McGuire, J. M. (1956), 'Vancomycin, a new antibiotic. I. Chemical and biologic properties', *Antibiol. Annual—1955–1956*, p. 606.

Modigliani, R. and Delchier, J. C. (1978), 'Vancomycin for antibiotic-induced colitis', *Lancet*, **1**, 97.

Nieto, M. and Perkins, H. R. (1971a), 'Physicochemical properties of vancomycin and

iodovancomycin and their complexes with diacetyl-L-lysyl-D-alanyl-D-alanine',
  Biochem. J., **123**, 773.
Nieto, M. and Perkins, H. R. (1971b), 'Modifications of the aceyl-D-alanyl-D-alanine
  terminus affecting complex-formation with vancomycin', *Biochem. J.*, **123**, 789.
Nieto, M. and Perkins, H. R. (1971c), 'The specificity of combination between
  ristocetins and peptides related to bacterial cell wall mucopeptide precursors',
  Biochem. J., **124**, 845.
Riley, H. D., Jr. (1961), 'Vancomycin and ristocetin', *Pediat. Clin. N. Amer.*, **8**, 1073.
Riley, H. D., Jr. (1970), 'Vancomycin and novobiocin', *Med. Clin. North America*, **54**,
  1277.
Rothenberg, H. J. (1959), 'Anaphylactoid reaction to vancomycin', *JAMA*, **171**, 1101.
Sande, M. A. and Johnson, M. L. (1975), 'Antimicrobial therapy of experimental en-
  docarditis caused by Staphylococcus aureus', *J. Infect. Dis.*, **131**, 367.
Sinha, R. K. and Neuhaus, F. C. (1968), 'Reversal of the vancomycin inhibition of pep-
  tidoglycan synthesis by cell walls', *J. Bacteriol.*, **96**, 374.
Spears, R. L. and Koch, R. (1960), 'The use of vancomycin in pediatrics', *Antibiot. An-
  nual*—1959–1960, p. 798.
Tedesco, F., Markham, R., Gurwith, M., Christie, D. and Bartlett, J. G. (1978), 'Oral
  vancomycin for antibiotic-associated pseudomembranous colitis', *Lancet*, **2**, 226.
Watanakunakorn, C. and Bakie, C. (1973), 'Synergism of vancomycin-gentamicin and
  vancomycin-streptomycin against Enterococci', *Antimicrob. Ag. Chemother.*, **4**,
  120.
Westenfelder, G. O., Paterson, P. Y., Reisberg, B. E. and Carlson, G. M. (1973),
  'Vancomycin-streptomycin synergism in Enterococcal endocarditis', *JAMA*, **223**,
  37.

Part II
Synthetic Antibacterial and Antiparasitic Drugs

Sulphonamides

Description

The first sulphonamide compound of clinical importance, 'Prontosil rubrum', was synthetized in Germany in 1932, and first used as a chemotherapeutic agent in 1935 initiating a new era in the treatment of infections. It was soon shown that the therapeutic action of this compound depended on its breakdown in the body into an inactive dye and an antibacterial substance called sulphanilamide. Since then many sulphonamides have been synthetized, and some of these have clinical uses other than for chemotherapy, such as the oral hypoglycaemic agent, tolbutamide (*Today's Drugs*, 1968). In addition, it had been observed that sulphanilamide could cause a metabolic acidosis and act as a diuretic, and this was later shown to be due to its sulphamoyl group ($-SO_2NH_2$). Subsequent chemical manipulations of sulphanilamide led to the development of the sulphamoyl diuretics, such as the carbonic anhydrase inhibitors (e.g. acetazolamide), the thiazides and frusemide (Feit, 1975).

The following classification of sulphonamides, useful for the treatment of infections, is based on their absorption and excretion patterns.

SHORT-ACTING SULPHONAMIDES: These compounds are readily absorbed from the gastro-intestinal tract and are rapidly excreted. They may be divided into several groups:

1. *Sulphanilamide, sulphacetamide, sulphapyridine and sulphathiazole.* These are now largely of historical interest, although sulphacetamide is still used in eye drops because of its high solubility. The first two have low antibacterial activity, and whilst sulphapyridine and sulphathiazole were once important because of their improved antibacterial activity, they are no longer used singly because of their toxicity.

2. *Sulphadiazine or sulphapyrimidine group.* This includes:

   (a) *Sulphadiazine (sulphapyrimidine).*
   (b) *Sulphamerazine (sulphamethylpyrimidine).*
   (c) *Sulphadimidine (sulphamezathine, sulphadimethylpyrimidine or sulphamethazine).*

Sulphadiazine is a potent antibacterial and penetrates well into the cerebrospinal fluid, but it has the disadvantage of low solubility in urine. It was once regarded as the sulphonamide of choice for treatment for meningococcal meningitis, but the sulphonamides are now rarely used for this disease. Sulphadimidine, being effective and soluble in urine, is still extensively used for most of the indications applicable to sulphonamides. Sulphamerazine, being more toxic and without special advantages, is no longer used singly.

A topical, non-absorbable drug, *silver sulphadiazine* has been introduced for chemoprophylaxis in burns (Fox, 1968).

3. *Sulphasomidine* (*sulphadimethine*, '*Elkosin*', '*Pepsilphen*'), *sulphafurazole* (*sulfisoxazole*, '*Gantrisin*') and *sulphamethizole* (*sulphamethylthiodiazole or 'Urolucosil*'). Because they are soluble in urine, of low toxicity, and rapidly excreted, these compounds are suitable for treatment of urinary tract infections. The first two have also been used for treatment of systemic infections, but sulphamethizole is not useful for this purpose, because it is very rapidly excreted.

4. *Triple sulphonamides*. Mixtures of the sulphonamides were introduced to avoid renal complications after it was shown that the solubility of a sulphonamide is not impaired by the presence of other sulphonamides in the urine, and that their antibacterial activity is probably additive (*Today's Drugs*, 1964; Pryles, 1970). For instance one 500 mg tablet of 'Sulphatriad' (May and Baker) contains 185 mg sulphathiazole, 185 mg sulphadiazine and 130 mg sulphamerazine. sulphamerazine.

5. *Sulphasalazine* (*Salazopyrin*). This combination of sulphapyridine and salicylic acid, originally introduced for the treatment of rheumatoid arthritis, is useful for ulcerative colitis (page 677).

6. *Marfanil* (*Mafenide*, '*Sulphamar' or 'Sulfamylon*'). This drug differs from the other short-acting sulphonamides in chemical structure, and it is also not inactivated by para-amino-benzoic acid or by pus. It is used as an 11·2 per cent mafenide acetate cream for the treatment of burns (page 678), being active against Pseudomonas aeruginosa in this concentration (Lowbury *et al.*, 1971; Pegg, 1972).

MEDIUM-ACTING SULPHONAMIDES: *Sulphamethoxazole* ('*Gantanol*', *Roche*) belongs to this group. This is well absorbed from the gastro-intestinal tract, but rather more slowly excreted, so that 12-hourly administration is adequate. Sulphamethoxazole is used in combination with trimethoprim as co-trimoxazole (page 687).

LONG-ACTING SULPHONAMIDES: Rapidly absorbed from the gastro-intestinal tract, but excreted slowly, these can be administered in single daily doses. The group includes the following:

1. *Sulphamethoxypyridazine* ('*Lederkyn*', '*Midicel*' or '*Kynex*'). The first of the long-acting sulphonamides, it has a serum half-life of about 40 h, and single daily doses of 0·5 g maintain adequate serum levels in adults.

2. *Sulphadimethoxine* ('*Madribon*'), *sulphaphenazole* ('*Orisul*'), and *sulphamethoxydiazine* ('*Durenate*', 'Bayrena', *or 'Kirocid*'). These are all rather similar to sulphamethoxypyridazine. Sulphamethoxydiazine is about 75 per cent serum protein bound, by contrast with the other long-acting sulphonamides which are 90–95 per cent protein bound.

3. *Sulphasymazine* ('*Prosul*', *Lederle*). This compund has a shorter plasma half-life of about 26 h, and is sometimes classified as a 'medium-acting sulphonamide'. It has been used either in a single daily dose of 0·5 g, or 0·5 g twice a day for the treatment of urinary tract infections in adults (Nanra *et al.*, 1969).

ULTRA-LONG-ACTING SULPHONAMIDES: Therapeutic serum and urine levels persist for up to seven days after a single oral dose of 1–2 g of these drugs. There are two compounds with this characteristic:

1. *Sulfadoxine* ('*Fanasil*'), which was previously known with the generic name of sulphormethoxine. This drug is commercially available in combination with pyrimethamine ('Fansidar') for the treatment of malaria (page 676).

2. *Sulfametopyrazine* (*Sulfalene*, '*Kelfizine*').

These drugs have been used as 'single-dose treatment' for urinary tract infections (Grüneberg and Brumfitt, 1967; Williams and Smith, 1970).

POORLY ABSORBED SULPHONAMIDES: Most of the orally administered dose of these drugs is excreted unchanged in the faeces, and their action is confined to the gut. These drugs are rarely used nowadays, and include:

1. *Sulphaguanidine.*
2. *Succinylsulphathiazole.*
3. *Phthalylsulphathiazole* ('*Thalazole*').

Sensitive Organisms

1. The sulphonamides originally had a wide range of activity, but this range has now been seriously restricted by acquired bacterial resistance. The microorganisms which were originally sensitive to sulphonamides are described first, and acquired bacterial resistance is discussed separately later in this section.

2. *Gram-positive bacteria*. Gram-positive cocci such as Staph. pyogenes, Strep. pyogenes, Strep. pneumoniae and Strep. viridans are sensitive, but Strep. faecalis is invariably resistant. Gram-positive bacilli such as B. anthracis, Cl. tetani and Cl. perfringens (welchii) are also sensitive.

Actinomyces are commonly sulphonamide-sensitive. The Nocardia, both N. asteroides and N. brasiliensis, are usually sensitive to a degree, but some strains are resistant to very high sulphonamide concentrations (Bach *et al.*, 1973; Berd, 1973). Other chemotherapeutic agents such as ampicillin (Orfanakis *et al.*, 1972), and trimethoprim (page 687) may potentiate the action of sulphonamides against the Nocardia.

3. *Gram-negative bacteria*. All the Enterobacteriaceae such as Esch. coli, the Enterobacter, Klebsiella, Proteus, Yersinia, Salmonella and Shigella spp. are sulphonamide-sensitive. This also applies to other Gram-negative bacteria, such as the pathogenic Neisseria (gonococci and meningococci) and B. pertussis. H. influenzae type b including ampicillin-resistant strains (page 102) is also sensitive and this organism can be inhibited by concentrations achievable in saliva (Bannatyne and Cheung, 1978). Most strains of Pseudomonas pseudomallei are sensitive (Eichoff *et al.*, 1970). Even some strains of Pseudomonas aeruginosa are susceptible. The Legionnaires' disease bacterium is inhibited by sulphadiazine (Lewis *et al.*, 1978).

It also appears that Bacteroides fragilis may be susceptible to sulphonamides, but the degree of sensitivity depends on the laboratory technique used (Phillips and Warren, 1976).

4. *Chlamydia*. The sulphonamides are active against the causative organisms of lymphogranuloma venereum, trachoma and inclusion body con-

junctivitis, but not against C. psittaci which causes psittacosis.

5. *Other microorganisms.* Most Mycobacteria, the Mycoplasmas, Treponemata (e.g. T. pallidum), Leptospirae, Rickettsiae and Coxiella burnetti are sulphonamide-resistant. The long-acting sulphonamide, sulphadimethoxine, has a bactericidal action against Mycobacterium leprae similar to that of dapsone. However, the inhibitory concentrations of sulphadimethoxine and sulphadoxine against M. leprae are much higher than the serum levels achieved by normal doses. Because these groups of drugs are chemically related, strains of M. leprae resistant to dapsone are also resistant to long-acting sulphonamides (Shepard *et al.*, 1976).

6. *Protozoa.* The Malaria and Toxoplasma organisms are also susceptible to the sulphonamides. The former may develop sulphonamide resistance.

7. *Silver sulphadiazine.* This agent has special activities of its own. At concentrations easily attainable by topical application, it is active against Ps. aeruginosa (Rosenkranz and Carr, 1972), and against a number of dermatophytes such as the Microsporum and Trichophyton spp. and Epidermophyton floccosum (Speck and Rosenkranz, 1974). At a concentration of 10 μg per ml, it inhibits Herpesvirus hominis types 1 and 2 *in vitro* (Chang and Weinstein, 1975b) and at this concentration it also prevents acute herpetic keratoconjunctivitis in rabbits (Chang and Weinstein, 1975c). Silver sulphadiazine also has activity against Treponema pallidum (Chang and Weinstein, 1975a).

8. *Acquired resistance.* This is now common among many of the bacterial species which are described above as 'classically' sulphonamide-sensitive.

(a) Some strains of all the Gram-positive bacteria are sulphonamide-resistant, and resistant strains may also emerge *in vivo* during treatment with the sulphonamides. Although resistance of Group A beta-haemolytic streptococci to sulphadiazine appeared and spread rapidly amongst military recruits at the end of World War II, this does not appear to be a problem now. Only 3 of 35 strains of beta-haemolytic streptococci isolated in 1972 were highly resistant (MIC > 25 μg per ml) to sulphamethoxazole (Finland *et al.*, 1976). None of 59 strains of beta-haemolytic streptococci (Groups A, B, C and G) isolated from patients in Belgium were resistant to sulphamethoxazole (Yourassowsky *et al.*, 1974).

(b) Sulphonamide-resistant strains of Esch. coli and of all other Enterobacteriaceae are now common, particularly in hospitals. For instance, 25 per cent of Esch. coli, 53 per cent of Klebsiella-Enterobacter spp. and 40 per cent of Proteus mirabilis strains isolated from patients with urinary tract infections in Sweden were sulphonamide-resistant (Burman, 1977). The majority of Shigella spp. strains are now resistant to sulphonamides. In one survey in North America 59 per cent of Sh. flexneri and 87 per cent of Sh. sonnei strains isolated from patients were sulphadiazine-resistant (Haltalin and Nelson, 1965). A similar survey in London showed that over 80 per cent of Sh. sonnei strains were resistant (Davies *et al.*, 1970). Sulphonamide-resistant shigellae are also common in Papua New Guinea (Morahan and Hawksworth, 1970). Salmonellae resistant to sulphonamides are apparently no longer rare. A survey in

California showed that 39·8 per cent of Salm. typhimurium and 16·5 per cent of Salm. typhi strains were sulphonamide-resistant (Bissett *et al.*, 1974). Of 1156 strains of Vibrio cholerae isolated in various parts of the world, only four, all from the Philippines, showed increased resistance to sulphonamides (O'Grady *et al.*, 1976). The resistance of many of these Gram-negative organisms to sulphonamides is mediated by R plasmids (*see* page 422).

(c) Sulphonamide-resistant gonococci became common among troops during the Second World War when these drugs were extensively used for treatment of gonorrhoea. Sulphonamide-resistant gonococci now appear to be less common, because penicillin G has been mainly used for the treatment of gonorrhoea. Nevertheless, in certain parts of the world such as South-East Asia, a high percentage of gonococcal strains are still resistant to sulphonamides (Report, 1978).

(d) Sulphonamide-resistant meningococci are common in many parts of the world. They have been particularly prevalent in both military (Millar *et al.*, 1963) and civilian populations in the United States of America. In an early study in Los Angeles, 36·9 per cent of strains isolated from civilian patients were sulphadiazine-resistant, but only 23·7 per cent of strains from pharyngeal carriers were resistant; resistant strains were defined as those with an MIC of 10 mg per 100 ml (100 μg per ml) or greater (Leedom *et al.*, 1967). Since 1969 meningococci of serogroup C have replaced those of serogroup B as the most frequent cause of disease in the United States. In the years 1972, 1973 and 1974 the percentage of these organisms resistant to sulphonamides were 82·3, 74·4 and 68·9, respectively (Jacobson *et al.*, 1975). In 1975, serogroup B again became the most prevalent serogroup in the United States and although only 4 per cent of these were sulphonamide resistant, 27 per cent of all isolates were resistant (Center for Disease Control, 1976).

Meningococci resistant to sulphonamides have been reported from Norway (Holten *et al.*, 1969; 1970), where in 1974–1975 an epidemic mainly due to serogroup B occurred, in which 94 per cent of strains tested had an MIC of $\geqslant$50 μg per ml and 88 per cent an MIC of $\geqslant$100 μg per ml (Bøvre *et al.*, 1977). Resistant strains have also been found in Sweden (Holmgren and Tunevall, 1973) and Africa (Wright and Plorde, 1970). In the Helsinki area of Finland during 1973–1974, an epidemic due to sulphonamide-resistant serogroup B strains occurred (Salmi *et al.*, 1976). In 1971 a large urban epidemic of meningococcal disease began in Saõ Paulo, Brazil, which was due to sulphonamide-resistant serogroup C strains (de Morais *et al.*, 1974). Resistant strains have been reported in the United Kingdom (WHO, 1971; 1974; Abbott and Graves, 1972; Leading article, 1974a) and the percentage of strains resistant rose from 6 in 1974 to 11 in 1975 and 13 per cent in 1976 (Epidemiology, 1977). During 1977 in England and Wales, serogroup B organisms predominated, especially in children and 7 per cent of strains tested were resistant to sulphonamides; serogroup A strains were more common in adults and 45 per cent of these which were tested were sulphonamide-resistant (WHO, 1978). In Melbourne, during the period from June 1967 to June 1977, 60 clinical isolates from patients at Fairfield

Hospital have been tested for sulphadizine sensitivity. Twenty-five of these strains were resistant to sulphadiazine in a concentration of 0·1 mg per cent (1 μg per ml), 9 of these 25 were also resistant to 1·0 mg per cent (10 μg per ml), and 2 were also resistant to 10 mg per cent (100 μg per ml).

9. *Bacterial sensitivity testing.* In clinical practice usually only one of the sulphonamides is used for these tests, and the results obtained are generally applicable to the others. The relative antibacterial activity of the various sulphonamides against the 'sensitive bacteria' varies to some extent. Of the commonly used short-acting sulphonamides, sulphadiazine appears to have the highest activity against most bacteria. The more recently introduced long-acting sulphonamides are said to have higher *in vitro* activity against Gram-positive cocci than the older compounds. These differences do not appear to have any practical significance. Garrod *et al.* (1973) tested the *in vitro* activity of the sulphonamides in current use, and concluded 'that there is very little indeed to choose between the antibacterial activities of the more potent sulphonamides'. In this investigation all tests were carried out under standard conditions. The results of *in vitro* tests obtained by different authors with the sulphonamides are often not comparable, because the findings are greatly influenced by the use of different media and techniques.

10. *Synergy with other drugs.* Sulphonamides potentiate the action of (or act synergistically with) other chemotherapeutic substances against certain pathogens. They may potentiate the action of the polymyxins against Ps. aeruginosa, Proteus spp. and Serratia marcescens (page 532), and their strong synergistic effect with trimethoprim on many bacteria is now well known (page 691). Similarly the sulphonamides potentiate the action of pyrimethamine ('Daraprim') on malarial parasites (McGregor *et al.*, 1963) (*see* page 700).

In Vitro Sensitivities

These vary according to the methods and media used for their estimation, and there are also variations between individual sulphonamides. Table 42 (page 693) shows the minimum inhibitory concentrations of sulphadiazine and sulphamethoxazole compared to trimethoprim.

Mode of Administration and Dosage

The sulphonamides are usually administered by mouth.

1. *Short-acting sulphonamides.* The usual adult oral dose of members of this group, such as sulphadiazine, sulphadimidine, sulphafurazole or triple sulphonamides is 2–3 g initially, followed by 1 g six-hourly. A dose of 0·5 to 1·0 g daily may be sufficient for long-term 'suppressive therapy' in chronic urinary tract infections.

The recommended doses for children are summarized in Table 41. Doses of up to 150 mg per kg per day can be used in children with severe infections.

Sulphamethizole ('Urolucosil') is the only compound of this group which was used in smaller doses, such as 100 to 200 mg six-hourly for adults, but now a dose of 1·0 g eight-hourly is recommended.

A parenteral preparation of sodium sulphadimidine is available as a 33·3

TABLE 41

Age	Initial dose	Six-hourly maintenance dose
6 months	0·5 g	0·25 g
1/2–4 years	1·0 g	0·50 g
5–7 years	1·5 g	0·50–0·75 g
8–12 years	2·0 g	0·75–1·0 g

per cent solution, marketed in 1 g (3 ml) ampoules. This can be administered intramuscularly or intravenously in similar doses to those recommended for oral administration. For severe infections 3–4·5 g can be given immediately, and then 1–2 g every 6 h. Intramuscular injections of this drug should be given deeply because this solution is irritating to tissues.

If intravenous administration is used, it is preferable to slowly inject the dose directly into the drip tubing every 6 h. This preparation should never be given intrathecally.

A parenteral preparation of sodium sulphadiazine (1 g in 4 ml) is also available, and is used in a similar dosage to parenteral sulphadimidine.

2. *Medium-acting sulphonamides.* The adult oral dose of sulphamethoxazole ('Gantanol') is 2 g initially, followed by 1 g twelve-hourly.

3. *Long-acting sulphonamides.* The usual oral adult doses of these compounds are as follows:

(a) *Sulphamethoxypyridazine* (*'Lederkyn', 'Midicel'*). 1 g initially, followed by 0·5 g daily.
(b) *Sulphadimethoxine* (*'Madribon'*). 1–2 g initially, followed by 0·5 to 1·0 g daily.
(c) *Sulphaphenazole* (*'Orisul'*). Initial dose 1 g twelve-hourly for one to two days, followed by 0·5 g twelve-hourly.
(d) *Sulphamethoxydiazine* (*'Durenate', 'Bayrena' or 'Kirocid'*). Initial dose 1–2 g followed by 0·5 g daily.
(e) *Sulphasymazine* (*'Prosul'*). Initial dose 1·0 g, followed by 0·5 g once or twice-daily.

4. *Ultra-long-acting sulphonamides.*

(a) *Sulfadoxine* (*'Fanasil'*). This compound is available as 200 mg and 0·5 g tablets and also as a solution for injection (1 g in 4 ml). The adult dose is 1–2 g once-weekly.
(b) *Sulfametopyrazine* (*sulfalene, 'Kelfizine'*). The usual adult oral dose is 2 g once a week.

5. *The poorly absorbed sulphonamides* (*sulphaguanidine, succinylsulphathiazole and phthalylsulphathiazole*). The adult oral dose of these drugs is 5–20 g daily given in four divided doses.

6. *Sulphasalazine* (*'Salazopyrin'*). The adult dose used for ulcerative colitis, is 1–2 g four- to six-hourly.

7. *Patients with renal failure.* It is difficult to formulate dosage schedules for these patients, as individual sulphonamides are excreted by different renal

mechanisms and at different rates. Williams *et al.* (1968) found that a fall of glomerular filtration rate did not significantly affect the renal clearance of sodium sulphadimidine, and concluded that this drug could be used in ordinary doses even in patients with terminal renal failure. They also noted that, in most uraemic patients, adequate urine concentrations of this drug were attained for the treatment of urinary tract infections. However these findings are at variance with those by most other investigators. Fischer (1972) observed the sulphadimidine clearance in uraemic patients to be significantly lower than that in patients with normal renal function. Also Adam and Dawborn (1970) and Adam *et al.* (1973) in studies on sulphadiazine, sulphamethizole and sulphadimidine found that with moderate doses both the free drugs and their conjugated derivatives accumulated in the plasma of uraemic patients. In some patients the high serum levels appeared to cause side-effects. Furthermore they showed that the urine concentration of free sulphonamides was low in uraemic patients. These authors concluded that sulphonamides are unlikely to be useful for the treatment of urinary tract infections in patients with serum creatinine levels exceeding 5 mg per cent ($0\cdot4$ mmol/l), and that for patients with lesser degrees of renal failure a reduced sulphonamide dose may be required to avoid toxicity. In addition sulphonamides such as sulphafurazole or sulphamethoxazole, which have lower inhibitory concentrations for common urinary pathogens, and are less readily conjugated, may be preferable to sulphadimidine for the treatment of urinary tract infections in uraemic patients (Adam *et al.*, 1973).

For treatment of systemic infections, the sulphonamides can probably be safely used in most patients with renal disease, but regular estimations of the serum concentrations of both free and acetylated sulphonamide seem advisable. The various sulphonamides are handled by the kidney in different ways (*see* excretion, page 666), and the rate of acetylation of sulphonamides in the body varies in individual patients. For these reasons in some uraemic patients it may be impossible to select a dose which will give adequate serum levels of the free active drug, yet not lead to accumulation of toxic levels of the acetylated compounds. The relationship between toxicity and serum levels in the case of the sulphonamides is not well defined, but some patients with a total serum level of greater than 10 mg per 100 ml show toxic effects (Adam and Dawborn, 1970).

8. *Newborn and premature infants.* The sulphonamides are contraindicated in these patients (*see* toxicity, page 670).

9. *Intraperitoneal administration.* Sulphadimidine, in a concentration of 100 μg per ml, has been administered intraperitoneally during peritoneal dialysis for four to five days without any adverse effects (Adam *et al.*, 1973).

Availability

Nearly all the sulphonamides are available as $0\cdot5$ g tablets. Sulphamethizole ('Urolucosil') is also marketed in 100 mg and 250 mg tablets and sulfadoxine ('Fanasil') is also available as 200 mg tablets. Sulfametopyrazine ('Kelfizine') is available only as 200 mg and 2 g tablets. Most of these drugs are also marketed as oral suspensions for administration to children. The parenteral preparations available have already been described.

Serum Levels in Relation to Dosage

1. All the sulphonamides, except sulphaguanidine and the other two compounds of that group (page 659) are well absorbed after oral administration. After absorption these drugs are partly conjugated with acetate in the liver, and the proportion conjugated varies with different sulphonamides. Sulphonamide conjugates are inactive therapeutically. Serum levels of sulphonamides are usually estimated by a colorimetric method (Bratton and Marshall, 1939), which enables the measurement of either the total sulphonamide level or the free active (unconjugated) drug level.

2. About 60 per cent of sulphadimidine is present in the serum in an active free form after usual therapeutic doses. Following a single oral dose of 4 g of this drug, a peak free drug serum concentration of 8–10 mg per 100 ml (80–100 μg per ml) is attained after 2–3 h (Fig. 32). This serum level falls rapidly, and the serum half-life of this drug is about 2–3 h. Therapeutic levels can be maintained by using an oral dose of 1 g six-hourly. Serum levels after parenteral administration are similar, but the peak concentration is achieved more rapidly.

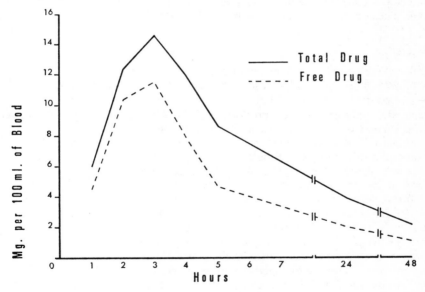

FIG. 32. Average free and total sulphadimidine serum concentrations after single oral dose of 4 g in adults. (Redrawn after Bullowa and Ratish, 1944.)

Other short-acting sulphonamides are also well absorbed after oral administration, but differ from sulphadimidine in both the serum levels attained and in the proportion of drug acetylated. Thus after a 4 g oral dose of sulphadiazine to adults, the peak free drug level is lower (40–60 μg per ml), but about 90–95 per cent of this drug is in the active form (Bullowa and Ratish, 1944).

3. The medium-acting sulphonamide sulphamethoxazole is also well ab-

sorbed (*see* Fig. 34, page 697). The peak serum levels are similar to those obtained with an identical dose of sulphadimidine, and 75–85 per cent exists in serum in a free non-acetylated form. In addition the serum levels of this drug are more prolonged, because it is more slowly excreted by the kidneys (*see* page 658).

4. The long-acting sulphonamides also give high serum levels after oral administration. After a single oral dose of 4 g of sulphamethoxypyridazine ('Lederkyn') to adults, peak total serum levels of 110–118 μg per ml are attained at 5 h, and these are maintained for the next 3 h. Very little acetylation of this drug occurs during the first 3 h after administration, but subsequently about 5–22 per cent becomes acetylated. Total serum levels of 20–50 μg per ml are still detectable 105 h later (Weinstein *et al.*, 1960).

After administration of a 2 g dose of sulphadimethoxine ('Madribon') to adults, a total drug level of 50–70 μg per ml is attained in 2 h, and this is maintained for 24 h. With an initial dose of 2 g followed by 1·0 g daily in adults, serum levels are maintained between 50–100 μg per ml.

5. The ultra-long-acting sulphonamides—sulfadoxine ('Fanasil'), and sulfametopyrazine ('Kelfizine') also give high serum levels after oral administration. The serum half-life of the former is 150–200 h, and the latter about 65 h.

Excretion

URINE: Free and conjugated sulphonamides are excreted mainly via the kidney. About 73–85 per cent of an orally administered dose of sulphadimidine can be recovered from the urine, but because individuals vary in their ability to acetylate sulphonamides, the proportion of this which is in a free unconjugated form varies from 15–70 per cent (Bullowa and Ratish, 1944).

Sulphonamides and their acetylated conjugates are excreted both by glomerular filtration and tubular secretion. Some of the drug secreted by tubules is again reabsorbed. Different sulphonamides and their conjugates are handled by the kidney in different ways. Some compounds such as sulphafurazole are rapidly excreted in urine where high concentrations are attained. By contrast the excretion of the long-acting sulphonamides is slow, so that their serum levels are maintained for long periods, and only low concentrations are attained in urine. The long-acting sulphonamides are more extensively bound to serum proteins, and the bound fraction is not excreted through the glomeruli. This factor together with more complete tubular reabsorption is responsible for the maintenance of prolonged serum levels of the long-acting sulphonamides (Newbould and Kilpatrick, 1960).

The pH of the urine influences the renal clearance of all sulphonamides. Sulphonamide clearance is increased in the presence of alkaline urine (Williams *et al.*, 1968), apparently because there is less tubular reabsorption (Nanra *et al.*, 1969). This effect is pronounced with the newer long-acting sulphonamide, sulphasymazine. Furthermore all the sulphonamides and their acetylated conjugates are more soluble in alkaline urine. The solubility in urine of the various sulphonamides and their conjugates varies considerably. Sulphadimidine and its acetylated form are very soluble compared to other sulphonamides, such as sulphadiazine.

BILE: Only small amounts of the sulphonamides are excreted via the biliary tract, and they are not concentrated in bile.

INACTIVATION IN BODY: A percentage of the absorbed sulphonamide is acetylated in the liver, producing inactive conjugates. Individuals vary in their capacity to acetylate sulphonamides. Active acetylators of sulphadimidine also rapidly inactivate isoniazid and *vice versa*, because a similar enzyme is involved in the processing of both of these drugs. If a patient is given a test dose of sulphadimidine, and the proportion of acetylated drug is less than 25 per cent in the serum or less than 70 per cent in the urine, he may be considered to be a slow sulphonamide acetylator and will also usually be a slow isoniazid inactivator (Rao *et al.*, 1970) (*see also* page 804).

Some of the sulphonamides are also converted to inactive metabolites in the liver by glucuronidation. This process is particularly marked with sulphadimethoxine, and about 80 per cent of this drug is excreted as a very soluble glucuronide in the urine (Busch and Lane, 1967).

Distribution of the Drugs in Body

1. After absorption the sulphonamides become widely distributed throughout the body. The short-acting sulphonamides, especially sulphadiazine, readily penetrate into the normal cerebrospinal fluid, where this drug may attain a concentration of about half that present in the serum at the time. The drugs also penetrate the aqueous humour of the eye, and cross the placenta, fetal serum concentrations reaching about half of those found in the maternal blood at the time. High concentrations also occur in saliva.

2. All the sulphonamides are bound to serum albumin, but the degree varies with different sulphonamides. Sulphadiazine is only about 20 per cent protein bound, but most other short-acting sulphonamides such as sulphadimidine and sulphafurazole are 40–80 per cent bound. The medium-acting sulphonamide, sulphamethoxazole, is about 65 per cent protein bound. The long-acting sulphonamides are more highly bound to serum proteins, sulphamethoxypyridazine and sulphadimethoxine being about 90 per cent protein bound, but sulphamethoxydiazine is only about 75 per cent bound. The percentage of each sulphonamide bound to serum proteins is not constant, and similar to the antibiotics (page 86), decreases as the total serum concentration of the drug increases.

The degree of sulphonamide protein binding influences the rate of renal excretion of these drugs (*see* page 666). The protein bound drug does not penetrate into some body compartments such as the subarachnoid space, but this may not apply if the meninges are inflamed. It is not yet clear whether a high degree of protein binding helps or prevents the sulphonamides to penetrate into inflammatory exudates (*Today's Drugs*, 1968). Newbould and Kilpatrick (1960) considered that protein bound sulphonamide has no antibacterial activity, and therefore higher total serum levels of the newer long-acting highly protein bound sulphonamides are required to obtain comparable diffusible concentrations and an equivalent therapeutic effect. Madsen *et al.* (1963) compared the sulphonamide concentration and antibacterial activity in serum of two long-acting sulphonamides, sulphadimethoxine and sulphamethoxypyridazine, with sulphadiazine. These authors found that these three sulphonamides all produced about the same antibacterial activity in the serum. In all of their experiments there was a close correlation between the total sulphonamide concentration and the antibacterial activity regardless of the degree of protein binding. The highly protein bound long-acting sulphonamides also penetrated well into extravascular fluids and exudates, particularly when these were of a high protein content.

Mode of Action

Folic acid derivatives are essential for purine and ultimately DNA synthesis in both humans and bacteria. Bacterial cells appear to be impermeable to folic acid, and synthetize it from para-amino-benzoic acid, whereas humans absorb preformed folic acid from their diet. The sulphonamides, being structurally related to para-amino-benzoic acid, act by competitive blocking of the enzyme dihydrofolic acid synthetase, necessary for the conversion of para-amino-benzoic acid to dihydrofolic acid (*see* trimethoprim, page 700). Their action on the malaria parasites is similar. Sulphonamide resistance probably occurs because mutants arise, which are either capable of over-production of para-amino-benzoic acid, or develop a structural change in the enzyme dihydrofolic acid synthetase, giving it a lowered affinity for sulphonamides.

Toxicity

1. *Nausea, vomiting and diarrhoea.* These side-effects were common with earlier compounds such as sulphapyridine, but are uncommon with the newer sulphonamides.

2. *Headache and dizziness* similarly were common with the older sulphonamides, but are rare with the newer compounds.

3. *Drug fever.* This was also frequent with the earlier sulphonamides, but is rare with commonly used short-acting sulphonamides such as sulphadimidine and sulphafurazole. Drug fever has been occasionally observed with the long-acting sulphonamide, sulphamethoxypyridazine (Grieble and Jackson, 1958).

4. *Hypersensitivity reactions.* Allergic rashes are fairly frequent complications of sulphonamide therapy. Similar to the penicillins, these usually occur after one week's treatment, but may appear earlier with prior sulphonamide sensitization. The most common types of rashes are maculopapular or urticarial, but erythema nodosum, exfoliative dermatitis or rarely Stevens–Johnson syndrome may occur. Photosensitivity can also result. These rashes may be accompanied by features of a 'serum sickness-like illness' such as fever and joint pains.

Erythema multiforme exudativum or Stevens–Johnson syndrome is the most serious form of hypersensitivity reaction to sulphonamides. In its most extensive form this syndrome consists of erythema multiforme, and ulceration of the mucous membranes of the eyes, mouth and urethra, which can be very severe and sometimes fatal. This complication has been described in association with all sulphonamides, but the long-acting ones, sulphamethoxypyridazine and sulphadimethoxine, have been particularly implicated (Salvaggio and Gonzalez, 1959; Rallison *et al.*, 1961; Claxton, 1963). The United States Food and Drug Administration collected reports of 116 cases of Stevens–Johnson syndrome associated with long-acting sulphonamide administration from 1957 to 1965 from all parts of the world (Carroll *et al.*, 1966). This series included 79 children with 20 deaths and 37 adults with 9 deaths. The median time of appearance of this complication was about the tenth day of treatment. Only one patient was known to be rechallenged with the sulphonamide, and Stevens–Johnson syndrome promptly recurred. It was estimated that there had been about one or two cases reported for every 10 million doses of these drugs which had been distributed. This report suggested that this syndrome may be more common in children. Nine cases of Stevens–Johnson syndrome in children with three fatalities were reported from one Sydney hospital during the period 1962–1964 (Beveridge *et al.*, 1964). During the years 1950 to 1968 inclusive, 106 patients with Stevens–Johnson syndrome have been admitted to Fairfield hospital, Melbourne. Fifty-eight of these patients (55 per cent) were aged less than 14 years. In 32 patients (30 per cent) the disease was associated with prior sulphonamide administration, and in 11 of these one of the long-acting sulphonamides was implicated. Corticosteroids are successful in the treatment of many of the severe cases.

The risk of Stevens–Johnson syndrome appears to be the main reason why the long-acting sulphonamides have not become more popular for general use (Annotation, 1967; Pryles, 1970). Some authors have used these compounds extensively for the treatment of urinary tract infections, but have not encountered this complication (Brumfitt, 1970). Drugs other than sulphonamides may also cause this syndrome, and in addition there is evidence to suggest that the underlying infection for which the drugs are given, may sometimes be responsible for Stevens–Johnson syndrome. A variety of infectious agents such as Mycoplasma pneumoniae (Ludlam *et al.*, 1964) and Herpesvirus hominis (Ström, 1969) have an aetiological role in this syndrome. However the aetiological role of the sulphonamides is beyond doubt in many cases. Ström (1962) used provocative tests with suspected drugs (sulphonamides and others) in 29 patients who had had Stevens–Johnson syndrome, and obtained positive reactions in nineteen.

A generalized hypersensitivity reaction has been described in one young man after a three-week course (60 g) of sulphasalazine (Mihas *et al.*, 1978). This resulted in fever, skin rash, arthralgia, lymphadenopathy and hepatitis, and it was accompanied by decreased complement levels and circulating immune complexes.

Hypersensitivity manifestations following topical sulphonamide therapy are common, and this form of treatment is now only rarely used. Stevens–Johnson syndrome has been described following the use of sulphonamide eye drops (Gottschalk and Stone, 1976).

There is usually cross-allergy between all the sulphonamides, and it is unwise to administer any sulphonamide to a patient with a previous history of allergy to one of these drugs. There are no satisfactory tests available for sulphonamide allergy.

5. *Systemic lupus erythematosus and polyarteritis nodosa.* Systemic lupus has been observed in patients receiving sulphonamides, particularly the long-acting drugs (Rallison *et al.*, 1961; Alarćon–Segovia, 1969). A lupus-like syndrome has been reported in a patient with ulcerative colitis who was treated with sulphasalazine (Griffiths and Kane, 1977). Polyarteritis nodosa has also been reported in patients who had received sulphonamides, but their

aetiological role in this disease has not been clearly established (Rose and Spencer, 1957).

6. *Blood dyscrasias*. These are important complications of sulphonamide therapy. The most common manifestation is acute agranulocytosis; aplastic anaemia, haemolytic anaemia, megaloblastic anaemia and thrombocytopenia also have been described.

Agranulocytosis was apparently fairly common with the older sulphonamides, such as sulphapyridine, but is rare with the currently used drugs. It is reversible and recovery usually occurs within one week after stopping the drug, provided that supervening septicaemia can be controlled. The compound of sulphapyridine and salicyclic acid (sulphasalazine) is absorbed, and acute agranulocytosis due to this drug has been reported in two patients, both of whom died with septicaemia (Thirkettle *et al.*, 1963).

Fatal aplastic anaemia has been attributed to sulphonamides, but less commonly than aplastic anaemia due to chloramphenicol.

Acute haemolytic anaemia is another rare complication, and is sometimes due to prior sensitization to sulphonamides (Weinstein *et al.*, 1960). In addition these drugs can induce haemolysis in patients with glucose-6-phosphate dehydrogenase deficient red cells, producing a 'Heinz body anaemia' with intravascular haemolysis and haemoglobinuria. This type of anaemia may also occur in the fetus or premature infant whose red cells are normally deficient in glucose-6-phosphate dehydrogenase (*Today's Drugs*, 1968).

Megaloblastic anaemia responding to therapy with folic acid has been described in two patients with ulcerative colitis, who were being treated with sulphasalazine (Schneider and Beeley, 1977; Kane and Boots, 1977).

Thrombocytopenia alone is a rare complication of sulphonamide therapy (Weinstein *et al.*, 1960). In one case induced by sulfisoxazole an immune mechanism was demonstrated (Hamilton and Sheets, 1978). The patient was a farmer who presumably had become sensitized by drinking cow's milk contaminated by sulphonamides. Thrombocytopenia recurred with a small challenge dose of sulfisoxazole and a serum factor was detected which caused platelet agglutination in the presence of sulfisoxazole.

Cyanosis due to the formation of either methaemoglobin or sulphaemoglobin was fairly common with the earlier sulphonamides, but is now rare with the currently used compounds (*Today's Drugs*, 1964).

7. *Jaundice and kernicterus in the newborn*. Sulphonamides compete with a number of substances, including bilirubin, for albumin binding sites (Odell, 1959). For this reason infants, born to mothers treated with sulphonamides, may develop jaundice with high free serum bilirubin levels or even kernicterus, especially if there is also increased haemolysis (Leading article, 1968). This may also occur in newborn or premature infants treated with sulphonamides. To avoid this complication sulphonamides should not be given to pregnant women near term or to newborn or premature infants. The administration of the long-acting sulphonamides to women near term has an added danger because they give prolonged blood levels, which may persist in the baby, despite cessation of the drug at the onset of labour.

8. *Hepatotoxicity*. Dujovne *et al.* (1967) reported a patient who developed hepatocellular jaundice after a second course of sulphamethoxazole. The serum transaminase was raised and liver biopsy revealed areas of liver cell necrosis.

An associated eosinophilia suggested a hypersensitivity mechanism. Liver damage reappeared with a further test dose of sulphonamide and the authors noted that the phenomenon had occurred in two other reported cases. Dujovne *et al.* (1967) also reviewed 106 cases of sulphonamide hepatotoxicity reported during the preceding 30 years. The majority of these had occurred before 1947, which is probably a reflection of the greater hepatotoxicity of the older sulphonamides.

9. *Renal damage.* Crystalluria causing renal damage is the 'classical sulphonamide complication' which was common with earlier sulphonamides such as sulphapyridine, because these drugs are excreted in urine in high concentrations, in which the drugs themselves and their acetyl conjugates are relatively insoluble (Lehr, 1957). Crystalluria may cause pain and haematuria, and anuria can occur if the renal pelvis or the ureters become completely occluded. A high fluid intake and alkalinization of urine minimizes this side-effect. The currently used short-acting sulphonamides such as sulphadimidine and sulphafurazole and their acetyl conjugates are very soluble in urine. However crystalluria may occur with sulphadiazine, which is still in current use, and therefore it is important to maintain a high fluid intake and alkalinize the urine when this drug is used. Craft *et al.* (1977) reported a three-year-old girl who developed acute renal failure and also hypoglycaemia whilst receiving treatment with an excessively high dose of sulphadiazine for meningococcal septicaemia. The medium- and long-acting sulphonamides, which being slowly excreted, do not attain high concentrations in the urine, rarely cause crystalluria. However Buchanan (1978) reported two patients who developed crystalluria and oliguric renal failure following intravenous co-trimoxazole (page 696) therapy. The medium-acting sulphonamide, sulphamethoxazole, is a component of co-trimoxazole. Both these patients were hypoproteinaemic and most of the sulphamethoxazole in their serum was in the free rather than protein bound form. It was therefore postulated that crystalluria ensued secondary to the massive renal load of the free drug. The author recommends that co-trimoxazole should be used with caution in hypoalbuminaemic patients.

Hypersensitivity reactions due to sulphonamide therapy may cause renal damage as may sulphonamide-induced haemolysis and haemoglobinuria (Appel and Neu, 1977). The nephrotic syndrome has been described following topical silver sulphadiazine therapy (Owens *et al.*, 1974). Renal damage may also occur in association with co-trimoxazole administration (*see* pages 696, 704).

10. *Cardiomyopathy*, apparently due to sulphonamide hypersensitivity, has been reported in a twelve-year-old African boy (MacSearraigh and Patel, 1968). A few other cases of apparent sulphonamide induced 'hypersensitivity myocarditis' have been previously reported (Weinstein *et al.*, 1960).

11. *Pulmonary reactions.* These occur in association with the use of a variety of drugs, including sulphonamides (*Brit. med. J.*, Leading article, 1969), but the sulphonamide-induced type is rare (Tydd and Dyer, 1976). An acute syndrome (pulmonary eosinophilia) usually results, which is characterized by fever, dyspnoea, cough, eosinophilia and patchy radiological pulmonary opacties. Symptoms and radiological abnormalities rapidly disappear when the drug is stopped. Sulphasalazine, in addition to this acute syndrome, may produce fibrosing alveolitis or a bronchial asthmatic reaction. Salicylates can also cause

pulmonary reactions, and either the salicyclic acid or the sulphonamide component of sulphasalazine may be responsible. The abnormalities again usually disappear when sulphasalazine is stopped (Leading article, 1974b).

12. *Teratogenicity*. Several sulphonamides can cause fetal abnormalities in experimental animals (Leading article, 1965), but sulphonamide teratogenicity has not been observed in humans.

13. *Miscellaneous reactions*. Other rare side-effects have been described following sulphonamide administration. These include hypothyroidism and disturbances of the nervous system such as drowsiness, fatigue, insomnia, nightmares, confusion, depression, vertigo, ataxia, peripheral neuritis and acute psychosis (Weinstein *et al.*, 1960). Benign intracranial hypertension has also been observed to follow sulphamethoxazole administration in two patients (Ch'ien, 1970). Lisander (1970) reported a patient who on three occasions developed intense myalgia in the arms and legs following the administration of sulphamethoxydiazine. Another patient developed recurrent fever, meningitis, pancreatitis and a leucocytosis in association with administration and readministration of sulphamethizole (Barrett and Thier, 1963). Sulphonamides decrease the ability of human neutrophils to kill certain Candida spp. and some bacteria, but whether this is of any significance even in patients susceptible to systemic candidiasis, is unknown (Lehrer, 1971).

14. *Drug interactions*. Christensen *et al.* (1963) reported hypoglycaemic attacks in several diabetic patients who were treated by both tolbutamide and sulphaphenazole. These patients had greatly increased serum tolbutamide levels, and it appeared that sulphaphenazole interfered with oxidation and excretion of tolbutamide. The metabolism by liver microsomal enzymes of other drugs such as diphenylhydantoin (phenytoin) and warfarin (and tolbutamide) are inhibited by usual therapeutic doses of sulphaphenazole, sulphadiazine and sulphamethizole. Co-trimoxazole also increases the diphenylhydantoin half-life in patients by decreasing its metabolism (Hansen *et al.*, 1975). By contrast, sulphadimethoxine, sulphamethoxypyridazine and sulphamethoxydiazine do not affect phenytoin metabolism.

Barnett and Hancock (1975) described one case in which co-trimoxazole (page 706) potentiated warfarin by apparently inhibiting its metabolism. Hassall *et al.* (1975) detected six patients in whom potentiation of warfarin occurred two to six days after commencement of co-trimoxazole therapy. One of these patients had a gastro-intestinal haemorrhage requiring intravenous vitamin K_1 therapy, whilst in the others the thrombin ratio was corrected by either reducing the warfarin dosage or withdrawing it for several days. In two of these patients serum warfarin levels were low; this suggested that sulphamethoxazole may displace protein bound warfarin, thus increasing both its intrinsic action and its rate of metabolism and excretion. Circumstances in another case also suggested that co-trimoxazole may interact with warfarin by displacing it from its plasma albumin binding sites (Tilstone *et al.*, 1977). These authors considered that co-trimoxazole was not contraindicated in patients receiving warfarin, because this interaction is only likely to occur in patients receiving high warfarin doses and who have low plasma albumin concentrations. Whatever the mechanism involved it is obvious that co-trimoxazole may on occasions potentiate the action of warfarin.

Clinical Uses of the Drugs

There are now very few specific indications for sulphonamide therapy because of the wide range of available antibiotics. The emergence of sulphonamide resistance among many bacterial species has also made these drugs unsuitable for the treatment of many diseases, for which they have been successfully used in the past. The combination of sulphonamides with trimethoprim however is highly effective in many diseases (page 706). This section describes the clinical uses of the sulphonamides alone, or their use in combination with drugs other than trimethoprim.

1. *Urinary tract infections*. The sulphonamides alone are often successful for treatment of acute uncomplicated urinary tract infections. They are still extensively used to treat such infections in domiciliary practice, because of their cheapness (Brumfitt, 1970). The ultra-long-acting sulphonamide sulfametopyrazine has been used as a single dose of 2 g and as two 2 g doses given four days apart, to treat bacteriuria in pregnancy (Reeves, 1975). Results in terms of cure rate were not superior to that obtained with other agents when the organism was sensitive to sulphonamides, but side-effects with this drug were infrequent. Lidin-Janson (1977) also used sulfametopyrazine to treat Esch. coli urinary tract infections in non-pregnant women; a loading dose of 0·4 g was given which was followed by 0·1 g daily for 21 days. This was compared to conventional treatment with the short-acting sulphonamide, sulphasomidine. Both regimens were effective for simple cystitis caused by sulphonamide-sensitive organisms, but both also favoured selection of sulphonamide-resistant Esch. coli strains in faecal flora (*see also* page 707). In a prospective study in young women, Sellin *et al.* (1975) found that novobiocin-resistant micrococci (Staph. saprophyticus) were the second commonest cause after Esch. coli of acute urinary infections; these infections all responded to treatment with sulphadimidine but the organisms persisted and were responsible for clinical relapse in two of seven patients. Sulphonamides are not usually effective in chronic and recurrent infections or in hospital acquired infections.

2. *Respiratory tract infections*. The role of sulphonamides for these infections is controversial (Camp, 1969). These drugs have been used for treatment of Strep. pyogenes throat infections (Nunnelly, 1960; Alban, 1965). Penicillin G remains the drug of choice for these infections, and safe effective alternative antibiotics are available for penicillin-allergic patients. In one controlled trial, sulfisoxazole suspension in a dose of 0·5 g twice-daily was effective in the prevention of recurrent otitis media in children (Perrin *et al.*, 1974). Sulphonamides have been used for treatment of pneumococcal pneumonia and other lower respiratory tract bacterial infections, but safer and more effective chemotherapeutic agents are available.

3. *Rheumatic fever chemoprophylaxis*. Sulphonamides have been used for this purpose as alternatives to penicillin for penicillin-allergic patients. Nowadays erythromycin (page 507) is probably a better alternative. Nevertheless the American Heart Association has recommended sulphadiazine 1 g daily as an alternative to penicillin (page 60) for this purpose (Leading article, 1977b). Sulphonamides may be unreliable, because sulphonamide-resistant Strep. pyogenes strains can emerge.

4. *Meningococcal infections*. Formerly the sulphonamides were extensively and successfully used for the treatment of meningococcal meningitis and septicaemia, for prevention of meningococcal disease in contacts, and for eradication of the chronic meningococcal carrier state. Sulphonamide-resistant meningococci are still common (page 661), and these drugs are usually no longer suitable for these clinical situations. There is currently no problem in the treatment of meningococcal disease, because ampicillin, chloramphenicol and especially penicillin G are very effective for these infections. The use of parenteral penicillin G is also probably effective for the prevention of meningococcal disease in contacts, but oral phenoxypenicillin may be ineffective for this purpose (Holten *et al.*, 1970). However, none of the currently available antibiotics, except perhaps rifampicin (page 573) or minocycline (page 628), are as effective in eradicating the nasopharyngeal meningococcal carrier state as the sulphonamides were in the past (Leedom *et al.*, 1965; 1967; Holten *et al.*, 1970). Rifampicin is currently recommended as the chemoprophylactic agent of choice for meningococcal infections in the United States (*see* page 573). However in some circumstances, such as the localised epidemic of serogroup B sulphonamide-sensitive meningococcal disease which occurred in Alabama during 1975–1976, chemoprophylaxis with sulphonamides has been used with effect (Jacobson *et al.*, 1977). In the United Kingdom, where the incidence of sulphonamide-resistant meningococci is of the order of 10–15 per cent, treatment with sulphadiazine in full dosage for 24 h has still been recommended for chemoprophylaxis (Leading article, 1974c).

5. *Bacterial meningitis other than meningococcal*. Although the sulphonamides have been combined with chloramphenicol for the treatment of H. influenzae meningitis, and occasionally with penicillin G for the treatment of pneumococcal meningitis, there is no evidence that the sulphonamide contributes to the therapeutic success of such treatment. Sulfisoxazole has been used with streptomycin to treat H. influenzae meningitis successfully (*see* page 303).

6. *Intestinal infections*. Both the non-absorbed sulphonamides such as sulphaguanidine and the well absorbed short-acting sulphonamides (e.g. sulphadiazine or sulphadimidine) have been used extensively in the past for treatment of shigella dysentery. These drugs are no longer useful for this disease, because most strains of Shigella spp. are now sulphonamide-resistant (page 660). There is considerable doubt whether any chemotherapeutic substance shortens the clinical illness or eradicates the carrier state in Sh. sonnei infections (page 413). Shigella flexneri dysentery, which is often more severe, may be helped by chemotherapy, and sulphonamides can be useful, provided the organism is sensitive (Kerr Grant *et al.*, 1969). The sulphonamides have never been useful for treatment of salmonellosis.

The long-acting sulphonamide sulfadoxine in a single oral dose of 0·5–2·0 g (according to the patient's age) has been compared to treatment with oral tetracycline 0·25–0·5 g (according to age) 12-hourly for three days for reducing transmission of cholera infection among contacts of cholera patients (Deb *et al.*, 1976). Tetracycline was effective in significantly reducing the number of infections from the second to the sixth day, while sulfadoxine was effective from the third to the sixth day after treatment.

7. *Chemoprophylaxis in abdominal surgery.* The poorly absorbed sulphonamides have been used for this purpose. Nowadays other agents are preferred, such as gentamicin (page 345), clindamycin (page 485) and metronidazole (page 774).

8. *Chlamydial infections.* Various serotypes of Chlamydia trachomatis are the aetiological agents of trachoma, paratrachoma, genital infection and lymphogranuloma venereum. Hyperendemic trachoma is transmitted from eye to eye and paratrachoma is transmitted sexually. Paratrachoma includes TRIC ophthalmia neonatorum, inclusion conjunctivitis, TRIC punctate keratoconjunctivitis and endemic trachoma, which are all usually transmitted from the genital tract to the eye (Leading article, 1977a). For treatment of trachoma, topical tetracycline (page 626) or rifampicin eye ointment (page 574) three times a day for five or six weeks is usually preferred to topical sulphonamides. Systemic therapy is necessary in paratrachoma to encompass the associated genital infection; tetracycline 1 g daily, doxycycline 100 mg daily (page 626) or 2–3 g daily of a short-acting sulphonamide, all administered for three weeks, are recommended (Leading article, 1977a). Both Chlamydia trachomatis and Ureaplasma urealyticum (T-strain Mycoplasma) are important causes of non-specific (non-gonococcal) urethritis. Bowie *et al.* (1976) showed that non-gonococcal urethritis caused by C. trachomatis responds better to sulphafurazole than that due to U. urealyticum, for which sulphonamides are relatively inactive. Conversely, non-gonococcal urethritis due to U. urealyticum responds to the aminocyclitols streptomycin (page 304) and spectinomycin (page 589), which are relatively inactive against C. trachomatis. A dose of 0·5 g sulphafurazole (sulfisoxazole) four times a day for 10 days is effective for non-specific urethritis (Schachter, 1978). Sulphonamides are effective for the treatment of lymphogranuloma venereum (Willcox, 1977), but the tetracyclines (page 626) are usually preferred. Psittacosis does not respond to sulphonamide therapy.

9. *Chancroid.* This venereal infection responds to treatment with sulphonamides, tetracycline (page 627), streptomycin (page 304) and chloramphenicol (page 445) (Willcox, 1977). By contrast to the latter three antibiotics, sulphonamides are not effective for granuloma inguinale.

10. *Nocardiosis.* Various drugs have been reported to be effective *in vitro* against the Nocardia spp., but these findings do not correlate well with clinical results. One of the sulphonamides, possibly in combination with other drugs, remains the best treatment (Weinstein *et al.*, 1960; Cohen *et al.*, 1971; Orfanakis *et al.*, 1972; Berd, 1973). Various antibiotics such as streptomycin, kanamycin, penicillin G, ampicillin, tetracycline, chloramphenicol and cycloserine have been used in combination with sulphonamides for this purpose. The combination of a sulphonamide with trimethoprim may also be satisfactory (page 713). Therapy with sulphonamides should be prolonged and continued for several months after apparent cure in patients whose immune system is comprised (Idriss *et al.*, 1975; Krick *et al.*, 1975).

11. *Toxoplasmosis.* If treatment is considered necessary, a combination of pyrimethamine ('Daraprim') (page 687) and a sulphonamide is recommended for this disease (Wettingfeld *et al.*, 1956; Boughton 1970; Roth *et al.*, 1971). This combination is effective in murine toxoplasmosis. Mahmoud and Warren (1977) recommended a loading dose of 4 g sulphadiazine followed by 1 g four

times a day, plus pyrimethamine in a 100 mg loading dose and then 25 mg daily for a period of six weeks. Folinic acid 6 mg daily should also be given, because pyrimethamine is a folic acid antagonist. A combination of pyrimethamine (25 mg) and sulfadoxine (500 mg) in 'Fansidar' tablets has been used in pregnant women with serological evidence of toxoplasmosis. The usual dose was two tablets weekly for periods of 4–24 weeks. No side-effects were observed and a satisfactory therapeutic effect was considered to be achieved because of a good outcome of pregnancy, and a reduction of toxoplasma antibody titres in the patients (Barbosa and Ferreira, 1978). A sulphonamide-trimethoprim combination may also be effective in this disease (page 714). However the efficacy of any drug therapy for the various forms of toxoplasmosis has not been confirmed by clinical trials (Krogstad *et al.*, 1972).

12. *Malaria*. It was demonstrated by Fairley and his co-workers at Cairns, Australia, during the Second World War, that the sulphonamides have an action upon parasites, and that these drugs are more effective against Plasmodium falciparum than P. vivax infections (Fairley, 1945). It is now known that sulphonamides potentiate the action of pyrimethamine on malarial parasites. McGregor *et al.* (1963) reported that this combination was effective for the treatment of P. falciparum malaria, which was resistant to pyrimethamine alone. Laing (1964) used the ultra-long-acting sulphonamide, sulfadoxine (then known as sulphormethoxine), in field trials in Africa. He found that this drug used by itself in a weekly dose of 0·5 g was just as effective as a schizonticide, as when given together with 25 mg pyrimethamine weekly. At that time it was suggested that this sulphonamide may be mainly useful as a suppressive, because its action would be too slow for the treatment of falciparum malaria.

Strains of P. falciparum resistant to chloroquine are present in certain parts of South-East Asia, Central and South America, and Africa. Combined drug therapy, usually containing a long-acting sulphonamide, is recommended for these infections (Hall *et al.*, 1975; Hall, 1976; Leading article, 1976; Hall *et al.*, 1977; Bruce-Chwatt, 1977). Triple drug regimens advocated consist of quinine, pyrimethamine (page 687) and a long-acting sulphonamide (sulfadoxine or sulfametopyrazine). Pyrimethamine, like trimethoprim (page 700), interferes with the synthesis of folinic acid in the malarial parasite at a point immediately succeeding that where sulphonamide acts. It irreversibly combines with the enzyme dihydrofolate reductase, thereby inhibiting its action of reducing dihydrofolate to tetrahydrofolate (folinic acid). Tablets containing sulfadoxine (0·5 g) and pyrimethamine (25 mg) are available commercially under the trade name of 'Fansidar' (Roche). Ampoules (2·5 ml) containing 0·5 g sulphadoxine and 25 mg pyrimethamine are also available for intramuscular administration. The regimen now recommended for the treatment of chloroquine-resistant P. falciparum malaria is at least four doses of quinine (each equivalent to 10 mg quinine base per kg) at intervals of 8 or 12 h (equivalent to a total of 2 g quinine base for an adult), followed by a single dose of three tablets of 'Fansidar'. Corresponding doses of 'Fansidar' for children are two tablets for those aged 9–14 years, one tablet for those aged 4–8 years and half a table if aged less than four years. 'Fansidar' is not recommended in pregnancy because of the possibility of teratogenicity (page 705), but this must be assessed against the risk of malaria in the patient. This regimen of quinine and 'Fansidar' results in a very high cure-rate which is nearly as good as a regimen using quinine followed by mefloquine. 'Fansidar' is the most effective chemosuppressant drug against P. falciparum strains resistant to chloroquine, being more effective than dapsone-pyrimethamine combinations (Pearlman *et al.*, 1977). It is effective when given every one, two or four weeks, but the standard adult dose is two tablets ($\frac{1}{2}$–2 tablets according to age for children) every two weeks. For semi-immune subjects the recommended dosage interval is two tablets every four weeks (Bergson, 1977). 'Fansidar' has been given for periods of up to 12 months for chemosuppression, without serious toxicity (Leading article, 1976), 'Fansidar' is also an effective chemosuppressive against P. vivax (Pearlman *et al.*, 1977) and P. malariae malaria.

13. *Pneumocystis carinii pneumonia.* Pentamidine isothionate was considered the only effective agent for the treatment of this disease, but because of its toxicity a combination of pyrimethamine (page 687) and sulphadiazine was tried. This combination is effective in the treatment and prophylaxis of P. carinii pneumonia in experimental animals. Kirby *et al.* (1971) also obtained a satisfactory clinical response when it was used in courses lasting 10–28 days to treat three consecutive patients with biopsy-proven P. carinii pneumonia. A combination of sulfadoxine and pyrimethamine was effective in a small trial in preventing P. carinii infection in an orphanage. Treatment with this combination at least twice-monthly was recommended for all babies between the age of two and six months, who are at risk from this infection (Post *et al.*, 1971). Present evidence indicates that co-trimoxazole is the best combination for the treatment and prevention of P. carinii pneumonia (*see* page 715).

14. *Ulcerative colitis and Crohn's disease.* Originally introduced for this purpose in Sweden (Svartz, 1942), the compound of sulphapyridine and salicyclic acid (sulphasalazine, 'Salazopyrin', is of proven value in ulcerative colitis. Baron *et al.* (1962) in a double blind trial on patients with mild ulcerative colitis found that sulphasalazine gave significantly better results than a placebo. However combined local and systemic corticosteroid therapy is more effective than sulphasalazine for the treatment of acute episodes of ulcerative colitis (Truelove *et al.*, 1962). Sulphasalazine, given in a maintenance dose of 0·5 g four times a day, is also effective in reducing the number of relapses of this disease (Misiewicz *et al.*, 1965). A small trial has indicated that sulphasalazine given as a rectal enema (two tablets or 1 g in a glass of water) was also effective in inducing remissions of active ulcerative colitis of the rectum and descending colon (Serebro *et al.*, 1977).

The pharmacokinetics of sulphasalazine in the body are now well understood (Goldman and Peppercorn, 1975). Absorbed in the upper gastrointestinal tract, the drug is detectable in the blood 1–2 h after oral administration. Most of it is then returned to the gut via the biliary system and little is excreted in urine. The intestinal bacteria then split the drug into its two constituents, 5-aminosalicyclic acid and sulphapyridine. Sulphapyridine is then absorbed and appears in the blood 3–5 h after oral administration; this is excreted in the urine either as the free drug or its metabolites. In contrast, 5-aminosalicyclic acid tends to remain in the colon and is excreted in the faeces with some unchanged sulphasalazine. Some acetylated derivatives of 5-aminosalicyclic acid are also excreted in urine and faeces.

In one study, patients with faecal stasis proximal to active distal colitis, who were receiving sulphasalazine, only went into remission when treated with hydrophilic colloid or bran. This suggested that the metabolites of sulphasalazine must be delivered in the faeces to the lumen of the diseased colon (Cowan *et al.*, 1977). Another study in which 5-aminosalicylic acid, sulphapyridine and sulphasalazine were given separately to patients with ulcerative colitis by retention enema suggested that the active moiety of sulphasalazine is 5-aminosalicylic acid, and that sulphapyridine only functions as a carrier ensuring that 5-aminosalicylic acid is liberated within the colon (Azad Khan *et al.*, 1977). A similar investigation in which sulphapyridine and 5-aminosalicyclic acid were given as rectal suppositories to patients with ulcerative colitis supports this contention (Van Hees *et al.*, 1978).

The side-effects of the sulphonamides, including those peculiar to sulphasalazine (page 671), tend to occur in patients receiving 4·0 g or more per day of sulphasalazine; mild side-effects can be managed by withdrawal of the drug for a few days and its subsequent readministration in a lower dosage (Goldman and Peppercorn, 1975). Most patients whose ulcerative colitis is maintained in remission have a serum sulphapyridine concentration greater than 20 μg per ml (Cowan *et al.*, 1977). This level was achieved in rapid acetylators (*see* page 667) by doses of 3·0–4·0 g sulphasalazine daily, whereas slow acetylators are likely to get side-effects at this dosage, because their serum sulphapyridine concentration will rise to over 50 μg per ml. These authors therefore suggested that slow acetylators of sulphapyridine should only be given 2·5–3·0 g of sulphasalazine daily.

The results of a number of studies, particularly in Scandinavia, suggest that sulphasalazine is also useful for the treatment of Crohn's disease (Leading article, 1975).

15. *Burns*. Certain sulphonamides, applied topically, are of benefit in the management of burns. Mafenide ('Sulphamylon') was used in Germany for the topical therapy of war wounds in the 1940's. Because this topical therapy was effective in suppressing Ps. aeruginosa infection in burned rats, it was used with similar results for the treatment of burns in humans (Lindberg *et al.*, 1965). Many studies have since confirmed that an 11·2 per cent cream of mafenide can significantly reduce sepsis in burned patients (Lowbury *et al.*, 1971; Pegg, 1972). However these applications are usually painful and mafenide is absorbed through burned areas. Mafenide and its breakdown products are strong acids and also carbonic anhydrase inhibitors, so that if large quantities of the drug are used, a metabolic acidosis may result, but this is usually compensated for by hyperventilation (Pegg, 1972). Silver nitrate in an 0·5 per cent solution is another popular topical application for burned patients (Lowbury *et al.*, 1971).

The topical use of the compound silver sulphadiazine (page 658) has also been very effective for the prevention and treatment of sepsis in burn wounds (Stanford *et al.*, 1969; Lowbury *et al.*, 1971; McDougall, 1972). This drug has been used extensively at the Royal Children's Hospital, Melbourne, since 1970, and after 1971 has been combined with 0·2 per cent chlorhexidine. As a result the incidence of sepsis due to Gram-negative organisms and also that due to Staph. pyogenes has been considerably reduced (Clarke, 1975). Controlled trials indicate that 0·5 per cent silver nitrate compresses, one per cent silver sulphadiazine cream, and a cream containing 0·5 per cent silver nitrate and 0·2 per cent chlorhexidine digluconate are all about equally effective in protecting burns from infection; silver nitrate was, however, less active than the other two preparations against less common Gram-negative bacilli (Lowbury *et al.*, 1976). Unfortunately in one burns unit, sulphonamide-resistant Gram-negative bacilli became predominant during a trial of silver sulphadiazine cream, and the effectiveness of the preparation was reduced. It became necessary to suspend silver sulphadiazine and replace it with silver nitrate and chlorhexidine cream (Lowbury, *et al.*, 1976; Bridges and Lowbury, 1977). In another burns unit, *in vitro* tests suggested that extensive use of parenteral gentamicin and replacement of topical mafenide ointments by silver sulphadiazine cream favoured the emergence of Providencia stuartii over Ps. aeruginosa as the predominant colonizing organism (Wenzel *et al.*, 1976).

16. *Umbilical cord care.* Silver sulphadiazine cream has been compared to washing with castile soap and triple dye for controlling neonatal bacterial colonization. Triple dye and silver sulphadiazine inhibited bacterial colonization, the former being better for Staph. pyogenes, but silver sulphadiazine was superior in inhibiting Group B streptococci and Gram-negative organisms (Speck *et al.*, 1977).

17. *Chronic granulomatous disease.* Johnson *et al.* (1975) noted a decrease in the frequency and severity of bacterial infections in four of five children with chronic granulomatous disease, on long-term sulphonamide therapy, which was out of proportion to the anticipated antibacterial effect of the drug. These authors showed that the killing of sulfisoxazole-resistant Esch. coli and Staph. pyogenes by leucocytes of patients with this disease was enhanced in the presence of the sulphonamide. The explanation for this effect of sulphonamides is unknown.

18. *Dermatitis herpetiformis.* Prolonged administration of sulphapyridine or the long-acting sulphonamide sulphamethoxypyridazine, is often useful for the control of this disease. Diaminodiphenylsulphone (dapsone), a drug used for the treatment of leprosy, is also usually helpful in dermatitis herpetiformis (Leading article, 1971). The reason for the beneficial effect of these drugs in this disease of unknown aetiology is not understood.

REFERENCES

Abbot, J. D. and Graves, J. F. R. (1972), 'Serotype and sulphonamide sensitivity of meningococci isolated from 1966 to 1971', *J. clin. Path.*, **25**, 528.

Adam, W. R. and Dawborn, J. K. (1970), 'Urinary excretion and plasma levels of sulphonamides in patients with renal impairment', *Aust. Ann. Med.*, **19**, 250.

Adam, W. R., Brown, D. J., Hales, P. and Dawborn, J. K. (1973), 'The use of sulphadimidine (sulphamethazine) in patients with renal failure', *Med. J. Aust.*, **1**, 936.

Alarćon-Segovia, D. (1969), 'Drug-induced lupus syndromes', *Mayo Clin. Proc.*, **44**, 664.

Alban, J. (1965), 'Treatment of B-haemolytic streptococcal infection. A study of the pediatric use of sulfamethoxazole', *Amer. J. Dis. Child.*, **109**, 304.

Annotation (1967), 'Long-acting sulphonamides', *Lancet*, **1**, 150.

Annotation (1969), 'Resistant falciparum malaria', *Lancet*, **1**, 246.

Appel, G. B. and Neu, H. C. (1977), 'The nephrotoxicity of antimicrobial agents (third of three parts)', *New Engl. J. Med.*, **196**, 784.

Azad Khan, A. K., Piris, J. and Truelove, S. C. (1977), 'An experiment to determine the active therapeutic moiety of sulphasalazine', *Lancet*, **2**, 892.

Bach, M. C., Sabath, L. D. and Finland, M. (1973), 'Susceptibility of Nocardia asteroides to 45 antimicrobial agents *in vitro*', *Antimicrob. Ag. Chemother.*, **3**, 1.

Bannatyne, R. M. and Cheung, R. (1978), 'Susceptibility of Haemophilus influenzae type b to rifampicin and sulfisoxazole', *Antimicrob. Ag. Chemother.*, **13**, 969.

Barbosa, J. C. and Ferreira, I. (1978), 'Sulfadoxine-pyrimethamine (Fansidar) in pregnant women with toxoplasma antibody titres'. In Siegenthaler, W. and Lüthy, R. (Ed.), *Current Chemotherapy: Proceedings of the 10th International Congress of Chemotherapy*, Zurich/Switzerland, 1977. American Society for Microbiology, Washington, D.C., p. 134.

Barnett, D. B. and Hancock, B. W. (1975), 'Anticoagulant resistance: An unusual case', *Brit. med. J.*, **1**, 608.

Baron, J. H., Connell, A. M., Lennard-Jones, J. E. and Avery Jones, F. (1962), 'Sulphasalazine and salicylazosulphadimidine in ulcerative colitis', *Lancet*, **1**, 1094.

Barrett, P. V. D. and Thier, S. O. (1963), 'Meningitis and pancreatitis associated with sulfamethizole', *New Engl. J. Med.*, **268**, 36.

Berd, D. (1973), 'Nocardia brasiliensis infection in the United States: A report of nine cases and a review of the literature', *Amer. J. Clin. Path.*, **59**, 254.

Bergson, V. (1977), 'Chemoprophylaxis of malaria', *Brit. med. J.*, **1**, 447.

Beveridge, J., Harris, M., Wise, G. and Stevens, L. (1964), 'Long-acting sulphonamides associated with Stevens–Johnson syndrome', *Lancet*, **2**, 593.

Bissett, M. L., Abbott, S. L. and Wood, R. M. (1974), 'Antimicrobial resistance and R factors in Salmonella isolated in California (1971–1972)', *Antimicrob. Ag. Chemother.*, **5**, 161.

Boughton, C. R. (1970), 'Toxoplasmosis', *Med. J. Aust.*, **2**, 418.

Bøvre, K., Holten, E., Vik-Mo, H., Brøndbo, A., Bratlid, D., Bjark, P. and Moe, P. J. (1977), 'Neisseria meningitidis infections in Northern Norway: An epidemic in 1974–1975 due mainly to Group B organisms', *J. Infect. Dis.*, **135**, 669.

Bowie, W. R., Alexander, E. R., Floyd, J. F., Holmes, J., Miller, Y. and Holmes, K. K. (1976), 'Differential response of chlamydial and ureaplasma-associated urethritis to sulphafurazole (sulfisoxazole) and aminocyclitols', *Lancet*, **2**, 1276.

Bratton, A. C. and Marshall, E. K., Jr. (1939), 'A new coupling component for sulfanilamide determination', *J. biol. Chem.*, **128**, 537.

Bridges, K. and Lowbury, E. J. L. (1977), 'Drug resistance in relation to use of silver sulphadiazine cream in a burns unit', *J. clin. Path.*, **30**, 160.

Bruce-Chwatt, L. J. (1977), 'Prevention and treatment of malaria', *Trop. Doct.*, **7**, 17.

Brumfitt, W. (1970), 'Some basic concepts underlying the chemotherapy of urinary infections', *Aspects of Infection. Proc. Symp. Auckland, Sydney and Melbourne*, p. 59.

Buchanan, N. (1978), 'Sulphamethoxazole, hypoalbuminaemia, crystalluria, and renal failure', *Brit. med. J.*, **2**, 172.

Bullowa, J. G. M. and Ratish, H. D. (1944), 'A therapeutic and pharmacological study of sulfadiazine, monomethylsulfadiazine and dimethylsulfadiazine in lobar pneumonia', *J. Clin. Investig.*, **23**, 676.

Burman, L. G. (1977), 'Apparent absence of transferable resistance to nalidixic acid in pathogenic Gram-negative bacteria', *J. Antimicrob. Chemother.*, **3**, 509.

Busch, H. and Lane, M. (1967), *Chemotherapy*, Year Book Medical Publishers, Inc., p. 106.

Camp, B. W. (1969), 'Treatment of streptococcal infection with sulfamethoxazole and penicillin', *Amer. J. Dis. Child.*, **117**, 663.

Carroll, O. M., Bryan, P. A. and Robinson, R. J. (1966), 'Stevens–Johnson syndrome associated with long-acting sulfonamides', *JAMA*, **195**, 691.

Center for Disease Control (1976), 'Analysis for endemic meningococcal disease by serogroup and evaluation of chemoprophylaxis', *J. Infect. Dis.*, **134**, 201.

Chang, T. W. and Weinstein, L. (1975a), 'Inactivation of Treponema pallidum by silver sulfadiazine', *Antimicrob. Ag. Chemother.*, **7**, 538.

Chang, T. W. and Weinstein, L. (1975b), '*In vitro* activity of silver sulfadiazine against Herpesvirus hominis', *J. Infect. Dis.*, **132**, 79.

Chang, T. W. and Weinstein, L. (1975c), 'Prevention of Herpes keratoconjunctivitis in rabbits by silver sulfadiazine', *Antimicrob. Ag. Chemother.*, **8**, 677.

Ch'ien, L. T. (1970), 'Intracranial hypertension and sulfamethoxazole', *New Engl. J. Med.*, **283**, 47.

Christensen, L. K., Hansen, J. M. and Kristensen, M. (1963), 'Sulphaphenazole-induced hypoglycaemic attacks in tolbutamide-treated diabetics', *Lancet*, **2**, 1298.

Clarke, A. M. (1975), 'Topical use of silver sulphadiazine and chlorhexidine in the prevention of infection in thermal injuries', *Med. J. Aust.*, **1**, 413.

Claxton, R. C. (1963), 'A review of 31 cases of Stevens–Johnson syndrome', *Med. J. Aust.*, **1**, 963.

Cohen, M. L., Weiss, E. B. and Monaco, A. P. (1971), 'Successful treatment of Pneumocystis carinii and Nocardia asteroides in a renal transplant patient', *Amer. J. Med.*, **50**, 269.

Cowan, G. O., Das, K. M. and Eastwood, M. A. (1977), 'Further studies of sulphasalazine metabolism in the treatment of ulcerative colitis', *Brit. med. J.*, **2**, 1057.

Craft, A. W., Brocklebank, J. T. and Jackson, R. H. (1977), 'Acute renal failure and hypoglycaemia due to sulphadiazine poisoning', *Postgrad. Med. J.*, **53**, 103.

Davies, J. R., Farrant, W. N. and Uttley, A. H. C. (1970), 'Antibiotic resistance of Shigella sonnei', *Lancet*, **2**, 1157.

Deb, B. C., Sengupta, P. G., De, S. P., Sil, J., Sikdar, S. N. and Pal, S. C. (1976), 'Effect of sulfadoxine on transmission of Vibrio cholerae infection among family contacts of cholera patients in Calcutta', *Bull. Wld. Hlth. Org.*, **54**, 171.

De Morais, J. S., Munford, R. S., Risi, J. B., Antezana, E. and Feldman, R. A. (1974), 'Epidemic disease due to serogroup C Neisseria meningitidis in Saõ Paulo, Brazil', *J. Infect. Dis.*, **129**, 568.

Dujovne, C. A., Chan, C. H. and Zimmerman, H. J. (1967), 'Sulfonamide hepatic injury. Review of the literature and report of a case due to sulfamethoxazole', *New Engl. J. Med.*, **277**, 785.

Eickhoff, T. C., Bennett, J. V., Hayes, P. S. and Feeley, J. (1970), 'Pseudomonas pseudomallei: Susceptibility to chemotherapeutic agents', *J. Infect. Dis.*, **121**, 95.

Epidemiology (1977), 'Meningococcal meningitis', *Brit. med. J.*, **1**, 1671.

Fairley, N. H. (1945), 'Chemotherapeutic suppression and prophylaxis in malaria', Transactions of the Royal Society of Tropical Medicine and Hygiene, **38**, 311.

Feit, P. W. (1975), 'Structure-activity relationships of sulphamoyl diuretics', *Postgrad. Med. J.* (Suppl. 6), **51**, 9.

Finland, M., Garner, C., Wilcox, C. and Sabath, L. D. (1976), 'Susceptibility of beta-hemolytic streptococci to 65 antibacterial agents', *Antimicrob. Ag. Chemother.*, **9**, 11.

Fischer, E. (1972), 'Renal excretion of sulphadimidine in normal and uraemic subjects', *Lancet*, **2**, 210.

Fox, C. L. (1968), 'Silver sulfadiazine—a new topical therapy for Pseudomonas in burns', *Arch. Surg.*, **96**, 184.

Garrod, L. P., Lambert, H. P. and O'Grady, F. (1973), *Antibiotic and Chemotherapy*, 4th edn., Churchill and Livingstone, Edinburgh and London, p. 14.

Goldman, P. and Peppercorn, M. A. (1975), 'Drug therapy: Sulfasalazine', *New Engl. J. Med.*, **293**, 20.

Gottschalk, H. R. and Stone, O. J. (1976), 'Stevens–Johnson syndrome from ophthalmic sulfonamide', *Arch. Dermatol.*, **112**, 513.

Grieble, H. G. and Jackson, G. G. (1958), 'Prolonged treatment of urinary-tract infections with sulfamethoxypyridazine', *New Engl. J. Med.*, **258**, 1.

Griffiths, I. D. and Kane, S. P. (1977), 'Sulphasalazine-induced lupus syndrome in ulcerative colitis', *Brit. med. J.*, **2**, 1188.

Grüneberg, R. N. and Brumfitt, W. (1967), 'Single-dose treatment of acute urinary tract infection: A controlled trial', *Brit. med. J.*, **3**, 649.

Hall, A. P., Doberstyn, E. B., Mettaprakong, V. and Sonkom, P. (1975), 'Falciparum malaria cured by quinine followed by sulfadoxine-pyrimethamine', *Brit. med. J.*, **2**, 15.

Hall, A. P. (1976), 'The treatment of malaria', *Brit. med. J.*, **1**, 323.

Hall, A. P., Doberstyn, E. B., Karnchanachetanee, C., Samransamruajkit, S., Laixuthai, B., Pearlman, E. J., Lampe, R. M., Miller, C. F. and Phintuyothin, P. (1977), 'Sequential treatment with quinine and mefloquine or quinine and pyrimethamine-sulfadoxine for Falciparum malaria', *Brit. med. J.*, **1**, 1626.

Haltalin, K. C. and Nelson, J. D. (1965), '*In vitro* susceptibility of shigellae to sodium sulfadiazine and to eight antibiotics', *JAMA*, **193**, 705.

Hamilton, H. E. and Sheets, R. F. (1978), 'Sulfisoxazole-induced thrombocytopenic purpura. Immunologic mechanism as cause', *JAMA*, **239**, 2586.

Hansen, J. M., Siersbaek-Nielsen, K., Skovsted, L., Kampmann, J. P. and Lumholtz, B. (1975), 'Potentiation of warfarin by co-trimoxazole', *Brit. med. J.*, **2**, 684.

Hassall, C., Feetam, C. L., Leach, R. H. and Meynell, M. J. (1975), 'Potentiation of warfarin by co-trimoxazole', *Lancet*, **2**, 1155.

Holmgren, E. B. and Tunevall, G. (1973), 'Five cases of meningitis due to sulfonamide-resistant meningococci', *Scand. J. Infect. Dis.*, **5**, 75.

Holten, E., Vaage, L., Neess, C., Midtvedt, T. and Jyssum, K. (1969), 'Sulphonamide-resistant meningococci after sulphonamide prophylaxis among naval recruits in Norway', *Scand. J. Infect. Dis.*, **1**, 185.

Holten, E., Vaage, L. and Jyssum, K. (1970), 'Sulphonamide-resistant meningococci in Norwegian naval recruits', *Scand. J. Infect. Dis.*, **2**, 111.

Idriss, Z. H., Cunningham, R. J. and Wilfert, C. M. (1975), 'Nocardiosis in children: Report of three cases and review of the literature', *Pediatrics*, **55**, 479.

Jacobson, J. A., Weaver, R. E. and Thornsberry, C. (1975), 'Trends in meningococcal disease, 1974', *J. Infect. Dis.*, **132**, 480.

Jacobson, J. A., Chester, T. J. and Fraser, D. W. (1977), 'An epidemic of disease due to serogroup B Neisseria meningitidis in Alabama: Report of an investigation and community-wide prophylaxis with a sulfonamide', *J. Infect. Dis.*, **136**, 104.

Johnston, R. B., Jr., Wilfert, C. M., Buckley, R. H., Webb, L. S., DeChatelet, L. R. and McCall, C. E. (1975), 'Enhanced bactericidal activity of phagocytes from patients with chronic granulomatous disease in the presence of sulphisoxazole', *Lancet*, **1**, 824.

Kane, S. P. and Boots, M. A. (1977), 'Megaloblastic anaemia associated with sulphasalazine treatment', *Brit. med. J.*, **2**, 1287.

Kerr Grant, A., Purser, B. N. and Hazel, J. R. (1969), 'Shigella flexner dysentery in Australian forces in South Vietnam', *Med. J. Aust.*, **2**, 752.

Kirby, H. B., Kenamore, B. and Guckian, J. C. (1971), 'Pneumocystis carinii pneumonia treated with pyrimethamine and sulfadiazine', *Ann. Intern. Med.*, **75**, 505.

Krick, J. A., Stinson, E. B. and Remington, J. S. (1975), 'Nocardia infection in heart transplant patients', *Ann. Intern. Med.*, **82**, 18.

Krogstad, D. J., Juranek, D. D. and Walls, K. W. (1972), 'Toxoplasmosis. With comments on risk of infection from cats', *Ann. Intern. Med.*, **77**, 773.

Laing, A. B. G. (1964), 'Antimalarial effect of sulphorthodimethoxine (Fanasil)', *Brit. med. J.*, **2**, 1439.

Leading Article (1965), 'Teratogenic effects of sulphonamides', *Brit. med. J.*, **1**, 142.

Leading Article (1968), 'Some hazards of sulphonamides', *Brit. med. J.*, **1**, 658.

Leading Article (1969), 'Lung disease caused by drugs', *Brit. med. J.*, **3**, 729.

Leading Article (1971), 'Dermatitis herpetiformis', *Lancet*, **1**, 484.

Leading Article (1974a), 'Meningococcal infections', *Brit. med. J.*, **3**, 295.

Leading Article (1974b), 'Sulphasalazine-induced lung disease', *Lancet*, **2**, 504.
Leading Article (1974c), 'Chemoprophylaxis of meningococcal infections', *Lancet*, **2**, 1431.
Leading Article (1975), 'Sulphasalazine for Crohn's disease?', *Brit. med. J.*, **2**, 297.
Leading Article (1976), 'Chemoprophylaxis of malaria', *Brit. med. J.*, **2**, 1215.
Leading Article (1977a), 'Chlamydial infections of the eye', *Lancet*, **2**, 857.
Leading Article (1977b), 'Preventing endocarditis', *Brit. med. J.*, **2**, 1564.
Leedom, J. M., Ivler, D., Mathies, A. W., Thrupp, L. D., Portnoy, B. and Wehrle, P. F. (1965), 'Importance of sulfadiazine resistance in meningococcal disease in civilians', *New Engl. J. Med.*, **273**, 1395.
Leedom, J. M., Ivler, D., Mathies, A. W., Jr., Thrupp, L. D., Fremont, J. C., Wehrle, P. F. and Portnoy, B. (1967), 'The problem of sulfadiazine-resistant meningococci', *Antimicrob. Ag. Chemother.*—1966, p. 281.
Lehr, D. (1957), 'Clinical toxicity of sulfonamides', *Ann. New York Acad. Sci.*, **69**, 417.
Lehrer, R. I. (1971), 'Inhibition by sulphonamides of the candidacidal activity of human neutrophils', *J. Clin. Investig.*, **50**, 2498.
Lewis, V. J., Thacker, W. L., Shepard, C. C. and McDade, J. E. (1978), '*In vivo* susceptibility of the Legionnaires' disease bacterium to ten antimicrobial agents', *Antimicrob. Ag. Chemother.*, **13**, 419.
Lidin-Janson, G. (1977), 'Sulphonamides in the treatment of acute Escherichia coli infection of the urinary tract in women', *Scand. J. Infect. Dis.*, **9**, 211.
Lindberg, R. B., Moncrief, J. A., Switzer, W. E., Order, S. E. and Mills, W., Jr. (1965), 'The successful control of burn wound sepsis', *J. Trauma*, **5**, 601.
Lisander, B. (1970), 'Myalgia after sulphonamides', *Lancet*, **1**, 1062.
Lowbury, E. J. L., Jackson, D. M., Lilly, H. A., Bull, J. P., Cason, J. S., Davies, J. W. L. and Ford, P. M. (1971), 'Alternative forms of local treatment for burns', *Lancet*, **2**, 1105.
Lowbury, E. J. L., Babb, J. R., Bridges, K. and Jackson, D. M. (1976), 'Topical chemoprophylaxis with silver sulphadiazine and silver nitrate chlorhexidine creams: Emergence of sulphonamide-resistant Gram-negative bacilli', *Brit. med. J.*, **1**, 493.
Ludlam, G. B., Bridges, J. B. and Benn, E. C. (1964), 'Association of Stevens–Johnson syndrome with antibody for Mycoplasma pneumoniae', *Lancet*, **1**, 958.
Macsearraigh, E. T. M. and Patel, K. M. (1968), 'Cardiomyopathy as a complication of sulphonamide therapy', *Brit. med. J.*, **3**, 33.
Madsen, S. T., Øvsthus, Ø. and Bøe, J. (1963), 'Antibacterial activity of long-acting sulfonamides', *Acta Med. Scand.*, **173**, 707.
Mahmoud, A. A. F. and Warren, K. S. (1977), 'Algorithms in the diagnosis and management of exotic diseases. XX. Toxoplasmosis', *J. Infect. Dis.*, **135**, 493.
McDougall, I. A. (1972), 'Use of silver sulphadiazine in treatment of burns at Royal Perth Hospital', *Med. J. Aust.*, **1**, 979.
McGregor, I. A., Williams, K. and Goodwin, L. G. (1963), 'Pyrimethamine and sulphadiazine in treatment of malaria', *Brit. med. J.*, **2**, 728.
Mihas, A. A., Goldenberg, D. J. and Slaughter, R. L. (1978), 'Sulfasalazine toxic reactions, hepatitis, fever, and skin rash with hypocomplementemia and immune complexes', *JAMA*, **239**, 2590.
Millar, J. W., Siess, E. E., Feldman, H. A., Silverman, C. and Frank, P. (1963), '*In vivo* and *in vitro* resistance to sulfadiazine in strains of Neisseria meningitidis', *JAMA*, **186**, 139.
Misiewicz, J. J., Lennard-Jones, J. E., Connell, A. M., Baron, J. H. and Avery Jones, F. (1965), 'Controlled trial of sulphasalazine in maintenance therapy for ulcerative colitis', *Lancet*, **1**, 185.
Morahan, R. J. and Hawksworth, D. N. (1970), 'Antibiotic and sulphadiazine sensitivities of New Guinea salmonellas and shigellas', *Med. J. Aust.*, **2**, 222.

Nanra, R. S., Bailie, M. and Kincaid,-Smith, P. (1969), 'Sulphasymazine in recurrent urinary tract infection', *Med. J. Aust.*, **2**, 1258.

Newbould, B. B. and Kilpatrick, R. (1960), 'Long-acting sulphonamides and protein-binding', *Lancet*, **1**, 887.

Nunnelly, G. (1960), 'Sulfadimethoxine in upper respiratory infections', *JAMA*, **173**, 1020.

Odell, G. B. (1959), 'The dissociation of bilirubin from albumin and its clinical implications', *J. Pediatrics*, **55**, 268.

O'Grady, F., Lewis, M. J. and Pearson, N. J. (1976), 'Global surveillance of antibiotic sensitivity of Vibrio cholerae', *Bull. Wld. Hlth. Org.*, **54**, 181.

Orfanakis, M. G., Wilcox, H. G. and Smith, C. B. (1972), '*In vitro* studies of the combined effect of ampicillin and sulfonamides on Nocardia asteroides and results of therapy in four patients', *Antimicrob. Ag. Chemother.*, **1**, 215.

Owens, C. J., Yarbrough D. R., III, and Brackett, N. C., Jr. (1974), 'Nephrotic syndrome following topically applied sulfadiazine silver therapy', *Arch. Intern. Med.*, **134**, 332.

Pearlman, E. J., Lampe, R. M., Thiemanun, W. and Kennedy, R. S. (1977), 'Chemosuppressive field trials in Thailand. III. The suppression of Plasmodium falciparum and Plasmodium vivax parasitemias by a sulfadoxine-pyrimethamine combination', *Am. J. Trop. Med. Hyg.*, **26**, 1108.

Pegg, S. P. (1972), 'Adult burns: A three-year survey with assessment of sulfamylon', *Med. J. Aust.*, **1**, 350.

Perrin, J. M., Charney, E., MacWhinney, J. B., Jr., McInerny, T. K., Miller, R. L. and Nazarian L. F. (1974), 'Sulfisoxazole as chemoprophylaxis for recurrent otitis media. A double-blind crossover study in pediatric practice', *New Engl. J. Med.*, **291**, 664.

Phillips, I. and Warren, C. (1976), 'Activity of sulfamethoxazole and trimephoprim against Bacteroides fragilis', *Antimicrob. Ag. Chemother.*, **9**, 736.

Post, C., Fakouhi, T., Dutz, W., Bandahizadeh, B. and Kohout, E. E. (1971), 'Prophylaxis of epidemic infantile pneumocystosis with a sulfadoxine pyrimethamine combination', *Curr. Ther. Res.*, **13**, 273.

Pryles, C. V. (1970), 'The use of sulfonamides in urinary tract infections', *Med. Clin. North America*, **54**, 1077.

Rao, K. V. N., Mitchison, D. A., Nair, N. G. K., Prema, K. and Tripathy, S. P. (1970), 'Sulphadimidine acetylation test for classification of patients as slow or rapid inactivators of isoniazid', *Brit. med. J.*, **3**, 495.

Rallison, M. L., O'Brien, J. and Good, R. A. (1961), 'Severe reactions to long-acting sulfonamides. Erythema multiforme exudativum and lupus erythematosus following administration of sulphamethoxypyridazine and sulfadimethoxine', *Pediatrics*, **28**, 908.

Reeves, D. S. (1975), 'Laboratory and clinical studies with sulfametopyrazine as a treatment for bacteriuria in pregnancy', *J. Antimicrob. Chemother.*, **1**, 171.

Report of a WHO Scientific Group (1978), 'Neisseria gonorrhoeae and gonococcal infections', *Wld. Hlth. Orgn. techn. Rep. Ser.*, No. 616.

Rose, G. A. and Spencer, H. (1957), 'Polyarteritis nodosa', *Quart. J. Med.*, **26**, 43.

Rosenkranz, H. S. and Carr, H. S. (1972), 'Silver sulfadiazine: Effect on the growth and metabolism of bacteria', *Antimicrob. Ag. Chemother.*, **2**, 367.

Roth, J. A., Siegel, S. E., Levine, A. S. and Berard, C. W. (1971), 'Fatal recurrent toxoplasmosis in a patient initially infected via a leukocyte transfusion', *Amer. J. Clin. Path.*, **56**, 601.

Salmi, I., Pettay, O., Simula, I., Kallio, A.-K. and Waltimo, O. (1976), 'An epidemic due to sulphonamide-resistant Group A meningococci in the Helsinki area (Finland). Epidemiological and clinical observations', *Scand. J. Infect. Dis.*, **8**, 249.

Salvaggio, J. and Gonzalez, F. (1959), 'Severe toxic reactions associated with sulfamethoxypyridazine (kynex)', *Ann. Intern. Med.*, **51,** 60.

Schachter, J. (1978), 'Chlamydial infections (second of three parts)', *New Engl. J. Med.*, **298,** 490.

Schneider, R. E. and Beeley, L. (1977), 'Megaloblastic anaemia associated with sulphasalazine treatment', *Brit. med. J.*, **1,** 1638.

Sellin, M., Cooke, D. I., Gillespie, W. A., Sylvester, D. G. H. and Anderson, J. D. (1975), 'Micrococcal urinary-tract infections in young women', *Lancet*, **2,** 570.

Serebro, H., Kay, S., Javett, S. and Abrahams, C. (1977), "Sulphasalazine rectal enemas: Topical method of inducing remission of active ulcerative colitis affecting rectum and descending colon', *Brit. med. J.*, **2,** 1264.

Shepard, C. C., Ellard, G. A., Levy, L., de Araujo Opromolla, V., Pattyn, S. R., Peters, J. H., Rees, R. J. W. and Waters, M. F. R. (1976), 'Experimental chemotherapy in leprosy', *Bull. Wld. Hlth. Org.*, **53,** 425.

Speck, W. T. and Rosenkranz, H. S. (1974), 'Activity of silver sulphadiazine against dermatophytes', *Lancet*, **2,** 895.

Speck, W. T., Driscoll, J. M., Polin, R. A., O'Neill, J. and Rosenkranz, H. S. (1977), 'Staphylococcal and streptococcal colonization of the newborn infant. Effect of antiseptic cord care', *A. J. Dis. Child.*, **131,** 1005.

Stanford, W., Rappole, B. W. and Fox, C. L. (1969), 'Clinical experience with silver sulfadiazine, a new topical agent for control of Pseudomonas infections in burns', *J. Trauma*, **9,** 377.

Ström, J. (1962), 'The role of drugs in certain febrile mucocutaneous manifestations (syndroma mucocutaneum febrile) as illustrated by provocation of clinical and thrombocyte reactions', *Acta allergologica, XVII*, 232.

Ström, J. (1969), 'Herpes simplex virus as a cause of allergic mucocutaneous reactions (ectodermosis erosiva pluriorificalis, Stevens–Johnson's syndrome, etc.) and generalised infection', *Scand. J. Infect. Dis.*, **1,** 3

Svartz, N. (1942), 'Salazopyrin: A new sulphanilamide preparation', *Acta Med. Scand.*, **110,** 577.

Thirkettle, J. L., Gough, K. R. and Read, A. E. (1963), 'Agranulocytosis associated with sulphasalazine ('Salazopyrin') therapy', *Lancet*, **1,** 1395.

Tilstone, W. J., Gray, J. M. B., Nimmo-Smith, R. H. and Lawson, D. H. (1977), 'Interaction between warfarin and sulphamethoxazole', *Postgrad. Med. J.*, **53,** 388.

Today's Drugs (1964), 'Sulphonamides', *Brit. med. J.*, **1,** 419 and 483.

Today's Drugs (1968), 'Sulphonamides', *Brit. med. J.*, **2,** 674.

Truelove, S. C., Watkinson, G. and Draper, G. (1962), 'Comparison of corticosteroid and sulphasalazine therapy in ulcerative colitis', *Brit. med. J.*, **2,** 1708.

Tydd, T. F. and Dyer, N. H. (1976), 'Sulphasalazine lung', *Med. J. Aust.*, **1,** 570.

Van Hees, P. A. M., Van Tongeren, J. H. M., Bakker, J. H. and Van Lier, H. J. J. (1978), 'Active therapeutic moiety of sulphasalazine', *Lancet*, **1,** 277.

Weinstein, L., Madoff, M. A. and Samet, C. M. (1960), 'The sulphonamides', *New Engl. J. Med.*, **263,** 793, 842, 900 and 952.

Wenzel, R. P., Hunting, K. J., Osterman, C. A. and Sande, M. A. (1976), 'Providencia stuartii, a hospital pathogen: Potential factors for its emergence and transmission', *Amer. J. Epidemiol.*, **104,** 170.

Wettingfeld, R. F., Rowe, J. and Eyles, D. E. (1956), 'Treatment of toxoplasmosis with pyrimethamine (Daraprim) and triple sulfonamide', *Ann. Intern. med.*, **44,** 557.

WHO (1971), 'Meningococcal meningitis', *WHO Wkly. epidem. Rec.*, **46,** 381.

WHO (1974), 'Meningococcal infections', *WHO Wkly. epidem. Rec.*, **49,** 197.

WHO (1978), 'Meningococcal disease surveillance', *WHO Wkly. epidem. Rec.*, **53,** 261.

Willcox, R. R. (1977), 'How suitable are available pharmaceuticals for the treatment of sexually transmitted diseases? (2) Conditions presenting as sores or tumours', *Brit. J. vener. Dis.*, **53,** 340.

Williams, J. D. and Smith, E. K. (1970), 'Single-dose therapy with streptomycin and sulfametopyrazine for bacteriuria during pregnancy', *Brit. med. J.,* **4,** 651.

Williams, D. M., Wimpenny, J. and Asscher, A. W. (1968), 'Renal clearance of sodium sulphadimidine in normal and uraemic subjects', *Lancet,* **2,** 1058.

Wright, L. J. and Plorde, J. J. (1970), 'Group-A sulphadiazine-resistant Neisseria meningitidis in Ethiopia', *Lancet,* **2,** 1033.

Yourassowsky, E., Vanderlinden, M. P. and Schoutens, E. (1974), 'Sensitivity of Streptococcus pyogenes to sulphamethoxazole, trimethoprim, and cotrimoxazole', *J. clin. Path.,* **27,** 897.

Trimethoprim and Co-trimoxazole

Description

Trimethoprim or 2,4-diamino-5-(3,4,5-trimethoxybenzyl)-pyrimidine was synthetized in 1956 as a result of a planned systematic study carried out by Hitchings at the Wellcome Laboratories in the United States (Roth *et al.*, 1962). It has both antibacterial and antimalarial activity, whilst a chemically related compound, pyrimethamine, which was synthetized in 1951 (Russel and Hitchings, 1951), is mainly antimalarial (*see* page 676). Trimethoprim interrupts bacterial purine synthesis at a stage which immediately follows that blocked by the sulphonamides (page 700). The combination of these two drugs therefore has a synergistic effect against certain bacteria (Bushby and Hitchings, 1968; Darrell *et al.*, 1968). In the period 1968 till 1978, trimethoprim has only been available for general clinical use as a mixture with a particular sulphonamide. The medium-acting sulphonamide, sulphamethoxazole (page 658), was selected for commercial formulations, because its rate of absorption and excretion closely parallels that of trimethoprim. Commercial preparations presently available contain a mixture of sulphamethoxazole and trimethoprim in a fixed ratio of 5:1. The generic name of co-trimoxazole is used to describe this drug combination; it is marketed with the trade name of 'Septrin' or 'Septra' (Burroughs Wellcome) and 'Bactrim' (Roche). Co-trimoxazole was introduced to the United Kingdom in 1968, to Australia in 1969, and to the United States of America in 1974.

Sensitive Organisms

Trimethoprim has a wide range of antibacterial activity (Bushby, 1969; Bushby, 1973; Bach *et al.*, 1973b).

1. *Gram-positive bacteria*. Trimethoprim is active against pyogenic cocci such as Staph. pyogenes, including penicillin- and methicillin-resistant strains (Seligman, 1973), Staph. epidermidis, Strep. pyogenes, Strep. pneumoniae, Strep. viridans and also Strep. faecalis. Some Gram-positive bacilli such as C. diphtheriae are also susceptible, but the Clostridium spp. are resistant.

Trimethoprim has some activity against Nocardia but its MIC for this organism is usually 10–50 μg per ml (Bach *et al.*, 1973a). The results of studies using co-trimoxazole have usually demonstrated a synergistic effect of this combination against Nocardia (Beaumont, 1970; Bushby, 1973; Pavillard, 1973; Maderazo and Quintiliani, 1974), but others have been unsuccessful (Black and McNellis, 1970). It now appears that the demonstration of *in vitro* synergism of co-trimoxazole against Nocardia depends on the isolate, duration of incubation and the ratio of the component drugs used (Bennett and Jennings,

1978). Higher doses of trimethoprim than in commercially available co-trimoxazole are required to produce synergism.

2. *Gram-negative aerobic bacteria.* Most of the Enterobacteriaceae are susceptible to trimethoprim. These include Esch. coli and the Enterobacter, Proteus, Salmonella, Shigella, Providencia, Citrobacter, Hafnia, Edwardsiella and Arizona spp. and Serratia marcescens. Co-trimoxazole is active against most enterotoxogenic Esch. coli strains which have been isolated from different geographic locations (Dupont *et al.*, 1978). Yersinia enterocolitica is sensitive to trimethoprim (Gutman *et al.*, 1973), Y. pestis is sensitive to co-trimoxazole (Ai *et al.*, 1973) and probably also to trimethoprim alone, and Y. pseudotuberculosis is sensitive to co-trimoxazole (Brodie *et al.*, 1973). Klebsiella spp. are usually sensitive, but resistant strains were present before trimethoprim became available for clinical use (Hamilton-Miller and Grey, 1975). Co-trimoxazole is active against ampicillin-resistant shigellae (page 101) which may also be multiply-resistant to tetracyclines, chloramphenicol and sulphonamides (Rodriguez *et al.*, 1978).

H. influenzae including ampicillin-resistant strains (page 102) is sensitive to trimethoprim and when this is combined with sulphamethoxazole synergism is demonstrable against these organisms (Kirven and Thornsberry, 1974; McGowan *et al.*, 1976; Pelton *et al.*, 1977; Sinai *et al.*, 1978). B. pertussis and Pasteurella multocida are quite sensitive. Vibrio cholerae, both classical and El Tor biotypes, are also susceptible (Northrup *et al.*, 1972). The Brucella spp. (Robertson *et al.*, 1973) and the pathogenic Neisseria (meningococci and gonococci) are only moderately sensitive to trimethoprim.

Pseudomonas aeruginosa is resistant to trimethoprim, but conditions may be such in the urine that it may act synergistically with sulphamethoxazole against this organism. Grey and Hamilton-Miller (1977) divided Ps. aeruginosa strains into those which were 'highly resistant' (MIC $>$ 1000 μg per ml), and the majority (84 per cent) which were 'moderately resistant' (MIC $<$ 1000 μg per ml) to sulphamethoxazole. Trimethoprim was synergistic with sulphamethoxazole against the latter strains when these drugs were used in a ratio of 1:2; this approximates to the ratio of the concentration of these drugs achieved in urine after treatment with co-trimoxazole (page 698) and differs from the usual 1:19 ratio (1·25/23·75) used for testing synergy to these drugs (page 691). Pseudomonas cepacia (multivorans) is usually sensitive to trimethoprim (Moody and Young, 1975) and co-trimoxazole (Hamilton *et al.*, 1973; Rahal *et al.*, 1973; Moody and Young, 1975). By comparison, Ps. maltophilia is usually resistant to trimethoprim (MIC $>$ 32 μg per ml), but the majority of strains are sensitive to co-trimoxazole (Moody and Young, 1975). Although Pseudomonas pseudomallei is usually trimethoprim-resistant, some strains are sulphamethoxazole-sensitive and the majority can be inhibited by therapeutically achievable concentrations of trimethoprim/sulphamethoxazole (Beaumont, 1970; Bassett, 1971; Everett and Kishimoto, 1973). The Legionnaires' disease bacterium is sensitive to co-trimoxazole *in vitro* (Thornsberry *et al.*, 1978).

3. *Gram-negative anaerobic bacteria.* Results of sensitivity testing of these bacteria to trimethoprim and co-trimoxazole have been conflicting. Bushby (1973) found some Bacteroides spp. resistant to trimethoprim and susceptible to sulphamethoxazole, and could not demonstrate synergism between these

two drugs. Rosenblatt and Stewart (1974) tested a variety of anaerobes including Bacteroides, Fusobacterium and Clostridium spp., Peptococci, Peptostreptococci, Eubacterium limosum and Propionibacterium acnes; trimethoprim, sulphamethoxazole or their combination was inactive against the majority of these anaerobes. On the other hand, Okubadejo *et al.* (1973) reported inhibition of Bacteroides spp. including B. fragilis by co-trimoxazole. Similar results were obtained by Phillips and Warren (1974) who showed that B. fragilis was susceptible to sulphamethoxazole, and when used with trimethoprim, synergism could be demonstrated if greater amounts of trimethoprim than sulphamethoxazole was used, the reverse of the optimum ratio for most bacteria. More recently, Phillips and Warren (1976) suggested that these discrepancies were explicable by differences in techniques. They concluded that true resistance of B. fragilis to sulphamethoxazole was rare, and that its sensitivity to trimethoprim may be more or less than its sensitivity to sulphonamides, depending on the techniques used. Also synergism against B. fragilis could be demonstrated if these drugs were combined together in the ratio of their MIC's for this organism, as determined by the particular method used.

4. *Other microorganisms.* Trimethoprim may have an effect against some true fungi such as Histoplasma capsulatum (Macleod, 1970). It probably has no activity against the Treponemata (e.g. T. pallidum), Leptospirae, Chlamydia, Rickettsiae and Coxsiella burnetti, although one case report suggested that it might have been of benefit to a patient with Q fever endocarditis (Freeman and Hodson, 1972). Mycobacteria and Mycoplasmas are resistant.

5. *Malaria parasites.* These are sensitive to trimethoprim.

6. *Comparative antibacterial activity with sulphonamides.* Trimethoprim (although having a similar antibacterial spectrum) is more active than the sulphonamides against most bacterial species, with the exception of the Neisseria, Brucella and Nocardia spp. (*vide supra* and Table 42). Strep. faecalis, which is usually completely resistant to the sulphonamides, is sensitive to trimethoprim.

7. *Acquired resistance.* By contrast to the sulphonamides (page 660), trimethoprim-resistant strains of usually sensitive bacteria are still uncommon. It is possible that this has been partly because trimethoprim has always been combined with sulphamethoxazole. Should trimethoprim be used otherwise in the future, resistant strains may become more prevalent. If Gram-negative bacteria are passaged in increasing trimethoprim concentrations *in vitro*, drug resistance develops rapidly (Reisberg *et al.*, 1967). Laboratory studies with trimethoprim and sulphonamides suggest that if infections by bacteria initially sensitive to both are treated with these drugs together, trimethoprim-resistant strains are unlikely to emerge. However trimethoprim-sensitive but sulphonamide-resistant organisms become trimethoprim-resistant much more readily (Darrell *et al.*, 1968; Smith *et al.*, 1972).

Trimethoprim-resistant variants of many bacterial species have now been encountered. Nakhla (1972) tested 675 Staph. pyogenes strains isolated from hospital patients, and found that 1·6 per cent were trimethoprim-resistant. Of 623 multi-resistant Staph. pyogenes strains isolated from patients in England during 1975–1976, 12·6 per cent were resistant to co-trimoxazole (Chattopadhyay, 1977). A pneumococcus, resistant to trimethoprim, has also been reported (Howe and Wilson, 1972), and Strep. faecalis mutants, resistant to trimethoprim, readily appear if co-trimoxazole is used to treat urinary infections caused by this organism (Chattopadhyay, 1972; Lewis and Lacey, 1973). In this case only a one step mutation is required, as Strep. faecalis is always sulphonamide-resistant.

Gram-negative bacilli resistant to trimethoprim also occur (Lacey et al., 1972; Barker et al., 1972). According to most reports these are not increasing in prevalence. McAllister (1976) using urinary tract Esch. coli isolates in Glasgow as a marker, detected no significant increase in resistance to co-trimoxazole in the five-year period 1970–1974. When 711 'coliform' strains isolated from hospital and non-hospital patients in Bristol were tested, 16 strains (2·5 per cent) were trimethoprim-resistant (Lewis and Lacey, 1973). In 1977, 380 coliform isolates were examined at the same laboratory and 13·2 per cent were resistant to trimethoprim. However when a single strain of Klebsiella aerogenes, which was causing a hospital outbreak at the time, was excluded, only 2·4 per cent of isolates (Klebsiella and Escherichia spp.) were resistant to trimethoprim and 28·7 per cent resistant to sulphonamide (Marks et al., 1977). Brumfitt et al. (1977) examined resistance to trimethoprim of 3086 isolates from urine, which in descending order of frequency consisted of Esch. coli, Kl. aerogenes, Pr. mirabilis and Enterobacter spp. The overall frequency of acquired resistance was 4·3 per cent, but there was a higher percentage resistance amongst Kl. aerogenes (18·3 per cent) and Enterobacter spp. (12 per cent) than amongst Esch. coli (1·4 per cent) and Pr. mirabilis (2 per cent) strains. By contrast, Hart et al. (1977) in Liverpool found an increase from 7 to 17 per cent of urinary pathogens resistant to co-trimoxazole in 1977 compared to 1976. Brandberg et al. (1976) tested the susceptibility of 150 strains Klebsiella spp. and Esch. coli isolated from the blood of patients in Gothenburg, and found that 17 per cent were resistant to co-trimoxazole.

Resistance of the Enterobacteriaceae to trimethoprim or trimethoprim-sulphamethoxazole may be mediated by R plasmids (page 422) (Fleming et al., 1972; Pinney and Smith, 1973). This type of transferable resistance remains rare (Marks et al., 1977; Brumfitt et al., 1977). In only 8·3 per cent of all the resistant strains detected by Brumfitt et al. (1977) (vide supra) was resistance transferable. The remainder were presumed to have chromosomal resistance which seemed to be mainly due to the production of dihydrofolate reductase (page 700) with a diminished susceptibility to trimethoprim, and in addition some strains had increased activity of this enzyme.

The use of trimethoprim or co-trimoxazole in cultures can lead to the in vitro emergence of mutants of some Enterobacteriaceae, which do not utilise the tetrahydrofolate pathway (see page 700) leading to thymidine synthesis (Pinney and Smith, 1973). These strains utilise an exogenous source of thymine or thymidine for DNA synthesis and are unaffected by trimethoprim/sulphamethoxazole, which acts on the folate pathway. There is not sufficient thymine or thymidine in normal mammalian tissues, blood or urine for the survival of these mutants. They have been found in the urine of patients with renal calculi, the sputum of a patient with chronic lung sepsis and in pus from a patient with osteomyelitis (Maskell et al., 1976; Okubadejo and Maskell, 1977). It is possible that in these situations the breakdown of pus cells may act as a source of thymine. Special techniques are required to detect these thymine-requiring bacteria and if they are isolated from a patient, co-trimoxazole therapy should be discontinued (Tapsall *et al.*, 1974; Maskell *et al.*, 1976).

It appears that an earlier report of Haemophilus influenzae strains resistant to trimethoprim by May and Davies (1972) may have resulted from technical problems with the testing procedure (Kirven and Thornsberry, 1974; Pelton *et al.*, 1977). Nevertheless Howard *et al.* (1978) reported rare strains of H. influenzae in Britain which were resistant to trimethoprim. Resistant shigellae and salmonellae still appear to be rare. In surveys of Shigella strains in the United States of America, variants resistant to trimethoprim (Rudoy *et al.*, 1974) or co-trimoxazole (Byers *et al.*, 1976) have not been encountered. An epidemic strain of Salmonella heidelberg in Jamaica appeared to develop non-transferable trimethoprim resistance *in vivo* (French and Lowry, 1977). Transferable resistance to trimethoprim was demonstrated in one strain of Salm. typhimurium isolated from a patient in Canada, but this infection may have been acquired in South-East Asia (Finlayson and Jackson, 1978).

8. *Synergy with sulphonamides.* Trimethoprim and sulphonamides exert a strongly synergistic effect against some bacteria. When organisms sensitive to both drugs are tested *in vitro*, the addition of a subinhibitory concentration of one often reduces the minimum inhibitory concentration of the other by about eight-fold or more (Darrell *et al.*, 1968). For example, these authors found that a strain of Strep. pneumoniae was inhibited by a combination of $0\cdot12\,\mu$g per ml of trimethoprim and $1\cdot2\,\mu$g per ml of sulphafurazole, but the individual MIC's for this strain were $1\cdot0\,\mu$g per ml and $32\,\mu$g per ml respectively. This potentiation of trimethoprim by sulphonamides and *vice versa*, varies with bacterial species and also with individual strains. Darrell *et al.* (1968) found a high degree of potentiation with the gonococci and also most strains of Proteus spp., but the sulphonamide only potentiated the activity of trimethoprim about four- to eight-fold against most strains of staphylococci, streptococci, pneumococci, H. influenzae and Esch. coli. Maximum synergy usually occurs when trimethoprim and sulphamethoxazole are used together in a ratio of their MIC's (Table 42). This ratio is 1:19 for many organisms and is consequently used in co-trimoxazole disc testing. Darrell *et al.* (1968) found that some organisms such as gonococci were more sensitive to sulphonamides than trimethoprim, so that the optimal ratio was the reverse (Table 42). Nevertheless two groups of investigators in the United States showed that most N. gonorrhoeae strains, when tested against trimethoprim/sulphamethoxazole in a ratio of 1:19, were inhibited by concentrations of $2\cdot5\,\mu$g per ml or less of trimethoprim and $47\cdot5\,\mu$g per ml or less of sulphamethoxazole (Yoshikawa *et al.*, 1975; Prior *et al.*, 1976). In a study of 75 beta-lactamase producing gonococcal strains (page 8) isolated from patients in the United States or East Asia, all were sensitive to co-trimoxazole (Report, 1978). With some bacterial strains, synergy cannot be demonstrated despite sensitivity to both trimethoprim and sulphonamides (Lewis *et al.*, 1974).

With trimethoprim-sensitive but sulphonamide-resistant bacteria, the sulphonamides do not usually potentiate the action of trimethoprim. Reisberg *et al.* (1967) studied two strains of Esch. coli sensitive to low concentrations of trimethoprim, but resistant to sulfisoxazole, but were unable to demonstrate an additive effect. However with such sulphonamide-resistant bacteria, a synergistic effect can usually be demonstrated *in vitro*, if very high sulphonamide concentrations, which equal or exceed the MIC's of the organisms to sulphonamides, are used. Darrell *et al.* (1968) used a sulphafurazole/trimethoprim ratio of 2000:1 and demonstrated a four-fold potentiation of trimethoprim against sulphonamide-resistant Proteus and Staph. pyogenes strains. This finding is of no clinical importance, because such high sulphonamide concentrations cannot be safely attained *in vivo*. Synergy with trimethoprim can also be demonstrated against some strains of Ps. aeruginosa which are 'moderately resistant to sulphamethoxazole' (*see* page 688) and, because high concentrations of sulphonamides are attained in urine, this may be of significance in treating urinary tract infections. Similarly synergy may be attained in the urine of patients with sulphonamide-resistant Esch. coli treated by co-trimoxazole (Grüneberg, 1975).

In clinical practice the sensitivity of organisms to trimethoprim and sulphonamide should be tested separately. If the bacterial species is sensitive to both, a synergistic effect is likely, and treatment should be effective. However infections due to trimethoprim-sensitive, but sulphonamide-resistant bacteria, also usually respond to the combination and they would probably respond equally well to trimethoprim alone. On theoretical grounds it is possible that trimethoprim-resistant bacterial strains may emerge during the treatment of such infections, but this has not been a major problem so far (page 689).

9. *Synergy with other drugs*. Trimethoprim acts synergistically with rifampicin against a wide range of bacteria, particularly Gram-negative bacilli; in addition these two drugs are compatible pharmacologically (*see* page 555).

Trimethoprim also enhances the activity of the polymyxins against certain bacteria. The combination of a polymyxin, sulphamethoxazole and trimethoprim is more active than combinations of any two of these agents against a variety of Gram-negative bacilli (page 532).

A combination of trimethoprim and amikacin (page 379) is synergistic against some Gram-negative bacilli (Parsley *et al.*, 1977). Synergy was demonstrated against most strains of Klebsiella pneumoniae, Serratia marcescens and Esch. coli; trimethoprim had no antibacterial effect on strains of Pseudomonas aeruginosa and did not alter amikacin's activity against them.

In Vitro Sensitivities

The minimum inhibitory concentrations of trimethoprim compared to those of sulphadiazine and sulphamethoxazole are shown in Table 42. Trimethoprim is much more active than the sulphonamides against most bacterial species. Acquired bacterial resistance to the sulphonamides is common (page 660), therefore strains with higher minimum inhibitory concentrations to sulphonamides than those shown in this table will be encountered.

Mode of Administration and Dosage

1. *Adults*. Until recently trimethoprim has only been available for general use as a mixture with sulphamethoxazole. The commonly used tablets or capsules of co-trimoxazole each contain 80 mg of trimethoprim and 400 mg of sulphamethoxazole. The usual adult dose is two tablets given 12-hourly. For

TABLE 42

Compiled from data published by Bushby and Hitchings (1968) and Bushby (1969)

ORGANISM	MIC (μg per ml)		
	Tri-methoprim	Sulpha-diazine	Sulpha-methoxazole
Gram-positive bacteria			
Staph. pyogenes	0·2	4·0	4·0
Strep. pyogenes (Group A)	0·4	50·0	100($\pm$25)
Strep. pneumoniae (Dip. pneumoniae)	1·0	32($\pm$16)	32($\pm$16)
Strep. viridans spp.	0·25	8·0	8·0
Strep. faecalis (Enterococcus, Group D)	0·5	100·0	100·0
Clostridium perfringens	50·0	16($\pm$8)	16($\pm$8)
Corynebacterium diphtheriae	0·4	>100·0	>100·0
Nocardia asteroides	10·0	—	5·0
Gram-negative bacteria			
Escherichia coli	0·2	8·0	8·0
Enterobacter spp.	3·0	>100·0	>100·0
Klebsiella pneumoniae	0·5	16·0	16·0
Citrobacter freundii	0·1	3·0	3·0
Proteus spp.	1·0	4–16	8·0
Salmonella typhi	0·4	4·0	4·0
Salmonella typhimurium	0·3	10·0	10·0
Shigella spp.	0·4	4·0	4·0
Neisseria gonorrhoeae	12·0	0·8–3·2	1·6
Neisseria meningitidis	8·0	0·5	0·5
Haemophilus influenzae	0·12	>50·0	>50·0
Bordetella pertussis	1·0–3·0	100·0	100·0
Vibrio cholerae	0·8	32·0	32·0
Pseudomonas aeruginosa	>100·0	25·0	25·0

severe infections this dose may be increased to a total of six tablets a day, given in two or three divided doses. A dose of one tablet 12-hourly is sufficient for long-term therapy of chronic bronchial or urinary tract infections.

2. *Children.* A paediatric suspension containing 40 mg trimethoprim and 200 mg sulphamethoxazole per 5 ml is available. The doses for children are as follows: six weeks to five months of age, 20 mg trimethoprim and 100 mg sulphamethoxazole (2·5 ml) twice-daily; six months to five years, 40 mg of trimethoprim and 200 mg of sulphamethoxazole (5·0 ml) twice-daily; and for those aged five to twelve years, 80 mg trimethoprim and 400 mg sulphamethoxazole (10 ml) twice-daily (Fowle, 1973).

3. *Newborn and premature infants.* The use of trimethoprim/sulphamethoxazole is not recommended for infants during the first four weeks of life. Young babies should not be breast fed by mothers receiving the drug. However this combination has been occasionally used for treatment of severe infections in 2–3-week-old infants without encountering serious toxicity. Roy (1971) suggests that a dose of trimethoprim 8–10 mg per kg per day and sulphamethoxazole 40–50 mg

per kg per day may be suitable for infants, but this combination should only be used at this age when absolutely necessary. Sulphonamides can cause kernicterus (page 670), and for this reason it is inadvisable to use trimethoprim/sulphamethoxazole for prematures or for infants during the first one week of life.
or for infants during the first one week of life.

4. *Patients with renal failure.* Both trimethoprim and sulphamethoxazole are excreted via the kidney, but in addition both drugs are removed by non-renal mechanisms (page 698). Renal function has little influence on the serum half-life of active sulphamethoxazole until there is severe impairment, but the excretion of sulphonamide metabolites and active trimethoprim are more dependent on renal function (Bergan and Brodwall, 1976). The half-life of total sulphamethoxazole increases rapidly as the creatinine clearance deteriorates past 30–40 ml per min, and it increases rapidly at about 20–25 ml for trimethoprim. The half-life of total sulphamethoxazole becomes more prolonged relative to that of trimethoprim (Bergan and Brodwall, 1976), and the half-life of trimethoprim is usually less than that of active sulphamethoxazole (Craig and Kunin, 1973a; Bergan and Brodwall, 1976). There is considerable variation of these half-lives in individual patients with renal failure, being in the range 13·8–46·3 h for trimethoprim and 21·8–50·2 h for active sulphamethoxazole (Craig and Kunin, 1973a).

In patients with mild to moderate degrees of renal functional impairment these drugs do not accumulate, and the usual doses may be given. Patients with a creatinine clearance of 10–30 ml per min may be given an initial full loading dose of both drugs (160 mg trimethoprim and 800 mg sulphamethoxazole), and then half this dose twice-daily (Craig and Kunin, 1973a). In patients with anuria or severe uraemia (creatinine clearance less than 10 ml per min) a full loading dose may also be given, followed by half this dose once- or twice-daily. However in these patients independent adjustment of the dosage of each drug may be advisable, because the half-life of total sulphamethoxazole in the serum is greatly increased compared to that of trimethoprim. Welling *et al.* (1973) suggest that patients with severe renal failure should receive a normal initial loading dose, and that subsequent 12-hourly doses of sulphamethoxazole and trimethoprim be reduced to one-third and one-half of the usual dose respectively. Bergan and Brodwall (1976) consider that because of the possibility of an accumulation of sulphonamide metabolites, co-trimoxazole should not be used in patients with a creatinine clearance less than 15 ml per min, unless regular determinations of total sulphonamide can be made.

Both drugs are removed during haemodialysis, and patients undergoing this procedure should receive a full dose before and after dialysis (Craig and Kunin, 1973a).

Even in patients with severe renal failure urinary levels of both drugs usually exceed those required for the eradication of most urinary pathogens. In patients with severe renal failure, trimethoprim accumulates in the serum to a lesser extent than sulphamethoxazole (because it is more efficiently removed by non-renal mechanisms), but its excretion via the kidney is reduced to a greater extent than that of sulphamethoxazole (Craig and Kunin, 1973a). Thus the sulphamethoxazole/trimethoprim ratio in the urine of uraemic patients may approach 19:1, which appears to be optimal for antibacterial synergy against common urinary pathogens (Bushby, 1969; Adam *et al.*, 1973).

Denneberg *et al.* (1976) used co-trimoxazole for long-term treatment of acute and chronic pyelonephritis in 15 patients with impaired renal function in the following dosage schedule: two tablets (each containing 400 mg sul-sulphamethoxazole and 80 mg trimethoprim) twice a day for six days followed by two tablets daily for patients with a creatinine clearance of 30–75 ml per min (serum creatinine 1·3–5·0 mg per cent*), for those with creatinine clearance of 15–30 ml per min (serum creatinine 5·0–12·0 mg per cent) two tablets twice-daily for three days and then two tablets daily, and for patients with a creatinine clearance of <5·0–15·0 ml per min (serum creatinine >12·0 mg per cent) some of who were receiving maintenance haemodialysis, one tablet daily for three days then usually one tablet daily according to serum levels. Patients were treated for periods of up to two years and over; regular serum level monitoring showed that active sulphamethoxazole and trimethoprim levels remained acceptable and their bacteriological and clinical response to treatment was good. Bennett and Craven (1976) treated urinary tract infections in six patients with severe renal failure (creatinine clearance <30 ml per min) by co-trimoxazole in a dose of two tablets (each 80 mg trimethoprim, 400 mg sul-phamethoxazole) for 14 days. Mean serum levels of trimethoprim (3·1 μg per ml) and sulphamethoxazole (65 μg per ml) were higher than normal but un-associated with adverse effects. Mean urine trimethoprim levels were 28·6 μg per ml and, although in four patients the urine sulphamethoxazole level was less than 10 μg per ml, bacteriological cure was obtained in all patients.

Nevertheless, because co-trimoxazole may cause deterioration in renal function (*see* toxicity, page 704), probably due to the high serum concentrations of sulphamethoxazole metabolites, serum concentrations should be determined regularly in patients with a creatinine clearance below 20–30 ml per min (Denneberg *et al.*, 1976). The manufacturers recommend that treatment should be interrupted if the serum level of total sulphamethoxazole exceeds 150 μg per ml and that it should only be recommenced when the level falls below 120 μg per ml.

5. *Intravenous administration.* A preparation of co-trimoxazole suitable for intravenous administration was introduced for general use in the United Kingdom in 1974 and subsequently in other countries such as Australia. It is available in 5 ml ampoules each containing 80 mg trimethoprim and 400 mg sulphamethoxazole for addition to an intravenous infusion; this preparation is not suitable for intramuscular or intravenous injection. The contents of ampoules should be diluted immediately before use in the following volumes: one ampoule (5 ml) in 125 ml infusion solution, two ampoules (10 ml) in 250 ml and three ampoules (15 ml) in 500 ml infusion solution. Commonly used dextrose and/or sodium chloride intravenous solutions and various dextran solutions are suitable diluents, if other additives are not present. The recommended daily dosage is 6 mg trimethoprim and 30 mg sulphamethoxazole per kg body weight, given in two divided doses. The dose for adults and children over 12 years old is 10 ml (2 ampoules) twice-daily, but this may be increased to 15 ml twice-daily for severe infections. For children the dosage is 1·25 ml twice-daily for those aged six weeks to five months, 2·5 ml twice-daily for those aged six months to five years and 5·0 ml twice-daily when aged six to twelve years.

---

* For conversion of serum creatinine values from SI units, *see* page 333.

Where possible the duration of the infusion should not exceed 1·5 h. This intravenous preparation should only be used when the patient cannot take oral therapy, and currently it is recommended that it should not be given for more than three successive days. Crystalluria and acute renal failure has followed the use of intravenous co-trimoxazole in two patients with hypoalbuminaemia (page 671). Nevertheless this preparation has been used for periods of 10 days to treat patients with septicaemias and meningitis and this has been well tolerated (Sabel and Brandberg, 1975; Olćen and Eriksson, 1976).

6. Co-trimoxazole should not be used in patients with liver disease, blood dyscrasias, and patients with a history of hypersensitivity to sulphonamides. The simultaneous administration of trimethoprim with other 2,4-diaminopyrimidines such as pyrimethamine or proguanil should also be avoided (Fleming et al., 1974).

Because this drug may interfere with folate metabolism (page 701), regular full blood examinations should be performed on patients receiving long-term therapy and those who are predisposed to folate deficiency.

Availability

1. Tablets each containing 80 mg trimethoprim and 400 mg sulphamethoxazole.
2. Tablets each containing 160 mg trimethoprim and 800 mg sulphamethoxazole ('Bactrim D.S.', 'Septrin Forte').
3. Paediatric suspension: 5 ml containing 40 mg trimethoprim and 200 mg sulphamethoxazole.
4. Preparation for intravenous use: 5 ml ampoules containing trimethoprim 80 mg and sulphamethoxazole 400 mg in a vehicle containing propylene glycol ('Septrin for infusion').

Serum Levels in Relation to Dosage

1. Trimethoprim is well absorbed after oral administration. After the usual oral dose of 160 mg a peak serum level of about 2 μg per ml is reached in 1–2 h; this is maintained for about 6 h, and then falls progressively. The serum half-life of the drug is about 13 h, and detectable serum levels are still present 24 h after a dose of 160 mg (Bushby and Hitchings, 1968). Higher serum levels are attained when this dose is increased (Fig. 33).

2. Sulphamethoxazole is also well absorbed from the gastro-intestinal tract. After a 1200 ml oral dose a peak level of about 60 μg per ml of the active drug is attained 2 h after administration, which persists for about 6 h. The serum half-life of this drug is 9–12 h (Fig. 34).

3. Trimethoprim and sulphamethoxazole can be administered simultaneously because their half-lives are almost identical. The administration of these drugs in a 1:5 ratio as co-trimoxazole results in serum levels of these drugs in a ratio of about 1:20 to 1:30 when their peak levels are reached at about 2 h. This is the ratio at which maximum synergy occurs against many organisms (page 691). After peak levels this ratio falls gradually to between 1:10 and 1:20 at the end of the dosage interval. In patients with impaired renal function, the ratio at the time of peak serum levels falls from 1:20 to 1:10 after 12 h (Bergan and Brodwall, 1976).

4. If the individual dose of co-trimoxazole is increased, even up to 12 tablets (960 mg trimethoprim and 4800 mg sulphamethoxazole), peak serum levels of

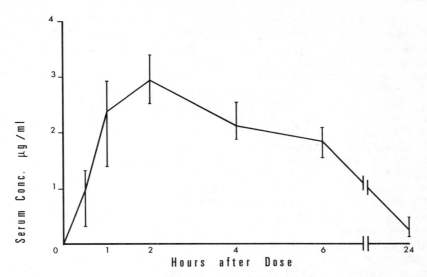

FIG. 33. Average trimethoprim serum levels in four volunteers after a 240 mg oral dose. (Redrawn after Brumfitt *et al.*, 1969.)

these drugs are increased linearly and their half-lives for elimination from the serum are prolonged (Fass *et al.*, 1977). Yoshikawa and Guze (1976) gave healthy volunteers nine tablets of co-trimoxazole (720 mg trimethoprim and 3600 mg sulphamethoxazole) as a single dose; resultant mean serum levels during the first 8 h were 6·12–8·32 μg per ml for trimethoprim and 98–120 μg per ml for sulphamethoxazole, and at 24 h the average levels of trimethoprim

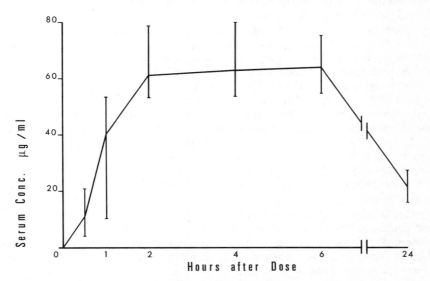

FIG. 34. Average serum levels of non-acetylated sulphamethoxazole in four fasting volunteers after a 1200 mg oral dose. (Redrawn after Brumfitt *et al.*, 1969.)

and sulphamethoxazole were 2·16 and 31·7 μg per ml respectively. When a 12-tablet dose of co-trimoxazole (960 mg trimethoprim and 4800 mg sulphamethoxazole) was given to volunteers, mean peak levels of trimethoprim and sulphamethoxazole at 2–4 h, were six-fold higher than those which occur after a two-tablet dose (Fass *et al.*, 1977). These mean peak serum levels were 9·2, 259·4 and 233·7 μg per ml for trimethoprim, total sulphamethoxazole and free sulphamethoxazole respectively; their corresponding elimination half-lives were 16·7, 14·6 and 12·9 h, so that mean serum concentrations at 24 h were approximately ten-fold higher than after a two-tablet dose.

5. Bushby and Hitchings (1968) studied serum levels in six adult volunteers after an intravenous dose of 100 mg of trimethoprim lactate. An average serum level of 1·4 μg per ml was obtained 5 min after injection, 1·0 μg per ml after 3 h and 0·95 μg per ml after 4·5 h. The average serum level was still 0·3 μg per ml at 24 h and the half-life of trimethoprim after intravenous injection was estimated to be 11–12 h. This does not differ significantly from the half-life of this drug after oral administration. According to the manufacturers, apart from initially higher serum levels following a co-trimoxazole infusion, subsequent serum levels are comparable to the serum levels of trimethoprim and sulphamethoxazole attained following oral co-trimoxazole. Franzén and Brandberg (1976) found that peak serum levels of trimethoprim and sulphamethoxazole immediately after an infusion of co-trimoxazole given over a period of 30 min were almost identical to the peak values obtained at 2 h when the same dose was given orally.

Excretion

URINE: Unchanged trimethoprim is mainly excreted by non-ionic renal diffusion and this is influenced by pH (Sharpstone, 1969; Craig and Kunin, 1973a). A considerable proportion of orally administered trimethoprim is excreted in the urine unchanged (Bushby and Hitchings, 1968; Bach *et al.*, 1973c). Approximately 10 per cent of the excreted drug is in the form of metabolites with little or no antibacterial activity. Urinary concentrations of about 100 μg per ml after the usual oral dose are approximately 100-fold higher than those attained in serum and remain high for about 24 h. Approximately 40–60 per cent of an orally administered dose of trimethoprim can be recovered from the urine in the active form within 24 h. However there is considerable individual variation in the amount of trimethoprim, which is excreted as the active drug (Sigel *et al.*, 1973). The amount of active trimethoprim excreted in urine during a 24-h period after intravenous administration, varies from 42 to 75 per cent of the administered dose (Bushby and Hitchings, 1968).

Sulphamethoxazole is also mainly excreted in the urine but about 70 per cent of this is in the form of its acetylated and other metabolites. The ratio of sulphamethoxazole to trimethoprim in the urine may vary from 1:1 to 5:1 (Grey and Hamilton-Miller, 1977; Fass *et al.*, 1977). Acidification of the urine results in increased urinary excretion of trimethoprim, but has no significant effect on that of active sulphamethoxazole. By contrast, alkalinization of the urine decreases urinary excretion of trimethoprim and increases the excretion of sulphamethoxazole. In acid urine the ratio of active sulphamethoxazole to trimethoprim is approximately one, whereas in alkaline urine the ratio is usually greater than five (Craig and Kunin, 1973a).

BILE: A small amount of trimethoprim appears to be eliminated via the bile. In patients without biliary obstruction, concentrations of the drug in bile are slightly higher than those in the serum 4 h after a dose, but these fall to levels lower than in the serum 24 h after a dose (Rieder, 1973).

INACTIVATION IN BODY: A significant proportion of administered trimethoprim is converted in the liver to antibacterially inactive metabolites. Five such metabolites have been identified, and all of these are also excreted in the urine (Sigel *et al.*, 1973).

Distribution of the Drug in Body

After absorption trimethoprim is rapidly distributed in the body, and animal experiments have shown that tissue levels are usually greater than those in the serum, except in brain, skin and fat. Particularly high tissue levels have been found in the kidney and liver (Craig and Kunin, 1973b).

In humans the drug is equally distributed between plasma and erythrocytes. Concentrations of trimethoprim in most tissues and body fluids, including sputum and pleural fluid, appear to be higher than corresponding serum levels. After co-trimoxazole administration, the trimethoprim concentration in sputum is about double that in serum but the sulphamethoxazole concentration is only about half the serum level (Hughes, 1976a). In addition, effective antibacterial concentrations of trimethoprim are attained in normal cerebrospinal fluid (Bach *et al.*, 1973c). Salmon *et al.* (1975) studied aqueous humour levels of patients receiving co-trimoxazole, who were undergoing cataract surgery. The mean ratio of the concentrations in aqueous humour to that of serum for trimethoprim and free sulphamethoxazole were 0·30 and 0·24 respectively. In general these ratios did not change with the time after the dose or with prolonged dosing with co-trimoxazole. Trimethoprim diffuses well into human vaginal fluid, reaching concentrations that sometimes are nearly three-fold simultaneous serum levels. By contrast, levels of sulphamethoxazole in vaginal fluid are often undetectable or very low after oral treatment with co-trimoxazole (Stamey and Condy, 1975). High levels of trimethoprim in vaginal fluid (and prostate) probably result from non-ionic diffusion into this more acid environment. When oral co-trimoxazole was given to healthy males, mean levels of 1·0–1·5 µg per ml of trimethoprim were detected in seminal fluid when their mean serum levels were 1·8–2·0 µg per ml (Gnarpe and Friberg, 1976). Pus obtained from a cerebral abscess of a patient receiving oral co-trimoxazole (160 mg trimethoprim, 800 mg sulphamethoxazole) twice-daily, contained trimethoprim and sulphamethoxazole levels of 1·6 and 15·47 µg per ml respectively (Greene *et al.*, 1975). Brain tissue from a Nocardial brain abscess contained a trimethoprim concentration of 5·1 µg per ml and a sulphamethoxazole concentration of 36 µg per ml, 6 h after an oral dose of 160 mg trimethoprim and 800 mg sulphamethoxazole (Maderazo and Quintiliani, 1974). Trimethoprim appears to be concentrated in the bile of patients with radiologically functioning gall bladders (Morran *et al.*, 1978).

With usual serum concentrations, trimethoprim is 42 to 46 per cent bound to serum proteins (Schwartz and Ziegler, 1969).

Mode of Action

Trimethoprim interferes with the action of dihydrofolic acid reductase, an enzyme which converts dihydrofolic to tetrahydrofolic acid, an essential stage in bacterial purine and, ultimately, DNA synthesis. This enzyme acts at a stage which immediately follows the enzyme conversion of para-amino-benzoic acid to dihydrofolic acid, which can be competitively blocked by sulphonamides (page 668). This sequential action of sulphonamides and trimethoprim explains the synergistic action of this combination against sensitive bacteria (Darrell *et al.*, 1968). The sulphonamides do not have an inhibitory effect on human folate metabolism because dihydrofolic acid is obtained directly from dietary folates (Fig. 35). The reduction of dihydrofolic to tetrahydrofolic acid in humans, similar to bacteria, is also catalysed by dihydrofolic acid reductase. However trimethoprim has at least 10 000 times more inhibitory effect on the bacterial enzyme than on the corresponding mammalian enzyme (Kahn *et al.*, 1968).

The inhibitory effect of trimethoprim on the dihydrofolic acid reductase of malarial parasites is about 2000 times greater than on the human enzyme, and trimethoprim can therefore be used for treatment of human malaria. The chemically related antimalarial drug, pyrimethamine, has a similar mode of action against dihydrofolic acid reductase of the malarial parasite (page 676), but this action is about 2000 times greater than its effect against either the mammalian or bacterial enzymes (Hichings, 1969). The sulphonamides potentiate the action of both trimethoprim and pyrimethamine against malaria parasites.

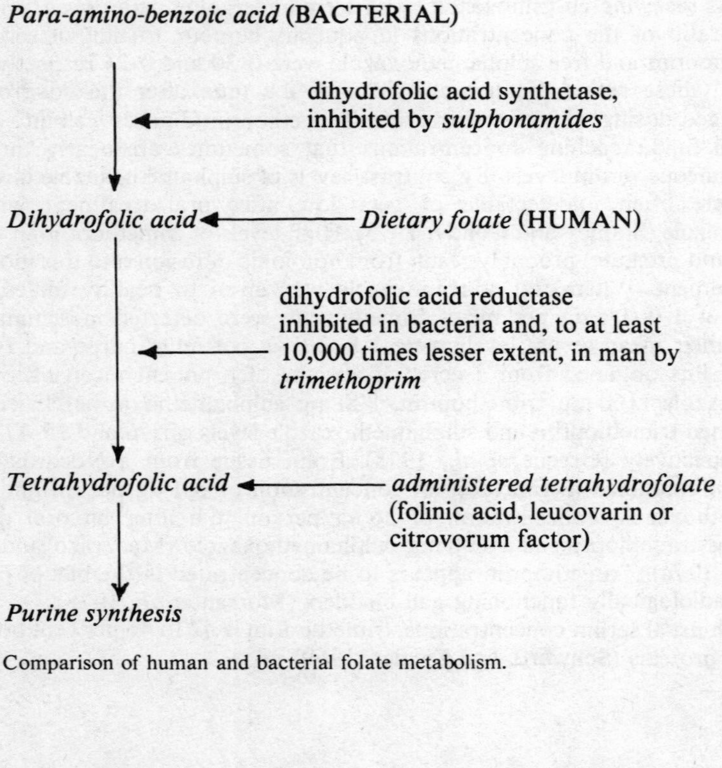

Para-amino-benzoic acid (BACTERIAL)

⟵ dihydrofolic acid synthetase, inhibited by *sulphonamides*

Dihydrofolic acid ⟵ *Dietary folate* (HUMAN)

⟵ dihydrofolic acid reductase inhibited in bacteria and, to at least 10,000 times lesser extent, in man by *trimethoprim*

Tetrahydrofolic acid ⟵ *administered tetrahydrofolate* (folinic acid, leucovarin or citrovorum factor)

Purine synthesis

Fig. 35. Comparison of human and bacterial folate metabolism.

It was predicted from studies of its mode of action that if depression of human folate metabolism due to trimethoprim therapy occurred, it would be reversed by administration of tetrahydrofolate compounds such as folinic acid. This was subsequently confirmed by clinical studies (*vide infra*). In addition on theoretical grounds, the administration of folinic acid should not interfere with the antibacterial action of trimethoprim, because bacteria cannot utilize preformed dihydrofolates or tetrahydrofolates. This has also been confirmed by both bacteriological (Grunberg *et al.*, 1970), and clinical studies (Kahn *et al.*, 1968; Jenkins *et al.*, 1970).

Whilst the components of co-trimoxazole, trimethoprim and sulphamethoxazole, have bacteristatic activity in clinically achievable concentrations, this combination is bactericidal when synergy is achieved (Bushby, 1968).

Toxicity

1. *Gastro-intestinal side-effects.* Trimethoprim can cause nausea and diarrhoea, and these were common in early clinical studies when doses as high as 1 g daily were given. The maximum recommended daily dose of trimethoprim is only 480 mg (six standard tablets of co-trimoxazole) with which gastro-intestinal side-effects are uncommon. Single oral doses of nine tablets of co-trimoxazole (720 mg trimethoprim and 3600 mg sulphamethoxazole) are usually well tolerated (Yoshikawa and Guze, 1976). However single oral doses of 12 tablets (960 mg trimethoprim and 4800 mg sulphamethoxazole) may cause malaise, nausea, headache and transient oliguria and crystalluria (Fass *et al.*, 1977).

2. *Haematological side-effects.* Because of its mode of action, it was anticipated that trimethoprim may interfere with human folate metabolism and hence haemopoiesis, especially if large doses were given over prolonged periods. The *in vitro* effect of various concentrations of trimethoprim has been studied on human bone marrow cultures. A sensitive indicator, which detects trimethoprim's effect on folate metabolism in such cultures, is interference of folate-dependent DNA-thymine synthesis by methylation of deoxyuridylate to thymidylate (Sive *et al.*, 1972; Koutts *et al.*, 1973). Only slight or no effect on folate metabolism was demonstrated by this method in normal bone marrow cells, if the trimethoprim concentrations used were similar to those attained in serum with usual doses. However ten-fold greater trimethoprim concentrations produced abnormalities of folate metabolism, which were only partially corrected by folic acid but were completely corrected by folinic acid (*vide supra*). In vitamin B_{12} or folate deficient marrow cultures, trimethoprim at therapeutic concentrations caused further disturbance in folate metabolism, which was not corrected by vitamin B_{12} or folic acid, but this was again completely reversed by folinic acid (Koutts *et al.*, 1973). Changes in folate metabolism have also been investigated in patients receiving co-trimoxazole by measuring the serum level of tetrahydrofolate, a specific indicator of dihydrofolate reductase activity (page 700). These serum levels remain normal in patients with otherwise normal haemopoiesis if trimethoprim is used in the usual doses (Davis and Jackson, 1973).

Clinical experience with co-trimoxazole supports the above experimental observations. If patients without a bone marrow disorder are treated with usual trimethoprim doses, haematological side-effects, although reported, appear to be uncommon (Salter, 1973; Frisch, 1973; Lawson and Henry, 1977). Reported abnormalities include aplastic anaemia (Frisch, 1973), neutropenia (Nielsen *et al.*, 1970; Frisch, 1973), acute agranulocytosis (Evans and Tell, 1969; Palva and Koivisto, 1971), and acute thrombocytopenia (Hammett, 1970; Rickard and Uhr, 1971; Raik and Vincent, 1973; Böse *et al.*, 1974). Thrombocytopenia appears to be more common in patients receiving long-term treatment with diuretics such as the thiazides or frusemide (Frisch, 1973). Whereas Salter (1973) found thrombocytopenia more frequent in patients over 70 years of age, others have observed this complication at all ages (Dickson, 1978). Pancytopenia has been described in a seven-month-old baby receiving oral co-trimoxazole (Tulloch, 1976). All these toxic effects, which indicate depression of haemopoiesis, appear to be more common following prolonged co-trimoxazole therapy (Dawborn *et al.*, 1973). It is possible that some of these reported side-effects may have been caused by sulphamethoxazole and not trimethoprim; in particular acute agranulocytosis, a well known complication of sulphonamides (Palva and Koivisto, 1971). Haemolytic anaemia has been rarely observed with co-trimoxazole therapy (Frisch, 1973). A patient with typhoid fever and glucose-6-phosphate dehydrogenase deficiency developed acute haemolysis when treated by co-trimoxazole (Owusu, 1972), but ten infants with the same defect were treated by co-trimoxazole for five days without haemolysis (Chan and Wong, 1975). Nevertheless haemolysis is a known complication of sulphonamides in such patients (page 670).

Jewkes *et al.* (1970) described a patient who developed megaloblastic erythropoiesis after a six month course of co-trimoxazole, given in usual doses for chronic bronchitis. Folic acid administration was of no benefit but the bone marrow reverted to normal within one week, despite continued administration of trimethoprim, when folinic acid was given in a daily dose of 60 μg by injection. This appears to be the only case in which megaloblastic changes have followed the administration of standard doses of a co-trimoxazole (Frisch, 1973), and even then, the causative relationship of trimethoprim in this case has been disputed (Girdwood, 1976). In many other patients who have developed megaloblastic anaemia while receiving this combination, an alternative explanation has been found for the blood dyscrasia (Girdwood, 1973). Hughes *et al.* (1975a) administered co-trimoxazole for long periods to 11 patients, one for 30 months and the remainder for periods of 3–16 months. A few of these patients appeared to develop at the most asymptomatic folate depletion as reflected by serial haematological investigations.

If trimethoprim is used in doses higher than normally recommended, bone marrow toxicity may result more commonly. Kahn *et al.* (1968) administered trimethoprim in a daily oral dose of 1·0 g for a period of four weeks to ten adult patients. Thirteen other adult patients were given the same dose of trimethoprim plus 4 g of sulfisoxazole daily, for periods varying from several months to over two years. Haematological abnormalities such as leucopenia, anaemia and thrombocytopenia were noted in several patients in both groups, but these abnormalities disappeared about two weeks after the drugs were stopped. In one patient thrombocytopenia and leucopenia were reversed by the administration of citrovorum factor (folinic acid), despite continued administration of trimethoprim (*see also* page 701). These haematological abnormalities also occur more frequently in patients with severe renal failure who are treated by usual doses, because they develop high serum levels of both trimethoprim and sulphamethoxazole (page 694). McPherson and Raik (1970) reported acute thrombocytopenia in two uraemic patients, who were treated with usual co-trimoxazole doses. Yuill (1973) described megaloblastic anaemia in a severely uraemic patient receiving this combination, but other factors such as dietary deficiency of folic acid were also contributory.

Patients with a pre-existing megaloblastic anaemia are seriously at risk if treated with trimethoprim/sulphamethoxazole (Annotation, 1973). Trimethoprim aggravates megaloblastic changes and prevents response to either vitamin B_{12} or folic acid (Koutts *et al.*, 1973). In addition it may cause neutropenia and thrombocytopenia in these patients (Chanarin and England, 1972). The drug is therefore contraindicated in all patients with a megaloblastic anaemia or in those who may possibly have megaloblastic bone marrow changes such as pregnant women, patients receiving anticonvulsant drugs and those with a raised mean red cell volume.

Girdwood (1976) considers that once the folate deficiency is corrected, there is no reason why co-trimoxazole should not be used.

Co-trimoxazole should also be used cautiously in patients with a predisposition to bone marrow depression, for example, those treated by trimethoprim-related drugs such as pyrimethamine (page 687) and those receiving immunosuppressive drug therapy. Ansdell *et al.* (1976) described a woman who developed a megaloblastic anaemia following a 14-day course of co-trimoxazole, whilst taking pyrimethamine for malarial prophylaxis. Hulme and Reeves (1971) reported four renal transplant patients receiving immunosuppressive therapy (prednisolone and azathioprine), who developed a marked leucopenia in association with a course of co-trimoxazole, given within the first 60 days after transplantation. Leucopenia was not observed in another ten patients who received identical therapy at a later stage after transplantation. It was concluded that co-trimoxazole should be used with extreme caution during the first 60 days after cadaveric renal transplantation. A large prospective study confirmed that the frequency of leucopenia in 94 antibiotic-treated patients, who were renal transplant recipients, was greater in the early weeks after transplantation. However, the frequency in a control group treated for urinary infections with antibiotics other than co-trimoxazole was not significantly different from those treated with co-trimoxazole. In eight patients leucopenia recovered when azathioprine was discontinued whilst co-trimoxazole was continued. Azathioprine was therefore considered to be the cause of leucopenia. This drug is partly excreted by the kidney and the patients who developed leucopenia, although receiving a similar dose of azathioprine as those that did not, had poorer renal function (Hall, 1974).

Despite all these reports trimethoprim bone marrow toxicity appears to be uncommon. Most of these side-effects can probably be avoided if the known contraindications and precautions are observed. Nevertheless it would seem advisable to perform regular blood examinations during prolonged trimethoprim administration.

3. *Immunosuppressive effect.* Co-trimoxazole inhibits DNA synthesis in lymphocytes cultured in the presence of phytohaemagglutinin. This effect

occurs with both trimethoprim and sulphamethoxazole separately, but it is more pronounced with the drug combination (Gaylarde and Sarkany, 1972). Furthermore Arvilommi *et al.* (1972) demonstrated that co-trimoxazole partially suppresses antibody response after tetanus vaccination. These observations suggest that co-trimoxazole may have some immunosuppressive effects, but the clinical significance of these is not yet clear.

4. *Nephrotoxicity.* During a four-year period, Kalowski *et al.* (1973) detected 16 patients who developed deterioration of renal function in association with co-trimoxazole treatment; most of these had antecedent renal functional impairment. The co-trimoxazole associated renal damage was reversible in most patients when the drug was discontinued, but three developed permanent impairment of renal function. The deterioration in renal function appeared to be due to an acute tubular necrosis, and the authors suggested that it may have resulted from an accumulation of conjugated sulphamethoxazole metabolites in the presence of renal failure, rather than trimethoprim. They therefore recommended that co-trimoxazole should not be used in patients with a serum creatinine greater than 2 mg per cent or 0·17 mmol/l (creatinine clearance less than 40 ml per min). Bailey and Little (1976) reported another four patients whose renal function deteriorated in association with co-trimoxazole therapy; one patient had recovering acute oliguric renal failure and the other three had chronic renal failure at the time of co-trimoxazole therapy; two of those with chronic disease had further permanent impairment of renal function. Some of the patients reported by these two groups may have received inordinately high doses of co-trimoxazole for the state of their renal function. Other studies have been unable to disclose deterioration in renal function following the use of co-trimoxazole in suitably reduced dosage for patients with renal disease. Tasker *et al.* (1975) treated urinary or respiratory infections in 20 patients with chronic renal failure with co-trimoxazole. Deterioration in renal function which occurred in only three of these patients was not considered to be due to co-trimoxazole. The drug has also been given for periods of up to two years to patients with chronic renal disease without evidence of deterioration in renal function (Denneberg *et al.*, 1976). Rosenfeld *et al.* (1975) treated 18 patients with a neurogenic bladder, all of whom had a creatinine clearance above 50 ml per min, with prophylactic co-trimoxazole; 18 patients were treated for 60–80 days and in seven the period was extended to 330–430 days; no significant differences between the creatinine clearance values of these patients taken before and after this therapy were demonstrable. Guignard *et al.* (1978) gave co-trimoxazole to 16 children for a period of six months after reconstructive surgery on the urogenital tract. These children had normal renal function pre-operatively, and after this treatment there was no evidence that co-trimoxazole interfered with renal function or with normal functional maturation of kidneys in babies. The findings of Shouval *et al.* (1978) are in contrast to these. They administered co-trimoxazole in a dose of two tablets (each containing 80 mg trimethoprim and 400 mg sulphamethoxazole) three times a day for periods of six to eight days; the recipients were two patients who had a decreased creatinine clearance during co-trimoxazole therapy three months previously, from which they had recovered, and four healthy volunteers. Significant falls in creatinine clearance, rises in serum creatinine and increases in sodium excretion occurred in all subjects, and these changes

all returned promptly to normal on cessation of the drug. A temporary rise in serum creatinine levels after five days treatment with co-trimoxazole was also noted by Lövestad et al. (1976).

Although there has been controversy about the significance of all these reports, it appears that co-trimoxazole can sometimes affect renal function and it should be used cautiously in patients with renal failure (page 694).

5. *Hypersensitivity reactions*. Rashes have been observed in 1·6 to 8 per cent of patients during clinical trials with co-trimoxazole (Frisch, 1973; Salter, 1973). Most of these were probably caused by the sulphonamide component but it is difficult to separate the side-effects of the two individual drugs. All the other well-known side-effects of sulphonamides (page 668) can be expected to occur from time to time when the combination is used. Long-acting sulphonamides are more prone to cause Stevens–Johnson syndrome (page 668), and sulphamethoxazole, the component in co-trimoxazole, is a medium-acting sulphonamide with serum half-life of 9–12 h. Six patients with Stevens–Johnson syndrome have been reported in association with co-trimoxazole therapy, all of whom recovered (Salter, 1973). Thorpe and Nysenbaum (1978) reported the death of a 48-year-old woman who developed a rash, fever, vomiting and abdominal pain 24 h after taking co-trimoxazole; necropsy revealed diffuse gastric and small-intestinal haemorrhagic ulceration with diffuse mucosal bullae characteristic of Stevens–Johnson syndrome. Apparently there have been 28 cases (including two fatalities) of this syndrome reported in the world in association with co-trimoxazole therapy (Bernstein and Cooper, 1978). Three of five patients with toxic epidermal necrolysis (Lyell's syndrome) ascribed to the combination have died (Salter, 1973). Other patients have been described with polymorphous rashes and fever in whom microscopic examination of skin lesions showed changes compatible with a necrotizing vasculitis (Wåhlin and Rosman, 1976); one such patient also developed reversible renal failure (Ramaiah et al., 1977).

6. *Miscellaneous side-effects*. Various other rare reactions have occurred during co-trimoxazole therapy. These include acute rheumatoid arthritis, anaphylaxis, angioneurotic oedema, glossitis, leg paraesthesiae, hallucinations, tremor, vertigo, visual disturbances, headache and depression (Hanley, 1969; Frisch, 1973). Jaundice, usually mild and cholestatic in type, has occurred in a number of patients. In one such patient rechallenge with the drug caused recurrence of jaundice, which rapidly disappeared when the drug was stopped (Frisch, 1973). Hepatic necrosis in an 80-year-old man has been attributed to co-trimoxazole (Colucci et al., 1975). Polyneuropathy associated with co-trimoxazole therapy has been described in one patient (Grossman et al., 1977), but this may have been a complication of cardiac surgery which the patient received (Vincent, 1977). Pseudomembranous colitis was reported in an 80-year-old woman who received co-trimoxazole (Cameron and Thomas, 1977). The significance of these anecdotal reports is not clear.

7. *Safety in pregnancy*. Large doses of trimethoprim are teratogenic in animals; this is to be expected because trimethoprim is a folic acid antagonist (page 700). Although this drug has been used in a small number of patients during the first 16 weeks of pregnancy (page 706) without encountering any fetal malformations, folate levels are often marginal in pregnant women. For this reason the use of co-trimoxazole should be avoided where possible during

pregnancy, particularly during the first trimester.

8. *Interaction with other drugs*. There have been several reports describing the potentiation of warfarin and phenytoin by co-trimoxazole (*see* page 672).

Clinical Uses of the Drug

Trimethoprim has been used mainly in combination with sulphamethoxazole as co-trimoxazole, although trimethoprim by itself or in combination with other drugs (page 692) may be suitable for the treatment of some infections.

1. *Urinary tract infections*. Co-trimoxazole has been used extensively for these diseases. It is effective and superior to either a sulphadimidine or an ampicillin regimen (Reeves *et al.*, 1969), and in other trials it has produced a higher cure rate than cephalexin (Gower and Tasker, 1976) and nitrofurantoin (Lövestad *et al.*, 1976). The combination is clearly superior to sulphamethoxazole alone (Grüneberg and Kolbe, 1969; Knudsen *et al.*, 1973; Harding and Ronald, 1973). In these studies many bacteria were sensitive to trimethoprim and resistant to sulphonamides, but the results of treatment with the combination were still quite good. In addition, trimethoprim alone is about as effective as co-trimoxazole for the treatment of various types of urinary tract infections (Brumfitt and Pursell, 1972; Kasanen *et al.*, 1974). Trimethoprim causes fewer side-effects than the combination, but its use alone has not been advocated, as it is anticipated that resistant bacterial strains may emerge more readily.

Co-trimoxazole treatment has also been successful in a high proportion of patients with chronic and recurrent urinary tract infections (Nanra *et al.*, 1971; Stratford and Dixson, 1971). It has also been used successfully in a lower dosage (one standard tablet every one or two nights) for prolonged treatment of patients with chronic bacteriuria (Cattell *et al.*, 1971; O'Grady *et al.*, 1973; Kincaid-Smith *et al.*, 1973; Chinn *et al.*, 1976). Its value for this purpose has been compared with several other chemotherapeutic agents. In one trial in which it was compared with methenamine mandelate (page 794) and sulphamethoxazole, co-trimoxazole in an adult dose of one tablet (80 mg trimethoprim, 400 mg sulphamethoxazole) was more effective in preventing reinfections in females (Harding and Ronald, 1974). In other trials a low dose of co-trimoxazole has proved to be more effective prophylactically than methenamine hippurate (Kalowski *et al.*, 1975) and nitrofurantoin macrocrystals (page 756) (Stamey *et al.*, 1977). A trial of co-trimoxazole was also carried out on 120 patients with bacteriuria of pregnancy (Williams *et al.*, 1969). In most patients bacteriuria was eradicated by a seven-day course, and in many of these prior treatment with other chemotherapeutic agents had already failed. Ten patients were treated during the first 16 weeks of pregnancy, and no fetal malformations were observed.

The superiority of co-trimoxazole in the prevention of recurrent urinary infections in females without underlying genito-urinary disease is mainly due to its effect of reducing intestinal Enterobacteriaceae, which colonize the periurethral or vaginal vestibule area, and which are responsible for reinfections (Harding and Ronald, 1974; Stamey and Condy, 1975; Stamey *et al.*, 1977). This is probably related to the high concentrations of trimethoprim attained in vaginal fluid (page 699). An added advantage of long-term co-trimoxazole therapy is that, so far, the frequency of resistant intestinal Enterobacteriaceae remains low; this may be the result of the differing actions of its two components (page 689). It is possible that trimethoprim alone may be effective in preventing recurrent urinary infections, but whether this is so and whether such therapy would also be accompanied by a low order of resistance in faecal organisms has yet to be determined (Stamey et al., 1977). One patient reported by Kunin et al. (1978), who had severe renal failure, chronic pyelonephritis and recurrent urinary infections due to Proteus mirabilis, was successfully managed by long-term prophylaxis with trimethoprim alone. Trimethoprim was given in a dose of 100 mg twice-daily for nearly six months, and then as a single daily dose of 100 mg for more than three years. Interestingly, very few aerobic enteric Gram-negative bacteria were found on rectal or vaginal swabs after three years of treatment; small numbers of Esch. coli detected on one occasion remained fully sensitive to trimethoprim.

Acute uncomplicated urinary tract infections in children usually respond well to co-trimoxazole (Bose et al., 1974). For the prevention of reinfections in children, Stansfield (1975) showed that a six-month course was not superior to a two-week course of co-trimoxazole. In a controlled trial, Ellerstein et al. (1977) found that the results of treatment of acute urinary tract infections in children with ampicillin or co-trimoxazole were comparable. In a reduced dosage co-trimoxazole is also valuable for long-term suppressive therapy in children with chronic or recurrent urinary tract infections (Hobday, 1971; Lirenman and Arnold, 1973). A dose of 2 mg trimethoprim combined with 10 mg sulphamethoxazole per kg body weight daily has proved effective for this purpose (Smellie et al., 1976; 1978). These authors noted that during such prophylaxis the number of rectal coliform bacilli was greatly and rapidly reduced, but at least 70 per cent of surviving coliform organisms remained sensitive to the two components of co-trimoxazole. When co-trimoxazole prophylaxis was stopped, rectal organisms rapidly returned to normal, and they were all again sensitive to trimethoprim and sulphamethoxazole (Grüneberg et al., 1976).

Chronic bacterial prostatitis responds poorly to any chemotherapeutic agent, but some data indicate that co-trimoxazole may sometimes be useful in this disease (Meares, 1973). Co-trimoxazole is effective in preventing bacteriuria after prostatectomy (Hills et al., 1976).

2. *Serious infections caused by Gram-negative bacilli.* Co-trimoxazole is a useful combination for the treatment of septicaemias due to Gram-negative bacilli. Alone or in combination with polymyxin, it is also often effective for hospital-acquired infections which are resistant to many other chemotherapeutic agents.

Early papers described the successful use of co-trimoxazole in Proteus septicaemia (Noall et al., 1962; Cooper and Wald, 1964) and septicaemias due to Esch. coli and Enterobacter aerogenes which had not responded to several antibiotics (Darrell et al., 1968). Other publications have confirmed the value of co-trimoxazole, particularly the parenteral preparation for septicaemias due to Gram-negative bacilli. Olćen and Eriksson (1976) treated 12 elderly patients with septicaemias due mainly to Esch. coli, Klebsiella or Enterobacter spp.; a good response was obtained in six and in the others, including one due to Yersinia enterocolitica, the response was poor or inconclusive. Co-trimoxazole was usually given intravenously for the first 10 days and thereafter by the oral route. The drug was used by Franzén and Brandberg (1976) to treat patients with septicaemias due to a variety of Gram-negative bacilli, many of whom had failed to respond to commonly used antibiotics; the drug was given intravenously until the patient was afebrile for three days and then orally. Favourable results were obtained with patients who had septicaemia due to Esch. coli, Klebsiella or Proteus spp. and also in one young man with a H. influenzae septicaemia. Grose et al. (1977) used oral co-trimoxazole to treat cancer patients with infections, many of whom had not responded to initial therapy which usually consisted of carbenicillin and an aminoglycoside. Their overall response compared favourably with that which had been reported with aminoglycosides, with the exception of patients with infections due to Klebsiella pneumoniae.

Co-trimoxazole alone or combined with polymyxin has been used to treat opportunist infections due to Pseudomonas cepacia and Ps. maltophilia, both of which are often resistant to many antibiotics. Endocarditis due to Ps. cepacia has responded to treatment with co-trimoxazole (Hamilton et al., 1973, Neu et al., 1973), but two cases treated by Seligman et al. (1973) relapsed after stopping treatment. Darby (1976) reported the case of an infant girl with a meningomyelocoele who developed Ps. cepacia meningitis; her meningitis which had failed to respond to a variety of antibiotics eventually responded to oral co-trimoxazole. Treatment with co-trimoxazole was successful in a patient reported by Fischer (1973), who developed endocarditis on a prosthetic valve due to Ps. maltophilia, and which had failed to respond to gentamicin. Rahal et al. (1973) showed that the addition of trimethoprim and a sulphonamide significantly lowered the MIC of polymyxin for strains of Ps. cepacia. Subsequently, Noriega et al. (1975) used the combination of trimethoprim, sulphamethoxazole and polymyxin B to treat Ps. cepacia endocarditis in five heroin addicts, which had failed to respond to treatment with chloramphenicol and kanamycin; two or these five patients recovered after valvulectomy or valve replacement. The in vitro synergistic effect of co-trimoxazole and polymyxins against Gram-negative bacilli (page 532) has also been used to treat another now common nosocomial infection, that due to Serratia marcescens. Thomas et al. (1976) used a daily dosage of 1600 mg of sulphamethoxazole and 320 mg of trimethoprim orally combined with 100–300 mg of colistin methane sulphonate parenterally to obtain clinical improvement in four of six patients. Possible renal toxicity occurred in two and the authors advise caution when using this combination, because both co-trimoxazole (page 704) and polymyxins (page 539) can cause nephrotoxicity.

Experience from the treatment of a small number of patients suggested that co-trimoxazole may give good results in the treatment of Bacteroides fragilis infections (Okubadejo, 1974). Intravenously administered, co-trimoxazole was used by Franzén and Brandberg (1976) to cure a young man with a septicaemia due to a Bacteroides species. A combination of trimethoprim (100 mg) and sulphadimidine (500 mg), given intravenously, has been used successfully for a patient with a Bacteroides septicaemia, and the same regimen with the addition of lincomycin was also used to cure another patient with B. fragilis septicaemia (Hanson and Woods, 1975).

3. *Plague.* Some studies had suggested that a 5–17 day course of co-

trimoxazole may be effective for the treatment of bubonic plague (Ai *et al.*, 1973; Butler *et al.*, 1974). Subsequently a small trial was carried out in Vietnam in 1975 in which streptomycin and co-trimoxazole treatments for Yersinia pestis infections were compared. Streptomycin was given intramuscularly in a dose of 0·5–1·0 g (depending on the patient's weight) twice-daily for 10 days and co-trimoxazole (160 mg trimethoprim, 800 mg sulphamethoxazole, and half this dose for children) was given intravenously for three to five days, then orally in the same dose to complete a 10-day course. Patients treated with streptomycin had a shorter median duration or fever and less complications than those treated by co-trimoxazole (Butler *et al.*, 1976).

4. *Melioidosis.* Several case reports indicate that co-trimoxazole may be a useful alternative to chloramphenicol (page 444), tetracycline (page 628) and other drugs, for the treatment of this disease. John (1976) obtained prompt resolution of cavitary pulmonary melioidosis occurring in a 21-year-old man by using oral co-trimoxazole. De Buse *et al.* (1975) used oral co-trimoxazole with kanamycin to cure a five-year-old child who presented with fever and jaundice, and who eventually developed multiple subcutaneous abscesses.

5. *Meningitis.* Co-trimoxazole has been used successfully in a few cases of neonatal meningitis due to Esch. coli (Morzaria *et al.*, 1969; Roy, 1971). Sabel and Brandberg (1975) treated ten infants aged between 8 days and 10 months with meningitis and/or septicaemia due to organisms such as Proteus morganii, Esch. coli and H. influenzae. Most of these infants had not responded to kanamycin, ampicillin and sulphonamides, but eight responded rapidly to intravenous co-trimoxazole, one only responded when kanamycin was added and one infant died. The authors considered that co-trimoxazole treatment was effective for infants with meningitis due to Gram-negative bacilli, but cautioned against its use in premature infants and infants in the first week of life (*see* page 693).

Intravenous co-trimoxazole has been used to treat four adults and one child with bacterial meningitis due to N. meningitidis or Strep. pneumoniae; the dose used was 10 mg of trimethoprim per kg body weight per day so that adults received 4–6 ampoules (each 80 mg trimethoprim, 400 mg sulphamethoxazole) daily given in four divided doses. Oral treatment was commenced on the fourth day and was continued for a total of eight days. In all of these patients clinical recovery was rapid and complete (Farid *et al.*, 1976). However, at present other drugs are preferable for these types of meningitis (*see* pages 33, 441).

In one patient with a brain abscess and meningitis, who eventually required surgical aspiration, the addition of co-trimoxazole to treatment may have contributed to his recovery (Green *et al.*, 1975).

6. *Bronchitis and pneumonia.* Co-trimoxazole has been extensively and successfully used in the treatment of acute bronchitis and bacterial pneumonia. In chronic bronchitis the results appear to be better than those obtained with either tetracycline or ampicillin (Hughes, 1969; Pines *et al.*, 1969), or doxycycline (Renmarker, 1976). Other studies indicate that co-trimoxazole is comparable to amoxycillin (page 142) for the treatment of acute bronchitis (Carroll *et al.*, 1977) and exacerbations of chronic bronchitis (Tandon, 1977). The common pathogens in bronchitis are pneumococci and H. influenzae, both of which are highly sensitive to this combination. Prolonged treatment with co-trimoxazole has also been used in patients with chronic bronchitis, and resis-

tant strains of H. influenzae do not emerge (Hughes, 1973). Co-trimoxazole (or amoxycillin) is only of marginal benefit for the treatment of presumed respiratory viral infections in children (Taylor *et al.*, 1977).

The respiratory tract of patients with chronic bronchitis, who have been treated by antibiotics, is often colonized by Gram-negative bacilli such as Esch. coli and Klebsiella spp. The presence of such organisms in sputum is usually not an indication for specific treatment, but in some debilitated patients they may cause 'suprainfection' evidenced not only by a positive sputum culture, but also by recurrence of fever, worsening of chest signs and increasing amounts of purulent sputum (Weinstein and Musher, 1969). Co-trimoxazole is effective against most of the bacteria which cause 'suprainfections' in patients with chronic bronchitis. This combination is also effective for the treatment of Klebsiella (Friedländer's) pneumonia.

7. *Staphylococcal and other Gram-positive coccal infections.* Co-trimoxazole is quite effective against staphylococcal infections, but other drugs are usually preferred. This combination has been used successfully to treat staphylococcal pneumonia (Darrell *et al.*, 1968), severe staphylococcal osteomyelitis (Craven *et al.*, 1970) and endocarditis (Bengtsson *et al.*, 1974). Co-trimoxazole may prove to be useful for the treatment of methicillin-resistant staphylococcal infections.

Two patients with a Strep. viridans septicaemia reported by Olcén and Eriksson (1976) responded to intravenous and then oral therapy with co-trimoxazole. Seligman *et al.* (1973) treated three patients with Strep. viridans endocarditis with oral co-trimoxazole; two treated for four weeks were cured, but the other patient, who was only treated for three weeks, relapsed three days after cessation of the drug.

Diseases such as streptococcal tonsillitis and pneumococcal lobar pneumonia also probably would respond well to co-trimoxazole. One study showed that although co-trimoxazole is effective for Strep. pyogenes pharyngitis and tonsillitis, it is inferior to penicillin G (Trickett *et al.*, 1973). Penicillin G is the preferred drug for these diseases and there are several other safe effective drugs available for use in penicillin-allergic patients.

8. *Gonorrhoea and other venereal diseases.* Co-trimoxazole is effective for the treatment of gonorrhoea (Csonka and Knight, 1967; Schofield *et al.*, 1971; Hatos and Tuza, 1972). Treatment regimens which have been used have varied from single daily doses given for one to five days to multiple doses for several days. In comparative studies using a total of 16–20 tablets of co-trimoxazole (each 80 mg trimethoprim and 400 mg sulphamethoxazole), cure rates are higher (92–100 per cent) when the daily dose consists of four to six tablets rather than one to three tablets (Austin *et al.*, 1973; Lawrence *et al.*, 1973; Svindland, 1973). Effective regimens have been four tablets twice-daily for two days (Lawrence *et al.*, 1973), five tablets daily for four days (Csonka, 1969) and six tablets daily for three days (Austin *et al.*, 1973). Good results have also been obtained by using two five-tablet doses separated by eight hours (Kristensen and From, 1975). This latter regimen also appeared to be satisfactory for rectal gonorrhoea in women, and tonsillar gonorrhoea which is less responsive to treatment. Single doses of nine tablets of co-trimoxazole are feasible for the treatment of gonorrhoea (page 701) but adverse reactions associated with a 12-tablet dose preclude its use (page 701). It is also possible that a

trimethoprim/sulphamethoxazole combination may be more effective for gonorrhoea if the present fixed ratio of 1:5 of these drugs was changed to 3:1, a ratio at which synergy is greater against N. gonorrhoeae (Austin *et al.*, 1973) (*also see* page 691). With the occurence of N. gonorrhoeae strains resistant to penicillin (page 7), tetracycline (page 596) and spectinomycin (page 586) and cross-resistance amongst multiple antibiotics, such as penicillin G, tetracycline, spectinomycin, chloramphenicol and erythromycin (page 8), co-trimoxazole may have an increasing role in the treatment of gonorrhoea. A single daily dose of nine tablets (each 80 mg trimethoprim and 400 sulphamethoxazole) for three consecutive days has been used in males with urethritis due to beta-lactamase-producing strains, with a failure rate of 9·1 per cent (Center for Disease Control, 1978). Co-trimoxazole is currently recommended as a possible alternative to spectinomycin (page 589) for the treatment of gonorrhoea in non-pregnant patients who are allergic to penicillin.

Csonka (1969) reported rapid clinical response to co-trimoxazole in three patients with lymphogranuloma venereum. Willcox (1977) considers that sulphonamides with or without trimethoprim are effective for this disease. Co-trimoxazole is ineffective in syphilis (Csonka, 1969; Lawrence *et al.*, 1973) and its use for gonorrhoea will not modify incubating syphilis (Svindland, 1973). The drug has been reported to be ineffective in non-specific urethritis (Csonka, 1969; Carroll and Nicol, 1970), but sulphonamides alone are effective in this disease when the agent is Chlamydia trachomatis (page 675). Although C. trachomatis is sensitive to co-trimoxazole, it is not known whether the above regimens, which are effective for gonorrhoea, will eradicate it from the genitalia or prevent post-gonococcal urethritis (Report, 1978).

9. *Typhoid fever and other salmonella infections.* It was first reported from Nigeria that co-trimoxazole is effective for the treatment of typhoid fever (Akinkugbe *et al.*, 1968). Subsequent reports confirmed this observation (Kamat, 1970; Farid *et al.*, 1970; Geddes *et al.*, 1971; Sardesai *et al.*, 1973). The results of some comparative trials have suggested that co-trimoxazole is more effective in relieving toxaemia in typhoid than chloramphenicol (Kamat, 1970; Sardesai *et al.*, 1973; Hassan *et al.*, 1975), whilst in others both drugs have been equally effective (Omer, 1975; Uwaydah *et al.*, 1975). Two small studies suggested that chronic carriers of Salm. typhi may be less frequent after treatment with co-trimoxazole than chloramphenicol (Geddes *et al.*, 1975; Jonsson, 1976). There have also been reports in which co-trimoxazole has not been satisfactory for the treatment of typhoid. Wicks and Stamps (1970) treated 50 typhoid fever patients with the combination; it was effective in the majority, but two patients with severe disease failed to respond, and a Salm. typhi strain resistant to co-trimoxazole was isolated from blood cultures of one of these. Scragg and Rubidge (1971) treated 103 children with typhoid fever by co-trimoxazole; their well-being rapidly improved, but fever often persisted and positive blood cultures were still obtained from many of these patients during the second or even third week of therapy. Snyder *et al.* (1973) compared the results of treatment with co-trimoxazole in 39 typhoid patients to 41 others treated with chloramphenicol. The majority of co-trimoxazole-treated patients responded as well as those treated by chloramphenicol; however, seven failed to respond after 11 or more days of co-trimoxazole treatment. The efficacy of chloramphenicol (parenteral and oral), parenteral ampicillin and oral co-

trimoxazole have been compared in clinical trials (Snyder *et al.*, 1976). Chloramphenicol, particularly when given orally, was more effective than the other two drugs in reducing the duration of fever. On the basis of all these observations, chloramphenicol (page 440) still remains the drug of choice for the treatment of typhoid fever due to sensitive strains, but co-trimoxazole is an effective alternative.

Co-trimoxazole is also a valuable drug for the treatment of typhoid fever due to chloramphenicol-resistant strains (page 423). Gilman *et al.* (1975) in Mexico found that orally administered co-trimoxazole was equally effective to oral amoxycillin in the treatment of disease due to chloramphenicol-resistant strains, but co-trimoxazole produced a more rapid lysis of fever than amoxycillin in infections due to chloramphenicol-sensitive strains. The resistance to chloramphenicol is mediated by an R plasmid (page 422) and this plasmid also confers resistance to sulphonamides, tetracycline and strep-tomycin. It was suggested that probably because of this resistance to sul-phonamides, co-trimoxazole does not exert synergism against chloramphenicol-resistant strains of Salm. typhi, and therefore trimethoprim alone may be effective for these infections (Gilman *et al.*, 1975). The findings in another smaller clinical trial in Vietnam are at variance to this (Butler *et al.*, 1977). Co-trimoxazole was compared to ampicillin for the treatment of patients with infections due to either chloramphenicol-resistant or -sensitive strains of Salm. typhi; each drug was given intravenously during the first three to five days and then, when improvement occurred, it was given orally. Both drugs were equally effective but treatment failures were more common in patients with chloramphenicol-sensitive than -resistant strains. Butler *et al.* (1977) demonstrated *in vitro* synergy with co-trimoxazole in a quarter of their chloramphenicol-resistant strains. This may occur if the sulphamethoxazole component reduces the synthesis of dihydrofolate (page 700) in sulphonamide-resistant organisms to a level that allows trimethoprim to reduce its conversion to tetrahydrofolate to a critically low level (Bushby, 1973). The format of these two trials (Gilman *et al.*, 1975; Butler *et al.*, 1977) differed in a number of aspects, which probably explains their contrasting results. Co-trimoxazole is probably also effective for the treatment of typhoid fever caused by chloramphenicol-resistant strains which, in addition, are resistant to ampicillin and amoxycillin (page 101).

Co-trimoxazole also appears to be a satisfactory drug for the treatment of paratyphoid fever (Franzén *et al.*, 1972) and for septicaemias due to other Salmonella spp. such as Salm. typhimurium (Jafary and Burke, 1970). A com-bination of trimethoprim and sulphadiazine given intravenously was used after therapy with various antibiotics to cure a four-month-old child with salmonella meningitis (Briggs and Robinson, 1975). There is also some evidence that co-trimoxazole may eradicate the chronic Salm. typhi and Salm. paratyphi carrier states (Brodie *et al.*, 1970). Although Chan *et al.* (1973) found that a two week course of treatment was unsatisfactory for this purpose, preliminary results reported by Pichler *et al.* (1973) using a three months course of co-trimoxazole appear promising. The efficacy of any antimicrobial agent in these carrier states is difficult to assess (page 115). Like other antimicrobials, co-trimoxazole is of no value in s̆almonella gastro-enteritis (Franzén *et al.*, 1972; Kazemi *et al.*, 1973).

10. *Shigella infections.* The use of co-trimoxazole in shigellosis causes a more rapid clinical recovery and also shortens the period during which shigellae are excreted (Franzén *et al.*, 1972; Lexomboon *et al.*, 1972). Co-trimoxazole is equally effective to ampicillin for the treatment of shigellosis in infants and children, and it is also effective when the disease is caused by ampicillin-resistant strains (Nelson *et al.*, 1976a; Nelson *et al.*, 1976b; Chang *et al.*, 1977). However Shigella dysentery, especially that caused by Sh. sonnei, is usually a self-limiting disease and chemotherapy is not generally indicated (page 115).

11. *Cholera.* A four- or five-day course of co-trimoxazole appears to be as effective as a similar course of tetracycline for the eradication of Vibrio cholerae, both classical and El Tor biotypes, from stools of patients with acute cholera (Gharagozloo *et al.*, 1970; Cash *et al.*, 1973). Rehydration is the most important measure in the treatment of this disease, but chemotherapy is also of proven value (page 624).

12. *Brucellosis.* There have been some reports of the successful use of co-trimoxazole in this disease (Lal *et al.*, 1970; Farid *et al.*, 1970). Further clinical trials are necessary to compare the effectiveness of this treatment to the commonly used streptomycin/tetracycline combination (pages 302, 623). Hassan *et al.* (1971) reported a good clinical response in eight patients with acute Brucella melitensis infection, treated by a three week course of co-trimoxazole. However, three of these patients relapsed after cessation of treatment and the authors suggested that a six weeks' course may be preferable. Daikos *et al.* (1973) treated 86 patients with brucellosis using co-trimoxazole for periods ranging from two weeks to two months. Clinical response was satisfactory in 78 patients. These authors concluded that prolonged treatment and higher initial doses (six standard tablets a day for the first two weeks) are advisable to improve results and prevent recurrences. Co-trimoxazole has also been used to treat chronic brucellosis; a dose of three tablets (each containing 80 mg trimethoprim and 400 mg sulphamethoxazole) twice-daily was given until fever subsided and then two tablets were given twice-daily for a total of two months. On this regimen, only two of twenty patients relapsed (Kontoyannis *et al.*, 1975).

13. *Meningococcal carrier state.* Co-trimoxazole is unsatisfactory for the eradication of sulphonamide-resistant meningococci from chronic nasopharyngeal carriers (Feldman, 1973a).

14. *Nocardiosis and Mycetoma.* Sulphonamides in combination with other drugs are usually regarded as the treatment of choice for nocardiosis (page 675). Successful treatment of several patients with nocardiosis by co-trimoxazole has been reported, suggesting that this combination may be more effective than previously available regimens (Baikie *et al.*, 1970; Marcovitch and Norman, 1970; Evans and Benson, 1971; Pavillard, 1973). Maderazo and Quintiliani (1974) described a patient who developed a brain abscess due to Nocardia asteroides during therapy with ampicillin and either sulphadiazine or sulfisoxazole for pulmonary nocardiosis. The pulmonary disease responded to this therapy, but the cerebral lesion required surgical excision and a three month course of co-trimoxazole. Poor penetration of ampicillin and sulfisoxazole into the CSF was demonstrated, but good concentrations of both trimethoprim and sulphamethoxazole were found in brain tissue (page 699). In

addition these drugs acted synergistically *in vitro* against the organism in-volved. *In vitro* studies suggest that higher doses of trimethoprim than those available in co-trimoxazole are necessary to obtain synergism against this organism (page 687). Treatment of nocardiosis usually lasts for months and the safety of prolonged high doses of trimethoprim has yet to be established (Bennett and Jennings, 1978). Dapsone therapy may be more effective than co-trimoxazole if the infecting organism is Nocardia caviae or Nocardia brasilien-sis, rather than Nocardia asteroides (Murray and Mahgoub, 1970).

Various drug combinations have been tested for *in vivo* and *in vitro* activity against the Actinomycetes (Streptomyces, Actinomadura and Nocardia spp.), which cause mycetoma in Sudan. The most effective treatments were dapsone plus streptomycin, and sulphamethoxazole/trimethoprime plus streptomycin (*see* page 303).

15. *Miscellaneous bacterial infections.* Mycobacterium marinum (pages 553, 833) may be sensitive to co-trimoxazole and it has been used to cure two patients with hand granulomata caused by this organism (Barrow and Hewitt, 1971; Kelly, 1976). Following the unusual occurrence of four cases of systemic Haemophilus influenzae type b infection in one pre-school day care centre, co-trimoxazole was used prophylactically for four days in the other children. This eradicated all H. influenzae type b strains which were carried in the nasopharynx of a high percentage of these children (Melish *et al.*, 1976). Co-trimoxazole has been suggested as the best drug to use for chemoprophylaxis in infants who have come in contact with whooping cough (Arneil and McAllister, 1977). It has also been used with clinical benefit in Whipple's dis-ease (Haeney and Ross, 1978) (*see also* pages 40, 630).

16. *Malaria.* Trimethoprim has sometimes been used in place of pyrimethamine in combination with quinine and a long-acting sulphonamide to provide triple drug treatment for chloroquine-resistant falciparum malaria (page 676). Trimethoprim in combination with a long-acting sulphonamide alone has also been used successfully for this purpose (Martin and Arnold, 1968). Nowadays a combination of the long-acting sulphonamide, sulfadoxine and pyrimethamine is preferred for treatment and chemoprophylaxis of chloroquine-resistant falciparum malaria (page 676). For treatment the addi-tion of quinine is also recommended.

17. *Toxoplasmosis.* Mossner (1969) suggested that co-trimoxazole may be effective in the treatment of human toxoplasmosis. Norrby *et al.* (1975) reported that patients with lymphonodular toxoplasmosis responded well to co-trimoxazole, but their studies were uncontrolled and the form of the disease was self-limiting. There have been conflicting reports of the effectiveness of trimethoprim and sulphonamide combinations for the treatment of murine toxoplasmosis. Feldman (1973b) found that neither trimethoprim nor sul-fisoxazole, alone or in combination, had any beneficial effect on mice infected with toxoplasmosis. In the same model Seah (1975) noted that sulphadiazine, sulphamethoxazole and pyrimethamine had therapeutic effects, but not trimethoprim. Although the effect of sulphamethoxazole was enhanced by the addition of trimethoprim, a trimethoprim/sulphamethoxazole combination was inferior to a pyrimethamine/sulphadiazine combination. Initial attempts by Remington (1976) failed to show trimethoprim/sulphamethoxazole synergism in mice but later, possibly because the method of drug administration was

changed, synergism was demonstrated (Grossman *et al.*, 1978). Another more recent study has also shown *in vitro* synergism and *in vivo* synergism in mice of a trimethoprim/sulphamethoxazole combination (Nguyen *et al.*, 1978). Treatment with sulphadiazine/pyrimethamine is still recommended for human toxoplasmosis (page 675), but because of the relative safety of trimethoprim as opposed to pyrimethamine, trials with a trimethoprim/sulphamethoxazole combination are warranted in humans (Grossman *et al.*, 1978).

18. *Pneumocystis carinii pneumonitis*. This infection mainly occurs in malnourished infants or in patients receiving immunosuppressive therapy. In the cortisone-treated rat model co-trimoxazole was as effective as pentamidine in the treatment of P. carinii pneumonitis, and also, when given prophylactically, it prevented infection (Hughes *et al.*, 1974). As a result of these findings co-trimoxazole was used to treat children with this infection complicating leukaemia (Hughes *et al.*, 1975b). Of 14 patients treated with a daily dose of 20 mg trimethoprim and 100 mg sulphamethoxazole per kg body weight per day, 12 recovered and two died; pentamidine was used to supplement the treatment of both patients who died and one who recovered. Six additional children were treated with about one-fourth of the dosage, four recovered (one also received pentamidine) and two died, both of whom also were given pentamidine. Lau and Young (1976) used a similar dosage to treat eight adult patients with P. carinii pneumonia; this amounted to 960–1200 mg trimethoprim and 4800–6000 mg sulphamethoxazole per day (12–15 standard tablets) for 9–16 days; when oral administration was not possible the intravenous route was used. Of the seven patients who could be evaluated, five were cured of their P. carinii infection. In a controlled trial involving 37 patients with P. carinii pneumonia, the results indicated that pentamidine and co-trimoxazole were equally effective (Hughes *et al.*, 1978). Experiences by Lau and Young (1976) and Miser *et al.* (1977) indicate that absorption of co-trimoxazole may not be adequate in critically ill patients with P. carinii pneumonia so that intravenous therapy is recommended for these. There have been case reports of the successful use of co-trimoxazole for this infection in infants (Rao *et al.*, 1977; Larter *et al.*, 1978) and in an adult (McLennan *et al.*, 1977). In view of the high prevalence of side-effects with pentamidine, co-trimoxazole currently seems to be the therapy of choice for P. carinii pneumonia (Hughes, 1976b). The therapeutic dosage schedule recommended by Hughes (1977) is 20 mg of trimethoprim and 100 mg of sulphamethoxazole per kg body weight daily, given orally in four divided doses.

Other studies by Hughes *et al.* (1977) indicate that co-trimoxazole is also very effective as a chemoprophylaxic drug for P. carinii pneumonitis. In a controlled study of 160 patients (children and young adults) who had either acute lymphoblastic leukaemia or some other form of malignancy being treated by cytotoxic drugs, half the patients were given co-trimoxazole and the remainder a placebo. Co-trimoxazole was given in a dose of 150 mg of trimethoprim and 750 mg of sulphamethoxazole per square metre body surface area (or 5 mg trimethoprim and 20 mg sulphamethoxazole per kg), per day, given in two divided doses. This was continued for a mean period of approximately one year, with 36 patients receiving the drug for periods of 13–24 months. Seventeen of the 80 patients receiving a placebo developed P. carinii pneumonitis, but none of those receiving co-trimoxazole. Bacterial sepsis, other forms of pneumonia, upper respiratory tract infection and cellulitis also occurred less frequently in the patients given the drug. Oral candidiasis was the only side-effect attributable to co-trimoxazole. In a smaller study Wolff and Baehner (1978) found that a two-week course of co-trimoxazole (20 mg trimethoprim and 100 mg sulphamethoxazole per kg per day) as prophylaxis in children with acute lymphoblastic leukaemia was unsatisfactory because it only delayed the onset of P. carinii pneumonitis.

19. *Histoplasmosis*. One case report has suggested that co-trimoxazole may be effective in this disease (Macleod, 1970).

20. *Q-fever*. Co-trimoxazole has been used to treat a few patients with chronic Q fever (Freeman and Hodson, 1972; Dathan and Heyworth, 1975). The value of this drug in Q fever has not been established and at this time either tetracycline or chloramphenicol is preferred.

21. *Chemoprophylaxis in biliary surgery*. The value of a single intravenous dose of co-trimoxazole (160 mg trimethoprim and 800 mg sulphamethoxazole) given by infusion over 60 min before operation in patients undergoing biliary surgery has been studied in a controlled trial (Morran *et al.*, 1978). There was a significant reduction in the frequency of wound sepsis and pulmonary complications in those patients who received co-trimoxazole.

22. *Prevention of infection in acute leukaemia*. Hughes *et al.* (1977) had observed that bacterial infections were less frequent in patients with acute leukaemia receiving co-trimoxazole as prophylaxis for P. carinii pneumonitis (*vide supra*). In a small trial on 30 neutropenic patients with acute leukaemia treated by cytotoxic drugs, 14 were allocated at random to receive treatment with co-trimoxazole (Enno *et al.*, 1978). Co-trimoxazole (160 mg trimethoprim and 800 mg sulphamethoxazole) was given orally twice a day in addition to oral non-absorbable antibiotics (framycetin sulphate 0·5 g, colistin sulphate 1·5 million units and nystatin 0·5 million units, all given every six hours). The other 16 patients only received the oral non-absorbable antibiotics. There was a significant reduction in the infection rate in those treated with co-trimoxazole (57 per cent) compared to control patients (94 per cent).

REFERENCES

Adam, W. R., Henning, M. and Dawborn, J. K. (1973), 'Excretion of trimethoprim and sulphamethoxazole in patients with renal failure', *Aust. N.Z. J. Med.*, **3**, 383.

Ai, N. V., Hanh, N. D., Dien, P. V. and Le, N. V. (1973), 'Co-trimoxazole in bubonic plague', *Brit. med. J.*, **4**, 108.

Akinkugbe, O. O., Lewis, E. A., Montefiore, D. and Okubadejo, O. A. (1968), 'Trimethoprim and sulphamethoxazole in typhoid', *Brit. med. J.*, **3**, 721.

Annotation (1973), 'Co-trimoxazole and Blood', *Lancet*, **2**, 950.

Ansdell, V. E., Wright, S. G. and Hutchinson, D. B. A. (1976), 'Megaloblastic anaemia associated with combined pyrimethamine and co-trimoxazole administration', *Lancet*, **2**, 1257.

Arneil, G. C. and McAllister, T. A. (1977), 'Whooping-cough in infants: Antimicrobial prophylaxis', *Lancet*, **2**, 33.

Arvilommi, H., Vuori, M. and Salmi, A. (1972), 'Immunosuppression by co-trimoxazole', *Brit. med. J.*, **3**, 761.

Austin, T. W., Brooks, G. F., Bethel, M., Roberts, F. L., Turck, M. and Holmes, K. K. (1973), 'Trimethoprim-sulfamethoxazole in the treatment of gonococcal urethritis:

Clinical and laboratory correlates', *J. Infect. Dis.* (Suppl.), **128**, 666.

Bach, M. C., Sabath, L. D. and Finland, M. (1973a), 'Susceptibility of Nocardia asteroides to 45 antimicrobial agents *in vitro*', *Antimicrob. Ag Chemother.*, **3**, 1.

Bach, M. C., Finland, M., Gold, O. and Wilcox, C. (1973b), 'Susceptibility of recently isolated pathogenic bacteria to trimethoprim and sulfamethoxazole separately and combined', *J. Infect. Dis. (Suppl.)*, **128**, 508.

Bach, M. C., Gold, O. and Finland, M. (1973c), 'Absorbtion and urinary excretion of trimethoprim, sulfamethoxazole, and trimethoprim-sulfamethoxazole: Results with single doses in normal young adults and preliminary observations during therapy with trimethoprim-sulfamethoxazole', *J. Infect. Dis. (Suppl.)*, **128**, 584.

Baikie, A. G., Macdonald, C. B. and Mundy, G. R. (1970), 'Systemic nocardiosis treated with trimethoprim and sulphamethoxazole', *Lancet*, **2**, 261.

Bailey, R. R. and Little, P. J. (1976), 'Deterioration in renal function in association with co-trimoxazole therapy', *Med. J. Aust.*, **1**, 914.

Barker, J., Healing, D. and Hutchison, J. G. P. (1972), 'Characteristics of some co-trimoxazole-resistant Enterobacteriaceae from infected patients', *J. clin. Path.*, **25**, 1086.

Barrow, G. I. and Hewitt, M. (1971), 'Skin infection with Mycobacterium marinum from a tropical fish tank', *Brit. med. J.*, **2**, 505.

Bassett, D. C. J. (1971), 'The sensitivity of Pseudomonas pseudomallei to trimethoprim and sulphamethoxazole *in vitro*', *J. clin. Path.*, **24**, 798.

Beaumont, R. J. (1970), 'Trimethoprim as a possible therapy for nocardiosis and melioidosis', *Med. J. Aust.*, **2**, 1123.

Bengtsson, E., Svanbom, M. and Tunevall, G. (1974), 'Trimethoprim-sulphamethoxazole treatment in staphylococcal endocarditis and Gram-negative septicaemia', *Scand. J. Infect. Dis.*, **6**, 177.

Bennett, W. M. and Craven, R. (1976), 'Urinary tract infections in patients with severe renal disease. Treatment with ampicillin and trimethoprim-sulfamethoxazole', *JAMA*, **236**, 946.

Bennett, J. E. and Jennings, A. E. (1978), 'Factors influencing susceptibility of Nocardia species to trimethoprim-sulfamethoxazole', *Antimicrob. Ag. Chemother.*, **13**, 624.

Bergan, T. and Brodwall, E. K. (1976), 'The pharmacokinetic profile of co-trimoxazole', *Scand. J. Infect. Dis.* (Suppl.), **8**, 42.

Bernstein, L. S. and Cooper, J. (1978), 'Co-trimoxazole and Stevens–Johnson syndrome', *Lancet*, **1**, 988.

Black, W.A. and McNellis, D. A. (1970), 'Systemic nocardiosis treated with trimethoprim and sulphamethoxazole', *Lancet*, **2**, 473.

Böse, W., Karama, A., Linzenmeier, G., Olbing, H. and Wellmann, P. (1974), 'Controlled trial of co-trimoxazole in children with urinary-tract infections. Bacteriological efficacy and haematological toxicity', *Lancet*, **2**, 614.

Brandberg, Å., Lindblom, G.-B. and Franzén, C. (1976), 'The resistance of 150 Klebsiella and E. coli strains isolated from patients suffering from bacteriaemia', *Scand. J. Infect. Dis.* (Suppl.), **8**, 103.

Briggs, A. E. and Robinson, M. F. (1975), 'Salmonella meningitis treatment with intravenous trimethoprim', *Aust. N.Z. J. Med.*, **5**, 364.

Brodie, J., Macqueen, I. A. and Livingstone, D. (1970), 'Effects of trimethoprim-sulphamethoxazole on typhoid and Salmonella carriers', *Brit. med. J.*, **3**, 318.

Brodie, M. J., Boot, P. A. and Girdwood, R. W. A. (1973), 'Severe Yersinia pseudotuberculosis infection diagnosed at laparoscopy', *Brit. med. J.*, **4**, 88.

Brumfitt, W. and Pursell, R. (1972), 'Double-blind trial to compare ampicillin, cephalexin, co-trimoxazole and trimethoprim in treatment of urinary infection', *Brit. med. J.*, **2**, 673.

Brumfitt, W., Hamilton-Miller, J. M. T. and Grey, D. (1977), 'Trimethoprim-resistant coliforms', *Lancet*, **2**, 926.

Bushby, S. R. M. and Hitchings, G. H. (1968), 'Trimethoprim, a sulphonamide potentiator', *Brit. J. Pharmacol. Chemother.*, **33**, 72.

Bushby, S. R. M. (1969), 'Combined antibacterial action *in vitro* of trimethoprim and sulphonamides', *Postgrad. Med. J.* (*Suppl.*), **45**, 10.

Bushby, S. R. M. (1973), 'Trimethoprim-sulfamethoxazole: *In vitro* microbiological aspects', *J. Infect. Dis.* (*Suppl.*), **128**, 442.

Butler, T., Bell, W. R., Linh, N. N., Tiep, N. D. and Arnold, K. (1974), 'Yersinia pestis infection in Vietnam. I. Clinical and haematological aspects', *J. Infect. Dis.* (*Suppl.*), **129**, 78.

Butler, T., Levin, J., Linh, N. N., Chau, D. M., Adickman, M. and Arnold, K. (1976), 'Yersinia pestis infection in Vietnam. II. Quantitative blood cultures and detection of endotoxin in the cerebrospinal fluid of patients with meningitis', *J. Infect. Dis.*, **133**, 493.

Butler, T., Linh, N. N., Arnold, K., Adickman, M. D., Chau, D. M. and Muoi, M. M. (1977), 'Therapy of antimicrobial-resistant typhoid fever', *Antimicrob. Ag. Chemother.*, **11**, 645.

Byers, P. A., Dupont, H. L. and Goldschmidt, M. C. (1976), 'Antimicrobial susceptibilities of shigellae isolated in Houston, Texas, in 1974', *Antimicrob. Ag. Chemother.*, **9**, 288.

Cameron, A. and Thomas, M. (1977), 'Pseudomembranous colitis and co-trimoxazole', *Brit. med. J.*, **1**, 1321.

Carroll, B. R. T. and Nicol, C. S. (1970), 'Trimethoprim/sulphamethoxazole in the treatment of non-gonococcal urethritis and gonorrhoea", *Brit. J. Vener. Dis.*, **46**, 31.

Carroll, P. G., Krejci, S. P., Mitchell, J., Puranik, V., Thomas, R. and Wilson, B. (1977), 'A comparative study of co-trimoxazole and amoxycillin in the treatment of acute bronchitis in general practice', *Med. J. Aust.*, **2**, 286.

Cash, R. A., Northrup, R. S. and Rahman, A. S. M. M. (1973), 'Trimethoprim and sulfamethoxazole in clinical cholera: Comparison with tetracycline', *J. Infect. Dis.* (*Suppl.*), **128**, 749.

Cattell, W. R., Chamberlain, D. A., Fry, I. K., McSherry, M. A., Broughton, C. and O'Grady, F. (1971), 'Long-term control of bacteriuria with trimethoprim-sulphonamide', *Brit. med. J.*, **1**, 377.

Center for Disease Control (1978), 'Penicillinase-(beta-lactamase-)producing Neisseria gonorrhoeae—worldwide', *Morbidity and Mortality Weekly Report*, **27**, 10.

Chan, A. C. H., Forrest, C. R. and Robertson, M. J. (1973), 'A fourteen-day treatment of typhoid carriers in Hong Kong with trimethoprim-sulphamethoxazole', *Med. J. Aust.*, **1**, 386.

Chan, M. C. K. and Wong, H. B. (1975), 'Glucose-6-phosphate dehydrogenase deficiency and co-trimoxazole', *Lancet*, **1**, 410.

Chanarin, I. and England, J. M. (1972), 'Toxicity of trimethoprim-sulphamethoxazole in patients with megaloblastic haemopoiesis', *Brit. med. J.*, **1**, 651.

Chang, M. J., Dunkle, L. M., Van Reken, D., Anderson, D., Wong, M. L. and Feigin, R. C. (1977), 'Trimethoprim-sulfamethoxazole compared to ampicillin in the treatment of shigellosis', *Pediatrics*, **59**, 726.

Chattopadhyay, B. (1972), 'Trimethoprim-sulphamethoxazole in urinary tract infection due to Streptococcus faecalis', *J. clin. Path.*, **25**, 531.

Chattopadhyay, B. (1977), 'Co-trimoxazole resistant Staphylococcus aureus in hospital practice', *J. Antimicrob. Chemother.*, **3**, 371.

Chinn, R. H., Maskell, R. Mead, J. A. and Polak, A. (1976), 'Renal stones and urinary infection: A study of antibiotic treatment', *Brit. med. J.*, **2**, 1411.

Colucci, C. F. and Cicero, M. L. (1975), 'Hepatic necrosis and trimethoprim-sulphamethoxazole', *JAMA*, **233**, 952.

Cooper, R. G. and Wald, M. (1964), 'Successful treatment of Proteus septicaemia with a new drug, trimethoprim', *Med. J. Aust.*, **2**, 93.

Craig, W. A. and Kunin, C. M. (1973a) 'Trimethoprim-sulfamethoxazole: Pharmacodynamic effects of urinary pH and impaired renal function', *Ann. Intern. Med.*, **78**, 491.

Craig, W. A. and Kunin, C. M. (1973b), 'Distribution of trimethoprim-sulfamethoxazole in tissues of rhesus monkeys', *J. Infect. Dis.* (Suppl.), **128**, 575.

Craven, J. L., Pugsley, D. J. and Blowers, R. (1970), 'Trimethoprim-sulphamethoxazole in acute osteomyelitis due to penicillin-resistant staphylococci in Uganda', *Brit. med. J.*, **3**, 201.

Csonka, G. W. and Knight, G. J. (1967), 'Therapeutic trial of trimethoprim as a potentiator of sulphonamides in gonorrhoea', *Brit. J. vener. Dis.*, **43**, 161.

Csonka, G. W. (1969), 'Therapeutic trial of some genital infections with trimethoprim-sulphamethoxazole', *Postgrad. Med. J.* (Suppl.), **45**, 77.

Daikos, G. K., Papapolyzos, N., Marketos, N., Mochlas, S., Kastanakis, S. and Papasteriadis, E. (1973), 'Trimethoprim-sulfamethoxazole in brucellosis', *J. Infect. Dis.* (Suppl.), **128**, 731.

Darby, C. P. (1976), 'Treating Pseudomonas cepacia meningitis with trimethoprim-sulfamethoxazole', *Am. J. Dis. Child.*, **130**, 1365.

Darrell, J. H., Garrod, L. P. and Waterworth, P. M. (1968), 'Trimethoprim: Laboratory and clinical studies', *J. clin. Path.*, **21**, 202.

Dathan, J. R. E. and Heyworth, M. F. (1975), 'Glomerulonephritis associated with Coxiella burnetti endocarditis', *Brit. med. J.*, **1**, 376.

Davis, R. E. and Jackson, J. M. (1973), 'Trimethoprim/sulphamethoxazole and folate metabolism', *Pathology*, **5**, 23.

Dawborn, J. K., Castaldi, P. A., Kilgour, A., Parkin, J. D. and Pattison, G. (1973), 'The prolonged use of trimethoprim/sulphonamide in urinary infection', *Med. J. Aust. Special Suppl.*, **1**, 52.

De Buse, P. J., Henderson, A. and White, M. (1975), 'Melioidosis in a child in Papua New Guinea. Successful treatment with kanamycin and trimethoprim-sulphamethoxazole', *Med. J. Aust.*, **2**, 476.

Denneberg, T., Ekberg, M., Ericson, C. and Hanson, A. (1976), 'Co-trimoxazole in the long-term treatment of pyelonephritis with normal and impaired renal function', *Scand. J. Infect. Dis.* (Suppl.), **8**, 61.

Dickson, H. G. (1978), 'Trimethoprim-sulphamethoxazole and thrombocytopenia', *Med. J. Aust.*, **2**, 5.

Dupont, H. L., West, H., Evans, D. G., Olarte, J. and Evans, D. J., Jr. (1978), 'Antimicrobial susceptibility of enterotoxigenic Escherichia coli', *J. Antimicrob. Chemother.*, **4**, 100.

Ellerstein, N. S., Sullivan, T. D., Baliah, T. and Neter, E. (1977), 'Trimethoprim/sulfamethoxazole and ampicillin in the treatment of acute urinary tract infections in children: A double-blind study', *Pediatrics*, **60**, 245.

Enno, A., Catovsky, D., Darrell, J., Goldman, J. M., Hows, J. and Galton, D. A. G. (1978), 'Co-trimoxazole for prevention of infection in acute leukaemia', *Lancet*, **2**, 395.

Evans, D. I. K. and Tell, R. (1969), 'Agranulocytosis after trimethoprim and sulphamethoxazole', *Brit. med. J.*, **1**, 578.

Evans, R. A. and Benson, R. E. (1971), 'Complicated nocardiosis successfully treated with trimethoprim and sulphamethoxazole', *Med. J. Aust.*, **1**, 684.

Everett, E. D. and Kishimoto, R. A. (1973), '*In vitro* sensitivity of 33 strains of Pseudomonas pseudomallei to trimethoprim and sulfamethoxazole', *J. Infect. Dis* (Suppl.), **128**, 539.

Farid, Z., Hassan, A., Wahab, M. F. A., Sanborn, W. R., Kent, D. C., Yassa, A. and Hathout, S. E. (1970), 'Trimethoprim-sulphamethoxazole in enteric fevers', *Brit. med. J.*, **3**, 323.

Farid, Z., Girgis, N. I., Yassin, W., Edman, D. C. and Miner, W. F. (1976), 'Trimethoprim-sulfamethoxazole and bacterial meningitis', *Ann. Intern. Med.*, **84**, 50.

Fass, R. J., Prior, R. B. and Perkins, R. L. (1977), 'Pharmacokinetics and tolerance of a single twelve-tablet dose of trimethoprim (960 mg)–sulfamethoxazole (4800 mg)', *Antimicrob. Ag. Chemother.*, **12**, 102.

Feldman, H. A. (1973a), 'Effects of trimethoprim and sulfisoxazole, alone and in combination, on growth and carriage of Neisseria meningitidis', *J. infect. Dis.* (Suppl.), **128**, 723.

Feldman, H. A. (1973b), 'Effects of trimethoprim and sulfisoxazole alone and in combination on murine toxoplasmosis', *J. Infect. Dis* (Suppl.), **128**, 774.

Finlayson, M. C. and Jackson, F. L. (1978), 'Trimethoprim-resistant salmonella', *Lancet*, **2**, 375.

Fischer, J. J. (1973), 'Pseudomonas maltophilia endocarditis after replacement of the mitral valve: A case study', *J. Infect. Dis.* (Suppl.), **128**, 771.

Fleming, A. F., Warrell, D. A. and Dickmeiss, H. (1974), 'Co-trimoxazole and the blood', *Lancet*, **2**, 284.

Fleming, M. P., Datta, N. and Grüneberg, R. N. (1972), 'Trimethoprim resistance determined by R factors', *Brit. med. J.*, **1**, 726.

Fowle, A. S. E. (1973), 'The dosage of septrin', *Med. J. Aust. Special Suppl.*, **1**, 26.

Franzén, C., Lidin-Janson, G. and Nygren, B. (1972), 'Trimethoprim-sulphamethoxazole in enteric infections', *Scand. J. Infect. Dis.*, **4**, 231.

Franzén, C. and Brandberg, Å. (1976), 'Co-trimoxazole in cases of Gram-negative septicaemia', *Scand. J. Infect. Dis.* (Suppl.), **8**, 96.

Freeman, R. and Hodson, M. E. (1972), 'Q fever endocarditis treated with trimethoprim and sulphamethoxazole', *Brit. med. J.*, **1**, 419.

French, G. L. and Lowry, M. F. (1977), 'Trimethoprim-resistant salmonella', *Lancet*, **2**, 1138.

Frisch, J. M. (1973), 'Clinical experience with adverse reactions to trimethoprim-sulfamethoxazole', *J. Infect. Dis.* (Suppl.), **128**, 607.

Gaylarde, P. M. and Sarkany, I. (1972), 'Suppression of thymidine uptake of human lymphocytes by co-trimoxazole', *Brit. med. J.*, **3**, 144.

Geddes, A. M., Fothergill, R., Goodall, J. A. D. and Dorken, P. R. (1971), 'Evaluation of trimethoprim-sulphamethoxazole compound in treatment of Salmonella infections', *Brit. med. J.*, **3**, 451.

Geddes, A. M., Pugh, R. N. H. and Nye, F. J. (1975), 'Treatment and follow-up studies with co-trimoxazole in enteric fever and in typhoid carriers', *J. Antimicrob. Chemother.*, **1**, 51.

Gharagozloo, R. A., Naficy, K., Mouin, M., Nassirzadeh, M. H. and Yalda, R. (1970), 'Comparative trial of tetracycline, chloramphenicol and trimethoprim/sulphamethoxazole in eradication of Vibro cholera El Tor', *Brit. med. J.*, **4**, 281.

Gilman, R. H., Terminel, M., Levine, M. M., Hernandez-Mendosa, P., Calderone, E., Vasquez, V., Martinez, E., Synder, M. J. and Hornick, R. B. (1975), 'Comparison of trimethoprim-sulfamethoxazole and amoxycillin in therapy of chloramphenicol-resistant and chloramphenicol-sensitive typhoid fever', *J. Infect. Dis.*, **132**, 630.

Girdwood, R. H. (1973), 'Trimethoprim/Sulphamethoxazole: Long-term therapy and folate levels', *Med. J. Aust. Special Suppl.*, **1**, 34.

Girdwood, R. H. (1976), 'The nature of possible adverse reactions to co-trimoxazole', *Scand. J. Infect. Dis.* (Suppl.), **8**, 10.

Gnarpe, H. and Friberg, J. (1976), 'The penetration of trimethoprim into seminal fluid and serum', *Scand. J. Infect. Dis.* (Suppl.), **8**, 50.

Gower, P. E. and Tasker, P. R. W. (1976), 'Comparative double-blind study of cephalexin and co-trimoxazole in urinary tract infections', *Brit. med. J.*, **1**, 684.

Greene, B. M., Thomas, F. E., Jr. and Alford, R. H. (1975), 'Trimethoprim-sulfamethoxazole and brain abscess', *Ann. Intern. Med.*, **82**, 812.

Grey, D. and Hamilton-Miller, J. M. T. (1977), 'Sensitivity of Pseudomonas aeruginosa to sulphonamides and trimethoprim and the activity of the combination trimethoprim: sulphamethoxazole', *J. Med. Microbiol.*, **10**, 273.

Grose, W. E., Bodey, G. P. and Rodriguez, V. (1977), 'Sulfamethoxazole-trimethoprim for infections in cancer patients', *JAMA*, **237**, 352.

Grossman, A. B., Braimbridge, M. V., Ross Russell, R. W. and Smith, S. E. (1977), 'Acute polyneuropathy possibly associated with co-trimoxazole', *Lancet*, **2**, 616.

Grossman, P. L., Krahenbuhl, J. L. and Remington, J. S. (1978), '*In vivo* and *in vitro* effects of trimethoprim and sulfamethoxazole on toxoplasma infection'. In Siegenthaler, W. and Lüthy, R. (Ed.), *Current Chemotherapy: Proceedings of the 10th International Congress of Chemotherapy*, Zurich/Switzerland, 1977. American Society for Microbiology, Washington, D.C., p. 135.

Grunberg, E., Prince, H. N. and de Lorenzo, W. F. (1970), 'The *in vivo* effect of folinic acid (citrovorum factor) on the potentiation of the antibacterial activity of sulfisoxazole by trimethoprim', *J. Clin. Pharmacol.*, **10**, 231.

Grüneberg, R. N. and Kolbe, R. (1969), 'Trimethoprim in the treatment of urinary infections in hospitals', *Brit. med. J.*, **1**, 545.

Grüneberg, R. N. (1975), 'The use of co-trimoxazole in sulphonamide-resistant Escherichia coli urinary tract infection', *J. Antimicrob. Chemother.*, **1**, 305.

Grüneberg, R. N., Smellie, J. M., Leakey, A. and Atkin, W. S. (1976), 'Long-term low-dose co-trimoxazole in prophylaxis of childhood urinary tract infection: Bacteriological aspects', *Brit. med. J.*, **2**, 206.

Grüneberg, R. N. and Emmerson, A. M. (1977), 'The interactions between rifampicin and trimethoprim: An *in vitro* study', *J. Antimicrob. Chemother.*, **3**, 453.

Guignard, J. P., Pippa, R. and Genton, N. (1978), 'Co-trimoxazole and creatinine clearance', *Lancet*, **1**, 712.

Gutman, L. T., Wilfert, C. M. and Quan, T. (1973), 'Susceptibility of Yersinia enterocolitica to trimethoprim-sulfamethoxazole', *J. Infect. Dis* (Suppl.), **128**, 538.

Haeney, M. R. and Ross, I. N. (1978), 'Whipple's disease in a female with impaired cell-mediated immunity unresponsive to co-trimoxazole and levamisole therapy', *Postgrad. Med. J.*, **54**, 45.

Hall, C. L. (1974), 'Co-trimoxazole and azathioprine: A safe combination', *Brit. med. J.*, **4**, 15.

Hamilton, J., Burch, W., Grimmett, G., Orme, K., Brewer, D., Frost, R. and Fulkerson, C. (1973), 'Successful treatment of Pseudomonas cepacia endocarditis with trimethoprim-sulfamethoxazole', *Antimicrob. Ag. Chemother.*, **4**, 551.

Hamilton-Miller, J. M. T. and Grey, D. (1975), 'Resistance to trimethoprim in Klebsiellae isolated before its introduction', *J. Antimicrob. Chemother.*, **1**, 213.

Hammett, J. F. (1970), 'Thrombocytopenia following administration of "bactrim"', *Med. J. Aust.*, **2**, 200.

Hanley, T. (1969), 'Adverse reactions to trimethoprim sulphamethoxazole', *Postgrad. Med. J.* (Suppl.), **45**, 85.

Hanson, G. C. and Woods, R. L. (1975), 'Intravenous trimethoprim/sulphadimidine in the treatment of Bacteroides septicaemia', *Postgrad. Med. J.*, **51**, 105.

Harding, G. K. M. and Ronald, A. R. (1973), 'Efficacy of trimethoprim-sulfamethoxazole in bacteriuria', *J. Infect. Dis.* (Suppl.), **128**, 641.

Harding, G. K. M. and Ronald, A. R. (1974), 'A controlled study of antimicrobial prophylaxis of recurrent urinary infection in women', *New Engl. J. Med.*, **291**, 597.

Hart, C. A., Gibson, M. F., Mulvihill, E. and Green, H. T. (1977), 'Co-trimoxazole resistant coliforms', *Lancet*, **2**, 1081.

Hassan, A., Erian, M. M., Farid, Z., Hathout, S. D. and Sorensen, K. (1971), 'Trimethoprim-sulphamethoxazole in acute brucellosis', *Brit. med. J.*, **3**, 159.

Hassan, A., Hathout, S., Safwat, Y., Erian, M. and Wahab, M. F. A. (1975), 'A comparative evaluation of the treatment of typhoid fever with co-trimoxazole and chloramphenicol in Egypt', *J. trop. Med. Hyg.*, **78**, 50.

Hatos, G. and Tuza, F. L. C. (1972), 'Treatment of gonorrhoea with trimethoprim-sulphamethoxazole and with rifampicin', *Med. J. Aust.*, **1**, 1197.

Hills, N. H., Bultitude, M. I. and Eykyn, S. (1976), 'Co-trimoxazole in prevention of bacteriuria after prostatectomy', *Brit. med. J.*, **2**, 498.

Hitchings, G. H. (1969), 'Species differences among dihydrofolate reductases as a basis for chemotherapy', *Postgrad. Med. J.* (Suppl.), **45**, 7.

Hobday, J. D. (1971), 'The prophylactic treatment of recurrent urinary tract infection with sulphamethoxazole-trimethoprim', *Aust. Paediat. J.*, **7**, 199.

Howard, A. J., Hince, C. J. and Williams, J. D. (1978), 'Antibiotic resistance in Streptococcus pneumoniae and Haemophilus influenzae. Report of a study group on bacterial resistance', *Brit. med. J.*, **1**, 1657.

Howe, J. G. and Wilson, T. S. (1972), 'Co-trimoxazole-resistant pneumococci', *Lancet*, **2**, 184.

Hughes, D. T. D. (1969), 'Single-blind comparative trial of trimethoprim-sulphamethoxazole and ampicillin in the treatment of exacerbations of chronic bronchitis', *Brit. med. J.*, **4**, 470.

Hughes, D. T. D. (1973), 'Use of combinations of trimethoprim and sulfamethoxazole in the treatment of chest infections', *J. Infect. Dis.* (Suppl.), **128**, 701.

Hughes, W. T., McNabb, P. C., Makres, T. D. and Feldman, S. (1974), 'Efficacy of trimethoprim and sulfamethoxazole in the prevention and treatment of Pneumocystis carinii pneumonitis', *Antimicrob. Ag. Chemother.*, **5**, 289.

Hughes, D. T. D., Jenkins, G. C. and Gurney, J. D. (1975a), 'The clinical, haematological and bacteriological effects of long-term treatment with co-trimoxazole', *J. Antimicrob. Chemother.*, **1**, 55.

Hughes, W. T., Feldman, S. and Sanyal, S. K. (1975b), 'Treatment of Pneumocystis carinii pneumonitis with trimethoprim-sulfamethoxazole', *Can. Med. Assoc. J.* (Suppl.), **112**, 47.

Hughes, D. (1967a), 'Chemoprophylaxis in chronic bronchitis', *J. Antimicrob. Chemother.*, **2**, 320.

Hughes, W. T. (1976b), 'Editorial. Treatment of Pneumocystis carinii pneumonitis', *New Engl. J. Med.*, **295**, 726.

Hughes, W. T. (1977), 'Pneumocystis carinii pneumonia', *New Engl. J. Med.*, **297**, 1381.

Hughes, W. T., Kuhn, S., Chaudhary, S., Feldman, S., Verzosa, M., Aur, R. J. A., Pratt, C. and George, S. L. (1977), 'Successful chemoprophylaxis for Pneumocystitis carinii pneumonitis', *New Engl. J. Med.*, **297**, 1419.

Hughes, W. T., Feldman, S., Chaudhary, S. C., Ossi, M. J., Cox, F. and Sanyal, S. K. (1978), 'Comparison of pentamidine isethionate and trimethoprim-sulfamethoxazole in the treatment of Pneumocystis carinii pneumonia', *J. Pediatrics*, **92**, 285.

Hulme, B. and Reeves, D. S. (1971), 'Leucopenia associated with trimethoprim-sulphamethoxazole after renal transplantation', *Brit. med. J.*, **3**, 610.

Jafary, M. H. and Burke, G. J. (1970), 'Antibiotics and Salmonella excretors', *Brit. med. J.*, **2**, 605.

Jenkins, G. C., Hughes, D. T. D. and Hall, P. C. (1970), 'A haematological study of patients receiving long-term treatment with trimethoprim and sulphonamide', *J. clin. Path.*, **23**, 392.

Jewkes, R. F., Edwards, M. S. and Grant, B. J. B. (1970), 'Haematological changes in a patient on long-term treatment with a trimethoprim-sulphonamide combination', *Postgrad. Med. J.*, **46**, 723.

John, J. F., Jr. (1976), 'Trimethoprim-sulfamethoxazole therapy of pulmonary melioidosis', *Amer. Rev. Resp. Dis.*, **114**, 1021.

Jonsson, M. (1976), 'The treatment of typhoid and paratyphoid fevers with co-trimoxazole in a comparative trial with chloramphenicol', *Scand. J. Infect. Dis.* (Suppl.), **8**, 81.

Kahn, S. B., Fein, S. A. and Brodsky, I. (1968), 'Effects of trimethoprim on folate metabolism in man', *Clin. Pharmacol. Ther.*, **9**, 550.

Kalowski, S., Nanra, R. S., Mathew, T. H. and Kincaid-Smith, P. (1973), 'Deterioration in renal function in association with co-trimoxazole therapy', *Lancet*, **1**, 394.

Kalowski, S., Nanra, R. S., Friedman, A., Radford, N., Standish, H. and Kincaid-Smith, P. (1975), 'Controlled trial comparing co-trimoxazole and methenamine hippurate in the prevention of recurrent urinary tract infections', *Med. J. Aust.*, **1**, 585.

Kamat, S. A. (1970), 'Evaluation of therapeutic efficacy of trimethoprim-sulphamethoxazole and chloramphenicol in enteric fever', *Brit. med. J.*, **3**, 320.

Kasanen, A., Toivanen, P., Sourander, L., Kaarsalo, E. and Aantaa, S. (1974), 'Trimethoprim in the treatment and long-term control of urinary tract infection', *Scand. J. Infect. Dis.*, **6**, 91.

Kazemi, M., Gumpert, T. G. and Marks, M. I. (1973), 'A controlled trial comparing sulfamethoxazole-trimethoprim, ampicillin, and no therapy in the treatment of salmonella gastroenteritis in children', *J. Pediatrics*, **83**, 646.

Kelly, R. (1976), 'Mycobacterium marinum infection from a tropical fish tank. Treatment with trimethoprim and sulphamethoxazole', *Med. J. Aust.*, **2**, 681.

Kincaid-Smith, P., Kalowski, S. and Nanra, R. S. (1973), 'Cotrimoxazole in urinary tract infection', *Med. J. Aust. Special Suppl.*, **1**, 49.

Kirven, L. A. and Thornsberry, C. (1974), '*In vitro* susceptibility of Haemophilus influenzae to trimethoprim-sulfamethoxazole', *Antimicrob. Ag. Chemother.*, **6**, 869.

Kontoyannis, P. A., Papapoulos, S. E. and Mortoglou, A. A. (1975), 'Co-trimoxazole in chronic brucellosis: A two-year follow-up study', *Brit. med. J.*, **2**, 480.

Koutts, J., Van der Weyden, M. B. and Cooper, M. (1973), 'Effect of trimethoprim on folate metabolism in human bone marrow', *Aust. N.Z. J. Med.*, **3**, 245.

Knudsen, J. B., Korner, B., Reinicke, V., Stahl, D. and Thomsen, Å. C. (1973), 'Treatment of urinary tract infections with a sulphamethoxazole/trimethoprim compound: A controlled, double blind, clinical trial', *Scand. J. Infect. Dis.*, **5**, 55.

Kristensen, J. K. and From, E. (1975), 'Trimethoprim-sulphamethoxazole in gonorrhoea. A comparison with pivampicillin combined with probenecid', *Brit. J. vener. Dis.*, **51**, 31.

Kunin, C. M., Craig, W. A. and Uehling, D. T. (1978), 'Trimethoprim therapy for urinary tract infection. Long-term prophylaxis in a uremic patient', *JAMA*, **239**, 2588.

Lacey, R. W., Gillespie, W. A., Bruten, D. M. and Lewis, E. L. (1972), 'Trimethoprim-resistant coliforms', *Lancet*, **1**, 409.

Lal, S., Modawal, K. K., Fowle, A. S. E., Peach, B. and Popham, R. D. (1970), 'Acute brucellosis treated with trimethoprim and sulphamethoxazole', *Brit. med. J.*, **3**, 256.

Larter, W. E., John, T. J., Sieber, O. F., Jr., Johnson, H., Corrigan, J. J., Jr. and Fulginiti, V. A. (1978), 'Trimethoprim-sulfamethoxazole treatment of Pneumocystis carinii penumonitis', *J. Pediatrics*, **92**, 826.

Lau, W. K. and Young, L. S. (1976), 'Trimethoprim-sulfamethoxazole treatment of Pneumocystis carinii pneumonia in adults', *New Engl. J. Med.*, **295**, 716.

Lawrence, A., Phillips, I. and Nicol, C. (1973), 'Various regimens of trimethoprim-sulfamethoxazole used in the treatment of gonorrhoea', *J. Infect. Dis.* (Suppl.), **128**, 673.

Lawson, D. H. and Henry, D. A. (1977), 'Fatal agranulocytosis attributed to co-trimoxazole therapy', *Brit. med. J.*, **2**, 316.

Lexomboon, U., Mansuwan, P., Duangmani, C., Benjadol, P. and M'cMinn, M. T. (1972), 'Clinical evaluation of co-trimoxazole and furazolidone in treatment of shigellosis in children', *Brit. med. J.*, **3**, 23.

Lewis, E. L. and Lacey, R. W. (1973), 'Present significance of resistance to trimethoprim and sulphonamides in coliforms, Staphylococcus aureus, and Streptococcus faecalis', *J. clin. Path.*, **26**, 175.

Lewis, E. L., Anderson, J. D. and Lacey, R. W. (1974), 'A reappraisal of the antibacterial action of cotrimoxazole *in vitro*', *J. clin. Path.*, **27**, 87.

Lirenman, D. S. and Arnold, W. J. D. (1973), 'Long-term use of trimethoprim-sulfamethoxazole in children with meningomyeloceles and recurrent urinary tract infections', *J. Infect. Dis.* (Suppl.), **128**, 636.

Lövestad, A., Sabel, G., Stefansson, M., Gästrin, B. and Lundström, R. (1976), 'Co-trimoxazole and nitrofurantoin in urinary-tract infections: A controlled clinical study', *Scand. J. Infect. Dis.* (Suppl.), **8**, 58.

Macleod, W. M. (1970), 'Treatment of histoplasmosis', *Lancet*, **2**, 363.

Maderazo, E. G. and Quintiliani, R. (1974), 'Treatment of nocardial infection with trimethoprim and sulfamethoxazole', *Amer. J. Med.*, **57**, 671.

Marcovitch, H. and Norman, A. P. (1970), 'Treatment of nocardiosis', *Lancet*, **2**, 362.

Marks, P. J., Bruten, D. M. and Speller, D. C. E. (1977), 'Trimethoprim-resistant coliforms', *Lancet*, **2**, 774.

Martin, D. C. and Arnold, J. D. (1968), 'Treatment of acute falciparum malaria with sulfalene and trimethoprim', *JAMA*, **203**, 476.

Maskell, R., Okubadejo, O. A. and Payne, R. H. (1976), 'Thymine-requiring bacteria associated with co-trimoxazole therapy', *Lancet*, **1**, 834.

May, J. R. and Davies, J. (1972), 'Resistance of Haemophilus influenzae to trimethoprim', *Brit. med. J.*, **3**, 376.

May, J. R. and Davies, J. (1973), 'Haemophilus influenzae apparently resistant to trimethoprim', *Brit. med. J.*, **3**, 407.

McAlister, T. A. (1976), 'Resistance to co-trimoxazole', *Scand. J. Infect. Dis.* (Suppl.), **8**, 29.

McGowan, J. E., Jr., Terry, P. M. and Nahmias, A. J. (1976), 'Susceptibility of Haemophilus influenzae isolates from blood and cerebrospinal fluid to ampicillin, chloramphenicol and trimethoprim-sulfamethoxazole', *Antimicrob. Ag. Chemother.*, **9**, 137.

McLennan, G., Antic, R., Seymour, A. E., Frith, P. A. and Clarkson, A. R. (1977), 'Pneumocystis carinii pneumonitis successfully treated with trimethoprim-sulphamethoxazole', *Aust. N.Z. J. Med.*, **7**, 299.

McPherson, V. J. and Raik, E. (1970), 'Thrombocytopenia following administration of "septrin"', *Med. J. Aust.*, **2**, 754.

Meares, E. M., Jr. (1973), 'Observations on activity of trimethoprim-sulfamethoxazole in the prostate', *Infect. Dis.* (Suppl.), **128**, 679.

Medical News (1974), 'Same drug combination works in pneumonitis, urinary infections', *JAMA*, **228**, 1508.

Melish, M. E., Nelson, A. J., Martin, T. E. and Norden, C. W. (1976), 'Epidemic spread of H. influenzae type B (HIB) in a day care center', *Pediatr. Res.*, **10**, 348.

Miser, J. S., Savitch, J. and Bleyer, W. A. (1977), 'Management of P. carinii pneumonia', *New Engl. J. Med.*, **296**, 47.

Moody, M. R. and Young, V. M. (1975), '*In vitro* susceptibility of Pseudomonas cepacia and Pseudomonas maltophilia to trimethoprim and 'rimethoprim-sulfamethoxazole', *Antimicrob. Ag. Chemother.*, **7**, 836.

Morran, C., McNaught, W. and McArdle, C. S. (1978), 'Prophylactic co-trimoxazole in biliary surgery', *Brit. med. J.*, **2**, 462.

Morzaria, R. N., Walton, I. G. and Pickering, D. (1969), 'Neonatal meningitis treated with trimethoprim and sulphamethoxazole', *Brit. med. J.*, **2**, 511.

Mossner, G. (1969), 'Clinical results with the combined preparation sulphamethoxazole + trimethoprim', *Proc. 6th International Congress Chemother., Tokyo.* A11–**2**, 250; quoted by Evaluations on New Drugs (1971).

Murray, I. G. and Mahgoub, E. S. (1970), 'Treatment of nocardiosis', *Lancet*, **2**, 362.

Nakhla, L. S. (1972), 'Resistance of Staphylococcus aureus to sulphamethoxazole and trimethoprim', *J. clin. Path.*, **25**, 708.

Nanra, R. S., Anderton, J. L., Evans, M., Fairley, K. F. and Kincaid-Smith, P. (1971), 'The use of trimethoprim and sulphamethoxazole in the management of chronic and recurrent upper and lower urinary tract infection', *Med. J. Aust.*, **1**, 25.

Nelson, J. D., Kusmiesz, H. and Jackson, L. H. (1976a), 'Comparison of trimethoprim-sulfamethoxazole and ampicillin therapy for shigellosis in ambulatory patients', *J. Pediatrics*, **89**, 491.

Nelson, J. D., Kusmiesz, H., Jackson, L. H. and Woodman, E. (1976b), 'Trimethoprim-sulfamethoxazole therapy for shigellosis', *JAMA*, **235**, 1239.

Neu, H. C., Garvey, G. J. and Beach, M. P. (1973), 'Successful treatment of Pseudomonas cepacia endocarditis in a heroin addict with trimethoprim-sulfamethoxazole', *J. Infect. Dis* (Suppl.), **128**, 768.

Nguyen, B. T., Stadtsbaeder, S. and Horvat, F. (1978), 'Comparative effect of trimethoprim and pyrimethamine, alone and in combination with a sulfonamide, on Toxoplasma gondii: *In vitro* and *in vivo* studies'. In Siegenthaler, W. and Lüthy, R. (Ed.), *Current Chemotherapy: Proceedings of the 10th International Congress of Chemotherapy*, Zurich/Switzerland, 1977. American Society for Microbiology, Washington, D.C., p. 137.

Nielsen, M. L., Laursen, H. and Strøyer, I. (1970), 'Short-term treatment of urinary tract infections with trimethoprim/sulphamethoxazole', *Scand. J. Infect. Dis.*, **2**, 211.

Noall, E. W. P., Sewards, H. F. G. and Waterworth, P. M. (1962), 'Successful treatment of a case of Proteus septicaemia', *Brit. med. J.*, **2**, 1101.

Noriega, E. R., Rubinstein, E., Simberkoff, M. S. and Rahal, J. J., Jr. (1975), 'Subacute and acute endocarditis due to Pseudomonas cepacia in heroin addicts', *Amer. J. Med.*, **59**, 29.

Norrby, R., Eilard, T., Svedhem, Å. and Lycke, E. (1975), 'Treatment of toxoplasmosis with trimethoprim-sulphamethoxazole', *Scand. J. Infect. Dis.*, **7**, 72.

Northrup, R. S., Doyle, M. A. and Feeley, J. C. (1972), '*In vitro* susceptibility of El Tor and classical Vibrio cholerae strains to trimethoprim and sulfamethoxazole', *Antimicrob. Ag. Chemother.*, **1**, 310.

O'Grady, F., Fry, I. K., McSherry, A. and Cattell, W. R. (1973), 'Long-term treatment of persistent or recurrent urinary tract infection with trimethoprim-sulfamethoxazole', *J. Infect. Dis* (Suppl.), **128**, 652.

Okubadejo, O. A., Green, P. J. and Payne, D. J. H. (1973), 'Bacteroides infection among hospital patients', *Brit. med. J.*, **2**, 212.

Okubadejo, O. A. (1974), 'Susceptibility of Bacteroides fragilis to co-trimoxazole', *Lancet*, **1**, 1061.

Okybadejo, O. A. and Maskell, R. (1977), 'Trimethoprim-resistant coliforms', *Lancet*, **2**, 926.

Olćen, P. and Eriksson, M. (1976), 'The intravenous infusion of co-trimoxazole in cases of septicaemia: Tolerance and results of treatment', *Scand. J. Infect. Dis.* (Suppl.), **8**, 91.

Omer, M. I. A. (1975), 'Trimethoprim-sulphamethoxazole in the treatment of enteric fever', *J. Trop. Med. Hyg.*, **78**, 162.

Owusu, S. K. (1972), 'Acute haemolysis complicating co-trimoxazole therapy for typhoid fever in a patient with G.-6-P.D. deficiency', *Lancet*, **2**, 819.

Palva, I. P. and Koivisto, O. (1971), 'Agranulocytosis associated with trimethoprim-sulphamethoxazole', *Brit. med. J.*, **4**, 301.

Parsley, T. L., Provonchee, R. B., Glicksman, C. and Zinner, S. H. (1977), 'Synergistic activity of trimethoprim and amikacin against Gram-negative bacilli', *Antimicrob. Ag. Chemother.*, **12**, 349.

Pavillard, E. R. (1973), 'Treatment of nocardial infection with trimethoprim/sulphamethoxazole', *Med. J. Aust. Special Suppl.*, **1**, 65.

Pelton, S. I., Shurin, P. A., Klein, J. O. and Finland, M. (1977), 'Quantitative inhibition of Haemophilus influenzae by trimethoprim/sulfamethoxazole', *Antimicrob. Ag. Chemother.*, **12**, 649.

Phillips, I. and Warren, C. (1974), 'Susceptibility of Bacteroides fragilis to trimethoprim and sulphamethoxazole', *Lancet*, **1**, 827.

Phillips, I. and Warren, C. (1976), 'Activity of sulfamethoxazole and trimethoprim against Bacteroides fragilis', *Antimicrob. Ag. Chemother.*, **9**, 736.

Pichler, J., Knothe, H., Spitzy, K. H. and Vielkind, G. (1973), 'Treatment of chronic carriers of Salmonella typhi and Salmonella paratyphi B with trimethoprim-sulfamethoxazole', *J. Infect. Dis.* (Suppl.), **128**, 743.

Pines, A., Greenfield, J. S. B., Raafat, H., Rahman, M. and Siddiqui, A. M. (1969), 'Preliminary experience with trimethoprim and sulphamethoxazole in the treatment of purulent chronic bronchitis', *Postgrad. Med. J.* (Suppl.), **45**, 89.

Pinney, R. J. and Smith, T. (1973), 'Joint trimethoprim and sulphamethoxazole resistance in bacteria infected with R factors', *J. Med. Microbiol.*, **6**, 13.

Prior, R. B., Fass, R. J. and Perkins, R. L. (1976), 'Regression-line analysis of trimethoprim-sulfamethoxazole activity against Neisseria gonorrhoeae', *Am. J. Clinic. Path.*, **66**, 605.

Rahal, J. J., Jr., Simberkoff, M. S. and Hymans, P. J. (1973), 'Pseudomonas cepacia tricuspid endocarditis: Treatment with trimethoprim, sulfonamide, and polymyxin B', *J. Infect. Dis.* (Suppl.), **128**, 762.

Raik, E. and Vincent, P. C. (1973), 'Thrombocytopenia with combined trimethoprim-sulphamethoxazole and allopurinol therapy', *Med. J. Aust.*, **2**, 468.

Ramaiah, R. S., Gallagher, M. A. and Biagi, R. W. (1977), 'Reactions to co-trimoxazole', *Lancet*, **1**, 604.

Rao, M., Steiner, P., Victoria, M. S., James, P., Fikrig, S., Goldenberg, L. and Kassner, E. G. (1977), 'Pneumocystis carinii pneumonia. Occurrence in a healthy american infant', *JAMA*, **238**, 2301.

Reeves, D. S., Faiers, M. C., Pursell, R. E. and Brumfitt, W. (1969), 'Trimethoprim-sulphamethoxazole: Comparative study in urinary infection in hospital', *Brit. med. J.*, **1**, 541.

Reisberg, B., Herzog, J. and Weinstein, L. (1967), '*In vitro* antibacterial activity of trimethoprim alone and combined with sulphonamides', *Antimicrob. Ag. Chemother.*—1966, p. 424.

Remington, J. S. (1976), 'Trimethoprim-sulfamethoxazole in murine toxoplasmosis', *Antimicrob. Ag. Chemother.*, **9**, 222.

Renmarker, K. (1976), 'A comparative trial of co-trimoxazole and doxycycline in the treatment of acute exacerbations of chronic bronchitis', *Scand. J. Infect. Dis.* (Suppl.), **8**, 75.

Report of a WHO Scientific Group (1978), 'Neisseria gonorrhoeae and gonococcal infections', *Wld. Hlth. Org. techn. Rep. Ser.*, No. 616.

Rickard, K. A. and Uhr, E. (1971), 'Acute thrombocytopenic purpura associated with "septrin"', *Med. J. Aust.*, **1**, 769.

Rieder, J. (1973), 'Excretion of sulfamethoxazole and trimethoprim into human bile', *J. Infect. Dis.* (Suppl.), **128**, 574.

Robertson, L., Farrell, I. D. and Hinchliffe, P. M. (1973), 'The sensitivity of Brucella abortus to chemotherapeutic agents', *J. Med. Microbiol.*, **6**, 549.

Rodriguez, W. J., Kahn, W. N., Ross, S., Controni, G. and Goldenberg, R. (1978), 'Trimethoprim-sulfamethoxazole in shigellosis'. In Siegenthaler, W. and Lüthy, R. (Ed.), *Current Chemotherapy: Proceedings of the 10th International Congress of Chemotherapy*, Zurich/Switzerland, 1977. American Society for Microbiology, Washington, D.C., p. 172.

Rosenblatt, J. E. and Stewart, P. R. (1974), 'Lack of activity of sulfamethoxazole and trimethoprim against anaerobic bacteria', *Antimicrob. Ag. Chemother.*, **6**, 93.

Rosenfeld, J. B., Najenson, T. and Grosswater, Z. (1975), 'Effect of long-term co-trimoxazole therapy on renal function', *Med. J. Aust.*, **2**, 546.

Roth, B., Falco, E. A., Hitchings, G. ... and Bushby, S. R. M. (1962), '5-benzyl-2,4-diaminopyrimidines as antibacterial agents. I Synthesis and antibacterial activity *in vitro*', *J. med. pharm. Chem.*, **5**, 1103; quoted by Darrell *et al.* (1968).

Roy, L. P. (1971), 'Sulphamethoxazole-trimethoprim in infancy', *Med. J. Aust.*, **1**, 148.

Rudoy, R. C., Nelson, J. D. and Haltalin, K. C. (1974), '*In vitro* susceptibility of Shigella strains to trimethoprim and sulfamethoxazole', *Antimicrob. Ag. Chemother.*, **5**, 439.

Russel, P. B. and Hitchings, G. H. (1951), '2,4-diaminopyrimidines as antimalarials III. 5-aryl-derivatives', *J. Amer. chem. Soc.*, **73**, 3763.

Sabel, K. G. and Brandberg, Å. (1975), 'Treatment of meningitis and septicaemia in infancy with a sulphamethoxazole/trimethoprim combination', *Acta. Paediatr. Scand.*, **64**, 25.

Salmon, J. D., Fowle, A. S. E. and Bye, A. (1975), 'Concentrations of trimethoprim and sulphamethoxazole in aqueous humour and plasma from regimens of co-trimoxazole in man', *J. Antimicrob. Chemother.*, **1**, 205.

Salter, A. J. (1973), 'The toxicity profile of trimethoprim/sulphamethoxazole after four years of widespread use', *Med. J. Aust. Special Suppl.*, **1**, 70.

Sardesai, H. V., Karandikar, R. S. and Harshe, R. G. (1973), 'Comparative trial of co-trimoxazole and chloramphenicol in typhoid fever', *Brit. med. J.*, **1**, 82.

Schofield, C. B. S., Masterton, G., Moffett, M. and McGill, M. I. (1971), 'Gonorrhoea in women: Treatment with sulfamethoxazole and trimethoprim', *J. Infect. Dis.*, **124**, 533.

Schwartz, D. E. and Ziegler, W. H. (1969), 'Assay and pharmacokinetics of trimethoprim in man and animals', *Postgrad. Med. J.* (Suppl.), **45**, 32.

Scragg, J. N. and Rubidge, C. J. (1971), 'Trimethoprim and sulphamethoxazole in typhoid fever in children', *Brit. med. J.*, **3**, 738.

Seah, S. K. K. (1975), 'Chemotherapy in experimental toxoplasmosis: Comparison of the efficacy of trimethoprim-sulfur and pyrimethamine-sulfur combinations', *J. Trop. Med. Hyg.*, **78**, 150.

Seligman, S. J. (1973), '*In vitro* susceptibility of methicillin-resistant Staphylococcus aureus to sulfamethoxazole and trimethoprim', *J. Infect. Dis.* (Suppl.), **128**, 543.

Seligman, S. J., Madhavan, T. and Alcid, D. (1973), 'Trimethoprim-sulfamethoxazole in the treatment of bacterial endocarditis', *J. Infect. Dis.* (Suppl.), **128**, 754.

Sharpstone, P. (1969), 'The renal handling of trimethoprim and sulphamethoxazole in man', *Postgrad. Med. J.* (Suppl.), **45**, 38.

Shouval, D., Ligumsky, M. and Ben-Ishay, D. (1978), 'Effect of co-trimoxazole on normal creatinine clearance', *Lancet*, **1**, 244.

Sigel, C. W., Grace, M. E. and Nichol, C. A. (1973), 'Metabolism of trimethoprim in man and measurement of a new metabolite: A new fluorescence assay', *J. Infect. Dis.* (Suppl.), **128**, 580.

Sinai, R., Hammerberg, S., Marks, M. I. and Pai, C. H. (1978), '*In vitro* susceptibility of Haemophilus influenzae to sulfamethoxazole-trimethoprim and cefaclor, cephalexin and cephradine', *Antimicrob. Ag. Chemother.*, **13**, 861.

Sive, J., Green, R. and Metz, J. (1972), 'Effect of trimethoprim on folate-dependent DNA synthesis in human bone marrow', *J. clin. Path.*, **25**, 194.

Smellie, J. M., Grüneberg, R. N., Leakey, A. and Atkin, W. S. (1976), 'Long-term low-dose co-trimoxazole in prophylaxis of childhood urinary tract infection: Clinical aspects', *Brit. med. J.*, **2**, 203.

Smellie, J. M., Katz, G. and Grüneberg, R. N. (1978), 'Controlled trial of prophylactic treatment in childhood urinary-tract infection, *Lancet*, **2**, 175.

Smith, D. D., Bell, S. M., Levey, J. M. and Loy, Y. T. (1972), 'The action of trimethoprim-sulphamethoxazole against urinary pathogens', *Med. J. Aust.*, **1**, 263.

Snyder, M. J., Perroni, J., Gonzalez, O., Palomino, C., Gonzalez, C., Music, S., Du Pont, H. L., Hornick, R. B. and Woodward, T. E. (1973), 'Trimethoprim-sulfamethoxazole in the treatment of typhoid and paratyphoid fevers', *J. Infect. Dis.* (Suppl.), **128**, 734.

Snyder, M. J., Perroni, J., Gonzalez, O., Woodward, W. E., Palomino, C., Gonzalez, C., Music, S. I., Dupont, H. L., Hornick, R. B. and Woodward, T. E. (1976), 'Comparative efficacy of chloramphenicol, ampicillin and co-trimoxazole in the treatment of typhoid fever', *Lancet*, **2**, 1155.

Stamey, T. A. and Condy, M. (1975), 'The diffusion and concentration of trimethoprim in human vaginal fluid', *J. infect. Dis.*, **131**, 261.

Stamey, T. A., Condy, M. and Mihara, G. (1977), 'Prophylactic efficacy of nitrofurantoin macrocrystals and trimethoprim-sulfamethoxazole in urinary infections. Biologic effects on the vaginal and rectal flora'. *New Engl. J. Med.*, **296**, 780.

Stansfeld, J. M. (1975), 'Duration of treatment for urinary tract infections in children', *Brit. med. J.*, **3**, 65.

Stratford, B. C. and Dixson, S. (1971), 'Results of treatment with trimethoprim plus sulphamethoxazole', *Med. J. Aust.*, **1**, 526.

Svindland, H. B. (1973), 'Treatment of gonorrhoea with sulphamethoxazole-trimethoprim. Lack of effect on concomitant syphilis', *Brit. J. vener. Dis.*, **49**, 50.

Tandon, M. K. (1977), 'A comparative trial of co-trimoxazole and amoxycillin in the treatment of acute exacerbations of chronic bronchitis', *Med. J. Aust.*, **2**, 281.

Tapsall, J. W., Wilson, E. and Harper, J. (1974), 'Thymine dependent strains of Escherichia coli selected by trimethoprim-sulphamethoxazole therapy', *Pathology*, **6**, 161.

Tasker, P. R. W., MacGregor, G. A., De Wardener, H. E., Thomas, R. D. and Jones, N. F. (1975), 'Use of co-trimoxazole in chronic renal failure', *Lancet*, **1**, 1216.

Taylor, B., Abbott, G. D., Kerr, N. McK., Ferguson, D. M. (1977), 'Amoxycillin and co-trimoxazole in presumed viral respiratory infections of childhood: Placebo-controlled trial', *Brit. med. J.*, **2**, 552.

Thomas, F. E., Jr., Leonard, J. M. and Alford, R. H. (1976), 'Sulfamethoxazole-trimethoprim-polymyxin therapy of serious multiple drug-resistant Serratia infections', *Antimicrob. Ag. Chemother.*, **9**, 201.

Thornsberry, C., Baker, C. N. and Kirven, L. A. (1978), '*In vitro* activity of antimicrobial agents on Legionnaires' disease bacterium', *Antimicrob. Ag. Chemother.*, **13**, 78.

Thorpe, J. A. C. and Nysenbaum, A. (1978), 'Co-trimoxazole fatality', *Lancet*, **1**, 276.

Trickett, P. C., Dineen, P. and Mogabgab, W. (1973), 'Trimethoprim-sulfamethoxazole versus penicillin G in the treatment of Group A beta-hemolytic streptococcal pharyngitis and tonsillitis', *J. Infect. Dis.* (Suppl.), **128**, 693.

Tulloch, A. L. (1976), 'Pancytopenia in an infant associated with sulfamethoxazole-trimethoprim therapy', *J. Pediatrics*, **88**, 499.

Uwaydah, M., Matossian, R. and Balabanian, M. (1975), 'Co-trimoxazole compared to chloramphenicol in the treatment of enteric fever', *Scand. J. Infect. Dis.*, **7**, 123.

Vincent, F. M. (1977), 'Acute polyneuropathy possibly associated with co-trimoxazole', *Lancet*, **2**, 980.

Wåhlin, A. and Rosman, N. (1976), 'Skin manifestations with vasculitis due to co-trimoxazole', *Lancet*, **2**, 1415.

Weinstein, L. and Musher, D. M. (1969), 'Antibiotic-induced suprainfection', *J. Infect. Dis.*, **119**, 662.

Welling, P. G., Craig, W. A., Amidon, G. L. and Kunin, C. M. (1973), 'Pharmacokinetics of trimethoprim and sulfamethoxazole in normal subjects and in patients with renal failure', *J. Infect. Dis* (Suppl.), **128**, 556.

Wicks, A. C. B. and Stamps, T. J. (1970), 'Trimethoprim-sulphamethoxazole in typhoid', *Brit. med. J.*, **4**, 52.

Willcox, R. R. (1977), 'How suitable are available pharmaceuticals for the treatment of sexually transmitted diseases? (2) Conditions presenting as sores or tumours', *Brit. J. vener. Dis.*, **53**, 340.

Williams, J. D., Brumfitt, W., Condie, A. P. and Reeves, D. S. (1969), 'The treatment of bacteriuria in pregnant women with sulphamethoxazole and trimethoprim. A microbiological, clinical and toxicological study', *Postgrad. Med. J.* (Suppl.), **45**, 71.

Wolf, L. J. and Baehner, R. L. (1978), 'Delayed development of Pneumocystis pneumonia following administration of short-term high-dose trimethoprim-sulfamethoxazole', *Am. J. Dis. Child.*, **132**, 525.

Yoshikawa, T. T., Miyamoto, S. and Guze, L. B. (1975), 'Comparison of *in vitro* susceptibility of Neisseria gonorrhoeae to trimethoprim-sulfamethoxazole on three different media', *Antimicrob. Ag. Chemother.*, **8**, 515.

Yoshikawa, T. T. and Guze, L. B. (1976), 'Concentrations of trimethoprim-sulfamethoxazole in blood after a single, large oral dose', *Antimicrob. Ag. Chemother.*, **10**, 462.

Yuill, G. M. (1973), 'Megaloblastic anaemia due to trimethoprim-sulphamethoxazole therapy in uraemia', *Postgrad. Med. J.*, **49**, 100.

Nalidixic Acid

Description

Nalidixic acid (1-ethyl-1, 4-dihydro-7-methyl-4-oxo-1, 8-naphthyridine-3-carboxylic acid) is one of a series of 1,8-naphthyridine derivatives, which are not chemically related to any other antibacterial agents. These synthetic chemotherapeutic drugs were first described by Lesher *et al.* (1962) and nalidixic acid was introduced into clinical use in 1964. It is commonly regarded as a urinary antiseptic, because initially it was thought that therapeutic concentrations of the drug are only consistently attained in urine. However therapeutic serum levels are also obtained, leading to the suggestion that nalidixic acid should not be solely classified as a urinary antiseptic similar to nitrofurantoin (page 750) and methenamine mandelate (Stamey *et al.*, 1969). Nevertheless in practice its other uses are limited.

Nalidixic acid is marketed with the trade name of 'Negram' (Winthrop).

Sensitive Organs

1. *Gram-negative bacteria*. Nalidixic acid is active against most of the Enterobacteriaceae such as Esch. coli, the Enterobacter, Klebsiella, all Proteus, Citrobacter, Serratia and Hafnia spp. The Salmonella and Shigella spp. are also usually sensitive (Lesher *et al.,* 1962).

Chromosomal mutations which lead to nalidixic acid resistance occur spontaneously with relatively high frequencies in Gram-negative bacteria (Burman, 1977), and resistance of these usually sensitive bacteria to nalidixic acid can easily be induced *in vitro* (Buchbinder *et al.*, 1962). The emergence of resistance *in vivo* during the treatment of patients has also been frequently observed (Buchbinder *et al.*, 1962; Barlow, 1963; Ronald *et al.*, 1966; Finegold *et al.*, 1967). Stamey and Bragonje (1976) consider that underdosage is the main reason why *in vivo* resistance to nalidixic acid has been a problem in treating urinary tract infections. They showed that the MIC of the infecting strain must be exceeded by at least ten-fold if the selection of resistant mutants is to be minimized. This is usually accomplished with an adult dose of 4 g per day which produces urinary concentrations of 50–500 μg per ml (page 734). With lower doses and in very young or very old patients (in whom absorption and excretion of the drug may be less), urinary concentrations are lower and they encourage selection of resistant mutants. Studies by Greenwood and O'Grady (1977) in which a bladder model was used, tend to support this view. Their results suggested that emergence of bacterial resistance should not be a major problem when nalidixic acid is used to treat uncomplicated urinary infection, but prolonged high dose therapy may be necessary for more complicated infections to avoid the development of bacterial resistance. Stamey and Bragonje (1976) found that when adequate dosage was used, resistance to nalidixic acid only developed in 7 per cent of patients, a frequency which is comparable with other effective antimicrobial agents. A similar low frequency (8 per cent) of emergence of resistant organisms during treatment was reported by Cederberg et al. (1974).

Nalidixic acid-resistant Gram-negative bacilli are still uncommon in both domiciliary and hospital infections. One study demonstrated that there had been no apparent increase in resistant strains of Esch. coli between the years 1962 to 1970 (Brumfitt and Pursell, 1971). Burman (1977) found nalidixic acid resistance in 9 per cent of strains of Gram-negative bacteria tested; this only occurred in 3 per cent of Esch. coli strains but it was more common amongst Proteus mirabilis and the Klebsiella and Enterobacter spp. After studying strains from urinary infections, Stamey and Bragonje (1976) concluded that with the exception of Ps. aeruginosa and Gram-positive cocci most urinary pathogens are sensitive to nalidixic acid, despite the presence of multiple drug resistance in more than one half of the strains. The reason for the continuing low frequency of nalidixic acid-resistant Gram-negative bacteria is that its resistance is not mediated by R plasmids (page 422), which are often involved with bacterial resistance to both antibiotics produced in nature, such as aminoglycosides, tetracyclines, chloramphenicol, beta-lactam compounds and the synthetic compounds trimethoprim and sulphonamides (Burman, 1977). Therefore resistance to nalidixic acid cannot be transferred in the bowel from one organism to another, and multiply-resistant Enterobacteriaceae remain sensitive to nalidixic acid. Nalidixic acid also induces less resistance amongst faecal Gram-negative bacilli than other antimicrobial agents used for urinary tract infections (Stamey and Bragonje, 1976). This may be important if reinfection occurs shortly after therapy, because faecal organisms are usually implicated.

Crumplin and Smith (1975) reported the paradoxical finding that with susceptible Gram-negative bacteria, when the bactericidal concentration for the strain was exceeded, the bactericidal effect of the drug was reduced and it became relatively bacteristatic. This phenomenon was explicable by the mode of action of nalidixic acid (page 735). At the higher concentrations of the drug which were used, RNA and protein synthesis were also inhibited and these are essential for the lethal action of the drug. Contrary to Stamey and Bragonje's opinion (vide supra), Crumplin and Smith (1975) considered that for some bacteria a 1 g oral dose of nalidixic acid may produce a urinary level which is in excess of the bactericidal level and be only bacteristatic; this could favour the emergence of resistant strains. This opinion has not been substantiated by clinical experience (vide supra).

Nalidixic acid often acts synergistically with kanamycin, gentamicin or colistin against most Enterobacteriaceae, whereas with chloramphenicol and tetracycline in vitro antagonism is not infrequent (Michel et al., 1973). Nalidixic acid is also antagonistic with nitrofurantoin in vitro. When it is combined with one of the penicillins or cephalosporins, there is usually neither synergism nor antagonism (Michel et al., 1973). In vitro nalidixic acid potentiates the action of metronidazole against Bacteroides fragilis (page 762).

The activity of this drug against other Gram-negative bacteria has not been extensively investigated. The Brucella spp. may be sensitive but Ps. aeruginosa is always resistant. Of 349 gonococcal strains collected from South-East Asia during the years 1968–71, 96 per cent were sensitive and 4 per cent moderately sensitive to nalidixic acid. In addition, beta-lactamase producing strains of N. gonorrhoeae (page 8) are inhibited by 2 μg per ml or less of the drug (Report, 1978).

2. *Gram-positive bacteria.* All bacteria of this group such as Staph. pyogenes, Strep. pneumoniae and Strep. faecalis are nalidixic acid-resistant (Lesher *et al.*, 1962; Barlow, 1963).

3. *Fungi.* Nalidixic acid can suppress the growth of Candida albicans in concentrations obtained in urine after normal doses of the drug (Sobieski and Brewer, 1976).

In Vitro Sensitivities

The minimum inhibitory concentrations of nalidixic acid against some selected bacterial species are shown in Table 43. For treatment of urinary tract infections, organisms with an MIC of 16 μg per ml or lower can be regarded as highly sensitive to this drug and those with an MIC of 16–50 μg per ml as of intermediate sensitivity (Barlow, 1963; Stamey and Bragonje, 1976).

TABLE 43

(After Lesher *et al.*, 1962)

ORGANISM	MIC (μg per ml)
Gram-negative bacteria	
Escherichia coli	5·0–12·5
Enterobacter aerogenes	1·6–25·0
Klebsiella pneumoniae	0·8–25·0
Proteus spp.	1·25–30·0
Salmonella spp.	3·2–50·0
Shigella spp.	0·8–3·2
Brucella spp.	7·5–10·0
Gram-positive bacteria	
Staph. pyogenes	50·0–100·0
Strep. pneumoniae (Dip. pneumoniae)	250·0

Mode of Administration and Dosage

1. *Adults.* Nalidixic acid is usually administered by the oral route in a dose of 4 g daily given in four divided doses. The dose may be reduced to 2 g daily for more prolonged treatment. A single daily dose of 1 g has been used for long-term suppressive therapy of chronic bacteriuria.

2. *Children.* The dosage is 50 mg per kg body weight daily, administered in four divided doses.

3. *Newborn and premature infants.* Infants under four weeks of age should not be treated by this drug. Kemball and Davies (1967) reported a premature infant weighing 1·72 kg, given nalidixic acid in a dose of 60 mg per kg daily, who developed deep sighing respirations, abdominal distension, muscle hypotonia, and a marked metabolic acidosis two days after commencement of

treatment. This infant recovered after cessation of nalidixic acid and treatment with sodium bicarbonate. The serum level of the drug 9 h after the last dose was 114 µg per ml, but the urinary level was only 20 µg per ml. Newborn infants apparently conjugate and excrete this drug much more slowly than older children and adults, and the high serum and low urine levels recorded in this case represent a reversal of the characteristic findings in the other age groups.

4. *Patients with renal failure*. In patients with moderate degrees of renal functional impairment (serum creatinine 4–6 mg per cent or 0·33–0·5 mmol/l) treated by usual doses of nalidixic acid, there is no accumulation of the active drug in the body, and adequate urinary concentrations (about 70 µg per ml) of the active drug are usually attained (Stamey *et al.*, 1969). It is therefore feasible to use this drug in ordinary doses for the treatment of urinary tract infections in moderately azotaemic patients. However inactive nalidixic acid metabolites (monoglucuronides) almost certainly accumulate in such patients, and may contribute to toxicity. For this reason treatment with nalidixic acid should be avoided in patients with renal failure whenever possible. Dosage reduction for such patients is not practicable because this would lead to inadequate urine levels of the active drug. In patients with severe renal failure, therapeutic urinary levels are unlikely to be achieved even with ordinary dosage.

5. *Intravenous administration*. The sodium salt of nalidixic acid is suitable for intravenous administration. This is prepared as a 10 per cent solution containing 1 g in each 10 ml ampoule, and although it is not generally available, it has been used by some clinical investigators. The 1 g dose of nalidixic acid is added to 500 ml of saline and administered to adults by slow intravenous infusion over 8 h. The dose in children is 15 mg per kg body weight every 8 h (Zinsser, 1970; Economou *et al.*, 1972). Intravenous nalidixic acid apparently does not cause any local or general adverse effects. It is incompatible with epsilon aminocaproic acid, and it may also precipitate in a 5 per cent dextrose solution (Economou *et al.*, 1972).

Availability

1. Tablets: 250 and 500 mg
2. Suspension: 50 mg per ml.

Serum Levels in Relation to Dosage

Early studies showed that serum concentrations could not be predicted after oral administration of nalidixic acid (Buchbinder et al., 1962; Gibbon *et al.*, 1965). Serum levels at 1, 2 and 4 h after a single 1·0 g oral dose of nalidixic acid varied widely from patient to patient. Some patients had high serum levels (10–40 µg per ml), but in others levels of only 1·0–2·0 µg per ml or even lower were recorded (Gibbon *et al.*, 1965). By contrast studies performed by Stamey *et al.* (1969) showed that adequate serum levels in a range of 21–50 µg per ml were always attained 2 h after a single oral dose of 1 g.

Nalidixic acid does not accumulate in the serum of patients with normal renal function if it is administered six-hourly in the usual recommended doses.

The mean serum levels attained after intravenous administration of the sodium salt of nalidixic acid, in a dose of 15 mg per kg eight-hourly, are in the range of 30–50 μg per ml (Zinsser, 1970).

Some nalidixic acid is converted in the body to a hydroxy metabolite, hydroxynalidixic acid, and this also has antibacterial activity. The serum levels of the drug, quoted above, include both nalidixic acid and its hydroxy metabolite, the latter accounting for about 30 per cent of the biologically active drug in the serum (Stamey, 1971).

Experiments in two volunteers have indicated that probenecid may prolong the serum half-life of nalidixic acid (Dash and Mills, 1976).

Excretion

Nalidixic acid and its active hydroxy metabolite are both rapidly conjugated in the liver to antibacterially inactive monoglucuronides, which are rapidly excreted via the kidney (Stamey et al., 1969). About 85–90 per cent of the drug excreted by the kidney is in the conjugated inactive form, but the remainder is excreted as unchanged nalidixic acid and its active hydroxy metabolite, producing therapeutically adequate urinary levels. Urine concentrations of these active drugs in adults are in the range of 25–250 μg per ml after a single oral dose of 0·5–1·0 g. These levels remain high (50 to 500 μg per ml) if a 1 g dose is administered orally, every 6 h (Buchbinder et al., 1962). The hydroxy metabolite of nalidixic acid accounts for about 85 per cent of the biologically active drug in the urine (Stamey, 1971).

Adequate urine levels of the active drugs are also usually attained in patients with moderate renal failure (Stamey et al., 1969). These do not accumulate in the serum of azotaemic patients, but their inactive monoglucuronides do and probably contribute to toxicity (Adam and Dawborn, 1971).

Nalidixic acid should be administered cautiously to patients with liver disease in whom conjugation of the drug may be impaired.

About 4 per cent of orally administered nalidixic acid is not absorbed and is excreted in the faeces.

Distribution of the Drug in Body

Animal experiments show that even after prolonged administration, this drug fails to accumulate in the tissues, where concentrations attained are usually lower than simultaneous serum levels. The kidney is the only organ in which tissue concentrations may exceed serum levels. The concentration of nalidixic acid attained in the human kidney has been studied in patients undergoing elective nephrectomy (Jameson, 1965). The drug is concentrated in the pyelonephritic kidney and in seven out of eleven patients renal tissue levels exceeded serum levels, after treatment for 24 h or longer. There was no significant difference between renal medullary and cortical tissue levels. Nalidixic acid was also present in the pus of one patient with a perinephric abscess. The concentration of the drug in this pus varied from 8 to 24 μg per ml on different days.

Nalidixic acid is highly (about 93 per cent) bound to serum proteins, but its active hydroxy metabolite is only about 63 per cent serum protein bound (Stamey, 1971).

Mode of Action

Early studies suggested that nalidixic acid interferes with bacterial deoxyribonucleic acid (DNA) synthesis (Goss *et al.*, 1964). Subsequent investigators have been unable to demonstrate inhibition of any known enzyme step in DNA biosynthesis (Winshell and Rosenkranz, 1970), and all known proteins involved in DNA replication are unaffected by the drug (Bourguignon *et al.*, 1973). A more recent study suggests that nalidixic acid interferes with the conversion of intermediate size DNA fragments into high molecular DNA in Esch. coli (Crumplin and Smith, 1976). It has been shown that a bactericidal effect can only occur in the presence of competent ribonucleic acid (RNA) and protein synthesis (Deitz *et al.*, 1966). This has been regarded as lethal unbalanced growth. Crumplin and Smith (1975) showed that when the bactericidal concentration of nalidixic acid for a susceptible organism is exceeded, its bactericidal effect is reduced. This occurs because at higher concentrations nalidixic acid also inhibits RNA and protein synthesis, which are essential for the lethal action of the drug. It was suggested that a second target for nalidixic acid in the bacterial cell may be messenger RNA.

Toxicity

1. *Gastro-intestinal side-effects*. Nausea, vomiting or diarrhoea are relatively infrequent complications and are usually not severe.

2. *Neurotoxicity*. This is uncommon and includes visual disturbances, excitement, depression, confusion and hallucinations. Headache, giddiness, drowsiness, syncope, sensory changes and grand mal attacks have also been described (Cahal, 1965). Convulsions have occurred in small numbers of patients (Fraser and Harrower, 1977). Acute reversible psychosis has also been observed in a patient treated with large doses of nalidixic acid (Finegold *et al.*, 1967). Similarly Kremer *et al.* (1967) described an adult patient with acute glomerulo-nephritis, who developed a paranoid state after treatment by nalidixic acid for superimposed coliform urinary infection.

Severe neurotoxic reactions due to nalidixic acid have usually occurred when this drug has been used in large doses. However it seems wise to use it cautiously in patients with pre-existing mental instability, epilepsy and cerebral arteriosclerosis.

3. *Intracranial hypertension*. This is a rare complication and most reported patients have been infants (Boréus and Sundström, 1967; Fisher, 1967). One of the best examples of this side-effect was the case of a six-months-old boy described by Boréus and Sundström (1967). This patient developed vomiting, a bulging fontanelle, papilloedema and widening of the skull sutures a few days after commencement of treatment with nalidixic acid in a dose of 100 mg given orally four times a day. This complication was observed on two separate occasions, when this drug was used for the treatment of urinary tract infection, and each time the signs resolved when it was discontinued. The causal relationship between nalidixic acid therapy and increased intracranial pressure was confirmed in this patient, when the condition was reproduced on a third occasion by the administration of the drug under carefully controlled conditions. Another patient, a five-year-old girl reported by Anderson *et al.* (1971), developed a sixth nerve palsy as well as papilloedema following the administra-

tion of nalidixic acid. When the drug was stopped, the papilloedema rapidly resolved and lateral rectus function improved, but the child was left with a permanent internal strabismus.

4. *Metabolic disturbances*. Islam and Sreedharan (1965) reported the interesting case of a fourteen-year-old girl, who took an overdose of nalidixic acid (13 tablets of 0·5 g). She developed convulsions, hyperglycaemia and glycosuria, which simulated diabetic ketosis, but her plasma ketones were not elevated. Treatment was successful with intravenous fluids without insulin, and the blood gluclose returned to normal after 24 h. A similar case was observed at Fairfield Hospital in 1974. A two-year-old girl with varicella was admitted to hospital because she had a convulsion 15 min after accidentally ingesting one 0·5 g tablet of nalidixic acid. At the time of admission she was alert but tachypnoeic, and biochemical investigations disclosed a metabolic acidosis (standard bicarbonate 13 mEq or mmol per litre) and hyperglycaemia (blood gluclose 220 mg per cent or 12·2 mmol/l), but no glycosuria. She was treated with intravenous dextrose/saline and in 12 h her respiration rate reverted to normal and within 48 h the biochemical abnormalities had disappeared. Her serum nalidixic acid level, estimated soon after admission to hospital, was 140 μg per ml. Hyperglycaemia was confirmed in these cases by the specific Sömogyi-Nelson method.

Fraser and Harrower (1977) reported a thirty-one-year-old woman who developed convulsions and hyperglycaemia two days after starting nalidixic acid in a dose of 1 g four times a day. This patient had no underlying neurological disease and she recovered after ceasing the drug. The authors suggested that convulsions and hyperglycaemia may occur in otherwise healthy people as a result of an idiosyncratic reaction.

Metabolic acidosis without hyperglycaemia has also been ascribed to nalidixic acid overdose. Dash and Mills (1976) described an eighteen-year-old man who ingested an unknown quantity of nalidixic acid, plus probenecid and a number of other drugs. He became stuporose and had a metabolic acidosis with a normal plasma glucose but markedly elevated nalidixic acid serum levels. The patient awoke gradually during 12 h, and it was considered that the concomitant administration of probenecid had prolonged the serum half-life of nalidixic acid (*see* page 734).

5. *Skin rashes*. Pruritus and rashes, usually urticarial in type, associated with eosinophilia have occurred in patients taking nalidixic acid. In addition severe photosensitivity reactions, involving exposed surfaces, have been reported (Zelickson, 1964; Burry and Crosby, 1966; Mathew, 1966; Brauner, 1975). Five patients described by Mathew (1966), developed bullous skin eruptions in the summer while receiving nalidixic acid therapy, three of whom had impaired renal function. The bullae slowly resolved two weeks to two months after cessation of the drug. One of these patients was treated with prednisolone without apparent beneficial effect. Mathew (1966) recommended that nalidixic acid therapy should be avoided during sunny weather, particularly in patients with impaired renal function. All patients receiving nalidixic acid should be warned to avoid sun exposure, and to cease the drug at the first sign of an abnormal skin reaction. Burry and Crosby (1966) consider that the reaction produced by nalidixic acid is a phototoxic reaction (which resembles excessive sun-burn and does not spread beyond areas exposed to light), and not a

photoallergic reaction (which looks like an allergic skin disease and spreads beyond areas exposed to light). Demethylchlortetracycline causes classical phototoxicity (page 615), while the sulphonamides (page 668) cause photoallergy. Brauner (1975) has pointed out that nalidixic acid photodermatitis is uncommon; its incubation period is up to several weeks and reactivity occurs irrespective of dosage and continues even when most of the drug has been cleared from the body. These features suggest photoallergy rather than phototoxicity.

6. *Haemolytic anaemia*. This appears to be a rare, but potentially serious complication of nalidixic acid therapy, particularly in newborn infants. Belton and Jones (1965) reported a two-week-old baby, who developed a haemolytic anaemia apparently as a result of drinking breast milk, whilst the mother was being treated with nalidixic acid. This baby's red cells were not deficient in glucose-6-phosphate dehydrogenase. However nalidixic acid does appear to be another drug, which can precipitate haemolytic crises in individuals with this red cell enzyme deficiency. This complication has been described in an older child with this defect (Mandal and Stevenson, 1970), and in an adult with the same deficiency who had an occupational exposure to nalidixic acid dust (Alessio and Morselli, 1972). An autoimmune haemolytic anaemia with a positive direct Coombs test, has been described in a woman aged 65 after she had received intermittent courses of nalidixic acid (Gilbertson and Jones, 1972). Therefore it seems that this drug may cause haemolytic anaemia by a variety of haematological mechanisms.

7. *Respiratory failure*. There is some evidence to suggest that nalidixic acid may precipitate acute respiratory failure in patients whose respiratory function is already impaired (*Today's Drugs*, 1967).

8. *Fetal toxicity*. No teratogenic effects have been noted in pregnant animals given nalidixic acid (Ward-McQuaid et al., 1963), and pregnant patients have received this drug without untoward effects (Wren, 1969). However many clinicians still have reservations about its use during the first trimester of pregnancy (Zinsser, 1970).

9. *Drug interactions*. Nalidixic acid can displace warfarin and other highly albumin-bound coumarins from their binding sites on serum albumin, so that excess anticoagulation may result if the drug is given to patients stabilized on warfarin (Hoffbrand, 1974; Koch-Weser and Sellers, 1976).

Nalidixic acid glucuronide conjugates may produce a false positive reaction for glucose in urine with clinitest or Benedict's test, but not with clinistix. Diabetic patients should be informed of this, if they are treated with nalidixic acid.

Clinical Uses of the Drug

1. *Urinary tract infections*. Nalidixic acid is useful for treatment of urinary tract infections caused by organisms such as Esch. coli and all species of Enterobacter, Klebsiella and Proteus. It has been used successfully for the treatment of acute, chronic and recurrent urinary tract infections (Barlow, 1963; Ward-McQuaid et al., 1963; Gibson and Potts, 1964; Ronald et al., 1966). The follow-up cure rate in patients with chronic infections is, similar to that with other antimicrobial agents, disappointing.

Nalidixic acid in a lower dosage is one of several drugs suitable for long-term suppressive therapy in patients with chronic bacteriuria. Such therapy may prevent recurrent bacteriuria in patients with chronic bacterial prostatitis, but it usually fails to eradicate bacteria from prostatic fluid (Stamey, 1971).

It has been used successfully for the treatment of urinary tract infections in childhood, particularly acute uncomplicated pyelonephritis, and also for the prolonged treatment of children with urinary infections associated with renal tract abnormalities (Kneebone, 1965). In the latter group bacterial strains resistant to nalidixic acid unfortunately emerge in a proportion of cases. Drugs such as nalidixic acid, oxolinic acid (page 742) and nitrofurantoin (page 750), which only produce low or therapeutically negligible blood and tissue levels, are better suited for the treatment of uncomplicated acute infections of the lower urinary tract, or for prophylaxis against ascending infection after retrograde instrumentation. For upper urinary infections and chronic bacteriuria associated with underlying urinary tract pathology, drugs which produce effective blood and tissue levels are preferable (Naumann, 1978).

The drug has been used occasionally for the treatment of urinary infections during pregnancy, and no teratogenic effects have been noted (Wren, 1969).

The antibacterial activity of nalidixic acid remains unchanged over the entire pH range of urine, and on this basis alone there is no need to regulate urinary pH, when the drug is used to treat urinary infections. However alkalinization of the urine markedly increases urine levels of the active drug, and therefore may enhance its clinical effect (Zinsser, 1970). The absorption of nalidixic acid from the gastro-intestinal tract and renal clearance of the active drug both appear to be increased by the concomitant administration of sodium bicarbonate (Adam and Dawborn, 1971).

Nalidixic acid should not be used together with nitrofurantoin, because these two drugs show antagonism *in vitro*.

2. *Systemic infections due to Gram-negative bacilli.* Nalidixic acid is not usually regarded as suitable for treatment of systemic infections such as septicaemia. The efficacy of nalidixic acid in acute pyelonephritis, a disease involving renal parenchyma, may be partly because the drug is concentrated in the pyelonephritic kidney (Jameson, 1965). Stamey *et al.* (1969) re-studied serum concentrations attained after oral administration of nalidixic acid, and found that they were adequate (page 733), and suggested that the orally administered drug may be effective in some systemic infections. Sharma (1965) had previously reported the successful treatment of four patients with brucellosis by oral nalidixic acid, but there appear to be no other reports on the efficacy of the oral drug in systemic infections.

The sodium salt of nalidixic acid has been used intravenously for the treatment of a small number of patients with septicaemias due to Enterobacter and Klebsiella species. Adequate serum levels were attained and clinical results appeared satisfactory (Zinsser, 1970). This intravenous preparation is not currently available for general use.

3. *Intestinal infections.* It has been suggested that orally administered nalidixic acid may be beneficial in Shigella sonnei dysentery (Moorhead and Parry, 1965), but it is now generally accepted that antimicrobial agents are not indicated for this disease (page 115). Similarly it was thought that this drug may have some place in the management of infantile gastro-enteritis due to

enteropathogenic Esch. coli (*Today's Drugs*, 1967), but it now seems that antimicrobial therapy is also unnecessary for this disorder. Recently nalidixic acid (or oxolinic acid page 742, or cinoxacin page 746) have been suggested as being worthy of trial for the prevention of traveller's diarrhoea due to enterotoxigenic Esch. coli (Dupont *et al.*, 1978). These drugs have the advantage that resistance to them is not mediated by R plasmids (page 731).

4. *Burns*. Experimental studies have shown that the topical application of 0·2 per cent nalidixic acid cream in conjunction with systemic carbenicillin can prevent death of mice with burns infected with a carbenicillin-sensitive virulent Pseudomonas and a carbenicillin-resistant avirulent Klebsiella. Systemic carbenicillin alone was ineffective. It was demonstrated that nalidixic acid inhibited bacterial conjugation which prevented the transfer of carbenicillin resistance from Klebsiella to Pseudomonas. Nalidixic acid, being a useful drug for the treatment of urinary tract infections, should probably not be used for the topical therapy of burns, as this may encourage the emergence of nalidixic acid-resistant bacilli. Other compounds, which prevent bacterial conjugation, but are not used for chemotherapy, may be more appropriate for this purpose (Roe and Jones, 1972).

REFERENCES

Adam, W. R. and Dawborn, J. K. (1971), 'Plasma levels and urinary excretion of nalidixic acid in patients with renal failure', *Aust. N.Z. J. Med.*, **1**, 126.

Alessio, L. and Morselli, G. (1972), 'Occupational exposure to nalidixic acid', *Brit. med. J.*, **4**, 110.

Anderson, E. E., Anderson, B., Jr. and Nashold, B. S. (1971), 'Childhood complications of nalidixic acid', *JAMA*, **216**, 1023.

Barlow, A. M. (1963), 'Nalidixic acid in infections of urinary tract', *Brit. med. J.*, **2**, 1308.

Belton, E. M. and Jones, R. V. (1965), 'Haemolytic anaemia due to nalidixic acid', *Lancet*, **2**, 691.

Boréus, L. O. and Sundström, B. (1967), 'Intracranial hypertension in a child during treatment with nalidixic acid', *Brit. med. J.*, **2**, 744.

Bourguignon, G. J., Levitt, M. and Sternglanz, R. (1973), 'Studies on the mechanism of action of nalidixic acid', *Antimicrob. Ag. Chemother.*, **4**, 479.

Brauner, G. J. (1975), 'Bullous photoreaction to nalidixic acid', *Amer. J. Med.*, **58**, 576.

Brumfitt, W. and Pursell, R. (1971), 'Observations on bacterial sensitivities to nalidixic acid and critical comments on the 6-centre survey', *Postgrad. Med. J. (September Suppl.)*, **47**, 16.

Buchbinder, M., Webb, J. C., Anderson, L. V. and McCabe, W. R. (1962), 'Laboratory studies and clinical pharmacology of nalidixic acid (WIN 18, 320)', *Antimicrob. Ag. Chemother.*, p. 308.

Burman, L. G. (1977), 'Apparent absence of transferable resistance to nalidixic acid in pathogenic Gram-negative bacteria', *J. Antimicrob. Chemother.*, **3**, 509.

Burry, J. N. and Crosby, R. W. L. (1966), 'A case of phototoxicity to nalidixic acid', *Med. J. Aust.*, **2**, 698.

Cahal, D. A. (1965), 'Reactions to nalidixic acid', *Brit. med. J.*, **2**, 590.

Cederberg, Å., Denneberg, T., Ekberg, M. and Juhlin, I. (1974), 'Nalidixic acid in urinary tract infections with particular reference to the emergence of resistance', *Scand. J. Infect. Dis.*, **6**, 259.

Crumplin, G. C. and Smith, J. T. (1975), 'Nalidixic acid: An antibacterial paradox' *Antimicrob. Ag. Chemother.*, **8**, 251.

Crumplin, G. C. and Smith, J. T. (1976), 'Nalidixic acid and bacterial chromosome replication', *Nature,* **260,** 643.

Dash, H. and Mills, J. (1976), 'Severe metabolic acidosis associated with nalidixic acid overdose', *Ann. Intern. Med.,* **84,** 570.

Deitz, W. H., Cook, T. M. and Goss, W. A. (1966), 'Mechanism of action of nalidixic acid on Escherichia coli', *J. Bacteriol.,* **91,** 768.

Dupont, H. L., West, H., Evans, D. G., Olarte, J., and Evans, D. J., Jr. (1978), 'Antimicrobial susceptibility of enterotoxigenic Escherichia coli', *J. Antimicrob. Chemother.,* **4,** 100.

Economou, G., Macis, R. and Ward-McQuaid, N. (1972), 'Nalidixic acid by intravenous infusion. A report of 50 cases', *Brit. J. Urol.,* **44,** 503.

Finegold, S. M., Miller, L. G., Posnick, D., Patterson, D. K. and Davis, A. (1967), 'Nalidixic acid: Clinical and laboratory studies', *Antimicrob. Ag. Chemother.*—1966, p. 189.

Fisher, O. D. (1967), 'Nalidixic acid and intracranial hypertension', *Brit. med. J.,* **3,** 370.

Fraser, A. G., and Harrower, A. D. B., (1977), 'Convulsions and hyperglycaemia associated with nalidixic acid', *Brit. med. J.,* **2,** 1518.

Gibbon, N. O. K., Benstead, J. G. and Misra, G. C. (1965), 'A comparative study of the levels of nalidixic acid in plasma and urine and its antibacterial activity in urinary infections in paraplegics', *Postgrad. Med. J.,* **41,** 501.

Gibson, G. R. and Potts, I. F. (1964), 'A clinical trial of nalidixic acid: A new antibacterial substance', *Med. J. Aust.,* **2,** 225.

Gilbertson, C. and Jones, D. R. (1972), 'Haemolytic anaemia with nalidixic acid', *Brit. med. J.,* **4,** 493.

Goss, W. A., Deitz, W. H. and Cook, T. M. (1964), 'Mechanism of action of nalidixic acid on Escherichia coli', *J. Bacteriol.,* **88,** 1112.

Greenwood, D. and O'Grady, F., (1977), 'Factors governing the emergence of resistance to nalidixic acid in treatment of urinary tract infections', *Antimicrob. Ag. Chemother.,* **12,** 678.

Hoffbrand, B. I. (1974), 'Interaction of nalidixic acid and warfarin', *Brit. med. J.,* **2,** 666.

Islam, M. A. and Sreedharan, T. (1965), 'Convulsions, hyperglycaemia, and glycosuria from overdose of nalidixic acid', *JAMA,* **192,** 1100.

Jameson, R. M. (1965), 'Tissue concentration of nalidixic acid in chronic pyelonephritis', *Brit. med. J.,* **2,** 621.

Kemball, M. L. and Davies, P. A. (1967), 'Nalidixic acid for the newborn', *Brit. med. J.,* **2,** 310.

Kneebone, G. M. (1965), 'A clinical appraisal of nalidixic acid in urinary tract infection in childhood', *Med. J. Aust.,* **2,** 947.

Koch-Weser, J. and Sellers, E. M. (1976), 'Binding of drugs to serum albumin. (Second of two parts)', *New Engl. J. Med.* **294,** 526.

Kremer, L., Walton, M. and Wardle, E. N. (1967), 'Nalidixic acid and intracranial hypertension', *Brit. med. J.,* **4,** 488.

Lesher, G. Y., Froelich, E. J., Gruett, M. D., Bailey, J. H. and Brundage, R. P. (1962), '1,8-naphthyridine derivatives. A new class of chemotherapeutic agents', *J. Med. Pharm. Chem.,* **5,** 1063.

Mandal, B. K. and Stevenson, J. (1970), 'Haemolytic crisis produced by nalidixic acid', *Lancet,* **1,** 614.

Mathew, T. H. (1966), 'Nalidixic acid', *Med. J. Aust.,* **2,** 243.

Michel, J., Luboshitzky, R. and Sacks, T. (1973), 'Bactericidal effect on combinations of nalidixic acid and various antibiotics on Enterobacteriaceae', *Antimicrob. Ag. Chemother.,* **4,** 201.

Moorhead, P. J. and Parry, H. E. (1965), 'Treatment of Sonne dysentery', *Brit. med. J.,*

2, 913.

Naumann, P. (1978), 'The value of antibiotic levels in tissue and in urine in the treatment of urinary tract infections', *J. Antimicrob. Chemother.*, **4**, 9.

Roe, E. and Jones, R. J. (1972), 'Effects of topical chemoprophylaxis on transferable antibiotic resistance in burns', *Lancet*, **2**, 109.

Report of a WHO Scientific Group (1978), 'Neisseria gonorrhoeae and gonococcal infections', *Wld. Hlth. Org. techn. Rep. Ser.*, No. 616.

Ronald, A. R., Turck, M. and Petersdorf, R. G. (1966), 'A critical evaluation of nalidixic acid in urinary-tract infections', *New Engl. J. Med.*, **275**, 1081.

Sharma, B. (1965), 'Treatment of brucellosis by nalidixic acid', *Lancet*, **1**, 1171.

Sobieski, R. J. and Brewer, A. R. (1976), 'Toxicity of nalidixic acid on Candida albicans, Saccharomyces cerevisiae, and Kluyveromyces lactis', *Antimicrob. Ag. Chemother.*, **9**, 485.

Stamey, T. A., Nemoy, N. J. and Higgins, M. (1969), 'The clinical use of nalidixic acid. A review and some observations', *Investigative Urology*, **6**, 582.

Stamey, T. A. (1971), 'Observations on the clinical use of nalidixic acid', *Postgrad. Med. J. (September Suppl.)*, **47**, 21.

Stamey, T. A. and Bragonje, J. (1976), 'Resistance to nalidixic acid. A misconception due to underdosage', *JAMA*, **236**, 1857.

Today's Drugs (1967), 'Nalidixic acid', *Brit. med. J.*, **1**, 741.

Ward-McQuaid, J. F. N. C., Jichlinski, D. and Macis, R. (1963), 'Nalidixic acid in urinary infections', *Brit. med. J.*, **2**, 1311.

Winshell, E. B. and Rosenkranz, H. S. (1970), 'Nalidixic acid and the metabolism of Escherichia coli', *J. Bacteriol.*, **104**, 1168.

Wren, B. G. (1969), 'Subclinical renal infection in pregnancy: Pathogenesis and drugs of choice', *Med. J. Aust.*, **2**, 895.

Zelickson, A. S. (1964), 'Phototoxic reaction with nalidixic acid', *JAMA*, **190**, 556.

Zinsser, H. H. (1970), 'Nalidixic acid in acute and chronic urinary tract infections', *Med. Clin. North America*, **54**, 1347.

Oxolinic Acid

Description

Oxolinic acid is a synthetic antimicrobial agent, chemically related to nalidixic acid (page 730), and has the chemical formula of 5-ethyl-5, 8-dihydro-8-oxo-1, 3-dioxolo (4,5-g) quinoline-7-carboxylic acid (Kaminsky and Meltzer, 1968). This drug, similar to nalidixic acid, is only suitable for the treatment of urinary tract infections, but it has the advantage of only requiring twice-daily medication. It is marketed by Warner with the trade names of 'Utibid' (Australia and United States) and 'Prodoxol' (United Kingdom).

Sensitive Organisms

1. *Gram-negative bacteria*. Oxolinic acid has a similar spectrum of activity against these bacteria to that of nalidixic acid (page 730) (Turner *et al.*, 1968; Atlas *et al.*, 1969; Kershaw and Leigh, 1975; Klein and Matsen, 1976). It is active against most of the Enterobacteriaceae such as Esch. coli, the Enterobacter, Klebsiella and all Proteus spp., the Hafnia, Citrobacter, Providencia, Shigella and Salmonella species. Chloramphenicol-resistant strains of Salm. typhi (page 423) are also sensitive (Sanford *et al.*, 1976). Oxolinic acid has considerably greater activity than nalidixic acid against Esch. coli, the Proteus and Klebsiella spp. (Turner *et al.*, 1968; Atlas *et al.*, 1969) and slightly greater activity against Shigella spp. (Gordon *et al.*, 1976).

Resistance of these usually sensitive bacteria can be induced *in vitro* and such strains show cross-resistance with nalidixic acid (Ringel *et al.*, 1968). Resistance may also develop *in vivo* but in one study this occurred to a lesser degree in patients with chronic bacteriuria treated by oxolinic acid (2·0 g per day) than in others treated by nalidixic acid (4·0 g per day). In addition, with most isolates cross-resistance between these drugs was not marked (Atlas *et al.*, 1969). Similar to nalidixic acid (page 731), oxolinic acid also shows *in vitro* antagonism with nitrofurantoin (Westwood and Hooper, 1975). Most urinary pathogens (Esch. coli, Proteus, Klebsiella and Enterobacter spp.) are inhibited by an oxolinic acid concentration of 2·5 μg per ml or less (Kershaw and Leigh, 1975).

Amongst other Gram-negative organisms, N. meningitidis and N. gonorrhoeae are very sensitive and the Acinetobacter spp. and, to a less extent the Brucella spp., are sensitive. Most strains of Pseudomonas aeruginosa are resistant.

2. *Gram-positive bacteria*. By contrast to nalidixic acid, Staph. pyogenes is frequently susceptible to concentrations of oxolinic acid which can be easily attained in the urine. Staph. epidermidis is also occasionally susceptible. The

drug has no significant activity against other Gram-positive organisms, including the micrococci which often cause urinary tract infections in young women (Meers, 1974).

Mode of Administration and Dosage

Oxolinic acid is given by the oral route and the recommended dose for adults is 750 mg twice-daily. This has been administered for periods of 14–28 days for the treatment of urinary tract infections (Guyer, 1974). The drug has also been given to children as a suspension, in a dose of 15–20 mg per kg body weight per day, in two divided doses (Shapera and Matsen, 1977). Apparently oxolinic acid does not accumulate in patients with impaired renal function, so that no dosage reduction is necessary in such patients (Guyer, 1974).

Availability

Tablets: 750 mg.

Serum Levels in Relation to Dosage

Oxolinic acid is poorly absorbed following oral administsration. Guyer (1974) recorded maximum serum levels of $2 \cdot 7$–$3 \cdot 2$ μg per ml, 3–4 h after a single oral dose of 750 mg. Kershaw and Leigh (1975) obtained lower levels when a similar dose was given to volunteers; a mean peak serum level of $0 \cdot 8$ μg per ml (range $0 \cdot 2$–$1 \cdot 1$ μg per ml) was reached after 2–6 h, and at 8 h the level was $0 \cdot 15$ μg per ml. The serum half-life of oxolinic acid is 6–7 h (Guyer, 1974).

Excretion

URINE: After a single 750 mg oral dose a\mean peak urinary concentration of $9 \cdot 1$ μg per ml (range $0 \cdot 4$–55) of the active drug is obtained 2–4 h later (Kershaw and Leigh, 1975). If this dose is repeated five times at 12-hourly intervals, a mean urinary concentration of $19 \cdot 7$ μg per ml (range $12 \cdot 5$–$35 \cdot 0$) occurs. A higher mean urinary concentration of 54 μg per ml (range 30–80) was recorded by Guyer (1974) with a dosage of 750 mg twice-daily. Only about one per cent of an administered dose is excreted in the urine in an active form over 8 h (Kershaw and Leigh, 1975).

FAECES: About 16 per cent of an oral dose is excreted in the faeces over a 48-h period (Guyer, 1974).

Distribution of the Drug in Body

There is no information available on tissue concentrations obtained with oxolinic acid. In view of the low serum levels obtained (*vide supra*), they are unlikely to be of any clinical value. Oxolinic acid is 80–85 per cent bound to serum proteins (Gordon *et al.*, 1976).

Mode of Action

Similar to nalidixic acid (page 735), oxolinic acid appears to exert its primary action on the synthesis of deoxyribonucleic acid (DNA) (Pianotti *et al.*, 1968).

Toxicity

Adverse reactions with oxolinic acid have been common and similar to those observed with nalidixic acid (page 735) (Atlas *et al.*, 1969; Guyer, 1974; Kershaw and Leigh, 1975; Guyer and Whitford, 1975; Pearson, 1975), but they are apparently milder in children (Shapera and Matsen, 1977).

Side-effects consist mainly of gastro-intestinal symptoms and CNS disturbances, particularly stimulation. These include nausea, vomiting, diarrhoea, pruritus, headache, insomnia, restlessness, dizziness, confusion, visual disturbances and paraesthesiae. The manufacturers advise against the use of oxolinic acid in pregnant patients, nursing mothers and infants. The drug should be used cautiously in patients with impaired renal function or in those with convulsive disorders. Similar to nalidixic acid, oxolinic acid may produce a false positive reaction for glucose in urine with Benedict's test and other tests based on copper sulphate, but not with 'Clinistix' or 'Testape'.

Clinical Uses of the Drug

Because of the low serum levels obtained after oral administration, oxolinic acid is only suitable for the treatment of urinary tract infections. Atlas *et al.* (1969) compared it to nalidixic acid for the treatment of patients with chronic bacteriuria. Although the emergence of resistant strains was less with oxolinic acid, the overall results with both drugs were similar. In another small trial, the results showed that oxolinic acid was superior to ampicillin (page 113) for the treatment of urinary tract infections (Guyer and Whitford, 1975). The drug has also been used in several other trials to treat urinary tract infections in adults (Guyer, 1974; Pearson, 1975) and children (Shapera and Matsen, 1975) with favourable results. However in these studies resistant strains emerged in 11–13 per cent of patients treated. Apart from the fact that oxolinic acid is administered only twice-daily, at present it does not seem to offer any advantages over nalidixic acid.

Seven young adult patients with typhoid fever due to chloramphenicol-resistant strains of Salm. typhi have been treated with oral oxolinic acid in a dose of 1·5 g twice-daily (approximately 75 mg per kg per day). Although blood cultures became negative in the majority in two to three days, all but one patient remained ill and febrile after four to nine days. This small study indicates that oxolinic acid is unsuitable for the treatment of typhoid fever (Sanford *et al.*, 1976).

REFERENCES

Atlas, E., Clark, H., Silverblatt, F. and Turck, M. (1969), 'Nalidixic acid and oxolinic acid in the treatment of chronic bacteriuria', *Ann. Intern. Med.*, **70**, 713.
Gordon, R. C., Stevens, L. I., Edmiston, C. E., Jr. and Mohan, K. (1976), 'Comparative *in vitro* studies of cinoxacin, nalidixic acid and oxolinic acid', *Antimicrob. Ag. Chemother.*, **10**, 918.
Guyer, B. M. (1974), 'Drug profile: Prodoxol (oxolinic acid)', *J. Int. Med. Res.*, **2**, 458.
Guyer, B. M. and Whitford, G. M. (1975), 'Oxolinic acid in urinary tract infections: A multi-centre trial', *Curr. Med. Res. Opin.*, **2**, 636.

Kaminsky, D. and Meltzer, R. I. (1968), 'Quinolone antibacterial agents, oxolinic acid and related compounds', *J. Med. Chem.,* **11,** 160.

Kershaw, N. J. and Leigh, D. A. (1975), 'The antibacterial and pharmacological activity of oxolinic acid (Prodoxol)', *J. Antimicrob. Chemother.,* **1,** 311.

Klein, D. and Matsen, J. M. (1976), '*In vitro* susceptibility comparison and recommendations for oxolinic acid', *Antimicrob. Ag. Chemother.,* **9,** 649.

Meers, P. D. (1974), 'Oxolinic acid in urinary infections', *Lancet,* **2,** 721.

Pearson, B. S. (1975), 'Urinary tract infection treated with oxolinic acid', *Med. J. Aust.* **1,** 140.

Pianotti, R. S., Mohan, R. R. and Schwartz, B. S. (1968), 'Biochemical effects of oxolinic acid on Proteus vulgaris', *J. Bact.,* **95,** 1622.

Ringel, S. M., Turner, F. J., Lindo, F. L., Roemer, S., Direnga, B. A., and Schwartz, B. S. (1968), 'Oxolinic acid, a new synthetic antimicrobial agent. II Bactericidal rate and resistance development', *Antimicrob. Ag. Chemother.* 1967, p. 480.

Sanford, J. P., Linh, N. N., Kutscher, E., Arnold, K. and Gould, K. (1976), 'Oxolinic acid in the treatment of typhoid fever due to chloramphenicol-resistant strains of Salmonella typhi, *Antimicrob. Ag. Chemother.,* **9,** 387.

Shapera, R. M. and Matsen, J. M., (1977), 'Oxolinic acid therapy for urinary tract infections in children', *Am. J. Dis. Child.,* **131,** 34.

Turner, F. J., Ringel, S. M., Martin, J. F., Storino, P. J., Daly, J. M. and Schwartz, B. S. (1968), 'Oxolinic acid, a new synthetic antimicrobial agent. 1. *In vitro* and *in vivo* activity', *Antimicrob. Ag. Chemother.—*1967, p. 475.

Westwood, G. P. C., and Hooper, W. L. (1975), 'Antagonism of oxolinic acid by nitrofurantoin', *Lancet,* **1,** 460.

Cinoxacin

Synthetized at Lilly Research Laboratories, cinoxacin has the chemical formula 1-ethyl-4 (1H) -oxo-(1,3) dioxolo (4,5-g) cinnoline-3-carboxylic acid (Wick *et al.*, 1973). This is another organic acid which is related chemically to nalidixic acid (page 730) and oxolinic acid (page 742). Its antibacterial spectrum is similar to that of nalidixic acid, but its activity against some bacterial species is somewhat greater (Wick *et al.*, 1973; Lumish and Norden, 1975; Kurtz and Turck, 1975; Giamarellou and Jackson, 1975; Jones and Fuchs, 1976; Mårdh *et al.*, 1977).

Cinoxacin is active against most of the Enterobacteriaceae which commonly cause urinary tract infection at concentrations which are easily attained in urine. It is most active against Esch. coli and all Proteus spp., but it is also active against most strains of Klebsiella, Enterobacter, Citrobacter and Serratia spp. Cinoxacin is also active against most Salmonella and Shigella spp. In comparative *in vitro* studies, cinoxacin (and nalidixic acid) are not as active as oxolinic acid against Shigella spp. (Gordon *et al.*, 1976). By comparison to ampicillin (page 100) and chloramphenicol (page 421), cinoxacin is more active *in vitro* against Salmonella spp. and Shigella sonnei, and its activity against Sh. flexneri and Sh. boydii is similar to chloramphenicol but greater than that of ampicillin (Rubinstein and Shainberg, 1977). Resistance to cinoxacin of organisms which are usually susceptible can be induced *in vitro* (Lumish and Norden, 1975; Giamarellou and Jackson, 1975). Cinoxacin has negligible activity against Pseudomonas aeruginosa and Gram-positive cocci including Staph. saphrophyticus (a micrococcus) (page 188).

After an oral dose of 250 mg, peak serum levels 2 h later are in the range of $<4-14\cdot8\,\mu$g per ml and urine concentrations at that time are in the range of $88-925\,\mu$g per ml. In the six-hour period after administration, 34 per cent of the dose is recoverable from the urine. Urinary concentrations appear to be decreased by impaired renal function (Panwalker *et al.*, 1976). When the drug is given orally in a dose of $0\cdot5$ g twice-daily, peak serum levels occur within 3 h and are in the range $2\cdot8-28\,\mu$g per ml (mean $16\cdot9\,\mu$g per ml). A mean peak urinary concentration of $766\,\mu$g per ml is attained and the mean excretion 12 h after a dose is 65 per cent (Colleen *et al.*, 1977). These authors also found that bladder and prostatic tissue concentrations of cinoxacin were 71 and 63 per cent of simultaneous serum levels respectively. Concentrations in renal tissue were in general higher than those in serum. If cinoxacin is given intravenously in a dose 250 mg per 70 kg body weight, over a period of 1 h, and then half this dose during a further 2 h, serum concentrations of about $10\,\mu$g per ml are maintained. Probenecid markedly inhibits cinoxacin excretion by the kidney (Rodriguez *et al.*, 1978). Wick *et al.* (1973) found that cinoxacin was 16 per cent protein bound but Gordon *et al.* (1976) reported a value of 77–83 per cent.

In a study using experimental pyelonephritis in rats, Holmes *et al.* (1974) showed that cinoxacin was more effective than either nalidixic acid or oxolinic acid, when all three were administered in the same dose. Panwalker *et al.* (1976) used the drug in an oral dose of 250 mg every 6 h for 10 days to treat 29 patients with urinary tract infections; a satisfactory cure rate was obtained and apart from one patient with renal insufficiency who developed severe nausea, vomiting and diarrhoea, no side-effects were observed. Other studies have confirmed cinoxacin's use in lower urinary tract infections (Elo *et al.*, 1978; Exaire, 1978). In comparative trials it has appeared slightly more effective and produced fewer side-effects than nalidixic acid (Wilson, 1978; Drylie, 1978) and it has been about as effective as co-trimoxazole (page 706) (Klastersky and Kahan-Coppens, 1978). The results of further clinical trials are needed before the role of this drug can be established.

REFERENCES

Colleen, S., Andersson, K.-E., and Màrdh, P.-A. (1977), 'Studies on cinoxacin 3. Concentrations of cinoxacin in serum, urine and tissues of urological patients', *J. Antimicrob. Chemother.*, **3**, 579.

Drylie, D. M. (1978), 'Comparison of cinoxacin and nalidixic acid in the treatment of urinary tract infections', In Siegenthaler, W. and Lüthy, R. (Ed.), *Current Chemotherapy: Proceedings of the 10th International Congress of Chemotherapy, Zurich/Switzerland, 1977.* American Society for Microbiology, Washington, D. C. p. 700.

Elo, J., Tallgren, L. G. and Sarna, S. (1978), 'Treatment of childhood urinary tract infection with cinoxacin', In Siegenthaler, W. and Lüthy, R. (Ed.), *Current Chemotherapy: Proceedings of the 10th International Congress of Chemotherapy, Zurich/Switzerland, 1977.* American Society for Microbiology, Washington, D. C. p. 693.

Exaire, E. (1978), 'Cinoxacin therapy of urinary tract infections'. In Siegenthaler, W. and Lüthy, R. (Ed.), *Current Chemotherapy: Proceedings of the 10th International Congress of Chemotherapy, Zurich/Switzerland, 1977.* American Society for Microbiology, Washington, D. C. p. 697.

Giamarellou, H. and Jackson, G. G. (1975), 'Antibacterial activity of cinoxacin *in vitro*', *Antimicrob. Ag. Chemother.*, **7**, 688.

Gordon, R. C., Stevens, L. I., Edmiston, C. E., Jr. and Mohan, K. (1976), 'Comparative *in vitro* studies of cinoxacin, nalidixic acid and oxolinic acid', *Antimicrob. Ag. Chemother.*, **10**, 918.

Holmes, D. H., Ensminger, P. W. and Gordee, R. S. (1974), 'Cinoxacin: Effectiveness against experimental pyelonephritis in rats', *Antimicrob. Ag. Chemother.*, **6**, 432.

Jones, R. N. and Fuchs, P. C. (1976), '*In vitro* antimicrobial activity of cinoxacin against 2968 clinical bacterial isolates', *Antimicrob. Ag. Chemother.*, **10**, 146.

Klastersky, J. and Kahan-Coppens, L. (1978), 'Comparative study of cinoxacin and co-trimoxazole in complicated urinary tract infections: A double-blind randomized study', In Siegenthaler, W. and Lüthy, R. (Ed.), *Current Chemotherapy: Proceedings of the 10th International Congress of Chemotherapy, Zurich/Switzerland, 1977.* American Society for Microbiology, Washington, D.C. p. 702.

748 THE USE OF ANTIBIOTICS

Kurtz, S. and Turck, M. (1975), '*In vitro* activity of cinoxacin, an organic acid antibacterial', *Antimicrob. Ag. Chemother.*, **7**, 370.

Lumish, R. M. and Norden, C. W. (1975), 'Cinoxacin: *In vitro* antibacterial studies of a new synthetic organic acid', *Antimicrob. Ag. Chemother.*, **7**, 159.

Mårdh, P.-A., Colleen, S. and Andersson, K.-E. (1977), 'Studies on cinoxacin. 1. *In vitro* activity of cinoxacin, as compared to nalidixic acid, against urinary tract pathogens', *J. Antimicrob. Chemother.*, **3**, 411.

Panwalker, A. P., Giamarellou, H. and Jackson, G. G. (1976), 'Efficiency of cinoxacin in urinary tract infections', *Antimicrob. Ag. Chemother.*, **9**, 502.

Rodriguez, N., Madsen, P. O. and Welling, P. G. (1978), 'Pharmacokinetics of cinoxacin after intravenous infusion: Influence of probenecid', In Siegenthaler, W. and Lüthy, R. (Ed), *Current Chemotherapy: Proceedings of the 10th International Congress of Chemotherapy,* Zurich/Switzerland, 1977. American Society for Microbiology, Washington, D.C., p. 692.

Rubinstein, E. and Shainberg, B. (1977), '*In vitro* activity of cinoxacin, ampicillin and chloramphenicol against shigella and nontyphoid salmonella', *Antimicrob. Ag. Chemother.*, **11**, 577.

Wick, W. E., Preston, D. A., White, W. A. and Gordee, R. S. (1973), 'Compound 64716, a new synthetic antibacterial agent', *Antimicrob. Ag. Chemother.*, **4**, 415.

Wilson, P. (1978), 'Comparative trial of cinoxacin and nalidixic acid in urinary tract infection', In Siegenthaler, W. and Lüthy, R. (Ed.), *Current Chemotherapy: Proceedings of the 10th International Congress of Chemotherapy,* Zurich/Switzerland, 1977. American Society for Microbiology, Washington, D.C. p. 699.

Nitrofurans: Nifuratel, Nitrofurazone, Furazolidone and Nitrofurantoin

Description

The nitroheterocyclic drugs consist of a primary nitro group joined to a heterocyclic ring. Three groups of these compounds are important in human therapeutics: the nitrothiazoles, the nitroimidazoles and the nitrofurans. The best known nitrothiazole is niridazole, which is used to treat bilharziasis; it is also useful for amoebiasis, dracontiasis and strongyloidiasis and is active against a variety of bacteria (Hamilton-Miller and Brumfitt, 1976). A number of nitroimidazole drugs are of clinical use and these include metronidazole (page 761), tinidazole (page 782) and nimorazole, ornidazole and carnidazole (page 789). Interest was first evoked in the nitrofurans as chemotherapeutic agents in the early 1940's, and since then thousands of nitrofuran compounds have been synthetized (Chamberlain, 1976). The most widely used nitrofurans at present are:

1. *Nifuratel ('Magmilor' in the United Kingdom)* has the same antibacterial spectrum as nitrofurantoin (*vide infra*), and it is also active against Candida spp. and Trichomonas vaginalis. It is more active *in vitro* than nitrofurantoin against Bacteroides and Fusobacterium spp. (Brumfitt *et al.*, 1975). Nifuratel is usually used as vaginal pessaries and tablets to treat vaginal trichomonal and candidal infections, but it has been used to treat urinary tract infections (Hamilton-Miller and Brumfitt, 1976). Nifuratel has also been used in an oral dose of 400 mg three times daily for a week, to treat candidal urinary tract infections (Grüneberg and Leakey, 1976).

2. *Nitrofurazone ('Furacin', Smith Kline and French)* is active *in vitro* against Staph. pyogenes, Strep. pyogenes, Esch. coli and the Clostridium, Salmonella and Shigella spp. It is less active against Proteus and Serratia spp. and virtually inactive against Pseudomonas aeruginosa (Chamberlain, 1976). Nitrofurazone is now mainly used for topical chemotherapy of wounds, burns, skin infections and for skin grafts. It has also been used as a bladder irrigant. A cream and an ointment containing 0·2 per cent nitrofurazone are available commercially. This drug is absorbed from the skin and 1·13 per cent of a daily dose applied to intact skin can be recovered in the urine (Chamberlain, 1976).

3. *Furazolidone ('Furoxone', Smith Kline and French)* is active *in vitro* against Staph. pyogenes, Strep. pyogenes, Strep. faecalis, Esch. coli, Vibrio cholerae and the Clostridium, Klebsiella, Enterobacter, Salmonella, Shigella and Bacteroides spp. It is also active against trichomonads and Giardia lamblia (Chamberlain, 1976). Furazolidone is recommended by the manufacturers for

749

the treatment of bacterial dysentery and giardiasis and is available commercially as 100 mg tablets and a suspension containing 25 mg per 5 ml. The dose used for adults is 100 mg given four times a day and appropriately lowered doses are recommended for children. It appears that very little, if any, furazolidone is absorbed after oral administration (Chamberlain, 1976). Side-effects include nausea, vomiting, headache, dizziness, drowsiness, drug fever, rashes and an 'antabuse' (disulfiram) like reaction to alcohol.

4. *Nitrofurantoin*. The sole use of this drug is for the treatment of urinary tract infections, because after oral or even intravenous administration, therapeutically active concentrations are attained only in urine. This urinary antiseptic has been available for clinical use in a crystalline form since 1953, and is marketed as 'Furadantin' (Smith Kline and French). A macrocrystalline form has been developed (Hailey and Glascock, 1977), which may produce fewer gastro-intestinal side-effects (page 753), and is marketed with the trade name of 'Furandantin MC'.

The following details only apply to nitrofurantoin.

Sensitive Organisms

1. Nitrofurantoin is active against most Gram-negative bacilli, which commonly cause urinary tract infections. Most strains of Esch. coli are sensitive but Enterobacter and Klebsiella spp. are less susceptible. Strains of Proteus spp. vary in their sensitivity but most are moderately resistant. Pseudomonas aeruginosa is usually resistant.

2. The drug is also active against those Gram-positive cocci which sometimes cause urinary tract infections, such as Strep. faecalis, Staph. pyogenes and Staph. epidermidis.

3. Nitrofurantoin has a broad spectrum of antibacterial activity. Gram-negative bacilli such as Salmonella, Shigella, Bacteroides and Neisseria spp. are often susceptible. Bacteroides fragilis is usually susceptible (Hamilton-Miller, 1975). Gram-positive bacteria such as Strep. pyogenes, Strep. pneumoniae and C. diphtheriae are also quite sensitive. However these organisms rarely, if ever, cause urinary tract infections and their susceptibility to nitrofurantoin is of little practical importance.

4. An important property of nitrofurantoin is that the usually sensitive microorganisms do not readily become resistant to the drug. Although resistance can be induced *in vitro*, there has been very little change in the resistance pattern of bacteria to nitrofurantoin over the years. Cross-resistance can occur between the nitrofurans but there is no cross-resistance between them and other chemotherapeutic agents. There is also no evidence that infectious transferable resistance (mediated by R plasmids, page 422) occurs with nitrofurantoin (Chamberlain, 1976).

In Vitro Sensitivities

Bacterial species with a minimum inhibitory concentration of 32 μg per ml or less can be regarded as highly sensitive to nitrofurantoin. Nitrofurantoin urine concentrations of at least 100 μg per ml can be easily attained with usual therapeutic doses. However if the causative enterobacteria are not sensitive to

32 μg per ml or less, the infection often persists or relapses shortly after cessation of treatment (Turck *et al.*, 1967). These authors found that 92 per cent of Esch. coli strains were highly sensitive to the drug, but only 32 per cent of other Gram-negative bacteria were in this category. The usual minimum inhibitory concentration of nitrofurantoin for Esch. coli is 16 μg per ml, while Kl. aerogenes is usually only inhibited by 100 μg per ml and Pr. mirabilis by 200 μg per ml. The minimum inhibitory concentrations of nitrofurantoin for the Gram-positive cocci are lower, being usually 4 μg per ml for Staph. pyogenes and 25 μg per ml for Strep. faecalis (Garrod *et al.*, 1973).

The activity of nitrofurantoin against all bacteria is increased in acid urine. Brumfitt and Percival (1967) demonstrated that the sensitivity of an Esch. coli strain decreased twenty-fold when the pH was changed from 5·0 to 8·0. Proteus mirabilis strains are less sensitive to nitrofurantoin than Esch. coli at any pH, and in addition Proteus spp. infections make the urine alkaline, further reducing the response of these infections to this drug.

Mode of Administration and Dosage

1. Nitrofurantoin is usually administered by mouth. The dosage is identical for both the crystalline and the macrocrystalline preparations; for adults it is 200–400 mg per day, given in four divided doses, and for children 5–7 mg per kg body weight per day, given in four divided doses.

Acute uncomplicated urinary tract infections due to Esch. coli usually respond well to the lower dose of 200 mg daily. For more severe, chronic or recurrent infections the higher dose of 400 mg daily is advisable, but this high dosage should not be continued for longer than two weeks.

For long-term suppressive therapy in adults a single daily dose of 50–100 mg (usually in the evening) is suitable. A long-term prophylactic dosage of 2–4 mg per kg body weight daily has been recommended for children with chronic infections (Marshall and Johnson, 1959). The lower dose of 2 mg per kg body weight per day is advisable if treatment is continued for longer than three months.

2. Nitrofurantoin can also be administered intravenously, but this is rarely used, and the parenteral preparation is not generally available. A limited study to define the clinical indications for intravenous nitrofurantoin was performed by Halliday and Jawetz (1962). The drug was administered intravenously in doses of up to 720 mg daily to ten patients with urinary tract infections. These authors concluded that intravenous nitrofurantoin is only indicated for the treatment of urinary tract infections in acutely ill patients, who are unable to take oral drugs because of nausea. Nowadays other parenteral drugs are used in this situation. Intravenous nitrofurantoin is unsuitable for the treatment of systemic infections of any kind.

Availability

(a) *Nitrofurantoin* ('*Furadantin*') tablets, each containing 50 mg or 100 mg.
(b) *Nitrofurantoin* ('*Furadantin*') *suspension,* containing 25 mg per 5 ml.
(c) *Nitrofurantoin macrocrystals* ('Furadantin MC') capsules, each containing 50 or 100 mg.

Serum Levels in Relation to Dosage

1. The crystalline and macrocrystalline nitrofurantoin preparations are both equally well absorbed from the gastro-intestinal tract, absorption occurring primarily in the small intestine. However the macrocrystalline form dissolves more slowly and is thus absorbed at a slower rate (Hailey and Glascock, 1967). Despite good absorption, therapeutically active serum levels are not obtained after the usual doses of oral nitrofurantoin (Richards *et al.*, 1955). Its serum half-life in humans with normal renal function is only about 20 min, the drug being both rapidly broken down in the tissues and rapidly excreted in urine (Reckendorf *et al.*, 1962). Nitrofurantoin also does not accumulate in the serum of patients with normal renal function if it is continuously administered in the recommended doses.

2. Intravenously administered nitrofurantoin sodium in doses of up to 720 mg per day in adults does not produce therapeutically effective serum levels.

3. Nitrofurantoin accumulates in the serum of patients with impaired renal function. Loughridge (1962) detected serum levels ranging from $5\cdot1$ to $6\cdot5$ μg per ml in one patient with uraemia (blood urea 300 mg per cent or 50 mmol/l), who was receiving 300 mg of oral nitrofurantoin daily. The elevated serum level of nitrofurantoin in this uraemic patient was associated with severe toxicity (*see* page 754). A mean serum level of only $1\cdot8$ μg per ml was demonstrated in twelve similarly treated patients with normal renal function.

4. Newborn and premature infants may also develop toxic serum levels and nitrofurantoin is contraindicated in this age group.

Excretion

URINE: Nitrofurantoin is rapidly excreted in urine, where about one-third of an orally or parenterally administered dose appears in a therapeutically active form (Reckendorf *et al.*, 1962). With the usual doses, urine levels vary from 50–250 μg per ml, provided renal function is normal. There is no difference between the excretion patterns of the crystalline and the macrocrystalline forms except that with the macrocrystalline form there is a slower rise of urinary concentrations (Hailey and Glascock, 1967).

Woodruff *et al.* (1961) studied urinary mechanisms of nitrofurantoin excretion in dogs. The drug is excreted by glomerular filtration, but a small part is also both secreted and reabsorbed by the tubules. Tubular reabsorption is enhanced by acid urine, and depressed by alkalinization of urine, the latter yielding higher active nitrofurantoin urine concentrations. Urine acidification therefore increases renal tissue levels of the drug, which may be advantageous when treating pyelonephritis. On the other hand, although alkalinization of the urine increases urine nitrofurantoin concentrations, this is of doubtful value for the treatment of lower urinary tract infections such as cystitis, as the antibacterial effect of the drug is reduced in alkaline urine (Brumfitt and Percival, 1967).

Uraemic patients excrete very little nitrofurantoin in the urine, where the levels attained are invariably therapeutically inadequate (Sachs *et al.*, 1968).

BILE: Animal studies show that nitrofurantoin is also eliminated via the bile, and biliary concentrations about 200 times higher than those in the serum have been detected. It was also noted that nitrofurantoin administration resulted in an increased rate of bile flow (Annotation, 1971).

INACTIVATION IN BODY: In patients with normal renal function a considerable proportion of a dose of nitrofurantoin is inactivated in the body. For this reason, even in patients with renal failure there is only a relatively minor rise in serum levels of the active drug, but these serum levels may cause severe toxicity (Kunin, 1968). Inactivation of nitrofurantoin apparently takes place in all body tissues, but the liver may play a major role. It is not known whether this drug accumulates in patients with liver disease.

Distribution of the Drug in Body

Therapeutically active concentrations of nitrofurantoin are not attained in most body tissues. Tissue levels in the renal medulla are usually about the same as those in the urine (Stamey *et al.*, 1965).

Mode of Action

The precise mode of action of nitrofurantoin is not known. The nitrofurans inhibit a number of bacterial enzymes (Chamberlain, 1976) and they may also damage DNA (McCalla, 1977). Inhibition of carbohydrate metabolism in human nervous tissues may be the mechanism responsible for nitrofurantoin neurotoxicity (Loughridge, 1962).

Toxicity

1. *Nausea and vomiting.* These are frequent complications and are dose related (Koch-Weser *et al.*, 1971). They can often be controlled by reducing the dose, but concomitant administration of food or milk is less effective. Nausea and vomiting may sometimes be severe enough to necessitate cessation of treatment, and they occur more commonly in women (Koch-Weser *et al.*, 1971). By comparison, diarrhoea is a rare side-effect. Nitrofurantoin induced nausea may result from the action of rapidly absorbed drug on the central nervous system, rather than from gastro-intestinal irritation. Intravenously administered nitrofurantoin also causes this effect (Halliday and Jawetz, 1962).

Some authors have shown that the newer macrocrystalline form, which is more slowly absorbed, evokes nausea and vomiting less frequently than crystalline nitrofurantoin in patients with a known history of nitrofurantoin intolerance (Hailey and Glascock, 1967). This was also demonstrated by Kalowski *et al.* (1974) in a double blind study of patients whose past experience with nitrofurantoin was not known. It is possible that these symptoms are related to the rate of absorption of the drug, and thus the more slowly absorbed macrocrystalline form may be less prone to cause nausea and vomiting. Despite its slower rate of absorption macrocrystalline nitrofurantoin appears to be therapeutically equally effective to the older crystalline drug (Hailey and Glascock, 1967; Kalowski *et al.*, 1974). Alternatively other authors have found that the administration of the macrocrystalline form does not prevent nausea, and consider that these symptoms are related more closely to the average serum level rather than to the rate of absorption of the drug

(Koch-Weser *et al.*, 1971).

2. *Hypersensitivity reactions*. Compared to gastro-intestinal side-effects these are relatively infrequent, and in one large series they were observed in 4·1 per cent of treated patients (Koch-Weser *et al.*, 1971). Common manifestations included skin rashes, eosinophilia and drug fever, which usually subsided rapidly when the drug was stopped. Asthma due to sensitization to the drug has been observed and anaphylaxis has been reported as a rare complication.

3. *Peripheral neuritis*. This is one of the most serious side-effects of nitrofurantoin therapy, and it usually occurs in patients with renal failure who develop toxic serum levels of the drug (Ellis, 1962; Loughridge, 1962). Six cases of nitrofurantoin neuropathy were reported by Ellis (1962). Three patients, in whom the drug was continued, died as a result of progressive polyneuritis, but the other three, in whom therapy was stopped soon after the onset of symptoms, made a slow partial recovery. Symptoms of nitrofurantoin peripheral neuritis usually begin within 45 days of starting treatment, and the clinical course is one of ascending motor and sensory polyneuropathy (Toole and Parrish, 1973). The degree of recovery is usually inversely related to the severity of the neuritis. This complication has also been reported in patients with normal blood urea levels, but who have had marginal renal functional impairment as evidenced by low creatinine clearance values (Craven, 1971). Neuritis may also develop in patients with normal renal function, especially in the elderly, if prolonged courses of nitrofurantoin are used. Changes in nerve conduction have been detected without clinical features of neuritis, after a two weeks' course of 400 mg nitrofurantoin daily in healthy volunteers (Toole *et al.*, 1968). Patients receiving nitrofurantoin should be warned to report early signs of neuritis such as paraesthesiae, and in this event the drug should be stopped.

4. *Pulmonary reactions*. Nitrofurantoin therapy has been associated with three types of pulmonary reaction:

(a) *Acute pneumonitis*. This is more common in elderly patients, and is characterized by a sudden onset of cough, fever and dyspnoea, and may simulate acute respiratory infection or pulmonary oedema (Dawson, 1966; Hailey *et al.*, 1969; Leading article, 1969; Simonson *et al.*, 1977). Pulmonary infiltrations may be present on radiological examination of the lungs. Symptoms may become evident within hours or days after starting nitrofurantoin therapy, but in some cases these have only occurred after a prolonged period of treatment. This pneumonitis is probably allergic in nature, and is often accompanied by eosinophilia. Clinical recovery rapidly ensues when the drug is discontinued. However corticosteroid treatment is beneficial and may be necessary in severe cases (Morgan, 1970). An accelerated and more severe pulmonary reaction typically occurs if the patient is rechallenged with the drug (Murray and Kronenberg, 1965; Murphy, 1966).

(b) *Subacute pneumonitis*. A more subacute reaction has been described in a patient, who presented with pulmonary symptoms of one month's duration having taken nitrofurantoin for one year (Sollaccio *et al.*, 1966). This patient recovered rapidly, when the drug was discontinued and prednisolone was administered.

(c) *Chronic pulmonary reactions*. Five patients described by Rosenow

(1968) and another patient reported by Israel *et al.* (1973), all gradually developed a diffuse interstitial pneumonitis with fibrosis in association with long-term nitrofurantoin therapy. These changes were only partially reversible when the drug was discontinued and corticosteroids were given. In two patients reported by Bäck *et al.* (1974), long-term nitrofurantoin administration was associated not only with pulmonary fibrosis, but also liver damage and the presence of autoimmune antibodies in the serum. Bone *et al.* (1976) described another two patients who developed diffuse interstitial lung disease after long-term nitrofurantoin therapy, and who on open lung biopsy had pathological changes typical of desquamative interstitial pneumonia. Both of these patients improved considerably with corticosteroid treatment. It seems that in these cases a causal relationship with nitrofurantoin exists, but this is difficult to prove (Harrow, 1969; Notes on Current Drugs, 1970).

5. *Hepatotoxicity.* It appears that both hepatocellular damage or cholestatic jaundice can on rare occasions be caused by nitrofurantoin administration. Ernaelsteen and Williams (1961) reported a patient, who developed prodromal fever, rash and eosinophilia, followed by an intrahepatic obstructive jaundice (confirmed by liver biopsy) similar to chlorpromazine jaundice, in association with nitrofurantoin therapy. Subsequently Murphy and Innis (1968) reported a sixty-five-year-old patient, who suddenly developed a severe toxic hepatitis with jaundice and haemorrhagic manifestations after treatment with nitrofurantoin for one month. This patient recovered but was very ill for one week, during which time an exchange transfusion was necessary to control bleeding. Another patient with mild toxic hepatitis, apparently caused by nitrofurantoin, has been reported by Bhagwat and Warren (1969). These authors surveyed all published reports on nitrofurantoin toxicity during the previous decade, and found only six cases of liver damage which were presumably caused by the drug.

Temporal circumstances in a small number of patients suggest that nitrofurantoin, particularly after prolonged administration, may cause chronic active hepatitis (Lindberg *et al.*, 1975; Strömberg and Wengle, 1976). In the two patients described by Strömberg and Wengle (1976), clinical and biochemical recovery occurred on withdrawal of nitrofurantoin, without treatment with immunosuppressive drugs.

6. *Haematological side-effects.* Three types of blood disorder have been reported in association with nitrofurantoin therapy:

   (a) *Haemolytic anaemia.* Nitrofurantoin is one of many drugs which can precipitate acute haemolysis in patients with glucose-6-phosphate dehydrogenase deficient red blood cells. The drug therefore should be used with caution in patients of Mediterranean origin, and it should be avoided in infants under one month of age, whose red cell enzyme systems are immature. Nitrofurantoin apparently can also precipitate a haemolytic anaemia in patients with erythrocytes deficient in other glycolytic enzymes. Stefanini (1972) described a patient with red blood cells deficient in the enzyme enolase and whose chronic haemolytic anaemia was exacerbated by nitrofurantoin.

   (b) *Megaloblastic anaemia.* Nitrofurantoin is chemically related to phenytoin, and similarly may cause, albeit rarely, a megaloblastic anaemia due to folic acid deficiency, particularly when repeated courses are used (Bass, 1963).

(c) *Bone marrow depression.* This complication has been observed in association with nitrofurantoin therapy, but a definite causal relationship has not been established (Notes on Current Drugs, 1966).

7. *Miscellaneous side-effects.* Permanent yellow discolouration of primary dentition, ascribed to nitrofurantoin, was observed in one 17-month-old infant (Ball and Ferguson, 1962). This child received the drug for a total of 68 days, and only those teeth which erupted during the period of nitrofurantoin administration were discoloured. It was postulated that the discolouration resulted from repeated direct contact between the drug and the erupting teeth, and that possibly the yellow nitrofurantoin can be taken up by early carious lesions in the enamel. However there have been very few additional reports of teeth discolouration reported to the manufacturers, so that if this effect is due to nitrofurantoin, it must be extremely rare.

Macdonald and Macdonald (1976) reported nitrofurantoin crystalluria in three patients. These patients were all elderly, had urinary catheters and were receiving long-term prophylaxis with nitrofurantoin against urinary infections. Their renal function and urinary output was normal and they were receiving the low recommended dosage. Crystalluria therefore seems to be a rare side-effect of the drug.

Benign intracranial hypertension has been described in a 10-month-old child following nitrofurantoin therapy, suggesting a possible causal relationship (Sharma and James, 1974).

Although the nitrofurans, including nitrofurantoin are mutagenic toward mammalian cells by damaging DNA (McCalla, 1977), there is no evidence that they are carcinogenic in humans. Nevertheless similar to metronidazole (page 769, it may be wise to use these drugs cautiously in pregnant patients.

8. *Drug interactions.* An 'antabuse' (disulfiram) reaction to alcohol may be produced by nitrofurans and nitroimidazoles (*see* page 769) by inhibiting the metabolism of acetaldehyde (Birkett and Pond, 1975). Nitrofurantoin can also interfere with the laboratory determinations of serum bilirubin, urine creatinine, blood urea and urine glucose.

Clinical Uses of the Drug

1. Nitrofurantoin is only suitable for treatment of urinary tract infections, particularly those caused by Esch. coli (Richards *et al.*, 1955; Turck *et al.*, 1967). It is useful for both acute uncomplicated infections and chronic bacteriuria and in the latter it has also been used for long-term suppressive therapy (Annotation, 1969). The use of nitrofurantoin for suppressive therapy has the advantages that it does not induce resistant strains in the urinary or intestinal tracts, and it is not implicated in transferable drug resistance (page 421). It may not be as efficient for this purpose as co-trimoxazole (page 706), because the latter also reduces colonization of the vaginal vestibule by pathogens responsible for recurrent urinary infections (Stamey *et al.*, 1977) *see also* page 706). The dose of nitrofurantoin for suppressive therapy is 50–100 mg once each evening, and this has been highly successful in reducing recurrences of infection and is almost free from side-effects (Bailey *et al.*,

1971). The drug can be used for urinary tract infections during pregnancy, because it has been widely used for over 25 years without being implicated as a cause of congenital abnormalities. Nevertheless the long-term use of nitrofurantoin in pregnancy may be unwise (*see* page 756). It is also suitable for these infections in children (Marshall and Johnson, 1959; Normand and Smellie, 1965). Nitrofurantoin macrocrystals in a dose of 1·2–2·4 mg per kg per day is a safe effective drug for the prevention of recurrent bacteriuria in girls (Lohr *et al.*, 1977). This drug is not recommended for premature babies and infants under one month of age (*see* page 752).

2. The drug is effective for the treatment of all infections localized to the urinary tract such as urethritis, prostatitis, cystitis and pyelonephritis. Although therapeutically active serum levels are not obtained, it is usually effective for renal infections, because renal medullary and urinary concentrations are almost identical (Stamey *et al.*, 1965). This use of nitrofurantoin in upper urinary tract infections has been questioned (Leading article, 1976, Naumann, 1978). If renal infection is associated with systemic signs of infection suggesting possible Gram-negative septicaemia, drugs such as the aminoglycosides, which produce therapeutic serum levels, are indicated. Nitrofurantoin also may not be effective in patients with upper urinary tract infections and in whom one kidney has poor function. In such cases, even though overall renal functions may be normal, effective concentrations of nitrofurantoin may not be reached in the urine of kidneys with a unilateral creatinine clearance of less than 20 ml per min. On these grounds, it has been recommended that nitrofurantoin should be restricted to the treatment of lower urinary tract infections in patients with normal renal function (Leading article, 1976). Nitrofurantoin is unsuitable for the treatment of systemic infections such as Esch. coli septicaemia.

3. It can also be used to treat urinary tract infections caused by Gram-positive cocci such as Strep. faecalis, Staph. pyogenes and Staph. epidermidis (albus). Other drugs which produce therapeutic serum levels, are usually preferred for these infections, particularly for those due to Staph. pyogenes, the presence of which in the urine often reflects disseminated infection.

4. Nitrofurantoin has been recommended for prophylactic purposes during urinary tract instrumentation and prostatectomy. This would be ineffective if Ps. aeruginosa or strains of Proteus or Klebsiella spp. resistant to nitrofurantoin, are introduced.

5. Nitrofurantoin is contraindicated in all patients with any degree of renal functional impairment (Sachs *et al.*, 1968), because in this situation therapeutic concentrations are not attained in urine, and toxic serum levels may occur (*see* Excretion, page 752 and Toxicity, page 754)

REFERENCES

Annotation (1969), 'Continuous chemotherapy in the prevention of recurrent bacteriuria', *Lancet,* **1,** 248.

Annotation (1971), 'Nitrofurantoin', *Lancet,* **2,** 1129.

Bäck, O., Lundgren, R. and Wiman, L.-G. (1974), 'Nitrofurantoin-induced pulmonary fibrosis and lupus syndrome', *Lancet,* **1,** 930.

Bailey, R. R., Roberts, A. P., Gower, P. E. and De Wardener, H. E. (1971), 'Prevention of urinary-tract infection with low-dose nitrofurantoin', *Lancet*, **2**, 1112.

Ball, J. S. and Ferguson, A. W. (1962), 'Permanent discoloration of primary dentition by nitrofurantoin', *Brit. med. J.*, **2**, 1103.

Bass, B. H. (1963), 'Megaloblastic anaemia due to nitrofurantoin', *Lancet*, **1**, 530.

Bhagwat, A. G. and Warren, R. E. (1969), 'Hepatic reaction to nitrofurantoin', *Lancet*, **2**, 1369.

Birkett, D. J. and Pond, S. M. (1975), 'Metabolic drug interactions—a critical review', *Med. J. Aust.*, **1**, 687.

Bone, R. C., Wolfe, J., Sobonya, R. E., Kerby, G. R., Strechschulte, D., Ruth, W. E. and Welch, M. (1976), 'Desquamative interstitial pneumonia following long-term nitrofurantoin therapy', *Amer. J. Med.*, **60**, 697.

Brumfitt, W. and Percival, A. (1967), 'Laboratory control of antibiotic therapy in urinary tract infection', *Ann. N.Y. Acad. Sci.*, **145**, 329.

Brumfitt, W., Reynolds, A. V. and Hamilton-Miller, J. M. T. (1975), 'Activity of nitrofurantoin and nifuratel against anaerobic Gram-negative bacilli', *Lancet*, **1**, 460.

Chamberlain, R. E. (1976), 'Chemotherapeutic properties of prominent nitrofurans', *J. Antimicrob. Chemother.*, **2**, 325.

Craven, R. S. (1971), 'Furadantin neuropathy', *Aust. N.Z. J. Med.*, **1**, 246.

Dawson, R. B. (1966), 'Pulmonary reactions to nitrofurantoin', *New Engl. J. Med.*, **274**, 522.

Ellis, F. G. (1962), 'Acute polyneuritis after nitrofurantoin therapy', *Lancet*, **2**, 1136.

Ernaelsteen, D. and Williams, R. (1961), 'Jaundice due to nitrofurantoin', *Gastroenterology*, **41**, 590.

Garrod, L. P., Lambert, H. P. and O'Grady, F. (1973), *Antibiotic and Chemotherapy*, 4th edn., Churchill Livingstone, Edinburgh and London, p. 405.

Grüneberg, R. N. and Leakey, A. (1976), 'Treatment of candidal urinary tract infections with nifuratel', *Brit. med. J.*, **2**, 908.

Hailey, F. J. and Glascock, H. W., Jr. (1967), 'Gastrointestinal tolerance to a new macrocrystalline form of nitrofurantoin: A collaborative study', *Curr. Ther. Res.*, **9**, 600.

Hailey, F. J., Glascock, H. W., Jr. and Hewitt, W. F. (1969), 'Pleuropneumonic reactions to nitrofurantoin', *New Engl. J. Med.*, **281**, 1087.

Halliday, A. and Jawetz, E. (1962), 'Sodium nitrofurantoin administered intravenously: A limited study to define its clinical indication', *New Engl. J. Med.*, **266**, 427.

Hamilton-Miller, J. M. T. (1975), 'Antimicrobial agents acting against anaerobes', *J. Antimicrob. Chemother.*, **1**, 273.

Hamilton-Miller, J. M. T. and Brumfitt, W. (1976), 'Leading article. The versatility of nitro compounds', *J. Antimicrob. Chemother.*, **2**, 5.

Harrow, B. R. (1969), 'Pulmonary reaction to nitrofurantoin', *New Engl. J. Med.*, **280**, 389.

Israel, K. S., Brashear, R. E., Sharma, H. M., Yum, M. N. and Glover, J. L. (1973), 'Pulmonary fibrosis and nitrofurantoin', *Amer. Rev. Resp. Dis.*, **108**, 353.

Kalowski, S., Radford, N. and Kincaid-Smith, P. (1974), 'Crystalline and macrocrystalline nitrofurantoin in the treatment of urinary-tract infection', *New Engl. J. Med.*, **290**, 385.

Koch-Weser, J., Sidel, V. W., Dexter, M., Parish, C., Finer, D. C. and Kanarek, P. (1971), 'Adverse reactions to sulfisoxazole, sulfamethoxazole, and nitrofurantoin', *Arch. Intern. Med.*, **128**, 399.

Kunin, C. M. (1968), 'More on antimicrobials in renal failure', *Ann. Intern. Med.*, **69**, 397.

Leading Article (1969), 'Pulmonary sensitivity to nitrofurantoin', *Brit. med. J.*, **4**, 704.

Leading Article (1976), 'Antibiotic treatment in kidneys of unequal function', *Brit.*

med. J., **1,** 4.

Lindberg, J., Lindholm, A., Lundin, P. and Iwarson, S. (1975), 'Trigger factors and HL—A antigens in chronic active hepatitis', *Brit. med. J.,* **4,** 77.

Lohr, J. A., Nunley, D. H., Howards, S. S. and Ford, R. F. (1977), 'Prevention of recurrent urinary tract infections in girls', *Pediatrics,* **59,** 562.

Loughridge, L. (1962), 'Peripheral neuropathy due to nitrofurantoin', *Lancet,* **2,** 1133.

Macdonald, J. B. and Macdonald, E. T. (1976), 'Nitrofurantoin crystalluria', *Brit. med. J.,* **2,** 1044.

Marshall, M. and Johnson, S. H. (1959), 'Use of nitrofurantoin in chronic and recurrent urinary tract infections in children', *JAMA,* **169,** 919.

McCalla, D. R. (1977), 'Biological effects of nitrofurans', *J. Antimicrob. Chemother.,* **3,** 517.

Morgan, L. K. (1970), 'Nitrofurantoin pulmonary hypersensitivity', *Med. J. Aust.,* **2,** 136.

Murphy, K. J. (1966), 'Pulmonary reaction to nitrofurantoin ('furadantin')", *Med. J. Aust.,* **2,** 607.

Murphy, K. J. and Innis, M. D. (1968), 'Hepatic disorder and severe bleeding diathesis following nitrofurantoin ingestion', *JAMA,* **204,** 396.

Murray, M. J. and Kronenberg, R. (1965), 'Pulmonary reactions simulating cardiac pulmonary edema caused by nitrofurantoin', *New Engl. J. Med.,* **273,** 1185.

Naumann, P. (1978), 'The value of antibiotic levels in tissue and in urine in the treatment of urinary tract infections', *J. Antimicrob. Chemother.,* **4,** 9.

Normand, I. C. S. and Smellie, J. M. (1965), 'Prolonged maintenance chemotherapy in the management of urinary infection in childhood', *Brit. med. J.,* **1,** 1023.

Notes on Current Drugs (1966), 'Nitrofurantoin', *Med. J. Aust.,* **1,** 1042.

Notes on Current Drugs (1970), 'A report from the Australian drug-evaluation committee: Pulmonary reactions to nitrofurantoin', *Med. J. Aust.,* **1,** 822.

Reckendorf, H. K., Castringius, R. G. and Spingler, H. K. (1962), 'Comparative pharmacodynamics, urinary excretion and half-life determinations of nitrofurantoin sodium', *Antimicrob. Ag. Chemother.,* p. 531.

Richards, W. A., Riss, E., Kass, E. H. and Finland, M. (1955), 'Nitrofurantoin: Clinical and laboratory studies in urinary tract infections', *Arch. Intern. Med.,* **96,** 437.

Rosenow, E. C., De Remee, R. A. and Dines, D. E. (1968), 'Chronic nitrofurantoin pulmonary reaction. Report of five cases', *New Engl. J. Med.,* **279,** 1258.

Sachs, J., Geer, T., Noell, P. and Kunin, C. M. (1968), 'Effect of renal function on urinary recovery of orally administered nitrofurantoin', *New Engl. J. Med.,* **278,** 1032.

Sharma, D. B. and James, A. (1974), 'Benign intracranial hypertension associated with nitrofurantoin therapy', *Brit. med. J.,* **4,** 771.

Simonson, W., Stennett, D. J. and Hall, C. A. (1977), 'Nitrofurantoin pneumonitis', *Drug. Intel. Clin. Pharm.,* **2,** 654.

Sollaccio, P. A., Ribaudo, C. A. and Grace, W. J. (1966), 'Subacute pulmonary infiltration due to nitrofurantoin', *Ann. Intern. Med.,* **65,** 1284.

Stamey, T. A., Govan, D. E. and Palmer, J. M. (1965), 'The localisation and treatment of urinary tract infections: The role of bactericidal urine levels as opposed to serum levels', *Medicine,* **44,** 1.

Stamey, T. A., Condy, M. and Mihara, G. (1977), 'Prophylactic efficiency of nitrofurantoin macrocrystals and trimethoprim-sulfamethoxazole in urinary infections. Biologic effects on the vaginal and rectal flora', *New Engl. J. Med.,* **296,** 780.

Stefanini, M. (1972), 'Chronic hemolytic anemia association with erythrocyte enolase deficiency exacerbated by ingestion of nitrofurantoin', *Amer. J. Clin. Path.,* **58,** 408.

Strömberg, A. and Wengle, B. (1976), 'Chronic active hepatitis induced by nitrofurantoin', *Brit. med. J.,* **2,** 174.

Toole, J. F., Gergen, J. A., Hayes, D. M. and Felts, J. H. (1968), 'Neural effects of nitrofurantoin', *Arch. Neurol.,* **18,** 680.

Toole, J. F. and Parrish, M. L. (1973), 'Nitrofurantoin polyneuropathy', *Neurology,* **23,** 554.

Turck, M., Ronald, A. R. and Petersdorf, R. G. (1967), 'Susceptibility of Enterobacteriaceae to nitrofurantoin correlated with eradication of bacteriuria', *Antimicrob. Ag. Chemother.*—1966, p. 446.

Woodruff, M. W., Malvin, R. L. and Thompson, I. M. (1961), 'The renal transport of nitrofurantoin. Effect of acid-base balance upon its excretion', *JAMA,* **175,** 1132.

Metronidazole

Description

Metronidazole is a nitroimidazole drug (page 749) similar to tinidazole (page 782), and nimorazole, ornidazole and carnidazole (page 782), and has the chemical formula of 1-(2-hydroxyethyl)-2-methyl-5-nitroimidazole. Following the discovery that azomycin, a nitroimidazole drug isolated from a Streptomyces species, was weakly active against Trichomonas vaginalis, many similar drugs were synthetized at Rhône-Poulenc Research Laboratories in France. One of these, metronidazole, was very active against experimental T. vaginalis infections (Cosar and Julou, 1959), and was soon shown to be useful for the systemic treatment of urogenital trichomoniasis in humans (Durel *et al.*, 1959). Animal studies suggesting that it may also be useful in amoebiasis (Cosar *et al.*, 1961) were subsequently confirmed in human infections (Powell *et al.*, 1966). In addition it was demonstrated to be effective in human Giardia lamblia infections (Fowler, 1960; Schneider, 1961).

The observation that metronidazole relieved acute ulcerative gingivitis in a patient being treated for trichomonal vaginitis, led to studies culminating in its use in anaerobic bacterial infections (Shinn, 1962). Subsequently it was confirmed that the drug was useful for the treatment of Vincent's stomatitis and that it inhibited Bacteroides necrophorus (Davies *et al.*, 1964). Based on experimental infections in mice, Freeman *et al.* (1968) suggested that metronidazole may be useful for the prevention of tetanus and gas gangrene. Finally Tally *et al.* (1972) showed that metronidazole was useful for the treatment of infections due to Bacteroides spp., and since then it has been used for a variety of anaerobic infections.

Metronidazole is marketed under the trade name of 'Flagyl' (May and Baker).

Sensitive Organisms

1. *Protozoa*. Metronidazole is active against the anaerobic protozoa Trichomonas vaginalis, Entamoeba histolytica, Giardia lamblia and Balantidium coli.

2. *Bacteria*. Only those bacteria with primarily anaerobic metabolism (obligate anaerobes) are susceptible to metronidazole. Various genera of these anaerobic bacteria are normally found in the oral cavity and the intestinal and female genital tracts; these have been increasingly implicated as pathogens in a variety of human infections. Metronidazole has no significant antibacterial activity against aerobes or facultative anaerobes, nor does it interfere with the ac-

tion of common antibacterial agents used against such organisms (Salem *et al.*, 1975).

Among Gram-negative organisms the Fusobacterium and Bacteroides species are the most sensitive of the anaerobes, the majority of their strains usually being susceptible to metronidazole (Chow *et al.*, 1975; Sutter and Finegold, 1976). In particular B. fragilis and B. melaninogenicus are nearly always sensitive. The Veillonella spp. are frequently sensitive. The 'microaerophilic anaerobe' Campylobacter fetus is also sensitive to metronidazole (Chow *et al.*, 1978). Of the Gram-positive organisms the Clostridium spp. are most sensitive, and Cl. perfringens is nearly always sensitive. The Peptococcus, Peptostreptococcus, Acidaminococcus and Eubacterium spp. are frequently sensitive, but the Propionibacterium, Bifidobacterium, Lactobacillus, Actinomyces and Arachnia spp., and anaerobic streptococci are less commonly sensitive. Metronidazole also has activity against Treponema pallidum (both Reiter and Nichol strains) and the oral spirochaetes.

Nalidixic acid potentiates the action of metronidazole against B. fragilis. Subinhibitory concentrations of spiramycin, clindamycin, rifampicin and tetracycline also reduce the MIC of metronidazole for this organism, but to a lesser extent (Salem *et al.*, 1975).

3. *Acquired resistance*. Until recently this was virtually unknown (Ingham *et al.*, 1975a). Ingham *et al.* (1978) isolated a metronidazole-resistant strain of B. fragilis from a patient's faecal fistula, at a time when infection relapsed during long-term prophylactic treatment with metronidazole. Thurner and Meingassner (1978) have reported a metronidazole-resistant strain of T. vaginalis.

In Vitro Sensitivities

The majority of Bacteroides spp. strains are inhibited *in vitro* by a concentration of 4–8 μg per ml of metronidazole (Sutter and Finegold, 1976). The values for Fusobacterium and Clostridium spp. are both <4·0 μg per ml. These concentrations can easily be attained in serum (page 764).

Mode of Administration and Dosage

1. *Oral administration*. Metronidazole is usually administered by this route, and the drug should be taken during or after a meal. The dosage schedule varies according to the infection treated (*see* clinical uses, page 769). For adults, doses range from 2·4 g as a single dose to 200–800 mg three times a day. A proportionately lower dose is used for children so that, for example, in the age group 1–3 years, one quarter of the adult dose is recommended. A dose of 400 mg three times daily for adults, or for children 7 mg per kg body weight three times daily, is recommended for the treatment of anaerobic infections. For prophylaxis against post-operative anaerobic infections in gynaecological patients, an adult dose of 2 g has been given on admission to hospital; this is followed by 200 mg three times a day as long as feasible pre-operatively, and it

is recommenced as soon as possible post-operatively and continued for another seven days.

2. *Rectal administration.* The use of rectal suppositories for adults and children is recommended whenever oral medication is inappropriate. For treatment, a 1 g suppository (0·5 g for children) should be administered three times daily. Giamarellou *et al.* (1977) used a loading dose of two suppositories (1 g) followed by one suppository every 8 h.

3. *Intravenous administration.* Metronidazole solution (0·5 g in 100 ml) has been given intravenously in a dose of 0·5 g eight-hourly, to adults. Each 100 ml of the solution should be administered over a period of 20 min (5·0 ml per min). Intravenous metronidazole can be used when the oral or rectal routes are not feasible.

In one adult patient intravenous metronidazole was given in a loading dose of 1·0 g and this was followed by a dose of 0·5 g eight-hourly until a total of 28·5 g had been administered (Chowcat and Wyllie, 1976). Eykyn and Phillips (1976) gave metronidazole intravenously to 40 patients, and in 22 this treatment was followed by oral therapy. In adults a dose of 0·5 g was infused every 8 h over a period of about 20 min. Two children received an intravenous dose of 250 mg every 8 h. The total intravenous dose given to these patients varied from 1·5 g to 29 g, and in half the total dose was 3·0–8·0 g. The drug was well tolerated by all patients and thrombophlebitis or other side-effects were not observed.

4. *Patients with renal failure.* The main route of clearance of metronidazole and its metabolites is via the kidney (page 765). Studies on three patients with renal impairment and one anephric patient showed that after a single oral dose of 0·5 g metronidazole, the peak serum level and rate of elimination of the drug was not significantly different from normal subjects (McHenry, 1977). However in another patient with renal failure, who was treated with an oral dose of 600 mg eight-hourly, there was accumulation of both metronidazole and particularly its inactive metabolites (page 764). When this patient was undergoing haemodialysis on alternate days, satisfactory serum levels were maintained by an oral dose of 600 mg twice-daily (Ingham *et al.*, 1975b). An intravenous dose of 0·5 g every 8 h was given to one patient recovering from acute renal failure and two others receiving haemodialysis; serum concentrations just before the infusion were 7·2, 13·0 and 19 μg per ml and peak levels, 30 min after completion of an infusion, were 13·0, 27·0 and 28·0 μg per ml respectively. These values fell within the ranges found when patients with normal renal function were treated in this way (Eykyn and Phillips, 1976) (*see also* page 764).

5. *Use in pregnancy.* According to the manufacturers metronidazole can be given at any stage of pregnancy and during lactation if it is indicated, but that in these circumstances short high dosage regimens (page 769) are not recommended. There is no evidence that the drug is teratogenic in experimental animals or in humans (Shepard and Fantel, 1977). However because metronidazole is mutagenic in certain bacterial test systems and it induces chromosome changes in human lymphocytes (page 768), its use during pregnancy should be carefully assessed. Furthermore the view has been expressed that metronidazole should not be used during the first trimester of pregnancy (Dykers, 1975b).

Availability

1. Tablets: 200 and 400 mg; 250 and 500 mg in the United States of America.
2. Rectal suppositories containing 0·5 or 1·0 g metronidazole.
3. Intravenous preparation: 0·5 g in 100 ml of a buffered isotonic solution.

Serum Levels in Relation to Dosage

1. *Oral administration.* Metronidazole is well absorbed when given by mouth. After a single oral dose of 200 mg, mean serum levels in 12 patients studied by Kane *et al.* (1961a) were 4·8, 4·5, 3·7, 2·9 and 0·8 μg per ml at 1, 2, 4, 8 and 24 h respectively. Ralph *et al.* (1974) gave metronidazole in single oral doses of 250 and 500 mg to 10 adult subjects and mean peak serum levels were 6·2 and 11·5 μg per ml respectively. However the rate of absorption in different individuals was quite variable; some developed high serum levels 15 min after administration, whilst in others peak levels occurred at 2–4 h. A mean peak serum level of 12·3 μg per ml was attained in four adult subjects given a single 750 mg dose of metronidazole (Schwartz and Jeunet, 1976). Following a single oral dose of 2·4 g. a mean peak serum level of 44·6 μg per ml (range 19·5–64·5) was obtained at 1 h and after 6 h the mean serum level was still 42 μg per ml (range 19·3–60·5) (McFadzean, 1969).

Wood and Monro (1975) performed serial chemical assays of metronidazole serum levels following a 2·0 g oral dose given to volunteers; the mean peak level at 1 h was 40 μg per ml, and this fell to 32 at 6 h, 5·7 at 24 h and to 0·9 μg per ml at 48 h. When bioassay was used, a mean peak serum level of 81 μg per ml was detected at 2 h. The reason for the discrepancy between the results obtained by chemical assay and bioassay is probably because the latter also estimates active metronidazole metabolites, which are present in serum for the first few hours after taking the drug (*see* page 765). Urtasun *et al.* (1976) administered large oral doses of 150 mg per kg body weight and serum concentrations of 180–200 μg per ml were obtained at 4 h. Furthermore, Deutsch *et al.* (1975) found a linear relationship between peak serum levels (102–340 μg per ml) when oral doses in the range of 80–190 mg per kg body weight were used. The serum half-life of metronidazole is about 8·5 h (Ralph *et al.*, 1974; Schwartz and Jeunet, 1076).

There have been a number of studies on the serum levels resulting from repeated oral doses of metronidazole. Kane *et al.* (1961b) gave two patients a dose of 200 mg six-hourly three times a day, for seven days; serum levels 2 h after the last dose were in the range of 6·1–9·8 μg per ml and there was no evidence of accumulation of the drug. Higher oral doses were used by Ralph *et al.* (1974) for 10 volunteers; dose regimens were 0·5 g four-hourly for four doses per day and 250 mg six-hourly for three doses a day. Serum levels with both of these dosage schedules increased progressively for the first few doses and then levelled off, with no accumulation evident between three and seven days. Maximal serum levels 12 h after the last dose each day were 3·9 and 13·1 μg per ml for the 250 mg and 0·5 g regimens respectively. Corresponding levels just prior to the last daily dose were 5·7 and 21·3 μg per ml respectively. It was considered that much higher peak serum levels would have been reached. Measurable serum levels of 0·41 and 0·54 μg per ml were still present in two volunteers 60 and 36 h respectively after stopping the drug; the former had received the drug in a dose of 2·0 g daily for six days and the latter 750 mg daily for six days. A dose of 1 g four times a day was used by Davies (1967) in three patients and this produced serum levels as high as 72·5 μg per ml.

2. *Intravenous administration.* Ingham *et al.* (1975a) studied serum levels in patients receiving 600 mg metronidazole intravenously over a period of 20 min. Levels at 60–90 min were in the range 20·7–48·2 (mean 35·2), at 4 h 16·3–48·9 (means 33·9) and at 8 h 16·5–27·5 (mean 23·7) μg per ml. Similar levels were observed by Eykyn and Phillips (1976) in 15 adult patients given a 0·5 g intravenous dose every 8 h; the drug was again infused over a period of 20 min and 30 min after its completion the mean serum level was 27·4 μg per ml (range 11·5–41·0); the mean trough concentration, taken just before an infusion, was 15·5 μg per ml (range 6·4–26·0). The drug appears to be eliminated from the serum in an approximately exponential fashion with a half-life of 4·25 h (Chowcat and Wyllie, 1976).

3. *Rectal administration.* After the insertion of a 1 g suppository into volunteers, a mean serum level of 2·3 μg per ml (range 1·0–4·8) was detected after 1 h and peak levels were usually reached after 4 h with a mean of 10·5 μg per ml (range 7·6–15·6) (Report, 1975). In another study, after rectal administration of a 0·5 g suppository to patients and volunteers, peak serum levels in the range 9–30 μg per ml occurred after 3–4 h and levels of 7–16 μg per ml persisted for 3 h after this peak. After a suppository dose of 1·0 g peak levels of 10–20 μg per ml were found (Giamarellou *et al.*, 1977).

Excretion

URINE: This is the main route by which metronidazole is eliminated from the body. Studies by Ings *et al.* (1966) indicated that 60–70 per cent of the ingested drug was excreted unchanged in the urine. However Ralph *et al.* (1974) were only able to recover 15–20 per cent of the administered dose in the urine as measured by microbiological assay, suggesting that significant amounts of the drug are excreted as its metabolites. Furthermore, they showed that the renal clearance of the drug 4 –8 h after administration was low, being only 10·2 ml per min per 1·73 square metre body surface, which accounts for its prolonged serum half-life of 8·7 h. Urinary concentrations of the drug during this period were in the range 15·7–67·0 μg per ml after an oral dose of 250 mg and in the range 76·4–115·0 μg per ml after a 0·5 g dose. Only 14·6 per cent of an administered dose is excreted unchanged in the first 24 h. Other studies using radioactively labelled metronidazole indicate that metabolites of the drug are eliminated at a slower rate than the parent drug (Schwartz and Jeunet, 1976). After a 750 mg oral dose, the percentage of unchanged drug in the serum was about 80 after 1 h and this fell progressively to about 17 after 48 h.

INACTIVATION IN BODY: Metronidazole is metabolized in the liver and a large proportion of an orally administered dose is excreted in the urine as nitroimidazole metabolites (Ralph *et al.*, 1974; Schwartz and Jeunet, 1976). These metabolites include a number of oxidative products of metronidazole and a glucuronic acid conjugate (Ings *et al.*, 1966; Stambaugh *et al.*, 1968). Based on microbiological assay studies of metronidazole excretion, Ralph *et al.* (1974) concluded that metronidazole metabolites are antibacterially inactive. Other studies indicate that some nitroimidazole metabolites excreted in the urine have antibacterial activity, and this may compromise the accuracy of microbiological assays (Wood and Monro, 1975; Speck *et al.*, 1976a). Metronidazole concentrations can be measured by a polarographic technique or by microbiological assay. Results obtained by these methods are comparable except for the estimation of urinary levels and the estimation of serum concentrations in patients with renal failure. In both of these situations the polarographic method gives falsely high values, because it measures both unchanged metronidazole and its metabolites (Ingham *et al.*, 1975a). Bioassay also gives higher serum levels than chemical assay in the first few hours after administration of metronidazole, because during this period this assay also probably estimates active metabolites (page 764). Using high-pressure liquid chromotography, Wheeler *et al.* (1978) have confirmed the presence of active metabolites in the serum. After intravenous administration of metronidazole in a dose of 13·6 mg kg given over one hour followed by a maintenance dose of 1·43 mg per kg per hour to patients, serum levels of metronidazole and its two principal metabolites were measured over succeeding days. Only very small amounts of its acid metabolite (1-acetic acid-2-methyl-5-metronidazole) was present but the serum ratio of the hydroxy metabolite (1-(2-hydroxyethyl-2-hydroxymethyl)-5-nitroimidazole) to unchanged metronidazole was 0·03–0·3. Ralph and Kirby (1975b) have shown that against Clostridium spp., the acid and hydroxy metabolites possess approximately 5 and 30 per cent respectively, of the activity of the parent compound.

FAECES: Only about 14 per cent of an orally administered dose of metronidazole is excreted in the faeces (Schwartz and Jeunet, 1976).

Distribution of the Drug in Body

Concentrations of the drug found in saliva and breast milk are comparable with those found in serum (Gray et al., 1961) whilst lower concentrations are detectable in semen and bone. Also in early studies much lower levels were found in embryonic tissue and the placenta. Therapeutic levels occur in bile and in the CSF (Tally *et al.*, 1972). Davies (1967) recorded CSF levels of 58 and 80·4 µg per ml respectively in two patients, who had received an oral dose of 1·0 g four times a day for a week. CSF levels of 13·9 and 11·0 µg per ml with simultaneous serum levels of 15·4 and 8·34 µg per ml respectively were detected 2 and 8 h after a 0·5 g oral dose in a patient receiving 1·0 g daily for Fusobacterium meningitis (O'Grady and Ralph, 1976). In volunteers given 2·4 g of metronidazole orally, CSF concentrations 90 min later varied between 6·0 and 22·7 µg per ml, being on the average 43 per cent of the simultaneous serum levels (Jokipii *et al.*, 1977). George and Bint (1976) found a concentration of 42 µg per ml in pus aspirated from a brain abscess of a three-year-old patient, who had received the drug in a dosage of 100 mg four times a day for one week. Concentrations of 35·0 and 34·4 µg per ml were detected in abscess cavities of two patients with a brain abscess receiving an oral dose of 400 mg every 8 h, at a time when concurrent serum levels were 11·5 and 35·1 µg per ml respectively. Abscess cavity concentrations of 20·7 and 45·0 µg per ml were obtained in two other patients receiving 400 and 600 mg respectively of the drug by the intravenous route every 8 h (Ingham *et al.*, 1977). In liver abscess pus, concentrations of the drug varying from nil to 24·0 µg per ml have been detected after a total oral dose of 5·8 g given over two days. A metronidazole level of 24·2 μg per ml was detected in drainage material from a lung empyema of a patient, who had received oral metronidazole in a dose of 400 mg six-hourly for the previous three-and-a-half days (Smith and Wellingham, 1976).

Ralph et al. (1974) could not detect any binding of metronidazole to serum proteins, whilst Schwartz and Jeunet (1976) using a different technique, found its binding to be less than 15 per cent.

Mode of Action

The mechanism of action of metronidazole has not yet been fully elucidated. Because it inhibits anaerobic protozoa and anaerobic bacteria (page 761) and because it has very limited activity against aerobic organisms or vertebrate cells in tissue culture, it was postulated that metronidazole interacts with biochemical pathways found only in anaerobes (Edwards et al., 1973; Ings et al., 1974).

Metronidazole diffuses into aerobic and anaerobic bacteria equally well, but in the former it remains unchanged whilst in the latter it is reduced. As a result of biochemical reduction in the cell, the concentration of unchanged drug is reduced and this probably creates a gradient which promotes further uptake of the drug into anaerobic organisms. The nitro group of metronidazole is reduced in anaerobic bacteria and protozoa by the pyruvate phosphoroclastic reaction, in which the drug acts as a preferential electron acceptor (Edwards and Mathison, 1970; Edwards et al., 1973). Oxygen markedly reduces the uptake of metronidazole in experiments using certain anaerobic protozoa, suggesting that this process depends on reducing power inside the cell (Müller and Lindmark, 1976). The selective uptake and specificity of metronidazole for anaerobes may be because their redox processes are different from those of aerobes; in anaerobes low-redox potential reactions involving ferridoxin- and flavodoxin-type electron transport proteins are important but they are absent or insignificant in aerobes. The products of metronidazole reduction within the cell have not yet been characterized; Ings et al. (1974) considered that the drug was most probably reduced to a hydroxylamine derivative whilst Plant and Edwards (1976) considered that an amino-derivative with the imidazole ring cleaved was more probable. It has been assumed that the product of reduction of the nitro group of metronidazole interacts with DNA with ultimate inhibition of nucleic acid synthesis and subsequent cell death (Ings and Constable, 1975). Moreover metronidazole has been shown to inhibit DNA synthesis and degrade existing DNA in Clostridium bifermentans (Plant and Edwards, 1976). Reduced metronidazole, but not the unreduced drug, affects DNA in vitro (Edwards, 1977). This ability of the reduced drug to induce changes in DNA may explain how it can cause mutations in bacteria resistant to its killing action (see page 768). Also the reported carcinogenicity of metronidazole in rodents (page 768) may be related to the fact that mammalian liver microsomes can reduce the drug (Edwards, 1977). The use of metronidazole as a radiosensitizer for hypoxic tumours (page 776) is in keeping with its action on DNA. It is also possible that radiation reduces metronidazole and induces binding to DNA only under hypoxic conditions (Edwards, 1977).

In studies using strains of Bacteroides fragilis and Clostridium perfringens, Ralph and Kirby (1975a) showed that metronidazole is more rapidly bactericidal than penicillin G, carbenicillin or clindamycin.

Toxicity

Since the early 1960's metronidazole has been used extensively for the treatment of certain protozoal infections, particularly Trichomonas vaginalis. The drug has been used in comparatively low dosage and for short periods of time for these infections, and this resulted in very few side-effects. More recently when metronidazole has been administered in higher doses and for more prolonged periods, side-effects have been more frequent.

1. *Gastro-intestinal side-effects.* Occasionally an unpleasant taste in the mouth, a furred tongue, nausea (rarely vomiting) and abdominal pain occur. Doses as high as 180 mg per kg body weight per day, when used in cancer patients as an adjunct to radiotherapy, produced slight but acceptable nausea; higher doses of up to 300 mg per kg body weight per day were progressively less well tolerated and produced severe anorexia, nausea and vomiting, which often persisted for 24–48 h after the last dose (Deutsch et al., 1975).

2. *Leucopenia.* A transient and reversible neutropenia has been occasionally observed during metronidazole therapy (Lefebvre and Hesseltine, 1975; Tally et al., 1975).

3. *Peripheral neuropathy.* This complication has been described in a number of patients, particularly those who have received prolonged treatment with relatively high doses of metronidazole (Ramsay, 1968; Ursing and Kamme, 1975; Ingham et al., 1975a; Bradley et al., 1977). Peripheral neuropathy is usually relatively mild and full recovery appears to occur when the drug is stopped or the dose decreased. In some patients sensory changes have persisted for months and even years after discontinuation of the drug (Karlsson and Hamlyn, 1977; Hishon and Pilling, 1977). Pathological investigation of the patient described by Bradley et al. (1977) showed that a major degree of nerve degeneration had occurred.

4. *Other side-effects.* Drowsiness, headache, depression, epilepsy, skin rashes, pruritus, vaginal and urethral burning, have all been reported. Clinical circumstances in three patients receiving high doses of metronidazole (in association with radiation for carcinoma) suggested that this was responsible for convulsions (Frytak et al., 1978). The urine of patients taking metronidazole may be coloured deep red-brown due to the presence of an azo-metabolite of the drug. Uneventful recovery has apparently occurred following attempts at suicide by the ingestion of up to 60 tablets (200 mg each).

5. *Mutagenicity and carcinogenicity.* Metronidazole can increase the spontaneous mutation rates of certain aerobic bacteria grown *in vitro* (Voogd et al., 1974; Lindmark and Müller, 1976), and urinary metabolites of patients taking metronidazole are also mutagenic when assayed in such bacterial test systems (Legator et al., 1975; Speck et al., 1976b). Furthermore, Mitelman et al. (1976) reported chromosomal abnormalities in the circulating lymphocytes of patients with Crohn's disease who had been taking metronidazole for 1–24 months, in an oral dose of 200–1200 mg per day.

A carcinogenic effect of very high doses of metronidazole in rodents has been reported (Rustia and Shubik, 1972; Rust, 1977), but this effect has not been confirmed in other experimental animals (Roe, 1977).

The extrapolation of these findings to humans is difficult, in whom to date there is no evidence that metronidazole is either teratogenic or carcinogenic. Nevertheless at this time it seems prudent to avoid using this drug in the first trimester of pregnancy where possible (page 763). In the context of carcinogenicity, Roe (1977) has pointed out that the use of metronidazole to eradicate Trichomonas vaginalis may actually reduce the risk of development of cancer of the uterine cervix.

6. *Interaction with other drugs.* Metronidazole can produce the 'antabuse syndrome' (Taylor, 1964). Similar to disulfiram (antabuse), metronidazole apparently affects the activity of hepatic enzymes involved with the metabolism of ethanol and acetaldehyde. When it is taken with alcohol it produces unpleasant symptoms, probably due to the accumulation of acetaldehyde in the blood (Birkett and Pond, 1975). In addition, a toxic psychosis has been described when metronidazole has been given to alcoholic patients receiving disulfiram (Rothstein and Clancy, 1969). Alcohol ingestion is therefore contraindicated in patients taking metronidazole.

The concomitant administration of metronidazole augments both the hypoprothrombinaemic effect and blood levels produced by commercial racemic sodium warfarin (coumadin sodium). O'Reilly (1976) showed that this was a stereoselective interaction, in that metronidazole augments the effects of racemic (a micture of laevowarfarin and dextrowarfarin) and S(-)-warfarin (laevowarfarin) and not R(+)-warfarin (dextrowarfarin). He suggested that this drug interaction can be lessened and even avoided if racemic warfarin is replaced by R(+) warfarin (dextrowarfarin). There is also some evidence that diphenylhydantoin, by its action of inducing enzymes, may increase the metabolism of metronidazole (Wheeler et al., 1978).

Clinical Uses of the Drug

1. *Trichomoniasis.* The oral administration of metronidazole is highly effective for the treatment of Trichomonas vaginalis infection of the genito-urinary tract in both males and females. The usually recommended oral dose for adult males and females is one tablet (200 or 250 mg) three times a day for 7–10 days. To prevent re-infection, the consort should receive a similar course of treatment concurrently. The recommended equivalent doses for children aged 7–10 years is half a tablet three times a day, for those aged 3–7 years half a tablet twice-daily, and for those aged 1–3 years, a quarter of a tablet three times daily. Shorter courses of treatment lasting only two to five days are also effective (McClean, 1971; Woodcock, 1972a; Davidson, 1973). A regimen of 800 mg given in the morning and 1200 mg given in the evening is often recommended (Davidson, 1973). Single dose treatment with 2 g metronidazole has also resulted in a high cure rate of trichomonal vaginitis (Csonka, 1971; Woodcock, 1972b; Ross, 1973; Dykers, 1975a). In a study of a small number of patients, single dose treatment with 1·5 g and even 1 g also appeared to be effective (Dykers, 1976).

2. *Amoebiasis.* Metronidazole is a most effective drug for the treatment of all forms of this disease. A great variety of treatment regimens have been used

in clinical trials to treat different amoebic infections. For intestinal infections and symptomless cysts passers, a regimen of 400–800 mg given orally three times a day for 5–10 days is now recommended. In some trials short courses of 2·0–2·4 g daily for one to three days have also resulted in a high cure rate. Appropriate dose reductions, similar to that used for the treatment of Trichomonal vaginalis infections (*vide supra*), is necessary for children. For amoebic liver abscess and other forms of extra-intestinal amoebiasis, a five-day course of 400 mg orally three times a day (with appropriate dose reduction for children) is recommended.

Many of these recommendations have been based on the extensive experience which has been gained in the treatment of amoebiasis at the King Edward VIII Hospital in Durban, South Africa. The current treatment for amoebiasis at that hospital has been summarized recently (Adams and MacLeod, 1977a and b). For amoebic dysentery metronidazole is preferred to tetracycline (page 629), because the former is effective against E. histolytica wherever it occurs, whilst tetracycline is a pure lumenal amoebicide and should also be combined with a tissue amoebicide. The dosage used is 800 mg three times a day for five days or single daily doses of 2 g for two to three days. Metronidazole in a dose of 800 mg three times a day for five days is also preferred to emetine for the treatment of amoebic liver abscess. Second courses are occasionally necessary. Aspiration of the amoebic liver abscess is also recommended for diagnosis and treatment. If progress is slow despite metronidazole and repeated aspirations, emetine is also used. If cysts are still passed after apparent cure of amoebic dysentery or an amoebic liver abscess, treatment with diloxanide furoate or diiodohydroxyquinoline is given.

Metronidazole is now generally accepted as the drug of choice for all forms of amoebiasis. In some situations treatment with an oral drug may not be feasible. This difficulty was overcome by administering metronidazole intravenously to a patient with severe amoebic colitis (Chowcat and Wyllie, 1976). The drug has also been used successfully by the intravenous route to treat amoebic liver abscess (Nair *et al.*, 1974).

Weber (1971) first reported the finding of an amoebic liver abscess after successful treatment of amoebic colitis with metronidazole. There have been several other reports describing failed treatment with metronidazole in amoebic liver abscess (Pittman, 1973; Fisher *et al.*, 1976). The patient described by Fisher *et al.* (1976) was treated with open surgical drainage and metronidazole for his amoebic liver abscess, but during therapy and while the original abscess was resolving, a second non-contiguous amoebic liver abscess developed; the second abscess responded to treatment with emetine, chloroquine and diiodohydroxyquinoline. The reasons why a few patients with amoebic liver abscess have failed to respond to metronidazole are unknown. The duration of metronidazole therapy may be important and the usually recommended five-day course may be inadequate for some severe infections. At Fairfield Hospital a small number of patients with moderately large liver abscesses have been treated successfully with metronidazole alone, given for several weeks. In some patients after this treatment, complete resolution, as monitored by serial liver scanning, has taken several months. It is apparent that wherever possible the course of an amoebic liver abscess should be followed by serial liver scans to ensure that complete resolution occurs. In addition, it does not necessarily follow that because clinical response occurs when a liver abscess is treated with metronidazole, it is amoebic in aetiology. Kane *et al.* (1976) described a man with a liver abscess who responded to metronidazole, and in whom amoebiasis could not be confirmed and susceptible anaerobic bacteria were probably the cause. The indications for either needle aspiration or open surgical drainage in amoebic abscess has been reduced by the use of metronidazole. It appears that large abscesses, particularly those in which there is a danger of rupture, still may require surgical intervention. This may also apply to amoebic liver abscesses which fail to respond to metronidazole; these should be additionally treated with emetine and chloroquine (Fisher *et al.*, 1976).

3. *Giardiasis.* The recommended dose for this infection is 2 g orally once a day, for three days. The equivalent dose for children aged 7–10 years is 1 g, for those aged 3–7 years 600 mg, and for those aged 1–3 years, 400 mg. This treatment schedule produces a higher parasitological cure rate than a standard course of mepacrine (Atabrine) (Wright *et al.*, 1977). Metronidazole also resulted in a higher cure rate than furazolidone (page 749) in another study (Levi *et al.*, 1977).

4. *Balantidium coli infection.* Metronidazole has been used to obtain clinical and parasitological cures of this infection (Garcia-Laverde and De Bonilla, 1975). A total dose of 5 g (children 2·5 g) given over five days or 12·5 g (children 7·5 g) given over 10 days was used.

5. *Dracunculus medinensis infection.* Studies by Antani *et al.* (1972) in which metronidazole was used to treat guinea worm infections (dracontiasis or dracunculiasis) were encouraging; the drug was given in a dose of 200 mg orally three times a day, for seven days. Subsequent studies have not been confirmatory (Kulkarni and Nagalotimath, 1975; Belcher *et al.*, 1975). These conflicting results may be due to differing criteria used to determine efficacy of treatment (Kale, 1977).

6. *Fasciola hepatica infection.* Nik-Akhtar and Tabibi (1977) used oral metronidazole for periods up to 28 days to treat four patients with fascioliasis successfully.

7. *Leishmaniasis.* Long (1973) successfully treated one patient with cutaneous leishmaniasis (Mexican type); an oral dose of 250 mg three times a day for two ten-day periods separated by 10 days was used. The drug is of no value in visceral leishmaniasis.

8. *Acute ulcerative gingivitis.* A number of controlled studies have demonstrated the effectiveness of metronidazole in this disease, in which anaerobic bacteria appear to be involved (Glenwright and Sidaway, 1966; Duckworth *et al.*, 1966) (*see also* page 761). The oral dose for adults is 200 mg three times a day for three days; equivalent doses for children 7–10 years is 100 mg three times a day, for those aged 3–7 years, 100 mg twice-daily and for those aged 1–3 years, 50 mg three times a day.

9. *Syphilis.* Davies (1967) used oral metronidazole in a dose of 1 g four times a day for periods of up to nine days to treat six patients with secondary syphilis. Local healing occurred and the treponemes disappeared from secondary syphilitic lesions. Metronidazole is not advocated as an alternative to penicillin G for the treatment of syphilis.

10. *Anaerobic bacterial infections.* Anaerobic bacteria may be involved in pyogenic infections particularly of the nervous, respiratory, biliary, intestinal,

urinary and female genital tracts. They are also important causes of septicaemia and endocarditis. The role of these bacteria as pathogens has become increasingly evident in the last decade, probably as a result of improved laboratory techniques for their isolation. Many anaerobic infections can be managed by surgery but others require chemotherapy sometimes in combination with surgery. Bacteroides fragilis is the most commonly encountered anaerobe and it is also one of the most resistant ones to penicillin G, cephalosporins, tetracyclines and erythromycin, antibiotics commonly used for infections in which anaerobes may be involved. The two most active chemotherapeutic agents against anaerobic organisms including B. fragilis are chloramphenicol (page 425), to which anaerobes are rarely resistant, and metronidazole which is active against virtually all obligately anaerobic bacteria of clinical significance (Finegold, 1977). Clindamycin (page 472) is also active against the anaerobes including B. fragilis. Present evidence indicates that metronidazole is a very effective drug for the treatment of human anaerobic infections. Many of these infections are mixed in that both aerobic and anaerobic organisms are implicated, so that it may be necessary to combine metronidazole with a suitable chemotherapeutic agent, which is active against aerobic bacteria.

Tally et al. (1972; 1975) first reported the oral use of metronidazole in 10 patients who had either septicaemia, necrotizing pneumonia, pulmonary abscess or osteomyelitis, caused by a variety of anaerobic organisms such as Fusobacterium, Eubacterium and Bacteroides spp.; six patients were cured and three had a good initial response. Willis and his co-workers described the successful use of oral metronidazole in four patients with non-clostridial anaerobic pelvic infections, one of which was due to Bacteroides fragilis (Report, 1974). Nineteen patients, who developed anaerobic infections in the pelvis or abdominal wound after hysterectomy or vaginal repair, were later described (Report, 1975). A variety of anaerobic organisms were isolated, particularly Bacteroides species. Metronidazole orally was used to treat nine of these patients; in seven it was curative and in two others the authors considered it helpful. Ledger et al. (1976) obtained favourable results in 20 of 25 women treated with metronidazole for post-partum pelvic infections.

Oral therapy was also successful for two patients reported by Ingham et al. (1975b). One had Bacteroides fragilis pyuria and septicaemia associated with a vesico-colic fistula, and the other an infected wound and septicaemia due to B. fragilis after the removal of an unsuccessful renal transplant. Other patients with septicaemia due to anaerobes have also been effectively treated with oral metronidazole. Mitre and Rotheram (1974) cured a patient with a septicaemia due to an unidentified anaerobe which was resistant to, and had not responded to treatment with gentamicin, tetracycline, chloramphenicol, clindamycin and penicillin G. Baron et al. (1975) used metronidazole successfully to treat two patients with B. fragilis septicaemia. Sharp et al. (1977) also described the cure of two patients with B. fragilis septicaemia, both of whom had failed to respond to treatment, one to clindamycin and the other to lincomycin, in spite of in vitro sensitivity of the organisms to these antibiotics. Metronidazole given orally in combination with ampicillin (page 99) and later amoxycillin (page 132) has also been used successfully to control Fusobacterium endocarditis in a patient who subsequently required valve replacement (Seggie, 1978).

Oral metronidazole in combination with aspiration and other antibiotics has been useful in the treatment of a number of adults (Ingham et al., 1975c; 1977) and one child (George and Bint, 1976), with a cerebral abscess. The drug was used to treat a 16-year-old boy with Fusobacterium meningitis and septicaemia, but success in this case could not be ascribed to metronidazole because chloramphenicol and other antibiotics were also used (O'Grady and Ralph, 1976). According to De Louvois et al. (1978), the majority of brain abscesses in which non-sporing anaerobes are implicated are otogenous in origin. Infection in these abscesses is often mixed in that aerobic organisms are also present. They consider that in these cases metronidazole may be of value in combination with other drugs or it may be used alone if only strict anaerobic bacteria have been cultured. Breast abscess (Hale et al., 1976), lung empyema (Smith and Wellington, 1976) and liver abscess (Bäck et al., 1978) have also been successfully treated with oral metronidazole.

There have been two publications reporting metronidazole treatment of comparatively large numbers of patients with anaerobic infections. Eykyn and Phillips (1976) described 50 patients. The majority had pelvic or intra-abdominal infection, but there were some with either osteomyelitis, leg abscess, gas gangrene or cholangitis. Of the 50 patients, 18 received the intravenous preparation, 10 the oral preparation and 22 intravenous followed by oral treatment. Twenty-six patients received other drugs as well. A wide range of anaerobes were isolated from pus and blood cultures taken from 44 patients, but the most common were Bacteroides and Clostridium spp.; in 39 patients these were also mixed with aerobic organisms. Satisfactory results were obtained in most patients; in 20 of the 24 treated with metronidazole alone there was a good response, but in 13 surgery formed an integral part of their management; overall 40 of the 50 patients showed clinical improvement. It was interesting that good results were obtained with metronidazole alone in those patients who had a mixture of aerobic and anaerobic organisms. It was observed that further cultures taken during treatment invariably yielded aerobic bacteria. One of their patients who was hypersensitive to penicillin, and who had gas gangrene, made excellent progress after amputation, when treated with hyperbaric oxygen and metronidazole alone. Giamarellou et al. (1977) described the use of orally (15 patients) or rectally (33 patients) administered metronidazole for the treatment of 50 anaerobic infections. These were mainly intra-abdominal or pelvic infections but there were also three cases of gas gangrene. In 18 patients penicillin and/or gentamicin were also administered (8 of the rectally treated group and 10 of the orally treated group). Thirty of the infections were purely anaerobic while the remaining were mixed. The majority of the anaerobes were Bacteroides spp., and others included Peptostreptococcus, Peptococcus, Fusobacterium and Clostridium spp. and microaerophilic cocci. Complete recovery occurred in 38 infections, a satisfactory response occurred in 9 and 3 were considered treatment failures. Thirteen of the 15 patients treated by the rectal route only had a complete recovery while the other two were considered to have a satisfactory response. In 5 cases obligate anaerobic cocci resistant to metronidazole were isolated as well as Bacteroides fragilis. In these cases penicillin was used in addition, whilst gentamicin was added to the therapy of the 20 cases in which aerobic Gram-negative bacteria were also isolated.

Present evidence suggests that antibiotic-associated colitis (pseudomem-branous colitis) may be caused by a clostridial toxin (page 482). Metronidazole has been used to treat four patients with antibiotic-associated pseudomem-branous colitis, all of whom had a rapid clinical response. This was attributed to activity of the drug against anaerobes (Dinh *et al.*, 1978; Matuchansky *et al.*, 1978).

11. *Chemoprophylaxis of anaerobic infections in surgical patients.* One study involving 202 gynaecological patients demonstrated that metronidazole is effective in reducing the frequency of post-operative non-clostridial anaerobic pelvic infection (Reports, 1974; 1975). One hundred patients received metronidazole as a single oral dose of 2 g if they were admitted to hospital 24 h before operation, or this dose followed by 200 mg three times on the day before operation, if they were admitted 48 h before operation. Both groups then received the drug in an oral dose of 200 mg three times a day until the end of the seventh post-operative day. Of these 100 patients, the vaginal-carriage rate of non-clostridial anaerobes was reduced from 49 to 6 per cent over the opera-tion period, whereas the same carriage rate rose from 44 to 66 per cent in 102 patients not receiving metronidazole over the same period. The anaerobes were Bacteroides spp. (particularly B. melaninogenicus and B. fragilis) and anaerobic cocci. During their stay in hospital and later in a convalescent home (average 14 days), anaerobic infection did not develop in any of the 100 patients who received metronidazole, but one did develop a pelvic abscess due to B. fragilis and an anaerobic streptococcus, 28 days post-operatively. By contrast, anaerobic infections developed in 19 control patients; mixed anaerobic infections predominated (18 of 19 patients) with the commonest isolates being B. melaninogenicus, B. fragilis, B. corrodens and anaerobic strep-tococci. Disc diffusion tests showed that all anaerobic isolates were sensitive to clindamycin (2 μg per ml) and metronidazole (5 μg per ml). In 7 of these 19 in-fections facultatively anaerobic pathogens such as Esch. coli and Proteus spp. were isolated as well as obligate anaerobic bacteria. In both the metronidazole treated group and those not receiving the drug, infections of the urinary tract and wound due to these facultative organisms also occurred.

The value of prophylactic metronidazole in elective large bowel surgery has also been studied. Goldring *et al.* (1975) investigated 50 patients undergoing elective colonic surgery; half were given oral kanamycin 1 g and oral metronidazole 200 mg every 6 h for three days before surgery. Examination of faecal specimens before treatment and at operation showed that in the an-tibiotic treated group Gram-negative aerobes (coliforms) and anaerobes (Bacteroides spp.) were greatly reduced, but they were virtually unchanged in those patients who had received mechanical bowel preparation alone. Eleven out of the 25 control patients but only 2 of the 25 patients in the antibiotic group, had a post-operative wound infection; these latter two were not due to Gram-negative organisms. One patient in the control group died from Bacteroides septicaemia. In another controlled trial of 46 patients undergoing elective colonic surgery, 27 received metronidazole and the remainder a placebo (Willis *et al.*, 1977). Metronidazole was given both as a 1 g oral dose 24 h pre-operatively and as a 1 g suppository just before the operation. The drug was then continued until the end of the seventh post-operative day in an oral dose of 200 mg three times daily, or as one suppository rectally or per colostomy, every 8 h until the drug could be taken orally. Patients in both groups were given a single intramuscular injection of 80 mg gentamicin as part of pre-operative medication (page 345). Within both groups there were several aerobic infections; anaerobic infections did not develop in any patients receiving metronidazole, but they occurred in 11 of the 19 control patients. These anaerobic infections produced foul-smelling wound discharges. In addition, in two patients wound breakdown occurred and another developed severe B. fragilis bacteraemia. The anaerobic infections were then treated with metronidazole in the same way as it was used prophylactically. In all cases the fever and wound discharges rapidly improved. Feathers et al. (1977) also showed the value of prophylactic gentamicin and metronidazole in colorectal surgery. Fourteen patients were given gentamicin and lincomycin parenterally, 14 parenteral gentamicin with metronidazole, and another 25 patients were not given antibiotics. Metronidazole was given as a 1 g suppository eight-hourly or, where this was impracticable, intravenously 0·5 g every 8 h. All chemotherapeutic agents were commenced with pre-medication and were given for five days. In the control group, the sepsis rate was 48 per cent, compared to 4 per cent (1 patient) in the treated group. These infections were mainly wound or deeper abscesses; the facultative anaerobes most commonly isolated were Esch. coli and Proteus spp., and Bacteroides spp. (particularly B. fragilis) were the most common anaerobes. All the obligate anaerobes were sensitive to metronidazole but three strains were resistant to lincomycin. Equally good results were obtained with combinations of gentamicin with either lincomycin or metronidazole, but with the former combination, pseudomembranous colitis (page 481) developed in two patients. For this reason the authors considered that lincomycin, unlike metronidazole, was unacceptable as a prophylactic agent in colorectal surgery.

Metronidazole has also proved of value in prevention and treatment of Bacteroides infections after appendicectomy (Willis et al., 1976). In a controlled trial 49 patients were given metronidazole as a 1 g suppository with pre-operative medication, and one suppository every 8 h after surgery, until oral metronidazole 200 mg three times a day could be given. Children under 12 years of age received suppositories containing 0·5 g metronidazole. Treatment with metronidazole was continued until the end of the seventh post-operative day. Forty-six other patients received placebo therapy. Within both groups of patients there were several infections due to facultative organisms (Esch. coli, enterococci and Staph. pyogenes). Anaerobic infection did not develop in any of the 49 patients who received metronidazole, but 9 (49 per cent) of the 46 controls developed fever and deep-seated infections due to non-sporing anaerobes. Five of these anaerobic infections were severe enough to warrant treatment with metronidazole (given in a similar way to its prophylactic use), and all had a rapid clinical response. In these 9 patients cultures also yielded facultative bacteria (Esch. coli, related coliform bacteria and enterococci) but in 7 obligate anaerobes were predominant, the commonest being B. fragilis and B. melaninogenicus. Therefore their infections responded to metronidazole alone, despite the presence of a minority of organisms insensitive to this drug.

12. *Crohn's disease.* Ursing and Kamme (1975) considered that bacterial overgrowth in the small intestine may contribute to abnormalities of absorption in Crohn's disease; in addition, intestinal anaerobes may be a source of antigen

for an immunological reaction involved in the pathogenesis of the disease. On this basis they gave metronidazole to five patients with Crohn's disease; a dose of 40 mg per kg body weight per day, later reduced to 30 mg per kg per day, resulted in improvement after two to four weeks' treatment in four patients; in the other patient improvement did not occur until after four months' treatment when corticosteroids were introduced. In three patients metronidazole was discontinued after 4–6 months of treatment, two patients remained quite well after further intervals of three and six months respectively, and the third was still free of symptoms but had laboratory evidence of disease activity.

13. *Rosacea*. In a small controlled trial involving 29 patients with rosacea, six weeks treatment with metronidazole in an oral dose of 200 mg twice-daily was therapeutically superior to treatment with a placebo (Pye and Burton, 1976). The drug was particularly effective against papules and pustules, but had relatively little effect on the erythema. The authors concluded that metronidazole was worth trying in patients with rosacea who have not responded to tetracycline (page 629).

14. *Glandular fever*. A small uncontrolled study has suggested that the use of metronidazole in an oral dose of 600–1200 mg daily may shorten the period of fever and tonsillitis in the anginose form of this disease (Hedström *et al.*, 1978). This effect was presumed to be due to the action of the drug on anaerobic bacteria.

15. *Radiosensitization*. Metronidazole sensitizes hypoxic cells to ionising radiation *in vitro* and *in vivo* in mice (Chapman *et al.*, 1973; Asquith *et al.*, 1974; Stone and Withers, 1974). Urtasun *et al.* (1976) used the drug in the high dose of 150 mg per kg in association with radiation to treat patients with supratentorial glioblastoma. Patients treated in this way survived longer compared to a group of patients treated by radiation alone.

16. *Topical therapy*. A solution of metronidazole (1 per cent in 0·6 per cent saline) applied as a wet dressing was found to be rapidly effective for the treatment of pressure sores, which are commonly infected with non-sporing anaerobes (Jones *et al.*, 1978). Similar treatment was also effective for diabetic ulcers, varicose ulcers and for large abscess cavities.

REFERENCES

Adams, E. B. and MacLeod, I. N. (1977a), 'Invasive amebiasis. I. Amebic dysentery and its complications', *Medicine,* **56,** 315.

Adams, E. B. and MacLeod, I. N. (1977b), 'Invasive amebiasis. II. Amebic liver abscess and its complications', *Medicine,* **56,** 325.

Antani, J. A., Srinivas, H. V., Krishnamurthy, K. R. and Borgaonkar, A. N. (1972), 'Metronidazole in dracunculiasis', *Amer. J. Trop. Med. Hyg.,* **21,** 178.

Asquith, H. C., Foster, J. L., Willson, R. L. and Study Group. (1974), 'Metronidazole ('Flagyl'). A radiosensitizer of hypoxic cells', *Br. J. Radiol.,* **470,** 474.

Bäck, E., Hermanson, J. and Wickman, M. (1978), 'Metronidazole treatment of liver abscess due to Bacteroides fragilis', *Scand. J. Infect. Dis.,* **10,** 152.

Baron, D., Drugeon, H., Nicolas, F. and Courtieu, A. L. (1975), 'Intérét du metronidazole dans les septicémias à Bactéroides fragilis: deux observations', *La Nouv. Presse Med.,* **4,** 667.

Belcher, D. W., Wunapa, F. K. and Ward, W. B. (1975), 'Failure of thiabendazole and metronidazole in the treatment and suppression of guinea worm disease', *Amer. J.*

Trop. Med. Hyg., **24,** 444.

Birkett, D. J. and Pond, S. M. (1975), 'Metabolic drug interactions—a critical review', *Med. J. Aust.,* **1,** 687.

Bradley, W. G., Karlsson, I. J. and Rassol, C. G. (1977), 'Metronidazole neuropathy', *Brit. med. J.,* **2,** 610.

Chapman, J. D., Reuvers, A. P. and Borsa, J. (1973), 'Effectiveness of nitrofuran derivatives in sensitizing hypoxic mammalian cells to X-ray'. *Brit. J. Radiol.,* **46,** 623.

Chow, A. W., Patten, V. and Guze, L. B. (1975), 'Susceptibility of anaerobic bacteria to metronidazole: Relative resistance of non-spore-forming Gram-positive bacilli', *J. Infect. Dis.,* **131,** 182.

Chow, A. W., Patten, V. and Bednorz, D. (1978), 'Susceptibility of Campylobacter fetus to twenty-two antimicrobial agents', *Antimicrob. Ag. Chemother.,* **13,** 416.

Chowcat, N. L. and Wyllie, J. H. (1976), 'Intravenous metronidazole in amoebic enterocolitis', *Lancet,* **2,** 1143.

Cosar, C. and Julou, L. (1959), 'Activité de L' (Hydroxy-2-éthyl)-1-méthyl-2-nitro-5-imidazole (8823 R.P.) vis-à-vis des infections expérimentales à trichomonas vaginalis', *Ann. Inst. Pasteur, Paris,* **96,** 238.

Cosar, C., Ganter, P. and Julou, L. (1961), 'Etude expérimentale due métronidazole (8823 R.P.). Activités trichomonacide et amoebicide. Toxicité et propriétes pharmacologiques générales', *Presse Méd.,* **69,** 1069.

Csonka, G. W. (1971), 'Trichomonal vaginitis treated with one dose of metronidazole', *Brit. J. vener. Dis.,* **47,** 456.

Davidson, F. (1973), 'Short term high-dose metronidazole for vaginal trichomoniasis', *J. Obstet. Gynaecol. Br. Commonw.,* **80,** 368.

Davies, A. H., McFadzean, J. A. and Squires, S. (1964), 'Treatment of Vincent's stomatitis with metronidazole', *Brit. med. J.,* **1,** 1149.

Davies, A. H. (1967), 'Metronidazole in human infections with syphilis', *Brit. J. vener. Dis.,* **43,** 197.

De Louvois, J., Gortvai, P. and Hurley, R. (1978), 'The role of Bacteroides fragilis in abscesses of the central nervous system: Implications for therapy', *J. Antimicrob. Chemother.,* **4,** 97.

Deutsch, G., Foster, J. L., McFadzean, J. A. and Parnell, M. (1975), 'Human studies with 'high dose' metronidazole: A non-toxic radiosensitiser of hypoxic cells', *Br. J. Cancer,* **31,** 75.

Dinh, H. T., Kernbaum, S. and Frottier, J. (1978), 'Treatment of antibiotic-induced colitis by metronidazole', *Lancet,* **1,** 338.

Duckworth, R., Waterhouse, J. P., Britton, D. E. R., Nuki, K., Sheiham, A., Winter, R. and Blake, G. C. (1966), 'Acute ulcerative gingivitis. A double-blind controlled clinical trial of metronidazole', *Br. Dent. J.,* **120,** 599.

Durel, P., Roiron, V., Siboulet, H. and Borel, L. J. (1959), 'Trial of an anti-trichomonal derivative of imidazole (8823 R.P.)', *Comptes Rendus de la Societé Française de Gynécologie',* **29,** 36.

Dykers, J. R., Jr. (1975a), 'Single-dose metronidazole for Trichomonas vaginitis. Patient and consort', *New Engl. J. Med.,* **293,** 23.

Dykers, J. R., Jr. (1975b), 'Hazards of metronidazole', *New Engl. J. Med.,* **293,** 454.

Dykers, J. R., Jr. (1976), 'Single-dose metronidazole for Trichomonas vaginitis: A follow up', *New Engl. J. Med.,* **295,** 395.

Edwards, D. I. and Mathison, G. E. (1970), 'The mode of action of metronidazole against Trichomonas vaginalis', *J. gen. Microbiol.,* **63,** 297.

Edwards, D. I., Dye, M. and Carne, H. (1973), 'The selective toxicity of antimicrobial nitroheterocyclic drugs', *J. gen. Microbiol.,* **76,** 135.

Edwards, D. I. (1977), 'The action of metronidazole on DNA', *J. Antimicrob. Chemother.,* **3,** 43.

Eykyn, S. and Phillips, I. (1976), 'Metronidazole and anaerobic sepsis', *Brit. med. J.*, **2**, 1418.

Feathers, R. S., Lewis, A. A. M., Sagor, G. R., Amirak, I. D. and Noone, P. (1977), 'Prophylactic systemic antibiotics in colorectal surgery', *Lancet*, **2**, 4.

Finegold, S. M. (1977), 'Therapy for infections due to anaerobic bacteria: An overview', *J. Infect. Dis.* (Suppl.), **135**, 25.

Fisher, L. S., Chow, A. W., Lindquist, L. and Guze, L. B. (1976), 'Failure of metronidazole in amebic liver abscess', *Amer. J. Med. Sci.*, **271**, 65.

Fowler, W. (1960), 'Flagyl in Trichomoniasis, (discussion at Medical Society for the study of venereal diseases), *Br. J. vener. Dis.*, **36**, 157.

Freeman, W. A., McFadzean, J. A. and Whelan, J. P. F. (1968), 'Activity of metronidazole against experimental tetanus and gas gangrene', *J. Appl. Bact.*, **31**, 443.

Frytak, S., Moertel, C. G., Childs, D. S. and Albers, J. W. (1978), 'Neurologic toxicity associated with high-dose metronidazole therapy', *Ann. Intern. Med.*, **88**, 361.

Garcia-Laverde, A. and De Bonilla, L. (1975), 'Clinical trials with metronidazole in human balantidiasis', *Amer. J. Trop. Med. Hyg.*, **24**, 781.

George, R. H. and Bint, A. J. (1976), 'Treatment of brain abscess due to Bacteroides fragilis with metronidazole', *J. Antimicrob. Chemother.*, **2**, 101.

Giamarellou, H., Kanellakopoulou, K., Pragastis, D., Tagaris, N. and Daikos, G. K. (1977), 'Treatment with metronidazole of 48 patients with serious anaerobic infections', *J. Antimicrob. Chemother.*, **3**, 347.

Glenwright, H. D. and Sidaway, D. A. (1966), 'The use of metronidazole in the treatment of acute ulcerative gingivitis', *Br. Dent. J.*, **121**, 174.

Goldring, J., Scott, A., McNaught, W. and Gillespie, G. (1975), 'Prophylactic oral antimicrobial agents in elective colonic surgery', *Lancet*, **2**, 997.

Gray, M. S., Kane, P. O. and Squires, S. (1961), 'Further observations on metronidazole (Flagyl)', *Brit. J. vener. Dis.*, **37**, 278.

Hale, J. E., Perinpanayagam, R. M. and Smith, G. (1976), 'Bacteroides: An unusual cause of breast abscess', *Lancet*, **2**, 70.

Hedström, S. A., Mardh, P.-A. and Ripa, T. (1978), 'Treatment of anginose infectious mononucleosis with metronidazole', *Scand. J. Infect. Dis.*, **10**, 7.

Hishon, S. and Pilling, J. (1977), 'Metronidazole neuropathy', *Brit. med. J.*, **2**, 832.

Ingham, H. R., Selkon, J. B. and Hale, J. H. (1975a), 'The antibacterial activity of metronidazole', *J. Antimicrob. Chemother.*, **1**, 355.

Ingham, H. R., Rich, G. E., Selkon, J. B., Hale, J. H., Roxby, C. M., Betty, M. J., Johnson, R. W. G. and Uldall, P. R. (1975b), 'Treatment with metronidazole of three patients with serious infections due to Bacteroides fragilis', *J. Antimicrob. Chemother.*, **1**, 235.

Ingham, H. R., Selkon, J. B., So, S. C. and Weiser, R. (1975c), 'Brain abscess', *Brit. med. J.*, **4**, 39.

Ingham, H. R., Selkon, J. B. and Roxby, C. M. (1977), 'Bacteriological study of otogenic cerebral abscesses: Chemotherapeutic role of metronidazole', *Brit. med. J.*, **2**, 991.

Ingham, H. R., Eaton, S., Venables, C. W. and Adams, P. C. (1978), 'Bacteroides fragilis resistant to metronidazole after long-term therapy', *Lancet*, **1**, 214.

Ings, R. M. J., Law, G. L. and Parnell, E. W. (1966), 'The metabolism of metronidazole', *Biochem. Pharmacol.*, **15**, 515.

Ings, R. M. J., McFadzean, J. A. and Ormerod, W. E. (1974), 'The mode of action of metronidazole in Trichomonas vaginalis and other micro-organisms', *Biochem. Pharmacol.*, **23**, 1421.

Ings, R. M. J. and Constable, F. L. (1975), 'An investigation into the effect of metronidazole on the morphology of Trichomonas vaginalis', *J. Antimicrob. Chemother.*, **1**, 121.

Jokipii, A. M. M., Myllylä, Hokkanen, E. and Jokipii, L. (1977), 'Penetration of the blood brain barrier by metronidazole and tinidazole', *J. Antimicrob. Chemother.*, **3**, 239.

Jones, P. H., Willis, A. T. and Ferguson, I. R. (1978), 'Treatment of anaerobically infected pressure sores with topical metronidazole', Lancet, **1**, 214.

Kale, O. O. (1977), 'Clinical evaluation of drugs for dracontiasis', *Trop. Doct.*, **7**, 15.

Kane, P. O., McFadzean, J. A., Squires, S., King, A. J. and Nicol, C. S. (1961a), 'Absorption and excretion of metronidazole. Part I. Serum concentration and urinary excretion after oral administration', *Brit. J. vener. Dis.*, **37**, 273.

Kane, P. O., McFadzean, J. A. and Squires, S. (1961b), 'Absorption and excretion of metronidazole, Part II. Studies on primary failures', *Brit. J. vener. Dis.*, **37**, 276.

Kane, J. G., Fossieck, B. E., Jr and Parker, R. H. (1976), 'Metronidazole and hepatic abscess. A false-positive response', *JAMA*, **236**, 2653.

Karlsson, I. J. and Hamlyn, A. N. (1977), 'Metronidazole neuropathy', *Brit. med. J.*, **2**, 832.

Kulkarni, D. R. and Nagalotimath, S. J. (1975), 'Guinea-worms and metronidazole', *Trans. roy. Soc. Trop. Med. Hyg.*, **69**, 169.

Ledger, W. J., Gee, C., Pollin, P. A., Lewis, W. L., Sutter, V. L. and Finegold, S. M. (1976), 'A new approach to patients with suspected anaerobic postpartum pelvic infections. Transabdominal uterine aspiration for culture and metronidazole for treatment', *Am. J. Obstet. Gynecol.*, **126**, 1.

Lefebvre, Y. and Hesseltine, H. C. (1965), 'The peripheral white blood cells and metronidazole', *JAMA*, **194**, 127.

Legator, M. S., Connor, T. H. and Stoeckel, M. (1975), 'Detection of mutagenic activity of metronidazole and niridazole in body fluids of humans and mice', *Science*, **188**, 1118.

Levi, G. C., de Ávila, C. A. and Neto, V. A. (1977), 'Efficacy of various drugs for treatment of giardiasis. A comparative study', *Am. J. Trop. Med. Hyg.*, **26**, 564.

Lindmark, D. G. and Müller, M. (1976), 'Antitrichomonad action, mutagenicity and reduction of metronidazole and other nitroimidazoles', *Antimicrob. Ag. Chemother.*, **10**, 476.

Long, P. I. (1973), 'Cutaneous leishmaniasis. Treated with metronidazole', *JAMA*, **233**, 1378.

Matuchansky, C., Aries, J. and Maire, P. (1978), 'Metronidazole for antibiotic-associated pseudomembranous colitis', *Lancet*, **2**, 580.

McClean, A. N. (1971), 'Treatment of trichomoniasis in the female with a 5-day course of metronidazole ('Flagyl')', *Br. J. vener. Dis.*, **47**, 36.

McFadzean, J. A. (1969), 'The absorption, distribution and metabolism of metronidazole', *Medicine Today*, **3**, 10.

McHenry, M. C. (1977), 'Use in impaired renal function', in press; quoted by Roe (1977).

Mitelman, F., Hartley-Asp, B. and Ursing, B. (1976), 'Chromosome aberrations and metronidazole', *Lancet*, **2**, 802.

Mitre, R. J. and Rotheram, E. B., Jr. (1974), 'Anaerobic septicaemia from thrombophlebitis of the internal jugular vein. Successful treatment with metronidazole', *JAMA*, **230**, 1168.

Müller, M. and Lindmark, D. G. (1976), 'Uptake of metronidazole and its effect on viability in Trichomonads and Entamoeba invadens under anaerobic and aerobic conditions', *Antimicrob. Ag. Chemother.*, **9**, 696.

Nair, K. G., Kothari, N. N. and Sheth, U. K. (1974), 'Intravenous metronidazole in amoebic liver abscess', *Lancet*, **1**, 1238.

Nik-Akhtar, B. and Tabibi, V. (1977), 'Metronidazole in fascioliasis. Report of four cases', *J. Trop. Med. Hyg.*, **80**, 179.

O'Grady, L. R. and Ralph, E. D. (1976), 'Anaerobic meningitis and bacteremia caused by Fusobacterium species', *Am. J. Dis. Child.,* **130,** 871.

O'Reilly, R. A. (1976), 'The stereoselective interaction of warfarin and metronidazole in man', *New Engl. J. Med.,* **295,** 354.

Pittman, F. E. (1973), 'Treatment of amoebic colitis', *Lancet,* **2,** 1325.

Plant, C. W. and Edwards, D. I. (1976), 'The effect of tinidazole, metronidazole and nitrofurazone on nucleic acid synthesis in Clostridium bifermentans', *J. Antimicrob. Chemother.,* **2,** 203.

Powell, S. J., Macleod, I., Wilmot, A. J. and Elsdon-Dew, R. (1966), 'Metronidazole in amoebic dysentery and amoebic liver abscess', *Lancet,* **2,** 1329.

Pye, R. J. and Burton, J. L. (1976), 'Treatment of rosacea by metronidazole', *Lancet,* **1,** 1211.

Ralph, E. D., Clarke, J. T., Libke, R. D., Luthy, R. P. and Kirby, W. M. M. (1974), 'Pharmacokinetics of metronidazole as determined by bioassay', *Antimicrob. Ag. Chemother.,* **6,** 691.

Ralph, E. D. and Kirby, W. M. M. (1975a), 'Unique bactericidal action of metronidazole against Bacteroides fragilis and Clostridium perfringens', *Antimicrob. Ag. Chemother.,* **8,** 409.

Ralph, E. D. and Kirby, W. M. M. (1975b), 'Bioassay of metronidazole with either anaerobic or aerobic incubation', *J. Infect. Dis.,* **132,** 587.

Ramsay, I. D. (1968), 'Endocrine ophthalmology', *Brit. med. J.,* **4,** 706.

Report by a Study Group (1974), 'Metronidazole in the prevention and treatment of Bacteroides infections in gynaecological patients', *Lancet,* **2,** 1540.

Report by a Study Group (1975), 'An evaluation of metronidazole in the prophylaxis and treatment of anaerobic infections in surgical patients', *J. Antimicrob. Chemother.,* **1,** 393.

Roe, F. J. C. (1977), 'Metronidazole: Review of uses and toxicity', *J. Antimicrob. Chemother.,* **3,** 205.

Ross, S. M. (1973), 'Single and triple dose treatment of trichomonas infection of the vagina', *Brit. J. vener. Dis.,* **49,** 475.

Rothstein, E. and Clancy, D. D. (1969), 'The toxicity of disulfiram combined with metronidazole', *New Engl. J. Med.,* **280,** 1006.

Rust, J. H. (1977), 'Tumorigenicity studies—mouse and rat', in press; quoted by Roe (1977).

Rustia, M. and Shubik, P. (1972), 'Induction of lung tumours and malignant lymphomas in mice by metronidazole', *J. Natl. Cancer Inst.,* **48,** 721.

Salem, A. R., Jackson, D. D. and McFadzean, J. A. (1975), 'An investigation of interactions between metronidazole ('Flagyl') and other antibacterial agents', *J. Antimicrob. Chemother.,* **1,** 387.

Schneider, J. (1961), 'Treatment of giardiasis (lambliasis) with metronidazole', *Bulletin de la Société de Pathologie Exotique,* **54,** 84.

Schwartz, D. E. and Jeunet, F. (1976), 'Comparative pharmacokinetic studies of ornidazole and metronidazole in man', *Chemotherapy,* **22,** 19.

Seggie, J. (1978), 'Fusobacterium endocarditis treated with metronidazole', *Brit. med. J.,* **1,** 960.

Sharp, D. J., Corringham, R. E. T., Nye, E. B., Sagor, G. R. and Noone, P. (1977), 'Successful treatment of Bacteroides bacteraemia with metronidazole, after failure with clindamycin and lincomycin', *J. Antimicrob. Chemother.,* **3,** 233.

Shepard, T. H. and Fantel, A. G. (1977), 'Is metronidazole teratogenic?', *JAMA,* **237,** 1617.

Shinn, D. L. S. (1962), 'Metronidazole in acute ulcerative gingivitis', *Lancet,* **1,** 1191.

Smith, B. J. D. and Wellingham, J. (1976), 'Metronidazole in treatment of empyema., *Brit. med. J.,* **1,** 1074.

Speck, W. T., Stein, A. B. and Rosenkranz, H. S. (1976a), 'Metronidazole bioassay', *Antimicrob. Ag. Chemother.,* **9,** 260.

Speck, W. T. A., Stein, A. B. and Rosenkranz, H. S. (1976b), 'Mutagenicity of metronidazole: Presence of several active metabolites in human urine', *J. Natl. Cancer Inst.*, **56**, 283.

Stambaugh, J. E., Feo, L. G. and Manthei, R. W. (1968), 'The isolation and identification of the urinary oxidative metabolites of metronidazole in man', *J. Pharmacol. exp. Therap.*, **161**, 373.

Stone, H. B. and Withers, H. R., (1974), 'Tumour and normal tissue response to metronidazole and irradiation in mice', *Radiology*, **113**, 441.

Sutter, V. L. and Finegold, S. M. (1976), 'Susceptibility of anaerobic bacteria to 23 antimicrobial agents', *Antimicrob. Ag. Chemother.*, **10**, 736.

Tally, F. P., Sutter, V. L. and Finegold, S. M. (1972), 'Metronidazole versus anaerobes. *In vitro* data and initial clinical observations', *Calif. Med.*, **117**, 22.

Tally, F. P., Sutter, V. L. and Finegold, S. M. (1975), 'Treatment of anaerobic infections with metronidazole', *Antimicrob. Ag. Chemother.*, **7**, 672.

Taylor, J. A. T. (1964), 'Metronidazole: A new agent for combined somatic and psychic therapy of alcoholism', *Bull Los. Angeles, Neurol. Soc.*, **29**, 158.

Thurner, J. and Meingassner, J. G. (1978), 'Isolation of Trichomonas vaginalis resistant to metronidazole', *Lancet*, **2**, 738.

Ursing, B. and Kamme, C. (1975), 'Metronidazole for Crohn's disease', *Lancet*, **1**, 775.

Urtasun, R., Band, P., Chapman, J. D., Feldstein, M. L., Mielke, B. and Fryer, C. (1976), 'Radiation and high-dose metronidazole in supratentorial glioblastomas', *New Engl. J. Med.*, **234**, 1364.

Voogd, C. E., Van Der Stel, J. J. and Jacobs, J. J. J. A. A. (1974), 'The mutagenic action of nitroimidazoles. 1. Metronidazole, nimorazole, dimetridazole and ronidazole', *Mutat. Res.*, **26**, 483.

Weber, D. M. (1971), 'Amebic abscess of liver following metronidazole therapy', *JAMA*, **216**, 1339.

Wheeler, L. A., De Meo, M., Halula, M., George, L. and Heseltine, P. (1978), 'Use of high-pressure liquid chromatography to determine plasma levels of metronidazole and metabolites after intravenous administration', *Antimicrob. Ag. Chemother.*, **13**, 205.

Willis, A. T., Ferguson, I. R., Jones, P. H., Phillips, K. D., Tearle, P. V., Berry, R. B., Fiddian, R. V., Graham, D. F., Harland, D. H. C., Innes, D. B., Mee, W. M., Rothwell-Jackson, R. L., Sutch, I., Kilbey, C. and Edwards, D. (1976), 'Metronidazole in prevention and treatment of Bacteroides infections after appendicectomy', *Brit. med. J.*, **1**, 318.

Willis, A. T., Ferguson, I. R., Jones, P. H., Phillips, K. D., Tearle, P. V., Fiddian, R. V., Graham, D. F., Harland, D. H. C., Hughes, D. F. R., Knight, D., Mee, W. M., Pashby, N., Rothwell-Jackson, R. L., Sachdeva, A. K., Sutch, I., Kilbey, C. and Edwards, D. (1977), 'Metronidazole in prevention and treatment of Bacteroides infections in elective colonic surgery', *Brit. med. J.*, **1**, 607.

Wood, B. A. and Monro, A. M. (1975), 'Pharmacokinetics of tinidazole and metronidazole in women after single large oral doses', *Brit. J. vener. Dis.*, **51**, 51.

Woodcock, K. R. (1972a), 'Two-day treatment with metronidazole in vaginal trichomoniasis', *Brit. J. vener. Dis.*, **48**, 383.

Woodcock, K. R. (1972b), 'Treatment of trichomonal vaginitis with a single oral dose of metronidazole', *Brit. J. vener. Dis.*, **48**, 65.

Wright, S. G., Tomkins, A. M. and Ridley, D. S. (1977), 'Giardiasis: Clinical and therapeutic aspects', *Gut*, **18**, 343.

Tinidazole

Description

Tinidazole is a nitroinmidazole drug similar to metronidazole (page 761), and nimorazole, ornidazole and carnidazole (page 789). It was synthetized in 1969 and *in vitro* studies showed that it was very effective against Trichomonas vaginalis (Howes *et al.*, 1970). It has the chemical formula of 1-(2-(ethylsulphonyl)ethyl)-2 methyl-5-nitroimidazole and is marketed with the trade name of 'Fasigyn' (Pfizer).

Sensitive Organisms

1. *Protozoa*. The minimum inhibitory concentration of tinidazole against Trichomonas vaginalis is similar to that of metronidazole (page 762), but its minimum trichomonicidal concentration is lower (Howes *et al.*, 1970; Forsgren and Wallin, 1974). Tinidazole is also active against Entamoeba histolytica and Giardia lamblia.

2. *Bacteria*. Reynolds *et al.* (1975) studied the *in vitro* sensitivity of 69 strains of obligately anaerobic Gram-negative rods (59 Bacteroides fragilis, 2 other Bacteroides spp. and 8 Fusobacterium spp.); all strains were sensitive to $2 \cdot 0 \mu g$ per ml or less of tinidazole. The drug was slightly more active than metronidazole, the two compounds having geometric mean MIC's of $0 \cdot 28$ and $0 \cdot 34 \mu g$ per ml respectively. Tinidazole is slightly less active than metronidazole against Clostridium spp. (Edwards *et al.*, 1973; Dornbusch and Nord, 1974).

The *in vitro* activity of various nitroimidazole drugs were tested by Wüst (1977) against 114 strains of anaerobes; these consisted of Bacteroides fragilis, B. melaninogenicus, Fusobacterium spp., Cl. perfringens, other Clostridium spp., Peptococcus, Peptostreptococcus, Veillonella and Eubacterium spp. and Propionibacterium acnes. With the exception of the isolates of Propionibacterium acnes, metronidazole and tinidazole inhibited all strains at a concentration of $3 \cdot 1 \mu g$ per ml or less and killed them at a concentration of $6 \cdot 3 \mu g$ per ml or less. When tested against clinical isolates of Bacteroides fragilis, metronidazole, tinidazole and ornidazole (page 789) are all active with a highest MIC value of $1 \cdot 0 \mu g$ per ml and a highest minimum bactericidal concentration of $2-4 \mu g$ per ml; tinidazole was statistically more active than the other two in both respects, but the average differences were less than two-fold (Jokipii and Jokipii, 1977). Clindamycin is more active than tinidazole against anaerobic bacteria, with the exception of the Clostridium spp. (Klastersky *et al.*, 1977).

Mode of Administration and Dosage

Tinidazole is administered by the oral route and dosage varies according to the protozoal infection. In trichomoniasis and giardiasis it has been used in a dose of 150 mg two or three times daily, for five to seven days, and also as a single dose of 2 g. In amoebiasis, doses ranging from 450–2400 mg given daily in divided doses have been used for five to ten days, and also single daily doses of 1–2 g given for two to six days. Pettersson (1975) used a single oral dose of 1 g to treat children with giardiasis, and a dose of 60 mg per kg body weight, for three days, has been used to treat children with intestinal amoebiasis (Scragg and Proctor, 1977). Tinidazole is insoluble in water and there is no parenteral preparation available.

The use of tinidazole is not recommended during the first trimester of pregnancy or for nursing mothers (*see also* metronidazole page 769).

Availability

Tablets, each containing 0·5 g tinidazole.

Serum Levels in Relation to Dosage

Following a single oral dose of 150 mg tinidazole to healthy female volunteers, a mean peak serum level of 4·91 μg per ml occurred at 3 h and the level after 24 h was still 1·56 μg per ml (Welling and Monro, 1972). When the drug was administered in a dose of 150 mg twice-daily, the average maximum serum concentration was 8·91 μg per ml and the average minimum level 4·64 μg per ml. In a cross-over study, comparable serum levels for metronidazole given in a dose of 200 mg twice-daily, were 7·07 and 2·47 μg per ml respectively. When a single oral dose of 2 g tinidazole was given to female volunteers, a mean serum level of 51 μg per ml was attained at 2 h, and this fell to 19·0 after 24 h, 4·2 after 48 h and 1·3 μg per ml at 72 h (Wood and Monro, 1975). These investigators also estimated metronidazole levels after a 2 g oral dose in a cross-over study; by bioassay metronidazole produced a higher peak level of 81 μg per ml, probably because of the presence of biologically active metabolites (*see* page 764), but by chemical assay its peak level of 40 μg per ml was lower. Four hours after administration, metronidazole serum levels fell much more rapidly, being a third of the tinidazole level at 24 h, a fifth of the tinidazole level at 48 h and undetectable at 72 h. These differences are due to the longer half-life of tinidazole which is 12·5 h.

Excretion

URINE: Following a single oral 250 mg dose, approximately 16 per cent of the drug can be recovered from the urine in an unchanged form (Taylor *et al.*, 1970).

INACTIVATION IN BODY: Apparently very little tinidazole is metabolized in humans. There is no significant difference between the peak serum level when estimated chemically or by bioassay, suggesting that all of the drug in the serum at that time is in the unchanged form (Wood and Monro, 1975).

Distribution of the Drug in Body

Detailed information on the distribution of tinidazole is unavailable. Apparently it crosses the placenta and is present in breast milk when administered to nursing mothers. Jokipii *et al.* (1977) estimated CSF concentrations of tinidazole in four patients without meningitis after a 2 g oral dose; these ranged from 17·0 to 39·0 μg per ml, corresponding to 88 per cent of the simultaneous serum concentrations. These CSF values were higher than those obtained using a 2·4 g oral dose of metronidazole (page 766).

Tinidazole is 12 per cent bound to serum proteins (Taylor *et al.*, 1970).

Mode of Action

The precise mode of action of tinidazole is unknown but presumably it is similar to that of metronidazole (page 767), because of its selective action against anaerobic organisms. Both metronidazole and tinidazole inhibit DNA synthesis and degrade existing DNA of Clostridium bifermentans (Plant and Edwards, 1976). Compared to metronidazole, tinidazole is a more rapid inhibitor of DNA and it has higher *in vitro* activity; both of these are probably because tinidazole penetrates the cell more rapidly (Miller *et al.*, 1970).

Like metronidazole (page 768), tinidazole can induce mutations in strains of Salmonella typhimurium (Lindmark and Müller, 1976).

Toxicity

As with metronidazole (page 768), side-effects with tinidazole therapy are usually mild and infrequent. If the drug is used for more prolonged periods than currently advocated, patients should be carefully observed for side-effects similar to those which have occurred with prolonged metronidazole therapy (page 768). Nausea, vomiting, anorexia and a metallic or bitter taste in the mouth are the most common side-effects. Malaise, vertigo, pruritis, headache, constipation and skin rashes have been reported. Dark urine has been observed in some patients after a single 2 g oral dose (Schmör, 1974; Jones and Enders, 1977; Swami *et al.*, 1977).

Because tinidazole causes motor inco-ordination in animals when given in high doses, it is not recommended for patients with central nervous system disease. It is also not recommended for patients with a past history of a blood dyscrasia because, like metronidazole (page 768), it may cause a leucopenia. Alcohol should be avoided during tinidazole therapy because it may cause the 'antabuse syndrome' similar to metronidazole (page 769).

Clinical Uses of the Drug

1. *Trichomoniasis.* Tinidazole is an effective drug when given orally for the treatment of urogenital trichomoniasis in both males and females. Wherever possible the patient's sexual partner should be treated simultaneously to prevent re-infection. A high cure rate was obtained when the drug was given in an oral dose of 150 mg twice-daily for seven days, or 150 mg three times daily for five days. Subsequent to the successful use of single-dose metronidazole treat-

ment for trichomoniasis (page 769), tinidazole is now also used in this manner. A single oral dose of 2 g tinidazole results in a cure rate usually in excess of 90 per cent (Wallin and Forsgren, 1974; Schmör, 1974; Dellenbach and Muller, 1974; Thavabalan and Oriel, 1974; Swarz, 1974; Ward, 1976; Jones and Enders, 1977; Hillström et al., 1977). Lower single doses of tinidazole are not as effective (Mílek and Nedělková, 1974). The cure rate with single-dose tinidazole therapy is comparable to that obtained with single-dose metronidazole but side-effects with tinidazole may be slightly less (Weidenbach and Leix, 1974). Single-dose therapy has the advantages of being more acceptable to the patient's sexual partner, and of requiring a shorter period of abstinence from sexual intercourse and intake of alcohol.

2. *Giardiasis*. Multiple and single-dose regimens have both been used successfully to treat this disease. Andersson et al. (1972) used tinidazole in an oral dose of 150 mg twice-daily for seven days, and obtained a high cure rate amongst students in Sweden. This seven-day regimen has been found to be slightly more effective than a similar regimen using metronidazole (Levi et al., 1977). Single-dose therapy using 2 g of tinidazole orally has also resulted in cure rates of 90–100 per cent (Farid et al., 1974; Pettersson, 1975; Levi et al., 1977). A lower single dose of 1 g for adults was also effective in one small study (Salih and Abdalla, 1977). Pettersson (1975) used a single oral dose of 1 g to treat successfully children with giardiasis. Gazder and Banerjee (1977) compared single oral doses of 50 mg per kg body weight of tinidazole and metronidazole for the treatment of giardiasis in children; clinical and parasitological cures were much higher in the children treated with tinidazole. Similarly Welch et al. (1978) found that single doses of 1·0–1·5 g (depending on the patient's weight) of tinidazole was as effective as a five-day course of metronidazole for eradicating G. lamblia from children aged 6–9 years; the same dose of tinidazole given for three consecutive days was somewhat more effective. Patients not cured by a first course of treatment usually respond to a second course of tinidazole.

3. *Amoebiasis*. Similar to metronidazole (page 769), tinidazole is also effective for the treatment of this disease. For the treatment of intestinal infection a dose for adults of 600 mg twice-daily, for a period of five or ten days, has been used (Misra and Laiq, 1974; Joshi and Shah, 1975). Three single daily oral doses of approximately 60 mg per kg body weight have been used for children with intestinal amoebiasis; this resulted in a high cure rate and was well tolerated (Scragg and Proctor, 1977). In two studies the efficacy of an oral dose of 2 g tinidazole given for three consecutive days has been compared with an identical metronidazole regimen for the treatment of intestinal amoebiasis. Both studies showed a cure rate in excess of 90 per cent with tinidazole and one of less than 60 per cent with metronidazole (Swami et al., 1977; Singh and Kumar, 1977). In another study tinidazole in a dose of 1·0–1·5 g given for three consecutive days, or even as a single dose, was somewhat more effective than a five-day course of metronidazole in clearing E. histolytica from the faeces of children aged 6–9 years (Welch et al., 1978). Powell and Eldson-Dew (1972) found that more patients continued to pass E. histolytica cysts in stools after tinidazole therapy than after metronidazole therapy.

Hatchuel (1975) used tinidazole in a dose of 800 mg three times a day for five days to obtain a high cure rate in patients with an amoebic liver abscess.

Tinidazole was compared with metronidazole in one small study in which 19 patients with an amoebic liver abscess were treated; both drugs were given in a dose of 2 g daily for two days. The authors claimed that complete recovery occurred in all 10 patients given tinidazole and in only five of nine patients given metronidazole (Khokhani *et al.*, 1977).

4. *Anaerobic bacterial infections.* Because tinidazole is active *in vitro* against anaerobic bacteria (page 782) and its serum concentrations are prolonged after oral administration, it may be of value in the treatment of infections due to these bacteria. In one small study equally favourable results were obtained with clindamycin and tinidazole for the treatment of anaerobic wound infections in cancer patients (Klastersky *et al.*, 1977).

REFERENCES

Andersson, T., Forssel, J. and Sterner, G. (1972), 'Outbreak of giardiasis: Effect of a new antiflagellate drug, tinidazole', *Brit. med. J.*, **1**, 449.

Dellenbach, P. and Muller, P. (1974), 'Single dose therapy of urogenital trichomoniasis with 2 grams tinidazole', *Curr. Med. Res. Opin.*, **3**, 142.

Dornbusch, K. and Nord, C.-E. (1974), '*In vitro* effect of metronidazole and tinidazole on anaerobic bacteria', *Med. microbiol. Immunol.*, **160**, 265.

Edwards, D. I., Dye, M. and Carne, H. (1973), 'The selective toxicity of antimicrobial nitroheterocycline drugs', *J. gen. Microbiol.*, **76**, 135.

Farid, Z., El-Masry, N. A., Miner, W. F. and Anwar Hassan (1974), 'Tinidazole in treatment of Giardiasis', *Lancet* **2**, 721.

Forsgren, A. and Wallin, J. (1974), 'Tinidazole—a new preparation for Trichomonas vaginalis infections. I. Laboratory evaluation', *Brit. J. vener. Dis.*, **50**, 146.

Gazder, A. J. and Banerjee, M. (1977), 'Single-dose treatment of giardiasis in children: A comparison of tinidazole and metronidazole', *Curr. Med. Res. Opin.*, **5**, 164.

Hatchuel, W. (1975), 'Tinidazole for the treatment of amoebic liver disease', *S.A. Medical Journal*, **49**, 1879.

Henderson, D. K., Chow, A. W. and Guze, L. B. (1977), 'Comparative susceptibility of anaerobic bacteria to ticarcillin, cefoxitin, metronidazole and related antimicrobial agents', *Antimicrob. Ag. Chemother.*, **11**, 679.

Hillström, L., Pettersson, L. and Pálsson, E. (1977), 'Comparison of ornidazole and tinidazole in single-dose treatment of trichomoniasis in women', *Brit. J. vener. Dis.*, **53**, 193.

Howes, H. L., Jr., Lynch, J. E. and Kivlin, J. L. (1970), 'Tinidazole, a new antiprotozoal agent: Effect on Trichomonas and other protozoa', *Antimicrob. Agents Chemother.* 1969, p. 261.

Jokipii, L. and Kokipp, A. M. M. (1977), 'Bactericidal activity of metronidazole, tinidazole and ornidazole against Bacteroides fragilis *in vitro*', *J. Antimicrob. Chemother.*, **3**, 571.

Jokipii, A. M. M., Myllylä, Hokkanen, E. and Jokipii, L. (1977), 'Penetration of the blood brain carrier by metronidazole and tinidazole', *J. Antimocrob. Chemother.*, **3**, 239.

Jones, R. and Enders, P. (1977), 'An evaluation of tinidazole as single-dose therapy for the treatment of Trichomonas vaginalis', *Med. J. Aust.* **2**, 679.

Joshii, H. D. and Shah, B. M. (1975), 'A comparative study of tinidazole and metronidazole in treatment of amoebiasis', *The Indian Practitioner*, **28**, 295.

Khokhani, R. C., Garud, A. D., Deodhar, K. P., Sureka, S. B., Kulkarni, M. and Damle, V. B. (1977), 'Comparative study of tinidazole and metronidazole in amoebic liver abscess', *Curr. Med. Res. Opin.*, **5**, 161.

Klastersky, J., Husson, M., Weerts-Ruhl, D. and Daneau, D. (1977), 'Anaerobic wound infections in cancer patients: Comparative trial of clindamycin, tinidazole, and doxycycline', *Antimicrob. Ag. Chemother.*, **12**, 563.

Levi, G. C., De Avila, C. A. and Neto, V. A. (1977), 'Efficacy of various drugs for treatment of giardiasis. A comparative study', *Amer. J. Trop. Med. Hyg.*, **26**, 564.

Lindmark, D. G. and Müller, M. (1976), 'Antitrichomonad action, mutagenicity, and reduction of metronidazole and other nitroimidazoles', *Antimicrob. Ag. Chemother.*, **10**, 476.

Mílek, E. and Nedělková, E. (1974), 'Single-dose therapy with tinidazole in trichomoniasis', *Curr. Med. Res. Opin.*, **3**, 169.

Miller, M. W., Howes, H. L. and English, A. R. (1970), 'Tinidazole, a potent new antiprotozoal agent', *Antimicrob. Agents Chemother.*—1969, p. 257.

Misra, N. P. and Laiq, S. M. (1974), 'Comparative trial of tinidazole and metronidazole in intestinal amoebiasis', *Curr. Ther. Res.*, **16**, 1255.

Pettersson, T. (1975), 'Single-dose tinidazole therapy for giardiasis', *Brit. med. J.*, **1**, 395.

Plant, C. W. and Edwards, D. I. (1976), 'The effect of tinidazole metronidazole and nitrofurazone on nucleic acid synthesis in Clostridium bifermentans', *J. Antimicrob. Chemother.*, **2**, 203.

Powell, S. J. and Elsdon-Dew, R. (1972), 'Some new nitro imidazole derivatives: Clinical trials in amoebic liver abscess.' *Am. J. Trop. Med. Hyg.*, **21**, 518.

Reynolds, A. V., Hamilton-Miller, J. M. T. and Brumfitt, W. (1975), 'A comparison of the *in vitro* activity of metronidazole, tinidazole and nimorazole against Gram-negative anaerobic bacilli', *J. clin. Path.*, **28**, 775.

Salih, S. Y. and Abdalla, R. E. (1977), 'Symptomatic giardiasis in Sudanese adults and its treatment with tinidazole', *J. Trop. Med. Hyg.*, **80**, 11.

Scragg, J. N. and Proctor, E. M. (1977), 'Tinidazole treatment of acute amoebic dysentery in children', *Am. J. Trop. Med. Hyg.*, **26**, 824.

Singh, G. and Kumar, S. (1977), 'Short course of single daily dosage treatment with tinidazole and metronidazole in intestinal amoebiasis: a comparative study', *Curr. Med., Res. Opin.*, **5**, 157.

Swami, B., Lavakusulu, D. and Sitha Devi, C. (1977), 'Tinidazole and metronidazole in the treatment of intestinal amoebiasis', *Curr. Med. Res. Opin.*, **5**, 152.

Swarz, H. (1974), 'International experience with a new single 2 gram dose of tinidazole ('Fasigyn')', *Curr. Med. Res. Opin.*, **3**, 181.

Taylor, J. A., Jr., Migliardi, J. R. and Von Wittenau, M. S. (1970), 'Tinidazole and metronidazole pharmacokinetics in man and mouse', *Antimicrob. Agents Chemother.* 1969, p. 267.

Thavabalan, P. B. and Oriel, J. D. (1974), 'Single-dose treatment of vaginal trichomonasis with tinidazole ('Fasigyn'), *Curr. Med. Res. Opin.*, **2**, 178.

Wallin, J. and Forsgren, A. (1974), 'Tinidazole—a new preparation for T. vaginalis infections. II. Clinical evaluation of treatment with a single oral dose', *Brit. J. vener. Dis.*, **50**, 148.

Ward, J. P. (1976), 'Tinidazole (Fasigyn)—single-dose therapy for Trichomonas vaginalis', *Med. J. Aust.*, **2**, 651.

Weidenbach, A. and Leix, H. (1974), 'Treatment of trichomonal vaginitis with a single dose of tinidazole', *Curr. Med. Res. Opin.*, **3**, 147.

Welch, J. S., Rowsell, B. J. and Freeman, C. (1978), 'Treatment of intestinal amoebiasis and giardiasis. Efficacy of metronidazole and tinidazole compared', *Med. J. Aust.*, **1**, 469.

Welling, P. G. and Monro, A. M. (1972), 'The pharmacokinetics of metronidazole and tinidazole in man', *Arzneim-Forsch*, **22**, 2128.

Wood, B. A. and Monro, A. M. (1975), 'Pharmacokinetics of tinidazole and metronidazole in women after single large oral doses', *Brit. J. vener. Dis.*, **51**, 51.

Wüst, J. (1977), 'Susceptibility of anaerobic bacteria to metronidazole, ornidazole, and tinidazole and routine susceptibility testing by standardized methods', *Antimicrob. Ag. Chemother.*, **11**, 631.

Nimorazole, Ornidazole and Carnidazole

These three drugs, similar to metronidazole (page 761) and tinidazole (page 782) are 5-nitroimidazole derivatives.

1. Nimorazole

Previously known as nitrimidazine, nimorazole has the chemical formula 1-(N-beta-ethylmorpholino)-5-nitroimidazole, and is marketed with the trade name of 'Nagoxin' (Carlo Erba). Similar to metronidazole and tinidazole it has antitrichomonal activity (de Carneri et al., 1969; Lindmark and Müller, 1976). For the treatment of trichomoniasis a single oral dose of 2 g is recommended (Willcox, 1977). Nimorazole is also used for the treatment of giardiasis with comparable effectiveness to metronidazole and tinidazole (Levi et al., 1977). The dosage used over five days was 250 twice-daily for adults, for children aged 6–10 years 125 mg three times a day, and for those aged 1–5 years 125 mg twice-daily. The only side-effects were minor gastro-intestinal symptoms. Nimorazole is also as effective as metronidazole in the treatment of acute ulcerative gingivitis (Lozdan et al., 1971). However it is about three-fold less active in vitro than tinidazole and metronidazole against obligately anaerobic Gram-negative bacilli (Reynolds et al., 1975).

2. Ornidazole

Ornidazole or alpha-(chloromethyl)-2-methyl-5-nitroimidazole-1-ethanol is marketed with the trade name of 'Tiberal' (Roche). An oral dose of 750 mg of ornidazole produces a mean peak serum level of $10 \cdot 9$ μg per ml after 2–4 h; its serum half-life is $14 \cdot 4$ h and it is excreted in the urine (Schwartz and Jeunet, 1976). After an oral dose of $1 \cdot 5$ g a mean peak serum level of $33 \cdot 2$ μg per ml is reached in 2 h, mean levels of $9 \cdot 2$, $2 \cdot 6$ and $0 \cdot 8$ μg per ml remaining at 24, 48 and 72 h respectively (Matheson et al., 1977). Ornidazole has been used to treat amoebiasis, giardiasis and vaginal trichomoniasis. Single oral dose treatment has been used successfully for trichomoniasis using either 2 g or $1 \cdot 5$ g (Sköld et al., 1977; Hillström et al., 1977). Ornidazole like tinidazole and metronidazole is also active against obligately anaerobic bacteria (Wüst, 1977; Jokipii and Jokipii, 1977). One disadvantage of this drug is that it has a higher frequency of side-effects, in particular dizziness when given as single dose of $2 \cdot 0$ or $1 \cdot 5$ g (Sköld et al., 1977; Matheson et al., 1977). An injectable form of ornidazole has recently been developed (Sankale et al., 1978). When $0 \cdot 5$ g of this preparation is administered by rapid intravenous injection over 5 min, peak serum levels of 13 ± 5 μg per ml are attained and the elimination half-life is

10·8 ± 2 h. Intravenous ornidazole in a daily dose of 1–2 g for five days is effective for the treatment of adults with amoebic colitis or amoebic liver abscess (Sankale *et al.*, 1978).

3. Carnidazole

This is a new nitroimidazole derivative which has the chemical formula (O-methyl (2-(2-methyl-5-nitro-1 H-imidazol-2-yl)ethyl) carbamothioate). This drug has been given in the form of enteric coated tablets to lessen side-effects (Notowicz *et al.*, 1977). An oral dose of 2 g has resulted in a high cure rate of vaginal trichomoniasis. Mild side-effects including nausea, vomiting, diarrhoea, gastric discomfort and dizziness, have been reported.

REFERENCES

de Carneri, I., Cantone, A., Emaneuli, A., Giraldi, P. N., Logemann, W., Meinardi, G., Monti, G., Nannini, G., Tosolini, G. and Vita, G. (1969), 'Nitrimidazine: A new systemic trichomonacide', *6th International Congress of Chemotherapy*, Tokyo (Kyoto).

Hillström, L., Pettersson, L., Pálsson, E. and Sandström, S. O. (1977), 'Comparison of ornidazole and tinidazole in single-dose treatment of trichomoniasis in women', *Brit. J. vener. Dis.*, **53**, 193.

Jokipii, L. and Jokipii, A. M. M. (1977), 'Bactericidal activity of metronidazole, tinidazole and ornidazole against Bacteroides fragilis *in vitro*'. *J. Antimicrob. Chemother.*, **3**, 571.

Levi, G. C., De Ávila, C. A. and Neto, V. A. (1977), 'Efficacy of various drugs for treatment of giardiasis'. *Amer. J. Trop. Med. Hyg.*, **26**, 564.

Lindmark, D. G. and Müller, M. (1976), 'Antitrichomonad action, mutagenicity and reduction of metronidazole and other nitroimidazoles', *Antimicrob. Ag. Chemother.*, **10**, 476.

Lozdan, J., Sheiham, A., Pearlman, B. A., Keiser, B., Rachanis, C. C. and Meyer, R. (1971), 'The use of nitrimidazine in the treatment of acute ulcerative gingivitis. A double-blind controlled trial', *Brit. Dent. J.*, **130**, 294.

Matheson, I., Hernborg Johannessen, K. and Bjørkvoll, B. (1977), 'Plasma levels after a single oral dose of 1·5 g ornidazole', *Brit. J. vener. Dis.*, **53**, 236.

Notowicz, A., Stolz, E. and De Koning, G. A. J. (1977), 'First experiences with single-dose treatment of vaginal trichomoniasis with carnidazole (R 25831)', *Brit. J. vener. Dis.*, **53**, 129.

Reynolds, A. V., Hamilton-Miller, J. M. T. and Brumfitt, W. (1975), 'A comparison of the *in vitro* activity of metronidazole, tinidazole, and nimorazole against Gram-negative anaerobic bacilli', *J. clin. Path.*, **28**, 775.

Sankale, M., Coly, D., Thomas, J., Courbil, L., Condat, M., Fernex, F. M. and Felix, H. (1978), 'Infectable ornidazole in severe amoebiasis' In Siegenthaler, W. and Lüthy, R. (Ed.), *Current Chemotherapy: Proceedings of the 10th International Congress of Chemotherapy*, Zurich/Switzerland, 1977. American Society for Microbiology, Washington, D.C., p. 140.

Schwartz, D. E. and Jeunet, F. (1976), 'Comparative pharmacokinetic studies of or-nidazole and metronidazole in man', *Chemotherapy*, **22**, 19.

Sköld, M., Gnarpe, H. and Hillström, L. (1977), 'Ornidazole: A new antiprotozoal compound for treatment of Trichomonas vaginalis infection', *Brit. J. vener. Dis.*, **53**, 44.

Willcox, R. R. (1977). 'How suitable are available pharmaceuticals for the treatment of sexually transmitted diseases? I. Conditions presenting as genitial discharges', *Brit. J. vener. Dis.*, **53**, 314.

Wüst, J. (1977), 'Susceptibility of anaerobic bacteria to metronidazole, ornidazole, and tinidazole and routine susceptibility testing by standardized methods', *Antimicrob. Ag. Chemother.*, **11**, 631.

Methenamine Mandelate and Methenamine Hippurate

Description

1. *Methenamine (hexamine, hexamethylenetetramine or urotropin)* was introduced into clinical use as a urinary antiseptic as long ago as 1894. The antiseptic action of this cyclic hydrocarbon depends on its hydrolysis to formaldehyde and ammonia. This process takes place in the urine and it only occurs to a significant degree when the urine is acid. *In vitro* studies suggest that an effective bacteristatic concentration of formaldehyde is likely to be achieved if the urine pH is less than 5·7–5·85 when recommended doses are used (Musher and Griffith, 1974). The drug is thereby entirely dependent for its effect on proper acidification of the urine (Kass, 1955). Formaldehyde is not released while methenamine circulates in the blood.

2. *Mandelic acid,* another urinary antiseptic, which is excreted unchanged in the urine, was introduced into clinical use by Rosenheim (1935). It is promoted as being antibacterial and also for making the urine more acid. However *in vitro* it (and hippuric acid, *vide infra*) has a minimal bacteristatic effect (Vainrub and Musher 1977), and in the doses used, there is no evidence that mandelic acid or hippuric acid significantly lower urine pH (Musher and Griffith, 1974).

3. *Methenamine mandelate and methenamine hippurate.* These two drugs are chemical combinations of methenamine with mandelic acid and hippuric acid respectively. It has been claimed that methenamine hippurate is effective in lower doses than methenamine mandelate and that additional urinary acidification is unnecessary (Gibson, 1970), but the latter has been refuted (*vide supra*).

In Australia only methenamine mandelate ('Mandelamine', Warner) and methenamine hippurate ('Hiprex', Riker) are available, but in the United States methenamine and methenamine sulfosalicylate are also available commercially.

Sensitive Organisms

As the antibacterial activity in the urine, produced by these compounds, is due to liberated formaldehyde (to which all microorganisms are susceptible), both methenamine mandelate and hippurate are active against all Gram-positive and Gram-negative bacteria and also against fungi. Urinary tract infections due to urea splitting organisms such as Proteus spp. will not respond to these drugs, because the urine cannot be acidified in the presence of these infections, and therefore formaldehyde is not liberated. The use of acetohydroxamic acid, a urease inhibitor, together with methenamine, has been suggested for the treatment of urinary infections by Proteus spp. (Musher *et al.*, 1976). Acquired resistance is never a problem with these compounds because bacteria and fungi do not become resistant to formaldehyde.

Mode of Administration and Dosage

These drugs are administered by the oral route. Enteric coated tablets are usually used to ensure that formaldehyde is not liberated in the acid containing stomach.

1. *Methenamine mandelate.* The dose of this drug for adults is 1·0 g six-hourly, and a total daily dose of six g should not be exceeded. For children the dose is 50–60 mg per kg body weight per day, administered in four divided doses. When methenamine mandelate is used, the urine pH should be ascertained from time to time, and if it is higher than 5·5, additional acidifying agents are recommended. Either ammonium chloride, ascorbic acid or methionine have been suggested in a dose of 3–6 g daily, but sometimes even higher doses have been used. For instance Zangwill *et al.* (1962) used doses as high as 8–18 g methionine daily for adults, but such doses of this substance may cause central nervous system and gastro-intestinal disturbances. Some authors therefore have preferred ascorbic acid as an acidifying agent (Holland and West, 1963). However Vainrub and Musher (1977) could not demonstrate any acidification when ascorbic acid was used in a dose of 4·0 g daily. They considered that even if urine acidification were achieved, it would be short-lived because of renal buffering mechanisms, and a lasting effect on urine pH would only result from doses that produce metabolic acidosis. Excessive fluid intake should be avoided when methenamine mandelate (or hippurate) are used, to avoid dilution of methenamine in the urine and to reduce frequency of micturition, thereby increasing the duration of exposure of bacteria to formaldehyde in the urine (*vide infra*).

2. *Methenamine hippurate.* The usual adult dose is 1·0 g twice-daily.

3. *Patients with renal failure.* In these patients the urinary excretion of methenamine salts is impaired, so that these drugs are usually contraindicated in the presence of renal failure. In mild cases of renal functional impairment it may be possible to use either of the methenamine salts in reduced doses, but with more severe renal failure, toxic serum levels and inadequate urine concentrations will result. The additional acid load due to these drugs may be particularly dangerous in uraemia (US Public Health, 1968).

Absorption and Excretion

Methenamine mandelate and hippurate are both rapidly absorbed from the gastro-intestinal tract (Knight *et al.*, 1952; Gibson, 1970). Antimicrobial activity is not achieved in the blood, as the methenamine moiety does not liberate formaldehyde in serum and mandelic or hippuric acid serum levels are too low to exert any antibacterial effect. Methenamine is rapidly excreted in urine, where some antibacterial activity is demonstrable within half-an-hour of administration; this activity is maintained for at least 6 h and over 90 per cent of an administered dose is excreted in the urine within 24 h. About 20 per cent of methenamine excreted in the urine is converted to formaldehyde, provided the urine pH is 5·0. At urinary pH levels higher than this, the proportion of formaldehyde liberated is less. Even in an acid medium (pH5–6), it takes 30 to 90 min to generate inhibitory concentrations of formaldehyde.

The mandelic or hippuric acid moieties are also rapidly excreted in the urine in active unchanged forms, by both glomerular filtration and tubular secretion.

Toxicity

Both methenamine salts are generally well tolerated, but some patients develop gastro-intestinal side-effects such as nausea, vomiting and diarrhoea. High doses or prolonged administration may lead to urinary tract irritation due to the liberated formaldehyde. This may result in frequency, dysuria, albuminuria and haematuria. One patient has been described who developed generalized oedema, urticaria and dyspnoea, which appeared to be a reaction to methenamine mandelate (US Public Health, 1968). No evidence of bone-marrow depression, liver damage or peripheral neuritis has been observed when these drugs have been used in the recommended doses (Gibson, 1970). The methenamine salts should be avoided in patients with gout because these drugs may precipitate urate crystals in their urine (US Public Health, 1968).

Clinical Uses of the Drugs

Methenamine mandelate or methenamine hippurate are only suitable for the treatment of urinary tract infections. They are nowadays rarely used because many other chemotherapeutic agents are available. In addition the use of drugs such as methenamine, nalidixic acid (page 737) and nitrofurantoin (page 756), which produce negligible therapeutic tissue levels, is questionable in anything other than uncomplicated lower urinary tract infections (see page 757). Because of the time taken to produce antibacterial concentrations of formaldehyde in urine (vide supra), methenamine would not be expected to be effective in upper urinary tract infections.

These drugs may still have a role in chronic bacteriuria, particularly if the infection is caused by highly resistant Gram-negative bacilli or by yeasts, because all such pathogens are susceptible to formaldehyde. Methenamine mandelate has also been used successfully for prolonged suppressive therapy in this condition (Zangwill et al., 1962; Holland and West, 1963; US Public Health, 1968). The usually recommended doses are used for long-term therapy. Nevertheless when used as long-term therapy in chronic bacteriuria in men, methenamine mandelate is less successful if underlying genito-urinary pathology is present (Freeman et al., 1975). Methenamine hippurate is not as effective as co-trimoxazole (page 706) in preventing recurrent urinary tract infections in patients with underlying abnormalities of the urinary tract (Kalowski et al., 1975). Vainrub and Musher (1977) investigated the effect of methenamine mandelate (and ascorbic acid) on bacteriuria in paraplegic and quadraplegic patients. The drug was of no value in preventing infection in patients with indwelling catheters (to be expected in view of the short duration of the drug in the urine), and those receiving intermittent catheterization. Even the prophylactic use of methenamine in women with recurrent urinary infections without underlying urinary tract abnormalities is in doubt; co-trimoxazole seems to have distinct advantages in this situation (page 706). It now appears that there are very few indications for the use of methenamine and its derivatives.

REFERENCES

Freeman, R. B., McFate Smith, W., Richardson, J. A., Hennelly, P. J., Thurm, R. H., Urner, C., Vaillancourt, J. A., Griep, R. J. and Bromer, L. (1975), 'Long-term therapy for chronic bacteriuria in men', U.S. Public Health Service Cooperative Study'. *Ann. Intern. Med.,* **83,** 133.

Gibson, G. R. (1970), 'A clinical appraisal of methenamine hippurate in urinary tract infections', *Med. J. Aust.,* **1,** 167.

Holland, N. H. and West, C. D. (1963), 'Prevention of recurrent urinary tract infections in girls', *Amer. J. Dis. Child.,* **105,** 560.

Kalowski, S., Nanra, R. S., Friedman, A., Radford, N., Standish, H., and Kincaid-Smith, P. (1975), 'Controlled trial comparing co-trimoxazole and methenamine hippurate in the prevention of recurrent urinary tract infections', *Med. J. Aust.,* **1,** 585.

Kass, E. H. (1955), 'Chemotherapeutic and antibiotic drugs in the management of infections of the urinary tract', *Amer. J. Med.,* **18,** 764.

Knight, V., Draper, J. W., Brady, E. A. and Attmore, C. A. (1952), 'Methenamine mandelate: Antimicrobial activity, absorption and excretion', *Antibiot. Chemother.,* **2,** 615.

Musher, D. M. and Griffith, D. P. (1974), 'Generation of formaldehyde from methenamine: Effect of pH and concentration, and antibacterial effect', *Antimicrob. Ag. Chemother.,* **6,** 708.

Musher, D. M., Griffith, D. P. and Templeton, G. B. (1976), 'Further observations on the potentiation of the antibacterial effect of methenamine by acetohydroxamic acid', *J. Infect. Dis.,* **133,** 564.

Rosenheim, M. L. (1935), 'Mandelic acid in the treatment of urinary infections', *Lancet,* **1,** 1032; quoted by Zangwill *et al.* (1962).

U.S. Public Health Service Cooperative Study (1968), 'Prevention of recurrent bacteriuria with continuous chemotherapy', *Ann. Intern. Med.,* **69,** 655.

Vainrub, B. and Musher, D. M. (1977), 'Lack of effect of methenamine in suppression of, or prophylaxis against, chronic urinary infection', *Antimicrob. Ag. Chemother.,* **12,** 625.

Zangwill, D. P., Porter, P. J., Kaitz, A. L., Cotran, R. S., Bodel, P. T. and Kass, E. H. (1962), 'Antibacterial organic acids in chronic urinary tract infection', *Arch. Intern. Med.,* **110,** 801.

Part III
Drugs Mainly for Tuberculosis

Isoniazid

Description

Isoniazid, isonicotinic acid hydrazide or INAH was discovered independently in 1952 at both Squibb and Roche Laboratories (Bernstein *et al.*, 1952; Fox, 1953). Animal studies showed that isoniazid was a very potent antituberculosis drug, and subsequent clinical trials confirmed its high efficacy for the treatment of human tuberculosis (An Interim Report, 1952). In addition, isoniazid is relatively non-toxic and cheap, and despite the development of other drugs, it remains one of the best drugs for the treatment of tuberculosis.

Activity against Mycobacteria

Isoniazid is highly active against Mycobacterium tuberculosis, most strains being inhibited by $0.05-0.20 \mu g$ per ml. The minimum inhibitory concentration for the standard H37 RV reference strain of M. tuberculosis is $0.05 \mu g$ per ml. Strains are considered to be isoniazid-sensitive if the MIC is $0.20 \mu g$ per ml or less i.e. a Resistance Ratio of 4 or less (*see* streptomycin, page 296).

Isoniazid-resistant strains of M. tuberculosis can be readily produced *in vitro,* and these also occur *in vivo* if this drug is used singly for treatment of tuberculosis. For instance, in an early clinical trial in which 173 patients were treated by isoniazid alone, resistant tubercle bacilli were found in 11 per cent of patients at the end of the first month, in 52 per cent at the end of the second, and in 71 per cent at the end of the third month (An Interim Report, 1952). Nowadays isoniazid is always used in combination with one or two other antituberculosis drugs, and this usually prevents emergence of isoniazid-resistant strains.

Occasionally strains of M. tuberculosis resistant to isoniazid are isolated from patients who have not received previous treatment with this drug. Such 'primary drug resistance' is relatively rare in developed countries such as Britain, North America and Australia, and in these areas it does not appear to be increasing in incidence. In a large survey in Britain in 1963 the incidence of primary isoniazid resistance (1.7 per cent) had not increased significantly during the previous seven years (Miller *et al.*, 1966). The situation regarding isoniazid resistance seems similar in Australia; during the five-year period 1972–1976, it had a mean incidence of 1.8 per cent (Commonwealth Dept. Health Australia, 1973–1977).

In North America the incidence of primary resistance is also generally low. In a co-operative study involving 22 hospitals in the United States during an eight-year period 1961 through 1968, the overall average resistance to isoniazid was 1.8 per cent and there was no indication that this was increasing

(Doster *et al.*, 1976). Similarly in a continuing study of drug resistance in veterans in the United States from 1969 to 1973, primary resistance to isoniazid remained less than 4·4 per cent and had not increased (Hobby *et al.*, 1971; 1974). In a smaller study in Massachusetts in 1972, Stottmeier and Burkes (1974) detected primary resistance in 3·46 per cent of strains; they also noted an increased incidence of resistance to two or three antituberculous drugs (including isoniazid) in residents of Boston who were addicted to alcohol or narcotics, or who were contacts of tuberculous relatives or friends. In 1975/76 the incidence of primary isoniazid resistance in Massachusetts was 2·65 per cent (Stottmeier and Baker, 1977) but in the Greater Boston area it was more than double the incidence in the rest of the state (Khan, 1977). A higher incidence of isoniazid resistance has also been detected in children of low socio-economic status (Steiner *et al.*, 1973). More recent studies in the United States suggest that there may be a significant variation in the rate of primary drug resistance from one geographic area to another (Glassroth *et al.*, 1977).

In certain Asian areas the incidence of primary drug resistance to isoniazid and other 'first-line' antituberculosis drugs, is quite high (Leading article, 1972). Although the level of primary resistance in developing countries is usually higher, it has not increased appreciably (WHO, 1975).

'Secondary (acquired) drug resistance' to isoniazid develops in patients who have been treated with the drug, either singly or in conjunction with other drugs, and is usually manifested clinically as failed chemotherapy or a relapse.

BCG (Bacille Calmette-Guérin) organisms are usually susceptible to the major antituberculosis drugs including isoniazid. A persisting finger infection due to accidental innoculation with BCG has been described which was caused by a strain resistant to isoniazid (Lorber *et al.*, 1977).

'Anonymous mycobacteria' (page 832) are usually isoniazid-resistant (Barter and Camens, 1968), but M. kansasii is sometimes sensitive (Pyle, 1970, Harris *et al.*, 1975). Isoniazid is inactive against M. ulcerans (Quinn and Crotty, 1963).

Mode of Administration and Dosage

1. *Daily administration*. Isoniazid is nearly always administered by the oral route. The usual adult dose for the treatment of pulmonary tuberculosis is 5–8 mg per kg body weight per day, administered preferably as a single dose but it may be given in two divided doses. A common adult dose is 300 mg daily or 150 mg twice a day. A single dose a day is somewhat more effective than two divided doses (Fox, 1977). For severely ill patients such as those with tuberculous meningitis or miliary tuberculosis, the dose is usually doubled to 10 mg per kg body weight per day, an adult dose of 150 mg every 6 h. In children a dose of 10–15 mg per kg per day is recommended for all forms of tuberculosis.

When the drug is administered daily, it is not necessary to determine whether patients are slow or rapid inactivators of isoniazid (page 804), because with standard daily doses results of treatment have been satisfactory in both groups, and also toxic effects have been uncommon.

2. *Intermittent administration*. Regimens of thrice-weekly, twice-weekly or even once-weekly administration of antituberculosis drugs, given under close supervision, have been introduced in an attempt to obviate the unreliable self-

administration of these drugs over prolonged periods, particularly in developing countries (Fox, 1971; Citron, 1972; Fox and Mitchison, 1975). Intermittent chemotherapy is equally effective to daily drug administration (page 811); it is usually cheaper and sometimes may be less toxic. The dose of isoniazid for a bi-weekly regimen is higher than the usual daily dose, and 15 mg per kg body weight is recommended (Fox, 1971; Tub. Chemother. Centre, 1973a).

Although the antituberculosis drugs pyrazinamide (page 842) and ethambutol (page 833) can be administered safely and effectively in greatly increased doses once a week, there have been difficulties in adapting isoniazid to such a regimen. For instance, isoniazid used in a dose of 13–17 mg per kg once a week has been unsatisfactory, because resistant organisms have emerged in some patients, especially in those who are rapid isoniazid inactivators (page 804) (Tub. Chemother. Centre, 1973b; WHO Prague, 1977). Alternatively increasing the once-weekly isoniazid dose to 30 mg per kg body weight may cause acute toxicity, especially in patients who inactivate the drug slowly. Where it is practicable to investigate the patient's inactivator status, streptomycin plus isoniazid can be administered once-weekly to slow inactivators and twice-weekly to rapid inactivators (Fox, 1968; WHO Prague, 1977). Slow-release isoniazid formulations (either enteric-coated tablets or isoniazid-matrix preparations) have been developed in an attempt to overcome these difficulties. Preliminary pharmacological studies in humans (Ellard et al., 1972; 1973; Sarma et al., 1975), studies with experimental tuberculosis in guinea pigs (Dickinson et al., 1973), and a trial on Indian patients with tuberculosis (Santha et al., 1976), indicate that the administration of a slow-release preparation of isoniazid (matrix isoniazid) once a week is feasible. Matrix isoniazid in a dose of 35 mg per kg body weight in slow inactivators and 50 mg per kg in rapid inactivators produces peak serum levels similar to those obtained with a nontoxic dose of ordinary isoniazid (15 mg per kg) in slow inactivators; matrix isoniazid in a lower dose of 30 mg per kg in rapid inactivators however produced substantially lower serum levels (Sarma et al., 1975). A six-month trial of matrix isoniazid in Indian patients with tuberculosis in a dose of 50 mg per kg for rapid inactivators (27 patients) and 35 mg per kg for slow inactivators (37 patients), each given weekly with streptomycin 1 g, demonstrated that this regimen was tolerated by most patients (Santha et al., 1976). Other studies using a slow release form of matrix isoniazid in Czechoslovakian patients have resulted in an unacceptable level of adverse reactions in both rapid and slow inactivators (WHO Prague, 1977). The efficacy and acceptability of a combination of ordinary isoniazid with a lower dose of the matrix preparation is currently being investigated.

Another approach is to use ordinary isoniazid in a dose of 15 mg per kg once-weekly for slow inactivators (in whom reasonably satisfactory results are obtained by this method), and to develop a slow-release preparation for use in rapid inactivators only. Eidus et al. (1974) studied a preparation consisting of 37 per cent ordinary isoniazid and 63 per cent of an isoniazid matrix component. A triple dose of this preparation (45 mg per kg) produced similar serum levels in rapid isoniazid inactivators to those attained in slow inactivators with 15 mg per kg of ordinary isoniazid, which is the usual dose for intermittent chemotherapy. It was suggested that this matrix formula may be suitable for once-weekly isoniazid administration to rapid inactivators of the drug. However there is considerable individual variation among the rapid inactivators, and therefore one standard isoniazid slow-release formula and dosage may not be suitable for all patients who inactivate the drug rapidly.

3. *Patients with renal failure.* Some active isoniazid is excreted via the kidney, so that the drug accumulates and some dosage reduction is necessary in patients with moderate or severe renal functional impairment (Kovnat *et al.*, 1973). Cheigh (1977) recommends that usual doses of 300–400 mg per day may be given to patients with mild renal failure or to patients undergoing dialysis; those with severe disease not receiving dialysis or those who are slow acetylators should be given 200–300 mg per day. However Usuda and Sekine (1978) found that most patients on dialysis treated with customary doses of isoniazid developed peripheral neuritis (page 806); they considered that a safe effective dose of isoniazid was 5 mg per kg per day, three times a week for patients on dialysis. Significant amounts of isoniazid are removed by peritoneal dialysis and haemodialysis (Bennett *et al.*, 1977). Where possible the dose of isoniazid should be adjusted according to monitored serum levels in patients with renal disease.

4. *Parenteral administration.* A solution containing 50 mg in 2 ml suitable for intramuscular or intravenous administration is available; this is effective and it is only rarely used, such as in circumstances when oral administration is not feasible.

Availability

1. Tablets: 50 and 100 mg.
2. Isoniazid is also available in various powders and granules combined with para-amino salicylic acid e.g. 150 mg isoniazid with 6 g PAS.
3. Isoniazid combined with rifampicin is also available, e.g. isoniazid 100 mg and rifampicin 150 mg.

Serum Levels in Relation to Dosage

Isoniazid is very well absorbed from the gastro-intestinal tract, and the peak serum level is reached 1–2 h after administration. After a single large dose of 12·5 mg per kg body weight (800–1000 mg in an adult), the peak level is 10–15 μg per ml. A similar peak serum level is attained by all patients at this time, but 4–6 h after administration serum levels differ according to whether the subject is a rapid or slow isoniazid inactivator. In the former, serum levels at 6 h approach zero, whilst in the latter a level of 5 μg per ml is still present (Fig. 36). The serum half-life of isoniazid in slow inactivators is 2–4 h and that in rapid inactivators 0·5–1·5 h (Bennett *et al.*, 1977).

Evans *et al.* (1960) studied isoniazid serum levels in 484 subjects 6 h after the administration of a single dose of 9·8–10 mg per kg body weight. The frequency-distribution curve for these values showed two peaks, separated by a trough (an antimode) at 2·5 μg per ml. Persons with serum isoniazid concentrations less than this value (most commonly about 1·0 μg per ml) were classified as 'rapid inactivators', whereas those with serum levels higher than 2·5 (most commonly 4·5 μg per ml) as 'slow inactivators'.

Serum levels are lower with the smaller doses which are commonly used for daily chemotherapy, and halving the dose approximately halves the serum

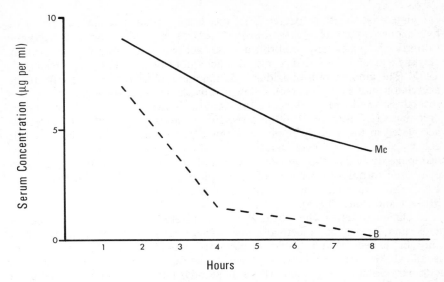

Fig. 36. Serum concentrations in patients after a single 800 mg isoniazid dose (MC-slow inactivator; B-rapid inactivator (Redrawn after Short, 1962.)

levels. Furthermore, the concomitant administration of aluminium hydroxide gel interferes with the gastro-intestinal absorption of isoniazid, resulting in lower serum levels. Therefore it has been recommended that isoniazid should be given at least one hour before the administration of antacids to patients receiving both forms of therapy (Hurwitz and Schlozman, 1974).

Excretion

URINE: Some unchanged active isoniazid is excreted via the kidney, and the amount excreted in the first 1–2 h after administration is about the same in all subjects. However 'slow inactivators' excreted about ten times more active isoniazid in the urine compared to 'rapid inactivators' from about the sixth hour after administration (Short, 1962). Approximately 70 per cent of administered isoniazid is excreted via the kidney, but most of this is in an inactive form. The main inactive substances excreted are acetyl isoniazid and isonicotinic acid, but there are others such as hydrazones of isoniazid (Robson and Sullivan, 1963). Fast inactivators excrete approximately 94 per cent of isoniazid as acetyl isoniazid and its metabolites and only 2·8 per cent and 3·6 per cent as free isoniazid and isoniazid hydrazone conjugates respectively. By contrast, slow inactivators excrete almost 37 per cent of the drug as either free isoniazid or its hydrazone conjugates and only 63 per cent as acetyl isoniazid and its metabolites of isonicotinic acid and acetylhydrazine (Mitchell et al., 1976).

INACTIVATION IN BODY: The metabolism of isoniazid has been extensively studied in man and animals (Hughes, 1953). The main method by which this drug is inactivated in man is acetylation in the liver by an enzyme N-acetyl transferase which converts it to acetyl isoniazid, which in turn is partly metabolized by hydrolysis to isonicotinic acid and acetylhydrazine. Non-acetylated isoniazid is excreted in the urine, either unchanged or as its hydrazone conjugates (*vide supra*). The rate at which humans acetylate isoniazid is genetically controlled, and accordingly they can be broadly classified as slow or rapid isoniazid inactivators or acetylators (Peters *et al.*, 1965). The amount of isoniazid acetylation metabolites in the urine reflects the acetylator status of the person. 'Slow inactivators' are autosomal homozygous recessives, and 'rapid inactivators' either heterozygous or homozygous dominants (Evans *et al.*, 1960; Harris, 1963). Isoniazid and sulphonamides are acetylated in the liver by similar enzymatic processes, and so an individual is either a slow or rapid inactivator of both of these drugs (Rao *et al.*, 1970) (*see also* page 667). Over 90 per cent of Orientals are genetically rapid inactivators compared to only 45 per cent of black and white Americans (Mitchell *et al.*, 1976). There are an equal number of slow and fast inactivators in Australia (Birkett and Pond, 1975).

In clinical practice when the drug is administered daily, there is little need to determine the patient's inactivator status (page 800). On theoretical grounds it may be expected that 'rapid inactivators' would require higher doses of isoniazid. Most studies, however, have shown that when isoniazid is combined with para-amino salicylic acid (PAS) in standard doses, the clinical results are not influenced by the patient's isoniazid inactivation phenotype (Harris, 1963). Also studies in children with primary tuberculosis, in whom isoniazid was used as a single drug prophylactically, show that results are about the same in both phenotypic groups (Mount *et al.*, 1961). Nevertheless peripheral neuritis due to isoniazid (page 806) appears to be related to high serum levels of the active drug, and is more common in slow isoniazid inactivators (Evans *et al.*, 1960; Harris, 1963), whilst rapid inactivators may be more prone to hepatotoxicity (*see* page 809).

If isoniazid is included in intermittent regimens, to ensure its effectiveness, it may be important to determine the patient's inactivator status (page 801). Several simple laboratory methods have been described for this purpose, such as various isoniazid urine analyses (Russell, 1970; Eidus and Hodgkin, 1973; Ellard and Gammon, 1973), and the sulphadimidine acetylation test (Rao *et al.*, 1970).

Higher active isoniazid serum levels have been demonstrated when PAS and isoniazid are administered together, suggesting that PAS may inhibit isoniazid acetylation (Lauener and Favez, 1959). These findings have not been confirmed by others (Robson and Sullivan, 1963). In any case it is now generally accepted that the therapeutic superiority of combined isoniazid/PAS therapy versus isoniazid alone is not attributable to the possible effect of PAS on isoniazid serum levels. It is due to the additional antituberculosis activity of PAS itself and its ability to prevent the emergence of isoniazid-resistant strains of M. tuberculosis.

Distribution of the Drug in Body

After absorption, isoniazid is widely distributed in body fluids and tissues (Harris, 1963; Robson and Sullivan, 1963). Concentrations of the drug in the cerebrospinal fluid of normal patients and those with tuberculous meningitis are approximately the same as those in the serum (Forgan-Smith *et al.*, 1973).

Adequate concentrations of isoniazid occur in pleural effusions and in all body tissues and are similar to serum levels. It readily penetrates caseous tissues, and by its entry into macrophages is active against intracellular tubercle bacilli. The drug also easily crosses the placenta and is excreted in human milk. The serum protein binding of isoniazid is less than 10 per cent (Bennett *et al.*, 1977).

Mode of Action

Since its discovery, the mode of action of isoniazid has been extensively studied. Early investigations suggested that the drug interfered with the formation of an essential metabolite for the tubercle bacillus (Barclay *et al.*, 1953). It was suggested that it interfered with the biosynthesis of nucleic acids (Wimpenny, 1967), but other data indicated that its lethal effect on tubercle bacilli precedes blocking of nucleic acid synthesis (Youatt, 1969). The drug also inhibits the synthesis of mycolic acids in M. tuberculosis by affecting an enzyme, mycolase synthetase, which is unique for the mycobacteria. The inhibitory concentration of isoniazid against this enzyme is very low and is comparable to the MIC of the drug against M. tuberculosis. However on the evidence available, it cannot be assumed that this is the main mechanism of action of isoniazid on tubercle bacilli (Takayama *et al.*, 1972; Wang and Takayama, 1972), and the drug's exact mode of action remains unknown (McDonald, 1974). Isoniazid has a bactericidal action on Mycobacterium tuberculosis.

Toxicity

Isoniazid is a drug of relatively low toxicity. Patients treated with it for periods of approximately two years rarely exhibit any untoward reactions. Extensive experience with this drug indicates that it can be safely used in pregnancy.

1. *Gastro-intestinal side-effects.* These are very uncommon, but nausea, vomiting and diarrhoea may occur if very large doses, such as 20 mg per kg body weight per day are given (Robson and Sullivan, 1963). Matrix isoniazid preparations may also cause gastro-intestinal symptoms (Parthasarathy *et al.*, 1976).

2. *Hypersensitivity reactions.* These occur, but much less frequently than with PAS (page 827) or streptomycin (page 300) (Joseph, 1973). Reactions usually take the form of fever and a maculopapular rash, and may occur in patients receiving two or three antituberculosis drugs. In this situation all drugs should be temporarily stopped, and the drug responsible determined by the cautious readministration of each drug separately in very small doses. If isoniazid is incriminated, and the reaction was not serious, then by contrast to PAS (page 828), desensitization is recommended because of the value of this particular drug. Previously, small but gradually increasing doses of isoniazid administered over a period of several weeks were used for desensitization. During this period of desensitization, two other effective antituberculosis drugs should also be administered to prevent the emergence of isoniazid-resistant organisms (*Today's Drugs,* 1963). Nowadays a more rapid method of desensitization is commonly used in which isoniazid and other antituberculosis drugs are continued in the usual doses. Reactions are suppressed by corticosteroids, which are usually administered in gradually reducing dosage for about two

months (Thompson, 1969). In severely ill patients, particularly those with tuberculous meningitis, in whom isoniazid is usually essential, the drug may be continued despite a severe hypersensitivity reaction, provided that high doses of corticosteroids are administered for a prolonged period. One patient who developed acute meningoencephalitis on readministration of isoniazid and in whom 'hypersensitivity meningitis' was postulated as the cause, has been described (Garagusi et al., 1976). Stevens–Johnson syndrome associated with isoniazid administration and which recurred when a test dose of the drug was given after the patient had fully recovered, has also been described (Bomb et al., 1976).

Febrile reactions without other manifestations of hypersensitivity occurring one to three weeks after commencement of treatment have been described when isonazid has been used alone for chemoprophylaxis (Davis and Stoler, 1977).

3. *Neurotoxicity*. Psychosis, confusion, coma and convulsions may occur if toxic serum levels of the active drug are attained, such as in attempted suicide, but these symptoms do not occur if the drug is used in usual doses. The highest non-toxic dose of the drug is 15 mg per kg per day. Studies on Indian patients showed that doses of 30 mg per kg of matrix isoniazid are well-tolerated. Higher doses of this preparation caused dizziness, which was dose-related, late in onset and usually present even 24 h later (Parthasarathy et al., 1976). The matrix preparation has also been given in doses of 50 and 35 mg per kg to rapid and slow inactivators respectively. Such a regimen was used for six months in a trial in Indian patients with tuberculosis, but the dosage had to be modified in small numbers of both types of patient because of giddiness (Santha et al., 1976).

Peripheral neuritis may occur with ordinary isoniazid doses, but it is more likely with higher doses. It rarely occurs with a dosage of 5 mg per kg body weight per day, but when this dose is doubled, 10–20 per cent of patients may develop this complication (*Today's Drugs*, 1968). In addition 'slow inactivators' develop this complication more frequently than 'rapid inactivators' with equivalent doses (Robson and Sullivan, 1963). In the preliminary studies with matrix isoniazid preparations described above, peripheral neuritis has not been observed in inactivators of either type so far (Santha et al., 1976). Adult patients receiving isoniazid excrete large amounts of pyridoxine (Vitamin B6), and the neuritis may be largely due to pyridoxine deficiency. The routine administration of pyridoxine to prevent this complication is not usually recommended, but it is advocated for adults receiving large doses of isoniazid, such as 10 mg per kg per day. In addition the routine administration of pyridoxine is advisable to patients who are predisposed to peripheral neuritis by conditions such as alcoholism. Pyridoxine has no effect on the antibacterial action or the serum concentration of active isoniazid (Riemensnider and Mitchell, 1960). By contrast to adults, children receiving moderately large doses of isoniazid do not develop pyridoxine deficiency or peripheral neuritis (Robson and Sullivan, 1963).

Peripheral neuritis due to isoniazid is usually completely reversible. In practice isoniazid therapy is discontinued, but when improvement occurs the drug can be resumed in lower doses. In addition pyridoxine therapy may be beneficial.

Minor neurotoxic symptoms such as muscle twitchings, restlessness and insomnia may occur with ordinary isoniazid doses. The drug may also precipitate convulsions in stabilized epileptics and urinary retention in the elderly. Loss of memory, sometimes quite disabling, has also been noted (Leading article, 1969).

4. *Hepatotoxicity*. Originally it was considered that liver damage due to isoniazid was rare, mild and transient. It is now apparent that isoniazid frequently causes asymptomatic hepatotoxicity and that it is an occasional cause of severe clinical hepatitis. Prior to the widespread use of isoniazid chemoprophylaxis, hepatotoxicity was probably attributed to other drugs such as PAS and streptomycin, which were used concomitantly with isoniazid.

Liver damage has been observed when isoniazid was administered together with other potentially hepatotoxic antituberculosis drugs. Isoniazid may also enhance rifampicin hepatotoxicity (page 563) and this may be more common in slow acetylators who have higher isoniazid serum levels. For example, Lees *et al.* (1971) observed an increased frequency of hepatotoxicity with rifampicin/isoniazid therapy compared to a combination of rifampicin plus ethambutol. More drug toxicity (including hepatotoxicity) was also noted when isoniazid/rifampicin was used to treat patients with pulmonary tuberculosis compared to others treated with isoniazid, streptomycin and ethambutol (Ravikrishnan *et al.*, 1977). In this study hepatotoxicity was more evident in alcoholics. Elevations of serum aspartate aminotransferase (SGOT) levels were recorded in 29 per cent of 63 patients treated by both rifampicin and isoniazid, and this appeared more common in those patients who were slow isoniazid inactivators (Lal *et al.*, 1972). In a similar study of patients treated with these two drugs, Smith *et al.* (1972) found that only those patients who had elevation of serum bilirubin in addition to elevation of serum transaminase were slow inactivators. By contrast, a study in Chinese patients, who also received daily rifampicin during the first four months of a six-month course of isoniazid and pyrazinamide, did not reveal an increased incidence of hepatotoxicity (Hong Kong/BMRC, 1976a).

'Isoniazid-associated hepatitis' has been described in patients receiving this drug alone for chemoprophylaxis. Garibaldi *et al.* (1972) reported 19 cases of 'hepatitis' amongst 2321 positive tuberculin reactors receiving isoniazid prophylactically. Thirteen of these were jaundiced and two died. Clinical features and pathological findings in these patients were indistinguishable from those found in viral hepatitis. In a matched control group of 2154 subjects who were not taking isoniazid, only one case of hepatitis occurred during the same nine-month period. Moss *et al.* (1972) reported 5 and Maddrey and Boitnott (1973) reported another 14 patients with hepatitis associated with isoniazid chemoprophylaxis. In the latter study three patients died from liver failure; on rechallenge of three other patients with isoniazid, two developed an accelerated recurrence of severe liver disease and the other only an elevated transaminase. Liver histology showed hepatocellular injury similar to viral hepatitis, and there was no evidence of cholestasis. These patients had a relatively long prodrome (about two weeks) before the onset of overt hepatitis, and the liver damage was thought to be due to hypersensitivity. Isoniazid-associated hepatitis, although described, is a rare occurrence in children (Brasfield *et al.*, 1976); fatal hepatic necrosis presumably due to isoniazid chemoprophylaxis has been reported in a

15-year-old girl (Vanderhoof and Ament, 1976).

A number of studies have now shown that isoniazid frequently causes hepatotoxicity as evidenced by abnormalities of serum enzymes, particularly the serum aspartate aminotransferase (serum glutamic-oxalacetic transaminase, SGOT). About 12 per cent of adult tuberculin-positive hospital employees receiving isoniazid developed moderately raised SGOT levels, compared to a control group in New Orleans (Bailey et al., 1974). Abnormalities in SGPT (serum glutamic-pyruvic transaminase) values were also detected in 10 per cent of adolescents receiving isoniazid; these occurred without jaundice usually within the first 10 weeks of isoniazid administration; treatment was continued in all patients (except one who had a very high SGPT level) and their transaminase levels fell spontaneously (Litt et al., 1976). Similarly 25 of 369 children (6·8 per cent) receiving isoniazid chemoprophylaxis developed a raised SGOT level two months after medication was begun. They had no other evidence of hepatotoxicity and in 21 of these children isoniazid administration was continued and the SGOT levels soon decreased (Beaudry et al., 1974). Other studies have also indicated that an asymptomatic rise in the SGOT may occur in 10–20 per cent of patients given isoniazid chemoprophylaxis (American Thoracic Society, 1974; Leading article, 1975).

It is now apparent that the commonest manifestation of isoniazid liver damage is asymptomatic transaminase elevation. This may occur one week or months after commencement of isoniazid therapy, it may persist without progression or resolve spontaneously, and in most patients resolution occurs when the drug is stopped (Mitchell et al., 1976). However overt hepatitis, clinically, biochemically and pathologically indistinguishable from viral hepatitis and which can be fatal, is one of isoniazid's most important side-effects. The overall frequency of overt hepatitis is approximately one per cent, but the risk increases in older age groups particularly in those aged greater than 35 years (Center for Disease Control, 1974; Black, 1974; Kopanoff et al., 1978). The probability of developing hepatitis during a year's treatment with isoniazid in the United States ranges from 2·4 per 1000 in persons aged less than 35 years, to 19·2 per 1000 among persons 55–64 years of age (Comstock and Edwards, 1975). Hepatitis is rare under the age of twenty years. It can occur at any time during isoniazid therapy, but is more common in the first two months of treatment (Black, 1974; Mitchell et al., 1976). Drinking alcohol, especially every day, seems to increase the risk of isoniazid hepatitis (Kopanoff et al., 1978). A retrospective study has suggested that isoniazid induced hepatitis is much less common in Australia, and that there is no evidence that isoniazid chemoprophylaxis (page 815) should be confined to patients aged less than 50 years of age (Thompson, 1978). The case fatality rate of isoniazid hepatitis is not known but may be of the order of 12–20 per cent depending on the initial severity of the liver disease (Mitchell et al., 1976; Brown, 1976).

The exact mechanism of isoniazid hepatotoxicity is not yet defined. Earlier suggestions that a hypersensitivity reaction was involved (Maddrey and Boitnott, 1973) have been disputed. Mitchell et al. (1976) noted that there was no correlation between SGOT levels and isoniazid induced antinuclear antibodies (see page 809), antibodies to isoniazid were not detected and associated features of hypersensitivity such as a rash or eosinophilia were uncommon. In addition the variable and often prolonged period of treatment with isoniazid before evidence of hepatotoxicity is not usual with hypersensitivity. Mitchell *et al.* (1976) suggested that acetylhydrazine (a metabolite of isoniazid, page 803) may act as a hepatotoxin because in animals this substance can be converted to a potent acylating agent which produces liver necrosis. They also provided evidence that 'rapid inactivators' (page 804) were more prone to liver disease, probably because they metabolized more isoniazid to acetylhydrazine than 'slow inactivators'. However the predilection of 'rapid inactivators' to isoniazid hepatitis has been disputed (Brown, 1976), and the findings of a small prospective study did not indicate that inactivator status is a risk factor in isoniazid hepatotoxicity (Dickinson *et al.*, 1977).

Bailey *et al.* (1973) suggested that patients receiving isoniazid should be biochemically monitored for hepatotoxicity. This is not practical because moderate rises of transaminase levels occur in many recipients of isoniazid and in most instances these subside despite continuation of the drug, so that clinical monitoring is ineffectual in predicting serious liver disease (Mitchell *et al.*, 1976). However isoniazid administration should be immediately discontinued in any patient who develops symptoms or signs of hepatitis (Black, 1974). A Tuberculosis Advisory Committee in the United States also recommends that isoniazid chemoprophylaxis should be restricted in patients greater than 35 years of age and tuberculin reactors in this age group should be individually assessed (Center for Disease Control, 1974; American Thoracic Society, 1974) (*see* page 816). It is also advisable to cease isoniazid chemoprophylaxis in patients more than 35 years of age who develop biochemical evidence of liver injury, unless the patients are critically ill with suspected tuberculosis (Mitchell *et al.*, 1976). Because the case fatality rate is high in patients developing high SGOT levels or in those with any rise of SGOT after eight weeks of therapy with isoniazid, it is advocated that the drug should be discontinued under these circumstances (Brown, 1976). The American Thoracic Society (1974) does not recommend the routine monitoring of serum enzymes, but advocates that all recipients of preventive therapy with isoniazid should be questioned at monthly intervals about symptoms or signs of hepatitis or other toxic effects of the drug. Should a raised serum enzyme level be detected for some other reason, and it does not exceed three times the normal value, isoniazid may be continued under careful observation.

If isoniazid hepatitis occurs and it is considered that because of the patient's clinical state antituberculosis therapy should continue, antituberculosis drugs with a propensity to cause hepatitis, particularly pyrazinamide and ethionamide to which isoniazid is chemically related and to which cross-sensitivity may occur, should be avoided (Leading article, 1975). Rifampicin can also cause liver damage and its use in this situation should be assessed according to the individual circumstances. Drugs which should be considered for such a patient include streptomycin (page 301), ethambutol (page 836), cycloserine (page 460) and capreomycin (page 851) (*see also* page 563).

5. *Miscellaneous side-effects.* Good *et al.* (1965) described seven patients who developed pain and contractures in the shoulders and arms, which appeared to be associated with isoniazid therapy. Acute arthritis, associated with fever and periorbital oedema has been described in a woman after nine days treatment with isoniazid; subsequently this arthritis rapidly recurred after one dose of isoniazid (Periman and Venkataramani, 1975). Antinuclear an-

tibodies occur in a large proportion of tuberculous patients treated with isoniazid for prolonged periods. This is usually asymptomatic but an occasional patient may develop overt systemic lupus erythematosis (Alarćon-Segovia et al., 1969; Alarćon-Segovia et al., 1971).

Theoretically there has been some concern that isoniazid may be carcinogenic because it can induce neoplasms in albino mice (Leading article, 1966). However there have been no indications of an increased risk of cancer in two follow-up studies of patients who have been treated with isoniazid 10–15 and about 20 years previously (Hammond et al., 1967; Stott et al., 1976).

A diffuse interstitial nephritis with similar features to that described with penicillin (page 29) and methicillin (page 72) has been observed in two patients, which may have been due to isoniazid and/or ethambutol therapy (Stone et al., 1976). Isoniazid has also been implicated as a cause of pubertal gynaecomastia (Leading article, 1976a).

6. *Drug interactions*. Inhibition of diphenylhydantoin (phenytoin) metabolism and associated diphenylhydantoin toxicity may occur due to isoniazid, particularly in slow inactivators in whom blood levels of isoniazid are relatively high (page 802) (Kutt et al., 1970). Symptoms similar to those of histamine poisoning have been observed in patients in Sri Lanka taking isoniazid after eating a particular variety of fish; the fish had a high histamine content and it was thought that isoniazid's action of inhibiting histaminase was a factor in producing the illness in these patients (Uragoda and Kottegoda, 1977). One case report has suggested that isoniazid administration may enhance the anticoagulant activity of warfarin (Rosenthal et al., 1977).

Clinical Uses of the Drug

1. *Standard chemotherapy for active pulmonary tuberculosis*. Isoniazid is a very effective 'first-line' drug, and is always used for the treatment of tuberculosis unless isoniazid resistance is demonstrated, or the patient suffers a serious reaction to the drug. Induced isoniazid resistance is common if this drug is used alone (page 799), so that combination chemotherapy is essential for the treatment of active disease. In addition, in countries such as Australia and Britain, about four per cent of previously untreated patients have M. tuberculosis strains resistant to one of the 'first-line' antituberculosis drugs. Resistance to two standard drugs in such countries is rare, and therefore to ensure that at least two effective antituberculosis drugs are given, initial chemotherapy with three 'first-line' drugs is advocated. Triple drug therapy is continued for two to four months and then two drugs are continued to complete a minimum course of 18–24 months. Nowadays the 'first-line' drugs used in most developed countries are isoniazid, rifampicin, streptomycin and ethambutol. PAS is rarely used because it is poorly tolerated (page 827). Since rifampicin is the most effective companion drug for isoniazid in the treatment of pulmonary tuberculosis (*see* page 568), in developed countries where cost is not such a significant factor, it is now nearly always included in initial therapy. Triple therapy consisting of isoniazid, rifampicin plus streptomycin or ethambutol is given for the first two to four months and this is followed by maintenance therapy with isoniazid and rifampicin. After initial therapy with isoniazid, rifampicin and ethambutol, continuation therapy for one year with

daily isoniazid and ethambutol is just as effective and acceptable as daily isoniazid and rifampicin for the same period (Lees *et al.*, 1977).

In the United States initial triple drug therapy is not always used; the most frequently used regimen is commencing treatment with isoniazid and ethambutot which are continued for eighteen months. This combination, instead of e rifampicin regimen, which can produce fetal abnormalities in animals (page 566), has also been preferred when treatment during pregnancy is necessary (Bailey *et al.*, 1977). If extensive cavitary disease is present or if the patient is from an area where drug-resistant tuberculosis is prevalent, daily strehtomycin may be used in addition for the first three months. However a combination of isoniazid and rifampicin is considered to be as effective as any such three drug regimen for treatment of extensive cavitary disease.

In Australia initial three drug therapy now consists of isoniazid, rifampicin and either streptomycin or ethambutol for the first two to four months of treatment. Continuation therapy is with isoniazid and rifampicin (if there is no evidence of drug resistance or other contraindications) for 18 months. If streptomycin is selected as a third drug, it is suggested that it be replaced by ethambutol after eight weeks to avoid injections (Commonwealth Dept. Health Australia, 1977).

2. *Intermittent chemotherapy for pulmonary tuberculosis.* In these regimens drugs are administered two or three times a week or occasionally once-weekly, but the individual doses used are higher than the usual daily doses (page 801). This method of treatment is not superior to standard daily regimens, but it is suitable for out-patients who cannot be relied on to take medication, provided that intermittent administration can be fully supervised (Fox, 1968; Proust, 1969; Citron, 1972). Intermittent regimens also cause fewer adverse reactions (Fox, 1971), and they can be effectively combined with short-course chemotherapy (Fox and Mitchison, 1975) (*vide infra*).

Optimally classical daily triple chemotherapy should be given in hospital for the first two or three months and then an intermittent regimen, usually consisting of two drugs, can be continued on an out-patient basis. If there are no contraindications, isoniazid is always included in such regimens. Two commonly used intermittent therapies are streptomycin 1 g intramuscularly plus isoniazid 15 mg per kg twice-weekly (Fox, 1971; BMRC, 1973; WHO, 1975), or PAS 12 g and isoniazid 15 mg per kg, administered twice-weekly (Tub. Chemother. Centre, 1973a). Studies in Czechoslovakia have shown that after an initial course of triple chemotherapy lasting 6 or 13 weeks, continuation therapy with twice-weekly streptomycin and isoniazid for a total duration of treatment of 12 months was just as effective as a similar regimen lasting for a total of 18 months (WHO Prague, 1976; 1977). Similarly twice-weekly oral regimens of isoniazid 15 mg per kg plus rifampicin 900 or 600 mg have been extensively used with success (Singapore/BMRC, 1975) (page 569). Isoniazid in this dose has also been combined with ethambutol 50 mg per kg on a twice-weekly basis (page 837). Albert *et al.* (1976) studied the outcome of 81 patients receiving supervised ambulatory treatment with twice-weekly isoniazid and ethambutol, after an initial course of daily therapy with isoniazid, streptomycin, ethambutol or PAS for 10–11 weeks; they concluded that twice-weekly isoniazid and ethambutol after an adequate phase of daily treatment is a highly effective and well tolerated regimen. Some drugs are suitable for once-weekly administration. Pyrazinamide (page 847) and ethambutol (page 833) in greatly increased doses and streptomycin in the usual dose of 1 g intramuscularly are used for this purpose. Ordinary isoniazid tablets cannot be used for once-weekly chemotherapy, especially in rapid inactivators (page 801), but matrix isoniazid preparations have been used weekly in preliminary studies (see page 801).

3. *Short-course chemotherapy for pulmonary tuberculosis.* A number of studies have now demonstrated that short courses of chemotherapy lasting nine or perhaps only six months are just as effective as standard regimens for the treatment of pulmonary tuberculosis. The advantages of short-course chemotherapy are numerous; it is cheaper, there is less chronic drug toxicity, patient co-operation is greater, there is less hazard to them if they default early from treatment, and the period of follow-up after treatment can be reduced (Fox and Mitchison, 1975). At this time the inclusion of rifampicin (page 569) in these regimens appears to be the most important factor in the success of short-course chemotherapy.

The back-ground studies leading up to the use of these regimens have been summarised by Fox and Mitchison (1975). Initial studies in East Africa and Zambia (East African/BMRC, 1972; 1973; 1974; Second East African/BMRC, 1974; 1976) showed that six-month regimens using streptomycin, isoniazid together with rifampicin or pyrazinamide were effective in the treatment of newly diagnosed African patients with pulmonary tuberculosis. Subsequently it was shown that a six-month regimen containing rifampicin and isoniazid was only marginally inferior to one which also contained streptomycin. In other trials intermittent short-course therapy was studied; in one of these it was shown that twice a week administration of isoniazid, pyrazinamide and streptomycin for four months, preceded by an initial two months course of daily therapy with four drugs (streptomycin, isoniazid, rifampicin and pyrazinamide), was also effective. Another study of Chinese patients in Hong Kong with smear-positive pulmonary tuberculosis investigated six- and nine-month regimens of streptomycin, isoniazid and pyrazinamide given daily, three times a week or twice a week from the start of treatment (Hong Kong/BMRC, 1975). Pyrazinamide was used in this trial instead of rifampicin, because it is cheaper and it does not cause immunological side-effects which occur with intermittent rifampicin therapy. At six months the twice-weekly regimen was marginally inferior in that it failed to produce complete bacteriological clearance in all patients with pretreatment drug-susceptible strains; this was considered to be unacceptable by comparison to the results obtained with daily regimens of standard duration. Relapse rates in the first six months after ceasing treatment were relatively high in the six-month regimens but were much lower in the nine-month regimens. The results of treatment of patients who had pretreatment drug-resistant strains were not satisfactory. Nevertheless, these studies showed that short-course regimens using intermittent chemotherapy from the start of treatment are effective for the treatment for pulmonary tuberculosis. More recently, preliminary results of a trial using short-course, intermittent chemotherapy with isoniazid and rifampicin in the United States have been published (Dutt *et al.*, 1977). Isoniazid 300 mg plus rifampicin 600 mg were used daily for one month and this was followed by twice-weekly treatment with isoniazid 900 mg and rifampicin 600 mg for eight months. Sputum conversion by culture occurred within three months in 77 of 87 patients (88 per cent) and within six months in 81 or 82 patients (98·8 per cent). The authors concluded that this regimen was highly effective for pulmonary tuberculosis, it was cheaper, and side-effects due to intermittent rifampicin therapy (page 563) did not appear to be a great problem. In another trial conducted in Roumania using short-course, intermittent therapy, rifampicin was only used for three months (Tuberculosis Res. Inst., 1977). Isoniazid (15 mg per kg) and rifampicin (15 mg per kg) were given twice-weekly for three months, followed by isoniazid (same dose) plus either streptomycin (1 g) or ethambutol (40 mg per kg) for six months. The results showed that this regimen was highly effective; 15 months after completion of treatment 5·6 per cent of patients had had a bacteriological relapse but the strains isolated were still sensitive to the drugs used. By contrast a similar regimen without rifampicin, but using isoniazid, streptomycin and ethambutol for the first three months, was not as satisfactory.

In other investigations on the efficacy of short-course daily regimens, rifampicin has been used daily throughout the duration of chemotherapy. A pilot study by Poppe de Figueiredo et al. (1974) demonstrated the efficacy of a six-month regimen of isoniazid, rifampicin and ethambutol. In France a study showed that six-, nine- and twelve-month courses of isoniazid plus rifampicin, supplemented by streptomycin or ethambutol daily in the first three months were also effective (Brouet and Roussel, 1974). A controlled study on British patients using a regimen of rifampicin plus isoniazid, supplemented in the first two months by ethambutol or streptomycin, was given for six, nine, 12 or 18 months (A Controlled Trial, 1976). The oral drugs were all taken together, in a single daily dose, on an empty stomach. These regimens all produced virtually complete bacteriological quiescence at the end of chemotherapy. Relapse rates assessed 33 months after the beginning of the trial were 1 per cent in the 12-month group, nil in the nine-month group and 5 per cent in those receiving therapy for only six months. Isoniazid and rifampicin were well tolerated, but there were significant adverse effects with streptomycin but none with ethambutol. It was concluded that a regimen of isoniazid plus rifampicin for nine months, supplemented by ethambutol in a dose of 25 mg per kg for the first two months, is acceptable as standard chemotherapy for pulmonary tuberculosis in Britain.

There is also evidence that the likelihood of late relapses following short-course chemotherapy for pulmonary tuberculosis is small (Fox and Mitchison, 1976), and even when this occurs, relapse is nearly always due to sensitive strains and retreatment of these relapses with standard first-line drugs is highly successful (Hong Kong/BMRC, 1976b). It has been suggested that there are two phases in the bactericidal activity of short-course regimens, the killing of actively growing organisms and the sterilizing action on organisms that are virtually dormant (Fox and Mitchison, 1975). Rifampicin is not only a potent drug in the initial elimination of organisms, including those resistant to isoniazid and/or streptomycin, but like pyrazinamide (page 847), it may have a role in the sterilizing phase.

There have also been trials of chemotherapy lasting only three or four months. One pilot study in France compared a daily regimen of streptomycin, isoniazid and rifampicin with one consisting of daily streptomycin plus isoniazid and rifampicin given three times a week, both administered for three months. There was an overall relapse-rate of 13 per cent (Kreis *et al.*, 1976). Further trials were carried out in Africa to determine the value of various four-month regimens (East African/BMRC, 1978). Two regimens preceded by a two-month course of streptomycin, isoniazid, rifampicin and pyrazinamide were followed by isoniazid, rifampicin with and without pyrazinamide for another two months. Both of these regimens had relatively low relapse-rates (8 per cent) after six months. In two other regimens the same four drugs given for two months were followed by isoniazid with or without pyrazinamide for two months. Surprisingly pyrazinamide was of no benefit when used in this continuation phase, and it may need to be used for more prolonged periods to be of value. It is possible that some of these four-month regimens may be of value in developing countries but their comparative efficacy has yet to be confirmed.

Fox and Mitchison (1975) have stated that 'it is just a matter of time before the standard durations of chemotherapy in general use, both in the technically advanced and developing countries, will be short'. The optimal durations of therapy for developed and developing countries must still be determined by further trials. Moreover there will always be a place for antituberculosis therapy which is designed for the clinical circumstances of the individual.

4. *Tuberculous meningitis and miliary tuberculosis*. In these acute forms of tuberculosis, drug treatment is similar to that for pulmonary disease, but higher doses of isoniazid are advocated. The results of treatment have been greatly improved since isoniazid has been used for tuberculous meningitis (Lepper and Spies, 1963; Sumaya *et al.*, 1975). This drug penetrates well into the CSF and its use in tuberculous meningitis has obviated the need for intrathecal streptomycin. The isoniazid dose recommended for miliary tuberculosis and meningitis is usually 10 mg per kg per day, and at this dosage pyridoxine should also be administered (page 806).

As for pulmonary tuberculosis, triple chemotherapy is advocated for these two forms of the disease during the first two to three months. This usually consists of isoniazid and streptomycin plus rifampicin or sometimes ethambutol. In certain situations where patients may have resistant strains, initial therapy with four antituberculosis drugs may be necessary. Steiner *et al.* (1974) reviewed the management and outcome of 26 children, mainly Negroes or Puerto Ricans who had primary isoniazid-resistant tuberculosis, many of whom had life-threatening disease such as miliary tuberculosis or meningitis. As a result they recommended that if the drug susceptibility pattern of the source strain is unknown, all patients with life-threatening tuberculosis should be initially treated with four drugs—isoniazid, streptomycin, ethambutol and rifampicin. Corticosteroids may also have an important role in the treatment of tuberculous meningitis during the first two months. Antituberculosis therapy must be continued for one to two years depending on response and extent of the disease.

5. *Other forms of tuberculosis*. Tuberculosis of the genitourinary tract (Riddle, 1971; Sutherland, 1976), of the spine (Jackson, 1971) or of other bones and joints and of the cervical lymph nodes (Newcombe, 1971) are treated by standard drug regimens similar to those used for pulmonary disease. Two to four months triple drug therapy is advocated, followed by treatment with a combination of two drugs for approximately two years. Isoniazid should always be included in such regimens. In some of these conditions, however, ap-

propriate surgical measures are also indicated. Nevertheless the results of trials in Rhodesia, Korea and Hong Kong indicate that patients with tuberculosis of the spine respond well to chemotherapy alone (Leading article, 1974b). Clinical and radiological healing occurred in patients treated with isoniazid and PAS for 18 months and the addition of streptomycin to the therapy made no significant difference.

Tuberculous lymphadenitis is a more benign infection and chemotherapy using isoniazid plus ethambutol, isoniazid and rifampicin or isoniazid alone has been used successfully (Neuhaus *et al.*, 1977). Treatment with isoniazid and either rifampicin or ethambutol (both regimens with an initial supplement of streptomycin) for 18 months produced comparable results in a study in the United Kingdom. This study also suggested that treatment of lymph node tuberculosis by chemotherapy alone had advantages over added biopsy or surgical excision (Campbell and Dyson, 1977).

6. *Tuberculosis chemoprophylaxis.* The use of isoniazid as a single drug is only recommended for this purpose. Chemoprophylaxis with isoniazid is of proven value in preventing subsequent tuberculous morbidity in primary tuberculosis, in contacts, tuberculin reactors and in those with presumed inactive disease (Leading article, 1974a). This reduction in tuberculosis risk is life-long when the risk of exogenous reinfection is virtually negligible (Comstock and Edwards, 1975). The use of isoniazid alone for the purpose of chemoprophylaxis has only rarely led to the emergence of resistant M. tuberculosis strains. Chemoprophylaxis in most instances is really preventive treatment in which it is presumed that the bacterial population in 'healed' or radiologically inapparent lesions is diminished by treatment. In fact, it has been suggested that many patients who are often followed at chest clinics with apparently inactive radiological lung lesions may well be better managed by receiving a 6–12 month course of isoniazid plus rifampicin or ethambutol (Leading article, 1974a).

Broadly speaking, any person who is judged to be at risk of developing active tuberculosis should be given isoniazid prophylactically. The recommended dose for prophylaxis is 5–10 mg per kg per day or 300 mg (maximum 400 mg) for adults, given as a single daily dose, which is usually continued for 12 months. Children tolerate isoniazid well and a dose range of 10–15 mg per kg per day is used. The precise definition of a person at risk of developing tuberculosis has been controversial. However, authorities in North America, Australia and Britain have published recommendations for isoniazid prophylaxis (American Thoracic Society, 1974; Bailey *et al.*, 1977; Commonwealth Dept. Health Australia, 1977; Joint Tub. Committee, 1973). It is generally agreed that the following categories of patients should be given or at least strongly considered for chemoprophylaxis:

(a) Recent tuberculin convertors of any age, particularly juveniles (Hsu, 1974).

(b) Positive tuberculin reactors under the age of 20 years, especially young children. If the patient has been a recent tuberculosis contact, the indication for isoniazid prophylaxis is very strong.

(c) Household contacts and close associates of patients with tuberculosis, both tuberculin-negative (especially children and particularly neonates) and tuberculin-positive are highly commended for isoniazid prophylaxis by the American authorities. The British recommendation for treatment in this situation is only for tuberculin-positive household contacts, while in Australia isoniazid prophylaxis is recommended only for juvenile tuberculin-positive contacts.

(d) Patients with inactive tuberculosis (or sometimes also positive tuberculin reactors), who are receiving long-term corticosteroids, cytotoxic or immunosuppressive drugs, therapeutic irradiation, and those who have had a recent gastrectomy or are about to undergo this operation.

Earlier fears that the use of corticosteroids for asthma in positive tuberculin reactors may cause reactivation of tuberculosis have been somewhat allayed by several studies. It appears that there is no indication for prophylactic chemotherapy when corticosteroids are used in asthma, because of positive tuberculin reactions alone (Leading article, 1976b).

As the risk of isoniazid hepatitis (page 808) increases with age, patients older than 35 years should be carefully assessed as to whether the risk of subsequent tuberculosis is sufficiently strong to warrant isoniazid prophylaxis (*see* page 809). By contrast younger patients can be treated much more readily if one of the above indications exists. In the United States chemoprophylaxis is considered mandatory for positive reactors up to the age of six years and it is highly recommended even in the absence of other risk factors for positive tuberculin reactors up to the age of 35 years.

There are other categories for which isoniazid prophylaxis may be considered, but about which there is no general agreement. These include the following groups of patients, in whom individual assessment is necessary:

(a) Known inactive tuberculosis in persons who have not had adequate chemotherapy, or who were treated in the pre-chemotherapy era.

(b) Inactive tuberculous lesions discovered on routine chest X-ray. The American authorities recommend isoniazid prophylaxis, especially if these patients are also positive tuberculin-reactors.

(c) Miscellaneous categories include patients with inactive pulmonary lesions who develop haematological or reticuloendothelial diseases such as leukaemia or Hodgkin's disease or unstable diabetes, pregnant women with an inactive pulmonary lesion, tuberculin-positive silicotics and tuberculin-positive children who develop whooping cough or measles or who receive measles vaccine. In Britain it has been suggested that chemoprophylaxis should be given to all Asian immigrants with a moderately or strongly positive tuberculin reaction, particularly those aged less than 18 years (Leading article, 1974a).

Chemoprophylaxis is contraindicated in patients who have had previous isoniazid hepatitis, or other severe adverse effects due to the drug, or in patients with acute liver disease of any aetiology (American Thoracic Society, 1974). Special care should be taken in patients receiving concurrent long-term medication, to avoid drug interactions e.g. diphenylhydantoin (*see* page 810). Patients taking alcohol daily and those with possible chronic liver disease should also be carefully assessed, because in these the risk of isoniazid hepatitis may be higher. Although isoniazid is not known to be harmful to the fetus, chemoprophylaxis in pregnancy is generally recommended to be delayed until delivery of the baby.

A rather special situation is the management of an infant, whose mother has active tuberculosis. In such a case vaccination with BCG is necessary, but if concurrent isoniazid prophylaxis is used, the development of immunity following BCG may be impaired. For this reason a special BCG vaccine containing strains resistant to isoniazid was developed. This vaccine produced satisfactory tuberculin conversion even when isoniazid was given concurrently (Gaisford and Griffiths, 1961).

Although a variable proportion of contacts of tuberculosis may be exposed to infection due to isoniazid-resistant M. tuberculosis strains (page 799), reports of failure of isoniazid chemoprophylaxis are infrequent (Fairshter et al., 1975). These authors suggested that in contacts of patients with isoniazid-resistant tuberculosis, other drugs should be used for prophylaxis such as either ethambutol or rifampicin alone.

Chemoprophylaxis with isoniazid has also been used to eradicate tuberculosis in isolated rural communities. Results of one such trial have been reported, in which all active cases were identified and treated conventionally, whilst healthy tuberculin reactors received isoniazid prophylaxis (Furcolow and Deuschle, 1973). These authors considered that the use of isoniazid in the latter group was beneficial.

Chemoprophylaxis using an intermittent regimen has also been used. Isoniazid in a dose of 10 mg per kg body weight (maximum 600 mg) and ethambutol 30 mg per kg body weight (maximum 2000 mg) given three times per week to Eskimo patients over the age of 10 years for a period of 18 months was very successful (Grzybowski et al., 1976).

7. *Other mycobacterial infections.* Isoniazid is sometimes used with streptomycin and ethambutol to treat M. kansasii infections (*see* page 838). Even though M. intracellulare is often resistant to all drugs except cycloserine, multiple drug regimens, usually including both isoniazid and rifampicin, may be effective (Bailey et al., 1977). Isoniazid is also usually very effective for the treatment of persistent local or the more rare disseminated infection due to BCG vaccination. Even when these complications occur in patients receiving BCG immunotherapy for malignancy, they respond rapidly to isoniazid (Aungst et al., 1975; Sparks, 1976). One physician, who developed a persisting ulcer on her finger after accidental innoculation with BCG despite isoniazid treatment, was shown to be infected with a strain resistant to isoniazid; the infection rapidly healed when treatment was changed to ethambutol and rifampicin (Lorber et al., 1977).

REFERENCES

A Controlled Trial by the British Thoracic and Tuberculosis Association (1976), 'Short-course chemotherapy in pulmonary tuberculosis', *Lancet,* **2,** 1102.

Alarcón-Segovia, D., Fishbein, E. and Betancourt, V. M. (1969), 'Antibodies to nucleoprotein and to hydrazide-altered soluble nucleoprotein in tuberculous patients receiving isoniazid', *Clin. exp. Immunol.,* **5,** 429.

Alarcón-Segovia, D., Fishbein, E. and Alcalá, H. (1971), 'Isoniazid acetylation rate and development of antinuclear antibodies upon isoniazid treatment', *Arthritis and Rheumatism,* **14,** 748.

Albert, R. K., Sbarbaro, J. A., Hudson, L. D. and Iseman, M. (1976), 'High-dose ethambutol: Its role in intermittent chemotherapy', *Amer. Rev. Resp. Dis.,* **114,** 699.

American Thoracic Society (1974), 'Preventive therapy of tuberculous infection', *Amer. Rev. Resp. Dis.*, **110**, 371.

An Interim Report to the Medical Research Council by Their Tuberculosis Chemotherapy Trials Committee (1952), 'The treatment of pulmonary tuberculosis with isoniazid', *Brit. med. J.*, **2**, 735.

Aungst, C. W., Sokal, J. E. and Jager, B. V. (1975), 'Complications of BCG vaccination in neoplastic disease', *Ann. Intern. Med.*, **82**, 666.

Bailey, W. C., Taylor, S. L., Dascomb, H. E., Greenberg, H. B. and Ziskind, M. M. (1973), 'Disturbed hepatic function during isoniazid chemoprophylaxis', *Amer. Rev. Resp. Dis.*, **107**, 523.

Bailey, W. C., Weill, H., deRouen, T. A., Ziskind, M. M., Jackson, H. A., and Greenberg, H. B. (1974), 'The effect of isoniazid on transaminase levels', *Ann. Intern. Med.*, **81**, 200.

Bailey, W. C., Raleigh, J. W. and Turner, J. A. P. (1977), 'Treatment of mycobacterial disease', *Amer. Rev. Resp. Dis.*, **115**, 185.

Barclay, W. R., Ebert, R. H. and Koch-Weser, D. (1953), 'Mode of action of isoniazid', *Amer. Rev. Tuberc. pulm. Dis.*, **67**, 490.

Barter, C. E. and Camens, I. M. H. (1968), 'Lung infection with anonymous mycobacteria', *Med. J. Aust.*, **1**, 408.

Beaudry, P. H., Brickman, H. F., Wise, M. B. and MacDougall, D. (1974), 'Liver enzyme disturbances during isoniazid chemoprophylaxis in children', *Amer. Rev., Resp. Dis.*, **110**, 581.

Bennett, W. M., Singer, I., Golper, T., Feig, P. and Coggins, C. J. (1977), 'Guidelines for drug therapy in renal failure', *Ann. Intern. Med.*, **86**, 754.

Bernstein, J., Lott, W. A., Steinberg, B. A. and Yale, H. L. (1952), 'Chemotherapy of experimental tuberculosis-isonicotinic acid hydrazide (nydrazid) and related compounds', *Amer. Rev. Tuberc.*, **65**, 357; quoted by Robson and Sullivan (1963).

Birkett, D. J. and Pond, S. M. (1975), 'Metabolic drug interactions—A critical review', *Med. J. Aust.*, **1**, 687.

Black, M. (1974), 'Editorial. Isoniazid and the liver', *Amer. Rev. Resp. Dis.*, **110**, 1.

Bomb, B. S., Purohit, S. D. and Bedi, H. K. (1976), 'Stevens-Johnson syndrome caused by isoniazid', *Tubercle*, **57**, 229.

Brasfield, D. M., Goodloe, T. B. and Tiller, R. E. (1976), 'Isoniazid hepatotoxicity in childhood', *Pediatrics*, **58**, 291.

British Medical Research Council Co-operative Study (1973), 'Cooperative controlled trial of a standard regimen of streptomycin, PAS and isoniazid and three alternative regimens of chemotherapy in Britain', *Tubercle*, **54**, 99.

Brouet, G. and Roussel, G. (1974), 'Modalités et bilan des traitements courts'. *XVII Congrès National de la Tuberculose et des Maladies Respiratoires*. Clermont-Ferrand., p. 27.

Brown, A. (1976), 'Risks of isoniazid therapy', *Ann. Intern. Med.*, **85**, 828.

Campbell, I. A. and Dyson, A. J. (1977), 'Lymph node tuberculosis: Comparison of various methods of treatment'. *Tubercle*, **58**, 171.

Center for Disease Control (1974), 'Isoniazid-associated hepatitis', *Morbidity and Mortality Weekly Report*, **23**, 97.

Cheigh, J. S. (1977), 'Drug administration in renal failure', *Amer. J. Med.*, **62**, 555.

Citron, K. M. (1972), 'Tuberculosis-chemotherapy', *Brit. med. J.*, **1**, 426.

Commonwealth Department of Health Australia (1973–1977), 'Tuberculosis statistics', Canberra.

Commonwealth Department of Health Australia (1977), *Treatment of Tuberculosis with particular reference to Chemotherapy*, 4th edn., Australian Government Publishing Service, Canberra.

Comstock, G. W. and Edwards, P. Q. (1975), 'Editorial. The competing risks of tuberculosis and hepatitis for adult tuberculin reactors', *Amer. Rev. Resp. Dis.*, **111**, 573.

Davis, R. S. and Stoler, B. S. (1977), 'Febrile reactions to INH', *New Engl. J. Med.*, **297**, 337.

Dickinson, J. M., Aber, V. R. and Mitchison, D. A. (1973), 'Studies on the treatment of experimental tuberculosis of the guinea-pig with intermittent doses of isoniazid', *Tubercle*, **54**, 211.

Dickinson, D. S., Bailey, W. C. and Hirschowitz, B. I. (1977), 'The effect of acetylation status on isoniazid (INH) hepatitis', *Amer. Rev. Resp. Dis.* (Suppl.), **115**, 395.

Doster, B., Caras, G. J. and Snider, D. E., Jr. (1976), 'A continuing survey of primary drug resistance in tuberculosis, 1961 to 1968', *Amer. Rev. Resp. Dis.*, **113**, 419.

Dutt, A. K., Jones, L. and Stead, W. W. (1977), 'Treatment of pulmonary tuberculosis with short-course, intermittent chemotherapy using rifampin-isoniazid', *Amer. Rev. Resp. Dis.* (Suppl.), **115**, 396.

East African/British Medical Research Councils (1972), 'Controlled clinical trial of short-course (6-month) regimens of chemotherapy for treatment of pulmonary tuberculosis', *Lancet*, **1**, 1079.

East African/British Medical Research Councils (1973), 'Controlled clinical trial of four short-course (6-month) regimens of chemotherapy for treatment of pulmonary tuberculosis. Second report', *Lancet*, **1**, 1331.

East African/British Medical Research Councils (1974), 'Controlled clinical trial of four short-course (6-month) regimens of chemotherapy for treatment of pulmonary tuberculosis. Third report', *Lancet*, **2**, 237.

East African/British Medical Research Councils (1978), 'Controlled clinical trial of five short-course (4-month) chemotherapy regimens in pulmonary tuberculosis', *Lancet*, **2**, 334.

Eidus, L. and Hodgkin, M. M. (1973), 'Screening of isoniazid inactivators', *Antimicrob. Ag. Chemother.*, **3**, 130.

Eidus, L., Hodgkin, M. M., Hsu, A. H. E. and Schaefer, O. (1974), 'Pharmacokinetic studies with an isoniazid slow-releasing matrix preparation', *Amer. Rev. Resp. Dis.*, **110**, 34.

Ellard, G. A., Aber, V. R., Gammon, P. T., Mitchison, D. A., Lakshminarayan, S., Citron, K. M., Fox, W. and Tall, R. (1972), 'Pharmacology of some slow-release preparations of isoniazid of potential use in intermittent treatment of tuberculosis', *Lancet*, **1**, 340.

Ellard, G. A., Gammon, P. T., Polansky, F., Viznerova, A., Havlik, I. and Fox, W. (1973), 'Further studies on the pharmacology of a slow-release matrix preparation of isoniazid (Smith & Nephew HS 82) of potential use in the intermittent treatment of tuberculosis', *Tubercle*, **54**, 57.

Ellard, G. A. and Gammon, P. T. (1973), 'Determination of the acetylator phenotype from the ratio of the urinary excretion of acetylisoniazid to acid-labile isoniazid: A study in Finnish Lapland', *Tubercle*, **54**, 201.

Evans, D. A. P., Manley, K. A. and McKusick, V. A. (1960), 'Genetic control of isoniazid metabolism in man', *Brit. med. J.*, **2**, 485.

Fairshter, R. D., Randazzo, G. P., Garlin, J. and Wilson, A. F. (1975), 'Failure of isoniazid prophylaxis after exposure to isoniazid-resistant tuberculosis', *Amer. Rev. Resp. Dis.*, **112**, 37.

Forgan-Smith, R., Ellard, G. A., Newton, D. and Mitchison, D. A. (1973), 'Pyrazinamide and other drugs in tuberculous meningitis', *Lancet*, **2**, 374.

Fox, H. H. (1952–1953), 'The chemical attack on tuberculosis', *Transact. N.Y. Acad. Sci.*, **15**, 234.

Fox, W. (1968), 'Changing concepts in the chemotherapy of pulmonary tuberculosis', *Amer. Rev. Resp. Dis.*, **97**, 767.

Fox, W. (1971), 'General considerations in intermittent drug therapy of pulmonary tuberculosis', *Postgrad. Med. J.*, **47**, 729.

Fox, W. and Mitchison, D. A. (1975), 'Short-course chemotherapy for pulmonary tuberculosis', *Amer. Rev. Resp. Dis.*, **111**, 325.

Fox, W. and Mitchison, D. A. (1976), 'Short-course chemotherapy for tuberculosis', *Lancet*, **2**, 1349.

Fox, W. (1977), 'Modern management and therapy of pulmonary tuberculosis', *Bull. Int. Un. Tuberc.*, **52**, 25.

Furcolow, M. L. and Deuschle, K. W. (1973), 'Modern tuberculosis control. A six-year follow-up in an Appalachian community', *Amer. Rev. Resp. Dis.*, **107**, 253.

Gaisford, W. and Griffiths, M. I. (1961), 'A freeze-dried vaccine from isoniazid-resistant B.C.G. A clinical investigation', *Brit. med. J.*, **1**, 1500.

Garagusi, V. F., Neefe, L. I. and Mann, O. (1976), 'Acute meningoencephalitis association with isoniazid administration', *JAMA*, **235**, 1141.

Garibaldi, R. A., Drusin, R. E., Ferebee, S. H. and Gregg, M. B. (1972), 'Isoniazid-associated hepatitis. Report of an outbreak', *Amer. Rev. Resp. Dis.*, **106**, 357.

Glassroth, J. L., Kilburn, J., Snider, D. E. and Kopanoff, D. (1977), 'A survey of primary drug resistance in tuberculosis', *Amer. Rev. Resp. Dis.* (Suppl.), **115**, 398.

Good, A. E., Green, R. A. and Zarafonetis, C. J. D. (1965), 'Rheumatic symptoms during tuberculosis therapy. A manifestation of isoniazid toxicity?', *Ann. Intern. Med.*, **63**, 800.

Grzybowski, S., Galbraith, J. D. and Dorken, E. (1976), 'Chemoprophylaxis trial in Canadian Eskimos', *Tubercle*, **57**, 263.

Hammond, E. C., Selikoff, I. J. and Robitzek, E. H. (1967), 'Isoniazid therapy in relation to later occurrence of cancer in adults and in infants', *Brit. med. J.*, **2**, 792.

Harris, H. W. (1963), 'Current concepts of the metabolism of antituberculous agents', *Ann. N.Y. Acad. Sci.*, **106**, 43.

Harris, G. D., Johanson, W. G., Jr. and Nicholson, D. P. (1975), 'Response to chemotherapy of pulmonary infection due to Mycobacterium kansasii', *Amer. Rev. Resp. Dis.*, **112**, 31.

Hobby, G. L., Johnson, P. M. and Boytar-Papirnyik, V. (1971), 'Primary drug resistance: A continuing study of drug resistance in tuberculosis in a veteran population within the United States. IX. September 1969–September 1970', *Amer. Rev. Resp. Dis.*, **103**, 842.

Hobby, G. L., Johnson, P. M. and Boytar-Papirnyik, V. (1974), 'Primary drug resistance: A continuing study of drug resistance in tuberculosis in a veteran population within the United States. X. September 1970 to September 1973', *Amer. Rev. Resp. Dis.*, **110**, 95.

Hong Kong Tuberculosis Treatment Services/British Medical Research Council (1975), 'Controlled trial of 6 and 9-month regimens of daily and intermittent streptomycin plus isoniazid plus pyrazinamide for pulmonary tuberculosis in Hong Kong', *Tubercle*, **56**, 81.

Hong Kong Tuberculosis Treatment Services/British Medical Research Council (1976a), 'Adverse reactions to short-course regimens containing streptomycin, isoniazid, pyrazinamide and rifampicin in Hong Kong', *Tubercle*, **57**, 81.

Hong Kong Tuberculosis Treatment Services and East African and British Medical Research Councils (1976b), 'First-line chemotherapy in the retreatment of bacteriological relapses of pulmonary tuberculosis following a short-course regimen', *Lancet*, **1**, 162.

Hsu, K. H. K. (1974), 'Isoniazid in the prevention and treatment of tuberculosis. A 20-year study of the effectiveness in children', *JAMA*, **229**, 528.

Hughes, H. B. (1953), 'On the metabolic fate of isoniazid', *J. Pharmacol. Exp. Ther.*, **109**, 444.

Hurwitz, A. and Schlozman, D. L. (1974), 'Effects of antacids on gastrointestinal absorption of isoniazid in rat and man', *Amer. Rev. Resp. Dis.*, **109**, 41.

Jackson, J. W. (1971), 'Spinal tuberculosis', *Postgrad. Med. J.*, **47**, 723.

Joint Tuberculosis Committee of the British Thoracic and Tuberculosis Association

(1973), 'Chemoprophylaxis against tuberculosis in Britain', *Tubercle*, **54**, 309.
Joseph, M. (1973), 'Hypersensitivity to anti-tuberculous drugs', *Aust. N.Z. J. Med.*, **3**, 311.
Khan, M. A. (1977), 'Primary drug-resistant tuberculosis in the Greater Boston area', *New Engl. J. Med.*, **297**, 397.
Kopanoff, D. E., Snider, D. E., Jr. and Caras, G. J. (1978), 'Isoniazid-related hepatitis. A U.S. Public Health Service cooperative surveillance study', *Amer. Rev. Resp. Dis.*, **117**, 991.
Kovnat, P., Labovitz, E. and Levison, S. P. (1973), 'Antibiotics and the kidney', *Med. Clin. North Amer.*, **57**, 1045.
Kreis, B., Pretet, S., Birenbaum, J., Guibout, P., Hazeman, J. J. Orin, E., Perdrizet, S. and Weil, J. (1976), 'Two three-month treatment regimens for pulmonary tuberculosis', *Bull. Un. int. Tuberc.*, **51**, 71.
Kutt, H., Brennan, R., Dehejia, H. and Verebely, K. (1970), 'Diphenylhydantoin intoxication. A complication of isoniazid therapy', *Amer. Rev. Resp. Dis.*, **101**, 377.
Lal, S., Singhal, S. N., Burley, D. M. and Crossley, G. (1972), 'Effect of rifampicin and isoniazid on liver function', *Brit. med. J.*, **1**, 148.
Lauener, H. and Favez, G. (1959), 'The inhibition of isoniazid inactivation by means of PAS and benzoyl-PAS in man', *Amer. Rev. Resp. Dis.*, **80**, 26.
Leading Article (1966), 'Isoniazid: How much a carcinogen?', *Lancet*, **2**, 1452.
Leading Article (1969), 'Isoniazid and loss of memory', *Brit. med. J.*, **1**, 461.
Leading Article (1972), 'Resistant tubercle bacilli', *Lancet*, **2**, 412.
Leading Article (1974a), 'Chemoprophylaxis against tuberculosis', *Brit. med. J.*, **4**, 63.
Leading Article (1974b), 'Tuberculosis of the spine', *Brit. med. J.*, **4**, 613.
Leading Article (1975), 'Antituberculous drugs and the liver', *Brit. med. J.*, **2**, 522.
Leading Article (1976a), 'Pubertal gynaecomastia', *Brit. med. J.*, **1**, 1238.
Leading Article (1976b), 'Tuberculosis in corticosteroid-treated asthmatics', *Brit. med. J.*, **2**, 266.
Lees, A. W., Allan, G. W., Smith, J., Tyrrell, W. F. and Fallon, R. J. (1971), 'Toxicity from rifampicin plus isoniazid and rifampicin plus ethambutol therapy', *Tubercle*, **52**, 182.
Lees, A. W., Allan, G. W., Smith, J. and Tyrrell, W. F. (1977), 'Ethambutol plus isoniazid compared with rifampicin plus isoniazid in antituberculosis continuation treatment', *Lancet*, **1**, 1232.
Lepper, M. H. and Spies, H. W. (1963), 'The present status of the treatment of tuberculosis of the central nervous system', *Ann. N.Y. Acad. Sci.*, **106**, 106.
Litt, I. F., Cohen, M. I. and McNamara, H. (1976), 'Isoniazid hepatitis in adolescents', *J. Pediatrics*, **89**, 133.
Lorber, B., Vonderheid, E. C., Swenson, R. M. and Cundy, K. R. (1977), 'Failure of isoniazid to cure localised BCG infection', *JAMA*, **238**, 55.
Maddrey, W. C. and Boitnott, J. K. (1973), 'Isoniazid hepatitis', *Ann. Intern. Med.*, **79**, 1.
McDonald, H. M. (1974), 'Antibiotics, antiseptics and tubercle bacilli', *Med. J. Aust.*, **2**, 41.
Medical News (1974), 'Risk of hepatitis remains problem in preventive isoniazid therapy', *JAMA*, **228**, 443.
Miller, A. B., Tall, R., Fox, W., Lefford, M. J. and Mitchison, D. A. (1966), 'Primary drug resistance in pulmonary tuberculosis in Great Britain: Second national survey, 1963', *Tubercle, Lond.*, **47**, 92.
Mitchell, J. R., Zimmerman, H. J., Ishak, K. G., Thorgeirsson, U. P., Timbrell, J. A., Snodgrass, W. R. and Nelson, S. D. (1976), 'Isoniazid liver injury: Clinical spectrum, pathology, and probable pathogenesis', *Ann. Intern. Med.*, **84**, 181.
Moss, J. D., Lewis, J. E. and Knauer, C. M. (1972), 'Isoniazid-associated hepatitis. A study of five cases', *Amer. Rev. Resp. Dis.*, **106**, 849.

Mount, F. W., Anastasiades, A. A. and Schnack, G. A. (1961), 'Control study of biologically active isoniazid in serum of children with primary tuberculosis', *Amer. Rev. Resp. Dis.,* **83,** 173.

Neuhaus, A., Ravikrishan, K. P., Muller, B. F. and Cramer, P. (1977), 'Tuberculous lymphadenitis in the modern chemotherapy era', *Amer. Rev. Resp. Dis.* (Suppl.), **115,** 405.

Newcombe, J. F. (1971), 'Tuberculous cervical lymphadenopathy', *Postgrad. Med. J.,* **47,** 713.

Parthasarathy, R., Devadatta, S., Fox, W., Krishnaswami, K. V., Radhakrishna, S., Somasundaram, P. R. and Tripathy, S. P. (1976), 'Studies of immediate adverse reactions to different doses of a slow-release preparation of isoniazid', *Tubercle,* **57,** 115.

Periman, P. and Venkataramani, T. K. (1975), 'Acute arthritis induced by isoniazid', *Ann. Intern. Med.,* **83,** 667.

Peters, J. H., Miller, K. S. and Brown, P. (1965), 'Studies on the metabolic basis for the genetically determined capacities for isoniazid inactivation in man', *J. Pharmacol. Exp. Ther.,* **150,** 298.

Poppe de Figueiredo, P., Brito, A. A., Valle, J. H. L., Tavares, P. M. and Trannin, P. L. (1974), 'Short duration chemotherapy of pulmonary tuberculosis: A pilot trial', Proceedings of the XXIInd International Tuberculosis Conference. *Bull. Int. Un. Tuberc.,* **49,** 382.

Proust, A. J. (1969), 'Intermittent chemotherapy in the treatment of tuberculosis. A review', *Med. J. Aust.,* **2,** 1052.

Pyle, M. M. (1970), 'Ethambutol and viomycin', *Med. Clin. North Amer.,* **54,** 1317.

Quinn, J. V. and Crotty, J. M. (1963), 'Mycobacterium ulcerans infections in the Northern Territory', *Med. J. Aust.,* **2,** 317.

Rao, K. V. N., Mitchison, D. A., Nair, M. G. K., Prema, K. and Tripathy, S. P. (1970), 'Sulphadimidine acetylation test for classification of patients as slow or rapid inactivators of isoniazid', *Brit. med. J.,* **3,** 495.

Ravikrishnan, K. P., Muller, B. F. and Neuhaus, A. (1977), 'Toxicity to isoniazid and rifampin in active tuberculosis patients', *Amer. Rev. Resp. Dis.* (Suppl.), **115,** 405.

Riddle, P. R. (1971), 'Urinary tuberculosis', *Postgrad. Med. J.,* **47,** 718.

Riemensnider, D. K. and Mitchell, R. S. (1960), 'The effect of pyridoxine on isoniazid serum concentrations in man', *Amer. Rev. Resp. Dis.,* **82,** 412.

Robson, J. M. and Sullivan, F. M. (1963), 'Antituberculosis drugs', *Pharmacol. Rev.,* **15,** 169.

Rosenthal, A. R., Self, T. H., Baker, E. D. and Linden, R. A. (1977), 'Interaction of isoniazid and warfarin', *JAMA,* **238,** 2177.

Russell, D. W. (1970), 'Simple method for determining isoniazid acetylator phenotype', *Brit. med. J.,* **3,** 324.

Santha, T., Fox, W., Nazareth, O., Prabhakar, R., Radhakrishna, S., Ramakrishnan, C. V., Sivasubramanian, S., Somasundaram, P. R. and Tripathy, S. P. (1976), 'Study of adverse reactions to a once-weekly regimen of streptomycin plus a slow-release preparation of isoniazid in high dosage for six months', *Tubercle,* **57,** 123.

Sarma, G. R., Kailasam, S., Mitchison, D. A., Nair, N. G. K., Radhakrishna, S. and Tripathy, S. P. (1975), 'Studies of serial plasma isoniazid concentrations with different doses of a slow-release preparation of isoniazid', *Tubercle,* **56,** 314.

Second East African/British Medical Research Council Study (1974), 'Controlled clinical trial of four short-course (6-Month) regimens of chemotherapy for treatment of pulmonary tuberculosis', *Lancet,* **2,** 1100.

Second East African/British Medical Research Council Study (1976), 'Controlled clinical trial of four 6-month regimens of chemotherapy for pulmonary tuberculosis. Second report', *Amer. Rev. Resp. Dis.,* **114,** 471.

Short, E. I. (1962), 'Studies on the inactivation of isonicotinyl acid hydrazide in normal subjects and tuberculous patients', *Tubercle, Lond.*, **43**, 33.

Singapore Tuberculosis Service/British Medical Research Council (1975), 'Controlled trial of intermittent regimens of rifampicin plus isoniazid for pulmonary tuberculosis in Singapore', *Lancet*, **2**, 1105.

Smith, J., Tyrrell, W. F., Gow, A., Allan, G. W. and Lees, A. W. (1972), 'Hepatotoxicity in rifampicin-isoniazid treated patients related to their rate of isoniazid inactivation', *Chest*, **61**, 587.

Sparks, F. C. (1976), 'Hazards and complications of BCG immunotherapy', *Med. Clin. North. Amer.* **60**, 499.

Steiner, M., Steiner, P., Rao, M., Padre, R. and Goldberg, R. (1973), 'Primary drug-resistant tuberculosis in children, 1961 to 1971', *Amer. Rev. Resp. Dis.*, **108**, 321.

Steiner, P., Rao, M., Victoria, M. and Steiner, M. (1974), 'Primary isoniazid-resistant tuberculosis in children', *Amer. Rev. Resp. Dis.*, **110**, 306.

Stone, W. J., Waldron, J. A., Dixon, J. H., Jr., Primm, R. K. and Horn, R. G. (1976), 'Acute diffuse interstitial nephritis related to chemotherapy of tuberculosis', *Antimicrob. Ag. Chemother.*, **10**, 164.

Stott, H., Peto, J., Stephens, R., Fox, W., Sutherland, I., Foster-Carter, A. F., Teare, H. D. and Fenning, J. (1976), 'An assessment of the carcinogenicity of isoniazid in patients with pulmonary tuberculosis', *Tubercle*, **57**, 1.

Stottmeier, K. D. and Burkes, J. (1974), 'Primary drug-resistant Mycobacterium tuberculosis isolated in Massachusetts in 1972', *J. Infect. Dis.*, **130**, 293.

Stottmeier, K. D. and Baker, S. (1977), 'Primary drug-resistant tuberculosis in Massachusetts, 1975/76', *New Engl. J. Med.*, **296**, 823.

Sumaya, C. V., Simek, M., Smith, M. H. D., Seidemann, M. F., Ferriss, G. S. and Rubin, W. (1975), 'Tuberculous meningitis in children during the isoniazid era', *J. Pediatrics*, **87**, 43.

Sutherland, A. M. (1976), 'The treatment of tuberculosis of the female genital tract with streptomycin, PAS and isoniazid', *Tubercle*, **57**, 137.

Takayama, K., Wang, L. and David, H. L. (1972), 'Effect of isoniazid on the *in vivo* mycolic acid synthesis, cell growth, and viability of Mycobacterium tuberculosis', *Antimicrob. Ag. Chemother.*, **2**, 29.

Thompson, J. E. (1969), 'The management of hypersensitivity reactions to antituberculosis drugs', *Med. J. Aust.*, **2**, 1058.

Thompson, J. E. (1978), 'How safe is isoniazid?', *Med. J. Aust.*, **1**, 165.

Today's Drugs (1963), 'Drugs for tuberculosis', *Brit. med. J.*, **1**, 1527.

Today's Drugs (1968), 'Drugs for tuberculosis', *Brit. med. J.*, **3**, 664.

Tuberculosis Chemotherapy Centre, Madras (1973a), 'Controlled comparison of oral twice-weekly and oral daily isoniazid plus PAS in newly diagnosed pulmonary tuberculosis', *Brit. med. J.*, **2**, 7.

Tuberculosis Chemotherapy Centre, Madras (1973b), 'A controlled comparison of two fully supervised once-weekly regiments in the treatment of newly diagnosed pulmonary tuberculosis', *Tubercle*, **54**, 23.

Tuberculosis Research Institute, Bucharest (1977), 'Trial of two intermittent short-course regimens (78 doses) in the initial treatment of pulmonary tuberculosis', *Tubercle*, **58**, 1.

Uragoda, C. G. and Kottegoda, S. R. (1977), 'Adverse reactions to isoniazid in ingestion of fish with a high histamine content', *Tubercle*, **58**, 83.

Usuda, Y. and Sekine, O. (1978), 'Chemotherapy of tuberculosis in patients on dialysis'. In Siegenthaler, W. and Lüthy, R. (Ed.), *Current Chemotherapy: Proceedings of the 10th International Congress of Chemotherapy*, Zurich/Switzerland, 1977. American Society for Microbiology, Washington, D.C., p. 241.

Vanderhoof, J. A. and Ament, M. E. (1976), 'Fatal hepatic necrosis due to isoniazid chemoprophylaxis in a 15-year-old girl', *J. Paediatrics*, **88**, 867.

Wang, L. and Takayama, K. (1972), 'Relationship between the uptake of isoniazid and its action on the *in vivo* mycolic acid synthesis in Mycobacterium tuberculosis', *Antimicrob. Ag. Chemother.*, **2**, 438.

WHO (1975), 'Tuberculosis control: Progress of the new strategy', *WHO Chronicle*, **29**, 123.

WHO Collaborating Centre for Tuberculosis Chemotherapy, Prague (1976), 'A study of two twice-weekly and a once-weekly continuation regimen of tuberculosis chemotherapy, including a comparison of two durations of treatment. 1. First report: The results at 18 months', *Tubercle*, **57**, 235.

WHO Collaborating Centre for Tuberculosis Chemotherapy, Prague (1977), 'A study of two twice-weekly and a once-weekly continuation regimen of tuberculosis chemotherapy, including a comparison of two durations of treatment. 2. Second report: The results at 36 months', *Tubercle*, **58**, 129.

Wimpenny, J. W. T. (1967), 'Effect of isoniazid on biosynthesis in Mycobacterium tuberculosis var. bovis BCG', *J. gen. Microbiol.*, **47**, 379.

Youatt, J. (1969), 'A review of the action of isoniazid', *Amer. Rev. Resp. Dis.*, **99**, 729.

Para-Amino Salicylic Acid (PAS)

Description

Para-amino salicylic acid was discovered as a result of a deliberate search for antituberculosis drugs. In 1941 Bernheim showed that salicylic and benzoic acids increase the oxygen consumption of the tubercle bacillus, and it was concluded that these acids were oxidized by the bacilli as metabolites. Subsequently Lehmann (1946) investigated many derivatives of these acids and discovered para-amino salicylic acid, and showed that it was beneficial for the treatment of human tuberculosis. Since then the antituberculous action of PAS has been amply confirmed (Robson and Sullivan, 1963), and for many years PAS has been widely used as one of the standard 'first-line' drugs for the treatment of tuberculosis.

Activity Against Mycobacteria

Sensitive strains of M. tuberculosis are inhibited by concentrations of PAS ranging from $0 \cdot 5$ to $2 \cdot 0 \mu g$ per ml. The MIC of the standard H37 RV strain of M. tuberculosis is $0 \cdot 5 \mu g$ per ml, and therefore strains with an MIC higher than $2 \cdot 0 \mu g$ per ml, have a Resistance Ratio (*see* page 296) higher than four, and for practical purposes are considered resistant to this drug.

Primary drug resistance to PAS occurs, but is uncommon in developed countries. In a nationwide survey in Britain in 1963, the incidence of this was only $0 \cdot 8$ per cent (Miller *et al.*, 1966). In Australia during the five-year period 1972–1976, its annual incidence has remained less than $1 \cdot 8$ per cent (Commonwealth Dept. Health, 1973–1977). The prevalence of primary drug resistance is also low in North America. The incidence of PAS resistance in Massachusetts in 1972 and 1975/76 were about one per cent and $0 \cdot 7$ per cent respectively (Stottmeier and Burkes, 1974; Stottmeier and Baker, 1977). A co-operative study involving 22 hospitals in the United States during the eight-year period 1961–1968 showed that primary resistance to PAS remained low (average of $0 \cdot 7$ per cent), and there was no evidence that it was increasing (Doster *et al.*, 1976). In a continuing study of patients admitted to United States Veterans' Administration hospitals from 1969 to 1973 the incidence of PAS resistance has remained below $4 \cdot 5$ per cent and also has not been increasing (Hobby *et al.*, 1971; 1974). Another study has suggested that there may be a significant variation in the frequency of primary drug resistance from one geographic area to another in America, and that certain subgroups are more likely to harbour resistant organisms (Glassroth *et al.*, 1977).

In certain Asian countries newly isolated strains of M. tuberculosis are more frequently resistant to PAS and to other 'first-line' antituberculosis drugs

(Leading article, 1972). However in recent years the level of primary resistance has not increased appreciably in developing countries (WHO, 1975).

In general the 'anonymous mycobacteria' (page 832) are resistant to para-amino salicylic acid (Barter and Camens, 1968) but some strains of M. kansasii have been reported to be sensitive (Pyle, 1970).

Mode of Administration and Dosage

1. *Oral administration*. Para-amino salicylic acid is usually administered by this route, and is available either as the sodium or calcium salt. The former is commonly used, but the latter may be more suitable for patients needing sodium restriction.

The total daily adult dose ranges from 10 to 20 g, and this is administered as a single dose or in two divided doses. The most common adult dose used is 12 g daily. The exact dose prescribed depends on the weight of the patient, the type of tuberculosis treated, the patient's tolerance of the drug and the type of concurrent antituberculosis therapy. For instance higher doses of PAS are required in a streptomycin/PAS combination than in an isoniazid/PAS combination, because streptomycin-resistant strains emerge more readily (*Today's Drugs*, 1963). If PAS is selected as a companion drug to isoniazid for intermittent therapy (page 829), it is usually administered in a dose of 10 to 12 g twice-weekly (Fox, 1971; Tub. Chem. Centre, 1973).

The dose in children is usually 0·20 to 0·25 g per kg body weight per day, over 2–4 h. Thrombophlebitis and hypersensitivity reactions (page 827) were

2. *Intravenous administration*. This route of administration is now rarely used. The usual daily dose was 15 g dissolved in 500 ml, which was infused over 2–4 h. Thrombophlebitis and hypersensitivity reactions (page 827) were common problems with this mode of administration (Sattler, 1962).

3. *Patients with renal failure*. If the drug is used in such patients, dosage reduction is necessary (Kovnat *et al.*, 1973). However it should be avoided in patients with renal failure because it may aggravate uraemic gastro-intestinal symptoms and acidosis (Cheigh, 1977). In end-stage renal disease the serum half-life of PAS is extended to 23 h. Significant amounts of PAS are removed by haemodialysis (Bennett *et al.*, 1977).

Availability

1. Sodium aminosalicylate: 0·5 g tablets, 1·5 g cachets.
2. Calcium aminosalicylate: 0·5 g tablets, 1·5 g cachets.
3. Sodium aminosalicylate combined with isoniazid is available as different strengths in packets containing powder or granules:

    e.g. PAS 2 g and INAH 50 mg
         PAS 6 g and INAH 150 mg
         PAS 12 g and INAH 300 mg

Serum Levels in Relation to Dosage

Para-amino salicylic acid is well absorbed from the gastro-intestinal tract. In adults after an oral dose of 4 g, a peak serum level of 7–8 μg per ml is reached in 1–2 h (Way *et al.*, 1948). Thereafter the serum level falls and after 6 h it is less than 1 μg per ml; the serum half-life being 0·75 h.

Excretion

URINE: PAS is rapidly excreted in the urine by both glomerular filtration and tubular secretion. Approximately 85 per cent of the dose can be recovered from the urine within seven hours of oral administration (Way *et al.*, 1948). However, only 14–33 per cent of the total dose is excreted in the urine as the active unchanged drug (Robson and Sullivan, 1963). The remainder is excreted as metabolites such as acetyl-para-amino salicylic acid, para-aminosalicyluric acid and other conjugated amines.

Probenecid ('Benemid') can partially block the renal tubular secretion of PAS and therefore enhance the serum levels of the drug (Boger and Pitts, 1950).

INACTIVATION IN BODY: PAS, like the sulphonamides (page 667) appears to be metabolized in the liver mainly by acetylation and inactive acetylated compounds are excreted in the urine (Harris, 1963). By contrast to isoniazid (page 804), phenotypic variation in PAS metabolism has not been demonstrated.

Distribution of the Drug in Body

After absorption para-amino salicylic acid is well distributed to various body fluids and tissues, but it does not penetrate into the cerebrospinal fluid of patients with uninflamed meninges. Animal experiments have shown that it penetrates readily into caseous tissue (Robson and Sullivan, 1963). The serum protein binding of PAS is 60–70 per cent (Bennett *et al.*, 1977).

Mode of Action

The mechanism of action of para-amino salicylic acid on M. tuberculosis is probably similar to the mode of action of sulphonamides on bacteria (page 668).

Toxicity

1. *Gastro-intestinal irritation.* This common side-effect is experienced by almost every patient to some degree. Symptoms include nausea, vomiting, anorexia, abdominal cramps and diarrhoea. These may be minimized by taking the drug with meals or by concomitant administration of antacids. However, in some patients the drug has to be discontinued because of intractable symptoms.

2. *Hypersensitivity reactions.* These occur in about 5–10 per cent of patients and usually become evident during the first five weeks of treatment. When streptomycin, isoniazid and PAS are used together, it is sometimes difficult to know which drug is causing the reaction (page 805). Cross-sensitivity may also occur between these three drugs, and apparently PAS can trigger reactions to streptomycin and isoniazid (Thompson, 1969). In a study of 7492 patients receiving antituberculosis therapy in Cape Town, drug reactions occurred in

nine per cent; PAS was the commonest cause of these (including hepatitis) compared with streptomycin, isoniazid, ethionamide and ethambutol (Rossouw and Saunders, 1975).

The most common manifestations of PAS hypersensitivity are fever, conjunctivitis, rash and pruritus. The rash is usually morbilliform, sometimes urticarial and rarely takes the form of exfoliative dermatitis (Simpson and Walker, 1960; Thompson, 1969; Rossouw and Saunders, 1975). The blood film may show an eosinophilia or atypical monocytes. Less common manifestations include lymphadenopathy, hepatosplenomegaly and joint pains. Pulmonary infiltrates associated with eosinophilia, similar to those produced by sulphonamides (page 671), have also been observed. Other rare, probably allergic manifestations include encephalopathy and myocarditis (Thompson, 1969), and a syndrome resembling lupus erythematosus has been described (Masel, 1967). Anaphylaxis is very rare.

Hepatitis which can be fatal has also been ascribed to PAS therapy and appears to be due to hypersensitivity (Simpson and Walker, 1960; Rossouw and Saunders, 1975; Leading article, 1975). This hepatitis usually becomes apparent within the first three months of PAS treatment and is commonly preceded by features of hypersensitivity to the drug, described above. This is in contrast to the hepatitis which occurs with other antituberculosis drugs such as rifampicin (page 562), isoniazid (page 807), pyrazinamide (page 844) and ethionamide (page 856), which are much less commonly associated with allergic manifestations. It is quite possible that a percentage of cases in which hepatotoxicity was ascribed to PAS were due to isoniazid used concomitantly (page 807).

If severe hypersensitivity reactions to PAS such as 'hepatitis' or exfoliative dermatitis occur, the drug should be stopped, and large doses of corticosteroids administered in conjunction with other antituberculosis drugs. In patients with milder reactions all tuberculosis chemotherapy is usually stopped, and when the reaction subsides the offending drug is identified by administering small test doses of each drug separately. If hepatitis develops in a patient with severe tuberculosis in whom the interruption of antituberculous therapy would be unjustified, then all the drugs mentioned above which can cause hepatitis should be avoided, and drugs such as streptomycin (page 294), ethambutol (page 832), cycloserine (page 457) and capreomycin (page 849) should be considered (Leading article, 1975).

A process of slow desensitization was used in the past for patients with PAS hypersensitivity, by administering gradually increasing doses of the drug and reaching full dosage in about five weeks. Success in desensitization has been obtained by continuing PAS and other drugs in full dosage and suppressing the allergic reactions with corticosteroids (Thompson, 1969). However occasionally severe reactions develop despite steroid administration or when they are withdrawn. Nowadays desensitization is no longer recommended for PAS hypersensitivity. In this situation it is simpler and safer to discontinue PAS and substitute ethambutol (page 836) or rifampicin (page 568) (Joseph, 1973). It has been suggested that patients suffering from active pulmonary tuberculosis, in which the erythrocyte sedimentation rate prior to treatment is low, may be more prone to hypersensitivity reactions due to 'first-line' antituberculosis drugs, particularly PAS (Thompson, 1973).

3. *Haematological side-effects.* Para-amino salicylic acid may rarely cause neutropenia or acute agranulocytosis. It may also precipitate acute haemolytic anaemia in patients with glucose-6-phosphate dehydrogenase deficiency. In addition MacGibbon *et al.* (1960) reported a patient who developed an acute autoimmune haemolytic anaemia associated with renal failure due to PAS sensitivity.

4. *Renal failure.* This is a rare complication of PAS therapy, and in most cases it has probably occurred in association with haemolysis (MacGibbon *et al.*, 1960) or hypersensitivity reactions (Sattler, 1962).

5. *Hypokalaemia.* The uncommon occurrence of hypokalaemia in patients receiving PAS therapy is largely due to gastro-intestinal disturbances caused by this drug (McIntyre, 1953).

6. *Sodium overload.* Fluid retention due to excess sodium may occur in patients suffering from heart disease if the sodium salt of PAS is used. This problem may be obviated by administering the calcium salt.

7. *Goitre.* Thyroid enlargement or even myxoedema have been observed on rare occasions after a prolonged course of PAS.

Clinical Uses of the Drug

For many years para-amino salicylic acid was one of the three 'first-line' drugs for treatment of all forms of tuberculosis. Classical initial treatment for bacteriologically positive cases of tuberculosis was the concurrent administration of streptomycin, isoniazid and PAS (page 810). These three drugs were continued for three or four months or longer until bacteriological conversion occurred, and then isoniazid and PAS alone were continued for a total period of eighteen months to two years (Citron, 1972).

In the past PAS was only deleted from this regimen if the M. tuberculosis strain was PAS-resistant, or the patient developed severe adverse effects. Nowadays rifampicin and ethambutol are commonly used 'first-line' drugs and are preferred to PAS. Such new regimens are usually more effective, and produce fewer side-effects and less interruptions of treatment. For these reasons PAS is being used less and less in developed countries, but its use is likely to be continued for some time in developing countries, because of its cheapness (Leading article, 1973). PAS is no longer included amongst the 'first-line' drugs for the treatment of tuberculosis in Australia (Commonwealth Dept. Health Australia, 1977).

PAS has also been used as one of the drugs in the intermittent chemotherapy regimens for tuberculosis (page 811). In India it was shown that PAS (0·2 g per kg body weight) and isoniazid (15 mg per kg body weight) administered twice-weekly were about as effective as a standard PAS/isoniazid combination administered daily to patients with pulmonary tuberculosis (Tub. Chem. Centre, 1973).

REFERENCES

Barter, C. E. and Camens, I. M. H. (1968), 'Lung infection with anonymous mycobacteria', *Med. J. Aust.*, **1,** 408.
Bennett, W. M., Singer, I., Golper, T., Feig, P. and Coggins, C. J. (1977), 'Guidelines

for drug therapy in renal failure', *Ann. Intern. Med.*, **86,** 754.

Bernheim, F. (1941), 'The effect of various substances on the oxygen uptake of the tubercle bacillus', *J. Bact.*, **41,** 387; quoted by Robson and Sullivan (1963).

Boger, W. P. and Pitts, F. W. (1950), 'Influence of p-(di-n-propylsulfamyl)-benzoic acid, "benemid", on para-amino-salicylic acid (PAS) plasma concentrations', *Ann. Rev. Tuberc. Pulm. Dis.*, **61,** 862.

Cheigh, J. S. (1977), 'Drug administration in renal failure', *Amer. J. Med.*, **62,** 555.

Citron, K. M. (1972), 'Tuberculosis-chemotherapy', *Brit. med. J.*, **1,** 426.

Commonwealth Department of Health Australia (1973–1977), *Tuberculosis Statistics,* Canberra.

Commonwealth Department of Health Australia (1977), *Treatment of Tuberculosis with Particular Reference to Chemotherapy*, 4th edn., Australian Government Publishing Service, Canberra.

Doster, B., Caras, G. J. and Snider, D. E., Jr. (1976), 'A continuing survey of primary drug resistance in tuberculosis, 1961 to 1968', *Amer. Rev. Resp. Dis.*, **113,** 419.

Fox, W. (1971), 'General considerations in intermittent drug therapy of pulmonary tuberculosis', *Postgrad. Med. J.*, **47,** 729.

Glassroth, J. L., Kilburn, J., Snider, D. E. and Kopanoff, D. (1977), 'A survey of primary drug resistance in tuberculosis', *Amer. Rev. Resp. Dis.* (Suppl.), **115,** 398.

Harris, H. W. (1963), 'Current concepts of the metabolism of antituberculous agents', *Ann. N.Y. Acad. Sci.*, **106,** 43.

Hobby, G. L., Johnson, P. M. and Boytar-Papirnyik, V. (1971), 'Primary drug resistance: A continuing study of drug resistance in tuberculosis in a veteran population within the United States. IX. September 1969–September 1970', *Amer. Rev. Resp. Dis.*, **103,** 842.

Hobby, G. L., Johnson, P. M. and Boytar-Papirnyik, V. (1974), 'Primary drug resistance: A continuing study of drug resistance in tuberculosis in a veteran population within the United States. X. September 1970 to September 1973', *Amer. Rev. Resp. Dis.*, **110,** 95.

Joseph, M. (1973), 'Hypersensitivity to anti-tuberculous drugs', *Aust. N.Z. J. Med.*, **3,** 311.

Kovnat, P., Labovitz, E. and Levison, S. P. (1973), 'Antibiotics and the kidney', *Med. Clin. North Amer.*, **57,** 1045.

Leading Article (1972), 'Resistant tubercle bacilli', *Lancet*, **2,** 412.

Leading Article (1973), 'PAS', *Tubercle*, **54,** 165.

Leading Article (1975), 'Antituberculous drugs and the liver', *Brit. med. J.*, **2,** 522.

Lehmann, J. (1946), 'Para-aminosalicylic acid in the treatment of tuberculosis', *Lancet*, **1,** 15.

MacGibbon, B., Loughridge, L., Hourihane, D. O'B and Boyd, D. W. (1960), 'Autoimmune haemolytic anaemia with acute renal failure due to phenacetin and p-aminosalicylic acid', *Lancet*, **1,** 7.

Masel, M. A. (1967), 'A lupus-like reaction to antituberculosis drugs', *Med. J. Aust.*, **2,** 738.

McIntyre, P. A. (1953), 'Hypokalaemia occurring during para-aminosalicylic acid therapy', *Bull. Johns Hopkins Hosp.*, **92,** 210.

Miller, A. B., Tall, R., Fox, W., Lefford, M. J. and Mitchison, D. A. (1966), 'Primary drug resistance in pulmonary tuberculosis in Great Britain: Second national survey, 1963', *Tubercle, Lond.*, **47,** 92.

Pyle, M. M. (1970), 'Ethambutol and viomycin', *Med. Clin. North Amer.*, **54,** 1317.

Robson, J. M. and Sullivan, F. M. (1963), 'Antituberculosis drugs', *Pharmacol. Rev.*, **15,** 169.

Rossouw, J. E. and Saunders, S. J. (1975), 'Hepatic complications of antituberculous therapy', *Q. J. Med.*, **44,** 1.

Sattler, A. (1962), 'The present status of PAS in tuberculosis therapy', *Amer. Rev.*

Resp. Dis., **85,** 927.

Simpson, D. G. and Walker, J. H. (1960), 'Hypersensitivity to para-aminosalicytic acid', *Amer. J. Med.*, **29,** 297.

Stottmeier, K. D. and Burkes, J. (1974), 'Primary drug-resistant Mycobacterium tuberculosis isolated in Massachusetts in 1972', *J. Infect. Dis.*, **130,** 293.

Stottmeier, K. D. and Baker, S. (1977), 'Primary drug-resistant tuberculosis in Massachusetts, 1975/76', *New Engl. J. Med.*, **296,** 823.

Thompson, J. E. (1969), 'The management of hypersensitivity reactions to antituberculosis drugs', *Med. J. Aust.*, **2,** 1058.

Thompson, J. E. (1973), 'The predictability of hypersensitivity to antituberculous drugs', *Aust. N.Z. J. Med.*, **3,** 239.

Today's Drugs (1963), 'Drugs for tuberculosis', *Brit. med. J.*, **1,** 1527.

Today's Drugs (1968), 'Drugs for tuberculosis', *Brit. med. J.*, **3,** 664.

Tuberculosis Chemotherapy Centre, Madras (1973), 'Controlled comparison of oral twice-weekly and oral daily isoniazid plus PAS in newly diagnosed pulmonary tuberculosis', *Brit. med. J.*, **2,** 7.

Way, E. L., Smith, P. K., Howie, D. L., Weiss, R. and Swanson, R. (1948), 'The absorption, distribution, excretion and fate of para-aminosalicylic acid', *J. Pharmac. exp. Ther.*, **93,** 368.

WHO (1975), 'Tuberculosis control: Progress of the new strategy', *WHO Chronicle*, **29,** 123.

Ethambutol

Description

This drug was discovered at Lederle Laboratories in 1961, when randomly selected synthetic compounds were being tested for antituberculosis activity. It was named ethambutol or dextro-2,2'-(ethylenediimino)-di-1-butanol dihydrochloride, and was shown to have a high degree of antituberculosis activity (Thomas *et al.*, 1961). Numerous clinical studies have now been carried out with ethambutol and it is now accepted as a 'first-line' drug for the treatment of human tuberculosis. It is marketed with the trade name of 'Myambutol' (Lederle).

Activity Against Mycobacteria

Ethambutol is only active against mycobacteria, all other bacteria being completely resistant (Wilson, 1967).

1. *Mycobacterium tuberculosis*. This is highly sensitive and the minimum inhibitory concentration is usually 1–2 μg per ml and seldom higher than 5 μg per ml (Karlson, 1961). The MIC of the standard H37 RV strain is 0·5–2·0 μg per ml. Strains with an MIC of 8 μg per ml (Resistance Ratio 4) are considered as sensitive, but those with higher MIC's as resistant. Ethambutol is active against M. tuberculosis strains resistant to isoniazid and/or other commonly used antituberculosis drugs (Robson and Sullivan, 1963). Ethambutol-resistant M. tuberculosis strains can be readily produced *in vitro* (Hobby and Lenert, 1972), and if it is used in the treatment of human tuberculosis without an adequate companion drug or drugs, resistant strains will emerge (Crofton, 1971). Primary ethambutol resistance is uncommon in developed countries. In a continuing study of patients admitted to United States Veterans' Administration hospitals the incidences each year of primary ethambutol resistance from 1969 to 1973 were 0·99, 1·6, 2·2 and 9·7 per cent respectively (Hobby *et al.*, 1971; 1974). The incidences of ethambutol resistance in Massachusetts in 1972 and 1975/76 were about 0·55 and 0·12 per cent respectively (Stottmeier and Burkes, 1974; Stottmeier and Baker, 1977). In Australia the incidence of primary ethambutol resistance is exceedingly low (Commonwealth Dept. Health Australia, 1973–1977). Acquired (secondary) resistance may occur as a result of inadequate chemotherapy.

2. *Other mycobacteria*. Some of the mycobacteria, previously referred to as anonymous, atypical or opportunist, appear to be ethambutol-sensitive *in vitro* (Thomas *et al.*, 1961; Karlson, 1961). At least ten of these organisms have been reported to cause human disease namely, Mycobacterium kansasii, M. avium, intracellulare and scrofulaceum (MAIS complex), M. xenopi, M. for-

tuitum, M. chelonei, M. simiae, M. szulgai, M. terrae and M. triviale (Runyon, 1974; Barksdale and Kim, 1977). The common clinical manifestations of infection with these mycobacteria are pulmonary disease and lymphadenitis, but disseminated disease or other organ involvement can occur. M. kansasii infections are more common in the United States and Europe than in Australia. This organism is commonly sensitive to ethambutol (Pyle, 1970; Harris *et al.*, 1975; Elder *et al.*, 1977) and to rifampicin (page 553). Mycobacteria of the 'anonymous group' are responsible for a significant number of mycobacterial infections in Australia (Commonwealth Dept. Health Australia, 1977), particularly in the Northern and Western parts of the country; M. intracellulare and to a lesser extent M. scrofulaceum and M. kansasii are most frequently involved. Some strains of M. intracellulare have been found to be ethambutol-sensitive *in vitro*. However *in vitro* sensitivity data do not always correlate with the results of ethambutol treatment for presumed infections with these mycobacteria (Evans and Thong, 1969; Elder *et al.*, 1977). Sometimes surgery is required for the pulmonary disease or lymphadenitis resulting from these mycobacterial infections.

Mycobacterium marinum (M. balnei) is not an uncommon cause of superficial infections (swimming pool or fish tank granuloma). This organism is usually resistant to most antituberculosis drugs but it may be sensitive to ethambutol (Barrow and Hewitt, 1971; Sage and Derrington, 1973), rifampicin (page 553) and co-trimoxazole (page 714). The place of chemotherapy for this infection is doubtful because it never assumes a serious form and resolves spontaneously in 6–30 months (Leading article, 1970).

Mycobacterium ulcerans is an important cause of disabling cutaneous ulceration in tropical and semi-tropical areas. Although some strains may be sensitive to ethambutol, streptomycin (page 294) is the only antibiotic to which this organism is consistently sensitive. In the absence of secondary bacterial infection it is doubtful whether any chemotherapeutic agents are of value for infections due to M. ulcerans, and surgical excision and skin grafting are the best forms of treatment (Quinn and Crotty, 1963; Lane, 1964; Report of Uganda Buruli Group, 1970; Radford, 1975).

Mode of Administration and Dosage

1. *Daily chemotherapy*. Ethambutol is administered by the oral route. The dose recommended is 25 mg per kg per day, administered in one dose, and an average daily adult dose is 1·2 to 1·6 g. After two months treatment the dose is reduced to 15 mg per kg per day (for adults 0·8 to 1·2 g per day), to reduce the frequency of ocular complications (page 835). In some European countries it is customary to continue the higher dosage of 25 mg per kg per day throughout the course of antituberculosis chemotherapy.

2. *Intermittent chemotherapy*. Ethambutol is suitable for fully supervised intermittent regimens (page 811), which have been used extensively, particularly in developing countries (Fox, 1971). For this purpose the drug may be given in a dose of 45–50 mg per kg twice-weekly (maximum dose 3·2 g) or 90 mg per kg once-weekly (Hong Kong, 1974; Sbarbaro and Hudson, 1974).

3. *Patients with renal failure*. As ethambutol is largely excreted via the kidney (page 834), these patients need dosage reduction (Kovnat *et al.*, 1973).

The normal serum half-life of ethambutol of 4 h is doubled in end-stage renal disease (Bennett *et al.*, 1977). The following dosage schedules have been recommended for patients with renal failure; for those with creatinine clearances of 50–25, 25–10 and less than 10 ml per min, daily oral doses of 25–15, 15–7·5 and 5 mg per kg respectively. A dose of 5 mg per kg per day is also recommended for patients undergoing haemodialysis or peritoneal dialysis, although significant amounts of the drug are removed by both forms of dialysis (Cheigh, 1977).

Availability

Ethambutol ('Myambutol' Lederle) is available as 100 and 400 mg tablets.

Serum Levels in Relation to Dosage

Ethambutol is well absorbed after oral administration, and following a dose of 25 mg per kg body weight, a peak serum level of about 5 μg per ml is reached in approximately 4 h (Peets *et al.*, 1965). Doubling the dose doubles the peak serum level (Place and Thomas, 1963). Thereafter the serum level slowly falls and 24 h after the dose it is usually less than 1·0 μg per ml. Administration with food does not impair ethambutol absorption. In the absence of renal disease ethambutol does not accumulate if daily doses of 25 mg per kg are used (Place and Thomas, 1963).

Excretion

URINE: Most of absorbed ethambutol (about 80 per cent) is excreted via the kidney as the active unchanged drug. This excretion occurs within 24 h of administration (Place and Thomas, 1963), and high concentrations of the active drug are attained in urine.

INACTIVATION IN BODY: Some 8–15 per cent of absorbed ethambutol is converted to various inactive metabolites, and these are also excreted in the urine (Peets *et al.*, 1965). The rate of ethambutol metabolism is similar in all individuals and it is not altered after prolonged administration.

FAECES: Unabsorbed ethambutol, about 20 per cent of an oral dose, is excreted unchanged in the faeces.

Distribution of the Drug in Body

Detailed data about the distribution of ethambutol in various body fluids and tissues are unavailable, but as the drug is therapeutically effective, it presumably reaches infected tissues in sufficient concentrations. Peets *et al.* (1965) have shown that ethambutol enters the red blood cells, where it accumulates against a concentration gradient. The erythrocytes may therefore serve as a depot for the drug.

Ethambutol does not enter the spinal fluid of patients with normal meninges (Place *et al.*, 1969), though very low levels have been found by some investigators (Pilheu *et al.*, 1971). In patients with tuberculous meningitis, some ethambutol enters the cerebrospinal fluid and with a daily dose of 25 mg per kg, CSF ethambutol concentrations of $1-2\,\mu g$ per ml have been reported (Place *et al.*, 1969; Bobrowitz, 1972). The serum protein binding of ethambutol is less than 10 per cent (Bennett *et al.*, 1977).

Mode of Action

Ethambutol appears to enter the cells of Mycobacterium tuberculosis in a passive manner, and the organisms do not accumulate the drug against a concentration gradient (Beggs and Auran, 1972). Its precise mechanism of action is not known, but it is probably an antimetabolite and may inhibit mycobacterial RNA synthesis (Forbes *et al.*, 1966). Ethambutol exerts its maximum inhibitory effect against mycobacteria at a neutral pH (Beggs and Andrews, 1974).

Toxicity

1. *Ocular complications*. Retrobulbar neuritis is the main complication of ethambutol therapy. Symptoms include blurred vision, central scotomata and colour blindness, but sometimes the only change is constriction of visual fields. These changes are usually completely reversible if treatment is stopped (Clarke *et al.*, 1972), though defective colour vision may persist for a prolonged period (Lees *et al.*, 1971). If the drug is continued after the onset of symptoms, optic atrophy with permanent impairment of vision may result. Rarely a haemorrhagic retinopathy has been observed.

Ocular complications due to ethambutol appear to be dose related (Leibold, 1966). Previously when a dose as high as 50 mg per kg per day was used, this complication occurred in 15 per cent of patients, but with a dose of 25 mg per kg per day continued longer than for two months, it occurred in about 5 per cent of patients. Aquinas and Citron (1972) treated 40 patients with daily rifampicin, ethambutol and capreomycin. Ethambutol was used in a dose of 25 mg per kg per day for six months and severe retrobulbar neuritis was observed in two patients, one of whom developed haemorrhagic retinopathy. These patients still had evidence of persistent eye damage 18 months after the drug was stopped. If ethambutol is used in a dose of 25 mg per kg for 60 days only, and then 15 mg per kg per day (as currently recommended), ocular complications are infrequent and commonly mild, but occasional severe cases still occur. The only changes usually noted with such dose regimens are diminution of visual acuity and red-green colour blindness, in most cases both completely reversible (Wilson, 1967). The intermittent ethambutol regimens of either 45 mg per kg twice-weekly or 90 mg per kg once-weekly also appear quite safe (Hong Kong, 1974).

Ocular complications sometimes can arise many months after the drug is started, but the total dose of ethambutol administered appears to have no relation to the frequency of these side-effects (Adel, 1969).

Patients treated by ethambutol should be instructed to report all ocular symptoms, and where possible it seems wise to perform base-line ophthalmological tests before treatment is started (Leading article, 1973). Most authorities now regard this as a satisfactory safeguard, but some still recommend the testing of visual fields, visual acuity and colour discrimination, every six weeks.

2. *Peripheral neuritis*. This is a rare side-effect. Tugwell and James (1972) described three patients who developed this complication during ethambutol therapy. One patient was treated by large doses (50 mg per kg per day) and also developed optic neuritis, but the other two patients received ethambutol in doses of less than 20 mg per kg per day. Two of these patients were receiving isoniazid as well, but it appeared that isoniazid was not responsible for this complication, because the neuritis only improved in all three patients when ethambutol was discontinued. Although this complication is rare, it is important to recognise that ethambutol as well as isoniazid (page 806) can cause peripheral neuropathy.

3. *Nephrotoxicity*. Circumstances relating to the occurrence and recovery of renal failure in two male patients aged 56 and 69 years suggested that ethambutol may rarely cause direct toxic damage to the kidneys (Collier *et al.*, 1976). A diffuse interstitial nephritis with similar features to that described with penicillin (page 29) and methicillin (page 72) has been observed in two patients, which may have been due to isoniazid and/or ethambutol therapy (Stone *et al.*, 1976).

4. *Other side-effects*. Allergic reactions with ethambutol appear to be very rare. The drug may decrease the renal clearance of uric acid in man thereby elevating serum urate concentrations (Postlethwaite *et al.*, 1972), and precipitation of acute gout has been observed. No other adverse effects such as gastrointestinal irritation or damage to the liver or bone marrow have been reported.

Polyarthritis, rash and hepatitis, associated with anti-native DNA antibodies and positive antinuclear factor, have been described in a nine-year-old boy after seven months continuous treatment with rifampicin and ethambutol (Grennan and Sturrock, 1976). It was considered that rifampicin was more likely to be the cause of these side-effects (page 568).

False-positive phentolamine tests for phaeochromocytoma have been observed in patients receiving ethambutol, presumably because of some interaction between these substances (Gabriel, 1972).

The drug also appears to be non-teratogenic to the human fetus (Pyle, 1970), and it can be used in pregnancy if indicated (Commonwealth Dept. Health Australia, 1977).

Clinical Uses of the Drug

1. *Initial treatment of pulmonary tuberculosis*. Ethambutol is one of the 'first-line' antituberculosis drugs (page 810). It is frequently used for the initial treatment of new patients with pulmonary tuberculosis, commonly as a substitute for PAS (page 829). Triple therapy with streptomycin, isoniazid and ethambutol may be used for the first two to four months, and thereafter an isoniazid/ethambutol regimen is continued to complete an 18 month to two-year course. Ethambutol containing regimens are as effective as those containing PAS for the treatment of new patients with pulmonary tuberculosis, and patients tolerate ethambutol better than PAS (Bobrowitz and Robins, 1967; Clarke *et al.*, 1972; Doster *et al.*, 1973; BMRC, 1973; Bobrowitz, 1974). However there is some evidence that ethambutol may not be quite as effective as PAS for the treatment of advanced cavitary tuberculosis (Citron, 1972). Ethambutol is also an acceptable replacement for streptomycin during

the first three to four months of triple therapy in patients in whom streptomycin is contraindicated. In Australia the recommended initial three drug therapy consists of isoniazid, rifampicin and either streptomycin or ethambutol for two to four months and in the absence of drug resistance or other contraindication, continuation therapy consists of isoniazid and rifampicin. If streptomycin is used, it is suggested that it be replaced by ethambutol after eight weeks to avoid infections (Commonwealth Dept. Health Australia, 1977). Standard chemotherapy of pulmonary tuberculosis in other developed countries is similar (see page 810).

Ethambutol is an important drug when used together with rifampicin and isoniazid for the short-course chemotherapy of pulmonary tuberculosis (page 812). It also has been used successfully for fully supervised intermittent chemotherapy of pulmonary tuberculosis (see page 811), most commonly combined with either isoniazid (page 811) or rifampicin (page 569).

2. *Retreatment of pulmonary tuberculosis.* Ethambutol is suitable for the retreatment of patients with pulmonary tuberculosis, who are excreting bacilli resistant to one or several of the older 'first-line' drugs, such as isoniazid, streptomycin and PAS. For this purpose ethambutol should be combined with at least one other drug to which the tubercle bacilli are still sensitive, otherwise ethambutol resistance will emerge within a few months (Pyle, 1970). For instance combined therapy with cycloserine is reasonably satisfactory, but the results with an ethambutol/ethionamide regimen are somewhat inferior (Pyle, 1970). Similarly an ethambutol/capreomycin regimen has been reported to be effective and well tolerated (Lim and Aquinas, 1969). The best results however are obtained when ethambutol is combined with rifampicin (page 569), a combination which is both effective and well tolerated (Somner *et al.*, 1971; 1973; Lees *et al.*, 1972). Some authors believe that where possible it is preferable to use three drugs initially to treat patients with drug-resistant tuberculosis. Aquinas and Citron (1972) added capreomycin to the rifampicin/ethambutol regimen for the first six months to treat 37 such patients successfully. Andrews *et al.* (1974) successfully treated 27 patients with isoniazid-resistant pulmonary tuberculosis by daily ethambutol and rifampicin for two years, but with the addition of daily capreomycin for the first four months.

Intermittent administration of ethambutol with rifampicin has also been satisfactory for the retreatment of tuberculosis. In a controlled trial in Hong Kong on Chinese adults with isoniazid-resistant pulmonary tuberculosis, favourable results were obtained when these drugs were used in once-weekly or bi-weekly regimens (Hong Kong, 1974; 1975). Similar results were obtained in studies carried out in Poland (A Cooperative Study, 1976).

3. *Tuberculous meningitis.* Ethambutol has been used for this disease, usually in combination with isoniazid and streptomycin (Place *et al.*, 1969; Bobrowitz, 1972; Girgis *et al.*, 1976).

4. *Other forms of tuberculosis.* Ethambutol can be combined with other antituberculosis drugs to treat tuberculosis of the genito-urinary tract or of the bones and joints. Drug regimens for these diseases are the same as those used in pulmonary tuberculosis.

5. *Tuberculosis chemoprophylaxis.* An intermittent regimen using isoniazid plus ethambutol has been used successfully for this purpose (Grzybowski *et al.*, 1976) (see page 817).

6. *Other mycobacterial infections.* Ethambutol has been used in combination with isoniazid and streptomycin to treat pulmonary infections due to M. kansasii successfully (*see* page 817). It has also been combined with rifampicin to treat M. marinum infections (page 572).

7. *Nocardia brasiliensis infections.* Ethambutol also has been reported to be effective in the treatment of mycetomas caused by this organism (Borelli and Leal, 1969; Berd, 1973).

REFERENCES

A Cooperative Tuberculosis Chemotherapy Study in Poland (1976), 'A comparative study of daily followed by twice- and once-weekly regimens of ethambutol and rifampicin in the retreatment of patients with pulmonary tuberculosis; Second report', *Tubercle*, **57**, 105.

Adel, A. (1969), 'Ophthalmological side-effects of ethambutol', *Scand. J. resp. Dis.* (Suppl.), **69**, 55.

Andrews, R. H., Jenkins, P. A., Marks, J., Pines, A., Selkon, J. B. and Somner, A. R. (1974), 'Treatment of isoniazid-resistant pulmonary tuberculosis with ethambutol, rifampicin and capreomycin: A co-operative study in England and Wales', *Tubercle*, **55**, 105.

Aquinas, M. and Citron, K. M. (1972), 'Rifampicin, ethambutol and capreomycin in pulmonary tuberculosis, previously treated with both first and second line drugs: The results of 2 years chemotherapy', *Tubercle*, **53**, 153.

Barksdale, L. and Kim, K. (1977), 'Mycobacteria', *Bacteriol. Rev.* **41**, 217.

Barrow, G. I. and Hewitt, M. (1971), 'Skin infection with Mycobacterium marinum from a tropical fish tank', *Brit. med. J.*, **1**, 505.

Barter, C. E. and Camens, I. M. H. (1968), 'Lung infection with anonymous mycobacteria', *Med. J. Aust.*, **1**, 408.

Beggs, W. H. and Auran, W. E. (1972), 'Uptake and binding of ^{14}C-ethambutol by tubercle bacilli and the relation of binding to growth inhibition', *Antimicrob. Ag. Chemother.*, **2**, 390.

Beggs, W. H. and Andrews, F. A. (1974), 'Chemical characterization of ethambutol binding to Mycobacterium smegmatis', *Antimicrob. Ag. Chemother.*, **5**, 234.

Bennett, W. M., Singer, I., Golper, T., Feig, P. and Coggins, C. J. (1977), 'Guidelines for drug therapy in renal failure', *Ann. Intern. Med.*, **86**, 754.

Berd, D. (1973), 'Nocardia brasiliensis infection in the United States: A report of nine cases and a review of the literature', *Amer. J. Clin. Path.*, **59**, 254.

Bobrowitz, I. D. and Robins, D. E. (1967), 'Ethambutol-isoniazid versus PAS-isoniazid in original treatment of pulmonary tuberculosis', *Amer. Rev. Resp. Dis.*, **96**, 428.

Bobrowitz, I. D. (1972), 'Ethambutol in tuberculous meningitis', *Chest*, **61**, 629.

Bobrowitz, I. D. (1974), 'Ethambutol-isoniazid versus streptomycin-ethambutol-isoniazid in original treatment of cavitary tuberculosis', *Amer. Rev. Resp. Dis.*, **109**, 548.

Borelli, D. and Leal, J. (1969), 'Mycetoma by Nocardia brasiliensis successfully treated with ethambutol', *Trans. R. Soc. Med. Hyg.*, **63**, 881; quoted by Berd (1973).

British Medical Research Council Co-operative Study (1973), 'Co-operative controlled trial of a standard regimen of streptomycin, PAS and isoniazid and three alternative regimens of chemotherapy in Britain', *Tubercle*, **54**, 99.

Cheigh, J. S. (1977), 'Drug administration in renal failure', *Amer. J. Med.*, **62**, 555.

Citron, K. M. (1972), 'Tuberculosis-chemotherapy', *Brit. med. J.*, **1**, 426.

Clarke, G. B. M., Cuthbert, J., Cuthbert, R. J. and Lees, A. W. (1972), 'Isoniazid plus ethambutol in the initial treatment of pulmonary tuberculosis', *Brit. J. Dis. Chest.*, **66**, 272.

Collier, J., Joekes, A. M., Philalithis, P. E. and Thompson, F. D. (1976), 'Two cases of ethambutol nephrotoxicity', *Brit. med. J.*, **2**, 1105.

Commonwealth Department of Health Australia (1977), *Treatment of Tuberculosis with Particular Reference to Chemotherapy*, 4th edn., Australian Government Publishing Service, Canberra.

Commonwealth Department of Health Australia (1973–1977), *Tuberculosis Statistics*, Canberra.

Crofton, J. (1971), 'Problems of drug resistance in tuberculosis—the newer anti-tuberculosis drugs', *Postgrad. Med. J.*, **47**, 748.

Davey, M. E. (1966), 'A preliminary report on the use of ethambutol in the treatment of infections due to 'anonymous' mycobacteria', *Med. J. Aust.*, **1**, 789.

Dawson, D. J., Reznikov, M., Blacklock, Z. M. and Leggo, J. H. (1974), 'Atypical mycobacteria isolated from clinical material in South-Eastern Queensland', *Pathology*, **6**, 153.

Doster, B., Murray, F. J., Newman, R. and Woolpert, S. F. (1973), 'Ethambutol in the initial treatment of pulmonary tuberculosis', *Amer. Rev. Resp. Dis.*, **107**, 177.

Elder, J. L., Edwards, F. G. B. and Abrahams, E. W. (1977), 'Tuberculosis due to Mycobacterium kansasii', *Aust. N.Z. J. Med.*, **7**, 8.

Evans, C. and Thong, K. L. (1969), 'A clinical trial of ethambutol plus capreomycin in the treatment of atypical tuberculosis', *Med. J. Aust.*, **2**, 744.

Forbes, M., Peets, E. A. and Kuck, N. A. (1966), 'Effect of ethambutol on mycobacteria', *Ann. N.Y. Acad. Sci.*, **135**, 726; quoted by Pyle (1970).

Fox, W. (1971), 'General considerations in intermittent drug therapy of pulmonary tuberculosis', *Postgrad. Med. J.*, **47**, 729.

Gabriel, R. (1972), 'Ethambutol and a false-positive screening test for phaeochromocytoma', *Brit. med. J.*, **3**, 332.

Girgis, N. I., Yassin, M. W., Sippel, J. E., Sorensen, K., Hassan, A., Miner, W. F., Farid, Z. and Abu El Ella, A. (1976), 'The value of ethambutol in the treatment of tuberculosis meningitis', *J. Trop. Med. Hyg.*, **79**, 14.

Grennan, D. M. and Sturrock, R. D. (1976), 'Polyarthritis, hepatitis and anti-native DNA antibodies after treatment with ethambutol and rifampicin', *Tubercle*, **57**, 259.

Grzybowski, S., Galbraith, J. D. and Dorken, E. (1976), 'Chemoprophylaxis trial in Canadian Eskimos', *Tubercle*, **57**, 263.

Harris, G. D., Johanson, W. G., Jr. and Nicholson, D. P. (1975), 'Response to chemotherapy of pulmonary infection due to Mycobacterium kansasii', *Amer: Rev. Resp. Dis.*, **112**, 31.

Hobby, G. L., Johnson, P. M. and Boytar-Papirnyik, V. (1971), 'Primary drug resistance: A continuing study of drug resistance in tuberculosis in a veteran population within the United States. IX. September 1969–September 1970', *Amer. Rev. Resp. Dis.*, **103**, 842.

Hobby, G. L. and Lenert, T. F. (1972), 'Observations on the action of rifampin and ethambutol alone and in combination with other antituberculous drugs', *Amer. Rev. Resp. Dis.*, **105**, 292.

Hobby, G. L., Johnson, P. M. and Boytar-Papirnyik, V. (1974), 'Primary drug resistance: A continuing study of drug resistance in tuberculosis in a veteran population within the United States. X. September 1970 to September 1973', *Amer. Rev. Resp. Dis.*, **110**, 95.

Hong Kong Tuberculosis Treatment Services/Brompton Hospital/British Medical Research Council Investigation (1974), 'A controlled clinical trial of daily and intermittent regimens of rifampicin plus ethambutol in the retreatment of patients with pulmonary tuberculosis in Hong Kong', *Tubercle*, **55**, 1.

Hong Kong Tuberculosis Treatment Services/Brompton Hospital/British Medical

Research Council (1975), 'A controlled trial of daily and intermittent rifampicin plus ethambutol in the retreatment of patients with pulmonary tuberculosis: Results up to 30 months', *Tubercle*, **56**, 179.

Karlson, A. G. (1961), 'The *in vitro* activity of ethambutol (dextro-2,2'-[ethylenediimino]-DI-1-butanol) against tubercle bacilli and other microorganisms', *Amer. Rev. Resp. Dis.*, **84**, 905.

Kovnat, P., Labovitz, E. and Levison, S. P. (1973), 'Antibiotics and the kidney', *Med. Clin. North Amer.*, **57**, 1045.

Lane, D. (1964), 'Mycobacterium ulcerans infection in Queensland', *Med. J. Aust.*, **1**, 124.

Leading Article (1970), 'Hazard from the home aquarium', *Brit. med. J.*, **1**, 438.

Leading Article (1973), 'Rifampicin or ethambutol in the routine treatment of tuberculosis', *Brit. med. J.*, **4**, 568.

Lees, A. W., Allan, G. W., Smith, J., Tyrrell, W. F. and Fallon, R. J. (1971), 'Toxicity from rifampicin plus isoniazid and rifampicin plus ethambutol therapy', *Tubercle*, **52**, 182.

Lees, A. W., Allan, G. W., Smith, J., Tyrrell, W. F. and Fallon, R. J. (1972), 'Retreatment of pulmonary tuberculosis with rifampin and ethambutol', *Amer. Rev. Resp. Dis.*, **105**, 129.

Leibold, J. E. (1966), 'The ocular toxicity of ethambutol and its relation to dose', *Ann. N.Y. Acad. Sci.*, **135**, 904.

Lim, B. T. and Aquinas, M. (1969), 'Ethambutol and capreomycin in the re-treatment of advanced pulmonary tuberculosis', *Amer. Rev. Resp. Dis.*, **99**, 792.

Marks, J. and Jenkins, P. A. (1971), 'The opportunist mycobacteria—a 20-year retrospect', *Postgrad. Med. J.*, **47**, 705.

Peets, E. A., Sweeney, W. M., Place, V. A. and Buyske, D. A. (1965), 'The absorption, excretion, and metabolic fate of ethambutol in man', *Amer. Rev. Resp. Dis.*, **91**, 51.

Pilheu, J. A., Maglio, F., Cetrangolo, R. and Pleus, A. D. (1971), 'Concentrations of ethambutol in the cerebrospinal fluid after oral administration', *Tubercle*, **52**, 117.

Pyle, M. M. (1970), 'Ethambutol and viomycin', *Med. Clin. North Amer.*, **54**, 1317.

Place, V. A. and Thomas, J. P. (1963), 'Clinical pharmacology of ethambutol', *Amer. Rev. Resp. Dis.*, **87**, 901.

Place, V. A., Pyle, M. M. and De la Huerga, J. (1969), 'Ethambutol in tuberculous meningitis', *Amer. Rev. Resp. Dis.*, **99**, 783.

Postlethwaite, A. E., Bartel, A. G. and Kelley, W. N. (1972), 'Hyperuricemia due to ethambutol', *New Engl. J. Med.*, **286**, 761.

Quinn, J. V. and Crotty, J. M. (1963), 'Mycobacterium ulcerans infections in the Northern Territory', *Med. J. Aust.*, **2**, 317.

Radford, A. J. (1975), 'Mycobacterium ulcerans in Australia', *Aust. N.Z. J. Med.*, **5**, 162.

Report II of the Uganda Buruli Group (1970), 'Clinical features and treatment of pre-ulcerative buruli lesions', *Brit. med. J.*, **1**, 390.

Robson, J. M. and Sullivan, F. M. (1963), 'Antituberculosis drugs', *Pharmacol. Rev.*, **15**, 169.

Runyon, E. H. (1974), 'Ten mycobacterial pathogens', *Tubercle*, **55**, 235.

Sage, R. E. and Derrington, A. W. (1973), 'Opportunistic cutaneous Mycobacterium marinum infection mimicking Mycobacterium ulcerans in lymphosarcoma', *Med. J. Aust.*, **2**, 434.

Sbarbaro, J. A. and Hudson, L. D. (1974), 'High dose ethambutol; An oral alternate for intermittent chemotherapy', *Amer. Rev. Resp. Dis.*, **110**, 91.

Somner, A. R., Selkon, J. B., Walton, M. and White, A. B. (1971), 'Drug resistant pulmonary tuberculosis treated with ethambutol and rifampicin in North East England', *Tubercle*, **52**, 266.

Somner, A. R., Selkon, J. B., Walton, M. and White, A. B. (1973), 'Drug resistant pulmonary tuberculosis treated with ethambutol and rifampicin in North East England', *Tubercle*, **54**, 141.

Stone, W. J., Waldron, J. A., Dixon, J. H., Jr., Primm, R. K. and Horn, R. G. (1976), 'Acute diffuse interstitial nephritis related to chemotherapy of tuberculosis', *Antimicrob. Ag. Chemother.*, **10**, 164.

Stottmeier, K. D. and Burkes, J. (1974), 'Primary drug-resistant Mycobacterium tuberculosis isolated in Massachusetts in 1972', *J. Infect. Dis.*, **130**, 293.

Stottmeier, K. D. and Baker, S. (1977), 'Primary drug-resistant tuberculosis in Massachusetts, 1975/76', *New Engl. J. Med.*, **296**, 823.

Thomas, J. P., Baughn, C. O., Wilkinson, R. G. and Shepherd, R. G. (1961), 'A new synthetic compound with antituberculous activity in mice: Ethambutol (dextro-2,2'-[ethylenediimino]-DI-1-butanol)', *Amer. Rev. Resp. Dis.*, **83**, 891.

Tugwell, P. and James, S. L. (1972), 'Peripheral neuropathy with ethambutol', *Postgrad. Med. J.*, **48**, 667.

Wilson, T. M. (1967), 'Current therapeutics. CCXL.—Capreomycin and ethambutol', *Practitioner*, **199**, 817.

Pyrazinamide

Description

Pyrazinamide, a derivative of nicotinamide, was synthetized in 1952 and shown to possess a higher degree of antituberculosis activity in man (Yeager *et al.*, 1952). In the past pyrazinamide has not been used as a 'first-line' drug for tuberculosis, but was mainly of value as a 'reserve drug' for treatment of patients in whom standard chemotherapy had failed. Recent studies suggest that this drug may be of value as a 'first-line' drug in the short-course chemotherapy of pulmonary tuberculosis (Fox and Mitchison, 1976).

Activity Against Mycobacteria

Pyrazinamide has a relatively low activity against Mycobacterium tuberculosis. The usual minimum inhibitory concentration is 20 μg per ml if this is tested at an acid pH of 5·5 (Stottmeier *et al.*, 1968), but pyrazinamide is almost completely inactive against M. tuberculosis at a neutral pH (Robson and Sullivan, 1963). *In vivo* studies however show that pyrazinamide is an effective bactericidal antituberculosis drug. It has been postulated that in human tuberculosis lesions the pH may be sufficiently low for the drug to be effective (McDermott and Tompsett, 1954).

As with other antituberculosis drugs, resistance to pyrazinamide develops rapidly if it is used alone to treat human tuberculosis.

The 'anonymous mycobacteria' (page 832) are pyrazinamide-resistant (Barter and Camens, 1968).

Mode of Administration and Dosage

1. *Standard daily administration.* Pyrazinamide is administered by the oral route. The recommended dose is 40 mg per kg body weight per day, administered in two or three divided doses. A common adult dose is 1 g twice-daily or a lower dose of 0·5 g three times a day. A slightly lower dose of 20 to 30 mg per kg of body weight per day has been used in various studies in developing countries, where pyrazinamide has been combined with streptomycin and/or PAS (Fox and Mitchison, 1975).

2. *Intermittent administration.* Pyrazinamide is suitable for intermittent therapy of tuberculosis (page 811). It has been used in a dose of 90 mg per kg once-weekly for this purpose (Fox, 1971). It may also be given in doses of 2·0–2·5 g three times weekly or 3·0–3·5 g twice-weekly, according to the weight of the patient.

Availability

Tablets 0·5 g.

Serum Levels in Relation to Dosage

The absorption of pyrazinamide from the gastro-intestinal tract is rapid and virtually complete. Peak serum levels occur within 2 h; these and the urinary excretion of pyrazinamide and its metabolite pyrazinoic acid are proportional to the dosage used, over a range of 0·5–3·0 g pyrazinamide (Ellard, 1969). Peak serum levels in one subject reached 33 μg per ml after 1·5 g and 59 μg per ml after 3·0 g of pyrazinamide; these then fell exponentially during the period 3–48 h after administration, with a serum half-life of 9–10 h. If pyrazinamide is given in a dose of 0·5 g three times a day, a serum concentration of 5 μg per ml is maintained for about 90 per cent of the time, but a level of 20 μg per ml is only briefly reached. When a dose of 3·0 g is given every second day, serum levels of 30 μg per ml or higher are maintained for 7 h, but a level of 5 μg per ml is only present for about 23 h.

Excretion

URINE: About 3–4 per cent of administered pyrazinamide is excreted as such in the urine and 30–41 per cent as pyrazinoic acid (Ellard, 1969; Ellard and Haslam, 1976). Urinary concentrations of pyrazinamide, similar to serum levels, reach a peak in about 2 h then fall exponentially from 3–48 h after a dose. The half-life of the drug in the urine is about 9 h. The ratio of urinary to serum concentrations of pyrazinamide after a single dose is fairly constant; after a dose of 1·5 g urinary concentrations are about 44 per cent higher and after 3·0 g about 85 per cent higher. About 98 per cent of pyrazinamide filtered by the kidneys is reabsorbed but very little pyrazinoic acid appears to be reabsorbed. Urinary levels of pyrazinoic acid after a single dose of pyrazinamide reach a maximum after about 12 h and fall exponentially from 16–50 h.

BILE: Animal experiments suggest that pyrazinamide may also be excreted and concentrated in the bile (Stottmeier et al., 1968).

INACTIVATION IN BODY: The most important metabolites of pyrazinamide (pyrazinoic acid amide) are pyrazinoic acid and its metabolite 5-hydroxypyrazinoic acid. The failure to recover the whole of an administered dose of pyrazinamide from the urine suggests there may be other metabolites (Ellard and Haslam, 1976). It is possible that pyrazinamide is metabolized in the liver, because the drug accumulates in jaundiced patients receiving the usual doses (Stottmeier et al., 1968).

Distribution of the Drug in Body

Animal experiments have shown that tissue concentrations of 15 to 20 μg per g may be attained in the liver, lungs and kidneys, but concentrations reached in other tissues such as the spleen, bone marrow and skeletal muscle are much less. Pyrazinamide apparently penetrates the cell wall of macrophages, indicating that it may have a high activity against phagocytosed tubercle bacilli (Stottmeier et al., 1968).

A pyrazinamide concentration of 15 μg per g of lung tissue has also been demonstrated in one patient treated for pulmonary tuberculosis (Stottmeier *et al.*, 1968).

Pyrazinamide appears to penetrate into the cerebrospinal fluid, at least in patients with tuberculous meningitis. In one such patient who was investigated during the first month of treatment, the CSF concentration 5 h after each dose averaged 50 μg per ml which was identical to the serum concentration at the time (Forgan-Smith *et al.*, 1973).

Mode of Action

The precise mechanism of action of pyrazinamide on tubercle bacilli is apparently not known. Its metabolite which is less active *in vitro* may possibly be involved in the *in vivo* activity of pyrazinamide (Ellard, 1969).

Toxicity

1. *Hepatotoxicity*. This is the most important toxic effect of this drug. Its frequency appears to be related to the dose and duration of pyrazinamide administration. In one study in which pyrazinamide was used in a dose of either 25 or 50 mg per kg daily (combined with isoniazid), liver damage was observed in 2–3 per cent of patients during a period of twelve weeks treatment. When pyrazinamide in a dose of 50 mg per kg daily was continued for 24 weeks in these patients, the frequency of hepatotoxicity increased to 6 per cent (A Public Hlth. Trial, 1959). McDermott *et al.* (1954) had a similar experience when treating 55 patients with pyrazinamide in a dose of 50 mg per kg per day, plus isoniazid in a dose of 5 mg per kg per day. Six of their patients developed hepatotoxicity, four of whom became jaundiced. In three of these the 'toxic hepatitis' was severe and one died from liver failure. In some series the frequency of pyrazinamide hepatotoxicity has been as high as 20 per cent (Robson and Sullivan, 1963).

Pyrazinamide's reputation as a toxic drug may have been exaggerated because of the circumstances in which it has been used (Fox and Mitchison, 1975; Hong Kong/BMRC, 1976). In earlier studies it was administered in moderately high dosage for prolonged periods, often with other toxic drugs such as ethionamide (page 854) and/or cycloserine (page 457) in retreatment regimens. Furthermore, pyrazinamide was usually given to middle-aged and elderly patients who are more vulnerable to toxic effects, and who may have already experienced toxic effects in failed primary chemotherapy. In addition, it is often very difficult to distinguish which antituberculosis drug is causing hepatotoxicity when multiple drugs are used. Evidence for pyrazinamide hepatotoxicity in many reports has depended on elevation of serum transaminases but this also frequently occurs with isoniazid (page 807) and rifampicin (page 562) therapy. When pyrazinamide has been used in moderate daily doses (20–30 mg per kg of body weight), combined with streptomycin or streptomycin plus PAS, toxicity has not been a major problem. Moreover even when pyrazinamide is used in high dosage in intermittent regimens (maximum of 90 mg per kg weekly) combined with streptomycin or streptomycin plus isoniazid, hepatotoxicity is uncommon.

Pyrazinamide toxicity has been investigated in Chinese adults with pulmonary tuberculosis, treated by short-course antituberculosis regimens in Hong Kong (Hong Kong/BMRC, 1976). One study investigated streptomycin, isoniazid plus pyrazinamide given daily, three times a week or twice a week. Another study compared daily streptomycin, isoniazid plus pyrazinamide with a daily regimen of streptomycin, isoniazid and PAS. The frequencies of adverse reactions in these studies were not high and they usually occurred during the first three months of treatment. Serum transaminase levels were higher during treatment with pyrazinamide regimens than those containing PAS, but these were often transient even when the regimen remained unchanged. A total of 668 patients received a pyrazinamide regimen and five (0·7 per cent) became jaundiced; four of these were receiving daily pyrazinamide and the other one received it three times weekly. The frequency of these hepatic reactions was not related to the pyrazinamide dosage corrected for body weight. In this study rifampicin was also added to the pyrazinamide regimen in a small number of patients; this did not appear to increase the frequency of hepatotoxicity.

Pyrazinamide hepatotoxicity somewhat resembles isoniazid hepatotoxicity (page 807). Further studies are necessary to confirm the low frequency of hepatotoxicity with short-course intermittent chemotherapy, demonstrated by the Hong Kong study. As with isoniazid, all patients receiving pyrazinamide should be warned to report symptoms suggestive of hepatitis, and should grossly elevated serum transaminase levels be detected, the drug should be discontinued.

2. *Gastro-intestinal side-effects.* Symptoms such as nausea, vomiting and diarrhoea may occur in the absence of hepatotoxicity (Robson and Sullivan, 1963), but liver function should always be checked in such patients.

3. *Hypersensitivity reactions.* Allergic rashes are rare and occasionally photosensitivity has been observed (*Today's Drugs*, 1963).

4. *Arthralgia and gout.* In the earliest report on the use of pyrazinamide in pulmonary tuberculosis, Yeager *et al.* (1952) noted the occurrence of pain and restricted joint movement without evidence of arthritis in a quarter of patients treated. Cullen *et al.* (1956) observed that the serum uric acid was elevated in patients receiving pyrazinamide, and some of these developed clinical gout. Pyrazinamide suppresses the urinary excretion of uric acid by attenuating its tubular secretion, and this is mediated by its metabolite, pyrazinoic acid (Gutman *et al.*, 1969). After a 3 g dose of pyrazinamide the urinary excretion of uric acid is maximally suppressed for 24 h and partially reduced for a further 24 h (Ellard and Haslam, 1976). Also prolonged exposure to pyrazinoic acid results in a net reduction of uric acid excretion suggesting that intermittent administration of pyrazinamide may cause less retention of uric acid.

In the Hong Kong trials in which various pyrazinamide regimens were studied (page 846), the commonest symptom attributed to this drug was arthralgia. The serum uric acid concentrations were higher in patients receiving daily pyrazinamide than in those receiving intermittent therapy, and they were also higher in patients with arthralgia receiving daily pyrazinamide than in matched controls. These results suggest that renal uric acid retention due to pyrazinoic acid is responsible for arthralgia in patients receiving daily pyrazinamide. Serum uric acid concentrations in patients receiving the drug intermittently, and who developed arthralgia, were lower and the same as matched controls, suggesting a different mechanism for the arthralgia. Acute gouty arthritis was not observed in the Hong Kong studies; arthralgia responded to analgesics, anti-inflammatory or uricosuric agents or to allopurinol, with or without temporary cessation of pyrazinamide administration.

A number of complex interactions occur when pyrazinamide and probenecid are given to patients with gout (Yü *et al.*, 1977). Pretreatment with pyrazinamide results in prolongation of the half-life of probenecid. As the rate of probenecid metabolism is decreased, its uricosuric action tends to be prolonged and the effect of pyrazinamide is lessened. After probenecid-induced uricosuria, pyrazinamide has a greater effect in suppressing urate excretion; this may be because it lessens the capacity of probenecid to inhibit tubular urate reabsorption while it continues to exert an inhibition on tubular urate secretion. When pyrazinamide and probenecid are co-administered, urinary excretion of urate depends on the relative doses and the times at which the drugs are administered.

Clinical Uses of the Drug

1. *Reserve drug for retreatment of pulmonary tuberculosis.* Pyrazinamide, especially if combined with isoniazid, is quite effective in the treatment of tuberculosis. However, because of its tendency to cause hepatotoxicity, pyrazinamide has not been regarded as a 'first-line' drug (McDermott *et al.*, 1954; Zorini *et al.*, 1958). It has been used as one of the 'reserve drugs', which are sometimes included in the therapeutic regimens for retreatment of patients whose tubercle bacilli have become resistant to one or more of the 'first-line' drugs.

As five 'first-line' drugs are now available (page 810), pyrazinamide is now only rarely used in countries such as Britain, North America and Australia. The position is different in developing countries, because resistant tubercle bacilli are more commonly encountered, and also expensive drugs like rifampicin often cannot be used on a wide scale. In one study in Africa, 103 patients with pulmonary tuberculosis who had failed to respond to standard regimens, such as an isoniazid/thiacetazone combination (page 859), were treated by a pyrazinamide containing regimen. During the first six months, treatment consisted of daily oral doses of PAS 15 g and pyrazinamide 2 g, plus streptomycin 1 g intramuscularly daily, and then PAS and pyrazinamide were continued alone to complete an 18-months course of treatment (East African/BMRC, 1971; 1973). The results of treatment were considered to be satisfactory, and drug toxicity was not a major problem. This retreatment regimen is still recommended because it remains effective and has relatively low toxicity, when isoniazid, thiacetazone and streptomycin constitute the usual standard regimen (WHO, 1975).

In Hong Kong, where drug-resistant tuberculosis is fairly common, Horsfall (1972) reported the results of treatment of 270 patients with drug combinations often including pyrazinamide. The drug was sometimes combined with both ethionamide and cycloserine, sometimes with ethionamide alone. Satisfactory results were obtained with the pyrazinamide regimens, but side-effects were frequent.

2. *Intermittent chemotherapy for pulmonary tuberculosis.* Pyrazinamide is suitable for this type of treatment because it can be safely given in greatly increased doses once-weekly (page 842). Intermittent chemotherapy (*see* page 811), if fully supervised, is particularly useful for patients who cannot be relied on to take medication; it is also convenient for the treatment of large numbers of patients in developing countries. Pyrazinamide given intermittently together with isoniazid and streptomycin has been effective for the treatment of pulmonary tuberculosis and has been successfully combined with short-course chemotherapy (*see* page 812).

3. *Short-course chemotherapy for pulmonary tuberculosis.* Developments in the use of courses of treatment for pulmonary tuberculosis lasting only nine months or for even shorter periods are described on page 812. Pyrazinamide has been used successfully in such courses when given daily or intermittently. Both pyrazinamide and rifampicin seem valuable in the short-course chemotherapy of pulmonary tuberculosis, because they may have special sterilizing actions against bacilli relatively unaffected by other drugs (Fox and Mitchison, 1975). Studies to date indicate that a nine-month course of daily rifampicin plus isoniazid (supplemented by ethambutol or streptomycin initially) is satisfactory for the treatment of pulmonary tuberculosis (*see* page 569). It is possible that the duration of chemotherapy may be reduced to less than nine months by the addition of pyrazinamide (Fox and Mitchison, 1976). In addition it will probably be unnecessary to administer rifampicin for the whole course of treatment which would be a significant cost advantage. The efficacy and safety of other short-course regimens using pyrazinamide either daily or intermittently, are yet to be determined (page 814).

REFERENCES

A United States Public Health Service Tuberculosis Therapy Trial (1959), 'Hepatic toxicity of pyrazinamide used with isoniazid in tuberculous patients', *Amer. Rev. Resp. Dis.*, **80**, 371.

Barter, C. E. and Camens, I. M. H. (1968), 'Lung infection with anonymous mycobacteria', *Med. J. Aust.*, **1**, 408.

Cullen, J. H., Early, L. J. A. and Fiore, J. M. (1956), 'The occurrence of hyperuricemia during pyrazinamide-isoniazid therapy', *Am. Rev. Tuberc.*, **74**, 289.

East African/British Medical Research Council Retreatment Investigation (1971), 'Streptomycin plus PAS plus pyrazinamide in the retreatment of pulmonary tuberculosis in East Africa', *Tubercle*, **52**, 191.

East African/British Medical Research Council Retreatment Investigation (1973), 'Streptomycin plus PAS plus pyrazinamide in the retreatment of pulmonary tuberculosis in East Africa: Second report', *Tubercle*, **54**, 283.

Ellard, G. A. (1969), 'Absorption, metabolism and excretion of pyrazinamide in man', *Tubercle*, **50**, 144.

Ellard, G. A. and Haslam, R. M. (1976), 'Observations on the reduction of the renal elimination of urate in man caused by the administration of pyrazinamide', *Tubercle*, **57**, 97.

Forgan-Smith, R., Ellard, G. A., Newton, D. and Mitchison, D. A. (1973), 'Pyrazinamide and other drugs in tuberculous meningitis', *Lancet*, **2**, 374.

Fox, W. (1971), 'General considerations in intermittent drug therapy of pulmonary tuberculosis', *Postgrad. Med. J.*, **47**, 729.

848 THE USE OF ANTIBIOTICS

Fox, W. and Mitchison, D. A. (1975), 'Short-course chemotherapy for pulmonary tuberculosis', *Amer. Rev. Resp. Dis.*, **111,** 325.

Fox, W. and Mitchison, D. A. (1976), 'Short-course chemotherapy for tuberculosis', *Lancet*, **2,** 1349.

Guttman, A. B., Yü, T. F. and Berger, L. (1969), 'Renal function in gout III. Estimation of tubular secretion and reabsorption of uric acid by use of pyrazinamide (pyrazinoic acid)', *Amer. J. Med.*, **47,** 575.

Hong Kong Tuberculosis Treatment Services/British Medical Research Council (1976), 'Adverse reactions to short-course regimens containing streptomycin, isoniazid, pyrazinamide and rifampicin in Hong Kong', *Tubercle*, **57,** 81.

Horsfall, P. A. L. (1972), 'Treatment of resistant pulmonary tuberculosis in Hong Kong with regimens of second-line drugs', *Tubercle*, **53,** 166.

McDermott, W. and Tompsett, R. (1954), 'Activation of pyrazinamide and nicotinamide in acidic environments *in vitro*', *Amer. Rev. Tuberc.*, **70,** 748.

McDermott, W., Ormond, L., Muschenheim, C., Deuschle, K., McCune, R. M., Jr. and Tompsett, R. (1954), 'Pyrazinamide-isoniazid in tuberculosis', *Amer. Rev. Tuberc.*, **69,** 319.

Robson, J. M. and Sullivan, F. M. (1963), 'Antituberculosis drugs', *Pharmacol. Rev.*, **15,** 169.

Stottmeier, K. D., Beam, R. E. and Kubica, G. P., (1968), 'The absorption and excretion of pyrazinamide', *Amer. Rev. Resp. Dis.*, **98,** 70.

Today's Drugs (1963), 'Drugs for tuberculosis', *Brit. med. J.*, **1,** 1593.

WHO (1975), 'Tuberculosis control: Progress of the new strategy', *WHO Chronicle*, **29,** 123.

Yeager, R. L., Munroe, W. G. C. and Dessau, F. I. (1952), 'Pyrazinamide (aldinamide) in the treatment of pulmonary tuberculosis', *Amer. Rev. Tuberc.*, **65,** 523; quoted by McDermott *et al.* (1954).

Yü, T. F., Perel, J., Berger, L., Roboz, J., Israili, Z. H. and Dayton, P. G. (1977), 'The effect of the interaction of pyrazinamide and probenecid on urinary uric acid excretion in man', *Amer. J. Med.*, **63,** 723.

Zorini, A. O., Spina, G. and De Simoni, G. E. (1958), 'Clinical and biological investigations on the new antituberculosis drugs (pyrazinamide and cycloserine)', *Dis. Chest.*, **34,** 27.

Capreomycin

Description

Capreomycin, a polypeptide antibiotic (page 417), was isolated from Streptomyces capreolus in 1960. It consists of four microbiologically active compounds which are named capreomycin IA, IB, IIA and IIB (Herr and Redstone, 1966). For clinical purposes capreomycin is used as the sulphate, and trade names include 'Caprocin' and 'Capastat sulphate' (Eli Lilly).

Activity Against Mycobacteria

Capreomycin is only active against mycobacteria. M. tuberculosis is moderately sensitive and the minimum inhibitory concentration of the standard H37 RV strain is usually 10 μg per ml. Strains of M. tuberculosis with a MIC of up to 40 μg per ml (Resistance Ratio 4) can still be regarded as capreomycin-sensitive. Tubercle bacilli which have become resistant to isoniazid, PAS, streptomycin, rifampicin, ethambutol, cycloserine or ethionamide usually remain capreomycin-sensitive. However cross-resistance may occur between capreomycin and viomycin and between capreomycin and kanamycin (Sutton et al., 1966; Drug Commentary, 1973). Capreomycin-resistant variants of M. tuberculosis can be readily selected in vitro (Sutton et al., 1966), and also develop readily in vivo if the drug is used as a single agent for the treatment of tuberculosis (Wilson, 1967). Capreomycin has a bacteristatic action against M. tuberculosis.

This drug may also show in vitro activity against some of the other mycobacteria (page 832) such as M. kansasii (Sutton et al., 1966).

Mode of Administration and Dosage

1. *Adults*. Capreomycin is administered by the intramuscular route. The usual dose is 15–20 mg per kg per day given as a single injection. A common adult daily dose is 1·0 g, which is usually given for two to four months, and thereafter it is reduced to 1·0 g two or three times per week, for the remainder of the course of treatment.

In some treatment regimens the daily dose for adults has been adjusted according to age. The dose is 1·0 g for patients under 50 years, 0·75 g for those aged 50–59 years and 0·5 g for those aged 60 years or more (Andrews et al., 1974).

2. *Children*. The dose of 15 mg per kg per day may be suitable for children. However because of insufficient data the use of capreomycin in children is currently not recommended (Drug Commentary, 1973).

3. *Patients with renal failure.* Capreomycin accumulates in these patients, so that a reduced dosage and serum level monitoring is necessary. A similar dose reduction to that advocated for streptomycin (page 296) may be used because the two drugs are excreted by the kidney in a similar manner (Black *et al.*, 1966).

Availability

Capreomycin sulphate: 1·0 g vials.

Serum Levels in Relation to Dosage

Capreomycin is not absorbed after oral administration, but it is well absorbed from intramuscular injection sites. A peak serum level of 30–35 μg per ml is attained 1–2 h after an intramuscular dose of 1·0 g in adults. Thereafter the serum concentration gradually falls, being 10 μg per ml at 6 h and usually less than 1·0 μg per ml at 24 h (Black *et al.*, 1966; Morse *et al.*, 1966). These serum concentrations are similar to those attained after an intramuscular injection of 1·0 g of streptomycin (page 297). Capreomycin does not accumulate in the serum of patients with normal renal function, when repeated daily doses of 1·0 g are given for prolonged periods.

Excretion

URINE: About 50–60 per cent of an administered dose of capreomycin is excreted by glomerular filtration, producing high concentrations of the active unchanged drug in the urine (Black *et al.*, 1966). Most of this is excreted during the first 12 h after the dose.

INACTIVATION IN BODY: Capreomycin not excreted in the urine is probably inactivated in the body.

BILE: Animal studies suggest that small amounts of capreomycin may be eliminated via the bile (Black *et al.*, 1966).

Distribution of the Drug in Body

The distribution of capreomycin in various body fluids and tissues has not been studied. The drug probably does not penetrate into the cerebrospinal fluid of patients with normal meninges.

Mode of Action

The mode of action of capreomycin is apparently unknown.

Toxicity

1. *Nephrotoxicity.* This appears to be the most serious toxic effect of capreomycin therapy (Garfield *et al.*, 1966; Miller *et al.*, 1966; Hesling, 1969). Many patients develop proteinuria, and casts, red and white cells may be detected in their urine. If only these changes occur, capreomycin may be con-

tinued cautiously in a reduced dosage. However if there is a rise in blood urea and serum creatinine, the drug should be stopped. Capreomycin can also cause a renal tubular dysfunction with resultant alkalosis and potassium, calcium and magnesium depletion. Patients with this complication may develop lethargy, muscular weakness and tetany (Hesling, 1969), in which case the drug should be discontinued, and correction of electrolyte disturbances may be needed.

When the drug has only been used for periods of four to six months in the retreatment of tuberculosis, hypokalaemia has been uncommon. Aquinas and Citron (1972) monitored serum potassium regularly, and during six months therapy 2 of 36 patients with capreomycin-induced hypokalaemia were detected and both responded rapidly to oral potassium. Andrews *et al.* (1974) in their study did not observe any electrolyte changes when capreomycin was used for four months in a dosage adjusted for age.

2. *Ototoxicity.* Capreomycin treated patients may develop vertigo, tinnitus or deafness. These toxic effects are uncommon, provided that the drug is not given to patients with pre-existing hearing loss or to patients with renal functional impairment, Elderly patients also are more prone to ototoxicity, and should not receive prolonged courses of this drug. Three of 36 patients in Hong Kong who were treated with capreomycin for six months developed deafness or tinnitus (Aquinas and Citron, 1972), but these symptoms were not observed in 33 British patients treated with this drug for four months (Andrews *et al.*, 1974).

Capreomycin should not be administered in conjunction with other ototoxic drugs such as kanamycin and streptomycin (*Drug Commentary*, 1973).

3. *Hepatotoxicity.* Transient abnormalities in liver function tests have been noted during capreomycin therapy, but in most cases these were probably caused by companion drugs such as isoniazid or PAS, rather than capreomycin (Browning and Donnerberg, 1966; Miller *et al.*, 1966). Serious hepatotoxicity has not been reported.

4. *Other side-effects.* Leucopenia has been observed, but appears to be rare. Eosinophilia is more common and sometimes is associated with hypersensitivity rashes or drug fever (Miller *et al.*, 1966). Capreomycin does not appear to be cross-allergenic with streptomycin (Wilson, 1969).

Clinical Uses of the Drug

1. *Retreatment of pulmonary tuberculosis.* Capreomycin is an effective antituberculosis drug, but because of its toxicity, it is only used for the retreatment of patients in whom treatment with 'first-line' drugs has failed. If it is used for this purpose, capreomycin should be combined with at least one other antituberculosis drug to which the organism is still sensitive. Schless *et al.* (1966) found capreomycin and ethionamide to be an effective combination, while others have obtained good results with an ethambutol/capreomycin regimen (Donomae, 1968; Lim and Aquinas, 1969). Nowadays the less toxic drugs, rifampicin (page 569) and ethambutol (page 837) are usually preferred for the retreatment of tuberculosis, but three antituberculosis drugs are often advocated for an initial period and capreomycin has been used for this purpose. Aquinas and Citron (1972) used capreomycin in this way to treat 36 patients in Hong Kong; daily rifampicin and ethambutol were given for two years,

supplemented by daily capreomycin in a dose of 15 mg per kg of body weight for the first six months; sputum cultures of 33 of the 36 patients rapidly became negative and remained so during the two years of chemotherapy. Andrews *et al.* (1974) also used these three drugs to treat 33 patients with isoniazid-resistant pulmonary tuberculosis in Britain; daily rifampicin and ethambutol were given for two years and daily capreomycin in a dosage adjusted for age (*see* page 849) for the first four months; all patients on this therapy had negative sputum cultures after treatment for six months, one year and two years.

Capreomycin appears to be better tolerated for prolonged treatment of tuberculosis than kanamycin (page 319) or viomycin (page 862), and it is preferred to either of these two drugs (*Today's Drugs*, 1967).

2. *Other mycobacterial infections.* Some authors have reported encouraging results using a combination of capreomycin and ethambutol for the treatment of lung infections caused by mycobacteria other than M. tuberculosis (Evans and Thong, 1969). These results have not been confirmed by others.

REFERENCES

Andrews, R. H., Jenkins, P. A., Marks, J., Pines, A., Selkon, J. B. and Somner, A. R. (1974), 'Treatment of isoniazid-resistant pulmonary tuberculosis with ethambutol, rifampicin and capreomycin: A co-operative study in England and Wales', *Tubercle*, **55**, 105.

Aquinas, M. and Citron, K. M. (1972), 'Rifampicin, ethambutol, and capreomycin in pulmonary tuberculosis, previously treated with both first and second line drugs: The results of 2 years chemotherapy', *Tubercle*, **53**, 153.

Black, H. R., Griffith, R. S. and Peabody, A. M. (1966), 'Absorption, excretion and metabolism of capreomycin in normal and diseased states', *Ann. N.Y. Acad. Sci.*, **135**, 974.

Browning, R. H. and Donnerberg, R. L. (1966), 'Capreomycin-experiences in patient acceptance and toxicity', *Ann. N.Y. Acad. Sci.*, **135**, 1057.

Donomae, I. (1968), 'The combined use of capreomycin and ethambutol in retreatment of pulmonary tuberculosis', *Amer. Rev. Resp. Dis.*, **98**, 699.

Drug Commentary (1973), 'Evaluation of a new antituberculous agent. Capreomycin sulfate (capastat sulfate)', *JAMA*, **223**, 179.

Evans, C. and Thong, K. L. (1969), 'A clinical trial of ethambutol plus capreomycin in the treatment of atypical tuberculosis', *Med. J. Aust.*, **2**, 744.

Garfield, J. W., Jones, J. M., Cohen, N. L., Daly, J. F. and McClement, J. H. (1966), 'The auditory, vestibular and renal effects of capreomycin in humans', *Ann. N.Y. Acad. Sci.*, **135**, 1039.

Herr, E. B., Jr. and Redstone, M. O. (1966), 'Chemical and physical characterization of capreomycin', *Ann. N.Y. Acad. Sci.*, **135**, 940.

Hesling, C. M. (1969), 'Treatment with capreomycin, with special reference to toxic effects', *Tubercle, March Suppl.*, p. 39.

Lim, B. T. and Aquinas, M. (1969), 'Ethambutol and capreomycin in the re-treatment of advanced pulmonary tuberculosis', *Amer. Rev. Resp. Dis.*, **99**, 792.

Miller, J. D., Popplewell, A. G., Landwehr, A. and Greene, M. E. (1966), 'Toxicology studies in patients on prolonged therapy with capreomycin', *Ann. N.Y. Acad. Sci.*, **135**, 1047.

Morse, W. C., Sproat, E. F., Arrington, C. W. and Hawkins, J. A. (1966), 'M. tuberculosis *in vitro* susceptibility and serum level experiences with capreomycin', *Ann.*

N.Y. Acad. Sci., **135**, 983.

Schless, J. M., Allison, R. F. and Inglis, R. M. (1966), 'Capreomycin-ethionamide as a retreatment regimen for pulmonary tuberculosis', *Ann. N.Y. Acad. Sci.*, **135**, 1085.

Sutton, W. B., Gordee, R. S., Wick, W. E. and Stanfield, L. V. (1966), '*In vitro* and *in vivo* laboratory studies on the antituberculous activity of capreomycin', *Ann. N.Y. Acad. Sci.*, **135**, 947.

Today's Drugs (1967), 'New drugs against tuberculosis', *Brit. med. J.*, **1**, 37.

Wilson, T. M. (1967), 'Current therapeutics. CCXL.—Capreomycin and ethambutol', *Practitioner,* **199,** 817.

Wilson, T. M. (1969), 'Capreomycin, ethambutol and rifampicin. Clinical experience in Manchester', *Scand. J. resp. Dis.* (Suppl.), **69,** 33.

Ethionamide and Prothionamide

Description

Ethionamide (alpha-ethyl thioisonicotinamide) is a derivative of isonicotinic acid, which was synthetized in France in 1956, and soon after shown to be an effective antituberculosis agent. Because of its toxicity, it has not been used as a 'first-line' drug, and has been reserved for retreatment of patients in whom initial chemotherapy has failed. Prothionamide is the n-propyl derivative of ethionamide, which was originally thought to be less toxic. However subsequent studies showed that the toxicity of the two compounds is about the same, so that for practical purposes the two drugs are identical. The following details relating to ethionamide also apply to prothionamide.

Activity Against Mycobacteria

Ethionamide is active against Mycobacterium tuberculosis. The MIC for the standard H37 RV strain is usually 10.0μg per ml, and most other strains are inhibited by $10–20 \mu$g per ml. Ethionamide-resistant strains of M. tuberculosis can rapidly be induced *in vitro* and they also emerge *in vivo* if the drug is used as a single agent for the treatment of human tuberculosis (Robson and Sullivan, 1963). M. tuberculosis strains which have become resistant to drugs such as isoniazid, streptomycin and PAS remain ethionamide-sensitive, but ethionamide may show cross-resistance with thiacetazone (*Today's Drugs*, 1968).

Ethionamide may also show *in vitro* activity against some of the other mycobacteria which produce disease similar to that caused by M. tuberculosis (page 832) (Dreisin *et al.*, 1976), but this does not appear to have a clinical application. Some strains of M. ulcerans are sensitive to ethionamide (Radford, 1975) (*see* page 833).

In kinetic studies using animals, depending on the dosage used, ethionamide has bacteristatic and bactericidal activity against Mycobacterium leprae (Shepard *et al.*, 1976).

Mode of Administration and Dosage

Ethionamide is administered by the oral route in a dose of 15 mg per kg body weight per day. The maximum daily adult dose is 1.0 g, but many patients cannot tolerate this, and more commonly a smaller daily dose of 500–750 mg is prescribed. Ethionamide is often given as a single daily dose, prior to retiring at night, to minimize gastro-intestinal side-effects. Alternatively it can be given in two divided doses.

Availability

Ethionamide: 125 mg and 250 mg tablets.
Prothionamide: 125 mg and 250 mg tablets.

Serum Levels in Relation to Dosage

There have been wide discrepancies in the reported serum concentrations after the oral administration of ethionamide (Weinstein *et al.*, 1962). Enteric-coated ethionamide tablets used in the past were poorly absorbed (*Today's Drugs*, 1968), and this may explain some of these differences. It appears that ethionamide administered in uncoated or sugar coated tablets is well absorbed, provided it does not cause gastro-intestinal disturbance.

After an oral dose of 1·0 g a peak serum concentration of about 20 μg per ml is attained in 3 h. Thereafter the serum level slowly falls and the drug is undetectable 20–24 h after the dose (Robson and Sullivan, 1963).

Excretion

Knowledge about the excretion of ethionamide is incomplete. Only about 1 per cent of an administered dose is excreted in the urine as the active drug (Robson and Sullivan, 1963); the remainder is presumably metabolized in the body. Animal experiments suggest that most of this inactivation occurs in the liver (Hamilton *et al.*, 1962).

Distribution of the Drug in Body

After absorption ethionamide appears to be widely distributed in the body. It penetrates well into the cerebrospinal fluid both in patients with tuberculous meningitis and in those with normal meninges, and CSF concentrations approximate to serum levels at the time (Hughes *et al.*, 1962). Animal studies indicate that ethionamide is quickly distributed to various organs in the body such as the liver, kidneys and spleen (Hamilton *et al.*, 1962).

Toxicity

1. *Gastro-intestinal side-effects.* Symptoms such as a metallic taste, nausea, vomiting, anorexia, abdominal pain and sometimes diarrhoea are very common, and occur to some degree in the majority of patients treated by ethionamide (Weinstein *et al.*, 1962; Schwartz, 1966). Such symptoms are often severe enough to necessitate cessation of treatment. These disturbances may be partly due to an effect of the drug on the central nervous system, because parenterally administered ethionamide also causes gastro-intestinal symptoms (*Today's Drugs*, 1968). Prothionamide is probably a little less prone to cause these disturbances.

Fox *et al.* (1969) performed a study amongst African patients to compare side-effects of ethionamide and prothionamide after a single dose of each drug as large as 1·75 g. The principal side-effects of both drugs were gastro-intestinal, giddiness and headache; males had more side-effects due to ethionamide than prothionamide, but there were no differences in females;

there were more side-effects in females than in males with both drugs.

2. *Hepatotoxicity*. Liver damage due to ethionamide is relatively uncommon. Jaundice usually of the hepatocellular type with a raised serum aspartate aminotransferase (SGOT) may occur (Phillips and Tashman, 1963). It is not known whether hepatotoxicity is due to a hypersensitivity reaction or to a direct toxic effect of the drug on the liver. Following cessation of ethionamide, the jaundice usually resolves, but it reappears if the drug is resumed (Pernod, 1965).

3. *Neurotoxicity*. Various types of mental disturbance may be caused by ethionamide, such as depression (Weinstein *et al.*, 1962), intense anxiety (Lees, 1967) and acute psychosis (Lees, 1965; Narang, 1972). In addition, dizziness, visual disturbances and peripheral neuritis have been reported (Lees, 1965). A pellagra-like encephalopathy has also been described in three patients receiving ethionamide therapy and two of these patients also developed a myelopathy. All three patients improved when ethionamide was stopped, but they were also treated by nicotinamide and other B group vitamins (Swash *et al.*, 1972). These authors considered that vitamin therapy had aided recovery, and suggested that nicotinamide should be administered to patients receiving ethionamide if any alteration of intellectual function occurs during therapy.

4. *Other side-effects*. Excessive salivation, gynaecomastia, skin rashes, photodermatitis, acne and alopecia have been described in association with ethionamide therapy (*Today's Drugs*, 1968).

5. *Teratogenicity*. The drug is teratogenic in experimental animals and its use during human pregnancy is not advised.

Clinical Uses of the Drug

1. *Retreatment of pulmonary tuberculosis*. Although it is effective for tuberculosis, because of its toxicity, ethionamide is only used as a 'reserve drug' for retreatment of patients in whom standard chemotherapy has failed (Schwartz, 1966). It should always be combined with at least one other antituberculosis drug to which the tuberculosis bacilli are still sensitive. Drug-resistant tuberculosis has been successfully treated with ethionamide/cycloserine combinations (Riddell *et al.*, 1960). In a study in Hong Kong, where drug-resistant tuberculosis is common, 270 patients were treated by various regimens. Some received triple therapy consisting of ethionamide, pyrazinamide and cycloserine, some a combination of ethionamide and pyrazinamide, and the remainder other combinations. The overall results obtained were satisfactory, but side-effects were frequent (Horsfall, 1972). Because of the development of safer effective drugs such as ethambutol and rifampicin, ethionamide has only a very limited, if any, role in the chemotherapy of tuberculosis, especially in developed countries.

2. *Leprosy*. In a small trial, ethionamide in a dose of 250 mg three times a day appeared as effective as dapsone in a dosage of 50 mg daily (Shepard *et al.*, 1976). It is very unlikely that this drug will be used extensively for this disease because of its toxicity.

REFERENCES

Dreisin, R. B., Scoggin, C. and Davidson, P. T. (1976), 'The pathogenicity of Mycobacterium fortuitum and Mycobacterium chelonei in man: A report of seven cases', *Tubercle*, **57**, 49.

Fox, W. Robinson, D. K., Tall, R. Mitchison, D. A., Kent, P. W. and MacFadyen, D. M. (1969), 'A study of acute intolerance to ethionamide, including a comparison with prothionamide, and of the influence of a vitamin B-complex additive in prophylaxis', *Tubercle*, **50**, 125.

Hamilton, E. J., Eidus, L. and Little, E. (1962), 'A comparative study *in vivo* of isoniazid and alpha-ethylthioisonicotinamide', *Amer. Rev. Resp. Dis.*, **85**, 407.

Horsfall, P. A. L. (1972), 'Treatment of resistant pulmonary tuberculosis in Hong Kong with regimens of second-line drugs', *Tubercle*, **53**, 166.

Hughes, I. E., Smith, H. and Kane, P. O. (1962), 'Ethionamide: Its passage into the cerebrospinal fluid in man', *Lancet*, **1**, 616.

Lees, A. W. (1965), 'Ethionamide, 750 mg daily, plus isoniazid, 450 mg daily, in previously untreated cases of pulmonary tuberculosis', *Amer. Rev. Resp. Dis.*, **92**, 966.

Lees, A. W. (1967), 'Ethionamide, 500 mg. Daily, plus isoniazid, 500 mg or 300 mg daily in previously untreated patients with pulmonary tuberculosis', *Amer. Rev. Resp. Dis.*, **95**, 109.

Narang, R. K. (1972), 'Acute psychotic reaction probably caused by ethionamide', *Tubercle*, **53**, 137.

Pernod, J. (1965), 'Hepatic tolerance of ethionamide', *Amer. Rev. Resp. Dis.*, **92**, 39.

Phillips, S. and Tashman, H. (1963), 'Ethionamide jaundice', *Amer. Rev. Resp. Dis.*, **87**, 896.

Radford, A. J. (1975), 'Mycobacterium ulcerans in Australia', *Aust. N.Z. J. Med.*, **5**, 162.

Riddell, R. W., Stewart, S. M. and Somner, A. R. (1960), 'Ethionamide', *Brit. med. J.*, **2**, 1207.

Robson, J. M. and Sullivan, F. M. (1963), 'Antituberculosis drugs', *Pharmacol. Rev.*, **15**, 169.

Schwartz, W. S. (1966), 'Comparison of ethionamide with isoniazid in original treatment cases of pulmonary tuberculosis', *Amer. Rev. Resp. Dis.*, **93**, 685.

Shepard, C. C., Ellard, G. A., Levy, L., de Araujo Opromolla, V., Pattyn, S. R., Peters, J. H., Rees, R. J. W. and Waters, M. F. R. (1976), 'Experimental chemotherapy in leprosy', *Bull. Wld. Hlth. Org.*, **53**, 425.

Swash, M., Roberts, A. H. and Murnaghan, D. J. (1972), 'Reversible pellagra-like encephalopathy with ethionamide and cycloserine', *Tubercle*, **53**, 132.

Today's Drugs (1963), 'Drugs for tuberculosis', *Brit. med. J.*, **1**, 1593.

Today's Drugs (1968), 'Drugs for tuberculosis', *Brit. med. J.*, **3**, 664.

Weinstein, H. J., Hallett, W. Y. and Sarauw, A. S. (1962), 'The absorption and toxicity of ethionamide', *Amer. Rev. Resp. Dis.*, **86**, 576.

Thiacetazone

Description

Thiacetazone is one of many thiosemicarbazones discovered by Domagk and his co-workers in Germany in 1946. Of several compounds from this group exhibiting antituberculosis activity, thiacetazone was the most promising for human therapeutics. Initially it was considered to be too toxic for widespread clinical use (Hinshaw and McDermott, 1950). However, because there was a need for another cheap and effective antituberculosis drug in developing countries, it was tried with success initially in East Africa (Leading article, 1963). It is now established as a 'first-line' drug for the treatment of pulmonary tuberculosis in many developing countries of the world, but it is only rarely, if at all, used in Britain, North America and Australia.

Activity Against Mycobacterium Tuberculosis

Thiacetazone is quite active against M. tuberculosis, most strains being inhibited by a concentration of $1\cdot0$ μg per ml. However, 'pre-treatment strains' in various parts of the world may vary in their degree of sensitivity to thiacetazone. For instance, strains isolated in East Africa are usually more sensitive (MIC $0\cdot4$ μg per ml) than those found in Southern India, Hong Kong and Singapore (Citron, 1972; Ellard et al., 1974). There are a few areas in Africa where thiacetazone-resistant strains (M. africanum) are so common as to make regimens containing this drug unsuitable (WHO, 1975). As with other antituberculosis drugs, thiacetazone resistance may emerge in patients during treatment unless at least one other effective drug is used concurrently (East African/BMRC, 1970).

Mode of Administration and Dosage

Thiacetazone is administered by the oral route, as a single daily dose of 150 mg to adults. The size of the individual dose appears to be critical; larger doses cause toxicity whilst lower doses are often ineffective (Leading article, 1963; Citron, 1972). Thiacetazone in a dose of 450 mg is well tolerated and therefore suitable for intermittent chemotherapy (Fox et al., 1974).

Absorption and Excretion

Thiacetazone is well absorbed following oral administration. After a 150 mg dose to adults, a peak serum level of $1\cdot0$ to $2\cdot0$ μg per ml is attained 4–5 h later. Doubling the dose approximately doubles the serum concentrations, but when a dose as high as 600 mg is given the peak level is attained at 6 h or later. The drug's serum half-life is approximately 12 h (Ellard *et al.*, 1974).

About 20 per cent of an orally administered thiacetazone dose is excreted in the urine in an unchanged form. Some metabolites of the drug are also eliminated via the kidney (Ellard *et al.*, 1974). Thiacetazone would presumably accumulate in patients with renal failure.

Toxicity

1. *Gastro-intestinal side-effects*. Thiacetazone can cause symptoms such as nausea, vomiting or diarrhoea, and their frequency and severity are similar to those caused by PAS (Miller *et al.*, 1966).

2. *Hepatotoxicity*. Severe liver damage with jaundice, resulting in occasional fatalities, apparently due to thiacetazone have been reported (Miller *et al.*, 1966). However, most of these patients had also received isoniazid simultaneously (*see* page 807).

3. *Haematological side-effects*. Bone marrow depression, thrombocytopenia and agranulocytosis have been caused by thiacetazone therapy (Miller *et al.*, 1966). Haemolytic anaemia has also been reported and according to Masel and Johnston (1968) minor degrees of haemolysis can be commonly detected in patients receiving thiacetazone.

4. *Ototoxicity*. Symptoms such as dizziness, vertigo, ataxia, tinnitus and even deafness can result from thiacetazone therapy. This drug also potentiates streptomycin ototoxicity (Miller *et al.*, 1966).

5. *Hypersensitivity*. Rashes, often trivial, frequently occur during thiacetazone therapy, and fatal exfoliative dermatitis has been described occasionally (Ferguson *et al.*, 1971). When a thiacetazone rash is observed, it is advisable to stop the drug.

6. *Side-effects in different ethnic groups*. The frequency of rashes varies widely in different geographical areas. In one large international study rashes were found to be common in patients from Singapore and Malaysia, less common in those from Czechoslovakia and non-existent in patients from Ethiopia (Ferguson *et al.*, 1971). Gastro-intestinal irritation and ototoxicity are more common in patients from Hong Kong than in those from Africa (Miller *et al.*, 1966). These differences probably result from environmental factors and from variations in recording and interpretation of side-effects. The patient's ethnic origin *per se* does not appear to be an important factor, because if patients from different racial groups are treated together in one hospital, the frequency of side-effects in all groups is about the same (Miller *et al.*, 1972). Nevertheless it has been suggested that sample population groups should be investigated for thiacetazone toxicity prior to its widespread use in a new community.

Clinical Uses of the Drug

1. *Pulmonary tuberculosis*. Because of its cheapness, thiacetazone has been extensively used as a 'first-line' drug, usually in combination with isoniazid for the treatment of pulmonary tuberculosis in many countries, particularly in Asia and Africa. It is only rarely used in developed countries, where other less toxic 'first-line' drugs are readily available. Isoniazid 300 mg and thiacetazone

150 mg given in one daily dose in a single tablet is recommended as effective and of low toxicity for patients weighing 35 kg or more (WHO, 1975). Results with this therapy are improved if intramuscular streptomycin in a dose of 1 g daily is added during the first eight weeks of treatment (East African/BMRC, 1970; 1973). A comparative trial of thiacetazone 150 mg and isoniazid 300 mg in a once-daily dose and a combination of PAS 12 g with isoniazid 300 mg daily in divided doses was carried out on 72 selected patients with pulmonary tuberculosis in Nigeria. It was concluded that thiacetazone was equally effective to PAS as a companion drug for isoniazid and was preferable because of its relative cheapness and once-a-day administration (Onadeko and Sofowora, 1975). Thiacetazone regimens have not been satisfactory in some countries. In Singapore, a combination of thiacetazone 150 mg plus isoniazid 300 mg daily was found to be rather ineffective and too toxic, and a second regimen, which contained streptomycin 1 g daily in addition for the first six months, although effective, was also too toxic (Singapore/Brompton Hospital/BMRC, 1971; 1974).

This drug has also been used in regimens for intermittent chemotherapy (*see* page 811) of pulmonary tuberculosis in East Africa. Thiacetazone 450 mg plus isoniazid 15 mg per kg body weight given twice-weekly has been used to complete a two-year course after an initial phase of streptomycin 1 g with thiacetazone 150 mg plus isoniazid 300 mg daily for four or eight weeks (East African/BMRC, 1974b). These regimens were fairly effective but were somewhat inferior to continuation therapy with a daily regimen of these drugs.

The efficacy of short-course regimens (*see* page 812) for the treatment of pulmonary tuberculosis, which contain thiacetazone, have not been satisfactory (East African/BMRC, 1972; 1974a).

2. *Leprosy*. Thiacetazone has been considered as a possible companion drug for dapsone in the treatment of leprosy. It is unlikely to be acceptable for long-term use because of its side-effects (Ellard, 1975).

REFERENCES

Citron, K. M. (1972), 'Tuberculosis-chemotherapy', *Brit. med. J.*, **1,** 426.

East African/British Medical Research Council Fifth Thiacetazone Investigation (1970), 'Isoniazid with thiacetazone (thioacetazone) in the treatment of pulmonary tuberculosis in East Africa—fifth investigation', *Tubercle*, **51,** 123.

East African/British Medical Research Councils (1972), 'Controlled clinical trial of short-course (6-month) regimens of chemotherapy for treatment of pulmonary tuberculosis', *Lancet*, **1,** 1079.

East African/British Medical Research Council Fifth Thiacetazone Investigation—Third Report (1973), 'Isoniazid with thiacetazone (thioacetazone) in the treatment of pulmonary tuberculosis in East Africa. Third report of fifth investigation', *Tubercle*, **54,** 169.

East African/British Medical Research Councils (1974a), 'Controlled clinical trial of four short-course (6-month) regimens of chemotherapy for treatment of pulmonary tuberculosis. Third report', *Lancet*, **2,** 237.

East African/British Medical Research Council Intermittent Thiacetazone Investigation (1974b), 'A pilot study of two regimens of intermittent thiacetazone plus isoniazid in the treatment of pulmonary tuberculosis in East Africa', *Tubercle*, **55,** 211.

Ellard, G. A., Dickinson, J. M., Gammon, P. T. and Mitchison, D. A. (1974), 'Serum concentrations and antituberculosis activity of thiacetazone', *Tubercle*, **55**, 41.

Ellard, G. A. (1975), 'The treatment of tuberculosis and leprosy', *Lepr. Rev.*, **46**, 149.

Ferguson, G. C., Nunn, A. J., Fox, W., Miller, A. B., Robinson, D. K. and Tall, R. (1971), 'A second international co-operative investigation into thiacetazone side-effects: Rashes on two thiacetazone-containing regimens', *Tubercle*, **52**, 166.

Fox, W. *et al.* (1974), 'A study of adverse reactions to high dosage intermittent thiacetazone', *Tubercle*, **55**, 29.

Hinshaw, H. C. and McDermott, W. (1950), 'Thiosemicarbazone therapy of tuberculosis in humans', *Amer. Rev. Tuberc.*, **61**, 145; quoted by Robson and Sullivan (1963).

Leading Article (1963), 'Thiacetazone in tuberculosis', *Lancet*, **2**, 817.

Masel, M. A. and Johnston, N. G. (1968), 'Haemolytic anaemia in a patient taking thiacetazone', *Med. J. Aust.*, **2**, 840.

Miller, A. B., Fox, W. and Tall, R. (1966), 'An international co-operative investigation into thiacetazone (thioacetazone) side-effects', *Tubercle*, **47**, 33.

Miller, A. B., Nunn, A. J., Robinson, D. K., Fox, W., Somasundaram, P. R. and Tall, R. (1972), 'A second international co-operative investigation into thiacetazone side effects', *Bull. Wld. Hlth. Org.*, **47**, 211.

Onadeko, B. O. and Sofowora, E. O. (1975), 'Comparative trial of thiacetazone with isoniazid and paraaminosalicylic acid (PAS) with isoniazid in the treatment of pulmonary tuberculosis in Nigerians', *J. Trop. Med. and Hyg.*, **78**, 201.

Singapore Tuberculosis Services/Brompton Hospital/British Medical Research Council Investigation (1971), 'A controlled clinical trial of the role of thiacetazone-containing regimens in the treatment of pulmonary tuberculosis in Singapore', *Tubercle*, **52**, 88.

Singapore Tuberculosis Services/Brompton Hospital/British Medical Research Council Investigation (1974), 'A controlled clinical trial of the role of thiacetazone-containing regimens in the treatment of pulmonary tuberculosis in Singapore: Second report', *Tubercle*, **55**, 251.

WHO (1975), 'Tuberculosis control: Progress of the new strategy', *WHO Chronicle*, **29**, 123.

Viomycin

This is a polypeptide antibiotic (page 417), which has been used as a 'reserve drug' for the treatment of drug-resistant tuberculosis since 1950. Viomycin is now only very rarely prescribed, because there are safer and more effective drugs available. For this reason only a brief outline of this drug is included.

The activity of viomycin against M. tuberculosis is only about a quarter that of streptomycin (Robson and Sullivan, 1963). It is usually active against organisms resistant to streptomycin and other antituberculosis drugs with the exception that it shows complete cross-resistance with capreomycin (McClatchy *et al.*, 1977).

Viomycin is administered by the intramuscular route. After a 1 g dose in adults the serum levels attained and the excretion patterns of this drug are similar to those of streptomycin (page 297).

The toxic effects of viomycin are like those of capreomycin (page 850); nephrotoxicity with associated electrolyte imbalance and ototoxicity being the main adverse effects. Viomycin appears to be more toxic than capreomycin.

To avoid toxicity, viomycin is usually only administered in an adult dose of 1·0–2·0 g daily for short periods of two or three weeks. Thereafter the dose is reduced to 2·0 g twice-weekly (Pyle, 1970).

For treatment of tuberculosis, the drug is always administered in conjunction with two or even more other antituberculosis drugs. However the combination of viomycin with other nephrotoxic and ototoxic drugs such as streptomycin, kanamycin and capreomycin should be avoided.

The drug is marketed as viomycin sulphate in 1 g vials.

REFERENCES

McClatchy, J. K., Kanes, W., Davidson, P. T. and Moulding, T. S. (1977), 'Cross-resistance in M. tuberculosis to kanamycin, capreomycin and viomycin', *Tubercle*, **58**, 29.

Pyle, M. M. (1970), 'Ethambutol and viomycin', *Med. Clin. North Amer.*, **54**, 1317.

Robson, J. M. and Sullivan, F. M. (1963), 'Antituberculosis drugs', *Pharmacol. Rev.*, **15**, 169.

Part IV
Antifungal Drugs

Amphotericin B

Description

Amphotericin is a member of the polyene group of antifungal agents (Hamilton-Miller, 1973), and it was isolated from Streptomyces nodosus found in soil (Gold *et al.*, 1956). There are two forms of amphotericin, A and B; the latter, being more active, is used clinically. Amphotericin B is very insoluble, and for parenteral administration it is supplied as a colloidal suspension using sodium desoxycholate as a dispersing agent. It is marketed with the trade names of 'Fungizone' (intravenous preparation), and 'Fungilin' (various topical preparations) by Squibb.

A methyl ester derivative of amphotericin has also been prepared (Mechlinski and Schaffner, 1972); it is less toxic and produces comparatively higher serum levels in animals (Keim *et al.*, 1976; Jagdis *et al.*, 1977) and is much more soluble in aqueous solutions. *In vitro*, amphotericin B methyl ester has a slightly lower activity than amphotericin B against pathogenic fungi (Howarth *et al.*, 1975; Bannatyne and Cheung, 1977; Huston and Hoeprich, 1978), and in experimental murine infections due to Histoplasma capsulatum, Blastomyces dermatitidis, Cryptococcus neoformans, Candida albicans and Coccidioides immitis, it is less effective than the parent compound (Bonner *et al.*, 1975; Lawrence and Hoeprich, 1976; Gadebusch *et al.*, 1976). Amphotericin B methyl ester also has an antiviral effect against viruses such as Herpesvirus hominis types 1 and 2, Sindbis and Vaccinia (Jordan and Seet, 1978).

As yet amphotericin B methyl ester has not been used in humans, and the following details only apply to amphotericin B.

Sensitive Organisms

1. *Pathogenic yeasts*. Cryptococcus neoformans (Torula) is usually considered to be sensitive to amphotericin B, but Hoeprich and Huston (1975) by their methodology found about one-third of clinical isolates resistant.

2. *Pathogenic yeast-like fungi*. It has been generally accepted that Candida albicans (Monilia) is quite sensitive although about one-half of the clinical isolates tested by Hoeprich and Huston (1975) were considered resistant. Other Candida spp. such as C. tropicalis are sensitive to a lesser degree (Stieritz *et al.*, 1973). Torulopsis glabrata is also susceptible.

3. *Dimorphic fungi*. Sporotrichum schenckii (causative agent of sporotrichosis), Blastomyces dermatitidis (causative agent of North American blastomycosis), Paracoccidioides brasiliensis (causative agent of South American blastomycosis), Histoplasma capsulatum and Coccidioides immitis

are all sensitive to amphotericin B. In one *in vitro* study of clinical isolates at least one-fifth of C. immitis strains were considered to be resistant (Hoeprich and Huston, 1975), but in experimental murine infections amphotericin B in clinically attainable concentrations was uniformly effective against C. immitis strains, including some of those studied by Hoeprich and Huston (Collins and Pappagianis, 1977).

4. *Moulds or filamentous fungi.* Aspergillus, the Cladosporium spp. (causative agents of cladosporiosis), Phialophora spp. (causative agents of chromoblastomycosis) and the Madurella spp. are all usually sensitive. Species of the genera Mucor, Rhizopus, Absidia, Entomophthora and Basidiobolus (causative agents of mucormycosis or phycomycosis) are often sensitive. The dermatophytes or ringworm fungi such as the Microsporum, Trichophyton and Epidermophyton spp. are usually resistant (Gold *et al.*, 1956).

5. *Actinomycetes.* Bacteria such as the Actinomyces and Nocardia spp. which may produce diseases resembling the mycoses, unlike the fungi, are amphotericin B-resistant.

6. *Prototheca spp.* These organisms which appear to be achloric algae and resemble fungi can be rare causes of human infection (protothecosis), characterized by chronic, persistent granulomata which may be cutaneous or disseminated (Davies *et al.*, 1964; Nosanchuk and Greenberg, 1973). Prototheca spp. are usually sensitive to amphotericin B (Segal *et al.*, 1976).

7. *Naegleria.* These amoeboflagellates, in particular N. fowleri, which causes primary amoebic meningoencephalitis in humans, are usually sensitive to amphoterin B, but resistant to commonly used anti-amoebic drugs such as emetine and metronidazole (Carter, 1969; Schuster and Rechthand, 1975).

8. *Acanthamoebae.* Fresh water amoebae such as Acanthamoeba polyphaga, A. castellanii can cause suppurative corneal and intraocular infections resembling those due to fungi; these protozoa are also susceptible *in vitro* to amphotericin B (Nagington and Richards, 1976).

9. *Synergism with other drugs.* Antibiotics such as rifampicin (page 556) and tetracyclines (page 598), normally inactive against fungi, act synergistically when combined with amphotericin B, because the latter by its action on the fungal cytoplasmic membrane (page 871) allows penetration of the other antibiotics into the cell.

A combination of amphotericin B and rifampicin is synergistic *in vitro* against Aspergillus spp. (Kitahara *et al.*, 1976a), Candida spp. (Medoff *et al.*, 1972; Beggs *et al.*, 1974; 1976), Coccidioides immitis (Rifkind *et al.*, 1974; Huppert *et al.*, 1976) and Histoplasma capsulatum and Blastomyces dermatitidis (Kobayashi et al., 1972; 1974). This combination is also more effective for murine infections due to Aspergillus fumigatus (Arroyo *et al.*, 1977), Histoplasma capsulatum and Blastomyces dermatitidis (Kitahara *et al.*, 1976b), but not for those due to Coccidioides immitis (Huppert *et al.*, 1976).

Tetracyclines act synergistically with amphotericin B *in vitro* against Histoplasma capsulatum (Kwan *et al.*, 1972) and this combination is also more effective in murine coccidioidomycosis (Huppert *et al.*, 1974). When used in conjunction with amphotericin B, tetracycline increases the survival rate of mice infected with Naegleria fowleri (Thong *et al.*, 1978). Polymyxin B, which also affects the cell cytoplasmic membrane (*see* page 533), enhances the activity of amphotericin B against Coccidioides immitis *in vitro* (Collins and Pappagianis, 1975).

The action of amphotericin B on the cytoplasmic membrane also renders yeast cells more susceptible to 5-fluorocytosine (page 886) (Medoff *et al.*, 1971). Together these two drugs frequently exert an *in vitro* synergistic effect against Candida spp. (Shadomy *et al.*, 1975). Sometimes synergy occurs even when the strain is resistant to 5-fluorocytosine (Montgomerie *et al.*, 1975). These two drugs often have an enhanced effect when used to treat experimental infections due to Candida albicans in mice (Titsworth and Grunberg, 1973; Ravinovich *et al.*, 1974). The combination of amphotericin B and 5-fluorocytosine also shows *in vitro* synergism against a proportion of isolates of Cryptococcus neoformans (Medoff *et al.*, 1972; Shadomy *et al.*, 1975) and enhanced efficacy in cryptococcal murine infections (Block and Bennett, 1973). Synergism is not demonstrable with all isolates of yeast-like organisms, and *in vitro* antagonism has sometimes been demonstrated when the two drugs have been used against Candida albicans (Hoeprich and Finn, 1972) and Cryptococcus neoformans (Hoeprich and Finn, 1972; Hamilton and Elliot, 1975). Amphotericin B together with 5-fluorocytosine shows synergism *in vitro* against some clinical isolates of Aspergillus (Kitahara *et al.*, 1976a). In addition Arroyo *et al.* (1977) found that suboptimal doses of amphotericin B in combination with 5-fluorocytosine was better than single-drug therapy in the treatment of disseminated Aspergillus fumigatus infection in mice.

Weak inhibitory concentrations of clotrimazole (page 899) may also enhance the action of amphotericin B against some Candida strains. The combination of amphotericin B with miconazole (page 907) has been reported to be antagonistic when used against Candida albicans *in vitro* and this may possibly occur *in vivo* in humans (Schacter *et al.*, 1976).

Notwithstanding these *in vitro* synergistic effects of amphotericin B and other drugs, drug combinations should be carefully assessed before use in any fungal infection (Medoff and Kobayashi, 1975). Not all fungi respond to the same drug combinations; drugs in combination with amphotericin B may have enhanced toxicity and amphotericin B may alter the host's immune response (page 873).

10. *Acquired resistance.* Although amphotericin B-resistant strains of C. albicans and C. immitis can be induced in the laboratory (Sorensen *et al.*, 1959; Athar and Winner, 1971), amphotericin B resistance of the usually sensitive fungi has not be a frequent problem in clinical practice.

In Vitro Sensitivities

Table 44 shows the minimum inhibitory concentrations of amphotericin B against some selected fungal species. Fungi with MIC's of less than $1 \cdot 0$ μg per ml are considered highly sensitive to this drug.

Mode of Administration and Dosage

1. *Intravenous administration.* Amphotericin B is poorly absorbed after oral administration (Louria, 1958) and from intramuscular sites. For this reason it is given intravenously for the treatment of systemic fungal infections. To avoid side-effects it is given by a slow intravenous infusion, the daily dose

ABLE 44

Compiled from data published by Gold *et al.* (1956), Seabury and Dascomb (1960) and Brandsberg and French (1972)

ORGANISM	MIC (μg per ml)
Cryptococcus neoformans	0·03– 0·6
Candida albicans	0·5 – 3·7
Sporotrichum schenckii	0·07– 0·5
Blastomyces dermatitidis	0·05– 0·5
Histoplasma capsulatum	0·04– 0·9
Coccidioides immitis	0·4 – 0·5
Aspergillus fumigatus	0·14– 0·6
Microsporum canis	7·3 –30·0
Trichophyton mentagrophytes	2·4 –14·0

being dissolved in 5 per cent dextrose (1000 ml for adults) and delivered over 4–6 h. Commercial preparations of 5 per cent dextrose usually have a pH level about 4·2; if the level is less than 4·2, the dextrose should be suitably buffered before it is used to dilute the concentrated solution of amphotericin. Since intravenous amphotericin B is in the form of a colloid suspension (page 865), membrane filters should not be used in the infusion line because they may remove significant amounts of the drug. Heparin (1000 units) and a corticosteroid (5–50 mg hydrocortisone) are often added to the flask (1000 ml) of infusion fluid in an attempt to decrease phlebitis and systemic reactions (Hickie and Walker, 1964). At the commencement of amphotericin B therapy, a test dose of 1 mg should be given by slow infusion, thereafter the daily infusion dose can be increased by 5–10 mg per day, until optimal dosage is reached. The recommended dose is 1·0–1·5 mg per kg body weight per day, or 50–100 mg for adults. Many patients cannot tolerate this dosage because of side-effects, chiefly nephrotoxicity (page 872); in this situation a reduced daily dose or less frequent administration of amphotericin B may be necessary. Daily amphotericin B infusions appear to be therapeutically superior to less frequent administration (Utz *et al.*, 1959; Seabury and Dascomb, 1960). However, Bindschadler and Bennett (1969) considered that alternate day therapy is satisfactory. They showed that minimum serum levels of the drug obtained with daily infusion were not significantly different from those when double the recommended dose was given on alternate days.

Drutz *et al.* (1967; 1968) have advocated that the dosage of amphotericin B should be adjusted in individual patients according to the *in vitro* sensitivity of the fungus involved. They manipulated the daily intravenous dose to produce, one hour after infusion, a peak serum level of about twice the MIC for the fungus. Such treatment was given for ten weeks to each of 15 patients who had cryptococcosis, histoplasmosis or blastomycosis, with satisfactory results and little toxicity. These authors suggested that a daily amphotericin B dose of 1·0 mg per kg may be too large for many patients, and considered that the total duration of therapy may be more important than high daily doses.

Solutions of amphotericin B are light sensitive. However there is no appreciable loss of drug activity if such solutions are exposed to light for 8 h, and therefore there is no need to take elaborate precautions to protect infusion solutions from light under normal hospital conditions (Shadomy *et al.*, 1972).

2. *Patients with renal failure*. Amphotericin B may cause renal failure (page 872), in which case the drug may have to be discontinued. In patients with pre-existing renal failure it should be avoided, if possible, because it may aggravate their disease. If amphotericin B therapy is imperative in such patients, it can be administered in the usual dosage. The excretion and serum concentrations of this drug are unaffected by renal failure (Bindschadler and Bennett, 1969). Even in anephric patients, the decline in its serum levels is similar to that in patients with normal renal function. Amphotericin B is not removed by haemodialysis (Feldman *et al.*, 1973; Block *et al.*, 1974).

3. *Intrathecal and intraventricular administration*. These modes of administration may occasionally be indicated in patients with severe torula meningitis, not responding to intravenous therapy (Littman and Walter, 1968).

The adult intrathecal dose is 0·5 mg given two to three times a week, each dose being first dissolved in 5 ml of cerebrospinal fluid. Severe arachnoiditis can follow this procedure. Animal experiments have shown that this complication can probably be minimized if the amphotericin B is administered in 10 per cent dextrose in water and the patient is placed in the Trendelenburg position after intrathecal injection (Alazraki *et al.*, 1974). It appears that with this technique amphotericin B moves from the lumbar space to the basal cisterns more rapidly. Nevertheless it is probably preferable to administer a similar dose of the drug intraventricularly. This may be conveniently done by using a subcutaneous Ommaya reservoir in the scalp (Witorsch *et al.*, 1965; Diamond and Bennett, 1973; Posner, 1973). Amphotericin B may be given intraventricularly each day if a low adult dose of 0·3 mg is infused over a period of one hour (Atkinson and Bindschadler, 1969). If an Ommaya reservoir is *in situ*, specimens of cerebrospinal fluid for laboratory tests should be taken by lumbar puncture, because fluid from the reservoir often shows low cell counts, and normal protein and glucose values which do not reflect the findings in the lumbar CSF (Goldstein *et al.*, 1972; Holt *et al.*, 1972).

4. *Intraperitoneal administration*. For the purpose of either treatment or prevention of Monilia infection during peritoneal dialysis, amphotericin B can be added to peritoneal dialysis fluid. The recommended dose is 1·0 mg added to 1000 ml of dialysis fluid (a concentration of 1·0 μg per ml).

5. *Bladder instillation or irrigation*. Monilial cystitis has been treated by instilling 15 mg of amphotericin B into the bladder daily (Goldman *et al.*, 1960). Wise *et al.* (1973) treated ten patients with Monilia bladder infections with daily instillations in a dose of 50 mg amphotericin B. No evidence of drug toxicity was observed.

6. *Topical therapy*. Amphotericin B is available as a lotion, cream and ointment for the treatment of cutaneous candidal infections, as a cream or tablets for treatment of vaginal moniliasis and as lozenges for the treatment of oral moniliasis. Tablets and a suspension are also available for oral administration to treat gastro-intestinal moniliasis.

Availability

Amphotericin B ('Fungizone' Squibb)

Vials containing lyophilised powder, providing 50 mg amphotericin B and 41 mg sodium desoxycholate and 25·2 mg sodium phosphate as buffer, which is ready for reconstitution in 10 ml sterile water for injection. This is suitable for intravenous, intraventricular and intraperitoneal use, and for instillation into the bladder.

Amphotericin B (*'Fungilin' Squibb*)

  (a) Vaginal tablets (50 mg) and a vaginal cream (100 mg per 4 g dose).
  (b) Oral tablets: 100 mg.
  (c) Lozenges: 10 mg.
  (d) Oral suspension: 100 mg per ml.
  (e) Lotion, cream and ointment (3 per cent).

Serum Levels in Relation to Dosage

1. If an amphotericin B dose of 0·65 mg per kg is given by intravenous infusion over a period of 4–6 h, a peak serum level of 1·8–3·5 μg per ml is reached during the first hour after infusion (Louria, 1958). This level is maintained for 6–8 h, and then gradually falls to about half the peak level 20 h after the infusion. The drug does not accumulate in the serum if this dosage is used daily (Bindschadler and Bennett, 1969). More recent pharmacokinetic studies in humans indicate that after an amphotericin infusion there is a rapid initial elimination of the drug (half-life of 24–48 h) from central and rapidly equilibrating peripheral compartments of the body (Atkinson and Bennett, 1978). In about six days this is followed by a final elimination phase which has a half-life of about 15 days; this implies that it takes a long time before a pharmacokinetic steady state is obtained, because there is a slowly equilibrating peripheral compartment in the body. The central compartment may be the blood and the rapidly equilibrating peripheral one is probably the extravascular compartment consisting of the interstitial fluid of tissues with discontinuous capillaries such as liver, spleen and intestine. The slowly equilibrating peripheral extravascular compartment probably consists of the interstitial fluid of tissues with continuous capillaries, such as skeletal muscle and skin.

2. The absorption of amphotericin B from the gastro-intestinal tract is poor. Louria (1958) showed that if a large oral dose of 3 g is administered to an adult, some of the drug is absorbed producing a serum level ranging from 0·04 to 0·5 μg per ml.

Excretion

URINE: Only about 5 per cent of a total daily dose of amphotericin B is excreted in the urine as the active drug (Louria, 1958). Pre-existing renal dysfunction has no effect on amphotericin B excretion (Bindschadler and Bennett, 1969).

INACTIVATION IN THE BODY: The fate of most of an infused dose of amphotericin B is not known. Presumably some of it is inactivated in the body, but no metabolites have been identified. Some of the drug also appears to be stored in the body (*vide supra*), because after treatment is stopped, serum concentrations continue to fall slowly over several weeks (Bindschadler and Bennett, 1969).

Distribution of the Drug in Body

Intravenously administered amphotericin B reaches the cerebrospinal fluid, but in patients with uninflamed meninges CSF levels are 30 to 50 times lower than simultaneous serum levels (Louria, 1958). In seven patients with cryptococcal meningitis studied by Utz *et al.* (1975), the drug was not detected in the CSF of four, and was less than 10 per cent of the serum values in the other three. Bindschadler and Bennett (1969) demonstrated a concentration of $1\cdot0\,\mu$g per ml in the pleural fluid of one patient, whose simultaneous serum level was $1\cdot8\,\mu$g per ml. The concentrations of amphotericin B in many other body fluids and tissues have not been well studied in humans. In one report, a level of less than $0\cdot5\,\mu$g per ml was detected in human aqueous humour when the serum level was $0\cdot6\,\mu$g per ml after intravenous administration of $0\cdot8$ mg per kg body weight and also topical application of amphotericin B to the eye (Richards *et al.*, 1969). In dogs, the drug penetrates into bronchial secretions poorly (Pennington *et al.*, 1974). Amphotericin B is highly ($>$90 per cent) bound to serum proteins (Block *et al.*, 1974).

Mode of Action

Amphotericin B and other polyene antifungal drugs such as nystatin (page 925), act on sensitive fungi by damaging the osmotic barrier formed by their plasma membrane. These drugs bind to a sterol, which is present in this plasma membrane (Kinsky, 1970), thereby interfering with its permeability. Amphotericin B potentiates the antifungal effect of 5-fluorocytosine and other drugs, probably by facilitating their penetration through the fungal cytoplasmic membrane (Kwan *et al.*, 1972) (*see also* page 890). The plasma membrane of the mammalian cell also contains sterols, mainly cholesterol, whilst the fungal plasma membrane contains mainly ergosterol (Gale, 1973). Mammalian cells are less susceptible than yeast cells to amphotericin B because it appears that the drug has a higher affinity for ergosterol than cholesterol (Kotler-Brajtburg *et al.*, 1974). However most of the toxic effects of amphotericin B in humans, are probably caused by a similar action of amphotericin B on human cell cytoplasmic membranes (Hsuchen and Feingold, 1973). For instance human red blood cells can be destroyed by amphotericin B *in vitro*, probably because the drug binds to sterol groups on the surface of erythrocytes (Carter and McCarthy, 1966).

Amphotericin B-resistant Candida strains have an altered sterol in their plasma membrane (Woods *et al.*, 1974). This is not the only possible mechanism of resistance. In one study, induced mutants of Cryptococcus neoformans resistant to amphotericin B seemed to be resistant not by alteration of sterols, but perhaps by impairment of permeability to amphotericin B (Kim *et al.*, 1975).

Toxicity

Intravenously administered amphotericin B is very toxic, and numerous side-effects have been described.

1. *Side-effects which may occur during intravenous infusion.* These include

fever, chills, headache, anorexia, nausea and vomiting. Sometimes hyperthermia may be marked (Bennett, 1974). Thrombophlebitis is also a common problem. Some of these symptoms can be minimized if heparin and hydrocortisone are added to the infusion and the use of oral or intramuscular antihistamines or chlorpromazine may also be of value (Utz et al., 1964).

2. *Nephrotoxicity.* This is common and the most important side-effect of parenteral amphotericin B. The drug causes some impairment of renal function in almost all patients treated. This is evidenced by rises in blood urea and serum creatinine, decrease in creatinine clearance, and the appearance of red and white blood cells, albumin and casts in the urine. If the patient's blood urea rises to levels higher than 100 mg per cent (16·7 mmol/l) or the serum creatinine to higher than 2·0 mg per cent (0·17 mmol/l), the drug should be stopped for several days until renal function returns to normal. Although nephrotoxicity frequently limits the duration of treatment with amphotericin B, the drug can usually be continued until the above limits of renal function are reached (Forgan-Smith and Darrell, 1974). Such renal damage is usually completely reversible. Occasionally permanent impairment can occur, which appears to be partially related to the total dose of amphotericin B used, because some degree of renal impairment has been demonstrated in 40 per cent of patients who had received more than 4 g of the drug (McCurdy et al., 1968). Irreversible renal failure may also occur if large doses of the drug are used (Takacs et al., 1963). However the possibility of severe amphotericin nephrotoxicity should not preclude its use in patients with potentially fatal systemic fungal infections, if this is the only suitable drug available. Temporary severe renal failure may be treated by dialysis and even irreversible renal failure may be successfully managed (Symmers, 1973).

The mechanism of the nephrotoxic effect of amphotericin B has been extensively studied (McCurdy et al., 1968; Douglas and Healy, 1969; Burgess and Birchall, 1972). The drug appears to cause vasoconstriction with resultant cortical ischaemia and a fall in the glomerular filtration rate. There is also an increased clearance of uric acid by the proximal tubule, and a more marked effect on the distal renal tubule, where excessive potassium, bicarbonate and water losses occur. In some patients a syndrome similar to renal tubular acidosis has developed. It has been suggested that as in idiopathic renal tubular acidosis, early recognition and alkali therapy may help to prevent nephrocalcinosis and renal failure in these patients. Potassium supplements are required for most patients receiving amphotericin B because of the excessive renal losses. Animal experiments have shown that concomitant administration of intravenous mannitol reduces amphotericin B nephrotoxicity (Bennett, 1974). Uncontrolled studies of a small number of patients suggested that the use of mannitol may also reduce nephrotoxicity in humans (Olivero et al., 1975; Rosch et al., 1976). A double-blind study was conducted by Bullock et al. (1976) of eleven patients with systemic mycotic infections, who were receiving amphotericin B in a dose of 1 mg per kg on alternate days; in five who also had mannitol in a dose of 1·0 g per kg added to the amphotericin infusion, there was no reduction in nephrotoxicity.

3. *Haematological side-effects.* A normochromic normocytic anaemia may be associated with amphotericin B therapy. Bone marrow examination in these cases shows reduced erythropoiesis. The changes are usually reversible on

cessation of the drug, but on occasions the anaemia may be severe enough to require treatment by blood transfusion. This anaemia may be due to a disturbance of red cell iron metabolism (Windom *et al.*, 1961), but it is more likely to be due to reversible bone marrow suppression (Utz *et al.*, 1964; Butler, 1966). Drutz *et al.* (1968) reported two patients in whom a pure red blood cell aplasia developed during amphotericin B therapy.

Thrombocytopenia has been occasionally noted, but leucopenia appears to be very rare.

4. *Hepatotoxicity*. Liver function abnormalities are rarely detected during amphotericin B therapy. However acute liver failure due to liver cell necrosis has been reported (Carnecchia and Kurtzke, 1960). This complication is so rare that doubt has been cast on its relation to amphotericin B therapy (Bennett, 1974).

5. *Cardiovascular side-effects*. Cardiac arrest has been reported with a rapid amphotericin B infusion, in which 28 mg of the drug was infused within 40 min (Hildick-Smith *et al.*, 1964). A temporary increase in the heart size has been noted in another patient treated by amphotericin B (Utz *et al.*, 1959).

6. *Neurotoxicity*. This is rare with intravenous amphotericin B therapy. One case of severe peripheral neuropathy associated with intravenous administration of the drug has been reported (Haber and Joseph, 1962).

Intrathecal administration can produce peripheral nerve pain, paraesthesiae, nerve palsies, paraplegia, convulsions and a chemical meningitis. Intraventricular administration is less likely to cause chemical meningitis (*see* page 869).

7. *Allergic reactions*. Anaphylactic reactions have been reported but are very rare. Hypersensitivity rashes occur but are uncommon (Bennett, 1974; Lorber *et al.*, 1976).

8. *Effect on fetus*. Amphotericin B has been given to pregnant women with serious fungal infections. Several of these have recovered and given birth to normal infants (Kuo, 1962; Frey and Durie, 1970; Philpot and Lo, 1972). However, the safety of amphotericin B during the first trimester of pregnancy has not been established.

9. *Immunosuppression*. *In vitro* studies show that in therapeutic concentrations (<3 μg per ml), human lymphocyte stimulation is only slightly or not at all inhibited by amphotericin B (Tärnvik and Ånsehn, 1974). Results of animal experiments suggests that amphotericin B can act as an adjuvant and either stimulate or suppress host resistance, depending on the dosage and timing of administration of the drug (Medoff and Kobayashi, 1975).

Clinical Uses of the Drug

1. *Cryptococcosis (Torulosis)*. This fungal disease may occur in otherwise healthy patients, but unfortunately it commonly occurs in patients with other diseases, particularly in those with an associated defect in cellular immunity. Cryptococcosis may affect most parts of the body, but the meninges and the lungs are most frequently involved (Lewis and Rabinovich, 1972). If a cryptococcal lung abscess is the only manifestation, it can usually be satisfactorily treated by surgery alone (Hammerman *et al.*, 1973). Cryptococcal meningitis always needs chemotherapy, because untreated the disease was almost uni-

formly fatal. With the use of amphotericin B more than 50 per cent of patients recover (Littman and Walter, 1968). Prolonged treatment is usually required but toxicity (page 872) often necessitates interruptions. This treatment is less likely to succeed in patients who have an underlying malignancy such as a reticulosis. Other unfavourable prognostic features appear to be a high initial cerebrospinal fluid pressure, a low CSF glucose level, a CSF with less than 20 leucocytes per mm^3 and cryptococci seen in smear, the isolation of cryptococci from other sites, particularly blood, and high cryptococcal antigen titres in the serum and CSF (Diamond and Bennett, 1974). A substantial proportion of patients with cryptococcosis fail to respond to amphotericin B, others relapse after completion of therapy and the complications, particularly nephrotoxicity, of this treatment are often serious. For these reasons amphotericin B has been used in combination with 5-fluorocytosine. *In vitro* and *in vivo* synergism has been demonstrated with these two drugs against C. neoformans (page 867). and the use of 5-fluorocytosine may allow lower doses of amphotericin B to be used, thereby reducing its toxicity. A prospective study by Utz *et al.* (1975) on 20 consecutive patients with disseminated cryptococcosis (15 with culturally confirmed meningitis) indeed indicated that a regimen using these two drugs was safe and as efficacious as single drug therapy. A shorter period of hospitalization was required and there was reduced amphotericin B toxicity. Amphotericin B was given intravenously in a dose of 20 mg daily with 5-fluorocytosine orally in a dose of 150 mg per kg per day for six weeks. Similar encouraging results have been obtained by the use of low doses of amphotericin B and 5-fluorocytosine; ten patients with cryptococcosis (eight with meningitis) after renal transplantation (Schröter *et al.*, 1976) and two other patients with cryptococcal meningitis complicating Hodgkin's disease (Tobias *et al.*, 1976) have been treated in this way.

Intravenous administration of amphotericin B is usually sufficient for most cases of torula meningitis, but intraventricular or intrathecal therapy may be indicated in special circumstances (*see* page 869). The duration of therapy depends on the nature and severity of the infection, and the side-effects of the drug. In most patients a minimum of about ten weeks treatment is usually indicated (Drutz *et al.*, 1968). It is usually not advisable to exceed a total adult dose of 3 g in one course of treatment (*see* page 872).

2. *Disseminated monilial infections.* Amphotericin B, 5-fluorocytosine (page 892) and possibly miconazole (page 913) are the only useful drugs available for systemic Candida albicans infections such as fungaemia, endocarditis and meningitis. Amphotericin B is also useful for Candida infections of the eye (*vide infra*). The decision to use amphotericin B, a relatively toxic drug, should be based on adequate evidence that a systemic Candida infection is present. This organism is often isolated from open sites such as the upper respiratory tract of debilitated patients treated by antibiotics, and this may only indicate colonization and not suprainfection.

If systemic therapy with amphotericin B is necessary, the drug should be used intravenously, in the same doses as for torula meningitis, but the duration of therapy can often be shorter. For instance, Roe and Haynes (1972) reported a child who recovered from Candida albicans meningitis after therapy with amphotericin B for 43 days. A course of amphotericin B as short as two weeks has also often been effective in treating systemic candidiasis in patients with burns (Gauto *et al.*, 1977). Amphotericin B has been used to treat C. albicans osteomyelitis, although this infection may heal without treatment (Edwards *et al.*, 1975). Arthritis due to C. tropicalis has been successfully treated by amphotericin B. Poplack *et al.* (1975) described an eleven-year-old girl with acute lymphoblastic leukaemia, whose C. tropicalis arthritis was only suppressed by systemic amphotericin B therapy, but it was cured when intra-articular injections of amphotericin B were also used. Similarly parenteral amphotericin B together with joint aspiration was used successfully to eradicate the infection in a man aged 77 years with C. tropicalis arthritis (Murray *et al.*, 1976). Clinical improvement was also noted by Pittard *et al.* (1976) who used systemic and intra-articular amphotericin B for neonates with C. albicans arthritis. Candida endocarditis often associated with prosthetic valves has a high mortality; immediate treatment by removal of the infected valve, irrigation of the infected site with amphotericin B (1·0 g per litre of Ringer's solution) followed by a prolonged course of amphotericin B intravenously, three times weekly, has been recommended (Editorial, 1975).

Peritoneal lavage with amphotericin B (1 μg per ml) was used successfully to treat peritonitis due to C. tropicalis in a 14-year-old girl, who was a renal transplant recipient (Bortolussi *et al.*, 1975). Similar treatment using amphotericin B intraperitoneally and/or short-term, low dose systemic treatment was useful for adult patients with unremitting Candida peritonitis (Bayer *et al.*, 1976).

Combined treatment using amphotericin B and 5-fluorocytosine which may show *in vitro* synergism (page 867) has been used to treat human candidal infections successfully. A patient reported by Fass and Perkins (1971) had Candida endocarditis in association with an aortic valve prosthesis. The combination of 5-fluorocytosine and amphotericin B, together with surgical replacement of the prosthesis, was successful. Chesney *et al.* (1976) treated two children with Candida albicans meningitis successfully; therapy consisted of 9–13 days treatment with amphotericin B given intravenously, combined with, or followed by six to nine weeks of oral 5-fluorocytosine. These two antifungal drugs were used concomitantly to treat several fungal infections by Eilard *et al.* (1976); they obtained good results in two cases of Candida endophthalmitis with invasion into the vitreous body, in one case of endocarditis on a prosthetic valve due to Torulopsis glabrata resistant to 5-fluorocytosine, and in one case of Candida fungaemia associated with an aorto-coronary graft. Keller *et al.* (1977) used amphotericin B and 5-fluorocytosine in association with appropriate surgical measures to treat a four-and-a-half-month-old infant successfully who had Candida albicans renal fungus balls and C. albicans arthritis.

Lou *et al.* (1977) used a combination of amphotericin B and rifampicin to cure Candida albicans endophthalmitis, which complicated candidaemia in a 14-year-old girl receiving intravenous hyperalimentation. Rifampicin was preferred to 5-fluorocytosine as a companion drug, because it is more consistently synergistic with amphotericin B against Candida albicans (page 866) and there is less chance of enhanced drug toxicity. Treatment consisted of a peribulbar injection of amphotericin B (125 μg in 0·3 ml of water), and a ten-day course of amphotericin B (dose rapidly increased to 1·0 mg per kg per day) with rifampicin 15 mg per kg per day.

3. *Histoplasmosis*. Amphotericin B is the drug of choice for the treatment of

this disease. For chronic pulmonary histoplasmosis, a total dose of 1·5 g administered intravenously, daily or on alternate days, over a period of ten weeks is satisfactory (Sutliff, 1972). In progressive disseminated histoplasmosis, a larger total dose of amphotericin B administered over a longer period is often necessary (Smith and Utz, 1972; Edmonson et al., 1974). By contrast, acute pulmonary histoplasmosis is usually a benign self-limiting infection which requires no chemotherapy. Nevertheless acute histoplasmosis, particularly if disseminated, may be a severe illness in infants and young children. Fosson et al. (1975) used amphotericin B to gain a favourable therapeutic response in six children with this form of the disease; a maximum dose of the drug (1 mg per kg per day) was reached rapidly by the third day and this was continued for only short periods of 7–19 days. Amphotericin B has also been used together with rifampicin (page 866) to treat disseminated histoplasmosis.

4. *Coccidioidomycosis*. Chemotherapy is usually not required for the milder forms of this disease such as primary infection. However disseminated, meningeal and chronic pulmonary coccidioidomycosis with cavitation require treatment, and amphotericin B is the drug of choice. For treatment of meningitis, intraventricular as well as intravenous administration may be required (Goldstein et al., 1972; Le Clerc and Giammona, 1975).

5. *North American Blastomycosis*. Amphotericin B is the most useful drug for the treatment of this disease. The total intravenous dose for a course should be at least 1·5 g, otherwise relapses are common (Parker et al., 1969).

6. *South American Blastomycosis*. Patients with this disease only rarely recover without intravenous amphotericin B therapy (Hildick-Smith et al., 1964).

7. *Sporotrichosis*. Intravenous amphotericin B is indicated for the treatment of disseminated sporotrichosis (Hildick-Smith et al., 1964), but milder cutaneous forms usually respond to orally administered potassium iodide (O'Donnell, 1962; Baum and Schwarz, 1974).

8. *Aspergillosis*. If surgical resection of a pulmonary aspergillosis lesion is not possible, intravenous amphotericin B therapy is recommended (Meyer et al., 1973). This treatment is usually ineffective in patients with severe underlying pulmonary disease, who have been colonized with Aspergillus either with or without aspergilloma formation (Hammerman et al., 1974). Burton et al. (1972) reported the successful use of amphotericin B in four renal transplant recipients who developed pulmonary aspergillosis. Therapy of pulmonary aspergillosis in patients with neoplastic diseases of the haemopoietic system is usually refractory. Pennington (1976) however described the successful use of parenteral amphotericin B in two adult patients with lymphoma who had Aspergillus fumigatus pneumonia. Aspergillus endocarditis, which usually occurs on prosthetic heart valves, has a high mortality; one patient has been described who was cured with a combination of surgery, amphotericin B, and long-term therapy with 5-fluorocytosine (Carrizosa et al., 1974). Combination of amphotericin B and 5-fluorocytosine may be more effective for this disease than either drug used alone (see page 894).

9. *Leishmaniasis*. Intravenous amphotericin B has been used, apparently sometimes with success, in visceral leishmaniasis (Kala-azar) in patients who have failed to respond to conventional chemotherapy (Moškovskij and Southgate, 1971). This form of therapy is also an effective alternative to antimony treat-

ment for muco-cutaneous leishmaniasis (Yesudian and Thambiah, 1974; Singer *et al.*, 1975; Crofts, 1976).

10. *Primary amoebic meningoencephalitis.* This is a rapidly fatal infection, and intravenous amphotericin B appears to be the only promising treatment. Most results of treatment have been poor (Symmers, 1969; Duma *et al.*, 1971), although occasional successes have been reported (Anderson and Jamieson, 1972). The demonstration of synergy between amphotericin B and tetracycline in mice infected with this organism (Thong *et al.*, 1978), indicates that this combination is worthy of trial in humans. Miconazole (pages 908, 914) and rifampicin (page 554) may also prove to be useful in this disease.

11. *Fungal infections of the eye* (*oculomycosis*). These infections may be superficial (keratomycosis) or invade the interior of the eye (endophthalmitis) and can be caused by a great variety of fungi (Jones, 1975). Candida albicans and various Aspergillus spp. are the commonest fungi causing eye infections in the United States and Europe, whilst Fusarium solani is common in West Africa (Editorial, 1976). Amphotericin B is active against Candida spp. and a small proportion of other fungi causing ocular infections. Topical administration of amphotericin B to the eyes is not recommended because of its poor penetration; it is also highly irritant and soon leads to epithelial erosions and ulcers (Jones, 1975). Subconjunctival injections of the drug are painful and like intraocular injections may cause tissue damage. Intravenous amphotericin B however seems to have a place in the treatment of orbital phycomycosis (*vide infra*) and other ocular fungal infections. Candida endophthalmitis may respond to intravenous amphotericin B, despite the fact that this drug penetrates poorly into the non-inflamed eye (Haning *et al.*, 1973) (*see* page 871). Meyers *et al.* (1973) preferred amphotericin B to 5-fluorocytosine (page 893) for this infection. Jones (1975) considers that 5-fluorocytosine is the drug of choice for intraocular and deep corneal infections caused by Candida spp. provided that the strain is sensitive, but that amphotericin B still probably has a place as a companion drug. Amphotericin B has been used successfully in combination with 5-fluorocytosine or rifampicin to treat candida endophthalmitis (*see* page 875).

12. *Mucormycosis* (*Phycomycosis*). This fungal infection may respond to amphotericin B therapy (Prout and Goddard, 1960; Burrow *et al.*, 1963).

13. *Mycetoma due to Petriellidium boydii* (*Allescheria boydii; Monosporium apiospermum*). This fungus is resistant to concentrations of both amphotericin B and 5-fluorocytosine (page 913) which can be safely attained by their systemic administration (Lutwick *et al.*, 1976). Nevertheless there have been some encouraging reports when amphotericin B was injected directly into the lesions of patients with mycetoma due to this fungus. Hayden *et al.* (1977) described a six-year-old boy with a monoarticular arthritis of the knee due to Petriellidium boydii, which responded to treatment by intra-articular injections of amphotericin B.

14. *Topical use of amphotericin B.* Amphotericin B, like nystatin (page 925) and natamycin (page 928), is available in tablets, a suspension for oral administration, lozenges and vaginal cream and tablets, all for the treatment of superficial or bowel Candida infections. In one trial amphotericin B vaginal tablets were found to be superior to natamycin vaginal tablets (Corkill and McCarthy, 1972). In general however amphotericin B, nystatin and natamycin

have a similar efficacy in topical use. Amphotericin B, like nystatin, is also marketed in combination with tetracycline (*see* page 613).

REFERENCES

Alazraki, N. P., Fierer, J., Halpern, S. E. and Becker, R. W. (1974), 'Use of a hyperbaric solution for administration of inthrathecal amphotericin B', *New Engl. J. Med.*, **290**, 641.

Anderson, K. and Jamieson, A. (1972), 'Primary amoebic meningoencephalitis', *Lancet*, **1**, 902.

Arroyo, J., Medoff, G. and Kobayashi, G. S. (1977), 'Therapy of murine aspergillosis with amphotericin B in combination with rifampin or 5-fluorocytosine', *Antimicrob. Ag. Chemother.*, **11**, 21.

Athar, M. A. and Winner, H. I. (1971), 'The development of resistance by Candida species to polyene antibiotics *in vitro*', *J. Med. Microbiol.*, **4**, 505.

Atkinson, A. J., Jr. and Bindschadler, D. D. (1969), 'Pharmacokinetics of intrathecally administered amphotericin B', *Amer. Rev. Resp. Dis.*, **99**, 917.

Atkinson, A. J., Jr. and Bennett, J. E. (1978), 'Amphotericin B pharmacokinetics in humans', *Antimicrob. Ag. Chemother.*, **13**, 271.

Bannatyne, R. M. and Cheung, R. (1977), 'Comparative susceptibility of Candida albicans to amphotericin B and amphotericin B methyl ester', *Antimicrob. Ag. Chemother.*, **12**, 449.

Baum, G. L. and Schwarz, J. (1974), 'Diagnosis and treatment of systemic mycoses', *Med. Clin. North. Amer.*, **58**, 661.

Bayer, A. S., Blumenkrantz, M. J., Montgomerie, J. Z., Galpin, J. E., Coburn, J. W. and Guze, L. B. (1976), 'Candida peritonitis. Report of 22 cases and review of the English literature', *Amer. J. Med.*, **61**, 832.

Beggs, W. H., Sarosi, G. A. and Andrews, F. A. (1974), 'Synergistic action of amphotericin B and rifampin on Candida albicans', *Amer. Rev. Resp. Dis.*, **110**, 671.

Beggs, W. H., Sarosi, G. A. and Walker, M. I. (1976), 'Synergistic action of amphotericin B and rifampin against Candida species', *J. Infect. Dis.*, **133**, 206.

Bennett, J. E. (1974), 'Chemotherapy of systemic mycoses (first of two parts), *New Eng. J. Med.*, **290**, 30.

Bindschadler, D. D. and Bennett, J. E. (1969), 'A pharmacologic guide to the clinical use of amphotericin B', *J. Infect. Dis.*, **120**, 427.

Block, E. R. and Bennett, J. E. (1973), 'The combined effect of 5-fluorocytosine and amphotericin B in the therapy of murine cryptococcosis', *Proc. Soc. Exp. Biol. Med.*, **142**, 476.

Block, E. R., Bennett, J. E., Livoti, L. G., Klein, W. J., Jr., MacGregor, R. R. and Henderson, L. (1974), 'Flucytosine and amphotericin B: Hemodialysis effects on the plasma concentration and clearance. Studies in man', *Ann. Intern. Med.*, **80**, 613.

Bonner, D. P., Tewari, R. P., Solotorovsky, M., Mechlinski, W. and Schaffner, C. P. (1975), 'Comparative chemotherapeutic activity of amphotericin B and amphotericin B methyl ester', *Antimicrob. Ag. Chemother.*, **7**, 724.

Bortolussi, R. A., MacDonald, M. R. A., Bannatyne, R. M. and Arbus, G. S. (1975), 'Treatment of Candida peritonitis by peritoneal lavage with amphotericin B', *J. Pediatrics*, **87**, 987.

Brandsberg, J. W. and French, M. E. (1972), '*In vitro* susceptibility of isolates of aspergillus fumigatus and Sporothrix schenckii to amphotericin B', *Antimicrob. Ag. Chemother.*, **2**, 402.

Bullock, W. E., Luke, R. G., Nuttall, C. E. and Bhathena, D. (1976), 'Can mannitol reduce amphotericin B nephrotoxicity? Double-blind study and description of a new vascular lesion in kidneys', *Antimicrob. Ag. Chemother.*, **10**, 555.

Burgess, J. L. and Birchall, R. (1972), 'Nephrotoxicity of amphotericin B, with emphasis on changes in tubular function', *Amer. J. Med.*, **53**, 77.

Burrow, G. N., Salmon, R. B. and Nolan, J. P. (1963), 'Successful treatment of cerebral mucormycosis with amphotericin B, *JAMA*, **183**, 370.

Burton, J. R., Zachery, J. B., Bessin, R., Rathbun, H. K., Greenough, W. B., III, Sterioff, S., Wright, J. R., Slavin, R. E. and Williams, G. M. (1972), 'Aspergillosis in four renal transplant recipients', *Ann. Intern. Med.*, **77**, 383.

Butler, W. T. (1966), 'Pharmacology, toxicity, and therapeutic usefulness of amphotericin B', *JAMA*, **195**, 371.

Carnecchia, B. M. and Kurtzke, J. F. (1960), 'Fatal toxic reaction to amphotericin B in cryptococcal meningo-encephalitis', *Ann. Intern. Med.*, **53**, 1027.

Carrizosa, J., Levison, M. E., Lawrence, T. and Kaye, D. (1974), 'Cure of Aspergillus ustus endocarditis on a prosthetic valve', *Arch. Intern. Med.*, **133**, 486.

Carter, R. F. (1969), 'Sensitivity to amphotericin B of a Naegleria sp. isolated from a case of primary amoebic meningo-encephalitis', *J. clin. Path.*, **22**, 470.

Carter, W. and McCarthy, K. S. (1966), 'Molecular mechanisms of antibiotic action', *Ann. Intern. Med.*, **64**, 1087.

Chesney, P. J., Teets, K. C., Mulvihill, J. J., Salit, I. E. and Marks, M. I. (1976), 'Successful treatment of Candida meningitis with amphotericin B and 5-fluorocytosine in combination', *J. Pediatrics*, **89**, 1017.

Collins, M. S. and Pappagianis, D. (1975), 'Inhibition of Coccidioides immitis *in vitro* and enhancement of anticoccidioidal effects of amphotericin B by polymyxin B', *Antimicrob. Ag. Chemother.*, **7**, 781.

Collins, M. S. and Pappagianis, D. (1977), 'Uniform susceptibility of various strains of Coccidioides immitis to amphotericin B', *Antimicrob. Ag. Chemother.*, **11**, 1049.

Corkill, B. M. and McCarthy, N. J. (1972), 'Comparative trial of fungilin (amphotericin B) and pimafucin (natamycin) pessaries in the treatment of vaginal candidiasis', *Med. J. Aust.*, **2**, 33.

Crofts, M. A. J. (1976), 'Use of amphotericin B in mucocutaneous leishmaniasis', *J. Trop. Med. Hyg.*, **79**, 111.

Davies, R. R., Spencer, H. and Wakelin, P. O. (1964), 'A case of human protothecosis', *Trans. Roy. Soc. Trop. Med. Hyg.*, **58**, 448.

Diamond, R. D. and Bennett, J. E. (1973), 'A subcutaneous reservoir for intrathecal therapy of fungal meningitis', *New Engl. J. Med.*, **288**, 186.

Diamond, R. D. and Bennett, J. E. (1974), 'Prognostic factors in Cryptococcal meningitis. A study in 111 cases', *Ann. Intern. Med.*, **80**, 176.

Douglas, J. B. and Healy, J. K. (1969), 'Nephrotoxic effects of amphotericin B, including renal tubular acidosis', *Amer. J. Med.*, **46**, 154.

Drutz, D. J., Spickard, A. and Koenig, M. G. (1967), 'New approach to therapy with amphotericin B', *Antimicrob. Ag. Chemother.*—1966, p. 202.

Drutz, D. J., Spickard, A., Rogers, D. E. and Koenig, M. G. (1968), 'Treatment of disseminated mycotic infections. A new approach to amphotericin B therapy', *Amer. J. Med.*, **45**, 405.

Duma, R. J., Rosenblum, W. I., McGehee, R. F., Jones, M. M. and Nelson, E. C. (1971), 'Primary amoebic meningoencephalitis caused by Naegleria. Two new cases, response to amphotericin B, and a review', *Ann. Intern. Med.*, **74**, 923.

Editorial (1975), 'Candida endocarditis', *Brit. Med. J.*, **2**, 264.

Editorial (1976), 'Direct fungal infection of the eye and its prevention', *Brit. J. Ophthal.*, **60**, 605.

Edmonson, R. P. S., Eykyn, S., Davies, D. R., Fawcett, I. W. and Phillips, I. (1974), 'Disseminated histoplasmosis successfully treated with amphotericin B', *J. clin. Path.*, **27**, 308.

Edwards, J. E., Jr., Turkel, S. B., Elder, H. A., Rand, R. W. and Guze, L. B. (1975),

'Hematogenous Candida osteomyelitis. Report of three cases and review of the literature', *Amer. J. Med.*, **59**, 89.

Eilard, T., Beskow, D., Norrby, R., Wåhlén, P. and Alestig, K. (1976), 'Combined treatment with amphotericin B and flucytosine in severe fungal infections', *J. Antimicrob. Chemother.*, **2**, 239.

Fass, R. J. and Perkins, R. L. (1971), '5-Fluorocytosine in the treatment of Cryptococcal and Candida mycoses', *Ann. Intern. Med.*, **74**, 535.

Feldman, H. A., Hamilton, J. D. and Gutman, R. A. (1973), 'Amphotericin B therapy in an anephric patient', *Antimicrob. Ag. Chemother.*, **4**, 302.

Forgan-Smith, R. and Darrell, J. H. (1974), 'Amphotericin pharmacophobia and renal toxicity', *Brit. med. J.*, **1**, 244.

Fosson, A. R. and Wheeler, W. E. (1975), 'Short-term amphotericin B treatment of severe childhood histoplasmosis', *J. Pediatrics*, **86**, 32.

Frey, D. and Durie, E. B. (1970), 'Deep mycoses reported from Australia and New Guinea during the years 1956 to 1969', *Med. J. Aust.*, **2**, 1117.

Gadebusch, H. H., Pansy, F., Klepner, C. and Schwind, R. (1976), 'Amphotericin B and amphotericin B methyl ester ascorbate. I. Chemotherapeutic activity against Candida albicans, Cryptococcus neoformans, and Blastomyces dermatitidis in mice', *J. Infect. Dis.*, **134**, 423.

Gale, E. F. (1973), 'Perspectives in chemotherapy', *Brit. med. J.*, **4**, 33.

Gauto, A., Law, E. J., Holder, I. A. and MacMillan, B. G. (1977), 'Experience with amphotericin B in the treatment of systemic candidiasis in burn patients', *Amer. J. Surg.*, **133**, 174.

Gold, W., Stout, H. A., Pagano, J. F. and Donovick, R. (1956), 'Amphotericin A and B, antifungal antibiotics produced by a streptomycete', *Antibiot. Annual 1955–56*, p. 579.

Goldman, H. J., Littman, N. L., Oppenheimer, G. D. and Glickman, S. I. (1960), 'Monilial cystitis—effective treatment with instillations of amphotericin B', *JAMA*, **174**, 97.

Goldstein, E., Winship, M. J. and Pappagianis, D. (1972), 'Ventricular fluid and the management of coccidioidal meningitis', *Ann. Intern. Med.*, **77**, 243.

Haber, R. W. and Joseph, M. (1962), 'Neurological manifestations after amphotericin B therapy', *Brit. med. J.*, **1**, 230.

Hamilton, J. D. and Elliott, D. M. (1975), 'Combined activity of amphotericin B and 5-fluorocytosine against Cryptococcus neoformans *in vitro* and *in vivo* in mice', *J. Infect. Dis.*, **131**, 129.

Hamilton-Miller, J. M. T. (1973), 'Chemistry and biology of the polyene macrolide antibiotics', *Bacteriol. Rev.*, **37**, 166.

Hammerman, K. J., Powell, K. E., Christianson, C. S., Huggin, P. M., Larsh, H. W., Vivas, J. R. and Tosh, F. E. (1973), 'Pulmonary cryptococcosis: Clinical forms and treatment', *Amer. Rev. Resp. Dis.*, **108**, 1116.

Hammerman, K. J., Sarosi, G. A. and Tosh, F. E. (1974), 'Amphotericin B in the treatment of saprophytic forms of pulmonary aspergillosis', *Amer. Rev. Resp. Dis.*, **109**, 57.

Haning, H. A. L., Johnston, R., Touloukian, R. and Margolis, C. Z. (1973), 'Successfully treated Candida endophthalmitis in a child', *Pediatrics*, **51**, 1027.

Hayden, G., Lapp, C. and Loda, F. (1977), 'Arthritis caused by Monosporium apiospermum treated with intra-articular amphotericin B', *Am. J. Dis. Child.*, **131**, 927.

Hickie, J. B. and Walker, T. (1964), 'Cryptococcosis (torulosis): Some problems in diagnosis and management', *Aust. Ann. Med.*, **13**, 229.

Hildick-Smith, G., Blank, H. and Sarkany, I. (1964), *Fungus Diseases and Their Treatment*, J. and A. Churchill Ltd, p. 403.

Hoeprich, P. D. and Finn, P. D. (1972), 'Activity of combinations of antifungal agents against Candida albicans and Cryptococcus neoformans' (abstract). In *Proceedings of the 72nd Meeting of the American Society for Microbiology*, Washington, D.C., 1972, p. 135.

Hoeprich, P. D. and Huston, A. C. (1975), 'Susceptibility of Coccidioides immitis, Candida albicans and Cryptoccus neoformans to amphotericin B, flucytosine and clotrimazole', *J. Infect. Dis.*, **132**, 133.

Holt, J. E., Gray, J. E. and Lerner, W. L. (1972), 'Coccidioidal meningitis', *Ann. Intern. Med.*, **77**, 814.

Howarth, W. R., Tewari, R. P. and Solotorovsky, M. (1975), 'Comparative *in vitro* antifungal activity of amphotericin B and amphotericin B methyl ester', *Antimicrob. Ag. Chemother.*, **7**, 58.

Hsuchen, C. C. and Feingold, D. S. (1973), 'Selective membrane toxicity of the polyene antibiotics: Studies on natural membranes', *Antimicrob. Ag. Chemother.*, **4**, 316.

Huppert, M., Sun, S. H. and Vukovich, K. R. (1974), 'Combined amphotericin B—tetracycline therapy for experimental coccidioidomycosis', *Antimicrob. Ag. Chemother.*, **5**, 473.

Huppert, M., Pappagianis, D., Sun, S. H., Gleason-Jordan, I., Collins, M. S. and Vukovich, K. R. (1976), 'Effect of amphotericin B and rifampin against Coccidioides immitis *in vitro* and *in vivo*', *Antimicrob. Ag. Chemother.*, **9**, 406.

Huston, A. C. and Hoeprich, P. D. (1978), 'Comparative susceptibilities of four kinds of pathogenic fungi to amphotericin B and amphotericin B methyl ester', *Antimicrob. Ag. Chemother.*, **13**, 905.

Jagdis, F. A., Hoeprich, P. D., Lawrence, R. M. and Schaffner, C. P. (1977), 'Comparative pharmacology of amphotericin B and amphotericin B methyl ester in the non-human primate, Macaca mulatta', *Antimicrob. Ag. Chemother.*, **12**, 582.

Jones, B. R. (1975), 'Principles in the management of oculomycosis', *Trans. Am. Acad. Ophthalmol. Otolaryngol.*, **70**, OP-15.

Jordan, G. W. and Seet, E. C. (1978), 'Antiviral effects of amphotericin B methyl ester', *Antimicrob. Ag. Chemother.*, **13**, 199.

Keall, D. D., Wilkie, J. A. and Binns, C. (1968), 'Cryptococcosis: A survey of cases diagnosed in Western Australia with a report of two cases', *Med. J. Aust.*, **2**, 665.

Keim, G. R., Jr., Sibley, P. L., Yoon, Y. H., Kulesza, J. S., Zaidi, I. H., Miller, M. M. and Poutsiaka, J. W. (1976), 'Comparative toxicological studies of amphotericin B methyl ester and amphotericin B in mice, rats, and dogs', *Antimicrob. Ag. Chemother.*, **10**, 687.

Keller, M. A., Sellers, B. B., Jr., Melish, M. E., Kaplan, G. W., Miller, K. E. and Mendoza, S. A. (1977), 'Systemic candidiasis in infants. A case presentation and literature review', *Am. J. Dis. Child.*, **131**, 1260.

Kim, S. J., Kwon-Chung, K. W., Milne, G. W. A., Hill, W. B. and Patterson, G. (1975), 'Relationship between polyene resistance and sterol compositions in Cryptococcus neoformans', *Antimicrob. Ag. Chemother.*, **7**, 99.

Kinsky, S. C. (1970), 'Antibiotic interactions with model membranes', *Annual Rev. Pharmacol.*, **10**, 119, quoted by Kwan et al. (1972).

Kitahara, M., Seth, V. K., Medoff, G. and Kobayashi, G. S. (1976a), 'Activity of amphotericin B and rifampicin combined in treatment of murine histoplasmosis and blastomycosis', *J. Infect. Dis.*, **133**, 663.

Kitahara, M., Kobayashi, G. S. and Medoff, G. (1976b), 'Enhanced efficacy of amphotericin B and rifampicin combined in treatment of Murine Histoplasmosis and Blastomycosis', *J. Infect. Dis.*, **133**, 663.

Kobayashi, G. S., Medoff, G., Schlessinger, D., Kwan, C. N. and Musser, W. E. (1972), 'Amphotericin B potentiation of rifampicin as an antifungal agent against the yeast phase of Histoplasma capsulatum', *Science*, **177**, 709.

Kobayashi, G. S., Cheung, S. C., Schlessinger, D. and Medoff, G. (1974), 'Effects of rifampicin derivatives, alone and in combination with amphotericin B, against Histoplasma capsulatum', *Antimicrob. Ag. Chemother.*, **5**, 16.

Kotler-Brajtburg, J., Price, H. D., Medoff, G., Schlessinger, D. and Kobayashi, G. S. (1974), 'Molecular basis for the selective toxicity of amphotericin B for yeast and filipin for animal cells', *Antimicrob. Ag. Chemother.*, **5**, 377.

Kuo, D. (1962), 'A case of torulosis of the central nervous system during pregnancy', *Med. J. Aust.*, **1**, 558.

Kwan, C. N., Medoff, G., Kobayashi, S., Schlessinger, D. and Raskas, H. J. (1972), 'Protentiation of the antifungal effects of antibiotics by amphotericin B', *Antimicrob. Ag. Chemother.*, **2**, 61.

Lawrence, R. M. and Hoeprich, P. D. (1976), 'Comparison of amphotericin B and amphotericin B methyl ester: Efficacy in murine coccidioidomycosis and toxicity', *J. Infect. Dis.*, **133**, 168.

Le Clerc, M. and Giammona, S. T. (1975), 'Coccidioidal meningitis. The use of amphotericin B intravenously and intrathecally by repeated lumbar punctures', *West. J. Med.*, **122**, 251.

Lewis, J. L. and Rabinovich, S. (1972), 'The wide spectrum of cryptococcal infections', *Amer. J. Med.*, **53**, 315.

Littman, M. L. and Walter, J. E. (1968), 'Cryptococcosis: Current status', *Amer. J. Med.*, **45**, 922.

Lorber, B., Cutler, C. and Barry, W. E. (1976), 'Allergic rash due to amphotericin B', *Ann. Intern. Med.*, **84**, 54.

Lou, P., Kazdan, J., Bannatyne, R. M. and Cheung, R. (1977), 'Successful treatment of Candida endophthalmitis with a synergistic combination of amphotericin B and rifampin', *Am. J. Ophthalmol.*, **83**, 12.

Louria, D. B. (1958), 'Some aspects of the absorption, distribution, and excretion of amphotericin B in man', *Antibiotic Med. Clin. Ther.*, **5**, 295.

Lutwick, L. I., Galgiani, J. N., Johnson, R. H. and Stevens, D. A. (1976), 'Visceral fungal infections due to Petriellidium boydii (Allescheria boydii). *In vitro* drug sensitivity studies', *Amer. J. Med.*, **61**, 632.

McCurdy, D. K., Frederic, M. and Elkinton, J. R. (1968), 'Renal tubular acidosis due to amphotericin B', *New Engl. J. Med.*, **278**, 124.

Mechlinski, W. and Schaffner, C. P. (1972), 'Polyene macrolide derivatives. I. N-acylation and esterification reactions with amphotericin B', *J. Antibiot.* (Tokyo), **25**, 256.

Medoff, G., Comfort, M. and Kobayashi, G. S. (1971), 'Synergistic action of amphotericin B and 5-fluorocytosine against yeast-like organisms (35943)', *Proc. Soc. Exper. Biol. Med.*, **138**, 571.

Medoff, G., Kobayashi, G. S., Kwan, C. N., Schlessinger, D. and Venkov, P. (1972), 'Potentiation of rifampicin and 5-fluorocytosine as antifungal antibiotics by amphotericin B', *Proc. Natl. Acad. Sci. U.S.A.*, **69**, 196.

Medoff, G. and Kobayashi, G. S. (1975), 'Amphotericin B. Old drug, new therapy', *JAMA*, **232**, 619.

Meyers, B. R., Lieberman, T. W. and Ferry, A. P. (1973), "Candida endophthalmitis complicating candidemia", *Ann. Intern. Med.*, **79**, 647.

Meyer, R. D., Young, L. S., Armstrong, D. and Yu, B. (1973), "Aspergillosis complicating neoplastic disease", *Amer. J. Med.*, **54**, 6.

Montgomerie, J. Z., Edwards, J. E., Jr. and Guze, L. B. (1975), 'Synergism of amphotericin B and 5-fluorocytosine for Candida species', *J. Infect. Dis.*, **132**, 82.

Moškovskij, S. D. and Southgate, B. A. (1971), 'Clinical aspects of leishmaniasis with special reference to the USSR', *Bull. Wld. Hlth. Org.*, **44**, 491.

Murray, H. W., Fialk, M. A. and Roberts, R. B. (1976), 'Candida arthritis. A manifestation of disseminated candidiasis', *Amer. J. Med.*, **60**, 587.

Nagington, J. and Richards, J. E. (1976), 'Chemotherapeutic compounds and acanthamoebae from eye infections', *J. clin. Path.*, **29**, 648.

Nosanchuk, J. S. and Greenberg, R. D. (1973), 'Protothecosis of the olecranon bursa caused by achloric algae', *Am. J. Clin. Pathol.*, **59**, 567.

O'Donnell, J. M. (1962), 'A case of sporotrichosis', *Med. J. Aust.*, **1**, 517.

Olivero, J. J., Lozano-Mendez, J., Ghafary, E. M., Eknoyan, G. and Suki, W. N. (1975), 'Mitigation of amphotericin B nephrotoxicity by mannitol', *Brit. med. J.*, **1**, 550.

Parker, J. D., Doto, I. L. and Tosh, F. E. (1969), 'A decade of experience with blastomycosis and its treatment with amphotericin B', *Amer. Rev. Resp. Dis.*, **99**, 895.

Pennington, J. E., Block, E. R. and Reynolds, H. Y. (1974), '5-Fluorocytosine and amphotericin B in bronchial secretions', *Antimicrob. Ag. Chemother.*, **6**, 324.

Pennington, J. E. (1976), 'Successful treatment of Aspergillus pneumonia in hematologic neoplasia', *New Engl. J. Med.*, **295**, 426.

Philpot, C. R. and Lo, D. (1972), 'Cryptococcal meningitis in pregnancy', *Med. J. Aust.*, **2**, 1005.

Pittard, W. B., III, Thullen, J. D. and Fanaroff, A. A. (1976), 'Neonatal septic arthritis', *J. Pediatrics*, **88**, 621.

Poplack, D. G. and Jacobs, S. A. (1975), 'Candida arthritis treated with amphotericin B', *J. Pediatrics*, **87**, 989.

Posner, J. B. (1973), 'Editorial. Reservoirs for intraventricular chemotherapy', *New Engl. J. Med.*, **288**, 212.

Prout, G. R., Jr. and Goddard, A. R. (1960), 'Renal mucormycosis. Survival after nephrectomy and amphotericin B therapy', *New. Engl. J. Med.*, **263**, 1246.

Ravinovich, S., Shaw, B. D., Bryant, T. and Donta, S. T. (1974), 'Effect of 5-fluorocytosine and amphotericin B on Candida albicans infection in mice', *J. Infect. Dis.*, **130**, 28.

Richards, A. B., Jones, B. R., Whitwell, J. and Clayton, Y. M. (1969), 'Corneal and intra-ocular infection by Candida albicans treated with 5-fluorocytosine', *Trans. Ophthal. Soc. U.K.*, **29**, 867.

Rifkind, D., Crowder, E. D. and Hyland, R. N. (1974), '*In vitro* inhibition of Coccidioides immitis strains with amphotericin B plus rifampin', *Antimicrob. Ag. Chemother.*, **6**, 783.

Roe, D. C. and Haynes, R. E. (1972), 'Candida albicans meningitis successfully treated with amphotericin B', *Amer. J. Dis. Child.*, **124**, 926.

Rosch, J. M., Pazin, G. J. and Fireman, P. (1976), 'Reduction of amphotericin B nephrotoxicity with mannitol', *JAMA*, **235**, 1995.

Schacter, L. P., Owellen, R. J., Rathbun, H. K. and Buchanan, B. (1976), 'Antagonism between miconazole and amphotericin B', *Lancet*, **2**, 318.

Schröter, G. P. J., Temple, D. R., Husberg, B. S., Weil, R., III and Starzl, T. E. (1976), 'Cryptococcosis after renal transplantation: Report of ten cases', *Surgery*, **79**, 268.

Schuster, F. L., and Rechthand, E. (1975), '*In vitro* effects of amphotericin B on growth and ultrastructure of the amoeboflagellates Naegleria gruberi and Naegleria fowleri', *Antimicrob. Ag. Chemother.*, **8**, 591.

Seabury, J. H. and Dascomb, H. E. (1960), 'Experience with amphotericin B', *Ann. N.Y. Acad. Sci.*, **89**, 202.

Segal, E., Padhye, A. A. and Ajello, L. (1976), 'Susceptibility of Prototheca species to antifungal agents', *Anticrob. Ag. Chemother.*, **10**, 75.

Shadomy, S., Brummer, D. L. and Ingroff, A. V. (1972), 'Light sensitivity of prepared solutions of amphotericin B', *Amer. Rev. Resp. Dis.*, **107**, 303.

Shadomy, S., Wagner, G., Espinel-Ingroff, A. and Davis, B. A. (1975), '*In vitro* studies with combinations of 5-fluorocytosine and amphotericin B', *Antimicrob. Ag. Chemother.*, **8**, 117.

Singer, C., Armstrong, D., Jones, T. C. and Spiro, R. H. (1975), 'Imported mucocutaneous leishmaniasis in New York City. Report of a patient treated with amphotericin B', *Amer. J. Med.*, **59**, 444.

Smith, J. W. and Utz, J. P. (1972), 'Progressive disseminated histoplasmosis. A prospective study of 26 patients', *Ann. Intern. Med.*, **76**, 557.

Sorensen, L. J., McNally, E. G. and Sternberg, T. H. (1959), 'The development of strains of Candida albicans and Coccidioides immitis, which are resistant to amphotericin B', *Antibiot. Annual, 1958–59*, p. 920.

Stieritz, D. D., Law, E. J. and Holder, I. A. (1973), 'Speciation and amphotericin B sensitivity studies on blood isolates of Candida from burned patients', *J. clin. Path.*, **26**, 405.

Sutliff, W. D. (1972), 'Histoplasmosis cooperative study. V. Amphotericin B dosage for chronic pulmonary histoplasmosis', *Amer. Rev. Resp. Dis.*, **105**, 60.

Symmers, W. St. C., Sen. (1969), 'Primary amoebic meningoencephalitis in Britain', *Brit. med. J.*, **4**, 449.

Symmers, W. St. C., Sen. (1973), 'Amphotericin pharmacophobia', *Brit. med. J.*, **4**, 460.

Takacs, F. J., Tomkiewicz, Z. M. and Merrill, J. P. (1963), 'Amphotericin B nephrotoxicity with irreversible renal failure', *Ann. Intern. Med.*, **59**, 716.

Tärnvik, A. and Ånséhn, S. (1974), 'Effect of amphotericin B and clotrimazole on lymphocyte stimulation', *Antimicrob. Ag. Chemother.*, **6**, 529.

Thong, Y. H., Rowan-Kelly, B., Ferrante, A. and Shepherd, C. (1978), 'Synergism between tetracycline and amphotericin B in experimental amoebic meningoencephalitis', *Med. J. Aust.*, **1**, 663.

Titsworth, E. and Grunberg, E. (1973), 'Chemotherapeutic activity of 5-fluorocytosine and amphotericin B against Candida albicans in mice', *Antimicrob. Ag. Chemother.*, **4**, 306.

Tobias, J. S., Wrigley, P. F. M. and Shaw, E. (1976), 'Combination antifungal therapy for cryptococcal meningitis', *Postgrad. Med. J.*, **52**, 305.

Utz, J. P., Bennett, J. E., Brandriss, M. W., Butler, W. T. and Hill, G. J. (1964), 'Amphotericin B toxicity. Combined clinical staff conference at the National Institutes of Health', *Ann. Intern. Med.*, **61**, 334.

Utz, J. P., Treger, A., McCullough, N. B. and Emmons, C. W. (1959), 'Amphotericin B: Intravenous use in 21 patients with systemic fungal diseases', *Antibiot. Annual, 1958–59*, p. 628.

Utz, J. P., Garriques, I. L., Sande, M. A., Warner, J. F., Mandell, G. L., McGehee, R. F., Duma, R. J. and Shadomy, S. (1975), 'Therapy of cryptococcosis with a combination of flucytosine and amphotericin B', *J. Infect. Dis.*, **132**, 368.

Windom, R. E., Sanford, J. P., Pritchard, J. A., Abernathy, R. S. and Muchmore, H. G. (1961), 'The hemotoxicity of amphotericin B', *Clin. Res.*, **9**, 47; quoted by Hildick-Smith *et al.* (1964).

Wise, G. J., Wainstein, S., Goldberg, P. and Kozinn, P. J. (1973), 'Candidal cystitis. Management by continuous bladder irrigation with amphotericin B', *JAMA*, **224**, 1636.

Witorsch, P., Williams, T. W., Jr., Ommaya, A. K. and Utz, J. P. (1965), 'Intraventricular administration of amphotericin B. Use of subcutaneous reservoir in four patients with mycotic meningitis', *JAMA*, **194**, 699.

Woods, R. A., Bard, M., Jackson, I. E. and Drutz, D. J. (1974), 'Resistance to polyene antibiotics and correlated sterol changes in two isolates of Candida tropicalis from a patient with an amphotericin B-resistant funguria', *J. Infect. Dis.*, **129**, 53.

Yesudian, P. and Thambiah, A. S. (1974), 'Amphotericin B therapy in dermal leishmanoid', *Arch. Dermatol.*, **109**, 720.

5-Fluorocytosine (5-Flucytosine)

Description

5-Fluorocytosine or 5-flucytosine (5-FC; RO 2-9915) is a fluorinated pyrimidine, which was synthetized in 1957 at Roche Laboratories as a cytosine anti-metabolite for the treatment of leukaemia. The drug proved ineffective for this purpose as it had no cytotoxic activity. That this drug had selective antifungal activity was first demonstrated by Grunberg et al. (1964). Many studies have confirmed that 5-fluorocytosine is effective in the treatment of several human fungal infections. It is marketed with the trade names of 'Ancotil' and 'Ancobon' by Roche.

Sensitive Organisms

5-Fluorocytosine has a relatively narrow spectrum of antifungal activity. Varying results from *in vitro* susceptibility testing with this drug have been reported, because there are no universally accepted testing methods (Kitahara et al., 1976; Bennett, 1977).

1. *Pathogenic yeasts. In vitro* 5-fluorocytosine is active against Cryptococcus neoformans and the yeast-like fungus Candida albicans (Shadomy, 1969; Shadomy et al., 1973). Other Candida spp. such as C. krusei, C. tropicalis and C. parapsilosis are usually sensitive (Steer et al., 1972; Shadomy et al., 1973, Segal et al., 1975). Another less common pathogenic yeast, Torulopsis glabrata is generally susceptible to 5-fluorocytosine (Utz, 1972; Shadomy et al., 1973).

Published results on the prevalence of resistance of naturally occurring yeast to 5-fluorocytosine vary, but overall it is probably low. Cryptococcus neoformans strains, previously unexposed to the drug, are nearly always 5-fluorocytosine-sensitive (Shadomy, 1970). Natually-occurring resistant Candida albicans strains have been encountered frequently by some authors (Shadomy, 1970), but only rarely by others (Speller and Davies, 1973; Jones, 1975). Studies at the National Institutes of Health (USA) showed that 99 per cent of 93 pre-treatment isolates of Cryptococcus neoformans, and 88 per cent of 58 pre-treatment Candida isolates were sensitive to less than 5 μg per ml of 5-fluorocytosine (Bennett, 1977).

Serogroup B strains of Candida albicans, which are more frequently isolated in Africa, are more commonly resistant to 5-fluorocytosine (85 per cent) than serogroup A strains (<1 per cent) which are more common in Europe and appear to have a different cell wall ultrastructure (Montplaisir et al., 1976).

2. *Moulds or filamentous fungi.* Aspergillus spp. are occasionally sensitive to 5-fluorocytosine, but in general they are moderately or highly resistant

(Shadomy, 1969; Holt and Newman, 1973). Three of seven Aspergillus strains tested by Steer *et al.* (1972) had an MIC of 3·9 μg per ml or less, and the remainder an MIC greater than 100 μg per ml. The Cladosporium spp., especially Cladosporium trichoides, appear to be 5-fluorocytosine-sensitive (Block *et al.*, 1973), as are the Phialophora spp. (Vandevelde *et al.*, 1972), the causative agents of chromoblastomycosis. The Madurella spp. and all the dermatophytes such as the Microsporum, Trichophyton and Epidermophyton spp. are resistant.

3. *Dimorphic fungi, which cause deep mycoses.* Sporotrichum schenckii is usually completely resistant, but occasional moderately susceptible strains have been isolated (Vandevelde *et al.*, 1972). Blastomyces dermatitidis, Paracoccidioides brasiliensis, Histoplasma capsulatum and Coccidioides immitis are all 5-fluorocytosine-resistant (Shadomy, 1969).

4. *Actinomyces and Nocardia spp.* These bacteria, unlike some of the true fungi, are 5-fluorocytosine-resistant. The drug has no effect on any other bacteria.

5. *Synergism with other drugs.* 5-Fluorocytosine acts synergistically with amphotericin B against many strains of Candida spp., Cryptococcus neoformans and Aspergillus spp. (*see* page 867). Weak inhibitory concentrations of clotrimazole may enhance the action of 5-fluorocytosine against some Candida strains (*see* page 899).

6. *Acquired resistance.* Strains of Candida spp. and Cryptococcus neoformans resistant to 5-fluorocytosine can be readily induced *in vitro* by successvie culture in the presence of increasing concentrations of the drug (Shadomy, 1969; Holt and Newman, 1973). 5-Fluorocytosine-resistant Cryptococcus neoformans strains frequently arise *in vivo* during treatment with the drug. This was exemplified by 14 patients with cryptococcosis reported by Shadomy (1970). Ten of these received 5-fluorocytosine in a dose of 100 mg per kg per day, and among them there were six therapeutic failures associated with the emergence of resistant cryptococci. The remaining four patients were treated by 150 mg per kg per day, and resistant organisms developed in only one of these. Resistant strains of Candida albicans can also emerge during therapy with 5-fluorocytosine. Cartwright *et al.* (1972) used the drug in a dose of 10 g daily to treat a patient with urinary candidiasis. The initial Candida strain isolated was sensitive to 0·25 μg per ml of 5-fluorocytosine, but after the infection relapsed, a strain resistant to more than 1000 μg per ml was isolated.

Hoeprich *et al.* (1974) described a heroin addict with endocarditis due to Candida parapsilosis who after an initial favourable response to 5-fluorocytosine, relapsed after 37 days treatment. The strain isolated was sensitive prior to treatment (MIC 6·5 μg per ml) but resistant after the relapse (MIC >129 μg per ml).

Torulopsis glabrata strains resistant to 5-fluorocytosine can also emerge both *in vitro* and *in vivo* (Normark and Schönebeck, 1972).

In Vitro Sensitivities

Table 45 shows the minimum inhibitory concentrations of 5-fluorocytosine against some selected fungal species. Fungi with MIC's of 6·25 μg per ml or less can be regarded as highly sensitive to this drug. Resistant variants (MIC's greater than 1000 µg per ml) of all these fungi can occur if they have been previously exposed to the drug.

TABLE 45

Compiled from data published by Shadomy (1969), Steer et al. (1972) and Vandevelde et al. (1972)

ORGANISM	MIC (µg per ml)
Cryptococcus neoformans	0·46–3·9
Candida albicans	0·46–3·9
Torulopsis glabrata	0·32
Aspergillus spp.	0·48–500
Phialophora spp.	3·12–6·25

Mode of Administration and Dosage

1. *Oral administration.* 5-Fluorocytosine is usually administered by the oral route in a dose of 100 to 150 mg per kg per day, in four divided doses at intervals of six hours. To prevent the emergence of resistant strains during therapy, it has been suggested that the higher dose of 150 mg per kg be used in all cases (Utz, 1972). Doses as high as 200 mg per kg per day have been used without encountering toxic effects (Webb *et al.*, 1970). A commonly used adult dose is 8 g per day administered in four divided doses.

2. *Infants and young children.* No definite dosage recommendations are available for infants under the age of four weeks. Burnell (1971) treated an infant aged nine weeks who had systemic candidiasis with 5-fluorocytosine. An initial dose of 250 mg per kg per day was used for 19 days, and then a reduced dose of 180 mg per kg per day was continued for a further 10 days. No effects attributable to 5-fluorocytosine toxicity were noted.

3. *Patients with renal failure.* Such patients need a reduced dosage schedule, because the drug is excreted almost entirely by glomerular filtration (page 888). Toxic effects are likely to occur if a peak serum level of 100 µg per ml is exceeded. A simple method has been devised to calculate the dosage for patients with renal failure. The usual individual doses are used, but the normal six-hourly interval between doses is increased by multiplying it by the value of the serum creatinine in mg per cent. For example an adult with moderate renal failure (serum creatinine 4 mg per cent) would be given 2 g of 5-fluorocytosine once every 24 (6 × 4) h (Dawborn *et al.*, 1973). (For conversion of serum creatinine value from SI units to mg per cent, *see* page 333). This calculation is only an approximation, and where possible, serum level monitoring is advisable in patients with impaired renal function. A rapid (4 h) microbiological serum 5-fluorocytosine assay has been described (Schiavone *et al.*, 1973). In severe renal failure it may be advisable in addition to reduce the initial loading dose of 5-fluorocytosine and subsequent maintenance doses to avoid toxic serum levels (Dawborn *et al.*, 1973). The drug is removed from the body by haemodialysis, and its clearance rate is the same as that of creatinine. In patients treated by maintenance haemodialysis every 48–72 h, therapeutic non-toxic serum levels of 5-fluorocytosine can usually be maintained by administering single doses of

25 to 50 mg per kg body weight, after each dialysis (Block *et al.*, 1974).

4. *Patients with liver disease.* This drug should be used with caution in such patients, because it may aggravate pre-existing liver disease. If it is used it may be administered in the usually recommended doses because hepatic function does not influence serum levels of 5-fluorocytosine (Block, 1973).

5. *Intravenous administration.* An intravenous preparation of 5-fluorocytosine (a 1 per cent solution) has been used in clinical trials. The intravenous dose is similar to the oral dose, i.e. 150 mg per kg per day or 2 g 6-hourly for adults. Some investigators have infused a 2 g dose safely into adults over 15 min (Wade and Sudlow, 1972), whilst others have infused the same dose slowly over six hours.

6. *Intrathecal administration.* 5-Fluorocytosine has been used intrathecally on rare occasions to treat patients with torula meningitis, but the precise indications for this form of therapy are not clear. A 10 ml dose of the 1 per cent solution has been administered to adults twice a week without producing chemical meningitis or other side-effects (Roche, 1972).

7. *Topical administration to the eyes.* The drug can be used in eye-drops (1·5 per cent) which are non-irritating. This may be effective for corneal lesions but intraocular penetration is poor.

Availability

Tablets and capsules: 0·5 g.

Serum Levels in Relation to Dosage

5-Fluorocytosine is well absorbed following oral administration. After a standard initial oral dose of 2 g in an adult, a peak serum level of about 45 μg per ml is reached within 2–6 h (Fig. 37). The serum level gradually declines over the next 6 h but some drug is still detectable 24 h after the dose. In patients with normal renal function there is slight accumulation of the drug during the first four days of treatment, but thereafter mean or peak serum levels remain much the same, even if therapy is continued for months (Block and Bennett, 1972). Peak serum levels are reached in a shorter period of 1–2 h in patients who have already received the drug for several days (Block and Bennett, 1972).

The serum half-life of 5-fluorocytosine is 3–4 h. This is prolonged in patients with impaired renal function.

After an intravenous infusion of 2 g of 5-fluorocytosine over 15 min, levels similar to those after oral administration are obtained, but the peak level (about 50 μg per ml) is attained immediately after the infusion (Wade and Sudlow, 1972).

Excretion

URINE: Nearly all of an oral dose of 5-fluorocytosine (85–95 per cent) is excreted unchanged via the kidney by glomerular filtration (Koechlin *et al.*, 1966; Wade and Sudlow, 1972). Very high urine levels of the active drug (>1000 μg per ml) are attained in patients with normal renal function. In patients with impaired renal function urine concentrations are lower (Davies and Reeves, 1971).

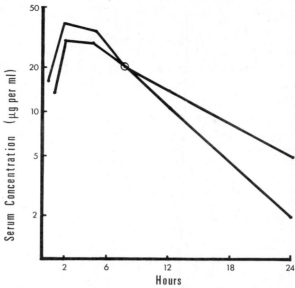

FIG. 37. Blood levels of 5-fluorocytosine in two patients after single oral doses of 2 g. (Redrawn after Koechlin *et al.*, 1966.)

INACTIVATION IN BODY: Earlier studies suggested that 5-fluorocytosine was not metabolized in the body (Koechlin *et al.*, 1966; Wade and Sudlow, 1972). Recently, using more sensitive tests, Diasio *et al.* (1978) showed that a small amount of the drug is converted to 5-fluorouracil (page 890) in the body and raised serum levels of this metabolite may account for the haematological toxicity associated with 5-fluorocytosine. Metabolic degradation may be more significant in patients with renal disease (*see* cephaloridine, page 206).

FAECES: Unabsorbed 5-fluorocytosine, usually less than 10 per cent, is excreted unchanged in the faeces (Koechlin *et al.*, 1966).

Distribution of the Drug in Body

5-Fluorocytosine is well distributed in body fluids and tissues. Tissue levels in liver, kidney, spleen, heart and lung are equal or greater than the serum levels at the time (Utz, 1972). The drug penetrates well into the CSF, at least in patients with torula meningitis. Cerebrospinal fluid 5-fluorocytosine levels, about half those of simultaneous blood levels, have been demonstrated in patients treated for fungal meningitis (Shadomy, 1970; Fass and Perkins, 1971; Block and Bennett, 1972). In eight patients with cryptococcal meningitis studied by Utz *et al.* (1975), concentrations of 5-fluorocytosine in the CSF were similar to their serum levels and exceeded the MIC of the patient's fungus with the exception of one patient. 5-Fluorocytosine penetrates well into infected exudates of peritoneum and joints (Bennett, 1977). In dogs it also penetrates well into bronchial secretions (Pennington *et al.*, 1974). In one human study, a level of 10 μg per ml of 5-fluorocytosine was found in the aqueous humour at a time when the blood level was 50 μg per ml (Richards *et al.*, 1969). Levels of 10 and 40 μg per ml have also been detected in the aqueous humour of patients receiving 5-fluorocytosine in an oral dose of 200 mg per kg per day (Jones, 1975).

Davies and Reeves (1971) estimated that 5-fluorocytosine is about 48 per cent serum protein bound, but most authors consider that it is not significantly bound to serum proteins (Wade and Sudlow, 1972; Block *et al.*, 1974).

Mode of Action

The precise mode of action of 5-fluorocytosine is not known. It appears that the drug enters the yeast cell via a permease system that recognizes several purines in addition to the natural analogue, cytosine. Inside the cell, 5-fluorocytosine is rapidly deaminated by an enzyme called cytosine deaminase to the anti-metabolite 5-fluorouracil (Polak and Scholer, 1973). In the normal cell, cytosine deaminase is also responsible for the metabolism of cytosine to uracil. 5-Fluorouracil is then incorporated instead of uracil into the fungal ribonucleic acid, the genetic code is misinterpreted and all growth stops. Cytosine deaminase is not present in mammalian cells, which explains the low toxicity of 5-fluorocytosine to humans. Cytosine arabinoside (page 940) appears to be a competitive inhibitor of 5-fluorocytosine (Bennett, 1974). Resistance of a strain of Candida parapsilosis which occurred during treatment with 5-fluorocytosine, appeared to result from a genetic block at cytosine deaminase (Hoeprich *et al.*, 1974).

Studies on Aspergillus spp. suggest that 5-fluorocytosine may exert its effect on fungi by another mechanism. It may be metabolized to fluorodeoxyuridine monophosphate, a strong inhibitor of thymidylate synthetase and thereby interfere with deoxyribonucleic acid synthesis (Wagner and Shadomy, 1976).

The synergistic effect of amphotericin B and 5-fluorocytosine against some fungi results from an action of amphotericin B on the plasma membrane (page 871), which allows the penetration of greater amounts of 5-fluorocytosine (Medoff *et al.*, 1971).

Toxicity

In contrast to amphotericin B (page 871), 5-fluorocytosine appears to be a drug of relatively low toxicity (Utz, 1972).

1. *Gastro-intestinal side-effects.* Nausea and diarrhoea may be caused by oral 5-fluorocytosine, but are uncommon. More severe symptoms may occur such as vomiting, abdominal pain and copious diarrhoea. In these cases procto-sigmoidoscopic findings are usually normal (Bennett, 1977). The findings in one fatal case resembled acute ulcerative colitis with multiple intestinal perforations and peritonitis (Robertson *et al.*, 1974).

2. *Hypersensitivity reactions.* Skin rashes have occasionally been observed.

3. *Haematological side-effects.* Many patients with serious fungal infections also have underlying haemopoietic disorders. In addition, 5-fluorocytosine is often administered in conjunction with other drugs such as amphotericin B, immunosuppressive agents and corticosteroids. For these reasons it has been difficult to assess possible effects of 5-fluorocytosine on the bone marrow. However, there are case reports indicating that occasionally 5-fluorocytosine *per se* can cause marrow toxicity. Meyer and Axelrod (1974) reported a fatal case of aplastic anaemia resulting from 5-fluorocytosine therapy. Record *et al.*

(1971) treated three cases of Candida endocarditis, two of whom died from bone marrow depression. Recent amphotericin B administration was probably responsible in one of these but in the other amphotericin B was discontinued three months prior to the onset of marrow depression, and therefore this complication was attributed to 5-fluorocytosine. Bryan and McFarland (1978) also described a patient who developed fatal bone marrow aplasia after a short course of 5-fluorocytosine, combined with amphotericin B for cryptococcal meningitis, but this patient also had multiple myeloma. Occasionally anaemia (Utz et al., 1969), neutropenia (Tassel and Madoff, 1968; Davies and Reeves, 1971), thrombocytopenia (Weese and Schope, 1972) and eosinophilia (Stanton and Sanderson, 1974) have been associated with 5-fluorocytosine therapy.

More recently Kauffman and Frame (1977) reported the occurrence of bone marrow toxicity in 4 of 15 patients with serious fungal infections treated with 5-fluorocytosine. Three of these patients had renal insufficiency and two received amphotericin B concomitantly. The maximum serum levels of 5-fluorocytosine preceding leucopenia in three patients was in the range $125-200\,\mu g$ per ml; leucopenia was readily reversed when the 5-fluorocytosine dosage and the subsequent serum levels were lowered. One patient with acute renal failure and prolonged high levels of 5-fluorocytosine (maximum 500 μg per ml) developed marrow aplasia and died of bacterial sepsis.

It now appears that bone marrow toxicity is more liable to occur with prolonged high serum levels ($100-150\,\mu g$ per ml) of 5-fluorocytosine. This is particularly likely if the patient has renal failure, or if amphotericin B is used concomitantly, a drug which frequently causes impairment of renal function (page 872). In the presence of renal failure, serum levels of 5-fluorocytosine should be monitored frequently (page 887). In rapidly progressive renal failure, very high levels of 5-fluorocytosine can occur and persist despite cessation of the drug. In this situation dialysis is recommended to remove accumulated drug (Kauffman and Frame, 1977). Regular blood examinations should be performed on all patients receiving 5-fluorocytosine.

4. *Hepatotoxicity.* Transient liver enlargement with associated elevation of serum aspartate aminotransferase (SGOT) levels has been noted in a few patients (Steer et al., 1972). Extensive liver cell necrosis together with fatal bone marrow depression has been reported in two patients (Record et al., 1971), but this appears to be very rare. It is probably advisable to monitor liver function tests regularly in patients receiving this drug. 5-Fluorocytosine is not contraindicated in patients with pre-existing liver disease (*see* page 888). Both hepatotoxicity and haemopoietic toxicity are probably dose related and more likely to occur when high serum levels ($>100\,\mu g$ per ml) are attained.

5. *Nephrotoxicity.* This has not been ascribed to 5-fluorocytosine therapy, and the drug apparently can be used safely in patients with pre-existing uraemia, provided appropriate dosage adjustments are made (page 887).

6. *Effect on fetus.* Philpot and Lo (1972) treated a woman in early pregnancy with 5-fluorocytosine without apparent ill-effect to the fetus. Similar experience has been recorded by Schönebeck and Segerbrand (1973), who used the drug successfully for the treatment of Candida fungaemia in a woman during the fourth month of pregnancy. However the safety of 5-fluorocytosine during pregnancy, especially the first trimester, has not been established. The drug is teratogenic in rats.

Clinical Uses of the Drug

1. *Cryptococcosis*. Many reports have confirmed the efficacy of 5-fluorocytosine in disseminated cryptococcal infections, particularly torula meningitis (Tassell and Madoff, 1968; Watkins *et al.*, 1969; Utz *et al.*, 1969; Fass and Perkins, 1971; Vandevelde *et al.*, 1972). It has also been used to cure a case of lymphonodular cryptococcosis; the patient was a five-year-old boy who presented with fever and painful enlargement of cervical lymph nodes and could not tolerate treatment with amphotericin B (Tolentino and Borrone, 1976). However 5-fluorocytosine has the disadvantage that resistant strains of Cryptococcus neoformans may emerge during treatment (Shadomy *et al.*, 1969). This is less likely to occur if higher doses of the drug (150 mg per kg per day) are used (Shadomy, 1970). Because of this possibility, the sensitivity of C. neoformans should be determined before therapy, and again if isolated during or after therapy (Utz, 1972).

Nowadays therapy with 5-fluorocytosine alone as initial therapy is not recommended; the possible development of secondary drug resistance may cause therapeutic failure and such resistant isolates do not show synergism with amphotericin B (page 867), negating the value of combination therapy (Bennett, 1977). Studies to date indicate that a combination of 5-fluorocytosine and amphotericin B is safe and efficacious for the treatment of disseminated cryptococcosis (*see* page 874). Secondary drug resistance has been very uncommon with this regimen, and it is possible that results of treatment may prove superior to single drug treatment because of the combination's synergistic effect. In addition, if these drugs are used in combination, amphotericin B can be used in a reduced dosage of 0·3 to 0·5 mg per kg body weight per day, resulting in less amphotericin B toxicity. Frequent adjustments to the dosage of 5-fluorocytosine are necessary if renal function is impaired due to amphotericin B, and in this way bone marrow and liver toxicity of 5-fluorocytosine may be reduced (*vide supra*).

2. *Candida infections*. 5-Fluorocytosine has been used as a single drug to treat systemic Candida infections. These infections usually occur in patients with severe underlying diseases, nevertheless some success has been obtained with 5-fluorocytosine treatment (Vandevelde *et al.*, 1972). Candida pyelonephritis has been eradicated in some instances, but in most patients it is difficult to treat because of the associated advanced abnormalities of the kidneys and urinary tract (Davies and Reeves, 1971; Steer *et al.*, 1972). Oral 5-fluorocytosine may be preferable to amphotericin B given either intravenously or by bladder wash out for the treatment of urinary candidiasis in children. Lines (1976) successfully treated two such children who developed this infection secondary to neurological bladder disease. The treatment of Candida endocarditis is also often unsuccessful. Record *et al.* (1971) treated three patients with 5-fluorocytosine; one of these, whose endocarditis was associated with aortic sclerosis, survived, but the other two, who had infections on prosthetic valves, died.

5-Fluorocytosine has been used alone to cure Candida fungaemia (Eilard *et al.*, 1974; Firkin, 1974), including fungaemia in an infant aged nine weeks (Burnell, 1971), Candida pulmonary mycetoma (Bartley 1973; Firkin, 1974), Candida thyroiditis (Robinson *et al.*, 1975) and Candida meningoencephalitis

(Nordström *et al.*, 1977). Treatment with this drug has also been successful in Candida albicans endophthalmitis (Robertson *et al.*, 1974; Harder and Hermans, 1975). Jones (1975) considers that 5-fluorocytosine (200 mg per kg weight per day and 1·5 per cent aqueous drops topically to the eye hourly) is the treatment of choice for intraocular and deep corneal infection due to Candida spp., provided that the fungus is sensitive. Nevertheless amphotericin B should probably be used in combination with 5-fluorocytosine for this infection (*see* page 877). 5-Fluorocytosine has also been reported to be effective in Candida albicans arthritis (Lindström and Lindholm, 1973), Candida parapsilosis arthritis (Imbeau *et al.*, 1977), and Candida osteomyelitis (Firkin, 1974; Edwards *et al.*, 1975), although the latter may heal without treatment. Candida peritonitis in a patient receiving haemodialysis, resolved after treatment with oral 5-fluorocytosine (Phillips *et al.*, 1973). Another patient with end-stage renal failure managed by peritoneal dialysis and who also developed Candida peritonitis was effectively managed by a continuous five-day peritoneal lavage containing 50 μg per ml of 5-fluorocytosine (Holdsworth *et al.*, 1975). When this drug is used for the treatment of systemic Candida infections, the sensitivity of the strain should be tested both before and during treatment, as in the case of cryptococcosis (Shadomy *et al.*, 1973).

Bennett (1977) has pointed out the difficulty in determining from such anecdotal case reports whether 5-fluorocytosine is of value in any of these Candida infections. He suggests that until its use is assessed by controlled trials, it should be reserved for Candida fungaemia or urinary tract infections which meet the following criteria; renal function is stable and not severely impaired, leucopenia and thrombocytopenia are absent, the Candida isolate can be promptly tested for susceptibility, and the infection is not immediately life-threatening.

Because the combination of amphotericin B and 5-fluorocytosine may show *in vitro* synergism (page 886), this combination has been used with apparent success to treat human Candida infections (*see* page 875). Until the situation becomes clearer, it seems reasonable to add 5-fluorocytosine whenever intravenous amphotericin B therapy is indicated (page 874), provided that the strain is not highly resistant to 5-fluorocytosine, when synergism is unlikely.

Superficial Candida infections should not be treated by topical 5-fluorocytosine, because the use of preparations such as vaginal tablets would encourage the emergence of resistant strains. Other satisfactory topical preparations such as nystatin (page 925) and amphotericin B (page 877) are available for this purpose.

3. *Torulopsis glabrata infections.* Systemic infections due to this less common human pathogen may respond to treatment with 5-fluorocytosine. Partial recovery was obtained when this drug was used to treat an adult suffering from Torulopsis glabrata meningitis (Wurzel *et al.*, 1972), and it has been used successfully in a dose of 200 mg per kg per day for ten days to treat a patient with Torulopsis glabrata fungaemia (Webb *et al.*, 1970). Torulopsis pyelonephritis similar to that due to Candida spp. (*vide supra*) is usually difficult to treat (Steer *et al.*, 1972), but some successes have been reported (Speller, 1974). Torulopsis glabrata strains resistant to 5-fluorocytosine may emerge (page 886), and sensitivity testing of this pathogen is important (Shadomy *et al.*, 1973).

4. *Chromoblastomycosis.* This disease caused by organisms of the Phialophora group has been successfully treated by 5-fluorocytosine. Vandevelde *et al.* (1972) found a 90-day course of 5-fluorocytosine to be effective in two patients with long-standing disease, in whom amphotericin B therapy had failed. This drug is the only one known to exert a beneficial effect in this infection (Bennett, 1977). Lopes *et al.* (1978) also showed that chromoblastomycosis due to Fonsecaea pedrosoi responded to 5-fluorocytosine but the fungus sometimes became resistant. They used a combination of 5-fluorocytosine with intravenous amphotericin B to cure a few patients and consider that this is the treatment of choice.

5. *Cladosporiosis.* Until the advent of 5-fluorocytosine, no effective chemotherapy was available for this condition (Emmons *et al.*, 1970). 5-Fluorocytosine is effective for the treatment of experimental Cladosporium trichoides infection in mice and may be the first useful drug available for the treatment of this disease in humans (Block *et al.*, 1973).

6. *Aspergillosis.* Aspergillus spp. are often relatively resistant to 5-fluorocytosine. In initial clinical trials with 5-fluorocytosine only a few patients with aspergillosis were treated and the results were inconclusive (Steer *et al.*, 1972; Vandevelde *et al.*, 1972). More encouraging results have been reported by Atkinson and Israel (1973), who treated twelve patients with pulmonary aspergillosis and one with aspergillus meningitis. Several of these patients including the one with meningitis, had a satisfactory response to 5-fluorocytosine. However it was noted that drug resistance, with resultant relapse of the infection, was a problem in those patients who had a pre-existing chronic lung disease. It was suggested that combined amphotericin B and 5-fluorocytosine therapy may prevent the development of resistance to 5-fluorocytosine in such patients. This combination is also advocated for the treatment of Aspergillus spp. endocarditis, which may develop in patients after cardiac surgery (Kammer and Utz, 1974). (*See also* page 876).

REFERENCES

Atkinson, G. W. and Israel, H. L. (1973), '5-Fluorocytosine treatment of meningeal and pulmonary aspergillosis', *Amer. J. Med.,* **55,** 496.

Bartley, P. C. (1973), 'Pulmonary candidiasis treated with 5-fluorocytosine', *Aust. N.Z. J. Med.,* **3,** 189.

Bennett, J. E. (1974), 'Chemotherapy of systemic mycoses (second of two parts)', *New Engl. J. Med.,* **290,** 320.

Bennett, J. E. (1977), 'Flucytosine', *Ann. Intern. Med.,* **86,** 319.

Block, E. R. and Bennett, J. E. (1972), 'Pharmacological studies with 5-fluorocytosine', *Antimicrob. Ag. Chemother.,* **1,** 476.

Block, E. R., Jennings, A. E. and Bennett, J. E. (1973), 'Experimental therapy of cladosporiosis and sporotrichosis with 5-fluorocytosine', *Antimicrob. Ag. Chemother.,* **3,** 95.

Block, E. R. (1973), 'Effect of hepatic insufficiency on 5-fluorocytosine concentrations in serum', *Antimicrob. Ag. Chemother.,* **3,** 141.

Block, E. R., Bennett, J. E., Livoti, L. G., Klein, W. J., Jr., MacGregor, R. R. and Henderson, L. (1974), 'Flucytosine and amphotericin B: Hemodialysis effects on the plasma concentration and clearance. Studies in man', *Ann. Intern. Med.,* **80,** 613.

Bryan, C. S. and McFarland, J. A. (1978), 'Cryptococcal meningitis. Fatal marrow aplasia from combined therapy', *JAMA*, **239**, 1068.

Burnell, R. H. (1971), 'Systemic candidiasis in an infant treated with 5-fluorocytosine', *Med. J. Aust.*, **2**, 859.

Cartwright, R. Y., Shaldon, C. and Hall, G. H. (1972), 'Urinary candidiasis after renal transplantation', *Brit. med. J.*, **2**, 351.

Davies, R. R. and Reeves, D. S. (1971), '5-Fluorocytosine and urinary candidiasis', *Brit. med. J.*, **1**, 577.

Dawborn, J. K., Page, M. D. and Schiavone, D. J. (1973), 'Use of 5-fluorocytosine in patients with impaired renal function', *Brit. med. J.*, **4**, 382.

Diasio, R. B., Lakings, D. E. and Bennett, J. E. (1978) 'Evidence for conversion of 5-fluorocytosine to 5-fluorouracil in humans: Possible factor in 5-fluorocytosine clinical toxicity', *Antimicrob. Ag. Chemother.*, **14**, 903.

Edwards, J. E., Jr., Turkel, S. B., Elder, H. A., Rand, R. W. and Guze, L. B. (1975), 'Hematogenous Candida osteomyelitis. Report of three cases and review of the literature', *Amer. J. Med.*, **59**, 89.

Eilard, T., Alestig, K., and Wahlén, P. (1974), 'Treatment of disseminated candidiasis with 5-fluorocytosine', *J. Infect. Dis.*, **130**, 155.

Emmons, C. W., Binford, C. H. and Utz, J. P. (1970), *Medical Mycology*, Lea & Febiger, Philadelphia, p. 426.

Fass, R. J. and Perkins, R. L. (1971), '5-Fluorocytosine in the treatment of Cryptococcal and Candida mycoses', *Ann. Intern. Med.*, **74**, 535.

Firkin, F. C. (1974), 'Therapy of deep-seated fungal infections with 5-fluorocytosine', *Aust. N.Z. J. Med.*, **4**, 462.

Grunberg, E., Titsworth, E. and Bennett, M. (1964), 'Chemotherapeutic activity of 5-fluorocytosine', *Antimicrob. Ag. Chemother.*—1963, p. 556; quoted by Holt and Newman (1973).

Harder, E. J. and Hermans, P. E. (1975), 'Treatment of fungal infections with flucytosine', *Arch. Intern. Med.*, **135**, 231.

Hoeprich, P. D., Ingraham, J., Kleker, E. and Winship, M. J. (1974), 'Development of resistance to 5-fluorocytosine in Candida parapsilosis during therapy', *J. Infect. Dis.*, **130**, 112.

Holdsworth, S. R., Atkins, R. C., Scott, D. F. and Jackson, R. (1975), 'Management of Candida peritonitis by prolonged peritoneal lavage containing 5-fluorocytosine', *Clinical Nephrology*, **4**, 157.

Holt, R. J. and Newman, R. L. (1973), 'The antimycotic activity of 5-fluorocytosine', *J. clin. Path.*, **26**, 167.

Imbeau, S. A., Hanson, J., Langejans, G. and D'Alessio, D. (1977), 'Flucytosine treatment of Candida arthritis', *JAMA*, **238**, 1395.

Jones, B. R. (1975), 'Principles in the management of oculomycosis', *Trans. Am. Acad. Ophthalmol. Otolaryngol.*, **70**, OP-15.

Kammer, R. B. and Utz, J. P. (1974), 'Aspergillus species endocarditis. The new face of a not so rare disease', *Amer. J. Med.*, **56**, 506.

Kauffman, C. A. and Frame, P. T. (1977), 'Bone marrow toxicity associated with 5-fluorocytosine therapy', *Antimicrob. Ag. Chemother.*, **11**, 244.

Kitahara, M., Seth, V. K., Medoff, G. and Kobayashi, G. S. (1976), 'Antimicrobial susceptibility testing of six clinical isolates of Aspergillus', *Antimicrob. Ag. Chemother.*, **9**, 908.

Koechlin, B. A., Rubio, F., Palmer, S., Gabriel, T. and Duschinsky, R. (1966), 'The metabolism of 5-fluorocytosine-2^{14}C and of cytosine-^{14}C in the rat and the disposition of 5-fluorocytosine-2^{14}C in man', *Biochemical Pharmacology*, **15**, 435.

Lindström, F. D. and Lindholm, T. (1973), 'Candida albicans arthritis treated with flucytosine', *Ann. Intern. Med.*, **79**, 131.

Lines, D. (1976), 'Childhood urinary candidiasis successfully treated with 5-fluorocytosine', *Aust. paediat. J.*, **12**, 49.

Lopes, C. F., Resende, M. A., Alvarenga, R. J., Moreira, Y. K. and Ferreira, I. (1978), '5-Fluorocytosine in the treatment of chromomycosis'. In Siegenthaler, W. and Lüthy, R. (Ed.), *Current Chemotherapy: Proceedings of the 10th International Congress of Chemotherapy,* Zurich/Switzerland, 1977. American Society for Microbiology, Washington, D.C., p. 219.

Medoff, G., Comfort, M. and Kobayashi, G. S. (1971), 'Synergistic action of amphotericin B and 5-fluorocytosine against yeast-like organisms', *Proc. Soc. Exper. Biol. Med.,* **138,** 571.

Meyer, R. and Axelrod, J. L. (1974), 'Fatal aplastic anaemia resulting from flucytosine', *JAMA,* **228,** 1573.

Montplaisir, S., Nabarra, B. and Drouhet, E. (1976), 'Susceptibility and resistance of Candida to 5-fluorocytosine in relation to the cell wall ultrastructure', *Antimicrob. Ag. Chemother.,* **9,** 1028.

Nordström, L., Öistämo, S. and Ölmebring, F. (1977), 'Candida meningoencephalitis treated with 5-fluorocytosine', *Scand. J. Infect. Dis.,* **9,** 63.

Normark, S. and Schönebeck, J. (1972), '*In vitro* studies of 5-fluorocytosine resistance in Candida albicans and Torulopsis glabrata', *Antimicrob. Ag. Chemother.,* **2,** 114.

Pennington, J. E., Block, E. R. and Reynolds, H. Y. (1974), '5-Fluorocytosine and amphotericin B in bronchial secretions', *Antimicrob. Ag. Chemother.,* **6,** 324.

Phillips, I., Eykyn, S., MacGregor, G. A. and Jones, N. F. (1973), 'Candida peritonitis treated with 5-fluorocytosine in a patient receiving hemodialysis', *Clinical Nephrology,* **1,** 271.

Philpot, C. R. and Lo, D. (1972), 'Cryptococcal meningitis in pregnancy', *Med. J. Aust.,* **2,** 1005.

Polak, A. and Scholer, H. J. (1973), 'Fungistatic activity, uptake and incorporation of 5-fluorocytosine in Candida albicans as influenced by pyrimidines and purines. II Studies on distribution and incorporation', *Pathol. Microbiol.,* **39,** 334.

Record, C. O., Skinner, J. M., Sleight, P. and Speller, D. C. E. (1971), 'Candida endocarditis treated with 5-fluorocytosine', *Brit. med. J.,* **1,** 262.

Richards, A. B., Jones, B. R., Whitwell, J. and Clayton, Y. M. (1969), 'Corneal and intra-ocular infection by Candida albicans treated with 5-fluorocytosine', *Trans. Ophthal. Soc. U.K.,* **29,** 867.

Robertson, D. M., Riley, F. C. and Hermans, P. E. (1974), 'Endogenous Candida oculomycosis. Report of two patients treated with flucytosine', *Arch. Ophthalmol.,* **91,** 33.

Robinson, M. F., Forgan-Smith, W. R. and Craswell, P. W. (1975), 'Candida thyroiditis- treated with 5-fluorocytosine', *Aust. N.N. J. Med.,* **5,** 472.

Roche, (1972), 'Data sheet on 5-fluorocytosine', Roche Research Department.

Schiavone, D. J., Page, M. D. and Dawborn, J. K. (1973), 'Rapid microbiological assay for 5-fluorocytosine', *Brit. med. J.,* **4,** 380.

Schönebeck, J. and Segerbrand, E. (1973), 'Candida albicans septicaemia during first half of pregnancy successfully treated with 5-fluorocytosine', *Brit. med. J.,* **4,** 337.

Segal, E., Romano, A., Eylan, E. and Stein, R. (1975), 'Experimental and clinical studies of 5-fluorocytosine activity in Candida ocular infections', *Chemotherapy,* **21,** 358.

Shadomy, S. (1969), '*In vitro* studies with 5-fluorocytosine', *Appl. Microbiol,* **17,** 871.

Shadomy, S. (1970), 'Further *in vitro* studies with 5-fluorocytosine', *Infect. Immunity,* **2,** 484.

Shadomy, S., Shadomy, H. J., McCay, J. A. and Utz, J. P. (1969), '*In vitro* susceptibility of Cryptococcus neoformans to amphotericin B, hamycin, and 5-fluorocytosine', *Antimicrob. Ag. Chemother.*—1968, p. 452.

Shadomy, S., Kirchoff, C. B. and Ingroff, A. E. (1973), '*In vitro* activity of 5-fluorocytosine against Candida and Torulopsis species', *Antimicrob. Ag. Chemother.,* **3,** 9.

Speller, D. C. E. and Davies, M. G. (1973), 'Sensitivity of yeasts to 5-fluorocytosine', *J. Med. Microbiol.*, **6**, 315.

Speller, D. C. E. (1974), 'Torulopsis glabrata urinary tract infection treated with 5-fluorocytosine', *J. clin. Path.*, **27**, 50.

Stanton, K. G. and Sanderson, C. R. (1974), 'The treatment of systemic cryptococcosis with 5-fluorocytosine', *Aust. N.Z. J. Med.*, **4**, 262.

Steer, P. L., Marks, M. I., Klite, P. D. and Eickhoff, T. C. (1972), '5-Fluorocytosine: An oral antifungal compound. A report on clinical and laboratory experience', *Ann. Intern. Med.*, **76**, 15.

Tassel, D. and Madoff, M. A. (1968), 'Treatment of Candida sepsis and Cryptococcus meningitis with 5-fluorocytosine., *JAMA*, **206**, 830.

Tolentino, P. and Borrone, C. (1976), 'Multiple lymphonodular cryptococcosis cured by 5-fluorocytosine', *Scand. J. Infect. Dis.*, **8**, 61.

Utz, J. P., Tynes, B. S., Shadomy, H. J., Duma, R. J., Kannan, M. M. and Mason, K. N. (1969), '5-Fluorocytosine in human cryptococcosis', *Antimicrob. Ag. Chemother.*—1968, p. 344.

Utz, J. P. (1972), 'Editorial. Flucytosine', *New Engl. J. Med.*, **286**, 777.

Utz, J. P., Garriques, I. L., Sande, M. A., Warner, J. F., Mandell, G. L., McGehee, R. F., Duma, R. J. and Shadomy, S. (1975), 'Therapy of cryptococcosis with a combination of flucytosine and amphotericin B', *J. Infect. Dis.*, **132**, 368.

Wade, D. N. and Sudlow, G. (1972), 'The kinetics of 5-fluorocytosine elimination in man', *Aust. N.Z. J. Med.*, **2**, 153.

Vandevelde, A. G., Mauceri, A. A. and Johnson, J. E., III (1972), '5-Fluorocytosine in the treatment of mycotic infections', *Ann. Intern. Med.*, **77**, 43.

Wagner, G. and Shadomy, S. (1976), 'Mode of action of flucytosine in Aspergillus species', *Chemotherapy* (Ed. Williams, J. D. and Geddes, A. M.), **3**, 211.

Watkins, J. S., Campbell, M. J., Gardner-Medwin, D., Ingham, H. R. and Murray, I. G. (1969), 'Two cases of cryptococcal meningitis, one treated with 5-fluorocytosine', *Brit. med. J.*, **3**, 29.

Webb, A. J., Speller, D. C. E. and Buckler, K. G. (1970), 'Torulopsis glabrata septicaemia treated with 5-fluorocytosine', *Lancet*, **1**, 839.

Weese, W. C. and Schope, R. W. (1972), '5-Fluorocytosine therapy', *Ann. Intern. Med.*, **77**, 1003.

Wurzel, B., Goldberg, P., Caroline, L., Bozza, A. T. and Kozinn, P. J. (1972), 'Torulopsis glabrata meningo-encephalitis treated with 5-flucytosine', *Ann. Intern. Med.*, **77**, 814.

Clotrimazole

Description

Clotrimazole (BAY b 5097) is an imidazole derivative (bis-phenyl-2-chlorophenyl-1-imidazolyl-methane) which was synthetized in the Bayer Research Laboratories in Germany in 1967 (Plempel *et al.*, 1969). Because it causes severe gastro-intestinal side-effects and results of its clinical use are inconsistent, oral treatment with clotrimazole has a very limited, if any, place for the treatment of systemic fungal infections. However the drug is valuable for the treatment of superficial fungal infections. It is marketed with the trade name of 'Canesten' (Bayer).

Sensitive Organisms

Clotrimazole has a wide range of antimycotic activity, most fungi pathogenic to man being susceptible (Plempel *et al.*, 1969; Shadomy, 1971; Waitz *et al.*, 1971; Holt and Newman, 1972b; Burgess and Bodey, 1972). Its activity against some of these (Coccidioides immitis, Candida albicans, Cryptococcus neoformans) is much greater than that of amphotericin B (page 865) or of 5-fluorocytosine (page 885) (Hoeprich and Huston, 1975). Clotrimazole is also active against Trichomonas vaginalis.

 1. *Moulds or filamentous fungi.* The dermatophytes or ringworm fungi such as the Microsporum, Trichophyton and Epidermophyton spp. which cause superficial infections are highly susceptible. The moulds which cause bronchopulmonary infections, such as the Aspergillus, Penicillium and Mucor spp. are also sensitive. Filamentous fungi of the Cladosporium and Phialophora spp., the latter causing chromoblastomycosis, are susceptible but the Madurella spp. (causative agents of mycetoma or Madura foot) are clotrimazole-resistant.

 2. *Pathogenic yeasts.* Cryptococcus neoformans (Torula histolytica) is usually sensitive.

 3. *Pathogenic yeast-like fungi.* Candida albicans (Monilia albicans), other Candida spp. such as Candida tropicalis and the less common human pathogen, Torulopsis glabrata, are all susceptible (Burgess and Bodey, 1972).

 4. *Dimorphic fungi, which cause deep infections.* Sporotrichum schenckii (causative agent of sporotrichosis), Blastomyces dermatitidis (causative agent of North American blastomycosis), Paracoccidioides brasiliensis (causative agent of South American blastomycosis), Histoplasma capsulatum and Coccidioides immitis are all clotrimazole-sensitive.

 5. *Nocardia spp.* Compared to the true fungi, this genus is considerably less sensitive to clotrimazole. The drug has also only limited activity against other

898

bacteria (Holt and Newman, 1972b).

6. *Naegleria*. The amoeboflagellate Naegleria fowleri which causes primary amoebic meningoencephalitis (page 877) is sensitive to clotrimazole *in vitro* (Jamieson and Anderson, 1974), but it is ineffective in protecting mice against the infection (Jamieson, 1975). Amphotericin B (page 877) is still the preferred drug for treatment of N. fowleri infections.

7. *Synergy with other drugs*. *In vitro* studies indicate that weak or partially inhibitory concentrations of clotrimazole can enhance the antifungal activity of both amphotericin B (page 867) and 5-fluorocytosine (page 886) against some strains of Candida albicans and Candida tropicalis (Beggs *et al.*, 1976).

8. *Acquired resistance*. It has been difficult to induce clotrimazole-resistant strains of Candida and Aspergillus spp. *in vitro*. Waitz *et al.* (1971) were able to produce clotrimazole-resistant Candida strains *in vitro* using prolonged incubation times, but normal sensitivity reappeared on subculture in drug-free media. It is not known whether resistant strains of other fungi may emerge more readily. The emergence of resistant strains of sensitive fungi during treatment has not been observed (Holt and Newman, 1972, a and b).

In Vitro Sensitivities

The minimum inhibitory concentrations of clotrimazole against various pathogenic fungal species are shown in Table 46. Most fungi are inhibited by a concentration of $1 \cdot 0 \, \mu$g per ml.

TABLE 46

(Condensed from Plempel *et al.*, 1969)

ORGANISM	MIC (μg per ml)
Trichophyton spp.	$1 \cdot 0$
Epidermophyton spp.	$< 1 \cdot 0$
Microsporum spp.	$1 \cdot 0$
Aspergillus spp.	$1 \cdot 0$
Madurella spp.	$> 20 \cdot 0$
Cryptococcus neoformans	$1 \cdot 0 – 4 \cdot 0$
Candida albicans	$1 \cdot 0$
Sporotrichum schenckii	$1 \cdot 0$
Paracoccidioides brasiliensis	$1 \cdot 0$
Histoplasma capsulatum	$1 \cdot 0$
Coccidioides immitis	$1 \cdot 0$
Nocardia spp.	$4 \cdot 0 – 10 \cdot 0$

Mode of Administration and Dosage

1. For systemic chemotherapy clotrimazole can only be administered orally. The drug is poorly soluble in water and parenteral administration is not feasible.

2. In clinical trials it has been used in a dosage ranging from 60 mg per kg body weight per day (Oberste-Lehn *et al.*, 1969) to 200 mg per kg per day (Marget and Adam, 1971). It appears that a dose of about 100 mg per kg per day, administered in two to four divided doses, is suitable for most purposes.

The dose for an average adult (weight 60 kg) is 6 g daily, given as 3 g 12-hourly or 1·5 g every 6 h. Doses higher than this are often not tolerated in adults.

Dosage regimens used in children have varied from 60–120 mg per kg body weight per day. The drug has been used on a long-term intermittent basis in one three-year-old child to obviate side-effects (Ipp *et al.*, 1977) (*see* page 903).

3. There are no dosage recommendations for patients with either renal or liver disease or for newborn infants. As urinary excretion of active clotrimazole is very low (Burgess and Bodey, 1972), the usual doses may well be safe in patients with renal failure.

4. Clotrimazole is suitable for topical chemotherapy. It is used as a one per cent cream for the treatment of superficial fungal infections, and as vaginal tablets for the treatment of vaginal candidiasis.

Availability

1. 0·5 g tablets for oral administration.
2. 100 mg vaginal tablets.
3. 1 per cent cream for topical use.

Serum Levels in Relation to Dosage

Clotrimazole is poorly absorbed after oral administration. After a 3 g dose in adults, a mean peak concentration of 1·29 μg per ml is attained after 2 h, and the serum level is still 0·78 μg per ml 6 h after administration (*see* Fig. 38).

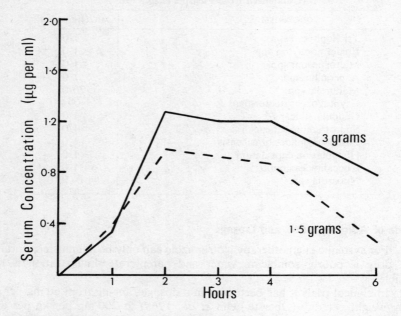

FIG. 38. Mean clotrimazole concentrations in serum after the administration of 1·5 and 3 g of the drug to eight adults. (Redrawn after Burgess and Bodey, 1972.)

Continued administration of the drug over several days results in a progressive decline in serum concentrations (Burgess and Bodey, 1972; Weuta, 1974). This is apparently because clotrimazole is a potent inducer of hepatic microsomal enzymes, resulting in accelerating metabolism of the drug with increasing duration of therapy (Burgess and Bodey, 1972; Bennett, 1974).

Much higher clotrimazole serum levels were reported by Plempel et al. (1969) and Marget and Adam (1969; 1971). For instance the former authors, using continuous medication in a dose of 76 mg per kg, administered three times daily, found serum levels as high as 17 μg per ml. However all of these authors used a photocolorimetric method for serum level assays, which estimates both the active drug and its antimycotically inactive metabolites. It appears that clotrimazole metabolites mainly account for the high serum concentrations obtained by this method.

Excretion

URINE: Very little of the active drug seems to be excreted by the kidney. Less than 1 per cent of an administered dose can be recovered from the urine (Burgess and Bodey, 1972). Urinary concentrations of the active drug are as low as 0·01–0·3 μg per ml (Holt and Newman, 1972b). Higher concentrations of inactive metabolites are excreted in urine (Plempel et al., 1969).

BILE AND OTHER ROUTES OF EXCRETION: It is not certain whether clotrimazole is excreted in the active form in humans by any other route such as the biliary tract (Plempel et al., 1969; Marget and Adam, 1971). In animals a considerable quantity of the drug is excreted in the faeces, sweat and other body secretions (Marget and Adam, 1969).

INACTIVATION IN BODY: The drug is largely metabolized to antimycotically inactive compounds in the body, presumably in the liver. In addition some of the drug is hydrolysed to inactive compounds by gastric juice before absorption (Plempel et al., 1969).

Distribution of the Drug in Body

Animal experiments have shown that clotrimazole is well distributed in tissues such as the heart, lungs and kidneys. There is some concentration of the drug in the liver, and particularly in adipose tissue (Plempel et al., 1969). Clotrimazole does not appear to penetrate into the cerebrospinal fluid of subjects with normal meninges.

The drug is about 50 per cent bound to serum proteins (Plempel et al., 1969).

Mode of Action

The imidazole antifungal agents, clotrimazole, miconazole (page 911) and econazole (page 917) all appear to act by damaging the fungal plasma membrane. When Candida albicans cells are exposed to relatively high concentrations of clotrimazole, leakage of potassium ions, amino acids, inorganic phosphate and nucleotides occurs from the cell. It appears that the imidazole antimycotics affect the fungal plasma membrane in a different way to the polyene antibiotics such as amphotericin B (page 871) and nystatin (page 925) (Yamaguchi, 1977).

Toxicity

1. *Gastro-intestinal side-effects*. Anorexia, nausea, vomiting, abdominal pain and diarrhoea may occur in patients taking oral clotrimazole (Oberste-Lehn *et al.*, 1969; Engelhardt, 1971). In early clinical trials these symptoms were found to be infrequent and relatively mild, but in later studies they have been more pronounced (Goldstein and Hoeprich, 1972; Weuta, 1974). These side-effects necessitated the cessation of treatment in 9 of 15 patients in one study (Burgess and Bodey, 1972).

2. *Hepatotoxicity*. Many clotrimazole treated patients show abnormalities in liver function tests such as bilirubin, serum aspartate aminotransferase (SGOT) and alkaline phosphatase elevations (Marget and Adam, 1969 and 1971; Weuta, 1974). These abnormalities usually disappear when the drug is stopped. As clotrimazole is metabolized in the liver, it is recommended that liver function tests be performed regularly during systemic clotrimazole therapy (Holt and Newman, 1972b).

3. *Other side-effects*. Excessive drowsiness and disorientation have been described in one patient who was treated by clotrimazole for urinary candidiasis, which developed after renal transplantation. This patient's mental state rapidly improved when the drug was discontinued (Cartwright *et al.*, 1972). Depression and other mental disturbances have also been reported.

No haematological or renal side-effects attributable to clotrimazole have been observed (Oberste-Lehn *et al.*, 1969; Marget and Adam, 1969; 1971; Engelhardt, 1971).

Clinical Uses of the Drug

Early studies of the use of oral clotrimazole for fungal infections were encouraging. Given in this way it was reported to be successful for the treatment of sycosis barbae caused by Candida albicans (Oberste-Lehn *et al.*, 1969), acne secondarily infected with Candida albicans (Engelhardt, 1971) and Candida fungaemia, pyelonephritis and dermatitis in children (Marget and Adam, 1971). Cartwright *et al.* (1972) used it successfully to treat urinary candidiasis in a patient who was a renal transplant recipient, and Holt and Newman (1972a) also obtained cures in children with Candida urinary tract infections and fungaemia. It was also used to effect a cure in a child with systemic candidiasis after cardiac surgery (Kozinn *et al.*, 1974). Early reports suggested that systemic clotrimazole may be of value in pulmonary aspergillosis (Oberste-Lehn *et al.*, 1969; Evans *et al.*, 1971). Milne (1974) however treated four patients with bronchopulmonary aspergillosis with clotrimazole for periods up to three months without improvement. It was also considered that the drug may be of some benefit in toxoplasmosis (Marget and Adam, 1971).

Because of its side-effects (*vide supra*), the progressively diminishing serum levels which occur with its continued administration (page 901) and the inconsistent results of other clinical studies, clotrimazole is now considered to have no specific indications in systemic fungal infections, except perhaps for desperately ill patients who have not responded to other antimycotic agents (Utz, 1975). The drug is useful for the treatment of the following superficial fungal infections.

1. *Superficial Candida infections.* Clotrimazole applied as a one per cent lotion or cream is very effective (comparable to nystatin) for the treatment of cutaneous candidiasis which is common on intertrigenous areas of the skin (Poleman, 1974; Fredriksson, 1974; Clayton and Connor, 1974; Zaias, 1975). Candidal balanitis also responds to treatment with one per cent clotrimazole cream for seven days (Waugh *et al.*, 1978). Clotrimazole pessaries and/or cream are effective alternatives to topical preparations of nystatin (page 925) or amphotericin B (page 877) for the treatment of vaginal candidiasis (Tamura *et al.*, 1973). In addition, a 28-day course of clotrimazole pessaries was effective for a patient with vaginal candidiasis in whom treatment with nystatin and amphotericin B preparations had failed (Cartwright, 1974). The use of two clotrimazole pessaries nightly for three consecutive nights results in about a 90 per cent cure rate for vaginal candidiasis (Masterton *et al.*, 1977).

Despite the disadvantages of oral clotrimazole administration (*vide supra*), this method of treatment is of value for chronic mucocutaneous candidiasis. Leikin *et al.* (1976) controlled skin and mucosal lesions in an eleven-year-old girl with this disease by continuous treatment with an oral dose of 120 mg per kg body weight per day (1 g twice-daily). An intolerable frequency of side-effects has been associated with the oral use of clotrimazole for some patients with chronic mucocutaneous candidiasis (Higgs, 1974). Effectiveness combined with minimum side-effects have been accomplished in other patients by using oral clotrimazole on an intermittent basis. Meade (1977) used oral clotrimazole (60 mg per kg body weight per day) to treat successfully a forty-year-old woman with chronic mucocutaneous candidiasis and then used it prophylactically in a dose of 2·5 g given once every 18 days; in this way recurrence was prevented for a period of 34 months. Ipp *et al.* (1977) used oral clotrimazole in a dose of 90 mg per kg body weight per day to treat a three-year-old girl with the disease. The drug was administered intermittently; it was given for two weeks and then discontinued for four weeks and then this cycle was repeated. Six months after starting clotrimazole the child's skin lesions had virtually cleared, and no recurrences occurred during a 20-month period of this treatment. Intermittent therapy as used in these two patients also lessens the effect of progressively declining serum levels, which occur with continuous oral use of clotrimazole (page 901).

2. *Trichomonas vaginitis.* This infection can be effectively treated by clotrimazole vaginal tablets (100 mg per day) for six days (Lohmeyer, 1974). The cure rate however is low compared to treatment with oral metronidazole (page 769). Local clotrimazole therapy also has the disadvantage that it cannot prevent renewed infection arising from the urethra and Bartholin's glands. Schnell (1974) suggested that clotrimazole vaginal tablets plus metronidazole oral tablets is a suitable combination for the treatment of suspected or proven vaginal mixed infections of trichomonads and yeasts.

3. *Superficial dermatophyte (ringworm) infections.* Skin ringworms and various forms of tinea caused by dermatophytes, such as Microsporum canis, Trichophyton mentagrophytes, T. rubrum, T. verrucosum and Epidermophyton floccosum, respond equally as well to one per cent clotrimazole

cream as to Whitfield's ointment and tolnaftate cream (Polemann, 1974; Fredriksson, 1974; Smith *et al.*, 1974; Clayton and Connor, 1974; Hall-Smith, 1974; Gip, 1974; Comaish, 1974; Male, 1974; Zaias, 1975). However griseofulvin is preferred for some dermatophyte infections for which topical therapy is not suitable (page 922). Tinea versicolor (caused by Pityrosporum orbicularis, also called Malassezia furfur) and erythrasma (caused by Corynebacterium minutissimum) also respond to treatment with clotrimazole cream.

4. *Fungal infections of the eye (oculomycosis)*. Jones (1975) considers that clotrimazole is the drug of choice for Aspergillus eye infections; it is given topically as oily eye drops or ointment every hour until clinical response is obtained, and is then continued four times daily for 8–12 weeks. Clotrimazole is also useful for Candida and a variety of other fungal eye infections. For severe intra-ocular fungal infections oral administration of clotrimazole may be desirable for the first two weeks.

REFERENCES

Beggs, W. H., Sarosi, G. A. and Steele, N. M. (1976), 'Inhibition of potentially pathogenic yeastlike fungi by clotrimazole in combination with 5-fluorocytosine or amphotericin B', *Antimicrob. Ag. Chemother.*, **9**, 863.

Bennett, J. E. (1974), 'Chemotherapy of systemic mycoses (second of two parts)' *New Engl. J. Med.*, **290**, 320.

Burgess, M. A. and Bodey, G. P. (1972), 'Clotrimazole (Bay b 5097): *In vitro* and clinical pharmacological studies', *Antimicrob. Ag. Chemother.*, **2**, 423.

Cartwright, R. Y., Shaldon, C. and Hall, G. H. (1972) 'Urinary candidiasis after renal transplantation', *Brit. med. J.*, **2**, 351.

Cartwright, R. Y. (1974), 'Clotrimazole in the treatment of acute and 'resistant' vaginal candidiasis', *Postgrad. Med. J.* (July Suppl.), **50**, 90.

Clayton, Y. M. and Connor, B. L. (1974), 'Clinical trial of clotrimazole in the treatment of superficial fungal infections', *Postgrad. Med. J.* (July Suppl.), **50**, 66.

Comaish, J. S. (1974), 'Double-blind comparisons of clotrimazole with Whitfield's and nystatin ointments', *Postgrad. Med. J.* (Suppl.), **50**, 73.

Engelhardt, A. W. (1971), 'Acne conglobata candidosa', *Mykosen*, **14**, 1.

Evans, E. G. V., Watson, D. A. and Matthews, N. R. (1971), 'Pulmonary aspergillomata in a child treated with clotrimazole', *Brit. med. J.*, **4**, 599.

Goldstein, E. and Hoeprich, P. D. (1972), 'Problems in the diagnosis and treatment of systemic candidiasis', *J. Infect. Dis.*, **125**, 190.

Fredriksson, T. (1974), 'Topical treatment of superficial mycoses with clotrimazole', *Postgrad. Med. J.* (Suppl.), **50**, 62.

Gip, L. (1974), 'The topical therapy of pityriasis versicolor with clotrimazole', *Postgrad. Med. J.* (Suppl.), **50**, 59.

Hall-Smith, P. (1974), 'Dermatomycoses: A brief history of therapy and initial results with clotrimazole', *Postgrad. Med. J.* (July Suppl.), **50**, 70.

Higgs, J. M. (1974), 'The use of clotrimazole in the treatment of chronic mucocutaneous candidiasis', *Postgrad. Med. J.* (Suppl.), **50**, 57.

Hoeprich, P. D. and Huston, A. C. (1975), 'Susceptibility of Coccidioides immitis, Candida albicans and Cryptococcus neoformans to amphotericin B, flucytosine and clotrimazole', *J. Infect. Dis.*, **132**, 133.

Holt, R. J. and Newman, R. L. (1972a), 'Urinary candidiasis after renal transplantation', *Brit. med. J.*, **2**, 714.

Holt, R. J. and Newman, R. L. (1972b), 'Laboratory assessment of the antimycotic drug clotrimazole', *J. clin. Path.,* **25,** 1089.

Ipp, M. M., Boxall, L. and Gelfand, E. W. (1977), 'Clotrimazole. Intermittent therapy in chronic mucocutaneous candidiasis', *Am. J. Dis. Child,* **131,** 305.

Jamieson, A. and Anderson, K. (1974), 'Primary amoebic meningoencephalitis', *Lancet,* **1,** 261.

Jamieson, A. (1975), 'Effect of clotrimazole on Naegleria fowleri', *J. clin. Path.* **28,** 446.

Jones, B. R. (1975), 'Principles in the management of oculomycosis', *Trans. Am. Acad. Ophthalmol. Otolaryngol.,* **70,** OP-15.

Kozinn, P. J., Lynfield, J. and Seelig, M. S. (1974), 'Successful treatment of systemic candidiasis following cardiac surgery', *Am. J. Dis. Child,* **128,** 106.

Leading Article (1971), 'Pulmonary aspergilloma', *Brit. med. J.,* **2,** 124.

Leikin, S., Parrott, R. and Randolph, J. (1976), 'Clotrimazole treatment of chronic mucocutaneous candidiasis', *J. Pediatrics,* **88,** 864.

Lohmeyer, H. (1974), 'Treatment of candidiasis and trichomoniasis of the female genital tract', *Postgrad. Med. J.* (Suppl.), **50,** 78.

Male, O. (1974), 'A double-blind comparison of clotrimazole and tolnaftate therapy of superficial dermatophytoses', *Postgrad. Med. J.* (Suppl.), **50,** 75.

Marget, W. and Adam, D. (1969), 'First experience with the broad-spectrum antimycotic BAY b 5097', *Medizinische Klinik,* **64,** 1235.

Marget, W. and Adam, D. (1971), 'BAY B 5097, a new orally applicable antifungal substance with broadspectrum activity. Preliminary clinical and laboratory experiences in children', *Acta Paediat. Scand.,* **60,** 341.

Masterton, G., Napier, I. R., Henderson, J. N. and Roberts, J. E. (1977), 'Three-day clotrimazole treatment in candidal vulvovaginitis', *Brit. J. vener. Dis.,* **53,** 126.

Meade, R. H., III (1977), 'Treatment of chronic mucocutaneous candidiasis', *Ann. Intern. Med.,* **86,** 314.

Milne, L. J. R. (1974), 'Mycological studies in the use of clotrimazole in bronchopulmonary aspergillosis and neonatal and vaginal candidiasis', *Postgrad. Med. J.* (July Suppl.), **50,** 20.

Oberste-Lehn, H., Baggesen, I. and Plempel, M. (1969), 'First clinical experience in systemic mycoses with a new oral antimycotic', *Deutsche Medizinische Wochenschrift,* **94,** 1365.

Plempel, M., Bartmann, K., Büchel, K. H. and Regel, E. (1969), 'Experimental findings with a new oral broad-spectrum antimycotic', *Deutsche Medizinische Wochenschrift,* **94,** 1356.

Polemann, G. (1974), 'Clinical experience in the local treatment of dermatomycoses with clotrimazole', *Postgrad. Med. J.* (Suppl.), **50,** 54.

Schnell, J. D. (1974), 'The incidence of vaginal Candida and Trichomonas infections and treatment of Trichomonas vaginitis with clotrimazole', *Postgrad. Med. J. (Suppl.),* **50,** 79.

Shadomy, S. (1971), '*In vitro* antifungal activity of clotrimazole (Bay b 5097)', *Infect. Immunity,* **4,** 143.

Smith, E. B., David, L. M. and Knox, J. M. (1974), 'Topical clotrimazole in dermatophytosis in a prison environment', *Postgrad. Med. J.* (Suppl.), **50,** 64.

Tamura, S., Kuramoto, H., Yamada, T., Majima, H. and Miyamoto, H. (1973), 'The therapy of Candida vaginitis and Candida vulvovaginitis with a new antimycotic substance, clotrimazole', *Curr. med. Res. Opin.,* **1,** 540.

Utz, J. P. (1975), 'New drugs for the systemic mycoses: Flucytosine and clotrimazole', *Bull. N.Y. Acad. Med.,* **51,** 1103.

Waitz, J. A., Moss, E. L. and Weinstein, M. J. (1971), 'Chemotherapeutic evaluation of clotrimazole (Bay b 5097,1(0-chloro-α-α-diphenylbenzyl) imidazole)', *Appl. Microbiol.,* **22,** 891.

Waugh, M. A., Evans, E. G. V., Nayyar, K. C. and Fong, R. (1978), 'Clotrimazole (canesten) in the treatment of Candidal balanitis in men', *Brit. J. vener. Dis.*, **54,** 184.

Weuta, H. (1974), 'Clinical studies with oral clotrimazole', *Postgrad. Med. J.* (July Suppl.), **50,** 45.

Yamaguchi, H. (1977), 'Antagonistic action of lipid components of membranes from Candida albicans and various other lipids on two imidazole antimycotics, clotrimazole and miconazole', *Antimicrob. Ag. Chemother.,* **12,** 16.

Zaias, N. (1975), 'Clotrimazole and miconazole', P.A.H.O. and W.H.O.: *Proceedings of the Third International Conference on the Mycoses,* São Paulo, Brazil, 27–29 August 1974. Scientific Publication No. 304, p. 241.

Miconazole

Description

Miconazole like clotrimazole (page 898) is an imidazole derivative which was synthetized at Janssen Pharmaceutical Research Laboratories in Belgium (Godefroi *et al.*, 1969). It is only slightly soluble in water and has the chemical formula of 1-{2, 4-dichloro-beta-((2,4-dichlorobenzyl) oxy)phenethyl} imidazole nitrate. Miconazole has a wide range of antifungal activity (Brugmans *et al.*, 1972; Van Cutsem and Thienpont, 1972). It is already established as a useful drug for the topical treatment of superficial fungal infections, and limited clinical studies suggest that it may be valuable for the treatment of certain systemic fungal infections.

Sensitive Organisms

1. *Pathogenic yeasts and yeast-like fungi.* Cryptococcus neoformans is quite sensitive to miconazole but the Candida spp., particularly Candida albicans, are much less sensitive. Depending when the test was read (48 or 24 h), 56 and 84 per cent respectively of C. albicans strains examined by Bannatyne and Cheung (1978) were sensitive to 4 µg per ml of miconazole. The combination of miconazole and amphotericin B (page 867) may show *in vitro* antagonism when tested against Candida albicans, and it is possible that this may also occur *in vivo* (Schacter *et al.*, 1976). For the treatment of experimental murine cryptococcosis, miconazole is much less effective than amphotericin B (Graybill *et al.*, 1978), but it is efficacious for treatment of disseminated candidiasis in rats (Balk *et al.*, 1978). Pityrosporum orbicularis (Malassezia furfur), the causative agent of tinea versicolor, is quite sensitive.

2. *Dimorphic fungi.* Histoplasma capsulatum, Paracoccidioides brasiliensis and Blastomyces dermatitidis are very sensitive. Coccidioides immitis is somewhat less sensitive to miconazole, but in experimental murine coccidioidomycosis it has a marked therapeutic effect (Levine *et al.*, 1975). Sporotrichum schenckii is usually only moderately sensitive.

3. *Moulds or filamentous fungi.* The Cladosporium spp. and the Phialophora spp. are usually sensitive, and whilst members of the Aspergillus spp. vary, they are commonly sensitive to miconazole. Some of the agents which cause fungal mycetoma such as Madurella mycetomii are quite sensitive. Lutwick *et al.* (1976) showed that some clinical isolates of Petriellidium boydii (Allescheria boydii; Monosporium apiospermum) were very sensitive (MIC <0·25 µg per ml). Miconazole is very active against the dermatophytes or ringworm fungi, particularly Trichophyton mentagrophytes, T. rubrum and Epidermophyton floccosum. Species of the genera Mucor, Rhizopus and Ab-

sidia are resistant, but those of the genera Basidiobolus and Entomphthora are sensitive.

4. *Actinomycetes*. Bacteria of this group which may cause disease resembling the mycoses are quite sensitive; these include Nocardia asteroides, N. brasiliensis, Actinomadura (Streptomyces) madurae, Streptomyces somaliensis and Actinomadura (Streptomyces) pelletierii.

5. *Other bacteria*. Gram-negative bacteria are resistant to miconazole, but some Gram-positive cocci and bacilli are quite sensitive. For instance, the MIC of miconazole for Strep. pyogenes has been reported to be 0·01 µg per ml (Van Cutsem and Thienpont, 1972).

6. *Prototheca spp*. Some species of these achloric algae which cause human infection (protothecosis) are sensitive (Segal *et al.*, 1976).

7. *Naegleria*. The growth of N. fowleri, the cause of primary amoebic meningoencephalitis in humans, is suppressed in culture by miconazole (Thong *et al.*, 1977).

8. *Acanthamoebae*. Fresh water amoebae such as Acanthamoeba polyphaga and A. castellanii can cause suppurative corneal and intra-ocular infections resembling those due to fungi; these protozoa are also suceptible *in vitro* to miconazole (Nagington and Richards, 1976).

9. *Trichomonas vaginalis*. Unlike clotrimazole (page 903), miconazole has no useful activity against this parasite.

10. *Acquired resistance*. Holt and Azmi (1978) reported the emergence of resistance to miconazole of Candida albicans during prolonged therapy for urinary candidiasis; the strain was equally resistant to clotrimazole (page 899) and econazole (page 917).

In Vitro Sensitivities

Table 47 shows the minimum inhibitory concentrations of miconazole against some selected fungal species. Serum concentrations of 2–4 µg per ml can be fairly easily attained by intravenous administration of the drug.

TABLE 47

(After Shadomy *et al.*, 1977)

ORGANISM	MIC (µg per ml)
Blastomyces dermatitidis	<0·25
Histoplasma capsulatum	<0·25
Coccidioides immitis	1·0–2·0
Sporotrichum schenckii	2·0–8·0
Cryptococcus neoformans	1·0
Candida albicans	1·0–>4·0
Torulopsis glabrata	0·5–>4·0
Cladosporium trichoides	2·0–>4·0
Phialophora spp.	1·0–2·0
Aspergillus fumigatus	4·0–>4·0
Aspergillus flavus	1·0–4·0
Aspergillus niger	1·0–4·0
Fusarium spp.	>4·0
Mucor	>4·0

Mode of Administration and Dosage

1. *Oral administration.* Miconazole is poorly absorbed after oral administration. A dose of 3 g per day for adults given in three divided doses has been well tolerated when given for several weeks (Brugmans *et al.*, 1972).

2. *Intravenous administration.* This mode of administration is preferred for the treatment of systemic infections because higher serum levels are attained (*vide infra*). In clinical studies various dosage schedules have been employed. A common intravenous dose for adults has been 600–1200 mg per day, given in three divided doses (Scheef *et al.*, 1974; Katz and Cassileth, 1977). The maximum daily dose usually recommended is 30 mg per kg body weight per day (about 2 g per day), but doses as high as 3·6 g per day for adults have been used for months (Stevens *et al.*, 1976). Each eight-hourly dose is diluted in 250–1000 ml of 5 per cent glucose, and infused over a period of one hour. Stevens *et al.* (1976) used an initial dose of 200 mg every 8 h which was gradually increased every two to seven days. No definite dosage recommendations are available for children. An intravenous dose of 15 mg per kg body weight, twice-daily, has been used in babies (Symoens, 1977). Initial intravenous doses of 30–60 mg per kg body weight per day, later reduced to 10–20 mg per kg per day, have been used in children (Fischer *et al.*, 1977).

3. *Administration direct into CSF.* Miconazole has been given directly into the CSF (lumbar, cisternal or ventricular), of four patients with fungal meningitis in a maximum total dose of 465 mg. After this form of administration (maximum individual dose 20 mg) the CSF miconazole concentration was 1·4 μg per ml after 24 h and 0·25 μg per ml after 48 h. The drug was well tolerated by this route (Deresinski *et al.*, 1976). Intrathecal therapy has been used for cryptococcal and coccidioidal meningitis (Symoens, 1977).

4. *Patients with renal failure.* The serum half-life of miconazole in patients with renal failure or in those undergoing haemodialysis is not significantly different from that in subjects with normal renal function. However, some patients with renal failure not undergoing haemodialysis may have elevated serum levels in the first four hours due to a reduction in the apparent volume of distribution (Lewi *et al.*, 1976).

5. *Use in pregnancy.* Although miconazole does not appear to be teratogenic in animals, its safety in human pregnancy has not been established.

6. *Topical therapy.* Miconazole is available as a vaginal cream for the treatment of vulvovaginal candidiasis. It is also available as a skin cream for the treatment of cutaneous dermatophytosis and candidiasis. Undiluted miconazole solution can be used for mouth washing, bladder instillation or for wound infiltration.

Availability

1. *Intravenous preparation.* Vials containing 10 mg of miconazole base in a colloidal suspension, stabilized with the detergent cremophor EL.
2. *Skin cream.* Two per cent miconazole nitrate in a 20 g tube ('Daktarin'—Janssen Pharmaceutica and Ethnor).
3. *Vaginal cream.* Two per cent miconazole nitrate in an 85 g tube with an applicator for delivery of 5 g into the vagina. It is also available as solid cream pessaries ('Gyno-Daktarin'—Janssen Pharmaceutica and Ethnor).

Serum Levels in Relation to Dosage

1. *Oral administration.* Miconazole is poorly absorbed from the gastro-intestinal tract, and peak serum levels are reached 4 h later (Brugmans *et al.*, 1972). After oral doses of 200 mg and 1 g, serum levels of 0·07–0·1 and 0·5–1·0 μg per ml, respectively, are reached and these persist for about 8 h. In one patient studied by Stevens *et al.* (1976), who received oral miconazole in a dose of 1 g three times a day, serum levels 2 and 12 h after the last dose were 0·3 and <0·1 μg per ml respectively. The serum half-life after oral administration is about 24 h.

2. *Intravenous administration.* After a 200 mg dose of miconazole is infused intravenously over a period of one hour, a peak serum level of about 1·6 μg per ml is reached at the end of the infusion (Shadomy *et al.*, 1977). In a patient treated by Hoeprich and Goldstein (1974), a 1 g dose infused over one hour produced serum levels of 5·1 and 0·9 μg per ml, 1 and 11 h after the infusion, respectively. Serum levels resulting from various miconazole doses given by one hour infusion have been studied in 14 adult patients by Stevens *et al.* (1976). After the initial peak serum level, there is a rapid early decay period with a half-life of approximately 30 min, and this is followed by a late flat phase with a serum half-life of about 20 h. Doses above 9 mg per kg body weight produce peak serum levels above 1·0 μg per ml in 71 per cent of patients, and levels of up to 7·5 μg per ml could be achieved in some.

Excretion

URINE: After oral administration about 10 per cent of the dose is excreted in the urine, largely as metabolites, only one per cent being in the form of the unchanged drug (Brugmans *et al.*, 1972). In four volunteers given 200 mg intravenously, no active drug was detected in the urine but about a quarter of the dose was present as a metabolite (Hoeprich and Goldstein, 1974).

INACTIVATION IN BODY: Miconazole is inactivated in the body to produce a number of metabolites; hydrolysis and N-deakylation appear to be the main metabolic pathways. This is the most important method by which miconazole is eliminated from the body. Metabolism of the drug or possible excretion in the faeces appears to account for the rapid fall of serum concentrations after intravenous administration (*vide supra*) (Lewi *et al.*, 1976).

FAECES: Following oral administration about 50 per cent of miconazole is excreted in the faeces mainly as the unchanged drug.

Distribution of the Drug in Body

Information concerning the distribution of miconazole in the tissues and body fluids is sparse. Penetration of the drug into the cerebrospinal fluid is poor (Hoeprich and Goldstein, 1974; Shadomy *et al.*, 1977). When a dose of 1 g every 12 h was given intravenously to an adult patient with disseminated coccidioidomycosis and meningitis, although a peak serum level of 5·1 μg per ml was reached, the concentration of miconazole in the lumbar CSF rose to only 0·26 μg per ml (Hoeprich and Goldstein, 1974). In another patient whose peak serum level was 2·5 μg per ml, the cisternal and lumbar CSF taken 15–30 min later showed levels of 0·4 and 0·27 µg per ml, respectively (Stevens *et al.*, 1976). They also described another patient without meningitis who had a CSF level of 0·1 µg per ml 30 min after a peak serum level of 2·0 µg per ml.

Penetration into the sputum also appears to be poor. Miconazole was undetectable in the sputum of a patient on two occasions, 30 min after the peak serum levels were 6·7 and 4·5 µg per ml (Stevens *et al.*, 1976). One estimation of the concentration of the drug in the vitreous humour of a patient 2·25 h after an infusion of 1 g miconazole was 0·6 µg per ml (Lutwick *et al.*, 1976). Very little of the unchanged drug is excreted in the urine (*vide supra*). The serum protein binding of miconazole is approximately 90 per cent (Stevens *et al.*, 1976).

Mode of Action

Miconazole damages the plasma membrane and cell wall of Candida albicans, thereby altering cellular permeability with resultant leakage of intracellular materials from the cell (Sreedhara Swamy *et al.*, 1974). Under electron microscopy the earliest changes observed in these fungi are at the plasma membrane. Then depending on the dose and duration of treatment with miconazole, the cells show progressive cytoplasmic deterioration and shape changes, finally resulting in cell necrosis (De Nollin and Borgers, 1975). Miconazole also binds strongly to erythrocyte membrane lipoproteins and can induce haemolysis of mammalian erythrocytes (Sreedhara Swamy *et al.*, 1976). It appears that the imidazole antimycotics (miconazole, clotrimazole, page 901 and econazole, page 917) effect the fungal plasma membrane in a different way to the polyene antibiotics such as amphotericin B (page 871) and nystatin (page 925) (Yamaguchi, 1977). The biochemical action of miconazole on Candida albicans may involve the enzymes peroxidase and catalase present in the yeast cell (De Nollin *et al.*, 1977).

Toxicity

In early studies miconazole was given orally; when doses of 1 g three times a day were given to volunteers for periods up to nine weeks, there were no significant side-effects (Brugmans *et al.*, 1972).

Although published reports on the intravenous use of miconazole for the treatment of human fungal disease are limited, the following side-effects have been observed.

1. *Haematological side-effects.* In three patients with coccidioidomycosis treated by Stevens *et al.* (1976), a fall in haematrocrit values was observed during treatment; these values returned to normal when the drug was stopped, and haematological investigations were unrevealing. Marmion *et al.* (1976) also recorded haematological changes in patients with active coccidioidomycosis treated by intravenous miconazole. All of six patients developed a normocytic, normochromic anaemia and progressive thrombocytosis, with increasing doses of miconazole. Changes were first observed after a dose ranging from 1·8 to 12·6 g had been administered. The lowest haemoglobin values (7·8–9·6 g per dl) coincided with maximal thrombocytosis (515–990 000 per cm²) and they were observed after miconazole had been administered for periods ranging from 5 to 23 days. Bone marrow studies in three

patients showed erythroid hypoplasia and increased or active platelet production; all other haematological investigations performed were normal, except for a prolonged Lee-White clotting time in one patient. Total miconazole doses given to these patients were in the range of 21·4 to 74·0 g; haematological changes appeared to be dose-related and reversible on cessation of the drug.

Other changes in the blood appear to be caused by the vehicle in which miconazole is available for intravenous use. Patients receiving intravenous miconazole therapy may develop high concentrations of serum cholesterol and triglycerides, and this is associated with an unusual pattern on paper lipoprotein electrophoresis. This hyperlipaemic state has been attributed to the carrier solution of miconazole, cremophor EL (polyethoxylated castor oil) (Bagnarello et al., 1977). Another unusual side-effect noted in patients receiving intravenous miconazole is marked rouleaux formation in peripheral blood smears (Stevens et al., 1976). This may also be due to an unusual surface active phenomenon related to the carrier solution cremophor EL (Niell, 1977). It is also possible that the anaemia and thrombocytosis (vide supra) described with intravenous miconazole is due to cremophor EL (Marmion et al., 1976).

In view of these reports, haematological monitoring should be carried out regularly on all patients receiving miconazole by oral or intravenous routes.

2. *Gastro-intestinal side-effects.* Nausea and vomiting, often transient, may accompany intravenous miconazole therapy. In one patient attempts to increase the dose above 600 mg once-daily resulted in malaise, chills, nausea and vomiting (Stevens et al., 1976). Diarrhoea, sometimes necessitating cessation of treatment, has been observed with oral doses of 1 g three times a day (Lima et al., 1977).

3. *Thrombophlebitis.* This was the most common side-effect, occurring in 10 of 14 patients treated by intravenous miconazole, described by Stevens et al., (1976). Infusion by central venous catheters seemed to circumvent this problem.

4. *Immunosuppression.* Miconazole in concentrations of 1–10 μg per ml inhibits mitogen-induced lymphocyte proliferative responses (Thong and Rowan-Kelly, 1978). The clinical significance of this observation is not yet known.

5. *Other side-effects.* Allergic rashes have been recorded during intravenous treatment (Stevens et al., 1976; Marmion et al., 1976; Fischer et al., 1977). Dryness of the eyes and knee arthralgias were recorded in one patient (Stevens et al., 1976). Of five patients including three children, treated by Fisher et al. (1977), some developed fever sometimes with pruritis and others transient mild rises in transaminases (SGOT and SGPT).

Clinical Uses of the Drug

1. *Systemic use for fungal infections.* Information relating to the clinical use of miconazole given intravenously for human fungal disease is limited. It has been used sporadically for a wide range of fungal infections with variable results (Symoens, 1977). These have included candidiasis, cryptococcosis, coccidioidomycosis, paracoccidioidomycosis, histoplasmosis and aspergillosis. According to the *in vitro* studies of Shadomy et al. (1977), infections due to B. dermatitidis and H. capsulatum should be susceptible, whilst the drug may be of value in some infections due to C. immitis, S. schenckii, C. neoformans,

some Candida spp., some Aspergillus spp. and some strains of Cladosporium.
Miconazole has been used to treat a number of patients with coccidioidomycosis. Hoeprich and Goldstein (1974) used it unsuccessfully for a
patient who had disseminated disease including meningitis, and in whom the
organism was resistant to amphotericin B. Presumably because of the poor
penetration of the drug into the CSF (page 910), at autopsy the organism was
recovered from the central nervous system but not from the lung and
peritoneum. Intravenous miconazole has also been used in another 14 patients
with coccidioidomycosis, many of whom had complicating diseases and/or had
failed to respond to amphotericin B (Stevens et al., 1976). Eight of these
patients showed objective evidence of response, three with chronic cavitary
lung disease had slight or equivocal responses, two could not be evaluated and
one was a treatment failure. There was evidence of persistence of the organism
after therapy in at least six patients. By contrast to the case described by
Hoeprich and Goldstein (1974), the CSF indices in one of their patients improved with therapy and at autopsy central nervous system cultures were
sterile, but the organisms persisted at another site of infection. Stevens et al.
(1976) concluded that miconazole may have a role in the treatment of
coccidioidomycosis.

Rohwedder and Archer (1976) reported the successful treatment of a patient
with pulmonary sporotrichosis by miconazole. The drug was used when drug
resistance and treatment failure occurred, after initial treatment with
amphotericin B and then with amphotericin B and 5-fluorocytosine in combination. Miconazole was used in a dose of 600–1000 mg three times a day intravenously; this produced clinical improvement despite serum drug levels
which were below or only transiently in excess of the MIC of the strain of S.
schenckii isolated from the patient.

Systemic Candida infections have been effectively treated by miconazole.
Scheef et al. (1974) used it intravenously in a dose of 200–400 mg thrice-daily,
for periods of 5–30 days, to successfully treat 14 patients with systemic candidiasis. Miconazole in a dose of 400 mg every 8 h, intravenously, for 14 days,
was also effective in eradicating disseminated Candida tropicalis from a patient
with acute leukaemia who had developed severe anaphylaxis to amphotericin B
(Katz and Cassileth, 1977). There are other reports of the successful use of intravenous miconazole in Candida infections (Wüst and Lennartz, 1977; Iwand
and Depperman, 1977; Verhaegen, 1977); in some of these therapy has been
supplemented by oral miconazole (Hatala, 1977). A favourable response was
obtained in four of five patients with chronic mucocutaneous candidiasis,
treated by miconazole given intravenously (Fischer et al., 1977). In this study
the dosage was adjusted to achieve lowest 'valley' concentration of the drug
which would inhibit the individual fungal isolate.

Paracoccidioidomycosis (South American blastomycosis) has responded to
oral or a combination of oral and intravenous treatment with miconazole. Lima
et al. (1977) used the drug in a dose of 1 g three times a day for three to eight
months for this purpose. Negroni et al. (1977) used 200–600 mg intravenously
plus 2·5–3·0 g orally per day, for 60 days, followed by 1·5 g orally per day for
periods up to two years.

Miconazole was used with success to treat one patient with sphenoidal
sinusitis caused by Petriellidium boydii (Allescheria boydii); this fungus was

resistant to amphotericin B and 5-fluorocytosine (Mader *et al.*, 1978).

In contradistinction to all of these optimistic reports, Fisher *et al.* (1978) described three patients in whom treatment with miconazole failed, although all the fungi involved showed *in vitro* susceptibility. The diseases treated were arthritis due to Sporothrix schenckii, cryptococcal meningitis and disseminated Aspergillus fumigatus infection.

2. *Superficial dermatophyte (ringworm) infections.* Various forms of tinea due to T. rubrum, T. mentagrophytes and Epidermophyton floccosum respond well to 2 per cent miconazole cream, applied twice-daily for two to four weeks (Mandy and Garrott, 1974; Fulton, 1975; Zaias, 1975). Tinea versicolor (caused by Pityrosporum orbicularis also called Malassezia furfur) also responds well to treatment with 2 per cent miconazole cream (Zaias, 1975). Oral therapy is less effective for these infections (Symoens, 1977).

3. *Superficial candida infections.* Miconazole vaginal cream (2 per cent) given in a 5 g dose each night by an applicator for 14 days is effective for the treatment of vaginal candidiasis (Morris and Sugrue, 1975), and results are comparable to those obtained with nystatin pessaries (Hilton *et al.*, 1978). Two per cent skin cream is also useful for the treatment of cutaneous candidiasis (Zaias, 1975). The drug has been used to treat oral candidiasis in debilitated patients, many of whom were granulocytopenic and were receiving immunosuppressive drugs and antibiotics. Given as one 250 mg tablet four times a day, which was allowed to melt slowly in the mouth and then swallowed, it was very effective for this infection (Brincker, 1976). Oral miconazole has also been used to reduce the intestinal yeast flora and to treat oral moniliasis (Symoens, 1977).

4. *Fungal infections of the eye* (*oculomycosis*). Topical one per cent miconazole eye drops are useful for some aspergillus and other fungal eye infections (Jones, 1975).

5. *Primary amoebic meningoencephalitis.* The recovery of a nine-year-old girl with this disease has been attributed to prompt diagnosis, and early treatment with miconazole and amphotericin B (both given intravenously and intrathecally), plus oral rifampicin (Center for Disease Control, 1978).

REFERENCES

Bagnarello, A. G., Lewis, L. A., McHenry, M. C., Weinstein, A. J., Naito, H. K., McCullough, A. J., Lederman, R. J. and Gavan, T. L. (1977), 'Unusual serum lipoprotein abnormality induced by the vehicle of miconazole', *New. Engl. J. Med.*, **296**, 497.

Balk, M. W., Crumrine, M. H. and Fischer, G. W. (1978), 'Evaluation of miconazole therapy in experimental disseminated candidiasis in laboratory rats', *Antimicrob. Ag. Chemother.*, **13**, 321.

Bannatyne, R. M. and Cheung, R. (1978), 'Susceptibility of Candida albicans to miconazole', *Antimicrob. Ag. Chemother.*, **13**, 1040.

Brincker, H. (1976), 'Treatment of oral candidiasis in debilitated patients with miconazole—a new potent antifungal drug', *Scand. J. Infect. Dis.*, **8**, 117.

Brugmans, J., van Cutsem, J., Heykants, J., Schuermans, V. and Thienpont, D. (1972), 'Systemic antifungal potential, safety, biotransport and transformation of miconazole nitrate', *Europ. J. Clin. Pharmacol.*, **5**, 93.

Center for Disease Control (1978), 'Primary amebic meningoencephalitis—California,

Florida, New York', *Morbidity and Mortality Weekly Report*, **27**, 343.

De Nollin, S. and Borgers, M. (1975), 'Scanning electron microscopy of Candida albicans after *in vitro* treatment with miconazole', *Antimicrob. Ag. Chemother.*, **7**, 704.

De Nolin, S., van Belle, H., Goosens, F., Thone, F. and Borgers, M. (1977), 'Cytochemical and biochemical studies of yeasts after *in vitro* exposure to miconazole', *Antimicrob. Ag. Chemother.*, **11**, 500.

Deresinski, S. C., Lilly, R. B., Levine, H. B., Galgiani, J. N. and Stevens, D. A. (1976), 'Treatment of fungal meningitis with miconazole', *Amer. Rev. Resp. Dis.* (Suppl.) **113**, 71.

Fischer, T. J., Klein, R. B., Kershnar, H. E., Borut, T. C. and Stiehm, E. R. (1977), 'Miconazole in the treatment of chronic mucocutaneous candidiasis: A preliminary report', *J. Pediatrics*, **91**, 815.

Fisher, J. F., Duma, R. J., Markowitz, S. M., Shadomy, S., Espinel-Ingroff, A. and Chew, W. H. (1975), 'Therapeutic failures with miconazole', *Antimicrob. Ag. Chemother.*, **13**, 965.

Fulton, J. E., Jr. (1975), 'Miconazole therapy for endemic fungal disease', *Arch. Dermatol.*, **111**, 596.

Godefroi, E. F., Heeres, J., van Cutsem, J. and Janssen, P. A. J. (1969), 'The preparation and antimycotic properties of derivatives of 1-phenethylimidazole', *J. Med. Chem.*, **12**, 784.

Graybill, J. R., Mitchell, L. and Levine, H. B. (1978), 'Treatment of experimental murine cryptococcosis: A comparison of miconazole and amphotericin B', *Antimicrob. Chemother.*, **13**, 277.

Hatalia, M. (1977), 'Miconazole in systemic candidosis', *Proc. roy. Soc. Med.* (Suppl. 1), **70**, 20.

Hilton, A. L., Warnock, D. W., Milne, J. D. and Scott, A. J. (1978), 'Treatment of vaginal candidosis with miconazole', *Curr. Med. Res. Opin.*, **5**, 295.

Hoeprich, P. D. and Goldstein, E. (1974), 'Miconazole therapy for coccidioidomycosis', *JAMA*, **230**, 1153.

Holt, R. J. and Azmi, A. (1978), 'Miconazole-resistant Candida', *Lancet*, **1**, 50.

Iwand, A. and Deppermann, D. (1977), 'Miconazole in systemic mycosis', *Proc. roy. Soc. Med.* (Suppl. 1), **70**, 43.

Jones, B. R. (1975), 'Principles in the management of oculomycosis', *Trans. Am. Acad. Opthalmol. Otolaryngol.*, **70**, OP-15.

Katz, M. E. and Cassileth, P. A. (1977), 'Disseminated candidiasis in a patient with acute leukaemia. Successful treatment with miconazole', *JAMA*, **237**, 1124.

Levine, H. B., Stevens, D. A., Cobb, J. M. and Gebhardt, A. E. (1975), 'Miconazole in coccidioidomycosis I. Assay of activity in mice and *in vitro*', *J. Infect. Dis.*, **132**, 407.

Lewi, P. J., Boelaert, J., Daneels, R., De Meyere, R., van Landuyt, H., Heykants, J. J. P., Symoens, J. and Wynants, J. (1976), 'Pharmacokinetic profile of intravenous miconazole in man. Comparison of normal subjects and patients with renal insufficiency', *Europ. J. Clin. Pharmacol.*, **10**, 49.

Lima, N. S., Teixeira, G., Miranda, J. and de Valle, A. C. F. (1977), 'Treatment of South American blastomycosis (Paracoccidioidomycosis) with miconazole by the oral route: An on-going study', *Proc. roy. Soc. Med.* (Suppl. 1), **70**, 35.

Lutwick, L. I., Galgiani, J. N., Johnson, R. H. and Stevens, D. A. (1976), 'Visceral fungal infections due to Petriellidium boydii ((Allescheria boydii). *In vitro* drug sensitivity studies', *Amer. J. Med.*, **61**, 632.

Mader, J. T., Ream, R. S. and Heath, P. W. (1978), 'Petriellidium boydii (Allescheria boydii) sphenoidal sinusitis', *JAMA*, **239**, 2368.

Mandy, S. J. and Garrott, T. C. (1974), 'Miconazole treatment for severe dermatophytoses', *JAMA*, **230**, 72.

Marmion, L. C., Desser, K. B., Lilly, R. B. and Stevens, D. A. (1976), 'Reversible thrombocytosis and anemia due to miconazole therapy', *Antimicrob. Ag. Chemother.,* **10,** 447.

Morris, D. F. and Sugrue, D. L. (1975), 'Miconazole nitrate compared with chlordantoin in the treatment of vaginal candidiasis', *Brit. J. vener. Dis.,* **51,** 123.

Nagington, J. and Richards, J. E. (1976), 'Chemotherapeutic compounds and Acanthamoebae from eye infection', *J. clin. Path.,* **29,** 648.

Negroni, R., Rubinstein, P., Herrmann, A. and Gimenez, A. (1977), 'Results of miconazole therapy in twenty-eight patients with paracoccidioidomycosis (South American blastomycosis)', *Proc. roy. Soc. Med.* (suppl. 1), **70,** 24.

Niell, H. B. (1977), 'Miconazole carrier solution, hyperlipidemia and hematologic problems', *New Engl. J. Med.,* **296,** 1479.

Rohwedder, J. J. and Archer, G. (1976), 'Pulmonary sporotrichosis: Treatment with miconazole', *Amer. Rev. Resp. Dis.,* **114,** 403.

Schacter, L. P., Owellen, R. J., Rathbun, H. K. and Buchanan, B. (1976), 'Antagonism between miconazole and amphotericin B', *Lancet,* **2,** 318.

Scheef, W., Symoens, J., van Camp, K., Daneels, R. and De Leeuw-Delvigne, C. (1974), 'Chemotherapy of candidiasis', *Brit. med. J.,* **1,** 78.

Segal, E., Padhye, A. A. and Ajello, L. (1976), 'Susceptibility of Prothotheca species to antifungal agents', *Antimicrob. Ag. Chemother.,* **10,** 75.

Shadomy, S., Paxton, L., Espinel-Ingroff, A. and Shadomy, H. J. (1977), '*In vitro* studies with miconazole and miconazole nitrate', *J. Antimicrob. Chemother.,* **3,** 147.

Sreedhara Swamy, K. H., Sirsi, M. and Ramananda Rao, G. (1974), 'Studies on the mechanism of action of miconazole: Effect of miconazole on respiration and cell permeability of Candida albicans', *Antimicrob. Ag. Chemother.,* **5,** 420.

Sreedhara Swamy, K. H., Joshi, A. and Ramananda Rao, G. (1976), 'Mechanism of action of miconazole: Labiliazation of rat liver lysosomes *in vitro* by miconazole', *Antimicrob. Ag. Chemother.,* **9,** 903.

Stevens, D. A., Levine, H. B. and Deresinski, S. C. (1976), 'Miconazole in coccidioidomycosis. II. Therapeutic and pharmacologic studies in man', *Amer. J. Med.,* **60,** 191.

Symoens, J. (1977), 'Clinical and experimental evidence on miconazole for the treatment of systemic mycosis: A review', *Proc. roy. Soc. Med.* (Suppl. 1), **70,** 4.

Thong, Y. H., Rowan-Kelly, B., Shepherd, C. and Ferrante, A. (1977), 'Growth inhibition of Naegleria fowleri by tetracycline, rifamycin, and miconazole', *Lancet,* **2,** 876.

Thong, Y. H. and Rowan-Kelly, B. (1978), 'Inhibitory effect of miconazole on mitogen-induced lymphocyte proliferative responses', *Brit. med. J.,* **1,** 133.

van Cutsem, J. M. and Thienpont, D. (1972), 'Miconazole, a broad-spectrum antimycotic agent with antibacterial activity', *Chemotherapy,* **17,** 392.

Verhaegen, H. (1977), 'Miconazole treatment in candidal oesophagitis', *Proc. roy. Soc. Med.* (Suppl. 1), **70,** 47.

Wüst, H. J. and Lennartz, H. (1977), 'Miconazole in systemic candidiasis', *Proc. roy. Soc. Med.* (Suppl. 1), **70,** 18.

Yamaguchi, H. (1977), 'Antagonistic action of lipid components of membranes from Candida albicans and various other lipids on two imidazole antimycotics, clotrimazole and miconazole', *Antimicrob. Ag. Chemother.,* **12,** 16.

Zaias, N. (1975), 'Clotrimazole and miconazole', P.A.H.O. and WHO: *Proceedings of the Third International Conference on the Mycoses,* São Paulo, Brazil, 27–29 August 1974. Scientific Publication No. 304, 1975, p. 241.

Econazole

Econazole, like clotrimazole (page 898) and miconazole (page 907), is another imidazole derivative which was developed at Janssen Pharmaceutica Research Laboratories in Belgium (Godefroi *et al.*, 1969). It has a wide range of antifungal activity (Thienpont *et al.*, 1975). Econazole has the chemical formula 1-{2,4-dichloro-beta-((p-chlorobenzyl)-oxy) penethyl} imidazole nitrate.

This drug has a high degree of activity against the dermatophytes such as Microsporum canis, Trichophyton spp. and Epidermophyton floccosum. Of the other filamentous fungi, Sporotrichum schenckii, Cladosporium spp. and most Aspergillus spp. are quite sensitive. The phycomycetes such as Absidia, Mucor and Rhizopus are resistant. Madurella mycetomii, one of the agents which cause fungal mycetoma, is quite sensitive.

The dimorphic fungi, Histoplasma capsulatum, Blastomyces dermatitidis and B. brasiliensis are very sensitive to econazole. The drug has an inhibitory effect on Coccidioides immitis *in vitro* and *in vivo* in mice (Levine, 1978). Pathogenic yeasts such as Cryptococcus neoformans and Candida spp. are much less sensitive.

Similar to miconazole (page 908), econazole is quite active against some bacteria. Of the actinomycetes, it is active against Actinomadura (Streptomyces) madurae, A. pelletierii, Streptomyces somaliensis and Nocardia asteroides. Econazole has no activity against Gram-negative bacteria, but it is highly active against some Gram-positive cocci and bacilli, including Strep. pyogenes and some strains of Staph. pyogenes.

Econazole is effective for the treatment of superficial dermatophyte and Candidal infections in experimental animals. It is now also available in various preparations for the treatment of human vaginal and cutaneous candidiasis. After a 250 mg oral dose, peak serum levels of about $3 \cdot 0$ μg per ml are reached in $2 \cdot 5$ h; the level then falls rapidly over the next 1–2 h (Cartwright, 1978). The value of econazole administered orally or by the intravenous route for the treatment of systemic mycoses has yet to be determined by clinical studies.

REFERENCES

Cartwright, R. Y. (1978), 'Absorption of econazole from the human gastrointestinal tract'. In Siegenthaler, W. and Lüthy, R. (Ed.), *Current Chemotherapy: Proceedings of the 10th International Congress of Chemotherapy*, Zurich/Switzerland, 1977. American Society for Microbiology, Washington, D.C., p. 231.

Godefroi, E. F., Heeres, J., van Cutsem, J. and Janssen, P. A. J. (1969), 'The preparation and antimycotic properties of derivatives of 1-phenethylimidazole', *J. Med. Chem.*, **12,** 784.

Levine, H. B. (1978), 'Econazole in experimental coccidioidomycosis'. In Siegenthaler,

W. and Lüthy, R. (Ed.), *Current Chemotherapy: Proceedings of the 10th International Congress of Chemotherapy*, Zurich/Switzerland, 1977. American Society for Microbiology, Washington, D.C., p. 233.

Thienpont, D., van Cutsem, J., van Nueten, J. M., Niemegeers, C. J. E. and Marsboom, R. (1975), 'Biological toxicological properties of econazole, a broad-spectrum antimycotic', *Arzneim. Forsch.* (Drug Res.), **25**, 3.

Griseofulvin

Description

Griseofulvin was isolated from Penicillium griseofulvium in 1939 (Oxford *et al.*, 1939), but it was not investigated further at that time because it lacked antibacterial activity. Although it was shown in 1947 that griseofulvin protected plants from fungal infections, its potential for the treatment of human infections was not realized until Gentles (1958) demonstrated that oral griseofulvin was effective in experimental Microsporum canis infection of guinea pigs. It was soon shown that the drug was also effective in human ringworm infections (Williams *et al.*, 1958; Blank *et al.*, 1959). Griseofulvin is now generally accepted as the drug of choice for treatment in the majority of these diseases.

Sensitive Organisms

1. *Dermatophytes or ringworm fungi.* All these fungi, including the Microsporum, Trichophyton and Epidermophyton spp., are highly sensitive to griseofulvin. Strains of dermatophytes resistant to griseofulvin have been produced *in vitro* (Roth, 1960), but resistant strains have not been isolated from patients receiving griseofulvin therapy (Grin and Nadaždin, 1965; Davies *et al.*, 1967).

2. *Other fungi.* Griseofulvin has no activity against other filamentous fungi such as Aspergillus and Phialophora spp. The drug also has no effect against yeasts (Cryptococcus neoformans) and yeast-like fungi (Candida spp.), nor against the dimorphic fungi such as Sporotrichum schenckii, Blastomyces dermatitidis, Paracoccidioides brasiliensis, Histoplasma capsulatum and Coccidioides immitis (Roth, 1960).

3. *Bacteria.* Griseofulvin has no activity against Actinomyces and Nocardia spp., and is also inactive against all other bacteria.

In Vitro Sensitivities

Minimum inhibitory concentrations of griseofulvin against sensitive fungi range from 0·18 to 0·42 μg per ml (Roth, 1960).

Mode of Administration and Dosage

1. *Adults.* Griseofulvin is administered by the oral route. The adult dose is 0·5 to 1·0 g daily, administered in one, or more commonly two, divided doses. For difficult chronic infections such as fungal paronychia a dose as high as 0·5 g three times a day has been used (Davies *et al.*, 1967). The drug should be

taken with meals, as its absorption is enhanced by fatty food in the stomach (*vide infra*).

2. *Children*. The dose for children is 10 mg per kg body weight per day, administered in one or two divided doses. A commonly used dose for children is 125 mg twice-daily. Grin and Nadaždin (1965) demonstrated that the optimal dose for children suffering from favus, a Trichophyton schoenleinii infection, was 25 mg per kg per day.

3. *Patients with renal failure*. Griseofulvin apparently can be given in the usual doses to such patients, because it does not accumulate in the presence of renal functional impairment.

4. *Topical griseofulvin therapy*. Goldman *et al.* (1960) used a 1·5 per cent griseofulvin suspension for topical therapy in various forms of tinea. Their results were not encouraging, probably because the topically applied drug does not diffuse into keratin. It is generally accepted that topical griseofulvin is of little value for the treatment of human ringworm (Comments, 1973).

Availability

Griseofulvin (fine particle) tablets of 125 mg and 500 mg.

Serum Levels in Relation to Dosage

After oral administration of 1·0 g to adults, a peak serum level of 1–2 μg per ml is reached in about 4 h in most patients. The level is slightly lower 8 h after administration, and at 12 h it is about half the peak serum level. There is considerable individual variation in the serum levels obtained after griseofulvin administration. Crounse (1961) studied 27 adult patients, each of whom received 1·0 g of the drug orally. Serum levels at 4 h ranged from 0–3·75 μg per ml, and at 8 h from 0·25–3·75 μg per ml. The average values were 1·31 and 1·19 μg per ml at 4 and 8 h, respectively. Crounse (1961) repeated these experiments over several months, and showed that patients who had high serum levels would consistently show high levels when retested, and those with low levels would consistently show low levels.

If the drug is taken with a fatty meal instead of in the fasting state, serum levels are approximately double. It appears that the presence of fat in the gut in some way enhances griseofulvin absorption (Crounse, 1961).

Excretion

URINE: Renal excretion does not play a significant role in the elimination of the active drug; less than 1 per cent of an administered dose of griseofulvin appears in the urine in an unchanged form (Roth, 1960).

INACTIVATION IN BODY: Animal experiments have shown that most absorbed griseofulvin is inactivated in the liver by dealkylation; the inactive metabolite, 6-demethylgriseofulvin, is then excreted in the urine. Griseofulvin inactivation appears to be enhanced by barbiturates, which induce the hepatic enzymes involved (Busfield *et al.*, 1964). The concomitant administration of griseofulvin and a barbiturate may reduce the efficacy of griseofulvin therapy, and significant lowering of griseofulvin serum levels has been demonstrated in volunteers when this drug combination was used (Busfield *et al.*, 1963).

FAECES: Unabsorbed griseofulvin, which constitutes a considerable proportion of the administered dose, appears unchanged in faeces.

Distribution of Drug in Body

In animals griseofulvin is distributed widely in body fluids and tissues and it is concentrated in liver, fat, and skeletal muscle (Roth, 1960).

Gentles *et al.* (1959) postulated that griseofulvin is deposited in the keratinous layer of the epidermis and also in newly formed keratin of hair-shafts. They confirmed this in guinea pigs by demonstrating presence of the drug in hair after oral therapy. Since then it has been accepted that griseofulvin reaches the skin, hair and nails where it is concentrated in keratinized tissues (Blank *et al.*, 1959), and this largely explains its therapeutic effects. New keratin formed during treatment with griseofulvin is resistant to invasion by fungus, but the drug does not destroy fungus which has infected the outer keratin layers. Therefore a dermatophyte infection will only be cured when new griseofulvin-containing keratin grows out completely and the infected portion of skin, hair or nail is shed.

Mode of Action

Griseofulvin impairs fungal growth, resulting in distortion of hyphae. Growing cultures of the dermatophyte Microsporum gypseum take up large amounts of griseofulvin from the medium, and the drug is concentrated intracellularly at levels 100 times greater than present in the medium (El-Nakeeb and Lampen, 1965). The exact mechanism of action of griseofulvin on sensitive fungi is not known. It has been suggested that it interferes with fungal DNA replication resulting in abnormal DNA production, which may arrest cellular division (Huber and Gottlieb, 1968).

Toxicity

Griseofulvin is a relatively non-toxic drug; there are no reports of renal, haemopoietic or liver toxicity.

1. *Gastro-intestinal side-effects.* A minority of patients develop thirst, nausea or diarrhoea, but these are rarely severe enough to necessitate cessation of therapy (Blank *et al.*, 1959). Heartburn, flatulence, angular stomatitis and a black furred tongue have also been described.

2. *Hypersensitivity rashes.* Maculopapular or urticarial rashes occur in a small percentage of patients and these disappear when the drug is stopped (Blank *et al.*, 1959; Roth, 1960). Photosensitivity rashes have been occasionally reported (*Today's Drugs*, 1967).

3. *Neurotoxicity.* Headaches have been described in association with griseofulvin therapy, but these often improve spontaneously without interruption to treatment. Other very rare side-effects include irritability, fatigue, confusion and difficulty in coordination (Hildick-Smith *et al.*, 1963). Peripheral neuritis, vertigo and blurred vision are other rare side-effects.

4. *Interference with porphyrin metabolism.* Griseofulvin has an effect on the porphyrin metabolism of normal subjects. This does not have any clinical

significance because it does not produce symptoms or abnormalities in liver function tests (Rimington et al., 1963). However, griseofulvin may aggravate acute intermittent porphyria (Redeker et al., 1964). Berman and Franklin (1965) described a woman aged 43 years with this form of porphyria, whose disease was acutely exacerbated following a ten-day course of griseofulvin therapy.

5. *Drug interactions.* Griseofulvin may reduce the anticoagulant effect of warfarin, presumably by acting as an inducer of the hepatic enzymes which metabolize warfarin (Cullen and Catalano, 1967). Griseofulvin augments the effects of alcohol but barbiturates diminish the effect of griseofulvin (Cartwright, 1978).

Clinical Uses of the Drug

Topical therapy alone may be effective for some Microsporum canis, Trichophyton mentagrophytes and M. audouinii skin lesions, provided they are limited in size and readily accessible. However, orally administered griseofulvin is the treatment of choice for the majority of dermatophyte (ringworm) infections of the skin, hair and nails.

Tinea capitis (scalp ringworm) is commonly caused by M. canis, T. mentagrophytes, T. rubrum and T. tonsurans (Donald, 1965). All of these infections respond well to a six to eight weeks course of griseofulvin. Tinea barbae, usually due to T. mentagrophytes or T. verrucosum infection, also responds to a similar griseofulvin course.

Tinea corporis, tinea cruris and tinea of the feet and hands are amenable to griseofulvin therapy. However, in some patients with ringworm of feet (tinea pedis), it may be necessary to combine oral griseofulvin with an appropriate topical fungicide (Hildick-Smith et al., 1964). In most of these tineas a three to four weeks course of griseofulvin may suffice, but the drug should be continued until complete cure has been obtained.

Tinea of the nails (onychomycosis) responds to griseofulvin, but prolonged therapy is needed. Davies et al. (1967) treated 122 patients with this disease and the duration of treatment necessary varied from six months to two years. Finger nail infections responded better than those of toe nails, and Trichophyton rubrum infections more favourably than those caused by T. mentagrophytes.

Before griseofulvin therapy is instituted for a presumed ringworm, scrapings from the lesions should be taken for laboratory confirmation of a dermatophyte infection. Many other chronic dermatological conditions, unresponsive to griseofulvin, resemble fungal skin infections (Goldman et al., 1960; Davies et al., 1967) and the drug may be misused under these circumstances (Green and Donald, 1973).

REFERENCES

Berman, A. and Franklin, R. L. (1965), 'Precipitation of acute intermittent porphyria by griseofulvin therapy', *JAMA*, **192**, 1005.
Blank, H., Smith, J. G., Jr., Roth, F. J., Jr. and Zaias, N. (1959), 'Griseofulvin for the systemic treatment of dermatomycoses', *JAMA*, **171**, 2168.

Busfield, D., Child, K. J., Atkinson, R. M. and Tomich, E. G. (1963), 'An effect of phenobarbitone on blood-levels of griseofulvin in man', *Lancet*, **2**, 1042.

Busfield, D., Child, K. J. and Tomich, E. G. (1964), 'An effect of phenobarbitone on griseofulvin metabolism in the rat', *Brit. J. Pharmacol.*, **22**, 137.

Cartwright, R. Y. (1978), 'Use of antibiotics', *Brit. med. J.*, **2**, 108.

Comments (1973), 'Griseofulvin', *Med. J. Aust.*, **2**, 756.

Crounse, R. G. (1961), 'Human pharmacology of griseofulvin: The effect of fat intake on gastrointestinal absorption', *J. Invest. Dermatol.*, **37**, 529.

Cullen, S. I. and Catalano, P. M. (1967), 'Griseofulvin-warfarin antagonism', *JAMA*, **199**, 582.

Davies, R. R., Everall, J. D. and Hamilton, E. (1967), 'Mycological and clinical evaluation of griseofulvin for chronic onychomycosis', *Brit. med. J.*, **3**, 464.

Donald, G. F. (1965), 'The current status of tinea', *Med. J. Aust.*, **2**, 837.

El-Nakeeb, M. A. and Lampen, J. O. (1965), 'Uptake of griseofulvin by the sensitive dermatophyte, Microsporum gypseum', *J. Bacteriol.*, **89**, 564.

Gentles, J. C. (1958), 'Experimental ringworm in guinea pigs: Oral treatment with griseofulvin', *Nature*, **182**, 476.

Gentles, J. C., Barnes, M. J. and Fantes, K. H. (1959), 'Presence of griseofulvin in hair of guinea pigs after oral administration', *Nature*, **183**, 256.

Goldman, L., Schwarz, J., Preston, R. H., Beyer, A. and Loutzenhiser, J. (1960), 'Current status of griseofulvin. Report on one hundred seventy-five cases', *JAMA*, **172**, 532.

Green, A. C. and Donald, G. F. (1973), 'The prescription of griseofulvin as a pharmaceutical benefit in South Australia', *Med. J. Aust.*, **2**, 760.

Grin, E. I. and Nadaždin, M. (1965), 'Experimental investigation into the therapeutic effect of griseofulvin in favus caused by Trichophyton schoenleinii', *Bull. Wld. Hlth. Org.*, **33**, 183.

Hildick-Smith, G., Blank, H. and Sarkany, I. (1964), *Fungus Diseases and Their Treatment*, J & A Churchill Ltd., pp. 100 and 454.

Huber, F. M. and Gottlieb, D. (1968), 'The mechanism of action of griseofulvin', *Can. J. Microbiol.*, **14**, 111.

Oxford, A. E., Raistrick, H. and Simonart, P. (1939), 'Studies in the biochemistry of micro-organisms. LX. Griseofulvin, $C_{17}H_{17}O_6Cl$, a metabolic product of Penicillium griseofulvum Diercks', *Biochem. J.*, **33**, 240; quoted by Roth (1960).

Redeker, A. G., Sterling, R. E. and Bronow, R. S. (1964), 'Effect of griseofulvin in acute intermittent porphyria', *JAMA*, **188**, 466.

Rimington, C., Morgan, P. N., Nicholls, K., Everall, J. D. and Davies, R. R. (1963), 'Griseofulvin administration and porphyrin metabolism', *Lancet*, **2**, 318.

Roth, F. J., Jr. (1960–61), 'Griseofulvin', *Ann. N.Y. Acad. Sci.*, **89**, 247.

Today's Drugs (1967), 'Griseofulvin', *Brit. med. J.*, **4**, 608.

Williams, D. I., Marten, R. H. and Sarkany, I. (1958), 'Oral treatment of ringworm with griseofulvin', *Lancet*, **2**, 1212.

Nystatin

Description

Nystatin, like amphotericin B (page 865) and natamycin (page 927), is a polyene antifungal antibiotic. It was isolated from Streptomyces noursei in 1950 and originally named 'fungicidin' (Hazen and Brown, 1951). Nystatin is not a single chemical compound, but a mixture of closely related substances (Chowdhry, 1976). It is a yellow powder which is insoluble in water and only sparingly soluble in methanol and ethanol. The drug was further developed by Squibb Research Laboratories (Dutcher *et al.*, 1954), and is marketed with their trade name of 'Mycostatin'. Nystatin is too toxic for parenteral administration (Hildick-Smith *et al.*, 1964), and it is only used for the treatment of superficial infections. For this reason the pharmacokinetics and toxic effects of parenteral nystatin are not described.

Sensitive Organisms

Nystatin has no antibacterial action, but it has a wide spectrum of antifungal activity. Yeasts (Cryptococcus neoformans) and yeast-like fungi such as Candida albicans and the other Candida spp. are susceptible. Moulds or filamentous fungi such as Aspergillus, Trichophyton, Epidermophyton and Microsporum spp. are also usually sensitive. The same applies to most of the dimorphic fungi which cause deep mycoses, such as Histoplasma capsulatum, Blastomyces dermatitidis, Coccidioides immitis and others. The minimum inhibitory concentrations of nystatin against these sensitive fungi are usually in the range of $1 \cdot 56$ to $6 \cdot 25$ μg per ml (Hazen and Brown, 1951).

Nystatin is now almost exclusively used for the topical treatment of candida infections and therefore there is considerable interest as to whether nystatin-resistant Candida strains occur. It appears that such strains can be produced in the laboratory, but they are either very rare or non-existent in human disease. In one study of over 2000 clinical isolates of Candida spp., no nystatin-resistant variants were found (Athar and Winner, 1971). However these authors showed that after gradual exposure to increased nystatin concentrations *in vitro*, nystatin resistance could be induced in isolates of seven Candida species. These nystatin-resistant strains were also resistant to other polyene antibiotics such as amphotericin B and natamycin. Such resistant variants were less pathogenic, and it was concluded that nystatin resistant Candida spp. are unlikely to become a problem in clinical practice.

Absorption of the Drug

Very little, if any, nystatin is absorbed from the gastro-intestinal tract. After a very large oral dose, such as 10 million units, some nystatin can be detected in the serum, but with ordinary oral doses there is insufficient absorption to produce either a systemic chemotherapeutic effect or any toxicity.

Mode of Action

Nystatin, like amphotericin B (page 871), acts by damaging the cytoplasmic membrane of sensitive fungi, apparently by binding to a specific sterol, which is only found in fungal plasma membranes (Kinsky, 1962).

Nystatin, presumably by its action of making the cytoplasmic membrane more permeable, potentiates the entry of 5-fluorocytosine (page 890) and tetracycline (page 598) into Candida albicans cells (Aszalos, 1975).

Toxicity

There are virtually no side-effects related to the topical use of nystatin. The drug does not cause irritation or allergic reactions when applied to skin or mucous membranes, but nausea and diarrhoea may occur following the administration of large oral doses.

Clinical Uses, Administration and Dosage

1. *Preparations available.* Many preparations of this drug are available such as oral tablets (500 000 units), an oral suspension (100 000 units per ml) and vaginal tablets (100 000 units). Vaginal and skin creams are also available. In addition, other creams and ointments are marketed in which nystatin is combined with antibiotics such as bacitracin, neomycin and polymyxin B. One milligram of nystatin is equivalent to 3500 units.

2. *Skin infections.* Topical nystatin is suitable for the treatment of superficial candida infections. Dermatophyte infections respond poorly if at all, and for these, oral griseofulvin is the drug of choice (page 922).

3. *Oral candidiasis ('thrush').* This condition can only be treated by local application of the drug to the oral cavity. Therefore treatment with nystatin tablets is unsatisfactory, but the oral infection responds well if the mouth is painted with a suspension of the drug or nystatin lozenges are sucked.

4. *Vaginal candidiasis.* This usually responds well to a 15-day course of nystatin pessaries, inserted high in the vagina either once or twice a day. A nystatin vaginal cream is also satisfactory for this purpose and may be more effective (Leading article, 1976).

5. *Candidiasis of the gastro-intestinal tract.* This can be treated by an oral dose of 500 000 units (1 tablet) every 8 h (Kane *et al.*, 1976). In debilitated patients receiving antibacterial chemotherapy, gastro-intestinal candidiasis may be anticipated. In these circumstances it is reasonable to use nystatin prophylactically, and this may also prevent Candida fungaemia, which may occur when the alimentary tract is heavily infected (page 614). Oral nystatin is also advisable to prevent Candida overgrowth whenever bowel sterilization is

attempted by oral non-absorbable antibacterial agents. Levi *et al.* (1973) administered oral nystatin with oral gentamicin and vancomycin to patients with acute leukaemia in an attempt to prevent infections during the period of induction therapy for their disease. They found that very large nystatin doses (4 000 000 units) six-hourly were needed in these patients to achieve consistent suppression of fungi in the gut. Nystatin has also been combined with oral colistin and framycetin to prevent infection in leukaemia (*see* page 413). (The routine use of nystatin with oral tetracyclines is discussed on page 613).

6. *Aspergillosis.* Some success has been claimed for the use of nystatin aerosols in pulmonary aspergillosis (Hazen and Brown, 1960). A dose of 30 000 to 500 000 units three times daily for a period of several months has been used.

REFERENCES

Aszalos, A. (1975), 'Differential potentiation by nystatin of the effect of antibiotics on yeast and mammalian cells', *Antimicrob. Ag. Chemother.*, **7**, 754.

Athar, M. A. and Winner, H. I. (1971), 'The development of resistance by Candida species to polyene antibiotics *in vitro*', *J. Med. Microbiol.*, **4**, 505.

Chowdhry, B. Z. (1976), 'Antifungal agents', *J. Antimicrob. Chemother.*, **2**, 102.

Dutcher, J. D., Boyack, G. and Fox, S. (1954), 'The preparation and properties of crystalline fungicidin (nystatin)', *Antibiot. Annual*—1953–1954, p. 191.

Hazen, E. L. and Brown, R. (1951), 'Fungicidin, and antibiotic produced by a soil actinomycete', *Proc. Soc. Exp. Biol.*, **76**, 93.

Hazen, E. L. and Brown, R. (1960), 'Nystatin', *Ann. N.Y. Acad. Sci.*, **89**, 258.

Hildick-Smith, G., Blank, H. and Sarkany, I. (1964), *Fungus Diseases and Their Treatment*, J. & A. Churchill Ltd., p. 380.

Kane, J. G., Chretien, J. H. and Garagusi, V. F. (1976), 'Diarrhoea caused by Candida', *Lancet,* **1**, 335.

Kinsky, S. C. (1962), 'Nystatin binding by protoplasts and a particulate fraction of Neurospora crassa, and a basis for the selective toxicity of polyene antifungal antibiotics', *Proc. Nat. Acad. Sci.*, **48**, 1049.

Leading Article (1976), 'Vaginal candidosis', *Brit. med. J.*, **1**, 357.

Levi, J. A., Vincent, P. C., Jennis, F., Lind, D. E. and Gunz, F. W. (1973), 'Prophylactic oral antibiotics in the management of acute leukaemia', *Med. J. Aust.*, **1**, 1025.

Natamycin (*Pimaricin*)

Description

Natamycin, another polyene antifungal agent, was isolated from Streptomyces natalensis (Struyk *et al.*, 1958). This antibiotic, like nystatin (page 924), is unsuitable for parenteral administration and is only used for the treatment of superficial infections. It is marketed with the trade name of 'Pimafucin' (Gist-Brocades).

Sensitive Organisms

Natamycin has a wide spectrum of antifungal activity. Yeasts and yeast-like fungi such as Cryptococcus neoformans, Candida albicans and other Candida spp. are quite sensitive. Filamentous fungi such as Aspergillus, Epidermophyton and Microsporum spp. are sensitive, but the Trichophyton spp. are moderately resistant. Most of the dimorphic fungi such as Histoplasma capsulatum, Blastomyces dermatitidis, Coccidioides immitis and Sporotrichum schenckii are also sensitive. The majority of sensitive fungi are inhibited by natamycin concentrations of 1 to 10 μg per ml (Struyk *et al.*, 1958). Acquired fungal resistance to this drug has not been a problem.

Unlike other polyene antifungal agents, natamycin is active against Trichomonas vaginalis (Struyk *et al.*, 1958).

Natamycin has no antibacterial activity.

Absorption of the Drug

Very little, if any, natamycin is absorbed from the gastro-intestinal tract when the drug is administered in the recommended doses.

Mode of Action

The mode of action of natamycin is probably similar to that of the other polyenes, amphotericin B (page 871) and nystatin (page 925).

Toxicity

There is virtually no toxicity from the topical use of natamycin, and it does not cause irritation or sensitization of skin or mucous membranes. Vomiting and diarrhoea may occur if an oral dose higher than 600 mg daily is given (Newcomer *et al.*, 1960), but the currently recommended maximum oral dose for adults is only 400 mg per day.

Clinical Uses, Administration and Dosage

1. *Preparations available.* Natamycin is marketed as 100mg oral tablets, and a 1 per cent oral suspension (50 mg in 5 ml). It is also available in 20 ml vials for aerosol use, each ml containing 25 mg (2·5 per cent). Vaginal tablets (25 mg) and various creams and ointments are marketed, some of which contain other antibiotics in addition.

2. *Skin infections.* Superficial infections may be treated by topical natamycin (2 per cent cream), but nystatin may be more effective for this purpose. Natamycin is also recommended for tinea including tinea versicolor.

3. *Oral candidiasis ('thrush').* Natamycin is effective for this disease and is used in a similar manner to nystatin (page 925).

4. *Vaginal candidiasis.* This can be satisfactorily treated by natamycin vaginal tablets (Don, 1967), but this treatment is not superior to nystatin therapy. Natamycin vaginal tablets, whilst having some effect on trichomonas infection, are perhaps not as effective as oral metronidazole for this condition (*see* page 769).

5. *Candidiasis of gastro-intestinal tract.* Natamycin, like nystatin (page 925), can be used for this infection and an adult dose of 100 mg three for four times a day is recommended.

6. *Systemic fungus infections.* Large oral doses of natamycin have been used in the past to treat systemic mycoses (Newcomer *et al.*, 1960). Clinical results were poor, and vomiting and diarrhoea accompanied doses greater than 600 mg per day. This drug is therefore not suitable for the treatment of systemic infections.

7. *Aerosol therapy for bronchopulmonary infections.* Administration of natamycin by aerosol has been used for pulmonary aspergillosis. Edwards and La Touche (1964) treated ten patients, using natamycin as a 2·5 per cent suspension diluted in an alkaline agent, and administered 2·5 mg doses by aerosol two or three times a day. These authors observed clinical improvement in seven of the ten patients after six weeks of therapy.

REFERENCES

Don, R. A. (1967), 'Pimafucin for treatment of moniliasis', *Med. J. Aust.*, **1**, 382.

Edwards, G. and LaTouche, C. J. P. (1964), 'The treatment of bronchopulmonary mycoses with a new antibiotic—pimaricin', *Lancet*, **1**, 1349.

Newcomer, V. D., Sternberg, T. H., Wright, E. T., Reisner, R. M., McNall, E. G. and Sorenson, L. J. (1960), 'The treatment of systemic mycoses with orally administered pimaricin: Preliminary report', *Ann. N.Y. Acad. Sci.*, **89**, 240.

Struyk, A. P., Hoette, I., Drost, G., Waisvisz, J. M., van Eek, T. and Hoogerheide, J. C. (1958), 'Pimaricin, a new antifungal antibiotic', *Antibiot. Annual*—1957–1958, p. 878.

Part V
Antiviral Drugs

Idoxuridine

Description

Idoxuridine (5-iodo-2'-deoxyuridine; IUdR; IDU)is one of several synthetic halogenated analogues of naturally occurring thymidine. It was synthetized in 1959 as a possible antitumour agent (Prusoff, 1959), and later shown to inhibit the growth of Herpesvirus hominis and Vaccinia virus in tissue culture (Herrmann, 1961). Subsequently it was reported to be useful for the treatment of Herpesvirus hominis keratitis in man (Kaufman, 1962), and this remains its main clinical indication. IDU is marketed with the trade names of 'Stoxil', 'Dendrid' and 'Herplex'.

Antiviral Activity

In vitro, IDU inhibits growth and replication of DNA viruses such as Herpesvirus hominis, Herpesvirus varicellae (Varicella-zoster virus), Cytomegalovirus and Vaccinia. The susceptibility of these viruses depends on the test system employed. For instance, *in vitro* activity of IDU against Herpesvirus hominis varies according to the virus inoculum, the tissue culture cell line and the strain of the virus (Marks, 1974). Moreover *in vitro* activity of the drug does not necessarily reflect its activity *in vivo* and varying results have been obtained when IDU has been used to treat experimental viral infections in animals (Kern *et al.*, 1973; Percy and Hatch, 1975; Lefkowitz *et al.*, 1976; De Clercq *et al.*, 1976; Steffenhagen *et al.*, 1976). In particular results of treatment of Herpesvirus hominis encephalitis in animals have been contradictory; in some it was of value (Tokumaru, 1967; Tomlinson and MacCallum, 1970), but in others results were discouraging (Kaufman, 1963; Cho *et al.*, 1973; Plummer and Ingerson, 1974; Marks, 1975). Factors probably determining the outcome of treatment of experimental Herpesvirus hominis encephalitis with IDU include the time treatment is commenced, dosage, pharmacology of the drug in the animal tested and particularly its ability to penetrate into the CSF and brain.

Mode of Administration and Dosage

1. *Topical administration to the eye*. The drug may be applied to the cornea either as an 0·1 per cent ophthalmic solution (1 mg per ml) or as an 0·5 per cent ophthalmic ointment (5 mg per g). If the solution is used, one drop is placed in the infected eye hourly during the day and every 2 h during the night; the frequency of instillation may be halved as improvement occurs. The ointment, which is more convenient for the patient, should be instilled every 4 h

during the day, with the last instillation at bedtime. Both forms of treatment should be continued for three to five days after healing becomes complete, but the total period of treatment should usually not exceed 21 days. Corticosteroids may be instilled into the eye with IDU, but they are contraindicated in uncomplicated keratitis. Antibiotics and atropine may be instilled together with IDU, if necessary.

2. *Topical application to the skin and mucous membranes.* (*See* clinical uses of the drug, page 934).

3. *Parenteral administration.* Therapeutic concentrations of IDU in the body are difficult to establish and maintain. Its solubility in neutral solutions is less than 0·1 mg per ml, but it is much more soluble in alkaline solutions (Juel-Jensen and MacCallum, 1972). The drug has been administered by intravenous infusion in a 5 per cent dextrose solution, suitably alkalinized by adding bicarbonate. IDU is rapidly metabolized in the body to iodouracil, uracil and iodide; these metabolites, which are neither antiviral nor toxic, are excreted in urine. Idoxuridine is not bound to serum proteins and inactivation occurs in the tissues, and not in the serum, CSF or urine (Lerner and Bailey, 1972). The urinary excretion of IDU is also very rapid. During a two-hour infusion, despite rapid inactivation, one-half to one-third of the drug is excreted in the active form (Calabresi, 1963). Very little active IDU remains in the body if it is infused slowly over 2 h. For this reason Lerner and Bailey (1972) advocated rapid infusion (50 mg per min), which produced transient concentrations of IDU in serum and CSF, comparable to *in vitro* minimum inhibitory concentrations of IDU for Herpesvirus hominis (Nolan *et al.*, 1973). IDU was not detected in serum, CSF or urine after slow intravenous infusion (4 mg per min). In addition when it is infused at this slow rate, in a dose of 60–80 mg per kg per day, no significant concentrations of IDU are detected in the brains of patients with Herpesvirus hominis encephalitis dying during or after therapy (Lauter *et al.*, 1975). Intrathecal administration of idoxuridine does not appear to be of any advantage (Clarkson *et al.*, 1967; Weinstein and Tang, 1973).

Treatment schedules of IDU for Herpesvirus hominis encephalitis have varied considerably; doses ranging from 1·5 to 125 mg per kg per day for periods of 2–19 days, have been used (Juel-Jensen and MacCallum, 1972). A dose commonly recommended was 80–100 mg per kg per day for five days (Weinstein and Chang, 1973).

Mode of Action

IDU inhibits the synthesis of DNA in normal human tissue cells and in DNA viruses. It appears to compete with thymidine, an essential constituent of DNA, and its phosphorylated derivatives may inhibit some of the enzymes concerned in DNA synthesis. The antiviral activity of IDU is reversed by thymidine. IDU is also incorporated into DNA. Mutant viruses resistant to IDU may develop both *in vitro* and *in vivo*. These strains are deficient in thymidine kinase-inducing activity (Renis and Buthala, 1965).

Toxicity

1. *Side-effects from ocular therapy.* Instillation in the eye may occasionally

cause allergy or inflammation with resultant pain and pruritus in the eye or eyelids. These manifestations appear to be becoming more common with the widespread use of IDU (Pavan-Langston, 1975; Amon and Hanifin, 1976). If IDU is instilled more frequently than recommended, small defects may appear on the cornea, in which case the drug should be discontinued. In addition, boric acid should not be used in the eye with idoxuridine because the combination may cause irritation. Ocular therapy is not recommended in pregnancy as this form of treatment may possibly be teratogenic in rabbits, presumably because of absorption of small amounts of the drug.

2. *Side-effects from topical therapy*. The 5 per cent solution of IDU in dimethyl sulphoxide (DMSO) (*see* page 934) should not be applied for more than four days, otherwise the skin may become macerated and secondary bacterial infection supervene. This solution must not be put into the eye. Rarely patients may develop skin irritation with oedema and urticarial vesicles as a result of DMSO application. Similarly in genital herpes, treatment with a 40 per cent solution of IDU in DMSO should not be continued for longer than three days, otherwise maceration of the skin may occur. No side-effects on hepatic, renal or bone marrow function have been observed following topical therapy.

Allergic contact dermatitis has resulted from the application of 5 per cent IDU in dimethylacetamide (a skin penetrant) to genital herpes and may be becoming more common with frequent use of the drug (Amon and Hanifin, 1976). Preparations containing 5 per cent IDU in dimethyl sulphoxide are only available commercially in the United Kingdom ('Herpid', W. B. Pharmaceuticals). The safety of 5 per cent IDU preparations for skin application has not been established in the United States. Because of the danger of contact dermatitis and other theoretical considerations, some authors suggest that the indiscriminate extraocular use of IDU should be avoided in the United States, until clinical trials prove its value (Green and Staal, 1976).

3. *Side-effects from parenteral administration*. IDU is potentially very toxic when administered parenterally, mainly because of its capacity to affect rapidly proliferating cells. Calabresi *et al.* (1961) observed leucopenia, stomatitis and alopecia when the drug was administered intravenously in high doses. Other side-effects include anorexia, nausea, vomiting, diarrhoea, glossitis, bone marrow depression including thrombocytopenia, abnormal liver function tests, jaundice, gastro-intestinal haemorrhage and loss of finger nails. Severe side-effects have also been observed in patients receiving IDU in the recommended dose of 100 mg per kg per day (Boston and NIAID Studies, 1975). Patients developed severe myelosuppression evidenced by leucopenia, thrombocytopenia and a falling haematocrit and some had liver function abnormalities. These side-effects predisposed to life-threatening infections and haemorrhagic complications in a number of patients. The dangers of such dose schedules had been recognized previously (Nolan *et al.*, 1973), who recommended that a safe dosage was 54 mg per kg per day for five days and the total dose given should never exceed 20 g. IDU tends to be concentrated in rapidly dividing cells and therefore it should not be used in pregnancy. The drug does not appear to be immunosuppressive (Sloan *et al.*, 1969).

Clinical Uses of the Drug

1. *Ocular keratitis*. Topical idoxuridine is an accepted form of treatment for keratitis due to Herpesvirus hominis and Vaccinia virus. It is particularly useful for acute dendritic ulcers, but is of no proven value for deep stromal ulcers. In such cases of stromal keratitis or keratouveitis, topical adenine arabinoside is preferable (Pavan-Langston, 1975) (*see* page 950). IDU is of no value for adenoviral keratoconjunctivitis, but it may be effective for herpes zoster keratitis (Pavan-Langston and McCulley, 1973). In these diseases the rapid synthesis of viral DNA in the superficial part of the cornea is more sensitive to IDU than DNA in the slowly proliferating corneal cells.

Idoxuridine is not the only form of treatment of ocular keratitis and in certain circumstances, cautery or other measures may be indicated (Juel-Jensen and MacCallum, 1972). Several controlled studies have shown the value of IDU in Herpesvirus hominis keratitis (Patterson *et al.*, 1963; Laibson and Leopold, 1964), but some authors consider it has no advantage over cautery (Jones, 1967). Prophylactic instillation of IDU into the eye may be indicated if herpes lesions are adjacent to the eye, and sometimes when topical corticosteroids are used in the eye for other purposes. Herpesvirus hominis strains may become resistant to idoxuridine *in vitro* and *in vivo* (Schabel and Montgomery, 1972), and this may explain the failure of this drug in the treatment of recurrent Herpesvirus hominis keratitis.

2. *Herpesvirus infections of the skin and mucous membranes*.
   (a) *Herpesvirus hominis lesions*. Initial controlled trials with IDU creams for the treatment of cutaneous Herpesvirus hominis infections (cold sores) were disappointing (Burnett and Katz, 1963; Juel-Jensen and MacCallum, 1964). The main reason for these failures seemed to be the insolubility of IDU and its inability in dilute solution to penetrate the skin. After a series of experiments in humans and animals, Juel-Jensen and MacCallum (1972) concluded that the best way to use IDU for the treatment of cutaneous lesions was to apply it as a 5 per cent solution in indiluted dimethyl sulphoxide (DMSO). This solution is stable for long periods but at low temperatures the idoxuridine may crystallize out. When this preparation was painted onto recurrent cold sores of recent onset, three times a day for three days, there was significant shortening of the duration of lesions (MacCallum and Juel-Jensen, 1966). In addition, recurrences at the same site became rare, but treated patients tended to get recurrences later at new sites (Dawber, 1972). More recently topical IDU in DMSO was compared to DMSO alone to treat recurrent genital herpes (Parker, 1977). Lesions treated with 20 per cent IDU healed more rapidly and shed virus for a shorter period than those treated with 5 per cent IDU, but the latter was still superior to the control.

   Other authorities are not convinced of the value of IDU for the treatment of cutaneous Herpesvirus hominis lesions (Weinstein and Chang, 1973). This form of treatment is not widely used or advocated in Australia, because these lesions are usually mild and self-limiting. There may be a place for topical IDU in the treatment of severe recurrent lesions.

Idoxuridine has also been used to treat Herpesvirus hominis stomatitis. Juel-Jensen and MacCallum (1972) claim that a 5 per cent solution in orabase (which adheres to the mucosa) is useful. They have also used 40 per cent IDU in DMSO painted onto the lesions, but patients may not tolerate the unpleasant taste of DMSO. Jaffe and Lehner (1968) showed an increased rate of healing when 0·1 per cent IDU was regularly painted onto mouth lesions, but the treatment schedule was cumbersome.

Herpetic whitlows have been treated by the continuous application of 40 per cent IDU in DMSO (Juel-Jensen and MacCallum, 1972). Genital Herpesvirus hominis lesions have also been managed by a similar regimen but type 2 virus infections are more resistant to treatment than type 1 virus infections (Juel-Jensen, 1973).

(b) *Herpes zoster.* Topical idoxuridine, applied continuously as a 40 per cent solution in DMSO has also been used in shingles (Juel-Jensen *et al.*, 1970). These authors showed that healing was accelerated and pain was relieved more rapidly by this treatment. Beneficial results in herpes zoster were also obtained using four-hourly applications of 5 per cent IDU in 100 per cent DMSO (Dawber, 1974), but Juel-Jensen and MacCallum (1974) maintain that a 35 or 40 per cent solution is more effective.

All of these uses of IDU may be indicated on occasions. However, cutaneous lesions of herpes zoster infections (and also those due to Herpesvirus hominis) vary considerably in severity and are usually self-limiting. Therefore it is unrealistic to advocate the use of IDU for all patients with these diseases, particularly since the frequent use of the drug may cause allergic contact dermatitis (*vide supra*).

3. *Herpesvirus hominis encephalitis.* The observation that patients receiving intravenous IDU for malignant disease were often resistant to infection with Vaccinia virus (Calabresi, 1965) suggested that systemic IDU may be useful for serious viral infections in man. Numerous cases have been described ascribing a beneficial action of IDU in Herpesvirus hominis encephalitis (Breeden *et al.*, 1966; Juel-Jensen and MacCallum, 1972; Rappel, 1973). Until comparatively recently it was considered that IDU may increase survival rate in this disease (Leading article, 1972; Jeul-Jensen and MacCallum, 1972). More critical appraisals of the value of IDU have since suggested that this treatment may not be superior to other forms of treatment (Upton, 1972; Rappel, 1973; Longson, 1977). There are many biases and difficulties in assessing the value of IDU (and other antiviral drugs) by retrospective studies (Rappel, 1973; Longson, 1977). Herpesvirus hominis is a common cause of sporadic encephalitis but the true incidence and the natural history of the disease are unknown. Undoubtedly many of the patients treated unsuccessfully with IDU have not been reported. The mortality of untreated patients is in the vicinity of 50–75 per cent, but these figures are probably biased because severe cases are admitted to hospital and the diagnosis is probably overlooked in milder forms of this disease. In addition, assessment by mortality alone may not be a true indication of the value of treatment, because survival time and the frequency of sequelae must be considered. There has been considerable difficulty in making comparisons between the results of published cases because of the

variety of IDU dosage schedules used. A number of reports suggested that the earlier treatment with IDU is instigated, the more favourable the result. This has theoretical appeal because if viral multiplication can be prevented early, recovery may occur, but complete recovery is unlikely when haemorrhagic necrosis of large areas of the brain has developed. Alternatively the beneficial effects of early instigation of treatment may be because milder cases are being treated. There is the additional difficulty of making an early diagnosis of Herpesvirus hominis encephalitis (Leading article, 1972). This usually involves brain biopsy, an investigation not without risk and which is difficult to advocate for patients with an early central nervous system infection.

In 1971 and 1972, two double-blind, placebo controlled, multicentre studies were commenced independently, to evaluate the use of parenteral IDU in patients with Herpesvirus hominis encephalitis, confirmed by brain biopsy (Boston and NIAID Studies, 1975). Both of these trials were terminated prematurely in 1973. In a number of patients receiving the drug there was histological evidence of continuing necrotizing encephalitis and no diminution in the amount of virus present in post-mortem brain tissue. In some patients side-effects due to IDU (*see* page 933) contributed to their death. In view of the results of these studies, which failed to show an antiviral effect of IDU, and which were associated with unacceptable side-effects of the drug, it is doubtful whether parenteral IDU can ever be justifiably used again in human viral infections.

4. *Cytomegalovirus and disseminated Herpesvirus hominis infections.* Parenteral IDU has been used for the treatment of Cytomegalovirus infections (Conchie *et al.*, 1968; Barton and Tobin, 1970) and disseminated Herpesvirus hominis infection of the newborn (Partridge and Millis, 1968; Tuffli and Nahmias, 1969; Golden *et al.*, 1969). It was also advocated for the treatment of disseminated Herpesvirus hominis infections in compromised hosts (Nahmias, 1970). In view of the experiences using IDU in Herpesvirus hominis encephalitis (*vide supra*), the parenteral use of IDU for these diseases is contraindicated.

REFERENCES

Amon, R. B. and Hanifin, J. M. (1976), 'Allergic contact dermatitis due to idoxuridine', *New Engl. J. Med.*, **294**, 956.

Barton, B. W. and Tobin, J. O'H. (1970), 'The effect of idoxuridine on the excretion of cytomegalovirus in congenital infection', *Ann. N.Y. Acad. Sci.*, **173**, 90.

Boston Interhospital Virus Study Group and the NIAID-Sponsored Cooperative Antiviral Clinical Study (1975), 'Failure of high dose 5-iodo-2'-deoxyuridine in the therapy of Herpes simplex virus encephalitis. Evidence of unacceptable toxicity', *New Engl. J. Med.*, **292**, 600.

Breeden, C. J., Hall, T. C. and Tyler, H. R. (1966), 'Herpes simplex encephalitis treated with systemic 5-iodo-2'-deoxyuridine', *Ann. Intern. Med.*, **65**, 1050.

Burnett, J. W. and Katz, S. L. (1963), 'A study of the use of 5-iodo-2'-deoxyuridine in cutaneous Herpes simplex', *J. Invest. Derm.*, **40**, 7.

Calabresi, P., Cardosa, S. S., Finch, S. C., Kligerman, M. M., von Essen, C. F., Chu, M. Y. and Welch, A. D. (1961), 'Initial clinical studies with 5-iodo-2'-deoxyuridine', *Cancer Res.*, **21**, 550.

Calabresi, P. (1963), 'Current studies of clinical investigations with 6-azauridine, 5-

iodo-2′-deoxyuridine, and related derivatives', *Cancer Res.,* **23,** 1260.

Calabresi, P. (1965), 'Clinical studies with systemic administration of antimetabolites of pyrimidine nucleosides in viral infections', *Ann. N.Y. Acad. Sci.,* **130,** 192.

Cho, C. T., Liu, C., Voth, D. W. and Feng, K. K. (1973), 'Effects of idoxuridine on Herpesvirus hominis encephalitis and disseminated infections in marmosets', *J. Infect. Dis.,* **128,** 718.

Clarkson, D. R., Oppelt, W. W. and Byvoet, P. (1967), 'The fate of 5-iodo-2′-deoxyuridine (IUdR) in plasma and cerebrospinal fluid of dogs', *J. Pharmacol. Exp. Ther.,* **157,** 581.

Conchie, A. F., Barton, B. W. and Tobin, J. O'H. (1968), 'Congenital cytomegalovirus infection treated with idoxuridine', *Brit. med. J.,* **4,** 162.

Dawber, R. P. R. (1972), 'Idoxuridine and erythema multiforme after Herpes simplex', *Brit. med. J.,* **4,** 300.

Dawber, R. (1974), 'Idoxuridine in herpes zoster: Further evaluation of intermittent topical therapy', *Brit. med. J.,* **2,** 526.

De Clercq, E., Luczak, M., Shugar, D., Torrence, P. F., Waters, J. A. and Witkop, B. (1976), 'Effect of cytosine arabinoside, iododeoxyuridine, ethyldeoxyuridine, thiocyanatodeoxyuridine, and rivavirin on tail lesion formation in mice infected with Vaccinia virus (39241)', *Proc. Soc. Exp. Biol. Med.,* **151,** 487.

Golden, B., Bell, W. E. and McKee, A. P. (1969), 'Disseminated herpes simplex with encephalitis in a neonate. Treatment with idoxuridine', *JAMA,* **209,** 1219.

Green, J. and Staal, S. (1976), 'Questionable dermatologic use of iododeoxyuridine', *New Engl. J. Med.,* **295,** 111.

Herrmann, E. C., Jr. (1961), 'Plaque inhibition test for detection of specific inhibitors of DNA containing viruses', *Proc. Soc. Exp. Biol. Med. (N.Y.),* **107,** 142.

Jaffe, E. C. and Lehner, T. (1968), 'Treatment of herpetic stomatitis with idoxuridine', *Brit. Dent. J.,* **124,** 392.

Jones, B. R. (1967), 'Prospects in treating viral disease of the eye', *Trans. Ophthal. Soc. (U.K.),* **87,** 537.

Juel-Jensen, B. E. and MacCallum, F. O. (1964), 'Treatment of Herpes simplex lesions of the face with idoxuridine: Results of a double-blind controlled trial', *Brit. med. J.,* **2,** 987.

Juel-Jensen, B. E., MacCallum, F. O., Mackenzie, A. M. R. and Pike, M. C. (1970), 'Treatment of zoster with idoxuridine in dimethyl sulphoxide. Results of two double-blind controlled trials', *Brit. med. J.,* **4,** 776.

Juel-Jensen, B. E. and MacCallum, F. O. (1972), *Herpes Simplex, Varicella and Zoster. Clinical Manifestations and Treatment,* London, William Heinemann Ltd.

Juel-Jensen, B. E. (1973), 'Herpes simplex and zoster', *Brit. med. J.,,* **1,** 406.

Juel-Jensen, B. E. and MacCallum, F. O. (1974), 'Idoxuridine in herpes zoster', *Brit. med. J.,,* **3,** 41.

Kaufman, H. E. (1962), 'Clinical cure of Herpes simplex keratitis by 5-iodo-2′-deoxyuridine', *Proc. Soc. Exp. Biol. Med. (N.Y.),* **109,** 251.

Kaufman, H. E. (1963), 'Chemotherapy of virus disease', *Chemotherapia,* **7,** 1.

Kern, E. R., Overall, J. C., Jr. and Glasgow, L. A. (1973), 'Herpesvirus hominis infection in newborn mice. 1. An experimental model and therapy with iododeoxyuridine', *J. Infect. Dis.,* **128,** 290.

Laibson, P. R. and Leopold, I. H. (1964), 'An evaluation of double-blind IDU therapy in 100 cases of herpetic keratitis', *Trans. Amer. Acad. Ophthal. Otolaryng.,* **68,** 22.

Leading Article (1972), 'Herpes encephalitis', *Brit. med. J.,* **1,** 582.

Lerner, A. M. and Bailey, E. J. (1972), 'Concentrations of idoxuridine in serum, urine and cerebrospinal fluid of patients with suspected diagnoses of Herpesvirus hominis enchephalitis', *J. Clin. Invest.,* **51,** 45.

Lauter, C. B., Bailey, E. J. and Lerner, A. M. (1975), 'Absence of idoxuridine and persistence of Herpes simplex virus in brains of patients being treated for encephalitis

(38966)', *Proc. Soc. Exp. Biol. Med.*, **150,** 23.

Lefkowitz, E., Worthington, M., Conliffe, McG. A. and Baron, S. (1976), 'Comparative effectiveness of six antiviral agents in Herpes simplex type 1 infection of mice (39392)', *Proc. Soc. Exp. Biol. Med.*, **152,** 337.

Longson, M. (1977), 'The treatment of Herpes encephalitis', *J. Antimicrob. Chemother.* (Suppl. A), **3,** 115.

MacCallum, F. O. and Juel-Jensen, B. E. (1966), 'Herpes simplex virus skin infection in man treated with idoxuridine in dimethyl sulphoxide. Results of double-blind controlled trial', *Brit. med. J.*, **2,** 805.

Marks, M. I. (1974), 'Variables influencing the *in vitro* susceptibilities of Herpes simplex viruses to antiviral drugs', *Antimicrob. Ag. Chemother.*, **6,** 34.

Marks, M. I. (1975), 'Evaluation of four antiviral agents in the treatment of Herpes simplex encephalitis in a rat model', *J. Infect. Dis.*, **131,** 11.

Nahmias, A. J. (1970), 'Disseminated herpes simplex virus infection', *New Engl. J. Med.*, **282,** 684.

Nolan, D. C., Lauter, C. B. and Lerner, A. M. (1973), 'Idoxuridine in herpes simplex virus (type 1) encephalitis. Experience with 29 cases in Michigan, 1966 to 1971', *Ann. Intern. Med.*, **78,** 243.

Parker, J. D. (1977), 'A double-blind trial of idoxuridine in recurrent genital herpes', *J. Antimicrob. Chemother.* (Suppl. A), **3,** 131.

Partridge, J. W. and Millis, R. R. (1968), 'Systemic herpes simplex infection in a newborn treated with intravenous idoxuridine', *Arch. Dis. Child.*, **43,** 377.

Patterson, A., Fox, A. D., Davies, G., Maguire, C., Holmes Sellers, P. J., Wright, P., Rice, N. S. C., Cobb, B. and Jones, B. R. (1963), 'Controlled studies of IDU in the treatment of herpetic keratitis', *Trans. ophthal. Soc.*, **83,** 583.

Pavan-Langston, D. and McCulley, J. P. (1973), 'Herpes zoster dendritic keratitis', *Arch. Ophthalmol.*, **89,** 25.

Pavan-Langston, D. (1975), 'Clinical evaluation of adenine arabinoside and idoxuridine in the treatment of ocular Herpes simplex', *Am. J. Ophthalmol.*, **80,** 495.

Percy, D. H. and Hatch, L. A. (1975), 'Experimental infection with Herpes simplex virus type 2 in newborn rats: Effects of treatment with iododeoxyuridine and cutosine arabinoside', *J. Infect. Dis.*, **132,** 256.

Plummer, G. and Ingerson, A. P. (1974), 'Iododeoxyuridine and Herpes-viral encephalitis: lack of inhibitory action against low-grade viral replication', *Antimicrob. Ag. Chemother.*, **5,** 672.

Prusoff, W. H. (1959), 'Synthesis and biological activities of iododeoxyuridine, an analogue of thymidine', *Biochem. biophys. Acta*, **32,** 295.

Rappel, M. (1973), 'The management of acute necrotizing encephalitis: A review of 369 cases', *Postgrad. Med. J.*, **49,** 419.

Renis, H. E. and Buthala, D. A. (1965), 'Development of resistance to antiviral drugs', *Ann. N.Y. Acad. Sci.*, **130,** 343.

Schabel, F. M., Jr. and Montgomery, J. A. (1972), Purines and pyrimidines, International Encyclopedia of Pharmacology and Therapeutics. Section 61. Chemotherapy of Virus Diseases. Vol. 1. New York, Pergamon Press, p. 231.

Sloan, B. J., Miller, F. A., Ehrlich, J., McLean, I. W. and Machamer, H. E. (1969), 'Antiviral activity of 9-β-D-arabinofuranosyladenine. iv. Activity against intracerebral herpes simplex virus infections in mice', *Antimicrob. Agents and Chemother.*—1968, p. 161.

Steffenhagen, K. A., Easterday, B. C. and Galasso, G. J. (1976), 'Evaluation of 6-azauridine and 5-iododeoxyuridine in the treatment of experimental viral infections', *J. Infect. Dis.*, **133,** 603.

Tokumaru, T. (1967), 'The protective effect of different immunoglobulins against herpetic encephalitis and skin infections in guinea pigs', *Arch. Gesamte Virusforsch.*, **22,** 332.

Tomlinson, A. H. and MacCallum, F. O. (1970), 'The effect of iododeoxyuridine on Herpes simplex virus encephalitis in animals and man', *Ann. N.Y. Acad. Sci.*, **173,** 20.

Tuffli, G. A. and Nahmias, A. J. (1969), 'Neonatal herpetic infection. Report of two premature infants treated with systemic use of idoxuridine', *Amer. J. Dis. Child.*, **118,** 909.

Upton, A. R. M. (1972), 'Herpes encephalitis', *Brit. med. J.*, **2,** 226.

Weinstein, L. and Chang, T. W. (1973), 'The chemotherapy of viral infections', *New Engl. J. Med.*, **289,** 725.

Cytarabine

Description

Cytarabine (cytosine arabinoside; 1-beta-D-arabinofuranosylcytosine; CA: Ara-C), similar to idoxuridine (page 931), is another pyrimidine nucleoside analogue. It differs from the normal nucleosides cytidine and deoxycytidine in that the sugar moiety is arabinose and not ribose or deoxyribose. Cytarabine was synthetized in 1959 (Walwick *et al.*, 1959) and originally introduced for the treatment of leukaemia, for which it is still used. Because of its action of interfering with pyrimidine synthesis, it was thought that it may be useful for the treatment of DNA virus infections. Cytarabine is marketed with the trade name of 'Cytosar' (Upjohn).

Antiviral Activity

Cytarabine has a similar antiviral spectrum to idoxuridine (page 931), being active in tissue culture against Vaccinia virus, Herpesvirus hominis, Herpesvirus varicellae and Cytomegalovirus (Underwood *et al.*, 1964; Buthala, 1964; Rapp, 1964). *In vitro*, cytarabine is a more effective inhibitor of Herpesvirus hominis types 1 and 2, Herpesvirus varicellae and Cytamegalovirus, than adenine arabinoside (page 947) and idoxuridine (page 931) (Walker *et al.*, 1971; Fiala *et al.*, 1972; Fiala *et al.*, 1974; Collins and Bauer, 1977). Similar to idoxuridine (page 931) a number of factors influence the *in vitro* susceptibility of a virus to this drug (Marks, 1974). Studies in tissue culture, showing that the therapeutic to toxic ratio of the drug approaches one, has cast doubts about its likely value in human infections (Lauter *et al.*, 1974).

The results following the use of cytarabine to treat various virus infections in experimental animals, have in general been disappointing (Tomlinson and MacCallum, 1973; Percy and Hatch, 1975; Marks, 1975; De Clercq *et al.*, 1976; Kelsey *et al.*, 1976) and in one study its use seemed to potentiate infection (Lefkowitz *et al.*, 1976).

Mode of Administration and Dosage

Because cytarabine is rapidly metabolized by both liver and intestines, it is always administered parenterally, usually by the intravenous route. After a single high intravenous dose, serum levels rapidly fall and become immeasurable in most patients within 15 min. This is because cytarabine is rapidly deaminated by an enzyme (cytidine deaminase), particularly in the liver and kidney, to the relatively inactive metabolite, arabinofuranosyl uracil (Kremer, 1975). Most of an intravenously administered dose (80 per cent) is excreted in

940

the urine within 24 h, mainly as the inactive metabolite. Active drug persists longer after intrathecal administration (half-life 2 h) because of low deaminase activity in the brain and CSF. If cytarabine is given by continuous infusion over a 2 h period, the CSF concentration is about 40 per cent of the simultaneous serum level (Ho and Frei, 1971).

The dosage schedules which have been used to treat Herpesvirus infections in humans have varied considerably. Some authors recommended that the daily dose should be given by rapid intravenous infusion (Juel-Jensen and MacCallum, 1972), whilst others preferred continuous infusion (Foerster and Hryniuk, 1971). Rapid intravenous administration was recommended to prevent inactivation by plasma enzymes before the drug reaches its target. Doses of 3–10 mg per kg per day or as expressed in many published reports 10–200 mg per square metre (m^2) body surface per day have been used for periods from one to seven days (Weinstein and Chang, 1973). Hryniuk et al. (1972) recommended a dose of 10–40 mg per m^2 per day because only mild myelotoxic effects were produced; they also used additional intrathecal therapy in a dose of 10 mg per m^2 in some cases of encephalitis.

Mode of Action

Cytarabine appears to inhibit the synthesis of DNA, by inhibiting the reduction of cytidilic acid to deoxycytidilic acid, thereby depleting the pool of phosphorylated derivatives of deoxycytidine available for incorporation into DNA (Cardeilhac and Cohen, 1965). It may also be partly incorporated into DNA and its phosphylated products may inhibit DNA polymerase (Goldenberg et al., 1968). Its action may be reversed by providing a competing concentration of deoxycytidine (Hirschman et al., 1969).

Toxicity

Side-effects following the intravenous use of cytarabine include nausea, vomiting, megaloblastosis, marrow depression (leucopenia, anaemia and thrombocytopenia), renal and hepatic damage, fever, rashes and stomatitis. Bone marrow depression is related to the dose and duration of treatment and thrombocytopenia is often the first sign of marrow damage (Geary, 1973). The drug should be used cautiously in patients with liver disease because a substantial amount of cytarabine is deaminated in the liver. Cytarabine also has potent humoral and cellular immuno-suppressive properties (Gray, 1973). It should not be used in pregnant patients.

Clinical Uses of the Drug

1. *Herpesvirus hominis keratitis*. Cytarabine has been used topically as a 5 per cent solution for this disease and is as effective as idoxuridine (Kaufman and Maloney, 1963). However, repeated instillation of a 0·5 or 1 per cent solution into the eyes causes a reversible speckling of the cornea due to distortion of the corneal epithelium (Elliot and Schut, 1965). For this reason either topical idoxuridine (page 934) or topical adenine arabinoside (page 950) is preferred for the treatment of Herpesvirus hominis keratitis.

2. *Herpesvirus hominis encephalitis*. A number of case reports suggested that cytarabine may be effective in this disease (Longson and Beswick 1971; Juel-Jensen and MacCallum, 1972; McAuley and Glasgow, 1974; Lagerkvist and Ekelund, 1975). Subsequently more critical reviews of published cases failed to show that this drug was of any value in this disease (Rappel, 1973; Longson, 1977). Because cytarabine is toxic to the immune and myeloid systems when used in the therapeutic doses required, it is doubtful whether it should ever be advocated for the treatment of any herpetic infection in humans (Alford and Whitley, 1976). This is based on observations that it not only has failed to be of value in some herpetic infections, but it also seems to potentiate them, particularly in immunosuppressed patients (*vide infra*). Longson (1977) has pointed out that the situation in herpes encephalitis is different because patients with this disease are not usually immuno-compromised. In addition if cytarabine is given by a daily rapid intravenous injection, even in high doses for five days, to a non-comprised patient, its toxic effects are only transient. However, the value of cytarabine in this disease is uncertain, and controlled trials are needed for its evaluation. Such a trial was begun in the United Kingdom in 1975 (*Lancet*, 1975) and cytarabine was not proven to be of any value in the treatment of herpes encephalitis (Longson, 1978).

3. *Other Herpesvirus hominis infections*. There have been reports suggesting that cytarabine has been beneficial in Herpesvirus hominis stomatitis, eczema herpeticum, genital herpes and generalized infections (Juel-Jensen and MacCallum, 1972; Hryniuk *et al.*, 1972). Studies by Juel-Jensen (1977) have indicated that cytarabine, administered in a non-toxic dose by rapid intravenous infusion, may reduce the duration of virus shedding in Herpesvirus hominis infections. Nevertheless, similar to Herpes encephalitis, the value of the drug in these conditions has not been proven, and potential dangers should preclude its use.

4. *Herpesvirus varicellae infections*. Cytarabine has been used in immunologically compromised hosts to treat varicella-zoster infections, which in these circumstances are sometimes fatal. Similar to the other herpetic infections described above, a series of favourable case reports, without evidence from controlled studies, was the basis for advocating cytarabine for these infections (McKelvey and Kwaan, 1969; Hall *et al.*, 1969; Hryniuk *et al.*, 1972; Juel-Jensen and MacCallum, 1972; Fortuny *et al.*, 1973; Pierce and Jenkins, 1973; Baron and Wechsler, 1975). Subsequently reports appeared which cast doubt on the value of cytarabine in preventing disseminated varicella-zoster infection in compromised hosts (Wilfert, 1971; Stevens *et al.*, 1972; Stevens and Merigan, 1972; Davis *et al.*, 1973). Of particular significance was a controlled trial conducted by Stevens *et al.* (1973) to assess the value of cytarabine in preventing disseminated varicella-zoster infections in patients with underlying cancer. Treatment was commenced within 48 h of the onset of dissemination, in a dose which produced inhibitory concentrations of the drug in the serum against Herpesvirus varicellae. There was greater dissemination in treated patients who also had depressed antibody formation, delay in vesicle interferon production, depression of local cellular response and greater haematological toxicity. The authors concluded that cytarabine prolongs disseminated varicella-zoster infections by further depressing host responses. In another controlled trial in which cytarabine was administered in a lower non-toxic dosage

to patients with cancer, it was of no value in localized Herpes zoster and it also failed to prevent dissemination of this disease (Schimpff et al., 1974). Cytarabine administered by the subcutaneous route to patients with localized Herpes zoster was also without benefit (Betts et al., 1975). Subcutaneous administration was chosen, amongst other reasons, because the pharmacology of the drug after this method of administration is similar to that resulting from rapid intravenous infusion (page 940). Also the serum levels reached after subcutaneous administration, exceed those necessary to inhibit Herpesvirus varicellae in vitro.

As a result of these controlled studies, it can now be concluded that cytarabine is of no benefit in the treatment of Herpesvirus varicellae infections.

5. *Cytomegalovirus infections.* In some reports clinical benefit has been attributed to the use of cytarabine in these infections (Plotkin and Stetler, 1970; Kraybill et al., 1972; McCracken and Luby, 1972). This has not been confirmed by controlled trials and the use of the drug should be discouraged because of possible potentiation of the infection.

6. *Smallpox.* Uncontrolled studies of the use of cytarabine in patients with variola major in Bangladesh appeared encouraging (Houssain et al., 1972). Subsequently a controlled trial conducted in that country failed to reveal any benefit in variola major from treatment with cytarabine; the mortality in the treated patients appeared to be higher than in those who were not treated (Monsur et al., 1975). These authors suggested that the drug lowered resistance to infection either by suppressing granulocytes or by interfering with other immune mechanisms. A small double-blind study on the effects of cytarabine in the treatment of Ethiopian patients with smallpox also showed that this disease is unaffected by such treatment (Dennis et al., 1974).

REFERENCES

Alford, C. A., Jr. and Whitley, R. J. (1976), 'Treatment of infections due to Herpesvirus in humans: A critical review of the state of the art', *J. Infect. Dis.* (Suppl.), **133**, 101.

Baron, M. and Wechsler, H. L. (1975), 'Low-dosage cytarabine therapy for herpes zoster with pneumonia', *Arch. Dermatol.*, **111**, 910.

Betts, R. F., Zaky, D. A., Douglas, R. G., Jr. and Royer, G. (1975), 'Ineffectiveness of subcutaneous cytosine arabinoside in localized herpes zoster', *Ann. Intern. Med.*, **82**, 778.

Buthala, D. A. (1964), 'Cell culture studies on antiviral agents. 1. Action of cytosine arabinoside and some comparisons with 5-iodo-2'-deoxyuridine', *Proc. Soc. Exper. Biol. and Med.*, **115**, 69.

Cardeilhac, P. T. and Cohen, S. S. (1965), 'Some metabolic properties of nucleotides of 1-beta-d-arabinofuranosylcytosine', *Cancer Res.*, **24**, 1595.

Collins, P. and Bauer, D. J. (1977), 'Comparison of activity of Herpes virus inhibitors', *J. Antimicrob. Chemother.* (Suppl. A), **3**, 73.

Davis, C. M., van Dersarl, J. V. and Coltman, C. A. (1973), 'Failure of cytarabine in varicella-zoster infections', *JAMA*, **224**, 122.

De Clercq, E., Luczak, M., Shugar, D., Torrence, P. F., Waters, J. A. and Witkop, B. (1976), 'Effect of cytosine arabinoside, iododeoxyuridine, ethyldeoxyuridine, thiocyanatodeoxyuridine, and ridavirin on tail lesion formation in mice infected with vaccinia virus (39241)', *Proc. Soc. Exp. Biol. Med.*, **151**, 487.

Dennis, D. T., Doberstyn, E. B., Awoke, S., Royer, G. L., Jr. and Renis, H. E. (1974), 'Failure of cytosine arabinoside in treating smallpox', *Lancet*, **2**, 377.

Elliot, G. A. and Schut, A. L. (1965), 'Studies with cytarabine HCl (CA) in normal eyes of man, monkey and rabbit', *Amer. J. Ophthol.*, **60**, 1074.

Fiala, M., Chow, A. and Guze, L. B. (1972), 'Susceptibility of Herpesviruses to cytosine arabinoside: Standardization of susceptibility test procedure and relative resistance of Herpes simplex type 2 strains', *Antimicrob. Ag. Chemother.*—1971, p. 354.

Fiala, M., Chow, A. W., Miyasaki, K. and Guze, L. B. (1974), 'Susceptibility of Herpesviruses to three nucleoside analogues and their combinations and enchancement of the antiviral effect at acid pH', *J. Infect. Dis.*, **129**, 82.

Foerster, J. and Hryniuk, W. (1971), 'Cytosine arabinoside and herpes zoster', *Lancet*, **2**, 712.

Fortuny, I. E., Weiss, R., Theologides, A. and Kennedy, B. J. (1973), 'Cytosine arabinoside in herpes zoster', *Lancet*, **1**, 38.

Geary, C. G. (1973), 'Haematological complications of therapy with pyrimidine analogues', *Postgrad. Med. J.*, **49**, 413.

Goldenberg, D. M., Biro, V., Elster, K., Schriker, K. T. and Sögtrop, H. H. (1968), 'Laboratory studies on the pharmacology, toxicology and antitumour action of cytosine arabinoside', *Arzneimittel-Forschung 19 Beiheft*, 31.

Gray, G. D. (1973), 'The immunosuppressive activity of ara-C (cytarabine) and derivatives', *Transplant Proc.* **5**, 1203.

Hall, T. C., Wilfert, C., Jaffe, N., Traggis, D., Lux, S., Rompf, P. and Katz, S. (1969), 'Treatment of varicella-zoster with cytosine arabinoside', *Trans. Am. Assoc. Physicians*, **82**, 201.

Henderson, D. A. (1974), Chief Smallpox Eradication Unit, WHO, Geneva, Personal Communication.

Hirschman, S. Z., Fischinger, P. J., Zaccari, J. J. and O'Connor, T. E. (1969), 'Effect of cytosine arabinoside on the replication of the Moloney sarcoma virus in 3T3 cell cultures', *J. Nat. Cancer Inst.*, **42**, 399.

Ho, D. H. W. and Frei, E. (1971), 'Clinical pharmacology of 1-β-D-arabinofuranosyl cytosine', *Clin. Pharmacol. Ther.*, **12**, 944.

Hossain, M. S., Foerster, J., Hryniuk, W., Israels, L. G., Chowdhury, A. S. and Biswas, M. K. (1972), 'Treatment of smallpox with cytosine arabinoside', *Lancet*, **2**, 1230.

Hryniuk, W., Foerster, J., Shojania, M. and Chow, A. (1972), 'Cytarabine for Herpesvirus infections', *JAMA*, **219**, 715.

Juel-Jensen, B. E. and MacCallum, F. O. (1972), *Herpes Simplex, Varicella and Zoster. Clinical Manifestations and Treatment*. London, William Heinemann Ltd.

Jeul-Jensen, B. (1977), 'Effects of cytarabine on virus shedding in Herpes simplex virus infections', *J. Antimicrob. Chemother.* (Suppl. A), **3**, 125.

Kaufman, H. E. and Maloney, E. D. (1963), 'IDU and cytosine arabinoside in experimental herpetic keratitis', *Arch. Ophthal.*, **69**, 626.

Kelsey, D. K., Kern, E. R., Overall, J. C., Jr. and Glasgow, L. A. (1976), 'Effect of cytosine arabinoside and 5-iodo-2'-deoxyuridine on a cytomegalovirus infection in newborn mice', *Antimicrob. Ag. Chemother.*, **9**, 458.

Kraybill, E. N., Sever, J. L., Avery, G. B. and Movassaghi, N. (1972), 'Experimental use of cytosine arabinoside in congenital cytomegalovirus infection', *J. Pediatrics*, **80**, 485.

Kremer, W. B. (1975), 'Cytarabine', *Ann. Intern. Med.*, **82**, 684.

Lagerkvist, B. and Ekelund, H. (1975), 'Cytarabine treatment of Herpes simplex encephalitis in infants and small children', *Scand. J. Infect. Dis.*, **7**, 81.

Lancet (1975), 'Cytarabine in Herpes encephalitis', **1**, 815.

Lauter, C. B., Bailey, E. J. and Lerner, A. M. (1974), 'Assessment of cytosine arabinoside as an antiviral agent in humans', *Antimicrob. Ag. Chemother.*, **6**, 598.

Lefkowitz, E., Worthington, M., Conliffe, McG. A. and Baron, S. (1976), 'Comparative effectiveness of six antiviral agents in Herpes simplex type 1 infection of mice (39392)', *Proc. Soc. Exp. Biol. Med.*, **152**, 337.

Longson, M. and Beswick, T. S. L. (1971), 'Dexamethasone treatment in Herpes-simplex encephalitis', *Lancet*, **1**, 749.

Longson, M. (1977), 'The treatment of Herpes encephalitis', *J. Antimicrob. Chemother.* (Suppl. A), **3**, 115.

Longson, M. (1978), Personal communication.

Marks, M. I. (1974), 'Variables influencing the *in vitro* susceptibilities of Herpes simplex viruses to antiviral drugs', *Antimicrob. Ag. Chemother.*, **6**, 34.

Marks, M. I. (1975), 'Evaluation of four antiviral agents in the treatment of Herpes simplex encephalitis in a rat model', *J. Infect. Dis.*, **131**, 11.

McAuley, D. L. and Glasgow, G. L. (1974), 'Herpes simplex virus encephalitis treatment with cytosine arabinoside', *Aust. N.Z. J. Med.*, **4**, 274.

McCracken, G. H., Jr. and Luby, J. P. (1972), 'Cytosine arabinoside in the treatment of congenital cytomegalic inclusion disease', *J. Pediatrics*, **80**, 488.

McKelvey, E. M. and Kwaan, H. C. (1969), 'Cytosine arabinoside therapy for disseminated herpes zoster in a patient with IgG pyroglobulinemia', *Blood*, **34**, 706.

Monsur, K. A., Hossain, M. S., Huq, F., Rahaman, M. M. and Haque, M. Q. (1975), 'Treatment of variola major with cytosine arabinoside', *J. Infect. Dis.*, **131**, 40.

Percy, D. H. and Hatch, L. A. (1975), 'Experimental infection with Herpes simplex virus type 2 in newborn rats: Effects of treatment with iododeoxyuridine and cytosine arabinoside', *J. Infect. Dis.*, **132**, 256.

Pierce, L. E. and Jenkins, R. B. (1973), 'Herpes zoster ophthalmicus treated with cytarabine', *Arch. Ophthalmol.*, **89**, 21.

Pierce, L. E. (1974), 'Cytosine arabinoside for herpes zoster', *New Engl. J. Med.*, **290**, 409.

Plotkin, S. A. and Stetler, H. (1970), 'Treatment of congenital cytomegalic inclusion disease with antiviral agents', *Antimicrob. Ag. Chemother.*—1969, p. 372.

Rapp, F. (1964), 'Inhibition by metabolic analogues of plaque formation by herpes zoster and Herpes simplex viruses', *J. Immunol.*, **93**, 643.

Rappel, M. (1973), 'The management of acute necrotizing encephaltis: A review of 369 cases', *Postgrad. Med. J.*, **49**, 419.

Renis, H. E. and Buthala, D. A. (1965), 'Development of resistance to antiviral drugs', *Ann. N.Y. Acad. Sci.*, **130**, 343.

Schimpff, S. C., Fortner, C. L., Greene, W. H. and Wiernik, P. H. (1974), 'Cytosine arabinoside for localized herpes zoster in patients with cancer: Failure in a controlled trial', *J. Infect. Dis.*, **130**, 673.

Seligman, B. R. and Rosner, F. (1970), 'Varicella and cytosine arabinoside', *Lancet*, **1**, 307.

Stevens, D. A. and Merigan, T. C. (1972), 'Uncertain role of cytosine arabinoside in varicella infection of compromised hosts', *J. Pediatrics*, **81**, 562.

Stevens, D. A., Waddell, T. F. and Merigan, T. C. (1972), 'Effect of cytosine arabinoside on disseminated herpes zoster and vesicle fluid interferon', *Ann. Intern. Med.*, **76**, 873.

Stevens, D. A., Jordan, G. W., Waddell, T. F. and Merigan, T. C. (1973), 'Adverse effect of cytosine arabinoside on disseminated zoster in a controlled trial', *New Engl. J. Med.*, **289**, 873.

Tomlinson, A. H. and MacCallum, F. O. (1973), 'Pyrimidine analogues in the treatment of experimental Herpes infections', *Postgrad. med. J.*, **49**, 416.

Underwood, G. E. (1962), 'Activity of 1-β-D-arabinofuranosylcytosine hydrochloride against Herpes simplex keratitis', *Proc. Soc. Exp. Biol. and Med.*, **8**, 660.

Underwood, G. E., Wisner, C. A. and Weed, S. D. (1964), 'Cytosine arabinoside (CA) and other nucleosides in Herpes virus infections', *Arch. Ophthal.*, **72**, 505.

Walker, W. E., Waisbren, B. A., Martins, R. R. and Batayias, G. E. (1971), '*In vitro* determination of viral susceptibility to drugs for possible clinical use', *Antimicrob. Ag. Chemother.*—1970, p. 380.

Walwick, E. R., Roberts, W. K. and Dekker, C. A. (1959), 'Cyclisation during the phosphorylation of uridine and cytidine by polyphosphoric acid. A new route to the O^2, $2'$-cyclonucleosides', *Proc. Chem. Soc.*, 84.

Weinstein, L. and Chang, T. W. (1973), 'The chemotherapy of viral infections', *New Engl. J. Med.*, **289,** 725.

Wilfert, C. M. (1971), 'Disseminated varicella in a patient with leukemia', *J. Pediatrics*, **79,** 172.

Adenine Arabinoside

Description

Adenine arabinoside (9-beta-D-arabinofuranosyladenine; vidarabine; adenosine arabinoside; ara-A) is a purine nucleoside analogue, which was originally synthetized as a potential anticancer agent (Lee *et al.*, 1960). It was subsequently discovered to be a naturally occurring nucleoside present in culture filtrates of Streptomyces antibioticus (Miller *et al.*, 1969). Adenine arabinoside has a broad antiviral spectrum, but it is primarily active against the herpes and pox viruses. By comparison to the pyrimidine analogues idoxuridine (page 931) and cytarabine (page 940), it has a low toxicity, its primary metabolite has high antiviral activity, it has a lower immunosuppressive effect and affects rapidly dividing cells to a lesser extent. It is of proven value in certain viral eye infections, but its place in other viral infections has yet to be determined by controlled trials.

Another drug adenine arabinoside 5'-monophosphate, which is the nucleotide precursor of adenine arabinoside, is being studied currently. It has the advantages of being highly soluble in water and of being slowly broken down in man, resulting in sustained serum and tissue levels of the fully active drug (Medical News, 1976).

The following details only apply to adenine arabinoside.

Antiviral Activity

In 1964 it was reported that adenine arabinoside was active *in vitro* against Herpesvirus hominis and Vaccinia virus (De Garilhe and De Rudder, 1964). Subsequently it was shown to be active *in vitro* against other DNA viruses such as Herpesvirus varicellae, Herpesvirus simiae and Cytomegalovirus and a single RNA virus (Rous sarcoma) (Schabel, 1968; Miller *et al.*, 1969). This activity, which has been confirmed in a variety of different types of cell culture, has also been extended to include other poxviruses such as Monkeypox and Tanapox and strains of Herpesvirus hominis types 1 and 2, which are resistant to idoxuridine (Shannon, 1975). It is doubtful whether adenine arabinoside has any activity against human adenoviruses. The drug has no activity against non-oncogenic RNA-containing viruses, but has a fairly broad spectrum of activity against RNA tumour viruses. More recently *in vitro* inhibitory action against the Epstein-Barr virus has been demonstrated (Coker-Vann and Dolin, 1977). If the rapid conversion of adenine arabinoside to ara hypoxanthine (*vide infra*) by adenosine deaminase in cell cultures is prevented by an inhibitor, minimum inhibitory concentration values against a number of these viruses, comparable to those obtained with idoxuridine (page 93) and cytarabine (page 940), are obtained. This observation is of doubtful clinical significance because rapid deamination of adenine arabinoside occurs *in vivo*. Strains of Herpesvirus hominis resistant to adenine arabinoside have been selected by passage of the virus in cell cultures containing increasing concentrations of the drug.

The activity of adenine arabinoside has also been extensively studied in a variety of experimental viral infections of animals (Sloan, 1975; Overall *et al.*, 1975; Griffith *et al.*, 1975). It has antiviral activity against Herpesvirus hominis and vaccinial keratitis, comparable to that obtained with idoxuridine (page 931), and it is also effective against skin lesions produced by these viruses. Adenine arabinoside increases the survival rate of animals with experimental Herpesvirus hominis (types 1 and 2) and vaccinial encephalitis. Human cytomegalovirus strains, sensitive *in vitro* to adenine arabinoside, when used to produce lethal infections in mice, failed to respond to high intraperitoneal doses of the drug (Overall *et al.*, 1976).

Depending on the experimental animal model studied, adenine arabinoside is effective when administered intraperitoneally, subcutaneously, perorally, intravenously, subconjunctivally, intracerebrally and by topical application. For a given chemotherapeutic effect, it has much less toxicity than either idoxuridine or cytarabine. In some animal experiments, adenine arabinoside only reduced viral replication sufficiently to allow normal host defence mechanisms to overcome the infection. In this context it is of interest that adenine arabinoside and human interferon are synergistic against Herpesvirus hominis type 1 in tissue culture (Lerner and Bailey, 1974). Also when it is used with humoral antibodies to Herpesvirus hominis, there is enhanced protection against Herpesvirus hominis infection in mice (Cho and Feng, 1977). These findings support the view that drugs such as adenine arabinoside can only reduce viral load in an acute illness, thereby assisting the host immune mechanisms to produce final cure (Alford and Whitley, 1976). This also explains the failure of the drug for the treatment of some viral infections in hosts with defective immune responses (*vide infra*).

Mode of Administration and Dosage

1. *Topical administration to the eyes.* Adenine arabinoside is available commercially as an ophthalmic ointment containing 3 per cent of the drug in an inert petrolatum base (Vira-A or Vidarabine ophthalmic ointment, Parke Davis and Company). Approximately one cm of the ointment should be put into the lower conjunctival sac five times daily at 3 h intervals. In keratitis, signs of improvement occur within seven days and complete re-epithelialization should occur by 21 days. After re-epithelialization, treatment should be continued for another seven days at a reduced dosage (twice-daily) to prevent recurrence. Gentamicin, erythromycin, chloramphenicol and corticosteroids may be administered into the eyes with adenine arabinoside ointment.

2. *Parenteral administration.* The drug is only used by the intravenous route, as intramuscular administration causes pain and muscle necrosis. Adenine arabinoside is relatively insoluble, 0·5 mg per ml of fluid or 500 mg per litre at 25°C. It is more soluble at 37°C (1·8 mg per ml of fluid). A concentration of 0·7 mg per ml or 700 mg per litre of intravenous fluid was used by Ch'ien *et al.* (1973), but sediment accumulated in the intravenous bottle so that

it had to be inverted and shaken every 2 h during infusion. Adenine arabinoside is compatible with all commonly used intravenous solutions but hypotonic saline solutions are recommended, without other added medications. It is incompatible with blood, plasma or plasma expanders.

The half-life of the drug in humans is about 3·5 h, so that it can be administered by continuous infusion without excessive drug accumulation. The total daily dose dissolved in an appropriate volume of fluid is usually infused intravenously over a 12-h period. Preliminary studies on the use of adenine arabinoside in human viral infections suggest that an appropriate dose is 10–20 mg per kg per day, for a maximum period of ten days.

Serum Levels, Excretion and Distribution in Body

When adenine arabinoside is administered by infusion in a dose of 10–20 mg per kg per day to humans, it is very rapidly deaminated by an enzyme adenosine deaminase, probably in the red cells, to a hypoxanthine derivative, ara hypoxanthine (Kinkel and Buchanan, 1975). Adenine arabinoside may also be metabolized by phosphorylation to various phosphate nucleotides, which are relatively stable to adenosine deaminase (Glazko et al., 1975). The maximum serum levels of adenine arabinoside and ara hypoxanthine at the end of a 12-h infusion are about 0·5 and 5·0 μg per ml respectively (Kinkel and Buchanan, 1975). In this study adenine arabinoside was not detectable in red blood cells or the CSF and it did not accumulate in a patient with impaired renal function. By contrast, ara hypoxanthine which did not accumulate in the dosage used in normal patients did accumulate in a patient with impaired renal function (serum level 77 μg per ml). Levels of ara hypoxanthine in red blood cells paralleled those in the serum and CSF levels were approximately 35 per cent of serum levels. Nearly all ara hypoxanthine is excreted in the urine and after the third day of infusion a steady amount (about 50 per cent of the daily dose) is excreted daily. The in vivo antiviral activity of adenine arabinoside therefore seems to be largely mediated by ara hypoxanthine, which has considerably less antiviral activity than adenine arabinoside (Sloan, 1975; Shannon, 1975; Bryson and Connor, 1976). Ara hypoxanthine seems to become widely distributed in human tissues and it has been detected in post-mortem specimens of kidney, liver and spleen, but lower levels were found in the brain, skeletal muscle and CSF. Nevertheless information on the persistence of adenine arabinoside and ara hypoxanthine in the body is very scanty.

Mode of Action

Adenine arabinoside selectively inhibits viral DNA synthesis but the exact biochemical mechanism is still unknown. It has been suggested that its triphosphate metabolite may inhibit viral DNA polymerase or virus induced ribonucleotide reductase (Le Page, 1973; Shannon, 1975; Sloan, 1975). In vitro adenine arabinoside triphosphate also inhibits mammalian cell DNA polymerases but to a lesser degree than its inhibition of viral DNA polymerase. It also can be incorporated into both cellular and viral DNA during DNA synthesis (Shannon, 1977; Müller et al., 1977). Other studies indicate that both adenine arabinoside and cytarabine (page 941) may act by a similar mechanism (Rashbaum and Cozzarelli, 1976), in that the triphosphate derivatives of both drugs have DNA polymerase as their primary target.

Toxicity

1. *Side-effects from ocular therapy*. Lacrimation, foreign-body sensation, conjunctivitis, burning, irritation, superficial punctate keratitis, pain, photophobia, punctal occlusion and hypersensitivity have been reported with adenine arabinoside ointment.

2. *Side-effects from parenteral administration*. In animals adenine arabinoside has a low toxicity and it does not appear to affect the haemopoietic system or the immune response (Le Page, 1973), but it is teratogenic in rats and rabbits and oncogenic in some animals (Kurtz, 1975). Preliminary studies in humans indicated that in the recommended doses it had virtually no effect on the liver, kidneys and haemopoietic system and its only consistent side-effect was nausea (Keeney, 1975). Adenine arabinoside also does not seem to interfere with normal cellular and humoral immune mechanisms in humans (Steele *et al.*, 1975; 1977). Haematologic toxicity, manifested by a fall in haematocrit and platelet and leucocyte counts, has been described when the drug was used to treat cytomegalovirus infection in renal allograft recipients (Rytel and Kauffman, 1976). It is possible that this resulted from high serum levels of the drug in association with impaired renal function. Myelosuppression evidenced by neutropenia and thrombocytopenia had been previously observed when adenine arabinoside was used to treat patients with metastatic cancer (Bodey *et al.*, 1975). In a study of 42 patients treated with adenine arabinoside, side-effects were noted more commonly in patients treated with the relatively higher dosage of 20 mg per kg per day (Ross *et al.*, 1976). Toxic effects were nausea and vomiting, weight loss, weakness (often with impaired ambulation), bone-marrow megaloblastosis, tremors and thrombophlebitis at the intravenous site. One of the patients with tremor had an abnormal encephalogram consistent with a toxic encephalopathy. All of these adverse reactions were reversible. The drug is not recommended in pregnancy unless there is some life-threatening indication for which its use can be justified.

Clinical Uses of the Drug

Similar to idoxuridine (page 934) and cytarabine (page 941), the original evidence for the efficacy of adenine arabinoside in various virus infections was by anecdotal case reports and uncontrolled trials. There is now accumulating evidence based on carefully planned trials, particularly in the United States, defining the place of this drug in antiviral chemotherapy.

1. *Ocular infections*. The efficacy of adenine arabinoside as compared to idoxuridine (page 934) has been studied in a double-blind trial in which both drugs were used topically to treat human viral keratoconjunctivitis (Pavan-Langston and Dohlman, 1972). Adenine arabinoside was as effective as idoxuridine for treatment of Herpesvirus hominis keratitis. It was also a suitable non-toxic alternative for treatment of cases resistant to IDU or with allergic or toxic reactions to IDU. Adenine arabinoside was as effective as IDU in the presence of corticosteroid medication for deep herpetic disease. Like

IDU, adenine arabinoside was of no value for adenoviral keratoconjunctivitis. Pavan-Langston and Dohlman (1972) also confirmed the findings of Hyndiuk *et al.* (1971) that adenine arabinoside appeared superior to IDU for treatment of vaccinial blepharoconjunctivitis. Further comparisons between IDU and adenine arabinoside have been made in the treatment of herpetic uveitis (Pavan-Langston *et al.*, 1975). Adenine arabinoside was only of value in those patients with defective corneal epithelium because this enabled its metabolite ara hypoxanthine to enter the eye; IDU was of no value, regardless of the corneal status, because although its metabolite uracil also penetrated the eye when the cornea was disrupted, it has no antiviral activity. Immune mechanisms are also involved in herpes uveitis and corticosteroids are often needed as well as antiviral therapy; topical adenine arabinoside in combination with topical corticosteroids has been used with benefit to treat stromal keratitis (Jones, 1975). Adenine arabinoside has also been given intravenously in a dose of 20 mg per kg per day for seven days to patients with herpetic keratouveitis. It was effective because the drug penetrated into the anterior chamber and this treatment was accompanied by only minimal side-effects (Abel *et al.*, 1975).

Numerous other studies have confirmed the value of adenine arabinoside in acute or recurrent herpes keratitis; it is as effective as IDU and preferable to that drug because of the intraocular penetration of its metabolite, its lack of tissue toxicity, its lesser allergenicity and also clinical resistance to the drug is very rare (Poirier *et al.*, 1975; Laibson and Krachmer, 1975; Hyndiuk *et al.*, 1975; Pavan-Langston, 1975; O'Day *et al.*, 1975; Jones, 1975). Adenine arabinoside also appears to be the prophylactic drug of choice in corneal transplant patients subject to cold sores and other herpetic lesions, because it results in healthier epithelial healing and is no more detrimental than IDU in slowing stromal repair (Langston *et al.*, 1975).

2. *Herpesvirus varicellae infections.* Juel-Jensen and MacCallum (1972) used adenine arabinoside to treat two patients with herpes zoster, who had an underlying reticulosis, with apparent beneficial effect. Other preliminary uncontrolled studies also suggested that this drug may be effective in certain varicella-zoster infections (Luby *et al.*, 1975). Adenine arabinoside appeared useful to control localized herpes zoster and also the disseminated disease in immuno-compromised patients; it did not seem to influence zoster encephalitis or complicated varicella in immuno-compromised patients. The results of one controlled study on the use of adenine arabinoside to treat herpes zoster in 87 immunodeficient patients have been published (Whitley *et al.*, 1976). One group of patients received an intravenous dose of 10 mg per kg per day of the drug for five days, followed by a placebo for five days, and the other group the reverse regimen. In spite of rapid natural healing of both localized and disseminated disease, patients who received adenine arabinoside for the first five days had more rapid clearance of virus from vesicles, cessation of new vesicle formation and the time taken to reach the vesicular stage was shortened. It was concluded that the drug is most efficacious when it is administered during the first six days of the disease and when the patient has reticuloendothelial neoplasia and is aged less than 38 years. Unfortunately, the long duration of disease (about seven days) before treatment, prevented an assessment of whether the drug can abort dissemination of infection; the cross-over design of the trial also did not enable study of the drug's effect on post-herpetic

neuralgia. Further controlled trials by this group are currently in progress to answer these and other questions (Merigan, 1976).

3. *Herpesvirus hominis infections*

(a) *Encephalitis.* To avoid the many biases associated with uncontrolled studies of antiviral drugs in this disease (*see* page 935), a collaborative controlled trial of adenine arabinoside in virologically confirmed Herpesvirus hominis encephalitis was instituted in the United States of America (Whitley *et al.*, 1977). In 28 cases (children and adults) proved by isolation of the virus (type 1) from a brain biopsy, treatment reduced the death rate from 70 to 28 per cent and over 50 per cent of treated survivors had no or only minor to moderately disabling neurologic sequelae. As could be expected, the most satisfactory outcome was obtained when treatment was given early in the course of infection. Treatment was not effective in patients with an encephalitis from whom virus could not be isolated from brain biopsy, although their encephalitis was clinically indistinguishable from those from whom the virus was grown. The drug was administered intravenously in a dose of 15 mg per kg per day, given over 12 h for ten days. Adverse drug effects were not observed. Even though the number of patients in this trial was comparatively small, the trial was terminated for ethical reasons, when the reduction of mortality resulting from treatment was considered to be significant. Taber *et al.* (1977) described the use of adenine arabinoside in five patients with Herpesvirus hominis encephalitis proven by brain biopsy; four of these patients survived with varying degrees of mental impairment.

Results of further experiences with adenine arabinoside in this disease are awaited to confirm these encouraging observations and to establish optimal dosage schedules.

(b) *Mucocutaneous infections.* Adenine arabinoside has been used to treat ten patients with severe mucocutaneous infections, most of whom were receiving immunosuppressive therapy. (Ch'ien *et al.*, 1975a). It appeared that the drug was of benefit in a dose of 5–10 mg per kg per day intravenously, particularly for lesions due to Herpesvirus hominis type 1. Clinical improvement was paralleled by a reduction in virus excretion from the throat and clinical lesions. Excretion of virus returned in some patients weeks after cessation of therapy, suggesting that the drug only reduces viral replication and recovery depends on the integrity of the host's immune system. Three patients with concomitant genital lesions due to type 2 virus showed no favourable response.

Topical treatment with 3 per cent adenine arabinoside has been studied in a controlled trial involving 55 men and 42 women with genital herpetic infection (Adams *et al.*, 1976). Treatment did not influence the course of either primary or recurrent genital infection. Similar results were obtained in a smaller controlled trial in which virologically proven episodes of herpes genitalis in 32 men were studied (Goodman *et al.*, 1975). Young *et al.* (1976) described a woman who developed disseminated type 2 genital infection in the 37th week of pregnancy, manifested by hepatitis, pancreatitis and genital lesions. Temporary improvement occurred following the delivery of a healthy infant by caesarian section, but on the third post-partum day she developed encephalitis, later complicated by myocarditis. Adenine arabinoside was administered intravenously for seven days in a dose of 20 reducing to 15 mg per kg per day, and the patient survived with mild neurologic sequelae.

(c) *Neonatal infections*. Adenine arabinoside was used to treat 13 neonates with Herpesvirus hominis infection, eight had disseminated disease, one localized central nervous system disease and in four infection was confined to the skin and eyes (Ch'ien *et al.*, 1975b). The drug was administered intravenously in a dose of 10–20 mg per kg per day within three to eight days after the appearance of skin vesicles, and was continued for 10–15 days. Treatment was delayed in one infant without skin vesicles and in four others whose skin lesions appeared after the occurrence of central nervous system damage. Of these five infants with disseminated disease, four died and one survived with severe neurological deficits. The eight other infants (four with disseminated disease and four with localized skin disease), who were treated within three days after the onset of neurologic signs, all survived with no neurologic deficit detectable at six months to one year of age.

4. *Cytomegalovirus infections*. Seventeen infants or young children with central nervous system involvement, disseminated congenital infection or cytomegalovirus pneumonitis have been treated (Baublis *et al.*, 1975). Adenine arabinoside was administered in a dose of 1–20 mg per kg per day intravenously, for 5–21 days. Although there was a temporary reduction in virus excretion in the urine and throat of some patients, the drug did not appear beneficial in any of these diseases.

Adenine arabinoside has also been used to treat adults with cytomegalovirus mononucleosis or with disseminated infection in renal transplant recipients on immunosuppressive therapy (Ch'ien *et al.*, 1974; Baublis *et al.*, 1975; Rytel and Kauffman, 1976). Equivocal results were obtained in patients with mononucleosis, and no improvement was noted in those receiving immunosuppressive therapy. On the basis of animal experiments (page 948), these results are not surprising.

Phillips *et al.* (1977) described two adult patients who were normal immunologically and who had acute encephalitis due to cytomegalovirus; their dramatic improvement was attributed to the use of adenine arabinoside intravenously.

5. *Smallpox*. A controlled study of the efficacy of adenine arabinoside in the treatment of variola major was conducted in Bangladesh (Koplan *et al.*, 1975). The drug was given in a dose of 20 mg per kg per day, intravenously for several days. The findings of this study suggested that adenine arabinoside is not effective in the chemotherapy of smallpox.

6. *Chronic hepatitis B*. Adenine arabinoside has been given in two patients with chronic active hepatitis B (Pollard *et al.*, 1978). An intravenous dose of 15 mg per kg per day was given for 9–14 days, in two courses separated by periods of 20 and 42 days respectively. In one patient both courses resulted in a temporary decrease in Dane particle-associated DNA polymerase. In the other patient this enzyme became undetectable after the second course and for

a follow-up period of 12 months; this was also associated with disappearance of hepatitis B core antigen and a fall in the level of hepatitis B surface antigen (HB$_s$Ag). In both patients no consistent changes in liver function test results occurred and, in both, the drug caused mild gastro-intestinal symptoms. Chadwick *et al.* (1978) also used the drug to treat four patients with chronic liver disease associated with persistent hepatitis B virus infection. A dose of 10 mg per kg per day was given for five consecutive days during each of two consecutive weeks. In all cases this treatment resulted in loss of serum DNA polymerase activity, but this returned in three patients after treatment ceased. In three of the patients who also had Dane particles and hepatitis B e antigen in their sera, no change was observed in these markers following treatment. The fourth patient who remained negative for DNA polymerase after treatment also had decreased serum levels of HB$_s$ Ag after treatment. A temporary reduction in DNA polymerase activity also only occurred in chimpanzees who were carriers of hepatitis B virus, when they were treated by adenine arabinoside (Zuckerman *et al.*, 1978).

The clinical significance of these findings are at present unknown. There is insufficient data to recommend the use of adenine arabinoside for any form of viral hepatitis.

REFERENCES

Abel, R., Jr., Kaufman, H. E. and Sugar, J. (1975), 'Effect of intravenous adenine arabinoside on Herpes simplex keratouveitis in humans'. In *Adenine Arabinoside: An Antiviral Agent* (Ed.), Pavan-Langston, D., Buchanan, R. A. and Alford, C. A., Jr., New York, Raven Press.

Adams, H. G., Benson, E. A., Alexander, E. R., Vontver, L. A., Remington, M. A. and Holmes, K. K. (1976), 'Genital herpetic infection in men and women: Clinical course and effect of topical application of adenine arabinoside', *J. Infect. Dis.* (Suppl.), **133**, A151.

Alford, C. A., Jr. and Whitley, R. J. (1976), 'Treatment of infections due to Herpesvirus in humans: A critical review of the state of the art', *J. Infect. Dis.* (Suppl.), **133**, A:101.

Baublis, J. V., Whitley, R. J., Ch'ien, L. T. and Alford, C. A., Jr. (1975), 'Treatment of Cytomegalovirus infection in infants and aults'. In *Adenine Arabinoside: An Antiviral Agent* (Ed.), Pavan-Langston, D., Buchanan, R. A. and Alford, C. A., Jr., New York, Raven Press.

Bodey, G. P., Gottlieb, J., McCredie, K. B. and Freireich, E. J. (1975), 'Adenine arabinoside in cancer chemotherapy'. In *Adenine Arabinoside: An Antiviral Agent* (Ed.), Pavan-Langston, D., Buchanan, R. A. and Alford, C. A., Jr., New York, Raven Press.

Bryson, Y. J. and Connor, J. D. (1976), '*In vitro* susceptibility of Varicella Zoster virus to adenine arabinoside and hypoxanthine arabinoside', *Antimicrob. Ag. Chemother.*, **9**, 540.

Chadwick, R. G., Bassendine, M. F., Crawford, E. M., Thomas, H. C. and Sherlock, S. (1978), 'HB$_s$ Ag-positive chronic liver disease: Inhibition of DNA polymerase activity by vidarabine', *Brit. med. J.*, **2**, 531.

Ch'ien, L. T., Cannon, N. J., Charamella, L. J., Dismukes, W. E., Whitley, R. J., Buchanan, R. A. and Alford, C. A., Jr. (1973), 'Effect of adenine arabinoside on severe Herpesvirus hominis infections in man', *J. Infect. Dis.*, **128**, 658.

Ch'ien, L. T., Cannon, N. J., Whitley, R. J., Diethelm, A. G., Dismukes, W. E., Scott,

C. W., Buchanan, R. A. and Alford, C. A., Jr. (1974), 'Effect of adenine arabinoside on Cytomegalovirus infections', *J. Infect. Dis.*, **130**, 32.

Ch'ien, L. T., Whitley, R. J., Charamella, L. J., Buchanan, R. A., Cannon, N. J., Dismukes, W. E. and Alford, C. A., Jr. (1975a), 'Clinical and virologic studies with systemic administration of adenine arabinoside in severe, progressive, mucocutaneous Herpes simplex virus infections'. In *Adenine Arabinoside: An Antiviral Agent* (Ed.), Pavan-Langston, D., Buchanan, R. A. and Alford, C. A., Jr., New York, Raven Press.

Ch'ien, L. T., Whitley, R. J., Nahmias, A. J., Lewin, E. B., Linnemann, C. C., Frenkel, L. D., Bellanti, J. A., Buchanan, R. A. and Alford, C. A., Jr. (1975b), 'Antiviral chemotherapy and neonatal Herpes simplex virus infection: A pilot study-experience with adenine arabinoside (ARA-A)', *Pediatrics*, **55**, 678.

Cho, C. T. and Feng, K. K. (1977), 'Interaction of adenine arabinoside on host defense factors in experimental infections due to Herpesvirus hominis', *J. Infect. Dis.*, **135**, 468.

Coker-Vann, M. and Dolin, R. (1977), 'Effect of adenine arabinoside on Epstein-Barr virus *in vitro*', *J. Infect. Dis.*, **135**, 447.

De Garilhe, P. and de Rudder, J. (1964), 'Effet de deux nucléosides de l'arabinose sur la multiplication des virus de l'herpès et de la vacine en culture cellulaise', *C.R. Acad. Sci.*, **259**, 2725.

Glazko, A. J., Chang, T., Drach, J. C., Mourer, D. R., Borondy, P. E., Schneider, H., Croskey, L. and Maschewske, E. (1975), 'Species differences in the metabolic disposition of adenine arabinoside'. In *Adenine Arabinoside: An Antiviral Agent* (Ed.), Pavan-Langston, D., Buchanan, R. A. and Alford, C. A., Jr., New York, Raven Press.

Goodman, E. L., Luby, J. P. and Johnson, M. T. (1975), 'Prospective double-blind evaluation of topical adenine arabinoside in male herpes progenitalis', *Antimicrob. Ag. Chemother.*, **8**, 693.

Griffith, J. F., Fitzwilliam, J. F., Casagrande, S. and Butler, S. R. (1975), 'Experimental Herpes simplex virus encephalitis: Comparative effects of treatment with cytosine arabinoside and adenine arabinoside', *J. Infect. Dis.*, **132**, 506.

yndiuk, R. A., Okumoto, M., Valenton, M. and Smolin, G. (1971), 'Effect of adenine arabinoside and rifampicin in experimental vaccinial keratitis'. Presented at Association for Research in Vision and Ophthalmology. Meeting, Sarasota, Florida, April 30, 1971.

Hyndiuk, R. A., Schultz, R. O. and Hull, D. S. (1975), 'Herpetic keratitis—clinical evaluation of adenine arabinoside and idoxuridine'. In *Adenine Arabinoside: An Antiviral Agent* (Ed.), Pavan-Langston, D., Buckanan, R. A. and Alford, C. A., Jr., New York, Raven Press.

Jones, D. B. (1975), 'Adenine arabinoside in Herpes simplex keratitis, treatment of idoxuridine-failure epithelial disease, and combined corticosteroid therapy in stromal keratitis'. In *Adenine Arabinoside: An Antiviral Agent* (Ed.), Pavan-Langston, D., Buchanan, R. A. and Alford, C. A., Jr., New York, Raven Press.

Juel-Jensen, B. E. and MacCallum, F. O. (1972), *Herpes Simplex, Varicella and Zoster. Clinical Manifestations and Treatment.* London, William Heinemann Ltd.

Keeney, R. E. (1975), 'Human tolerance of adenine arabinoside'. In *Adenine Arabinoside: An Antiviral Agent* (Ed.), Pavan-Langston, D., Buchanan, R. A. and Alford, C. A., Jr., New York, Raven Press.

Kinkel, A. W. and Buchanan, R. A. (1975), 'Human pharmacology'. In *Adenine Arabinoside: An Antiviral Agent* (Ed.), Pavan-Langston, D., Buchanan, R. A. and Alford, C. A., Jr., New York, Raven Press.

Koplan, J. P., Monsur, K. A., Foster, S. O., Huq, F., Rahaman, M. M., Huq, S., Buchanan, R. A. and Ward, N. A. (1975), 'Treatment of variola major with adenine arabinoside', *J. Infect. Dis.*, **131**, 34.

956 THE USE OF ANTIBIOTICS

Kurtz, S. M. (1975), 'Toxicology of adenine arabinoside'. In *Adenine Arabinoside: An Antiviral Agent* (Ed.), Pavan-Langston, D., Buchanan, R. A. and Alford, C. A., Jr., New York, Raven Press.

Laibson, P. R. and Krachmer, J. H. (1975), 'Controlled comparison of adenine arabinoside and idoxuridine therapy of human superficial dendritic keratitis'. In *Adenine Arabinoside: An Antiviral Agent* (Ed.), Pavan-Langston, D., Buchanan, R. A. and Alford, C. A., Jr., New York, Raven Press.

Langston, R. H. S., Pavan-Langston, D. and Dohlman, C. H. (1975), 'A comparison of the effect of adenine arabinoside and idoxuridine on corneal wound healing'. In *Adenine Arabinoside: An Antiviral Agent* (Ed.), Pavan-Langston, D., Buchanan, R. A. and Alford, C. A., Jr., New York, Raven Press.

Lee, W. W., Benitez, A., Goodman, L. and Baker, B. R. (1960), 'Potential anticancer agents. XL. Synthesis of the -anomer of 9-(D-arabinofuranosyl)-adenine', *J. Am. Chem. Soc.*, **82**, 2648.

LePage, G. A. (1973), 'Purines and purine nucleoside antagonists', *Transplant. Proc.*, **5**, 1157.

Lerner, A. M. and Bailey, E. J. (1974), 'Synergy of 9-β-D-arabinofuranosyladenine and human interferon against Herpes simplex virus, type 1', *J. Infect. Dis.*, **130**, 549.

Luby, J. P., Johnson, M. T., Buchanan, R., Ch'ien, L. T., Whitley, R. and Alford, C. (1975), 'Adenine arabinoside therapy of Varicella-zoster virus infections. Summary of Phase II studies'. In *Adenine Arabinoside: An Antiviral Agent* (Ed.), Pavan-Langston, D., Buchanan, R. A. and Alford, C. A., Jr., New York, Raven Press.

Medical News (1974), 'Viral inhibitor tests involve 17 centres', *JAMA*, **228**, 142.

Medical News (1976), 'Viderabine found effective against voial eye infections', *JAMA*, **236**, 13.

Merigan, T. C. (1976), 'Efficacy of adenine arabinoside in Herpes zoster', *New Engl. J. Med.*, **294**, 1233.

Miller, F. A., Dixon, G. J., Ehrlich, J., Sloan, B. J. and McLean, I. W., Jr. (1969), 'Antiviral activity of 9-β-D-arabinofuranosyladenine. I. Cell culture studies', *Antimicrob. Ag. Chemother.*—1968, p. 136.

Müller, W. E. G., Zahn, R. K., Bittlingmaier, K. and Falke, D. (1977), 'Inhibition of Herpesvirus DNA synthesis by 9-β-D-arabinofuranosyladenine in cellular and cell-free systems', *Ann. N.Y. Acad. Sci.*, **34**, 284.

O'Day, D. M., Poirier, R. H. and Elliot, J. H. (1975), 'Adenine arabinoside: Therapy in complicated herpetic keratitis'. In *Adenine Arabinoside: An Antiviral Agent* (Ed.), Pavan-Langston, D., Buchanan, R. A. and Alford, C. A., Jr., New York, Raven Press.

Overall, J. C., Jr., Kern, E. R. and Glasgow, L. A. (1975), 'Treatment of Herpesvirus hominis type 2 infections in mice with adenine arabinoside'. In *Adenine Arabinoside: An Antiviral Agent* (Ed.), Pavan-Langston, D., Buchanan, R. A. and Alford, C. A., Jr., New York, Raven Press.

Overall, J. C., Jr., Kern, E. R. and Glasgow, L. A. (1976), 'Effective antiviral chemotherapy in cytomegalovirus infection of mice', *J. Infect. Dis.* (Suppl.), **133**, A237.

Pavan-Langston, D. and Dohlman, C. H. (1972), 'A double blind clinical study of adenine arabinoside therapy of viral keratoconjunctivitis', *Am. J. Ophthalmol.*, **74**, 81.

Pavan-Langstron, D. (1975), 'Clinical evaluation of adenine arabinoside and idoxuridine in treatment of routine and idoxuridine-complicated Herpes simplex keratitis'. In *Adenine Arabinoside: An Antiviral Agent* (Ed.), Pavan-Langston, D., Buchanan, R. A. and Alford, C. A., Jr., New York, Raven Press.

Pavan-Langston, D., Dohlman, C. H., Geary, P. and Szulczewski, D. (1975), 'Intraocular penetration of adenine arabinoside and idoxuridine: Therapeutic implications in clinical herpetic uveitis'. In *Adenine Arabinoside: An Antiviral Agent*

(Ed.), Pavan-Langston, D., Buchanan, R. A. and Alford, C. A., Jr., New York, Raven Press.

Phillips, C. A., Fanning, L., Gump, D. W. and Phillips, C. F. (1977), 'Cytomegalovirus encephalitis in immunologically normal adults. Successful treatment with vidarabine', *JAMA*, **238**, 2299.

Poirier, R. H., Kinkel, A. W., Ellison, A. C. and Lewis, R. (1975), 'Intraocular penetration of topical 3% adenine arabinoside'. In *Adenine Arabinoside: An Antiviral Agent* (Ed.), Pavan-Langston, D., Buchanan, R. A. and Alford, C. A., Jr., New York, Raven Press.

Pollard, R. B., Smith, J. L., Neal, E. A., Gregory, P. B., Merigan, T. C. and Robinson, W. S. (1978), 'Effect of vidarabine on chronic hepatitis B virus infection', *JAMA*, **239**, 1648.

Rashbaum, S. A. and Cozzarelli, N. R. (1976), 'Mechanism of DNA synthesis inhibition by arabinosyl cytosine and arabinosyl adenine', *Nature*, **264**, 679.

Ross, A. H., Julia, A. and Balakrishnan, C. (1976), 'Toxicity of adenine arabinoside in humans', *J. Infect. Dis.* (Suppl.), **133**, A192.

Rytel, W. M. and Kauffman, H. M. (1976), 'Clinical efficacy of adenine arabinoside in therapy of cytomegalovirus infections in renal allograft recipients', *J. Infect. Dis.*, **133**, 202.

Schabel, F. M., Jr. (1968), 'The antiviral activity of 9-β-D-arabinosuranosyladenine (Ara-A), *Chemother*, **13**, 321.

Shannon, W. M. (1975), 'Adenine arabinoside: Antiviral activity *in vitro*'. In *Adenine Arabinoside: An Antiviral Agent* (Ed.), Pavan-Langston, D., Buchanan, R. A. and Alford, C. A., Jr., New York, Raven Press.

Shannon, W. M. (1977), 'Introductory remarks on adenine arabinoside', *Ann. N.Y. Acad. Sci.*, **3**, 284.

Sloan, B. J. (1975), 'Adenine arabinoside: Chemotherapy studies in animals'. In *Adenine Arabinoside: An Antiviral Agent* (Ed.), Pavan-Langston, D., Buchanan, R. A. and Alford, C. A., Jr., New York, Raven Press.

Steele, R. W., Chapa, I. A., Vincent, M. M., Hensen, S. A. and Keeney, R. E. (1975), 'Effects of adenine arabinoside on cellular immune mechanisms in man'. In *Adenine Arabinoside: An Antiviral Agent* (Ed.), Pavan-Langston, D., Buchanan, R. A. and Alford, C. A., Jr., New York, Raven Press.

Steele, R. W., Keeney, R. E., Brown, J., III and Young, E. J. (1977), 'Cellular immune responses to Herpesviruses during treatment with adenine arabinoside', *J. Infect. Dis.*, **135**, 593.

Taber, L. H., Greenberg, S. B., Perez, F. I. and Couch, R. B. (1977), 'Herpes simplex encephalitis treated with vidarabine (adenine arabinoside)', *Arch. Neurol.*, **34**, 608.

Whitley, R. J., Ch'ien, L. T., Dolin, R., Galasso, G. J., Alford, C. A., Jr. (Ed.), and The Collaborative Study Group (1976), 'Adenine arabinoside therapy of Herpes zoster in the immunosuppressed. NIAID collaborative antiviral study', *New Engl. J. Med.*, **294**, 1193.

Whitley, R. J., Soong, S. J., Dolin, R., Galasso, G. J., Ch'ien, L. T., Alford, C. A. and The Collaborative Study Group (1977), 'Adenine arabinoside therapy of biopsy-proved Herpes simplex encephalitis. National Institute of Allergy and Infectious Diseases collaborative antiviral study', *New Engl. J. Med.*, **297**, 289.

Young, E. J., Killam, A. P. and Greene, J. F. (1976), 'Disseminated Herpesvirus infection. Association with primary genital herpes in pregnancy', *JAMA*, **235**, 2731.

Zuckerman, A. J., Thornton, A., Howard, C. R., Tsiquaye, K. N., Jones, D. M. and Brambell, M. R. (1978), 'Hepatitis B outbreak among chimpanzees at the London zoo', *Lancet*, **2**, 652.

Amantadine

Description

Amantadine (1-adamantanamine; 1-aminoadamantane; 'Symmetrel') is a synthetic symmetrical three ringed amine which is used as its hydrochloride. Its precursor adamantane was sythetized in 1933 and 1-aminoadamantane was derived from it in 1941. Davies *et al.* (1964) reported that amantadine inhibited the multiplication of a number of myxoviruses in tissue culture; subsequently it was shown to have a virustatic effect which is entirely restricted to RNA viruses. This drug is a useful chemoprophylactic agent against Influenza A virus infections in humans. It has not been extensively used for this purpose, mainly because of the clinical difficulties in recognizing influenza and the drug's side-effects. Amantadine is also used for the treatment of Parkinson's disease and drug-induced extrapyramidal symptoms.

Antiviral Activity

The antiviral activity of amantadine has been demonstrated in tissue culture, *in ovo* (Davies *et al.*, 1964; Maassab and Cochran, 1964; Neumayer *et al.*, 1964) and in mouse infections (Davies *et al.*, 1964; Grunert *et al.*, 1965).

In vitro, it is active against Influenza A viruses, and in some culture systems it is also active against Rubella, Parainfluenza types 2 and 3 and Respiratory syncytial viruses, but Influenza B, Mumps and Newcastle disease viruses are resistant. The susceptibility of sensitive viruses varies according to the strain of virus used and the *in vitro* test system employed. Complete suppression of virus production has not been observed.

Amantadine is most consistently active against Influenza A viruses, but certain strains of this virus can develop resistance to the drug *in vitro* (Cochran *et al.*, 1965; Oxford *et al.*, 1970). This resistance is genetically controlled (Tuckova *et al.*, 1973). There is great variability in the susceptibility of different Influenza A strains tested under identical conditions (Oxford, 1975). Fortunately the most prevalent Influenza A viruses of recent years (those with haemagglutinin and neuraminidase subtypes of H2N2 or H3N2) are very susceptible to inhibition by amantadine in tissue culture studies, whereas classical strains (HON1) and swine influenza (presumably also A/New Jersey/8/76, Hsw1 N1) are only slightly inhibited. Nevertheless amantadine has a protective effect in mice and monkeys against type A/New Jersey/8/76 strains of influenza virus (Scott *et al.*, 1978).

In experimental mouse infections, oral or injected amantadine protects against the same spectrum of viruses as in tissue culture (Davies *et al.*, 1964; Cochran *et al.*, 1965; Wood, 1965). The drug is most effective when a relatively low infecting dose of virus is used and when treatment is begun at the time of the infection, but there is still some antiviral activity when treatment is delayed up to 72 h after infection. Inhibition of virus growth is not absolute, because surviving mice are immune to challenge with the original infecting virus. Amantadine does not protect mice completely, it only reduces the mortality or increases survival time.

Absorption, Excretion, Administration and Dosage

The pharmacokinetics of amantadine in man and animals has been studied by Bleidner *et al.* (1965). The drug is water soluble and very well absorbed from the gastro-intestinal tract. After a single oral dose, an average of 86 per cent of the drug is excreted in the urine within four days (average urinary excretion within 24 h is 56 per cent). The peak serum level is usually reached 1–4 h after an oral dose with maximal levels of $0 \cdot 3$ μg per ml after a dose of $2 \cdot 5$ mg per kg and of $0 \cdot 6$ μg per ml when the dose is 5 mg per kg (Couch and Jackson, 1976). Amantadine accumulates in the serum with repeated doses and the rate of excretion is dependent on the amount present in the body. It is possible to detect the drug in the urine one week after a single oral dose. The half-life of amantadine in man is about 15 h. The drug is excreted unchanged in the urine and there is no evidence that it is metabolized in man. In the recommended doses maximal concentrations of the drug are achieved in the tissues (particularly lungs, heart and brain) in about 48 h.

For prophylactic use amantadine should be commenced immediately influenza is known to be epidemic in the community, or immediately after the patient has come in contact with the disease. Amantadine is only effective during the period of its administration; prophylaxis should be continued for 10 days after a single exposure or for four weeks or more if repeated exposures occur during an epidemic. The usual dose for adults and older children is 200 mg daily by mouth, given in two divided doses with meals. The dose for children aged 1–9 years is 3 mg per kg daily, with a maximum dose of 150 mg per day.

Mode of Action

Amantadine acts at an early stage of replication of the influenza virus. It seems to inhibit or prevent penetration of the virus into susceptible cells and it may also affect the uncoating of penetrated virus particles (Hoffmann *et al.*, 1965; Oxford, 1975).

Toxicity

Amantadine may produce amphetamine-like effects. Symptoms such as nervousness, difficulty in concentration, dizziness, light headedness, slurred speech, ataxia, drowsiness and insomnia may occur. These may be transient and disappear spontaneously in a few days. Atropine-like side-effects consisting of blurring of vision, mouth dryness and palpitations can also occur. In one patient delirium and atropine-like effects associated with amantadine and haloperidol therapy were reversed by physostigmine (Casey, 1978). In view of these side-effects the drug should not be used for chemoprophylaxis in patients with pre-existing central nervous system symptoms (other than Parkinson's disease), or in those with epilepsy or patients taking stimulant drugs.

Indigestion, allergic skin rashes, ankle oedema, anorexia and urinary frequency have also been described in association with amantadine therapy. The drug is not advised during the first trimester of pregnancy and as it is secreted in breast milk, it should not be administered to nursing mothers. Amantadine is not as well tolerated by elderly people. It should be used cautiously in patients with renal disease in whom multiple doses can result in high serum and tissue levels with pronounced side-effects. Dialysis is not effective in such patients because of the relatively low concentration of the drug in the blood (Couch and Jackson, 1976).

The frequency of side-effects in healthy young adults appears to be of the order of 3–7 per cent (Couch and Jackson, 1976); about 10 per cent of healthy volunteers have mild reactions to an initial dose of 100 mg and 10–15 per cent react to an initial dose of 200 mg; these usually relate to the nervous system and are reversible on cessation of the drug. Extensive experience with amantadine in elderly patients with Parkinson's disease indicates that side-effects occur in 2–5 per cent. These usually appear after commencement of the drug or when its dose is increased. By contrast, livedo reticularis sometimes occurs as a side-effect between one month and a year after continuous therapy with the drug.

It is now generally accepted that amantadine is a relatively safe drug if used in the recommended dosage (Couch and Jackson, 1976; Jackson and Stanley, 1976). The use of the drug for mass prophylaxis, particularly in elderly patients, who are not only at greatest risk during an influenza outbreak, but who may also have undetected renal impairment and thereby be subject to more side-effects, is another matter (*vide infra*). Recent and as yet unconfirmed case reports indicating that amantadine may be teratogenic (Nora *et al.*, 1975), that it may induce heart failure (Vale and MacLean, 1977) and that it may cause temporary diminution of visual acuity (Pearlman *et al.*, 1977), are disquieting.

Clinical Uses of the Drug

Numerous trials in humans have demonstrated that amantadine is a useful chemoprophylactic agent against artificial and naturally acquired Influenza A (H2N2 and H3N2) virus infections.

Double-blind trials in which protection was judged by artificial challenge with influenza virus have been conducted (Jackson *et al.*, 1963; Stanley *et al.*, 1965; Tyrrell *et al.*, 1965; Schiff *et al.*, 1966; Hornick *et al.*, 1967; Togo *et al.*, 1968; Smorodintsev *et al.*, 1970a; Likar, 1970; Bloomfield *et al.*, 1970). With the exception of the trial conducted by Tyrell *et al.* (1965), all of these showed that amantadine had a protective value.

Many trials have also been carried out to study the protective value of amantadine in naturally occurring influenza (Wendel, 1964; Quilligan *et al.*, 1966; Finklea *et al.*, 1967; Knight *et al.*, 1969; Galbraith *et al.*, 1969 a and b; Nafta *et al.*, 1970; Smorodintsev *et al.*, 1970b; Oker-Blom *et al.*, 1970; O'Donohogue *et al.*, 1973). These trials were carried out on a variety of population groups including prison volunteers, school boys, children in institutions, family groups and general hospital patients. With the exception of one trial conducted by Galbraith *et al.* (1969b), all confirmed the efficacy of amantadine in protecting contacts against natural Influenza A (H2N2 and H3N2) virus infections. Various degrees of protection have been reported, but it seems that under field conditions amantadine provides about 50 per cent protection against influenzal infection and greater than 60 per cent protection against illness (Couch and Jackson, 1976). The protective value is evident after 48 h treatment with the drug but it ceases when amantadine is stopped (Muldoon *et al.*, 1976). Strains of influenza resistant to amantadine have not been selected in treated patients. Amantadine does not affect the immune response and patients given inactivated vaccines while receiving the drug have a normal antibody response. In this way amantadine can be given immediately after vaccination to provide protection during the 10–14 day period before antibodies are produced. Treatment has no effect on virus shedding. Some studies have suggested that for amantadine to be effective, it needs a back-ground of influenza antibody (Wink, 1975).

A number of studies have suggested that amantadine has a therapeutic effect in established influenza by reducing the duration of fever and amelioration of other symptoms (Wingfield *et al.*, 1969; Hornick *et al.*, 1969; Togo *et al.*, 1970; Galbraith *et al.*, 1971; Wink, 1975). In a study of natural influenza A infection in students, amantadine therapy appeared to be associated with resolution of peripheral airways dysfunction which occurs in uncomplicated influenza (Little *et al.*, 1976). Nevertheless, it is very doubtful whether amantadine is of practical therapeutic value (Stuart-Harris and Schild, 1976; Couch and Jackson, 1976).

Although amantadine has a proven chemoprophylactic effect, its place in clinical practice is difficult to define (Stuart-Harris and Schild, 1976; Leading article, 1976). There is the concern about possible side-effects and that these may be more common in elderly patients, particularly if they also have impaired renal function (page 960). It is in this age group that chemoprophylaxis would be most useful as influenza in the elderly may be a serious and even fatal disease. In general, influenza is not a serious illness and the mild side-effects which occur at the recommended doses must also be considered if amantadine is used as a routine for large population groups. Another problem is the early detection of influenza in a community. In the absence of a large epidemic, the clinical diagnosis of influenza is not always possible and presenting features may be diverse (Bennett, 1973). Because of this difficulty in early diagnosis, patients who require prophylaxis may not be identified in advance. It is also a difficult logistic problem to have supplies of amantadine readily available throughout a possible epidemic period, and delayed commencement or premature cessation of the drug nullifies its benefit. A more definite indication may be prophylaxis in already vaccinated health-care personnel when influenza is epidemic in the community (Couch and Jackson, 1976). Finally protection with amantadine is of the order of 60 per cent and the relative merits of chemoprophylaxis versus vaccination alone or perhaps vaccination combined with chemoprophylaxis have yet to be defined. There is insufficient evidence to recommend the use of amantadine for treatment of patients with severe influenza.

Amantadine has also been tried in adult male volunteers experimentally infected with type 1 Parainfluenza virus, but no beneficial effects were observed (Smith *et al.*, 1967).

Lymphocytic choriomeningitis (LCM) virus penetration into cells is prevented by amantadine and it also inhibits virus synthesis and release when viral replication has begun (Welsh *et al.*, 1971). LCM virus is an arenavirus, the group to which Lassa fever virus belongs, and amantadine may be of value in the treatment or prevention of this disease (Leading article, 1976).

REFERENCES

Bennett, N. McK. (1973), 'Diagnosis of influenza', *Med. J. Aust.*, (Spec. Suppl.), p. 19.

Bleidner, W. E., Harmon, J. B., Hewes, W. E., Lynes, T. E. and Hermann, E. C. (1965), 'Absorption, distribution and excretion of amantadine hydrochloride', *J. Pharmacol. exp. Ther.*, **150**, 484.

Bloomfield, S. S., Gaffney, T. E. and Schiff, G. M. (1970), 'A design for the evaluation of antiviral drugs in human influenza', *Amer. J. Epid.*, **91**, 568.

Casey, D. E. (1978), 'Amantadine intoxication reversed by physostigmine', *New Engl. J. Med.*, **298**, 516.

Cochran, K. W., Maasab, H. F., Tsunoda, A. and Berlin, B. S. (1965), 'Studies on the antiviral activity of amantadine hydrochloride', *Ann. N.Y. Acad. Sci.*, **130**, 432.

Couch, R. B. and Jackson, G. G. (1976), 'Antiviral agents in influenza—summary of influenza workshop VIII', *J. Infect. Dis.*, **134**, 516.

Davies, W. L., Grunert, R. R., Haff, R. F., McGahen, J. W., Neumayer, E. M., Paulshock, M., Watts, J. C., Wood, T. R., Hermann, E. C. and Hoffmann, C. E. (1964), 'Antiviral activity of l-adamantanamine HCl', *Science, N.Y.*, **144**, 862.

Finklea, J. F., Hennessy, A. V. and Davenport, F. M. (1967), 'A field trial of amantadine prophylaxis in naturally-occurring acute respiratory illness', *Amer. J. Epid.*, **85**, 403.

Galbraith, A. W., Oxford, J. S., Schild, G. C. and Watson, G. I. (1969a), 'Protective effect of 1-adamantanamine hydrochloride on influenza A2 infection in the family environment', *Lancet*, **2**, 1026.

Galbraith, A. W., Oxford, J. S., Schild, G. C. and Watson, G. I. (1969b), 'Study of l-adamantanamine hydrochloride used prophylactically during the Hong Kong influenza epidemic in the family environment', *Bull. Wld. Hlth. Org.*, **41**, 677.

Galbraith, A. W., Oxford, J. S., Schild, G. C., Potter, C. W. and Watson, G. I. (1971), 'Therapeutic effect of l-adamantanamine hydrochloride in naturally occuring influenza A2/Hong Kong infection. A controlled double-blind study', *Lancet*, **2**, 113.

Grunert, R. R., McGahen, J. W. and Davies, W. L. (1965), 'The *in vivo* antiviral activity of l-adamantanamine. 1. Prophylactic and therapeutic activity against influenza viruses', *Virology*, **26**, 262.

Hoffmann, C. E., Neumayer, E. M., Haff, R. F. and Goldsby, R. A. (1965), 'Mode of action of the antiviral activity of amantadine in tissue culture', *J. Bact.*, **90**, 623.

Hornick, R. B., Togo, Y., Dawkins, A. T. and Snyder, M. J. (1967), 'Clinical evaluation of amantadine HCL in the prophylaxis of induced influenza'. *Probleme der Verhütung von Viruskrankungen*, Berlin, Heidelberg, New York, Springer Verlag, p. 272.

Hornick, R. B., Togo, Y., Mahler, S. and Iezzoni, D. (1969), 'Evaluation of amantadine hydrochloride in the treatment of A2 influenzal disease', *Bull. Wld. Hlth. Org.*, **41**, 671.

Hornick, R. B., Togo, Y., Mahler, S. and Iezzoni, D. (1970), 'Evaluation of amantadine

AMANTADINE 963

hydrochloride in the treatment of A2 influenzal disease', *Ann. N.Y. Acad. Sci.*, **173**, 10.

Jackson, G. G., Muldoon, R. L. and Aker, L. W. (1963), 'Serologic evidence for prevention of influenza illness in volunteers by an antiinfluenzal drug, amantadine hydrochloride', *Antimicrob. Ag. Chemother.*–1962, p. 703.

Jackson, G. G. and Stanley, E. D. (1976), 'Prevention and control of influenza by chemoprophylaxis and chemotherapy, prospects from examination of recent experience', *JAMA*, **235**, 2739.

Knight, V., Fedson, D., Baldini, J., Douglas, R. G. and Couch, R. B. (1969), 'Amantadine therapy of epidemic influenza A2 Hong Kong', *Antimicrob. Ag. Chemother.*, **9**, 370.

Leading Article (1976), 'Amantadine and influenza', *Brit. med. J.*, **1**, 1552.

Likar, M. (1970), 'Effectiveness of amantadine in protecting vaccinated volunteers from an attenuated strain of influenza A/Hong Kong virus', *Ann. N.Y. Acad. Sci.*, **173**, 108.

Little, J. W., Hall, W. J., Douglas, R. G., Hyde, R. W. and Speers, D. M. (1976), 'Amantadine effect on peripheral airways abnormalities in influenza', *Ann. Intern. Med.*, **85**, 177.

Maassab, H. F. and Cochran, K. W. (1964), 'Rubella virus: Inhibition *in vitro* by amantadine HCl', *Science*, **145**, 1443.

Muldoon, R. L., Stanely, E. D. and Jackson, G. G. (1976), 'Use and withdrawal of amantadine chemoprophylaxis during epidemic influenza A', *Amer. Rev. Resp. Dis.*, **113**, 487.

Nafta, I., Turcanu, A. G., Braun, I., Companetz, W., Simionescu, A., Birt, E. and Florea, V. (1970), 'Administration of amantadine for the prevention of Hong Kong influenza', *Bull. Wld. Hlth. Org.*, **42**, 423.

Nora, J. J., Nora, A. H. and Way, G. L. (1975), 'Cardiovascular maldevelopment associated with maternal exposure to amantadine', *Lancet*, **2**, 607.

Neumayer, E. M., Haff, R. F. and Hoffmann, C. E. (1965), 'Antiviral activity of amantadine hydrochloride in tissue culture and in ovo', *Proc. Soc. Exp. Biol. (N.Y.)*, **119**, 393.

O'Donohogue, J. M., Ray, G. G., Terry, D. W., Jr. and Beaty, H. N. (1973), 'Prevention of nosocomial influenza infection with amantadine', *Amer. J. Epid.*, **97**, 276.

Oker-Blom, N., Hovi, T., Leinikki, P., Palosvo, T., Pettersson, R. and Sumi, J. (1970), 'Protection of man from natural infection with influenza A2 Hong Kong virus by amantadine: A controlled field trial', *Brit. med. J.*, **3**, 676.

Oxford, J. S., Logan, I. S. and Potter, C. W. (1970), 'Passage of influenza strains in the presence of aminoadamantane', *Ann. N.Y. Acad. Sci.*, **173**, 300.

Oxford, J. S. (1975), 'Specific inhibitors of influenza virus replication as potential chemoprophylactic agents', *J. Antimicrob. Chemother.*, **1**, 7.

Pearlman, J. T., Kadish, A. H. and Ramseyer, J. C. (1977), 'Vision loss associated with amantadine hydrochloride use', *JAMA*, **237**, 1200.

Quilligan, J. J., Jr., Hirayama, M. and Baernstein, H. D., Jr. (1966), 'The suppression of A2 influenza in children by the chemoprophylactic use of amantadine', *J. Pediatrics*, **69**, 572.

Schiff, G., Bloomfield, S. and Gaffney, T. (1966), 'The effects of amantadine HCL on experimental human influenza'. Annual meeting of the American Federation for Clinical Research, Atlantic City, N. J., May 1966. Abstracts. *Clinical Research*, **14**, 343.

Smith, C. B., Purcell, R. H. and Chanock, R. M. (1967), 'Effect of amantadine hydrochloride on parainfluenza type 1 virus infections in adult volunteers', *Amer. Rev. Resp. Dis.*, **95**, 689.

Smorodintsev, A. A., Slydnikov, D. M., Kiseleva, A. M., Romanov, J. A., Kazantsev, A. P. and Rumovsky, V. I. (1970a), 'Evaluation of amantadine in artificially induced

A2 and B influenza', *JAMA*, **213**, 1448.

Smorodintsev, A. A., Karpuchin, G. I., Zlydnikov, D. M., Malysheva, A. M., Burov, S. A., Chramtsova, L. M., Romanov, Y. A., Yu Taros, L., Ivannikov, Y. G. and Novoselov, S. D. (1970b), 'The prospect of amantadine for prevention of influenza A2 in humans (effectiveness of amantadine during influenza A2 Hong Kong epidemics in Jan.–Feb. 1969 in Leningrad)', *Ann. N.Y. Acad. Sci.*, **173**, 44.

Scott, G. H., Stephen, E. L. and Berendt, R. F. (1978), 'Activity of amantadine, rimantadine and ribavirin against swine influenza in mice and squirrel monkeys', *Antimicrob. Ag. Chemother.*, **13**, 284.

Stanley, E. D., Muldoon, R. E., Akers, L. W. and Jackson, G. G. (1965), 'Evaluation of antiviral drugs: The effect of amantadine on influenza in volunteers', *Ann. N.Y. Acad. Sci.*, **130**, 44.

Stuart-Harris, C. H. and Schild, G. C. (1976), *Influenza. The Viruses and the Disease*, London, Edward Arnold Ltd.

Togo, Y., Hornick, R. B. and Dawkins, A. T., Jr. (1968), 'Studies on induced influenza in man. I. Double-blind studies designed to assess prophylactic efficacy of amantadine hydrochloride against A2/Rockville/1/65 strain', *JAMA*, **203**, 1089.

Togo, Y., Hornick, R. B., Felitti, V. J., Kaufman, M. L., Dawkins, A. T., Kilpe, V. E. and Claghorn, J. L. (1970), 'Evaluation of therapeutic efficacy of amantadine in patients with naturally occurring A2 influenza', *JAMA*, **211**, 1149.

Tuckova, E., Vonka, V., Zavadova, H. and Kutinova, L. (1973), 'Sensitivity to 1-adamantanamine as a marker in genetic studies with influenza viruses', *J. biol. Stand.*, **1**, 341.

Tyrrell, D. A. J., Bynoe, M. L. and Hoorn, B. (1965), 'Studies on antiviral activity of 1-adamantanamine', *Br. J. exp. Path.*, **46**, 370.

Vale, J. A. and Maclean, K. S. (1977), 'Amantadine-induced heart-failure', *Lancet*, **1**, 548.

Welsh, R. M., Trowbridge, R. S., Kowalski, J. B., O'Connell, C. M. and Pfau, C. J. (1971), 'Amantadine hydrochloride inhibition of early and late stages of lymphocytic choriomeningitis virus—cell interactions', *Virology*, **45**, 679.

Wendel, H. A. (1964), 'Clinical and serologic effects in influenza of 1-adamantanamine HCl—a double-blind study', *Fed. Proc.*, **23**, 387.

Wingfield, W. L., Pollack, D. and Grunert, R. R. (1969), 'Therapeutic efficacy of amantadine HCl and rimantadine HCl in naturally occurring influenza A2 respiratory illness in man', *New Engl. J. Med.*, **281**, 579.

Wink, C. A. S. (Ed.) (1975), *Symmetrel in Virology*, Macclesfield, Geigy Pharmaceuticals.

Wood, T. R. (1965), 'Methods useful in evaluating 1-adamantanamine hydrochloride—a new orally active synthetic antiviral agent', *Ann. N.Y. Acad. Sci.*, **130**, 419.

Methisazone

Description

Methisazone (N-methylisatin-beta-thiosemicarbazone; 1-methylisatin 3-thio-semicarbazone; 'Marboran') is a thiosemicarbazone derivative. The thiosemicarbazones were originally introduced for the treatment of tuberculosis in Germany in 1946. They were largely abandoned for this disease because of their side-effects (*see* thiacetazone page 859). Hamre *et al*. (1950) discovered that one of these compounds, p-aminobenzaldehyde thiosemicarbazone, partially protected chick embryos or mice against infection with Vaccinia virus. Later, Thompson *et al*. (1953) found that isatin-beta-thiosemicarbazone (IBT) had greater activity against this infection in mice. Subsequently a considerable number of derivatives of IBT were synthetized and tested, and the N-methyl and N-ethyl derivatives were shown to have an even greater antiviral activity than the parent compound (Bauer and Sadler, 1960). The N-methyl compound (methisazone) was selected for further studies because of its ease of preparation. Bauer *et al*. (1962) showed that it possessed marked antiviral activity in mice infected intracerebrally with Variola virus; the following year it was shown to have a protective effect against this virus in humans (Bauer *et al*., 1963). The thiosemicarbazones were therefore the first antiviral agents to be discovered which were effective in experimental viral infections. Methisazone has a wide antiviral action, being active against a number of DNA and RNA viruses. Its use in man has been restricted to chemoprophylaxis against smallpox and for the treatment of some complications of smallpox vaccination.

Antiviral Activity

Methisazone and its analogues have a wide spectrum of antiviral activity in tissue culture (Bauer *et al*., 1970; Bauer, 1973; Levinson *et al*., 1974). They are active against DNA viruses such as Vaccinia, Variola major and minor (Alastrim), Cow-pox, some Adenoviruses, Herpesvirus varicellae and Herpesvirus hominis types 1 and 2. In addition, they inhibit some RNA viruses such as certain members of the poliovirus, echovirus, arbovirus and rhinovirus groups and Influenza A and B and Parainfluenza viruses. Methisazone is most effective *in vivo* against the poxviruses (Vaccinia and Variola) and the maximum effect occurs when treatment is started at the time of viral challenge. Drug dependent mutants of vaccinia virus have been obtained (Oxford, 1976).

Pharmacology

Methisazone is an orange-yellow powder which is only slightly soluble in water and there is no preparation of the drug which is suitable for parenteral administration. The drug is given orally in the form of a tablet or as a suspension. After oral administration, peak serum concentrations are reached in 4–6 h, and the drug is not detectable in the serum 10–12 h later. It is not well absorbed and both the rate of absorption and the proportion of a dose absorbed vary considerably in individuals. Methisazone is extensively metabolized in the body and its derivatives and the intact drug are excreted in the urine. Higher serum levels are found in infants, probably because the drug is less metabolized in this age group (Nimmo-Smith and Bauer, 1966). Methisazone does not appear to accumulate with continued therapy (Kempe *et al.*, 1965).

Mode of Action

Tissue culture studies on the antiviral action of the isatin-beta-thiosemicarbazones against pox viruses have shown that they act intracellularly. They do not halt the lethal effect of the virus on the host cell, there is normal synthesis of viral DNA and enzymes concerned in DNA synthesis, but immature appearing virus particles are produced, and there is inhibition of the synthesis of many viral antigens that are formed during the later stages of viral infection (Appleyard *et al.*, 1965; Magee and Bach, 1965, Sadler, 1965). These findings suggested that there was some interference with the synthesis or transcription of critical proteins late in the cycle of virus replication, so that the production of normal mature infective virus particles is virtually halted. Woodson and Joklik (1965) showed that in the case of Vaccinia virus, late protein synthesis was inhibited because viral messenger RNA formed late in the viral growth cycle becomes fragmented, causing dissolution of the polyribosome-late messenger RNA complex (the site of viral protein synthesis). Messenger RNA is also produced by RNA viruses and this explains why methisazone is also active against these viruses.

The antiviral activity of methisazone has been assessed by the inhibition of viral growth in tissue culture after the cells have been infected. In addition certain RNA tumour viruses can be inactivated before infection, because the drug inhibits the activity of ribonucleic acid (RNA)-dependent deoxyribonucleic acid (DNA) polymerase (reverse transcriptase). DNA-dependent RNA polymerase (transcriptase) of Vaccinia virus core is also inhibited by methisazone, but the intact virion is not susceptible because it seems to be inpenetrable to the drug. The lack of susceptibility of some RNA viruses, which possess a transcriptase, may also depend on whether the drug can penetrate the virion (Levinson *et al.*, 1974). Experiments by Levinson and Helling (1976) indicate that this activity of methisazone is mediated by its thiosemicarbazone moiety and copper is also required, and that DNA is one target for its action.

Toxicity

Gastro-intestinal symptoms, particularly nausea and vomiting, are the most common side-effects of methisazone. These were noted in 16·7–27·3 per cent of treated contacts (depending on the dosage used) by Bauer *et al.* (1969). In a trial in Brazil, do Valle *et al.* (1965) observed these symptoms in 66 per cent of patients. Landsman and Grist (1964) noted severe vomiting in medical students, who were given the drug during a trial. In one of the field studies by Heiner *et al.* (1971) vomiting occurred in 10·4 per cent of treated subjects. Dermatitis, jaundice, diarrhoea and alopecia have also been described.

Clinical Uses of the Drug

1. *Smallpox chemoprophylaxis*. Although methisazone is of no value for the treatment of smallpox, several studies have suggested that it is a useful chemoprophylactic agent for this disease. Bauer *et al.* (1969) summarized their results from the use of methisazone in 1963 in Madras, where the drug was used to prevent smallpox in close contacts of patients who were admitted to hospital. The drug was given to 2610 smallpox contacts and of these 18 (0·69 per cent) subsequently developed smallpox and four died. In a comparable group of 2710 untreated contacts from a similar environment, 113 (4·2 per cent) developed smallpox and 21 died. The incidence of disease was therefore reduced about six-fold. It was assessed that the majority of contacts had their treatment begun at about half-way through the incubation period. Four oral dose schedules were employed: a single dose of 3 g, two doses of 3 g separated by 8 h, 1·5 g twice-daily for four days and 3 g twice-daily for four days. Almost complete protection was obtained in patients treated with two doses of 3 g or the higher dosage schedules. This study has been criticized because it was uncontrolled and most of the contacts had been immunized during infancy and again shortly after identification of the index case of smallpox (Heiner *et al.*, 1971; Weinstein and Chang, 1973; Emond and McKendrick, 1974).

Do Valle *et al.* (1965) studied the action of small doses of methisazone in 976 contacts of patients with alastrim (variola minor) in São Paulo, Brazil. Of 406 contacts who had not previously been vaccinated and were not vaccinated after exposure, 187 were treated with an oral dose of 3 g or 6 g and 219 were left untreated as a control group. Seven cases of alastrim occurred amongst the treated contacts and 38 among the controls. These authors concluded that methisazone is effective in the prevention of alastrim in the doses employed. Rao *et al.* (1969) used methisazone in a small controlled trial between 1965 and 1967 to assess its value in prevention of variola major in previously unimmunized subjects in Madras. Two cases of smallpox developed in 17 subjects who received 5 g of the drug daily for five days, and 8 of 19 subjects who were given a placebo developed the disease. These results also suggested that the drug may be useful for smallpox prevention.

Other investigations into the use of thiosemicarbazones for the prevention of smallpox have not been so encouraging. Another thiosemicarbazone, 4-bromo-3-methylisothiazole-5-carboxaldehyde thiosemicarbazone (M & M 7714), has also been used in a prophylactic trial against smallpox in Madras (Rao *et al.*, 1966). This drug was used in an oral daily dose of 4 g for three days, with smaller doses for younger age-groups, and the trial was restricted to family contacts of smallpox patients who had not been previously vaccinated. Of 196 contacts who received the drug, there were 40 cases of smallpox with seven deaths, and in 201 contacts who were treated with a placebo, there were 60 cases with 12 deaths. There was therefore a significant difference in the frequency of smallpox, but there was no significant difference in case fatality rates. These authors did not recommend this drug for the routine prophylaxis of smallpox, because only a small reduction in case incidence was achieved and 74 per cent of those treated developed vomiting, which in 52 per cent was so severe that the subjects refused to complete the course of treatment.

Three field trials with methisazone as a prophylactic agent against smallpox carried out in West Pakistan between 1964 and 1970 failed to show a significant difference between the effects of the drug and placebo (Heiner *et al.*, 1971). Overall attack rates were 2·7 per cent (7 of 262 contacts) and 5 per cent (13 of 260 contacts), respectively, in drug and placebo groups. Previously vaccinated contacts showed low and almost identical secondary attack rates in the drug (1·2 per cent) and placebo (1·3 per cent) groups. Unvaccinated contacts had attack rates of 22·2 per cent (4 of 18) in the methisazone group and 45·5 per cent (10 of 22) in the placebo group, suggesting a possible protective effect of the drug. No differences in mortality or morbidity were noted between treated and placebo groups and there was no evidence of a suppressive effect of methisazone on the immunological response to vaccination. The drug was administered to adults as a single oral dose of 6 g suspended in 15 ml of a sucrose vehicle or 6 g in two divided doses separated by 4–6 h; children were given single doses ranging from 1–4 g depending on their age. Heiner *et al.* (1971) reviewed the results of all previous trials with methisazone and their own results. They concluded that in controlled studies the drug does exert a protective effect, although perhaps less than earlier studies had indicated. In addition, none of the studies has demonstrated a modification of disease or reduction of fatalities. They considered that the drug may be of use in contacts late in the incubation period, when vaccination would have no effect.

It is apparent that methisazone is of doubtful value as a prophylactic agent against smallpox. Vaccination still remains the prophylatic treatment of choice for contacts of smallpox, whether or not they have been vaccinated prior to exposure (Heiner *et al.*, 1971; Emond and McKendrick, 1974). In any case it now appears that the interruption of person-to-person transmission of smallpox in the world has been achieved (WHO, 1978).

2. *Treatment of complications of smallpox vaccination.* A small controlled study on 19 medical students suggested that methisazone, given two to four days after vaccination against smallpox, depresses the local reaction and may impair antibody response (Landsman and Grist, 1964). The dose used was 3 g orally twice-daily for three days but treatment was abandoned in all but one student after one to four doses, because of severe vomiting. Bauer *et al.* (1969) also found that the drug was associated with a slight reduction in the proportion of successful primary vaccinations and a significant reduction of successful revaccinations. However, no such effect was demonstrated by Heiner *et al.* (1971).

Bauer (1965) recommends methisazone for the treatment of eczema vaccinatum and vaccinia gangrenosa, possibly in conjunction with hyperimmune vaccinial immunoglobulin. For these infections he suggested a loading dose of 200 mg per kg followed by a further 400 mg per kg in divided doses, given orally over a total period of 48 h. There have been other reports of the successful use of methisazone to prevent or treat eczema vaccinatum and to treat vaccinia gangrenosa (Jaroszyńska-Weinberger and Mészáros, 1966; Adels and Oppé, 1966; Jaroszyńska-Weinberger, 1970; McLean, 1977). Many authors have reported isolated cases in which methisazone has been used for vaccinia gangrenosa. When these reports are reviewed collectively, it appears that treatment with methisazone reduces the usually high mortality of this disease to about 50 per cent. It is very difficult to assess the value of this drug for the treatment of complications of vaccination, because there have been no controlled studies on its use. Because of its doubtful efficacy and the high frequency of side-effects (page 966), methisazone is not used for the treatment of accidental vaccination or eczema vaccinatum at Fairfield Hospital. It may be worth considering in the rare potentially fatal complication of vaccinia gangrenosa.

REFERENCES

Adels, B. R. and Oppe, T. E. (1966), 'Treatment of eczema vaccinatum with N-methylisatin beta-thiosemicarbazone', *Lancet*, **1**, 18.

Appleyard, G., Hume, V. B. M. and Westwood, J. C. N. (1965), 'The effect of thiosemicarbazones on the growth of rabbit pox virus in tissue culture', *Ann. N.Y. Acad. Sci.*, **130**, 92.

Bauer, D. J. and Sadler, P. W. (1960), 'The structure-activity relationship of the antiviral chemotherapeutic activity of isatin β-thiosemicarbazone', *Brit. J. Pharmac. Chemother.*, **15**, 101.

Bauer, D. J., Dumbell, K. R., Fox-Hulme, P. and Sadler, P. W. (1962), 'The chemotherapy of variola major infection', *Bull. Wld. Hlth. Org.*, **26**, 727.

Bauer, D. J., St. Vincent, L., Kempe, C. H. and Downie, A. W. (1963), 'Prophylactic treatment of smallpox contacts with N-methylisatin β-thiosemicarbazone (compound 33T57, marboran)', *Lancet*, **2**, 494.

Bauer, D. J. (1965), 'Clinical experience with the antiviral drug marboran (1-methylisatin 3-thiosemicarbazone)', *Ann. N.Y. Acad. Sci.*, **130**, 110.

Bauer, D. J., St. Vincent, L., Kempe, C. H., Young, P. A. and Downie, A. W. (1969), 'Prophylaxis of smallpox with methisazone', *Amer. J. Epidemiol.*, **90**, 130.

Bauer, D. J., Apostolov, K. and Selway, J. W. T. (1970), 'Activity of methisazone against RNA viruses', *Ann. N.Y. Acad. Sci.*, **173**, 314.

Bauer, D. J. (1973), 'Antiviral chemotherapy: The first decade', *Brit. med. J.*, **3**, 275.

do Valle, L. A. R., de Melo, P. R., de Salles Gomes, L. F. and Proenca, L. M. (1965), 'Methisazone in prevention of variola minor among contacts', *Lancet*, **2**, 976.

Emond, R. T. D. and McKendrick, G. D. W. (1974), 'Vaccination of smallpox contacts', *Brit. med. J.*, **2**, 175.

Hamre, D., Bernstein, J. and Donovick, R. (1950), 'Activity of p-aminobenzaldehyde, 3-thiosemicarbazone on vaccinia virus in the chick embryo and in the mouse', *Proc. Soc. Exp. Biol. Med.*, **73**, 275.

Heiner, G. G., Fatima, N., Russell, P. K., Haase, A. T., Ahmad, N., Mohammed, N., Thomas, D. B., Mack, T. M., Khan, M. M., Knatterud, G. L., Anthony, R. L. and McCrumb, F. R., Jr. (1971), 'Field trials of methisazone as a prophylactic agent against smallpox', *Amer. J. Epidemiol.*, **94**, 435.

Jaroszyńska-Weinberger, B. and Mészáros, J. (1966), 'A comparison of the protective effect of methisazone and a hyperimmune antivaccinial gamma-globulin in primary smallpox vaccination carried out in the presence of contraindications', *Lancet*, **1**, 948.

Jaroszyńska-Weinberger, B. (1970), 'Treatment with methisazone of complications following smallpox vaccination', *Arch. Dis. Child.*, **45**, 573.

Kempe, C. H., Rodgerson, D. and Sieber, O. F., Jr. (1965), 'Measurement of N-methylisatin β-thiosemicarbazone serum levels', *Lancet*, **1**, 824.

Landsman, J. B. and Grist, N. R. (1964), 'Controlled trial of marboran on group vaccinated against smallpox', *Lancet*, **1**, 330.

Levinson, W., Coleman, V., Woodson, B., Rabson, A., Lanier, J., Whitcher, J. and Dawson, C. (1974), 'Inactivation of Herpes simplex virus by thiosemicarbazones and certain cations', *Antimicrob. Ag. Chemother.*, **5**, 398.

Levinson, W. and Helling, R. (1976), 'Inactivation of lambda phage infectivity and lambda deoxyribonucleic acid transfection by N-methyl-isatin β-thiosemicarbazone-copper complexes', *Antimicrob. Ag. Chemother.*, **9**, 160.

McLean, D. M. (1977), 'Methisazone therapy in pediatric vaccinia complications', *Ann. N.Y. Acad. Sci.*, **284**, 118.

Magee, W. E. and Bach, M. K. (1965), 'Biochemical studies on the antiviral activities of the isatin-β-thiosemicarbazones', *Ann. N.Y. Acad. Sci.*, **130**, 80.

Nimmo-Smith, R. H. and Bauer, D. J. (1966), 'Measuring methisazone serum-levels', *Lancet*, **2**, 346.

Oxford, J. S. (1976), 'Drug resistance and antiviral agents', *J. Antimicrob. Chemother.*, **2**, 223.

Rao, A. R., McKendrick, G. D. W., Velayudhan, L. and Kamalakshi, K. (1966), 'Assessment of an isothiazole thiosemicarbazone in the prophylaxis of contacts of variola major', *Lancet*, **1**, 1072.

Rao, A. R., Jacobs, E. S., Kamalakshi, S., Bradbury, and Swamy, A. (1969), 'Chemoprophylaxis and chemotherapy in variola major. Part 1. An assessment of CG 662 and marboran in prophylaxis of contacts of variola major', *Ind. Jour. Med. Res.*, **57**, 477.

Sadler, P. W. (1965), 'Antiviral chemotherapy with isatin-β-thiosemicarbazone and its derivatives', *Ann. N.Y. Acad. Sci.*, **130**, 71.

Thompson, R. L., Minton, S. A., Officer, J. E. and Hitchings, G. H. (1953), 'Effect of heterocyclic and other thiosemicarbazones on vaccinia infection in the mouse', *J. Immun.*, **70**, 229.

Weinstein, L. and Chang, T. W. (1973), 'The chemotherapy of viral infections', *New Engl. J. Med.*, **289**, 725.

WHO (1978), 'Smallpox surveillance', *Wkly. Epidem. Rec.*, **53**, 125.

Woodson, B. and Joklik, W. K. (1965), 'The inhibition of vaccinia virus multiplication by isatin β-thiosemicarbazone', *Proc. natn. Acad. Sci. U.S.A.*, **54**, 946.

Index

971